Core Curriculum for Pain Management Nursing

Second Edition

Barbara St. Marie, ANP, GNP, RN-BC, PhD Candidate
Editor

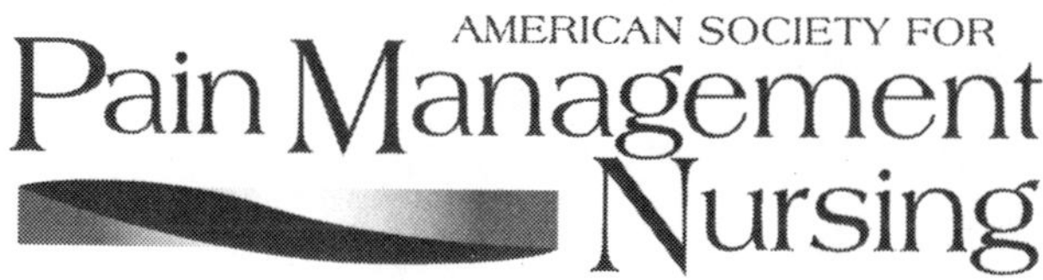

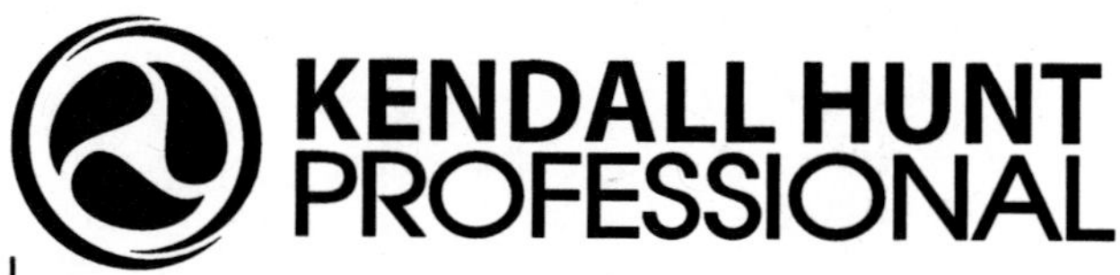

ISBN 978-0-7575-6613-4

Printed in the United States of America
10 9 8 7 6 5 4 3 2 1

I would like to dedicate this book to my parents, Gus and Isabel Cobb, who have supported me through my 30 years of clinical nursing practice. And to my husband, Daniel St. Marie, who has kept me focused and balanced throughout this project.

Contents

Presidential Foreword

It is truly an honor to be asked to write the foreword for the American Society for Pain Management Nursing (ASPMN) *Core Curriculum for Pain Management Nursing, 2009*, second edition. This edition is essentially a "new" text given the amount of updated information, advanced knowledge in pain management, and comprehensive coverage of pain management nursing. The new edition boasts a team of approximately 50 contributors, including three section editors, and has grown in size and depth of knowledge. It is remarkable that ASPMN nurses have embraced and contributed to the knowledge about pain and its management through research, clinical guidelines, and educational material. It is always a challenge to recognize that pain management knowledge is not just for nurses who practice pain management as a subspecialty but also for all nurses providing care to those interacting with the health care system. The editors were committed to providing the best available evidence when possible yet maintaining a practical clinical perspective for all frontline nurses. The mentoring provided by the editors and experienced authors to the numerous contributors speaks volumes to the commitment of pain management nurses to nursing education, the nursing profession, and ASPMN.

Pain management is the primary clinical challenge for nurses, and ASPMN is dedicated to meeting that challenge through nursing education. This book is intended to provide comprehensive knowledge to prepare the nurse for certification in pain management. ASPMN provides the expertise needed to collate the best practices and evidence needed through educational programs, practice modules, and publications (see http://www.aspmn.org). The promotion of pain management through the process of certification demonstrates the nurse's qualifications directly to the health care consumer.

To the authors and editors, you are to be commended for your dedication to improving patient care through your tireless efforts in promoting pain management knowledge. On behalf of ASPMN, congratulations to all current and future certified pain management nurses.

Nancy Eksterowicz, RN-BC, MSN, CNS
2009 ASPMN President
University of Virginia Health System
Department of Anesthesiology
Center for Excellence Comprehensive Pain Management Center
Charlottesville, Virginia

Preface

Pain management nursing has come a long way since the first edition of *Core Curriculum for Pain Management Nursing, 2002.* When the first edition was written, we did not have certification for nurses who called themselves specialists in pain management. We did not have trained master faculty teaching pain management nursing courses. And we had only a few products available for nurses to study pain management. Now, we have pain management as a specialty in nursing. We have multiple publications and position papers, we affect social policy through our work in advocacy, we have increasing numbers of nurses and advanced practice nurses who specialize in pain management, we have pain management and medication safety as a focus in undergraduate, graduate, and preceptor programs, and we have enhanced research that is further increasing our body of knowledge.

We can thank the many pain management nurses who have given us a strong foundation. We can thank the founders of the American Society for Pain Management Nursing who gathered together and inspired nurses to join the field of pain management. We can thank the current and past presidents of our organization who provide leadership in advancing the knowledge of nurses, advocating for our patients and the needs of our society, supporting nursing research, establishing networks of support for nurses in clinical practice, and responding to the changing field of pain management nursing.

As you read this second edition of the *Core Curriculum for Pain Management Nursing,* you see that our body of knowledge has grown since 2002, when the first edition was published. The bar has been elevated. Our expectations for further growth of our knowledge, skills, and performance are great. Your response to the first edition gave those who contributed a feeling of gratitude for your support, and we hope you find that the second edition further advances the art and science of pain management nursing and your promotion thereof.

The design of this edition of the *Core Curriculum for Pain Management Nursing* looks different in some ways from that of the first edition. At the beginning of each chapter are objectives to guide the reading experience. The chapters are organized by topics in four sections. Section 1 provides a foundation of knowledge on which the next three sections are built. Section 2 consists of the advocacy chapters and guides us in our continual advocacy for our patients at all levels of our society. Section 3 is the clinical domain of pain management nursing as we strive to manage individuals' pain across the life span. At the end of Section 3 is a subsection of four chapters called State of the Science. The selected topics in the State of the Science subsection are in the infancy of discovery and are meant to appeal to your curiosity to further research, read, and advocate. Section 4 conveys all the roles pain management nurses engage in our health care arena.

The research methods used to ensure the information in this second edition of *Core Curriculum for Pain Management Nursing* is up-to-date and evidence-based was accomplished by the individual authors, section editors, and editor. The databases used were Cumulative Index of Nursing and Allied Health Literature (CINAHL), Medline, ProQuest Nursing, and PsycINFO, using the subject headings in all topic areas pertinent to pain management nursing. A project of this size is never completed without the efforts of teams of individuals. Each author and editor donated exhaustive hours of research, review, writing, rewriting, emails, and phone calls through the calendar year to prepare this document that is intended to forward the knowledge and subsequent certification of pain management nurses. Janet Erdman, the medical librarian at Fairview Ridges Hospital and Fairview Southdale Hospital in Minneapolis, Minnesota, provided hundreds of articles and texts for me to review to ensure valid and reliable references. She played a solid role in creating a quality *Core Curriculum for Pain Management Nursing,* and her hard work is greatly appreciated.

We all place our efforts in an extraordinary and rapidly growing field where pain is no longer considered just a symptom that something is wrong but rather, in some cases, a disease itself. Pain can cause injury to organs, decrease longevity, and decrease quality of life, (See the chapter on Benefits of Proper Pain Management). The U.S. Congress passed into law a provision declaring 2001 to 2010 as the "Decade of Pain Control and Research" (Ashburn, 2002). And in 2006, the Centers for Disease Control and Prevention published a report stating 26% of all adults in the United States had pain for more than 24 hours in the month before the study. This information and "call to arms" has directed our attention to research and treatment, and we realize this is only the beginning.

As pain management nurses, we know our roles are changing, and we see an increase in our responsibility and accountability. It is our hope that the second edition of the *Core Curriculum for Pain Management Nursing* supports you in your practice, education, advocacy, and research.

Barbara St. Marie
Editor, *Core Curriculum for Pain Management Nursing, 2009*, second edition

References

Ashburn, M. A. (2002). *Decade of pain report, July 2002. American Pain Society Bulletin,* 12(4). Retrieved April 19, 2009, from http://www.ampainsoc.org/pub/bulletin/jul02/pres.htm.

Centers for Disease Control and Prevention. *(2006). New report finds pain affects millions of Americans.* Retrieved April 19, 2009, from http://www.cdc.gov/nchs/pressroom/06facts/hus06.htm.

Section Editors, Contributors, and Authors

Section Editors

Janette E. Elliott, RN-BC, MSN, AOCN

Theresa Di Maggio, PNP-BC, MSN, CRNP

Contributors

We would like to extend thanks and acknowledgment to those who contributed to *Core Curriculum for Pain Management Nursing, 2009,* second edition.

Annabel D. Edwards, RN, MSN, ANP, who wrote "Physiology of Pain" in the first edition.

Elaine Swope, RN-BC, MSN, CNP, who wrote "Benefits of Proper Pain Management" in the first edition.

Anna DuPen, MN, APRN, who wrote "The Role of the Nurse Practitioner in Pain Management" in the first edition.

Tom Nelson, PharmD, RPh, who reviewed the medication information in "Pediatric Pain Management" in the second edition.

Virginia Ghafoor, PharmD, RPh, who reviewed the medication information in all the chapters of the second edition.

Barbara Leary Dion, RN-C, MA, MSN, who reviewed "The Pain Management Nurse as an Educator" in the second edition.

Authors

Paul Arnstein, PhD, RN, CS
Clinical Nurse Specialist for Pain Relief
Massachusetts General Hospital
Boston, MA
Past President, American Society for Pain Management Nursing

Pamela Bennett, BSN, RN
Executive Director, Healthcare Alliance Development
Purdue Pharma L.P.
Stamford, CT
Past President, American Society for Pain Management Nursing

Barton T. Bobb, MSN, FNP-BC, ACHPN
Palliative Care and Pain Consult Team Nurse Practitioner
Massey Cancer Center, Thomas Palliative Care Unit
Medical College of Virginia Hospitals
Virginia Commonwealth University
Richmond, VA

Micke A. Brown, BSN, RN
Director of Communications/American Pain Foundation
Baltimore, MD
Past President, American Society for Pain Management Nursing

Patricia Bruckenthal, PhD, RN, ANP-C
Clinical Associate Professor
Stony Brook University School of Nursing
Stony Brook, NY
Nurse Practitioner
Pain and Headache Treatment Center
Manhasset, NY

Lynn M. Clark, MS, RN-BC, CPNP-PC
Pediatric Nurse Practitioner and Manager
Pediatric Pain Management Center
Children's Medical Center, Dallas
Dallas, TX

Christina L. Clyde, MS, RN-BC
Nurse Manager
University of Maryland Pain Management Center
Baltimore, MD

Alice E. Conway, PhD, RN, CRNP, FNP-BC
Professor
Edinboro University of Pennsylvania
Edinboro, PA

Donna Sipos Cox, MSN, ONC, CCRC, RN-BC
Clinical Nurse Associate
Winthrop Pain Management
Mineola, NY
Past President, American Society for Pain Management Nursing

Patrick J. Coyne, MSN, APRN, ACHPN, FAAN, FPCN
Clinical Director of Massey Cancer Center, Thomas Palliative Care Unit,
Medical College of Virginia Hospitals
Virginia Commonwealth University
Richmond, VA

Carol P. Curtiss, MSN, RN-BC
Clinical Nurse Specialist Consultant
Curtiss Consulting
Greenfield, MA

Michelle L. Czarnecki, MSN, RN-BC, CPNP-PC
Advanced Practice Nurse—Jane B. Pettit Pain and Palliative Care Center
Children's Hospital of Wisconsin
Milwaukee, WI

Yvonne D'Arcy, MS, CRNP, CNS
Pain Management and Palliative Care Nurse Practitioner
Suburban Hospital (a Johns Hopkins affiliate)
Bethesda, MD

Theresa J. Di Maggio, MSN, CRNP, PNP-BC
Pain Management Advanced Practice Nurse
Children's Hospital of Philadelphia
Philadelphia, PA

Debra J. Drew, MS, RN-BC, ACNS-BC
Clinical Nurse Specialist, Pain Management
University of Minnesota Medical Center, Fairview
Minneapolis, MN

Nancy Eksterowicz, RN-BC, MSN, CNS
Pain Services Coordinator
University of Virginia Health System
Charlottesville, VA
President, American Society for Pain Management Nursing

Janette E. Elliott, RN-BC, MSN, AOCN
Pain Management Clinical Nurse Specialist
Veterans Affairs Health Care System, Palo Alto
Palo Alto, CA

Virginia L. Ghafoor, PharmD, RPh
Clinical Pharmacy Specialist, Pain Management
University of Minnesota Medical Center, Fairview
Minneapolis, MN

Debra B. Gordon, RN-BC, MS, ACNS-BC, FAAN
Senior Clinical Nurse Specialist
UW Health University of Wisconsin Hospital and Clinics
Madison, WI

Theresa Grimes, MN, RN-BC, FNP-BC, CCRN
Associate Vice President for Nursing
Nurse Practitioner Pain Management
J. T. Mather Memorial Hospital
Port Jefferson, NY
President Elect, American Society for Pain Management Nursing

Karen P. Hall, MSHSA, RN-BC, NE-BC
Director of Patient Care Services for Emergency Department and Pain Management
Doctors Medical Center
Modesto, CA

Eleftheria T. Karapas, MS, RN-BC
Instructor, Medical-Surgical Nursing
College of Nursing and Health Professions
Lewis University
Romeoville, IL

Anne Marie Kelly, BSN, RN-BC, CHPN
Pain Management Educator and Consultant
Catholic Memorial Home
Fall River, MA

Nancy Kowal, MS, APRN, BC
Pain Consultant
Department of Anesthesia
University of Massachusetts Medical School
Worcester, MA
Past President, American Society for Pain Management Nursing

Kathleen Anne Kwiatkowski, BA, RN, L.Ac
Pain Management Nurse Consultant, Pain Management Services
University of Maryland Medical Systems
Baltimore, MD
Bayside Acupuncture and Healing Arts
Stevensville, MD

Connie Luedtke, MA, RN-BC
Nurse Supervisor
Mayo Clinic
Rochester, MN

John A. Menez, MS, RN-BC, CMSRN
Nursing Faculty
Rasmussen College Brooklyn Park Campus
Blaine, MN

Pamela J. Nelson, PhD, RN-BC
Clinical Nurse Specialist, Pain Management
Assistant Professor
Mayo Clinic
Rochester, MN

Susan O'Conner-Von, PhD, RN
Associate Professor
School of Nursing
University of Minnesota
Minneapolis, MN

Hob Osterlund, APRN, BC
Clinical Nurse Specialist, Pain and Palliative Care
The Queen's Medical Center
Honolulu, HI

Jerri Patterson, RN, MSN, APN, BC
Adult Nurse Practitioner
Pain Management Group of NC, LLC
Pinehurst, NC

Christine Peltier, BSN, RN-BC
Inpatient Pain Consult Service Coordinator
University of Minnesota Medical Center, Fairview
Minneapolis, MN

Rosemary C. Polomano, PhD, RN, FAAN
Associate Professor of Pain Practice
University of Pennsylvania School of Nursing
Associate Professor of Anesthesiology and Critical Care (Secondary)
University of Pennsylvania
Philadelphia, PA

Ann Quinlan-Colwell, RN-BC, FAAPM
Pain Management Clinical Nurse Specialist
New Hanover Regional Medical Center
Wilmington, NC
PhD Candidate
University of North Carolina, Greensboro
Greensboro, NC

Cheryl Rawe, RN, MS, CNS, BC
Clinical Nurse Specialist for Pain Services
Miami Valley Hospital
Dayton, OH

Marsha N. Rehm, MSN, RN-BC, FAAPM
Pain Management Clinical Nurse Specialist
Pitt County Memorial Hospital
Greenville, NC

Elizabeth Renaud, RN, MSN, CS, NP
Detroit Receiving Hospital
Anesthesia Pain Service
Detroit, MI

Diana L. Ruzicka, RN-BC, MSN, CNS
Chair, Disaster Health Services
Madison/Marshall County Chapter, American Red Cross
New Market, AL

Linda Shin, MN, ACNS-BC
Clinical Nurse Specialist, Staff Nurse
Swedish Medical Center
Seattle, WA

Melanie H. Simpson, PhD, RN-BC, OCN, CHPN
Pain Management Team Coordinator
The University of Kansas Hospital
Kansas City, KS

Barbara St. Marie, ANP, GNP, RN-BC
Nurse Practitioner, Supervisor
Pain and Palliative Care
Fairview Ridges Hospital
Minneapolis, MN
PhD Candidate
College of Nursing
University of Wisconsin, Milwaukee
Milwaukee, WI

Cathy D. Trame, RN-BC, MS, CNS
Coordinator, CNS Perioperative Pain Services
Miami Valley Hospital
Dayton, OH

Helen N. Turner, DNP, RN-BC, PCNS-BC
Clinical Nurse Specialist
Pediatric Pain Management Center
Doernbecher Children's Hospital
Oregon Health & Science University
Portland, OR

Barbara L. Vanderveer, MSN, RN-BC, ARNP
Clinical Coordinator
Acute & Cancer Pain Management
Department of Anesthesiology
UK HealthCare
Chandler Medical Center
University of Kentucky
Lexington, KY

Linda Vanni, RN, MSN, ACNS-BC, NP
Nurse Practitioner
Karmanos Pain Service
Karmanos Cancer Center
Detroit, MI

Michelle L. Witkop, FNP-BC, ACHPN
Palliative Care and Bleeding Disorders Nurse Practitioner
Munson Medical Center
Traverse City, MI

Mary Zaccagnini, DNP, RN, ACNS-BC, AOCN
Clinical Assistant Professor
University of Minnesota, School of Nursing
Minneapolis, MN

section

1

Foundation of Pain Management Nursing

chapter

1

Philosophy of Pain Management Nursing

Elizabeth Renaud, RN, MSN, CS, NP

Objectives

After studying this chapter, the reader should be able to:

1. Describe beliefs and values that contribute to the development of a philosophy of pain management nursing.
2. Review historical developments in nursing, health care, and society that support the role of nurses in management of pain.
3. Describe a personal philosophy of pain management to colleagues, other health care providers, and patients (including families, groups, and communities depending on the reader's area of practice).

I. Pain Management Nurses' Values and Beliefs

A. The nursing profession exists to serve the interests of society.

B. Nursing is obligated to self-regulate the profession's approach to nursing care, including pain management.

C. The values and beliefs that nurses hold guide their goals and actions for treatment of patients entrusted to their care.

1. Pain is one of the most universal and pervasive sources of human distress.
2. Pain is a subjective, multidimensional experience unique to the individual.

D. The nurse who provides pain management uses personal and professional codes of ethics to guide pain management practice that is characterized by respect for human dignity.

1. Nurses have a duty to prevent the harmful physiological and psychological effects of unrelieved pain.
2. At the most basic level, nursing care to provide pain relief is simply the right thing to do.
3. Relief of pain is a cornerstone of health care's humanitarian mission.
4. Pain is treatable.

II. Agency for Health Care Policy and Research (AHCPR)

A. AHCPR provided one of the first evidence-based national guidelines for acute pain in 1992 (Acute Pain Management Guidelines Panel, 1992).

1. With this widely publicized free guideline, information about pain management was made available to clinicians and consumers, including concepts such as the following:
   a. The most reliable indicator of the existence and intensity of acute pain and any resultant affective discomfort or distress is the patient's self-report.
   b. Neither behavior nor vital signs can substitute for a self-report. (Acute Pain Management Guidelines Panel, 1992, p. 11)

B. Institutional responsibility

1. Each institution should develop the resources necessary to provide the best and most modern pain relief appropriate to its patients.
2. Patients should have access to the best level of pain relief that may be safely provided. (Acute Pain Management Guidelines Panel, 1992, p. 71)
3. For nurses, physicians, and others treating acute pain, the common purpose is relief of patients' pain. The purpose should be explicit, and a commitment to this goal should be elicited from every provider who can influence the patient's pain. (Acute Pain Management Guidelines Panel, 1992, p. 72)

III. American Society for Pain Management Nursing (ASPMN)

A. ASPMN mission statement and goals

1. The ASPMN is a national organization of nurses dedicated to promoting and providing optimal care of the patient in pain.
2. The ASPMN mission is "to advance and promote optimal nursing care for people affected by pain by promoting best nursing practices" (http://www.aspmn.org/Organization/mission.htm).
   a. The ASPMN promotes education, standards, advocacy, and research in pain management nursing.
   b. All people will have access to health care services that provide quality pain management care.
   c. The history of ASPMN provides valuable insight into the beginnings of this group in 1990 (http://www.aspmn.org/Organization/history.htm).

B. The ASPMN (1998) *Standards of Clinical Practice for the Specialty of Pain Management Nursing.*

1. If pain cannot be eliminated, an attempt must be made to reduce suffering.
2. The core of pain management nursing involves prevention, assessment, diagnosis, treatment, evaluation, and rehabilitation considering the multidimensional aspects of pain, including sensory, emotional, cognitive, development, and behavioral components of pain.
3. The nurse who provides pain management
   a. Systematically collects, evaluates, records, and communicates comprehensive data regarding the patient's experience of pain.

b. Analyzes the comprehensive assessment data and formulates a nursing diagnosis or problem focus.
c. Identifies measurable, individualized, and comprehensive outcomes of pain care with and for the patient experiencing pain.
d. Develops a pain management plan in conjunction with the patient, significant others, and members of the health care team.
e. Implements the patient's pain management plan of care to achieve the identified outcomes.
f. Analyzes the patient's responses to the pain management plan and the progression toward the achievement of identified outcomes.

4. Pain management nursing involves close interaction with patients, families, and other health care providers to prevent pain whenever possible.
5. The nurse whose specialty is pain management
   a. Demonstrates clinical competency through a variety of mechanisms, which may include continuing education, certification, credentialing, and use of the ASPMN *Standards of Clinical Practice for the Specialty of Pain Management Nursing.*
   b. Facilitates the development, implementation, and ongoing evaluation of pain management practices to promote quality care.
   c. Seeks continuing education in the field of pain management.

C. In 2005, ASPMN and the American Nurses Association published their *Scope and Standards of Practice.*
   1. While pain management is best known in cancer, palliative, and end of life care, pain is also the nursing diagnosis most often used.
   2. Nurses who specialize in this interdisciplinary area work to optimize patient pain relief, function, and quality of life of the patient.
   3. This book contains the standards of care and professional practice and their measurement criteria for both general and advanced practice, and it describes the practice characteristics, settings, and roles, along with education and certification requirements, of pain management nursing.

D. ASPMN position statements (http://www.aspmn.org/Organization/position_papers.htm)
   1. ASPMN Position Statement on Promoting Pain Relief and Preventing Abuse of Pain Medications: A Critical Balancing Act (http://www.aspmn.org/pdfs/A_JOINT_STATEMENT_FROM_21_HEALTH_ORGANIZATIONS.pdf)
      a. Undertreatment of pain is a serious problem in the United States, including pain among patients with chronic conditions and those who are critically ill or near death.
      b. Effective pain management is an integral and important aspect of quality medical care, and pain should be treated aggressively.
      c. The critical roles of health care professionals and law enforcement personnel are to work toward balancing patient care and diversion prevention.
      d. Balancing patient care includes being cognizant of opioid abuse potential in certain individuals while realizing that focusing on abuse potential of opioids can impede legitimate use of opioids to treat pain (http://www.aspmn.org/pdfs/Balancing%20Pain%20Relief%20and%20Abuse.pdf).
   2. ASPMN Health Policy Guiding Principles (http://www.aspmn.org/pdfs/Health%20Policy%20Guiding%20Principles.pdf)
      a. The responsibility and obligation of pain management occurs across the life span.
      b. "ASPMN adheres to the ethical principles of beneficence (the duty to benefit another) and justice (the equal or comparative treatment of individuals) and oblige healthcare professionals to manage pain and provide humane care to all patients, including those patients known or suspected to have addictive disease."
      c. ASPMN advocates legitimate access to pain management care.
   3. ASPMN Position Statement for Pain Management in Patients with Addictive Disorders (http://www.aspmn.org/Organization/documents/addictions_9pt.pdf)
      a. Patients with addictive disease and pain have the right to be treated with dignity, respect, and the same quality of pain assessment and management as all other patients.

   b. Nurses are well positioned to advocate for their patients in pain when addictive disorders are present.
4. ASPMN Position Statement on Assisted Suicide (http://www.aspmn.org/pdfs/Assisted% 20 Suicide.pdf)
   a. ASPMN supports improved access for pain management services and other modalities that will benefit terminally ill patients and their families.
   b. Pain management nurses should advocate for health care environments that provide humane and dignified care of the dying.
5. ASPMN Position Statement on Pain Management at the End of Life (http://www.aspmn.org/Organization/documents/EndofLifeCare.pdf)
   a. End-stage disease is often accompanied by severe pain and other unpleasant symptoms that cause undue suffering.
   b. It is an ethical obligation for pain management nurses to advocate and provide for effective pain relief and symptom management to alleviate suffering for the patient receiving end-of-life care.
6. ASPMN Position Statement on the Use of Placebos in Pain Management (http://www.aspmn.org/pdfs/Use%20of%20Placebos.pdf)
   a. Placebos should not be used by any route of administration in the assessment or management of pain in any individual regardless of age or diagnosis.
   b. Placebos may be used only in institutional review board-approved clinical trials.

IV. Joint Commission on Accreditation of Healthcare Organizations (JCAHO, 2003, http://www.jcrinc.com)

A. History of JCAHO involvement in pain management
   1. In 1992, the JCAHO took a major step forward in promoting pain relief as a priority for patient care with the onset of standards requiring pain management as one of the rights of a dying patient.
   2. In 1994, the JCAHO indicated that, "that management of pain is appropriate for all patients, not just dying patients."
   3. In 1997, the JCAHO initiated the development of standards for pain management and planned to add these standards to the accreditation process for hospitals.
   4. In 2000, these pain management standards were published, establishing, for the first time, standards requiring that hospitals be held responsible for the provision of safe and effective management of pain for hospitalized patients.
   5. In 2001, the JCAHO began scoring for compliance with these pain management standards. Effective pain management for patients was no longer optional. The JCAHO standards for pain management set clear expectations about appropriate assessment and treatment of pain.

V. Connecting Philosophy and Practice (Pesut & McDonald, 2007)

A. Ideas ultimately shape what becomes acceptable practice.
   1. Scientific understandings are always shaped by human values, understandings, and choices.

B. McCaffery's definition of pain as "whatever the patient says it is" (1968) was truly revolutionary for nursing because of its capacity to lend credibility to the patient's pain experience.

C. The externalist perceptual view of pain considers pain as a perceptual experience, one that like any perceptual experience can be "misperceived" by the person having the experience.

D. The nonrepresentational view of pain considers pain as a holistic experience, one in which physical and existential aspects necessarily coincide.

E. Pain is an interpreted objective reality.
   1. The ability to discriminate among the various aspects of the pain experience and to treat them appropriately is fundamental to expert nursing care.

Summary

The problems within pain management care in our health care system can no longer be viewed as problems to be solved. Instead, they must be viewed as opportunities to change perspectives and further understanding of humanity, the environment, and the world. Nurses who specialize in pain management are dedicated to promoting and providing optimal care of patients with pain. Certification in pain management nursing validates nurses' knowledge of pain management concepts and practice, including knowledge of the physical, social, cultural, psychological, and spiritual dimensions of the pain experience. Goals for pain relief must be balanced with the necessity of providing safe nursing care, including monitoring patients' responses to treatment. Sir Francis Bacon stated that man prefers to believe what he prefers to be true (1620/1939). This statement provides us with a cautious note that acquisition of knowledge is not without influence of our beliefs, perspectives of truth, and motivation in seeking answers. The knowledge attained through scientific rigor cannot be denied the presence of bias. Rather, we must acknowledge its existence as a customary addition to the findings. It is important to recognize that standards of care change and need regular review and improvement.

References

Acute Pain Management Guideline Panel. (1992). *Acute pain management: operative or medical procedures and trauma.* Clinical Practice Guideline. (AHCPR Publication No. 92-0032). Rockville, MD: Agency for Health Care Policy and Research, Public Health Service, U.S. Department of Health and Human Services.

American Society for Pain Management Nursing. (1998). *Standards of clinical practice for the specialty of pain management nursing.* Pensacola, FL: Author.

American Nurses Association & American Society for Pain Management Nursing. (2005). *Scope and standards of practice.* (ANA Publication No. 9781558102262). Silver Spring, MD: American Nurses Association.

Bacon, F. (1939). Novum organum. In E. A. Burtt (Ed.). *The English philosophers from Bacon to Mill* (pp. 24–123). New York: Modern Library. (Original work published 1620)

Joint Commission on Accreditation of Healthcare Organizations. (2003). *Approaches to pain management: A guide for clinical leaders.* Oakbrook Terrace, IL: Joint Commission Resources.

McCaffery, M. (1968). *Nursing practice theories related to cognition, bodily pain, and man-environment interactions.* Los Angeles: University of California at Los Angeles Students' Store.

Pesut, B., & McDonald, H. (2007). Connecting philosophy and practice: implications of two philosophic approaches to pain for nurses' expert clinical decision making, *Nursing Philosophy, 8,* 256–263.

chapter

2

Taxonomy for Pain Management Nursing

Donna Sipos Cox, MSN, ONC, CCRC, RN-BC
Eleftheria T. Karapas, MS, RN-BC

Objectives

After studying this chapter, the reader should be able to:

1. Determine differences between pain and suffering.
2. List the characteristics of acute and chronic pain.
3. Demonstrate an understanding of key pain terms and diagnoses.

The taxonomy in pain management nursing is evolving. Clarifying what we mean when we use words to describe pain is an endeavor worth pursuing. We cannot take our words for granted, nor can we assume that others know what we mean when we use our words for pain or pain management. Pain management is a field of study that is specialized and has unique terms. Most of the following terms are generic, but some are specialized, used in the clinical practice, education, and research of pain management. You will read new terms and their meanings, as well as read new meanings for old terms. Looking at terms and their meanings helps improve our clinical and research value.

I. Pain

A. In Latin, the word *poena* means "punishment or penalty."

B. Pain is "an unpleasant sensory and emotional experience associated with actual or potential tissue damage or described in terms of such damage" (Mersky, 1986, p. S217). "Pain always is subjective" (American Pain Society [APS], 2008, p. 1; International Association for the Study of Pain [IASP], 2008).

C. Pain is "whatever the experiencing person says it is, existing whenever the experiencing person says it does" (McCaffery, 1968, p. 95).

D. "Pain perception is an inherent quality of life that appears early in ontogeny to serve as a signaling system for tissue damage" (Anand & Craig, 1996, p. 4).

E. The *Diagnostic and Statistical Manual of Mental Disorders,* fourth edition, text revision (DSM-IV-TR) includes three pain disorders associated with and without psychological factors (see VIII. Psychological Pain). The DSM-IV-TR relates comorbid conditions that "the essential feature of Pain Disorder is pain that is the predominant focus of the clinical presentation and is of sufficient severity to warrant clinical attention (Criterion A). The pain causes significant distress or impairment in social, occupational, or other important areas of functioning (Criterion B). Psychological factors are judged to play a significant role in the onset, severity, exacerbation, or maintenance of the pain (Criterion C). The pain is not intentionally produced or feigned as in Factitious Disorder or Malingering (Criterion D). Pain Disorder is not diagnosed if the pain is better accounted for by a Mood, Anxiety, or Psychotic Disorder, or if the pain presentation meets criteria for Dyspareunia (Criterion E)" (American Psychiatric Association [APA], 2000, p. 498).

II. Suffering

A. In Latin, the word *suffering* is divided into the Latin words *sub,* meaning "up under," and *fero,* meaning "to bear"—that is, to bear up under or undergo.

B. Suffering is an "individualized, subjective, and complex experience that involves the assignment of an intensely negative meaning to an event or a perceived threat" (Rodgers & Cowles, 1997, p. 1048).

C. Suffering is a "state of severe distress associated with events that threaten the intactness of the person" (Cassel, 1982, p. 640).

D. Suffering is a "state of anguish of one who bears pain, injury or loss" (Copp, 1974, p. 491).

E. Distinguishing pain and suffering

1. Suffering is the person's response to the sensation of pain. Pain is a primary response, and suffering is a secondary response (Beecher, 1957, as cited in Kahn & Steeves, 1986). Suffering is not a measure of pain or psychological distress (Kahn & Steeves, 1986).
2. "Suffering is the perception of serious threat or damage to the self, and it emerges when a discrepancy develops between what one expected of one's self and what one does or is. Some patients who experience sustained unrelieved pain suffer because pain changes who they are." (Chapman & Gavrin, 1999).

F. Ferrell and Coyle (2008, p. 246) propose 10 tenets concerning suffering:

1. Suffering is a loss of control that creates insecurity.
2. Suffering is associated with loss. The loss may be evident only in the mind of the sufferer, but it nonetheless leaves a person diminished and with a sense of brokenness.
3. Suffering is an intensely personal experience.
4. Suffering is accompanied by a range of intense emotions, including sadness, anguish, fear, abandonment, despair, and myriad other emotions.
5. Suffering can be linked deeply to recognition of one's own mortality.

6. Suffering often involves asking the question "why." Suffering people frequently seek to find meaning and answers for that which is unknowable.
7. Suffering often is associated with separation from the world.
8. Suffering often is accompanied by spiritual distress.
9. Suffering is not synonymous with pain but is closely associated with it.
10. Suffering occurs when an individual feels voiceless.

III. Acute pain: nociceptive pain

A. In Latin, the word *acer* means "sharp or swift."
B. Acute pain is a warning signal to the body that something is wrong or needs attention (Bonica, 1990).
C. Recent onset
   1. Follows an acute injury to the body.
   2. Abates as healing occurs (APS, 2008, p. 1).
   3. "Sometimes acute pain can evolve into chronic pain" (APS, 2008, p. 1).
D. Peripheral nociceptors are involved in transmission of sensation (Rosner, 1996).
E. Acute pain is often associated with the sympathetic portion of the autonomic nervous system responses—objective signs of pain (APS, 2008).
   1. Hypertension
   2. Tachycardia
   3. Diaphoresis
   4. Shallow respirations
   5. Agitation or restlessness
   6. Facial grimace
   7. Splinting or guarding behavior
   8. Pallor
   9. Mydriasis
   10. Hypotension as a sign and symptom of pain-related shock
G. Treatment is focused on the cause of the pain (Rosner, 1996).
H. Pain should be treated symptomatically while its source is investigated (APS, 2008).
I. Classifications of acute pain (Table 2-1) (Rosner, 1996).
   1. Acute
   2. Subacute
   3. Ongoing acute
   4. Recurrent acute
J. Bonica (1990) did not agree with the previously listed classifications of acute pain. He believed the definitions of *subacute, ongoing acute,* and *recurrent acute* are chronic pain syndromes.

IV. Persistent Pain: Chronic Pain

A. The term *persistent pain* may one day replace the use of the term *chronic pain.*
   1. Chronic pain "has become a label associated with negative images and stereotypes often associated with longstanding psychiatric problems, futility in treatment, malingering, or drug-seeking behavior" (American Geriatrics Society [AGS], 2002, p. S205).
   2. Persistent pain "may foster a more positive attitude by patients and professionals for the many effective treatments that are available to help alleviate suffering" (p. S205).
   3. Persistent pain is pain or discomfort that continues for an extended period of time. Some conditions cause pain that may come and go for months or years. In addition to physical discomfort, persistent pain can lead to depression, disability, difficulty with walking and sleep problems (AGS Foundation for Health in Aging, 2008).
   4. The term *persistent pain* was first identified and used in the AGS publication of 2002. Subsequently, other articles have been published in the literature using the term (Anand, 2007; Hartmann, Goldfarb, Kim, Nuthulaganti, & Seifeldin, 2003; Karp, Shega, Morone, & Weiner, 2008; Siddall & Cousins, 2004).

Table 2-1 Pain Classification by Duration of Symptoms (Rosner, 1996)

Acute	Subacute	Ongoing Acute	Recurrent Acute	Chronic Intractable Benign Pain Syndrome
Duration of 0 to 7 days	Duration of 7 days to 6 months	Any duration of time	Any duration of time	Duration of more than 6 months
Mild to severe	Mild to severe	Usually severe	Mild to severe	Mild to severe
Cause known or unknown; usually a single, fixable event	Cause as in acute pain	Due to ongoing tissue damage from neoplasms	Due to chronic organic nonmalignant pathology	Cause unknown
Input from nociceptors (peripheral pain receptors)	Input from nociceptors	Input from nociceptors	Input from nociceptors	No known nociceptive input
Treatment of causes and pain reduction: often urgent; analgesics are narcotic and nonnarcotic	Treatment of causes and pain reduction: usually not urgent; analgesics are narcotic and nonnarcotic	Treatment of causes and pain reduction: analgesics are narcotic and nonnarcotic	Treatment of causes and pain reduction: analgesics are nonnarcotic, and coanalgesics are used as first-line treatment; narcotics are sometimes indicated	Treatment aimed at pain reduction: analgesics are nonnarcotic, and coanalgesics are used; usually no indication for narcotics
Mild psychological contribution	Mild psychological contribution	Depression and anxiety common	Depression and anxiety common	Psychological factors important; psychotherapy indicated Patient may or may not have adequate coping mechanisms

From *A Practical Approach to Pain Management*, published by Lippincott, Williams & Wilkins. Reprinted by permission of the publisher.

5. The North American Nursing Diagnosis Association's (NANDA) *Nursing Diagnoses* defines chronic pain as "Unpleasant sensory and emotional experience arising from actual or potential tissue damage or described in terms of such damage (International Association for the Study of Pain); sudden or slow onset of any intensity from mild to severe, constant or recurring without an anticipated or predictable end and a duration of greater than 6 months" (NANDA International, 2005, p. 133).

B. Other terms for chronic pain are still used today. As our body of knowledge in pain continues to grow, these terms will be considered out of date.
   1. Chronic nonmalignant pain (Bonica, 1990; McCaffery & Beebe, 1989; Rosner, 1996)
   2. Chronic benign nonneoplastic pain (Bonica, 1990)
   3. Chronic intractable benign pain syndrome (Bonica, 1990; Rosner, 1996)
      a. The word *benign* suggests a mildness or gentleness and should not be used (Bonica, 1990; McCaffery & Beebe, 1989).

C. Chronic or persistent pain is pain persisting a month longer than the "usual course of an acute disease or that is associated with a chronic pathologic process that causes continuous pain or the pain recurs at intervals for months or years" (Bonica, 1990, p. 9).

D. Chronic or persistent pain lasts more than 6 months (APA, 2000, p. 499; Bonica, 1990; Doenges & Moorhouse, 1993; Dunajcik, 1999; McCaffery & Beebe, 1989; NANDA International, 2009; Rosner, 1996)
   1. This is an arbitrary time frame (Bonica, 1990).

E. Causes of chronic or persistent pain are
   1. Non-life threatening (Dunajcik, 1999; McCaffery & Beebe, 1989).
   2. Unknown (Rosner, 1996).

F. Treatment is focused on pain reduction (Rosner, 1996).
   1. Adjuvants are used primarily.
   2. Use of opioids is controversial.

G. The patient does not respond to current treatment methods (Dunajcik, 1999; McCaffery & Beebe, 1989; Rosner, 1996).

H. Treatment "may continue for the remainder of the patient's life" (Dunajcik, 1999, p. 468).

I. Other NANDA diagnoses associated with but not limited to chronic pain include the following (NANDA International, 2005, p. 133):
   1. Fear (p. 76)
   2. Fatigue (p. 75)
   3. Disturbed sleep pattern (p. 179)
   4. Self-care deficit (p. 160)

V. Cancer Pain

A. Cancer pain "can be acute or chronic (longer than 3 months' duration)" (APS, 2008, p. 1).

B. Cancer pain is a "multidimensional experience consisting of physiologic, sensory, affective, cognitive, behavioral, and sociocultural dimensions" (McGuire, 1995, p. 1).

C. Causes of cancer pain are
   1. Cancer itself (Mersky, 1986; Twycross, 1997, APS, 2008).
   2. Treatment of cancer (Mersky, 1986; Twycross, 1997, APS, 2008).
   3. Concurrent disease (Twycross, 1997).

D. With chronic cancer pain, the patient rarely has signs of sympathetic nervous system arousal (APS, 2008).

E. Breakthrough pain "is a transitory exacerbation, or flare of moderate-to-severe pain that occurs in patients on chronic opioid therapy with otherwise stable persistent pain (APS, 2008, p. 2).

VI. Neuropathic Pain

A. General terms for neuropathic pain and updates
   1. Criticism of the term *neuropathic pain* includes the following:
      a. The term is too vague conceptually and clinically (Backonja, 2003).
      b. It does not account for "different underlying mechanisms . . . that have a component of neurological dysfunction" (Backonja, 2003, p. 785).

c. The new definition proposed for the IASP pain terminology (2008) for neuropathic pain is "pain arising as a direct consequence of a lesion or disease affecting the somatosensory system." This definition was defended by the task force of Neuropathic Pain Special Interest Group: "This revised definition fits into the nosology of neurological disorders. The reference to the somatosensory system was derived from a wide range of neuropathic pain conditions ranging from painful neuropathy to central poststroke pain. Because of the lack of a specific diagnostic tool for neuropathic pain, a grading system of 'definite,' 'probable,' and 'possible' neuropathic pain was proposed. The grade 'possible' can only be regarded as a working hypothesis. The grades 'probable' and 'definite' require confirmatory evidence from a neurological examination." (IASP, 2008)

2. *Sensitization* is "increased responsiveness of neurons to their normal input or recruitment of a response to normally subthreshold inputs" (IASP, 2008). This is a new term, and the use of the term "may only be inferred indirectly from phenomena such as hyperalgesia or allodynia" (IASP, 2008).

B. Terms for central pain

1. *Central neuropathic pain* is "pain arising as a direct consequence of a lesion or disease affecting the central somatosensory system" (IASP, 2008).
2. *Poststroke syndrome (thalamic pain syndrome)* is a central pain syndrome that may occur when a stroke damages the thalamus or parietal lobe. This damage causes sensory neurons in these areas of the brain to misfire and can lead to constant disabling pain that may become more severe with time. About 9% of people who have a stroke develop central pain syndrome (which is also called poststroke pain syndrome). The pain can begin immediately after a stroke but sometimes does not appear until weeks, months, or even years later (Johns Hopkins Health Alert, 2008).
3. *Central sensitization* is "increased responsiveness of nociceptive neurons in the central nervous system to their normal or subthreshold afferent input" (IASP, 2008).
4. *Spinal cord injury pain* "is the development of chronic pain below the level of the lesion" (Defrin, Grunhaus, Zamir, & Zeilig, 2007, p. 1574).

C. Terms for peripheral pain

1. *Complex regional pain syndrome, type I (also referred to as CRPS-I or reflex sympathetic dystrophy)* is a "syndrome that usually develops after an initiating noxious event, is not limited to the distribution of a single peripheral nerve, and is apparently disproportionate to the inciting event. It is associated at some point with evidence of edema, changes in skin blood flow, abnormal sudomotor activity in the region of the pain, or allodynia or hyperalgesia" (Mersky & Bogduk, 1994, p. 41).
2. *Complex regional pain syndrome, type II (also referred to as CRPS-II or causalgia)* is a "burning pain, allodynia, and hyperpathia usually in the hand or foot after partial injury of a nerve or one of its major branches" (Mersky & Bogduk, 1994, p. 42).
3. *Peripheral neurogenic pain* is "pain initiated or caused by a primary lesion or dysfunction or transitory perturbation in the peripheral nervous system" (IASP, 2008).
4. *Peripheral neuropathic pain* is "pain arising as a direct consequence of a lesion or disease affecting the peripheral somatosensory system" (IASP, 2008).
5. *Peripheral neuropathy* is pain associated with damage to the "small fibers" of the sensory peripheral nervous system, especially A-delta and C fibers. There is sensory and motor dysfunction according to the sites of pathologic involvement. In peripheral neuropathy there is a stocking- or glovelike distribution. Patients describe their pain as burning, tingling, stabbing, or prickling. Causes are ischemia secondary to vasculitis, diabetes, musculoskeletal, or visceral (Brewer, 2008, p. 586).
6. *Peripheral sensitization* is "increased responsiveness and reduced threshold of nociceptors to stimulation of their receptive fields" (IASP, 2008).
7. *Radiculalgia* is "pain along the distribution of one or more sensory nerve roots" (Bonica, 1990, p. 21).
8. *Radiculopathy* is "a disturbance of function or pathologic change in one or more nerve roots" (Bonica, 1990, p. 21).
9. *Radiculitis* is "inflammation of one or more nerve roots" (Bonica, 1990, p. 21).

D. Terms for central and peripheral pain
   1. *Phantom limb pain* is "the sensation that the deafferented body part is still present" (Flor, 2002, p. 182).
      a. Nonpainful phantom sensations may include the following (Flor, 2002):
         (1) Specific position shape
         (2) Feelings of warmth or cold
         (3) Itching
         (4) Tingling
         (5) Electric sensations
         (6) Other paresthesias
      b. Pain may be exacerbated by physical and psychological factors.
   2. *Residual limb pain (also known as stump pain)* is "pain in the adjacent area of the amputated body part. This pain is different from phantom limb and different from pain at the wound site" (Flor, 2002, p. 182).
      a. Symptoms associated with residual limb pain are as follows (Flor, 2002):
         (1) Tingling
         (2) Itching
         (3) Cramping
         (4) Involuntary movement

VII. Myofascial Pain

A. *Fibromyalgia syndrome (formerly known as fibrositis)* (see the chapter on Persistent Pain) is "diffuse musculoskeletal aching and pain with multiple predictable tender points" (Mersky & Bogduk, 1994, p. 45). Although the exact etiology remains unclear, fibromyalgia is now categorized as a neuropathic syndrome because of the central pain processing abnormalities found in almost all patients studied (Staud & Domingo, 2001).
   1. According to the American College of Rheumatology (Wolfe et al., 1990) classification criteria, both of these are present for at least 3 months.
      a. History of widespread pain
         (1) Bilateral
         (2) Upper and lower body
         (3) Axial skeletal pain (cervical spine or anterior chest or thoracic spine or low back)
      b. Pain in 11 of 18 tender point sites on digital palpation.
B. *Myofascial pain syndrome* (see the chapter on Persistent Pain) is "localized muscle pain possibly accompanied by referred pain to another region. The extent of the pain . . . can be reliably provoked by palpatory stimulation of the trigger points of this muscle." (Bliddal & Curatolo, 2008, p. 335). All five major criteria and at least one minor criterion constitute the diagnosis.
   1. Major criteria
      a. Regional pain complaint
      b. Pain complaint or altered sensation in the expected distribution of referred pain from a myofascial trigger point
      c. Taut band palpable in an accessible muscle
      d. Exquisite spot tenderness at one point along the length of the taut band
      e. Some degree of restricted range of motion
   2. Minor criteria
      a. Reproduction of clinical pain complaint, or altered sensation, by pressure on the tender spot
      b. Elicitation of a local twitch response by transverse snapping palpation at the tender spot or by needle insertion into the tender spot in the taut band
      c. Pain alleviated by elongation (stretching) of the muscle or by injecting the tender spot (McCain, 1994)
C. A *trigger point* is "a hypersensitive area or site in muscle or connective tissue, usually associated with myofascial pain syndromes" (Bonica, 1990, p. 21).

VIII. Psychological Pain

A. DSM-IV definitions can be found at http://www.psych.org/MainMenu/Research/DSMIV/DSMV.aspx. The DSM-IV-TR is currently used to define features of pain disorders with and without psychiatric comorbidities. DSM-V will not be available until 2012.

1. *Pain disorder associated with psychological factors:* "Psychological factors are judged to have the major role in the onset, severity, exacerbation, or maintenance of the pain." (APA, 2000, p. 499).
2. *Pain disorder associated with psychological factors and a general medical condition:* "Both psychological factors and a general medical condition are judged to have the major role in the onset, severity, exacerbation, or maintenance of the pain." (APA, 2000, p. 499).
3. *Pain disorder associated with a general medical condition:* "[A] general medical condition has a major role in the onset, severity, exacerbation, or maintenance of the pain." (APA, 2000, p. 499)

B. Substance dependence (see the chapter on Coexisting Addiction and Pain)

1. The working group developing the DSM-V has been debating keeping the term *substance dependence* (O'Brien, Volkow, & Li, 2006). The rigor involved in discussions, research, and debates of terms will reduce misuse and misunderstandings. The term *addiction* is not used in the DSM-IV (APA, 2000; Erickson, 2007, pp. 14–15). The DSM-IV diagnostic criteria for substance dependence include a maladaptive pattern of substance use, leading to clinically significant impairment or distress, as manifested by three (or more) of the following occurring in a 12-month period (APA, 2000, pp. 192, 197).
   a. *Tolerance* is defined as either
      (1) Need for markedly increased amounts of the substance to achieve intoxication or desired effect.
      (2) Markedly diminished effect with continued use of the same amount of the substance (APA, 2000, p. 192).
   b. *Withdrawal* is defined as either
      (1) Characteristic withdrawal syndrome for the substance.
      (2) The same (or closely related) substance taken to relieve or avoid withdrawal symptoms.
   c. The substance often is taken in larger amounts over a longer period than was intended.
   d. Persistent desire occurs, or efforts to cut down or control substance use are unsuccessful.
   e. A great deal of time is spent in activities necessary to obtain the substance, use the substance, or recover from its effects.
   f. Important social, occupational, or recreational activities are given up or reduced because of substance use.
   g. Substance use is continued despite knowledge of having a persistent or recurrent physical or psychological problem that is likely to have been caused or exacerbated by the substance (Compton, Darakjian, & Miotto, 1998).

C. Substance abuse and substance dependence in chronic pain patients (see the chapter on Coexisting Addiction and Pain)

1. Realizing limitations of the DSM-IV diagnostic criteria, the American Society of Addiction Medicine developed its definition of addiction. The following are diagnostic criteria recommended when assessing the use of opioids in the context of pain treatment (American Academy of Pain Medicine, American Pain Society, & American Society of Addiction Medicine, 2001; Heit, 2003).
   a. *Physical dependence* is a physiologic state in which abrupt cessation of the opioid or administration of an opioid antagonist results in a withdrawal syndrome. Physical dependency on opioids is an expected occurrence in all individuals in the presence of continuous use of opioids for therapeutic or for nontherapeutic purposes. It does not, in and of itself, imply addiction.
   b. *Tolerance* is a form of a neuroadaptation to the effects of long-term opioid (or other medication) use that is indicated by the need for increasing or more frequent doses of the medication to achieve the initial effects of the drug. Tolerance may occur to the analgesic effects of opioids and to unwanted side effects, such as respiratory depression, sedation, or nausea. The occurrence of tolerance is variable, but it does not, in and of itself, imply addiction.

c. *Addiction* is characterized by a persistent pattern of dysfunctional opioid use that may involve any or all of the following:
   (1) Adverse consequences associated with the use of opioids
   (2) Loss of control over the use of opioids
   (3) Preoccupation with obtaining opioids despite the presence of adequate analgesia (Compton et al., 1998)
   (4) The term *addiction* may be misleading, and "stems partly from a desire to hold drug users accountable for their actions" (Erickson, 2007, p. 12).

D. *Chronic pain syndrome* is a "psychosocial disorder. Pain and suffering become the central focus for the patient and may exist without known organic pathology or known objective findings that are congruent with the pain reported. It can result in an endless pursuit of diagnoses and treatments, overuse of the medical system, and surgeries or procedures of questionable value. The patient's social situation typically supports him or her in these pursuits. The patient also may be depressed, anxious, consumed by pain problems, and no longer functioning in work, personal life, or society" (Dunajcik, 1999, p. 468).

E. *Drug-seeking* is "a set of behaviors in which an individual makes a directed and concerted effort to obtain a medication. Regarding opioid analgesics, behaviors may include 'clock watching', frequent requests for early refills, or hoarding opioid analgesics. These behaviors do not, in themselves, constitute addiction. When these behaviors are for the purpose of obtaining adequate pain relief, this is called *pseudoaddiction.* If the behaviors are for the purpose of using the drug for nonmedical purposes, they are suggestive of abuse or addiction" (Compton, 1999, p. 429).

F. *Factitious disorder:* "The essential feature of Factitious Disorder is the intentional production of physical or psychological signs and symptoms (Criterion A). The presentation may include fabrication of subjective complaints, . . . falsification of objective signs, . . . self inflicted condition, . . . exaggeration or exacerbation of pre existing general medical conditions, . . . or any combination or variation of these. The motivation for the behavior is to assume the sick role (Criterion B). External incentives for the behavior (e.g., economic gain, avoiding legal responsibility, or improving physical well-being, as in Malingering) are absent" (APA, 2000, p. 513).

G. *Malingering:* "The essential feature of Malingering is the intentional production of false or grossly exaggerated physical or psychological symptoms, motivated by external incentives such as avoid military duty, avoiding work, obtaining financial compensation, evading criminal prosecution, or obtain drugs" (APA, 2000, p. 739).

H. *Physical dependence* is "a neuroadaptive state resulting from chronic drug administration in which abrupt cessation of the drug, or administration of an antagonist to the drug, results in a drug-specific withdrawal syndrome." (Compton, 1999, p. 429).

I. *Pseudoaddiction* is a set of behaviors a person exhibits to obtain medication for adequate pain relief (Weissman & Haddox, 1989).

J. *Psychogenic pain disorder* is associated with psychological factors. It can be caused, increased or prolonged due to mental or emotional problems. The diagnosis is made when organic causes of pain are ruled out (Cleveland Clinic, 2005; Covington, 2000). Diagnosis is based on patient's signs and symptoms, not on etiology of pain. The patient responds to psychological treatment of this pain (Toda, 2007).

K. *Somatoform disorder* includes pain disorder. It is ". . . pattern of recurring, multiple, chronically significant somatic complaints. . . . The somatic complaints must begin before age 30 years and occur over a period of several years (Criterion A). . . . There must be a history of pain related to at least four different sites (e.g., head, abdomen, back, joints, extremities, chest, rectum) or functions (e.g., menstruation, sexual intercourse, urination) (Criterion B1). There must be a history of at least two GI symptoms other than pain (Criterion B2). . . . Symptoms are . . . of sufficient severity to warrant clinical attention. . . . [Pain disorder is] characterized by pain as the predominant focus of clinical attention. In addition, psychological factors are judged to have an important role in its onset, severity, exacerbation, or maintenance" (APA, 2000, pp. 485, 486, 498).

L. *Substance abuse* is a maladaptive pattern of substance use leading to clinically significant impairment or distress" (APA, 2000, p. 199). The criteria for substance abuse include the "harmful consequences of repeated use" but do not include withdrawal, tolerance, or compulsive use.

IX. General Terminology Used in Pain

A. *Algology* is "the science and study of pain phenomena. An algologist is a student, investigator, and practitioner of algology" (Bonica, 1990, p. 20).

B. *Dermatome* is "the sensory segmental supply to the skin and subcutaneous tissue" (Bonica, 1990, p. 21).

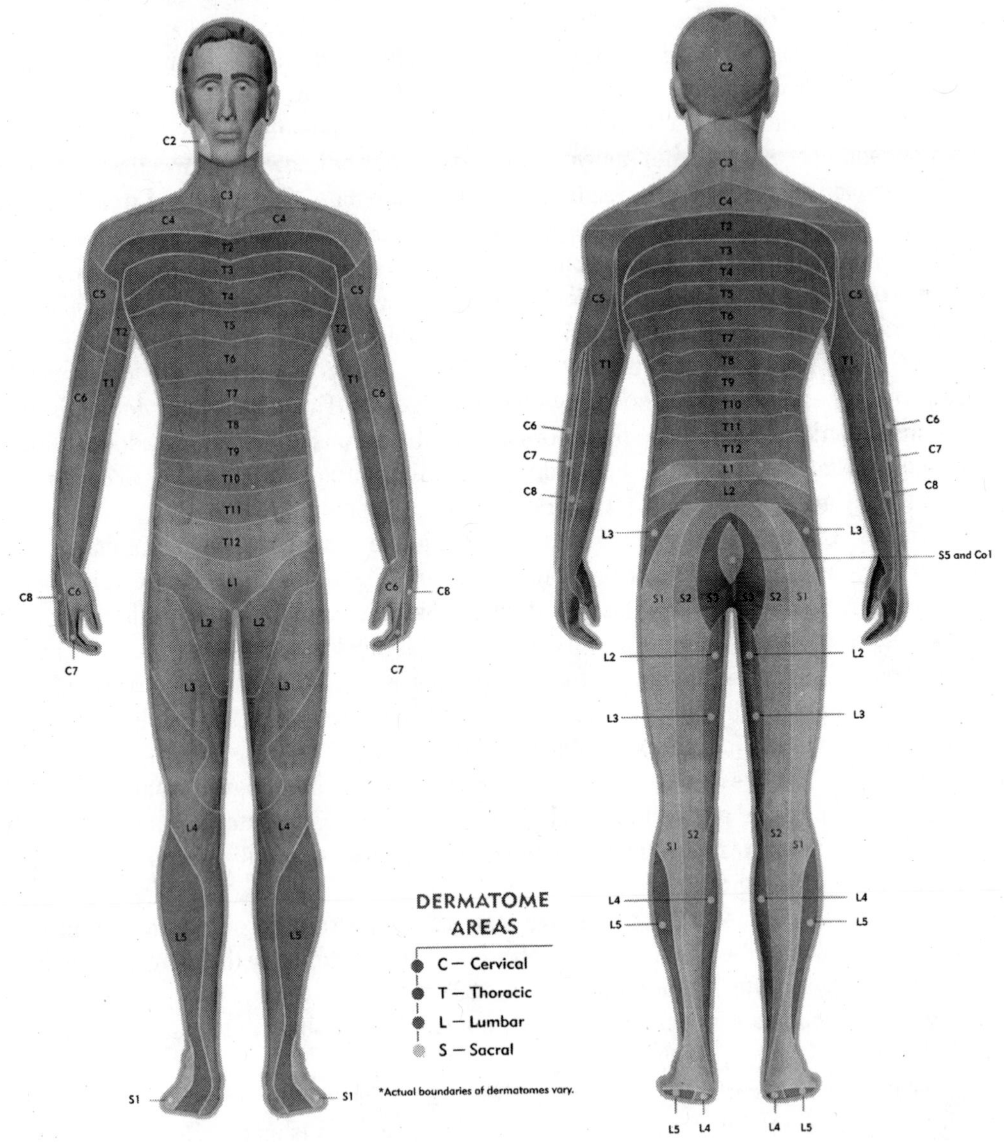

Image courtesy of Boston Scientific Corporation.

C. *Nociception* is "the neural processes of encoding and processing noxious stimuli" (IASP, 2008).

D. A *nociceptor:* is "a sensory receptor that is capable of transducing and encoding noxious stimuli" (IASP, 2008).

E. *Nociceptive pain* is "pain arising from activation of nociceptors" (IASP, 2008).

F. *Noxious stimulus* is "an actually or potentially tissue-damaging event transduced and encoded by nociceptors" (IASP, 2008).

G. The *pain intensity scale* is a tool used to communicate the intensity of pain and to guide treatment (APS, 2008, p. 1).

H. The *pain threshold* is "the minimal intensity of a stimulus that is perceived as painful" (IASP, 2008; for the older definition, see Mersky, 1986, p. S220).

I. The *pain tolerance level* is "the maximum intensity of a stimulus that evokes pain and that a subject is willing to tolerate in a given situation" (IASP, 2008 Mersky, 1986, p. S221).

J. A *receptor* is a component of an organism with which a chemical agent is presumed to interact (Ross, 1996).

X. Pain Descriptors and Types

A. *Allodynia* is "pain in response to a non-nociceptive stimulus" (IASP, 2008; Mersky, 1986, p. S217) (Table 2-2).

B. *Analgesia* is the "absence of pain in response to stimulation [that] would normally be painful" (Mersky, 1986, p. S218).

C. *Anesthesia* is the "absence of all sensory modalities" (Bonica, 1990, p. 20).

D. *Anesthesia dolorosa* is "pain in an area or region that is anesthetic" (IASP, 2008; Mersky, 1986, p. S218).

E. *Angina* is "derived from the Latin term *angor,* for strangling. [It is] usually employed for pain syndromes associated with cardiac disease and indicates a feeling of oppression or tightness of the throat" (Bonica, 1990, p. 20).

F. *Arthralgia* is "pain in a joint, usually due to arthritis or arthropathy" (Bonica, 1990, p. 20).

G. *Breakthrough pain* is "pain that increases above the pain addressed by the ongoing analgesics. [It] includes incident pain and end of dose failure" (Pasero, Portenoy, & McCaffery, 1999b, p. 162).

H. *Deafferentation pain* is "pain due to loss of sensory input into the central nervous system, as occurs with avulsion of the brachial plexus or other types of lesions of peripheral nerves or due to pathology of the central nervous system" (Bonica, 1990, pp. 20–21).

I. *Dysesthesia* is "an unpleasant abnormal sensation, whether spontaneous or evoked" (Mersky, 1986, p. S218).

J. *Hyperesthesia* is "increased sensitivity to stimulation, excluding the special senses" (Mersky, 1986, p. S218).

K. *Hyperalgesia* is "increased pain sensitivity" (IASP, 2008; for the older definition, see Mersky, 1986, p. S219). See opioid-induced hyperalgesia.

L. *Hyperpathia* is "a painful syndrome, characterized by increased reaction to a stimulus, especially a repetitive stimulus, as well as an increased threshold" (Mersky, 1986, p. S219) (Table 2-2).

M. *Hypoalgesia* is "diminished pain in response to normally painful stimulus" (Mersky, 1986, p. S219) (Table 2-2).

N. *Hypoesthesia* is "decreased sensitivity to stimulation, excluding the special senses" (Mersky, 1986, p. S219).

O. *Lancinating* is also called *tabetic pain.* It is "stabbing, knifelike" (Portenoy & McCaffery, 1999, p. 302).

P. *Neuralgia* is "pain in the distribution of a nerve or nerves" (Mersky, 1986, p. S220).

Q. *Neuritis* is "inflammation of a nerve or nerves" (Mersky, 1986, p. S220). This term is "not to be used unless inflammation is thought to be present" (IASP, 2008).

R. *Neuropathy* is "a disturbance of function or pathologic changes in a nerve; in one nerve, mononeuropathy; in several nerves, mononeuropathy multiplex; if diffuse and bilateral, polyneuropathy" (Mersky, 1986, p. S220).

Table 2-2 Pain Terminology

Term	Implications
Allodynia	Lowered threshold—stimulus and response mode differ
Hyperalgesia	Increased response—stimulus and response mode are the same
Hyperpathia	Raised threshold, increased response—stimulus and response mode may be the same or different
Hypoalgesia	Raised threshold, lowered response—stimulus and response mode are the same

Modified from Mersky, H. (Ed.). (1986). Classification of chronic pain: Descriptions of chronic pain syndromes and definitions of pain terms. *Pain* (suppl. 3, pt. II), S219.

S. *Paresthesia* is "an abnormal sensation, whether spontaneous or evoked" (Mersky, 1986, p. S221).

T. *Somatic* is a term "derived from the Greek word for 'body.' Somatosensory input refers to sensory signals from all tissues of the body, including skin, viscera, muscles, and joints. However, [it is] usually used for input for body tissue other than viscera" (Bonica, 1990, p. 21). *Somatic* refers to "pain of the musculoskeletal system" (Pasero, Paice, & McCaffery, 1999a, p. 16).

U. *Tabetic pain* is a synonym for *lancinating pain,* a "sharp, lightning type of pain" (Portenoy & McCaffery, 1999, p. 302).

V. *Visceral* is "pain of the body's internal organs" (Pasero et al., 1999a, p. 16).

XI. Pharmacologic Terms Used in Pain Management

A. *Agonists in pain management* are "drugs that bind to physiological receptors and mimic the regulatory effects of the endogenous signaling compounds" (Buxton, 2006, p. 23). Agonists are compounds that bind to mu (μ) or kappa (κ) receptors to produce analgesia (Jaffe & Martin, 1990).

B. *Analgesic* refers to "an agent that produces analgesia" (Bonica, 1990, p. 20).

C. An *anesthetic agent* is an agent that will block or temporarily take away a sensation (such as pain). This may allow the patient to undergo procedures or surgery without pain and distress (Salinas, Malik, & Benzon, 2008).

D. *Antagonists* are "compounds with no stimulatory action of their own that still may produce useful effects by inhibiting the action of an agonist (e.g., by competition for agonist-binding sites)" (Buxton, 2006, p. 23). This refers to the interference of one chemical with another. An μ-agonist binds with the μ-receptor, creating analgesia. When naloxone (an antagonist) is administered, it competes at the μ-receptor with the μ-agonist for the receptor site and reverses analgesia and side effects (Klaassen, 1996).

E. *Authorized agent–controlled analgesia* is "a method of pain control in which a consistently available and competent individual is authorized by a prescriber and properly educated to activate the dosing button of an analgesic infusion pump when a patient in unable, in response to that patient's pain" (Wuhrman et al., 2007, p. 6) This practice is supported by the American Society for Pain Management Nursing (2007) when the institution or agency has clear guidelines outlining the conditions in which the practice is implemented, monitored to ensure safe use of the therapy. The research on pediatric subjects is encouraging. The national patient safety goals hold us accountable for the education, monitoring, and safety of our patients, so pain management nurses are well positioned to continue to research this method of pain control for other populations measuring efficacy and safety of authorized agent–controlled analgesia. There are two types of authorized agents to control the analgesia:

1. Nurse-controlled analgesia, in which "the authorized agent is the nurse responsible for the patient" (Wuhrman et al., 2007, p. 6)
2. Caregiver-controlled analgesia, in which "the authorized agent is a nonprofessional individual (e.g., parent, significant other)" (Wuhrman et al., 2007, p. 6)

F. *Balanced analgesia* is "also referred to as continuous, multimodal analgesia" (Pasero et al., 1999b, p. 162) (described later). The preferred terms used in literature are *multimodal analgesia* (Kehlet & Dahl 1993; Maheshwari, Boutary, Yun, Sirianni, & Dorr, 2006) and *rational polypharmacy* (Gallagher, 2006).

G. *Hydrophilic* refers to the property of attracting or associating with water molecules (Benet, Kroetz, & Sheiner, 1996).

H. *Lipophilic* is "having an affinity for fat, . . . absorbing, dissolving or being dissolved in lipids . . ." (*Dorland's Illustrated Medical Dictionary,* 2007, p. 1079).

I. *Multimodal analgesia* is the combination of analgesics working on different sites in the peripheral and central nervous system (Maheshwari et al., 2006). It is "the administration of two analgesic agents that act by different mechanisms via a single route for providing superior analgesic efficacy with equivalent or reduced adverse effects. . . . The literature suggests that two routes of administration, when compared with a single route, may be more effective in providing perioperative analgesia" (American Society of Anesthesiologists Task Force, 2004, p. 1576). Multimodal analgesia also incorporates a multidisciplinary approach using nonpharmacological interventions (Moote, 1993; Polomano, Rathmell, Krenzischeck, & Dunwoody, 2008).

J. *N*-methyl-D-aspartate (NMDA)
   1. NMDA "represents one class of receptors for endogenous excitatory amino acid transmitters, which may include l-glutamate, l-aspartate, homocysteate, and cysteine sulfinic acid. NMDA receptors seem to be involved in synaptic transmission at a wide variety of sites in the [central nervous system] . . . [and] seem to be critically involved in synaptic formation and plasticity both during early development of the [central nervous system]" (Stone, 1993, p. 825).
   2. "NMDA receptor antagonists have been demonstrated to prevent morphine tolerance" (Wong, Cherng, Luk, Ho, & Tung, 1996, p. 27).

K. Narcotic
   1. "With the increasing use of the term in a legal context to refer to any substance that can cause dependence, the term 'narcotic' is no longer useful in a pharmacologic context" (Jaffe & Martin, 1990, p. 486).
   2. *Narcotic* is a "legal, not pharmacologic, term used in reference to all substances covered by the 1961 Single Convention on Narcotic Drugs, including synthetic and naturally occurring opioids and cocaine. Because the term covers a variety of substances with abuse potential, it is considered an obsolete term in the fields of addiction and pain management" (Compton, 1999, p. 429).

L. *Opiate* refers to medications derived from opium and semisynthetic morphine (Jaffe & Martin, 1990).

M. *Opioids* include all naturally occurring and synthetic agonists and antagonists with morphine-like activity (Reisine & Pasternak, 1996).

N. With *opioid-induced hyperalgesia (OIH),* the patient who receives opioids to control pain paradoxically may become more sensitive to pain as a direct result of opioid therapy (Angst & Clark, 2006).
   1. *OIH during maintenance and withdrawal:* Human studies illustrated aggravation of preexisting hyperalgesia by opioids during withdrawal (Angst & Clark, 2006; Compton, Athanasos, & Elashoff, 2003). In animals, hyperalgesia occurs between doses and withdrawal (Angst & Clark, 2006).
   2. *OIH with dose escalation and ultrahigh doses:* The condition is not reversed with an opioid antagonist, and increasing the opioid dose worsens condition. Dose reduction and substitution may decrease symptoms (Angst & Clark, 2006).
   3. *OIH with ultralow doses:* The dose is 1000-fold lower than antinociceptive effect. This type of OIH is shown to occur in an animal model; human studies are conflicting (Angst & Clark, 2006).

O. With *opioid-induced tolerance,* "a higher dose is required over time to maintain the same level of analgesia" (DuPen, Shen, & Ersek, 2007, p. 115).
   1. With *pharmacodynamic tolerance,* the decreased drug effect is due not to pharmacokinetic factors but to "changes in the response of the neural systems" (DuPen et al., 2007, p. 115).

P. *Partial agonists* are "agents that are only partly as effective as agonists no matter the amount employed" (Buxton, 2006, p. 23).

Q. *Patient-controlled analgesia (PCA)* is " a method of pain control designed to allow the patient to administer present doses of an analgesic, on demand, . . . using an analgesic infusion pump" (Wuhrman et al., 2007, p. 6). With PCA, the patient "has limited control of the dosing of opioid from an infusion pump within tightly mandated parameters. . . . The technique avoids delays in administration and permits greater dosing flexibility than other regimens, better adapting to individual differences in responsiveness to pain and to opioids. It also gives the patient a greater sense of control" (Gutstein & Aki, 2006, p. 581).

R. *PCA by proxy* is "a term that describes activation of the analgesic infusion pump by anyone other than the patient" (Wuhrman, et al., 2007, p. 6). In the ASPMN position statement (see the chapter on Pediatric Pain Management), this is an unauthorized activation of the pump that the patient only was intended to use. This position statement enforced that this is an unsafe practice (Wuhrman et al., 2007, p. 4). (See nurse-controlled analgesia and caregiver-controlled analgesia under XI. E. Authorized Agent-Controlled Analgesia).

S. *Preemptive analgesia* is "an intervention that is initiated before a nociceptive stimulus, and the intervention either lasts or is continued until nociceptive stimulus is abated. The intervention needs to significantly decrease or eliminate the usual immediate effect of the nociceptive stimulus." (Perkins & Washington, 2008, p. 336). Preemptive analgesia is "an antinociceptive intervention that starts before a surgical procedure and is more effective than the same intervention that starts after surgery" (Pogatzki-Zahn & Zahn, 2006, pp. 551). "Preemptive analgesia is a treatment that is initiated before the surgical incision and is operational during the surgical procedure in order to prevent the establishment of altered sensory processing that amplifies postoperative pain. Its effect on analgesic consumption or pain ratings after surgery needs to be greater compared with the same treatment initiated after surgery" (Pogatzki-Zahn & Zahn, 2006, pp. 553).

T. With ***preventive analgesia,*** "postoperative pain or analgesic consumption is reduced relative to another treatment, a placebo treatment or no treatment, as long as the effect is observed at a point in time that exceeds the expected duration of action of the target agent. The intervention may or may not be initiated before surgery" (Pogatzki-Zahn & Zahn, 2006, p. 553).

U. ***Rational polypharmacy*** involves "combining medications from different classes to affect different pathophysiologic mechanisms" (Gallagher, 2006, p. S1).

V. ***Rescue doses:*** The terms ***breakthrough*** and ***supplemental dose*** also are used interchangeably. An immediate-release opioid analgesic is used to treat breakthrough pain for a patient using around-the-clock opioid analgesics (Pasero et al., 1999b, p. 244).

References

American Academy of Pain Medicine, American Pain Society, & American Society of Addiction Medicine. (2001). *Definitions related to the use of opioids for the treatment of pain.* Retrieved October 22, 2007, from http://www.painmed.org/productpub/statements/pdfs/definition.pdf.

American Geriatrics Society. (2002). The management of persistent pain in older persons. *Journal of the American Geriatrics Society, 50*(6), S205–S224.

American Geriatrics Society Foundation for Health in Aging. (2008). *Public education.* Retrieved December 16, 2008, from http://www.healthinaging.org/public_education/pef/persistent_pain.php.

American Pain Society. (2008). *Principles of analgesic use in the treatment of acute pain and cancer pain* (6th ed.). Glenview, IL: Author.

American Psychiatric Association. (2000). *Diagnostic and statistical manual of mental disorders* (4th ed., text rev.) (DSM-IV-TR). Arlington, VA: Author.

American Society of Anesthesiologists Task Force. (2004). Practice guidelines for acute pain management in the perioperative setting. *Anesthesiology, 100,* 1573–1581.

Anand, K. J. S., & Craig, L. D. (1996). New perspectives on the definition of pain. *Pain, 67,* 3–6.

Anand, R. (2007). Neuropsychiatric management of persistent pain. *Internet Journal of Pain, Symptom Control & Palliative Care, 5*(2), 1-8.

Angst, M. S., & Clark, J. D. (2006). Opioid-induced hyperalgesia. *Anesthesiology, 104,* 570–587.

Backonja, M. M. (2003). Defining neuropathic pain. *Anesthesia & Analgesia,* 97, 785–790.

Benet, L. Z., Kroetz, D. L., & Sheiner, L. B. (1996). Pharmacokinetics: The dynamics of drug absorption, distribution, and elimination. In J. G. Hardman & L. E. Limbird (Eds.), *The pharmacological basis of therapeutics* (9th ed., pp. 3–41). New York: McGraw-Hill.

Bliddal, H., & Curatolo, M. (2008). Clinical manifestation of muscle and joint pain. In T. Graven-Nielsen, L. Arendt-Nielsen, & S. Mense (Eds.), *Fundamentals of musculoskeletal pain* (pp. 327-345). Seattle: IASP Press.

Bonica, J. J. (1990). Definitions and taxonomy of pain. In J. J. Bonica (Ed.), *The management of pain* (2nd ed., pp. 18–27). Philadelphia: Lea & Febiger.

Brewer, R. P. (2008). Pain in selected neurologic disorders. In H. T. Benzon, J. P. Rathmell, C. L. Wu, D. C. Turk, & C. E. Argoff (Eds.), *Raj's practical management of pain* (p. 586). Philadelphia: Mosby Elsevier.

Buxton, I. L. O. (2006). Pharmacokinetics and pharmacodynamics: The dynamics of drug absorption, distribution, action, and elimination. In L. L. Brunton, J. S. Lazo, & K. L. Parker (Eds.), *Goodman & Gilman's the pharmacological basis of therapeutics* (11th ed., p. 1–39). New York: McGraw-Hill.

Cassel, E. J. (1982). The nature of suffering and the goals of medicine. *New England Journal of Medicine, 306,* 639–645.

Chapman, C., & Gavrin, J. (1999, June 26). Suffering: the contributions of persistent pain. *Lancet, 353*(9171), 2233–2237.

Cleveland Clinic. (2005). *Health information: psychogenic pain.* Retrieved January 6, 2009, from http://my.clevelandclinic.org/services/pain_management/hic_psychogenic_pain.aspx.

Compton, P. (1999). Substance abuse. In M. McCaffery & C. Pasero (Eds.), *Pain: Clinical manual* (2nd ed., pp. 428–466). St. Louis: Mosby.

Compton, P., Athanasos, P., & Elashoff, D. (2003). Withdrawal hyperalgesia after acute opioid physical dependence in nonaddicted humans: A preliminary study. *Journal of Pain, 4,* 511–519.

Compton, P., Darakjian, J., & Miotto, K. (1998). Screening for addiction in patients with chronic pain and "problematic" substance use: Evaluation of a pilot assessment tool. *Journal of Pain and Symptom Management,* 16, 355–363.

Copp, L. A. (1974). The spectrum of suffering. *American Journal of Nursing, 74,* 491–495.

Covington, E. (2000). Psychogenic pain: what it means, why it does not exist, and how to diagnosis it. *Pain Medicine,* 1, 287–294.

Defrin, R., Grunhaus, L., Zamir, D., & Zeilig, G. (2007). The effect of a series of repetitive transcranial magnetic stimulations of the motor cortex on central pain after spinal cord injury. *Archives of Physical Medicine and Rehabilitation, 88,* 1574–1580.

Doenges, M. E., & Moorhouse, M. F. (1993). *Nurse's pocket guide: Nursing diagnoses with interventions* (4th ed.). Philadelphia: F. A. Davis.

Dorland's illustrated medical dictionary (31st ed.). (2007). Philadelphia: Saunders.

Dunajcik, L. (1999). Chronic nonmalignant pain. In M. McCaffery & C. Pasero (Eds.), *Pain: Clinical manual* (2nd ed., pp. 467–521). St. Louis: Mosby.

DuPen, A., Shen, D., & Ersek, M. (2007). Mechanisms of opioid-induced tolerance and hyperalgesia. *Pain Management Nursing, 8,* 113–121.

Erickson, C. K. (2007). *The Science of Addiction: From Neurobiology to Treatment.* New York: W. W. Norton.

Ferrell, B. R., & Coyle, N. (2008). The nature of suffering and the goals of nursing. *Oncology Nursing Forum, 35,* 241–247.

Flor, H. (2002). Phantom-limb pain: Characteristics, causes, and treatment. *Lancet, 1,* 182–189.

Gallagher, R. M. (2006). Analgesic selection in the management of chronic pain: Linking mechanisms & evidence-based research to clinical practice. *Clinical Journal of Pain* (Suppl. 1), S1.

Gutstein, H. B., & Aki, H. (2006). Opioid analgesics. In L. L. Brunton, J. S. Lazo, & K. L. Parker (Eds.), *Goodman & Gilman's the pharmacological basis of therapeutics* (11th ed., p. 547–590). New York: McGraw-Hill.

Hartmann, C. W., Goldfarb, N. I., Kim, S. S., Nuthulaganti, B. R., & Seifeldin, R. (2003). Care management for persistent pain: an introduction. *Disease Management, 6*(2), 103–110.

Heit, H. A. (2003). Addiction, physical dependence, and tolerance: Precise definitions to help clinicians evaluate and treat chronic pain patients. *Journal of Pain & Palliative Care Pharmacotherapy, 17*(1), 15–27.

International Association for the Study of Pain. (2008). *IASP proposed taxonomy changes.* Retrieved December 18, 2008, from http://www.iasp-pain.org/AM/Template.cfm?Section=Home&Template=/CM/ContentDisplay.cfm& ContentID=6633.

Jaffe, J. H., & Martin, W. R. (1990). Opioid analgesics and antagonists. In A. G. Goodman, T. W. Rall, A. S. Nies, & P. Tayler (Eds.), *Goodman and Gilman's the pharmacological basis of therapeutics* (pp. 485–521). New York: Pergamon Press.

Johns Hopkins Health Alert. (2008). *Understanding central pain syndrome.* Retrieved December 20, 2008, from http://www.johnshopkinshealthalerts.com/alerts/hypertension_stroke/JohnsHopkinsHealthAlertsHypertensionStroke_802-1.html.

Kahn, D. L., & Steeves, R. H. (1986). The experience of suffering: Conceptual clarification and theoretical definition. *Journal of Advanced Nursing, 11,* 623–631.

Karp, J. F., Shega, J. W., Morone, N. E., & Weiner, D. K. (2008). Advance understanding the mechanisms and management of persistent pain in older adults. *British Journal of Anaesthesia, 101,* 111–120.

Kehlet, H., & Dahl, J. B. (1993). The value of "multimodal" or "balanced analgesia" in postoperative pain treatment. *Anesthesia and Analgesia, 77,* 1048–1056.

Klaassen, C. D. (1996). Principles of toxicology and treatment of poisoning. In J. G. Hardman & L. E. Limbird (Eds.), *The pharmacological basis of therapeutics* (9th ed.). New York: McGraw-Hill.

Maheshwari, A. V., Boutary, M., Yun, A. G., Sirianni, L. E., & Dorr, L. D. (2006). Multimodal analgesia without routine parenteral narcotics for total hip arthroplasty. *Clinical Orthopaedics and Related Research, 453,* 231–238.

McCaffery, M. (1968). *Nursing practice theories related to cognition, bodily pain, and man–environment interactions.* Los Angeles: University of California at Los Angeles Students' Store.

McCaffery, M., & Beebe, A. (1989). *Pain: Clinical manual for nursing practice.* St. Louis: Mosby.

McCain, G. A. (1994). Fibromyalgia and myofascial pain syndromes. In P. Wall & R. Melzack (Eds.), *Textbook of pain* (3rd ed., pp. 475–493). London: Churchill Livingstone.

McGuire, D. B. (1995). The multiple dimensions of cancer pain: A framework for assessment and management. In D. B. McGuire, C. H. Yarbro, & B. R. Ferrell (Eds.), *Cancer pain management* (2nd ed., pp. 1–17). Boston: Jones & Bartlett.

Mersky, H. (Ed.). (1986). Classification of chronic pain: Descriptions of chronic pain syndromes and definitions of pain terms. *Pain* (Suppl. 3, Pt. 2), S215–S221.

Mersky, H., & Bogduk, N. (Eds.). (1994). *Classification of chronic pain: Descriptions of chronic pain syndromes and definitions of pain terms* (2nd ed.). Seattle: IASP Press.

Moote, C. (1993). Techniques for post-op pain management in the adult. *Canadian Journal of Anesthesia, 40,* R19–R28.

North American Nursing Diagnosis Association International. (2005). *NANDA nursing diagnoses: Definitions & classification, 2005–2006.* Philadelphia: Author.

O'Brien, C. P., Volkow, N., & Li, T-K. (2006). What's in a word? Addiction versus dependence in DSM-V. *American Journal of Psychiatry, 163*(5), 764–765.

Pasero, C., Paice, J. A., & McCaffery, M. (1999a). Basic mechanisms underlying the causes and effects of pain. In M. McCaffery & C. Pasero (Eds.), *Pain: Clinical manual* (2nd ed., pp. 15–34). St. Louis: Mosby.

Pasero, C., Portenoy, R. K., & McCaffery, M. (1999b). Opioid analgesics. In M. McCaffery & C. Pasero (Eds.), *Pain: Clinical manual* (2nd ed., pp. 161–299). St. Louis: Mosby.

Perkins, F., & Washington, T. (2008). Preemptive analgesia and prevention of chronic pain syndromes after surgery. In H. T. Benzon, J. P. Rathmell, C. L. Wu, D. C. Turk, & C. E. Argoff (Eds.), *Raj's practical management of pain* (pp. 335–341). Philadelphia: Mosby Elsevier.

Pogatzki-Zahn, E. M., & Zahn, P. K. (2006). From preemptive to preventive analgesia. *Current Opinion in Anaesthesiology, 19,* 551–555.

Polomano, R. C., Rathmell, M. D., Krenzischeck, D. A., & Dunwoody, C. J. (2008). Emerging trends and new approaches to acute pain management. *Pain Management Nursing, 9,* S33–S41.

Portenoy, R. K., & McCaffery, M. (1999). Adjuvant analgesics. In M. McCaffery & C. Pasero (Eds.), *Pain: Clinical manual* (2nd ed., pp. 300–361). St. Louis: Mosby.

Reisine, T., & Pasternak, G. (1996). Opioid analgesics and antagonists. In J. G. Hardman & L. E. Limbird (Eds.), *The pharmacological basis of therapeutics* (9th ed.). New York: McGraw-Hill.

Rodgers, B. L., & Cowles, K. V. (1997). A conceptual foundation for human suffering in nursing care and research. *Journal of Advanced Nursing, 25,* 1048–1053.

Rosner, H. L. (1996). The pharmacologic management of acute postoperative pain. In M. Lefkowitz & A. H. Lebovits (Eds.), *A practical approach to pain management.* Boston: Little, Brown.

Ross, E. M. (1996). Pharmacodynamics. In J. G. Hardman & L. E. Limbird (Eds.), *The pharmacological basis of therapeutics* (9th ed.). New York: McGraw-Hill.

Salinas, F. V., Malik, K., & Benzon, H. T. (2008). Local anesthetics for regional anesthesia and pain management. In H. T. Benzon, J. P. Rathmell, C. L. Wu, D. C. Turk, & C. E. Argoff (Eds.), *Raj's practical management of pain* (pp. 811–812). Philadelphia: Mosby Elsevier.

Siddall, P. J., & Cousins, M. J. (2004). Persistent pain as a disease entity: Implications for clinical management. *Anesthesia & Analgesia, 99,* 510–520.

Staud, R., & Domingo, M. (2001). Evidence for abnormal pain processing in fibromyalgia syndrome. *Pain Medicine, 2*(3), 208–215.

Stone, T. W. (1993). Subtypes of NMDA receptors. *General Pharmacology, 24,* 825–832.

Toda, K. (2007). The terms neurogenic pain and psychogenic pain complicate clinical practice. *Clinical Journal of Pain, 23,* 380.

Twycross, R. (1997). Cancer pain classification. *Acta Anaesthesiologica Scandinavica, 41,* 141–145.

Weissman, D. E., & Haddox, J. D. (1989). Opioid pseudoaddiction: an iatrogenic syndrome. *Pain, 36,* 363–366.

Wolfe, F., Smythe, H. A., Yunus, M. B., Bennett, R. M., Bombardier, C., Goldenberg, D. L., Tugwell, P., Campbell, S. M., Abeles, M., Clark, P., Fam. A.G., Farber, S.J., Fiechtner, J.J., Franklin, C.M., Gatter, R.A., Hamaty, D., Lessard, J., Lichtbroun, A.S., Masi, A.T., McCain, G.A., Reynolds, W.J., Romano, R.J., Russell, I.J., & Sheon, R.P. (1990). The

American College of Rheumatology 1990 criteria for the classification of fibromyalgia: Report of the Multicenter Criteria Committee. *Arthritis and Rheumatism 33,* 160–172.

Wong, C. S., Cherng, C. H., Luk, H. N., Ho, S. T., & Tung, C. S. (1996). Effects of NMDA receptor antagonists on inhibition of morphine tolerance in rats: binding at μ-opioid receptors. *European Journal of Pharmacology, 291,* 27–33.

Wuhrman, E., Cooney, M. F., Dunwoody, C. J., Eksterowicz, N., Merkel, S., & Oakes, L. I. (2007). Authorized and unauthorized ("PCA by proxy") dosing of analgesic infusion pumps: Position statement with clinical practice recommendations. *Pain Management Nursing, 8*(1), 4–11.

Suggested Reading

Scull, T., Motamed, C., & Carli, F. (1998). The stress response and pre-emptive analgesia. In M. A. Ashburn & L. J. Rice (Eds.), *The management of pain* (pp. 557–576). New York: Churchill Livingstone.

Stevens, B., Johnston, C., Franck, L., Petryshen, P., Jack, A., & Foster, G. (1999). The efficacy of developmentally sensitive interventions and sucrose for relieving procedural pain in very low birth weight neonates. *Nursing Research, 48,* 35–43.

Price, D., & Verne, G. (2002, March). Brain mechanisms of persistent pain states. The Fifth World Congress on Myofascial Pain and Fibromyalgia, MYOPAIN 2001, Portland, Oregon, USA, September 9–13, 2001. *Journal of Musculoskeletal Pain, 10*(1/2), 73–83.

chapter

3

Nursing Theories: Support of Pain Management Nursing

Alice E. Conway, PhD, RN, CRNP, FNP-BC

Objectives

After studying this chapter, the reader should be able to:

1. Recognize various theories and evaluate them for usefulness for pain management.
2. Compare and contrast various nursing conceptual models.
3. Select a theory relevant to individual pain management situations.
4. Relate middle-range theories to pain management.

"The systematic accumulation of knowledge is essential to progress in any profession. However, theory and practice must be constantly interactive. Theory without practice is empty and practice without theory is blind." (Cross, 1981, p. 110, as cited in Alligood & Tomey, 2006, p. 3)

This chapter provides an overview of various theories, particularly major nursing theories and their relevance, or lack thereof, to the management of pain.

I. Humanistic Theory: Maslow's Hierarchy of Needs

A. Overview
   1. In 1943, Maslow (1970) described a five-layer hierarchy that had physical needs on the bottom.
   2. Maslow's theory was that lower needs (physical) must be met before higher-level needs surface.

B. Underlying theoretical motivation for behavior
   1. Humans are motivated by two need systems.
      a. Basic or deficiency needs, such as food, water, and shelter, are imposed and rewarded by the environment.
      b. Growth needs, or *metaneeds,* such as needs for beauty and self-fulfillment, are motivated and reinforced internally (Maslow, 1970).
   2. These need systems are hierarchically arranged with lower-level needs assuming dominance over higher-level needs. When one level is satisfied, the next level becomes dominant.

C. Theoretical assumptions
   1. Theory is concerned with the uniqueness and the potential of individuals.
   2. It does not address shaping of human behaviors.

D. Use
   1. Explain behavior only in reference to need systems.
   2. Such systems are not intended for use in describing individuals or groups.

E. Usefulness for nursing
   1. The primary utility lies in awareness of the needs hierarchy.
   2. If basic needs are met, the individual can progress to the next level.

F. Usefulness for pain management nurses
   1. Freedom from pain is considered one of the physiological needs, and this addresses the dominance of this need before other and more self-fulfilling needs can be met (Fig. 3-1).
   2. The system helps the nurse prioritize needs.

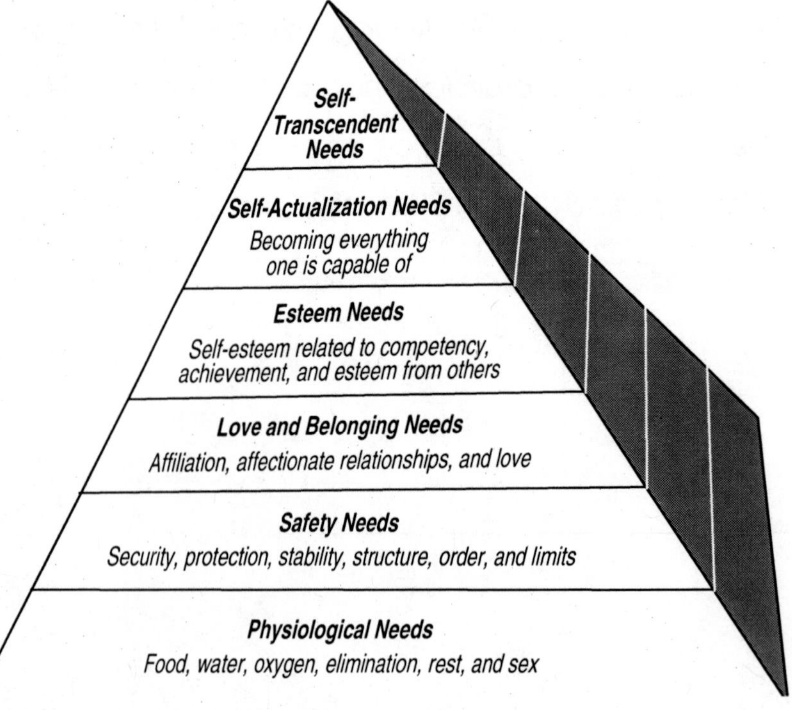

Figure 3-1 | Maslow's hierarchy of needs.

Adapted from Maslow, A. H. (1972). *The further reaches of human nature.* New York: Viking.

II. Psychosocial Development: Erikson's Theory of Personality Development

A. Overview
   1. In 1963, Erikson advanced a theory on personality development built on Freudian theory but emphasizing a healthy personality as opposed to a pathological approach.
   2. Erikson's theory embodies predictable age-related stages during which specific changes are assumed to take place.
   3. Erikson used the biological concepts of critical periods, describing key conflicts or core problems the individual has to master during critical periods of personality development.
   4. Successful completion or mastering of each of these core conflicts is built on the satisfactory completion or mastering of the previous core conflict.

B. Theoretical assumption
   1. At each stage of psychosocial development, humans are confronted with a unique problem requiring the integration of personal needs and skills with social demands and cultural expectations.
   2. Erikson referred to the individual's efforts to adjust as a *crisis;* this implies normal stresses as opposed to an extraordinary set of events.
   3. Each psychosocial stage has two components, the favorable and the unfavorable aspects of the core conflict. Progress to the next stage depends on the resolution of this conflict.
   4. No core conflict ever is mastered completely but remains a recurrent problem throughout life. No life situation ever is secure. Each new situation presents the conflict in a new form.

C. Use and usefulness for nursing
   1. Erikson's theory stresses the rational and adaptive nature of people but does not indicate clearly the kinds of experiences needed to cope with and resolve various cases. There is no concern for individual differences.
   2. The theory provides an excellent framework for explaining people, especially children in mastering developmental tasks.

D. Usefulness for pain management nurses
   1. Erikson's theory helps the nurse provide developmentally appropriate strategies that assist the patient, especially the child, cope more successfully with stressful experiences, such as pain.

III. Foundations of Mental Development: Piaget's Theory of Cognitive Development

A. Overview
   1. In 1969, Piaget described cognitive development that consisted of age-related changes that occur in mental activities as people grow.
   2. According to Piaget, intelligence enables individuals to make adaptations to the environment that increase the probability of survival, establishing and maintaining equilibrium with the environment.

B. Theoretical assumptions
   1. Piaget believed that there are four major stages in the development of logical thinking. Each is derived from and builds on the accomplishments of the previous stages in a continuous, orderly process.
   2. The course of intellectual development is maturational and sequential. Intellectual development can be divided into periods, subperiods, and stages.
   3. The mechanisms that enable children to adapt to new situations and to move from one stage to the next are assimilation and accommodation.
      a. By assimilation, children incorporate new knowledge, skill, ideas, and insights into cognitive schemas already familiar to them. Piaget used the term *schema,* which is a pattern of action, thought, or both.
      b. To new situations that do not fit into an established schema, children accommodate. They change and organize existing schemas to solve more difficult tasks and form new schemas.
   4. Understanding of a new experience is based on all relevant previous experiences.
   5. Children achieve an accurate understanding of reality and come to deal with increasingly complex problems in a more effective manner by applying schemas already available to them and accommodating those schemas.

C. Usefulness and use for nursing
   1. Piaget's theory provides one of the dominant frameworks for understanding children's thinking.
   2. It does not account for individual differences or for the concept of unconscious motivation and its impact on behavior.
   3. Piaget was conservative in his description of children's thinking; many children are capable of more advanced thought, especially preschoolers.

D. Usefulness for pain management nurses
   1. Knowledge of cognitive development assists the nurse to communicate about and prepare children more appropriately for upcoming stressful procedures (Table 3-1).

IV. Nursing Process

A. Definitions and scope
   1. The nursing process is a problem-solving approach used by nurses to meet the needs of the patient (Hall, 1955).
   2. It is a deliberative method that relies on the use of cognitive, interpersonal, and psychomotor skills.
   3. Yura and Walsh (1983) described the nursing process as a set of actions to assist patients in maintaining optimal wellness.
   4. Although the steps of the process are followed in a systematic order, the process is flexible, and the various steps of the process sometimes may take place concurrently.
   5. The nursing process is the guiding framework for nursing practice (American Nurses Association, 2005).

B. Steps of the nursing process (Black & Matassarin-Jacob, 1993; Waldman, 1997)
   1. *Assessment:* Collection of data about the patient from a variety of sources; it consists of several parts
      a. Establish a database by gathering objective and subjective information relative to the patient. This also includes review of diagnostic studies.
      b. After data have been gathered, data analysis is performed. This is the identification of actual or potential health care needs, problems, or both based on the assessment.
      c. The analysis phase involves examining information in the database so that it can be organized into a framework for nursing practice.
      d. After data have been analyzed, a diagnosis is made about the patient's condition.
      e. The conditions that nurses are educated to handle and licensed to treat are called ***nursing diagnoses.*** The North American Nursing Diagnosis Association (NANDA) has classified more than 100 nursing diagnoses approved for clinical use.
      f. Nursing diagnosis is a clinical assessment about individual, family, or community responses to actual and potential health problems and life processes that form the basis for selection of nursing interventions to achieve outcomes for which the nurse is accountable (NANDA International, 2003). These patient needs may be activities to promote healthy patient responses or to prevent, correct, or reduce unhealthy patient responses.
   2. *Planning:* Setting goals and outcomes for meeting patient needs and designing strategies to achieve these outcomes; the plan should be mutually agreeable and realistic
      a. Prioritize nursing diagnosis.
      b. Determine outcomes of care.
      c. Formulate outcome criteria.
      d. Develop plan of care and modify as necessary.
      e. Collaborate with other health care team members in designing strategies.
      f. Communicate plan of care.
   3. *Intervention:* Initiating and completing actions necessary to accomplish the defined goals and outcomes
      a. Organize and manage patient's care.
      b. Counsel and teach patient, significant others, and health care team members.

   c. Provide care to achieve established goal and outcomes for patient.
   d. Supervise and coordinate the delivery of the patient's care provided by nursing personnel.
   e. Communicate nursing intervention.
4. *Evaluation:* Determining the extent to which goals and outcomes have been achieved and interventions have been successful
   a. Compare actual outcomes with expected outcomes of care.
   b. Evaluate the patient's ability to implement self-care.
   c. Evaluate health care team members' ability to implement patient care.
   d. Communicate evaluation findings.
   e. Reassess as necessary. Begin the process over as needed.
5. For each NANDA International diagnosis there are accompanying nursing outcomes classification (NOC) links (Johnson, Bulechak, Dochterman, Maas & Moorhead, 2001).
   a. NOC outcomes are neutral concepts reflecting patient states and behaviors.
   b. Outcomes are nurse sensitive but not goals.
   c. Nurses can use these outcomes, along with specific indicators, to set goals.
6. Nursing intervention classifications (NIC)
   a. These classifications categorize nursing activities using standardized language.
   b. Priority interventions are research-based interventions developed by the Iowa Intervention Project team as the treatments of choice for a particular nursing diagnosis (Johnson, Maas, & Moorhead, 2000).
7. Implications for pain management nurses
   a. NANDA, NOC, and NIC have specific defining characteristics, outcomes, and interventions related to both acute and chronic pain.
   b. In addition, they cite nursing activities, patient–family teaching, and collaborative activities that the pain management nurse can use in developing and documenting a plan of care (Ackley & Ladwig, 2006).
8. The International Council of Nurses (ICN) has an updated position statement, the *Nurse's Role in Providing Care in Dying Patients and their Families* (2006), that discusses pain alleviation as a fundamental nursing responsibility. It is stated that nurses should be expertly trained in pain management.

V. Nursing Theories, Models, and Conceptual Systems as Related to Pain Management

A. Overview

1. "The focus of knowledge development in nursing is on the wholeness of life and experiences and the processes that support relationship, integration, and transformation." (Smith & Liehr, 2008, p. 3)
2. Theory-guided, evidence-based practice is the hallmark of any professional discipline. Nursing is a professional discipline (Donaldson & Crowley, 1978). Every discipline has a process of reasoning that is rooted in the philosophy, theories, and empirical generalizations that define it.
3. Nursing theories can be described in several ways. They can be described by their goals and purposes (descriptive, explanatory, prescriptive, or predictive) or by their level of abstraction. Levels of abstraction go from most abstract to least abstract: metatheory, grand, middle-range, and situation-specific or practice theories (Walker & Avant, 1988).
4. The terms *conceptual framework, conceptual model,* and *theoretical framework* have been used interchangeably in the nursing literature.
5. King's preference as "nursing moves into the 21st century is to use the term *conceptual system* because the word system is a symbol commonly used in all aspects of human activities, in science and in nursing" (1997, p. 22).
6. Fitzpatrick and Whall (1989) argued that most nursing conceptual models constitute a level of nursing theory. There is a range of specificity in the nursing models, however, with concomitant limits on generalizability.

Table 3-1 Nursing Interventions to Promote Coping Based on Psychosocial and Cognitive Development

Age	Cognitive Development (Based on Piaget)	Psychosocial Development (Based on Erikson)	Promotion of Coping
Overview of birth to 1 year	*Sensorimotor stage of development* Learns through gross and fine motor movement and use of senses. *Substage 1* *Use of reflexes (birth to 1 month)* Practices reflexes.	Developmental task: *Trust versus mistrust* Learns to trust by the meeting of basic needs in a consistent manner. Begins understanding of self as separate from others (body image).	Conserve infant's body heat. Assess while quiet.
1–4 months	*Substage 2* *Primary circular reactions* Can discriminate among various sensations. Follows moving objects with eyes. Does things for repetition. Begins to develop hand–eye coordination. Responds to parent with a social smile. Begins to vocalize–coos. Locates sounds by turning head.	Begins to bond with mother during alert periods–especially during feeding experiences. Learns to signal displeasure. Begins to discriminate strangers. Squeals.	Involve caretaker. Provide containment such as swaddling. Assist the infant with hand-to-mouth contact or non-nutritive sucking. Speak softly. Use bright objects, rattles, and bells to distract. Position infant 3 months and older on a parent's lap before and after procedure. Provide periods of rest between procedures and protect infant from noise and bright lights.
4–8 months	*Substage 3* *Secondary circular reactions* Begins to imitate sounds. Responds to own name. Claps hands. Intentional action.	Increases fear of strangers. Develops definite likes and dislikes. Responds to "no."	Same as above.

8–12 months	*Substage 4* *Coordination of secondary circular motions* Looks for hidden objects. Understands simple commands. Goal-directed activity. Can coordinate two behaviors to achieve desired outcome (push and grab).	Motility drive strong. Always moving. Clings to mom. Loves pat-a-cake and peek-a-boo. Likes to look at self in mirror. Fears separation from primary caregiver.	Be efficient and restrain for as short a period of time as possible. Allow infant to warm up to nurse before approaching. Reunite with parent as soon as possible. Provide a safe environment for exploration.
12–18 months	*Substage 5* *Tertiary circular reactions* Trial and error predominant method of learning. Evident object permanence. Increasing verbal ability.	Developmental task: *Autonomy versus shame and doubt* Establishes self-control. Strong independence drive: "me do it." Egocentric. Everything is "mine." Independence shown through negativism. Short attention span.	Be flexible. Begin slowly. Speak and involve caretaker, if appropriate. Explain in simple concrete terms before procedure what toddler will feel during the procedure. Allow choices when possible (blanket, teddy). Encourage toddler to squeeze parent's hand.
18–24 months	*Substage 6* *Invention of new means through deduction* Views self as separate from others in environment. Will imitate a model in environment that is important to self (pretends to shave like dad or to dust). *Preoperational period (2–7 years)* Big change in cognitive function—able to use symbols.	*Fears* Loss or separation from parent Dark Machines Bedtime Intrusive procedures	If separation from parent is essential, return as quickly as possible. Allow toddler to hold transitional object (blanket, stuffed animal). Provide hugs.
2–4 years	*Stage 1* *Preconceptual stage* Can use symbolic thought—one object can stand for something else (a block of wood can be a car). Attributes lifelike qualities to inanimate objects (apologizes to chair).		Can show child what will be done by demonstrating on a doll and let child comfort doll after procedure. Let child play after procedure.

continues

Table 3-1 Nursing Interventions to Promote Coping Based on Psychosocial and Cognitive Development *continued*

Age	Cognitive Development (Based on Piaget)	Psychosocial Development (Based on Erikson)	Promotion of Coping
4–6 years	*Stage 2*	Development task:	
	Perceptual or intuitive thought	*Initiative versus guilt*	
	Language skills increase greatly. Asks many questions: Why? How? What?	"I am what I imagine I can be." Boasts and brags. Family primary social group. Curious.	Introduce self to child. Establish rapport through play. Allow child to familiarize self with equipment. Show how equipment works.
	Uses fantasy to understand a problem.	Develops a conscience. Into everything.	
	Magical thinking present. Believes things can be made to happen just by thinking about them and the world exists for the child alone.	Explores the physical world with senses and all powers.	Use nonthreatening language, such as "fix" or "check" and "special medicine." Offer suggestions on how to master fear or pain; suggestions include "hold my hand" or "say ouch if it hurts." Reinforce coping by saying, "You are such a big help." Let the child hold the bandage. Use storytelling, distraction, counting, and singing songs as methods to help the child cope.
6–11 years	*Concrete operations stage of development*	Developmental task:	Explain all procedures and impact on body.
	Organized thought.	*Industry versus inferiority*	Encourage questioning and active participation. Explain by picture and models. Be honest and explain how they will feel; what they will see, hear and smell. Give choices as appropriate. Provide privacy.
	Reads. Focuses on concrete understanding.	Wants to engage in tasks and activities and carry them through to completion. Learns to compete and cooperate with others. Peers and school important. Learns the rules.	Allow time for questions. Tell how long it will take. Use guided imagery, self-talk, interactive storytelling, and distraction as nonpharmacological methods to assist coping.
	Thought becomes increasingly logical and coherent. Able to classify, sort order, and otherwise organize facts. Able to deal with many aspects of a situation at the same time but cannot deal with something abstract.		

		Sensitive to reactions of others. Seeks approval and recognition.	
		Fears Mutilation Death Immobility Rejection Failure	
12–18 years	***Formal operations stage of development***	Developmental task: ***Identity versus role confusion***	
	Characterized by adaptability and flexibility.	Values of peer group of prime importance.	Respect privacy. Accept expression of feelings.
	Can think in abstract terms. Can make hypotheses and test them.	Early adolescence: Characterized by rapid and marked physical changes. Trust in own body is shaken. Becomes preoccupied with what others think of appearance.	Encourage participation in decision-making process related to procedures or treatment whenever possible. Reaffirm the adolescent's normalcy. Accept questions and answer them honestly. Respect choice for a support person.
	Often confuses the ideal with the practical. Capable of analyzing own thinking. Can objectively assess a situation and ask lots of questions.	Peer pressure and role experimentation important to the development of identity.	
		Later adolescence: Integrates own concepts and values with those of society and comes to decisions regarding future occupations.	
		Fears Mutilation Body image changes Rejection by peers	

B. Definitions
   1. A *conceptual framework* is a general perspective of organizing and classifying concepts into a relevant structure (Kim, 1997).
   2. A *conceptual model* is a network of concepts in relationship that accounts for broad nursing phenomena; the term is synonymous with *conceptual framework* (Kramer, 1997).
   3. *Conceptual systems* are a set of concepts that are defined and linked by broad generalizations constructed by an individual for a purpose (King, 1997).
   4. A *paradigm* is a shared framework and a shared view held by members of a discipline about the discipline (Kuhn, 1970); it is also called a *disciplinary matrix* (Kuhn, 1977) or a *worldview* (Parse, 1987). "A paradigm is very powerful in the life of a society since it influences the way we think, how problems are solved, what goals we pursue and what we value" (Gablik, 1991, p. 2).
   5. A *metaparadigm* consists of the global concepts that identify the phenomena of interest to a discipline and the global propositions that state the relationships among these phenomena (Fawcett, 1997). The phenomena of interest to nursing are
      a. Person
      b. Environment
      c. Health
      d. Nursing
   6. A *paradigm shift* involves giving up of a present worldview within a discipline and taking on of a different worldview (e.g., shifting from the medical model to the holistic model). "Since cultural (and educational) conditioning strongly influences individual behavior and thought[,] to begin to move toward a different framework of assumptions that would change the basis of our experience is extremely difficult" (Gablik, 1991, p. 3).
   7. A *theory* is a set of theoretical statements that provides an understanding and explanation about a class or classes of phenomena (Kim, 1997). It can also be defined as an organized, coherent, and systematic articulation of a set of statements related to significant questions in a discipline that are communicated in a meaningful whole (McEwen & Wills, 2006). A theory provides a particular way of seeing phenomena of concern to a discipline in an organized way.
   8. *Nursing theory* is an inductively or deductively derived (or both) collage of coherent, creative, and focused nursing phenomena that frame, give meaning to, and help explain specific and selective aspects of nursing research and practice (Silva, 1997). "Theory informs the focus and content of practice as well as guides nursing action" (Fitzpatrick, 1997, p. 38).
   9. *Grand theories* are highly formal and global. Their concepts and statements that to relate them transcend specific events and populations. Grand theories provide universal understanding but not the particulars. They are frameworks consisting of concepts and relational statements that explicate abstract phenomena that are of concern to the profession of nursing (Fawcett, 2000).
   10. *Middle-range theories* are more specific and less formal than grand theories. They are more circumscribed, elaborating more concrete concepts and relationships such as uncertainty, self-efficacy, meaning, comfort, and pain. Middle-range theories contain concepts close to observed data, from which hypotheses may be logically derived and empirically tested. Middle-range theory can specifically derive a grand theory or can be directly related to a paradigm (Smith & Liehr, 2008).
   11. *Situation-specific or practice theories* relate specific populations to particular situations. Their scope is limited. They are socially and historically contexted (e.g., Taiwanese women experiencing menopause in the United States).

C. Beliefs about theory in nursing
   1. Theory exists to categorize and explain the world.
   2. Theory alone is not useful.
   3. "Theory exists in nursing to help professionals provide better nursing care" (Fitzpatrick, 1997, p. 38).
   4. Theories contribute to and assist in increasing the general body of knowledge within the discipline through the research implemented to validate them.

VI. Specific Nursing Conceptual Systems

A. This is not a comprehensive collection. It is a collection chosen because of historical significance or diversity in thought, which mirrors the diverse views of nurses.

B. Nightingale: an environmental adaptation conceptual system

1. Overview
    a. Environmental adaptation is the earliest model of nursing practice.
    b. It sees the function of nursing as a manipulation of the environment as it affects the patient's condition. Nursing is an art and science and a calling.
2. Major concepts and their relationships
    a. *Person:* The person was viewed as an individual, although families occasionally were mentioned. People were multidimensional and included biological, psychological, social, and spiritual elements. Nightingale stated that nurses take care of patients, not disease. The individual who is the recipient of nursing care may be ill or well because the maintenance and promotion of health are as important as recovery from disease.
    b. *Environment:* This was the core concept in Nightingale's model. Manipulating the environment affects the patient's condition. The environment consisted of physical attributes that could be altered and improve the patient's well-being. These elements included ventilation, light, clean water, warmth, noise control, and management of water and odors.
    c. *Health:* Health "is not only to be well, but to be able to use well every power we have to use" (Nightingale, 1859/1992, p. 26).
    d. *Nursing:* Nursing is "an art and a science. The purpose of nursing is to put the patient in the best possible condition for nature to act upon him" (Nightingale, 1859/1992, p. 75). Nursing is carried out by altering the environment in such a way as to implement the natural laws of health. The nurse can accomplish this by manipulation of the environment through knowledge gained by observation and study. Observation is the major route to determining the relationship between the patient and health (Fig. 3-2).
3. Relevance for pain management nurses
    a. Nightingale stated: "The reparative process which nature has instituted and which we call disease has been hindered by some want of knowledge or attention, in one or all of these things, and pain, suffering, or interruption of the whole process sets in" (Nightingale, 1859/1992, p. 5).
    b. Nightingale (1859/1992) also stated that doing away with pain and suffering allows nature's reparative processes to be successful.

C. Henderson: humanistic nursing conceptual system

1. Overview
    a. Humanistic nursing views nursing as focusing on the individual. The purpose is to assist the individual in maintaining health, recovering health, or achieving a peaceful death.
    b. A correlation with Maslow's hierarchy of needs is seen in Henderson's 14 components of nursing care, which begin with physical needs and progress to psychosocial components (Henderson & Nite, 1978).

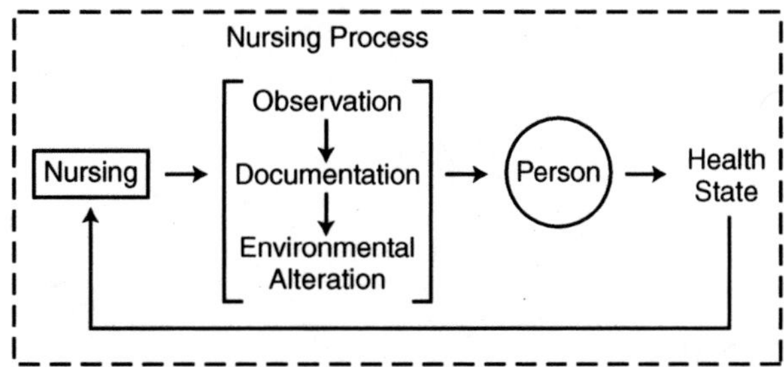

Figure 3-2 | Nightingale's model of nursing practice.

From McQuiston, C., & Webb, A. (Eds.). *Foundations of nursing theory* (p. 441). Thousand Oaks, CA: Sage Publications. Copyright 1995 by Sage Publications, Inc.

2. Major concept and relationships
    a. *Person:* An individual who requires assistance to achieve health and independence or peaceful death. Mind and body are inseparable. Patient and family are viewed as a unit.
    b. *Environment:* Henderson used the dictionary definition: "the aggregate of all the external conditions and influences affecting the life and development of an organism" (Henderson & Nite, 1978, p. 829).
    c. *Health:* Health is the individual's ability to function independently as stated in Henderson's components. These components are basic needs, and good health is a challenging goal for individuals—it is difficult for the nurse to help each person reach it (Henderson, 1960, p. 4).
    d. *Nursing:* The unique function of nursing is to help the individual, sick or well, in the performance of activities contributing to health that the individual would perform if he or she had strength, will, or knowledge.
    e. Henderson identified 14 basic needs of the patient, which are the components of nursing care. The needs range from breathing normally to learning and discovering what leads to health (Henderson & Nite, 1978).
    f. Henderson said the nurse must "get inside the skin of each of her patients in order to know what he needs." The needs must be validated with the patient (Henderson, 1964, p. 63).
3. Relevance for pain management nurses
    a. Although Henderson did not specify relief of pain as one of the basic needs, relief of pain can be assumed to meet the basic needs she outlined. For example, breathing normally, eating and drinking adequately, moving and maintaining desirable position, and sleeping and resting would be difficult to attain if the patient were experiencing either acute or chronic pain.

D. Orem: self-care deficit conceptual system (Fig. 3-3)
1. Overview
    a. Self-care deficit was based on maintaining or restoring the patient to self-care.
2. Major concepts and definitions
    a. Orem labeled her self-care deficit theory of nursing as a general theory composed of three related theories.
        (1) The *theory of self-care* describes and explains self-care—"the practice of activities that individuals initiate and perform on their own behalf in maintaining life, health and well-being" (Orem, 1991, p. 117).

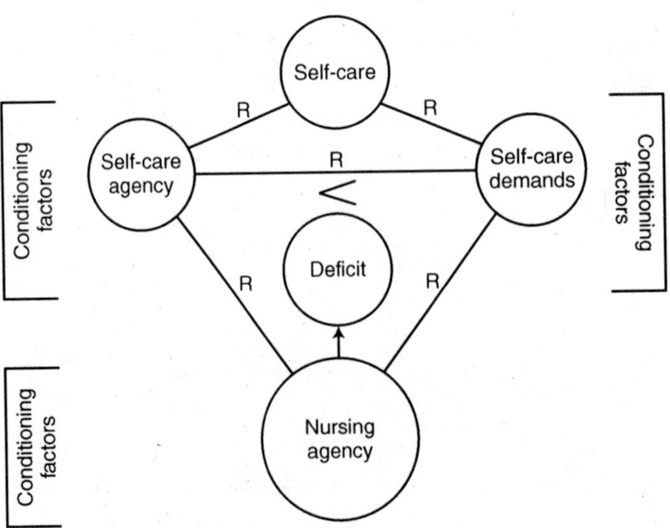

Figure 3-3 Conceptual framework for nursing. R, relationships; <, deficit relationship, current or projected.

From Orem, D. E. (2001). *Nursing concepts of practice* (6th ed., p. 491). St. Louis: Mosby.

(2) The *theory of self-care deficit* is a patient-focused concept that expresses a qualitative and quantitative relationship between two concepts: self-care agency and therapeutic self-care demand.

(3) The *theory of nursing systems* is "all the actions and interactions of nurses and patients in nursing practice situation" (Orem, 1985, p. 148). Nursing systems are wholly compensatory, partly compensatory, or supportive educative.

b. *Person:* People are called the ***human agency;*** they are capable and willing to perform care for self or dependent members of the family.

c. *Environment:* Environment is not defined, but Orem discussed environmental factors, elements, and conditions and development (Orem, 1985, pp. 140–141).

d. *Health:* Health is "a state of being whole and sound" (Orem, 1985, p. 176).

3. Relevance for pain management nurses

a. Orem's conceptual system is used widely. When the patient is unable to maintain self-care, such as when the patient is in pain, the nurse provides compensatory care to help the patient until self-care is restored. Nursing should support and educate patients so that they can function as independently as possible. For patients in chronic pain, their ability to perform self-care activities breaks down, and they develop self-care deficits. The nurse may use several methods of assisting the patient to move from a wholly compensatory system to a partly compensatory system.

E. Roy: adaptation conceptual system (Fig. 3-4)

1. Overview

a. Roy's system focuses on adaptive behaviors by the person and how these behaviors allow the person to cope with or adapt to stressors from the environment

2. Major concepts and relationships

a. Key concepts in the Roy adaptation model are person, goal, health, environment, and nursing activities.

b. *Person:* The person is the recipient of nursing care. People are holistic adaptive systems. The term ***adaptive*** means that "the human system has the capacity to adjust effectively to changes in the environment and, in turn, affect the environment" (Roy & Andrews, 1991, p. 7).

c. *Environment:* Environment consists of "all conditions, circumstances and influences that surround and affect the development and behavior of the person" (Roy & Andrews, 1991, p. 19).

d. *Health:* Health is "a state and process of being and becoming an integrated and whole person" (Roy & Andrews, 1991, p. 19).

e. *Nursing activities:* The nursing process includes six steps:

(1) Assessment of behavior
(2) Assessment of stimuli
(3) Nursing diagnosis
(4) Goal setting
(5) Intervention
(6) Evaluation

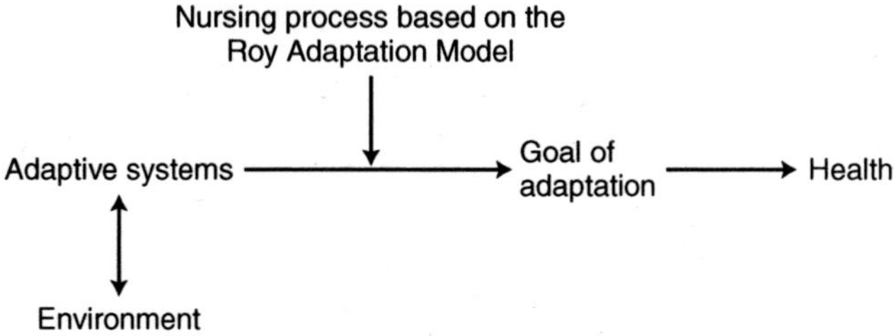

Figure 3-4 | Relationships between the key concepts of the Roy model.

From Roy, C. (1984). *Introduction to nursing: An adaptation model* (2nd ed.). Upper Saddle River, NJ: Pearson Education.

   f. *Goal:* The goal of nursing is to promote adaptation in four adaptive modes (physiological, self-concept, role function, and interdependence) and contribute to health.
3. Relevance for pain management nurses
   a. In Roy's model, the nurse's role is to assess the person's adaptive behavior, identify what is affecting this behavior (e.g., pain), and then manipulate the stimuli in such a way that the person is able to cope. The nurse uses knowledge of the four adaptive modes (physiological, self-concept, role function, and interdependence) to guide actions in promoting positive coping responses.

F. King: theory of goal attainment
1. Overview
   a. The theory of goal attainment is a dynamic interactive system model. The goal of nursing is a transaction between the nurse and the patient leading to attainment of the patient's goals.
   b. It is an open systems model composed of personal systems, interpersonal systems, and social systems.
2. Major concepts and relationships
   a. *Person:* The person is called a ***human being*** and is a complex, open living system that "copes with a wide variety of events, persons and things over time" (King, 1981, p. 6).
   b. *Environment:* The social system surrounding the concept in question is the environment. It can be external and internal (King, 1989).
   c. *Health:* Health is "a dynamic state of an individual in which change is constant and an ongoing process" (King, 1989, p. 152).
   d. *Nursing:* Nursing involves "recognition of presenting conditions; operations or activities related to the situations or conditions; and motivation to exert some control over the events in the situation to achieve goals" (King, 1981, p. 144).
   e. The focus of the theory is the interpersonal system because what nurses do with and for individuals is what makes the difference between nursing and any other health profession (King, 1989, pp. 154–155).
3. Relevance for pain management nurses
   a. King's theory defines outcomes in the form of individualizing the goals to be attained based on needs of the patient. The goal of relief from pain leading to an improvement of function is a goal that can be assessed and evaluated in determining effectiveness of nursing care.

G. Rogers: science of unitary humans (Rogers, 1970)
1. Overview
   a. The science of unitary humans is an abstract system that provides a worldview of the universe that is beyond current understanding or familiarity. It includes possibilities for the future and recognizes change as basic to existence. The building blocks of this abstract system include energy fields, openness, pandimensionality, and pattern. "The purpose of nurses is to promote health and well-being for all persons and groups wherever they are" (Rogers, 1990, p. 6).
2. Concepts and their relationships
   a. *Person:* People and their environment are the phenomena central to the focus of nursing. Humans are whole, and this wholeness is irreducible.
   b. *Environment:* The environmental field is whole with its own identity and is irreducible, indivisible, and differentiated by pattern. Human and environmental fields are integral to one another.
   c. *Health:* No explicit definition for health is given; Rogers considered ***health*** ambiguous and preferred the term ***human betterment.*** Health services are community based.
   d. *Nursing:* The term ***nursing*** is used as a noun—a learning profession. It is an organized body of abstract knowledge about people and their worlds. "Nursing is the study of unitary, irreducible, indivisible human and environmental fields" (Rogers, 1990, p. 6). The practice of

nursing in the future will be identified through noninvasive modalities with the purpose of promoting human betterment.

e. The fundamental guides to the practice of nursing are integrality, resonancy, and helicy.
   (1) *Integrality:* Human and environmental fields are a continuous and mutual process.
   (2) *Resonancy:* Manifestations of patterns characterizing human and environmental energy fields are changing continuously.
   (3) *Helicy:* Human and environmental field patterns are continuous, innovative, unpredictable, and increasing in diversity.
f. Nursing seeks to promote harmony of human and environmental energy fields to strengthen coherence and integrity of human fields and to participate in directing and redirecting patterning of human and environmental energy fields toward the goal of optimal health potential (Rogers, 1970).

3. Relevance for pain management nurses
   a. As Rogers' abstract system clarifies nursing, "it would be inappropriate to treat only a part of the whole person, such as the cardiovascular system. You could facilitate comfort during chest pain, however, with guided imagery and observe the changes in the duration of chest pains. Rogers viewed human bodies as manifestations of field" (Lutjens, 1995, p. 15). This view of humans and the purpose of nurses is distinct to Rogers' abstract system.

H. Leininger: cultural care diversity and universality theory
   1. Overview
      a. The theory is thought to be "the broadest and most holistic guide to study human beings with their lifeways, cultural values and beliefs, symbols, material and nonmaterial forms and living contexts" (Leininger, 1988, p. 155).
      b. Leininger maintained that culture and care are inextricably linked and that care and caring is the central concern for nurses. She is known for the sunrise model (Leininger, 1991).
   2. Major concepts and relationships
      a. *Person:* A person is called a ***human being*** in a culture. To be human is to be caring, and caring is culturally based.
      b. *Environment:* The environment is called the ***environmental context***—this refers to the totality of an event that gives meaning to human expressions in particular settings (Leininger, 1991).
      c. *Health:* Health is a state of well-being that is defined culturally.
      d. *Nursing:* The term ***nursing*** refers to a learned humanistic and scientific profession and discipline that is focused on human care phenomena (Leininger, 1991).
      e. *Caring:* The term ***caring*** refers "to actions and activities directed toward assisting, supporting or enabling another individual or group with evident or anticipated needs to ameliorate or improve a human condition or lifeway to face death" (Leininger, 1995, p. 390).
   3. Relevance for pain management nurses
      a. Leininger stated that the goal of her theory was ultimately "to provide culturally congruent nursing care" to improve nursing care to people of different or similar cultures (Leininger, 1991, p. 19). Pain is a culture-laden phenomenon. Nurses need to take into account the meaning of pain to the individual, the situation, and the meaning of pain in the person's culture to provide acceptable pain management strategies. Leininger's sunrise model depicts the theory of cultural care diversity and universality (Fig. 3-5).

I. Watson: philosophy and science of caring (Watson & Foster, 2003)
   1. Overview
      a. Watson developed a model of human care with human caring as the moral ideals of nursing. This model approach of nursing incorporates the concepts of soul and transcendence. This is a radical shift from traditional nursing models, moving beyond the scientific to a transcendent level. Watson based her theory for nursing practice on 10 carative factors (Watson, 1981).
   2. Major concepts and relationships
      a. *Person:* Nonreducible and interconnected with others and nature
      b. *Environment:* Interconnected with person and inseparable—includes external and internal

c. *Health:* An elusive, subjective external concept
d. *Nursing:* "A human science of persons and human health—illness experiences that are mediated by professional, personal, scientific, esthetic and ethical human care transactions" (Watson, 1985, p. 54), whose goal, through the caring process, is to help people gain a degree of harmony within themselves to promote self-healing
e. *Caring:* All the factors the nurse uses to deliver health care to patients

3. Relevance for pain management nurses
   a. One of Watson's carative factors is assistance with the gratification of human needs (Watson, 1979), which has to do with biophysical needs, including pain relief. Watson's conceptual system would use a "transpersonal relationship" (Watson, 1988, pp. 50–51) to assist the patient to develop strategies leading to pain relief. In this transpersonal caring relationship, a specific type of professional human-to-human contact is established. The goal is to restore the patient's experience of inner harmony. Both the nurse and the patient choose to engage in this transpersonal caring relationship. The ultimate guiding value of Watson's conceptual

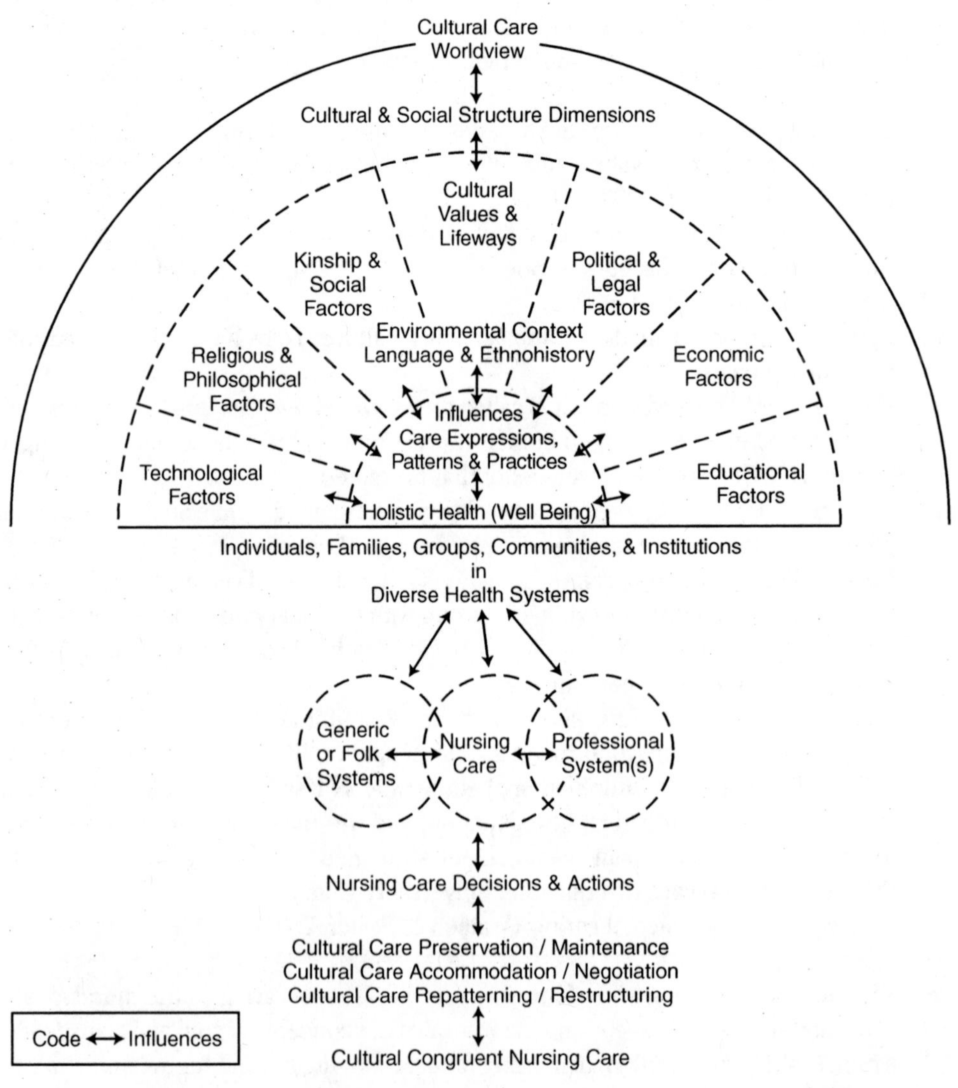

Figure 3-5 Leininger's sunrise model to depict the theory of cultural care diversity and universality.

From Leininger, M. (1991). *Culture care diversity and universality: A theory of nursing.* New York: National League for Nursing.

model is that "caring is presented as the moral ideal of nursing, with a concern for the preservation of humanity, dignity and fullness of self" (Watson, 1985, p. 73).

VII. Middle-Range Theories Related to Pain Management

A. Marion Good and Shirley Moore: middle-range theory that focuses on acute pain (1996) (Fig. 3-6)
   1. Overview
      a. Clinical practice guidelines were the source for the development of this middle-range theory and sought to illustrate the balance between analgesia and side effects.
      b. The authors synthesized a middle-range theory of acute pain management in adult patients from the Agency for Health Care Policy and Research publication *Acute Pain Management: Operative or Medical Procedures and Trauma* (Acute Pain Management Guideline Panel, 1992a).
   2. Major concepts and relationships
      a. Good and Moore used Walker and Avant's (1988) strategies for theory construction in developing their middle-range theory. They did this by writing three statements in a relational manner that they derived from the clinical practice guidelines:
         (1) "Giving adequate potent pain medication along with pharmacologic and nonpharmacologic adjuvants contribute to a balance between analgesia and side effects."
         (2) "Regular pain and side-effect assessment plus identification of inadequate pain relief and unacceptable side effects, plus a process of intervention, reassessment, and reintervention, contribute to a balance between analgesia and side effects."
         (3) "Patient teaching plus goal setting for pain relief contribute to a balance between analgesia and side effects." (Good & Moore, 1996, p. 76)
   3. Relevance for pain management nurses
      a. Use of this middle-range theory may demonstrate improved recovery and a lower incidence of extended pain, complications, length of stay, and cost.

B. Myra Huth and Shirley Moore: acute pain management in infants and children (1998) (Fig. 3-7)
   1. Overview
      a. This theory was derived from clinical practice guidelines from the Agency for Health Care Policy and Research for children (Acute Pain Management Guideline Panel, 1992b) that have logical and empirical usefulness and significance that can be tested.
      b. Previous work done by Good and Moore served as a basis for this theory development, as did Walker and Avant's strategies for theory development.
   2. Major concepts and relationships
      a. Three relational statements were developed and synthesized:
         (1) "An initial assessment consisting of past pain history, current pain assessment, assess-

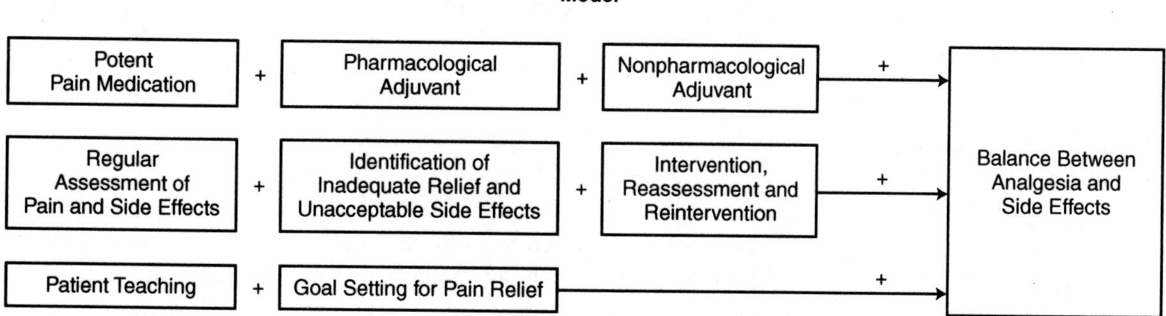

FIGURE 3-6 | Good and Moore theory on acute pain management.

Good, M., & Moore, S. M. (1996). Clinical practice guidelines as a new source of middle-range theory: Focus on acute pain. Nursing Outlook, 44(2), 74–79.

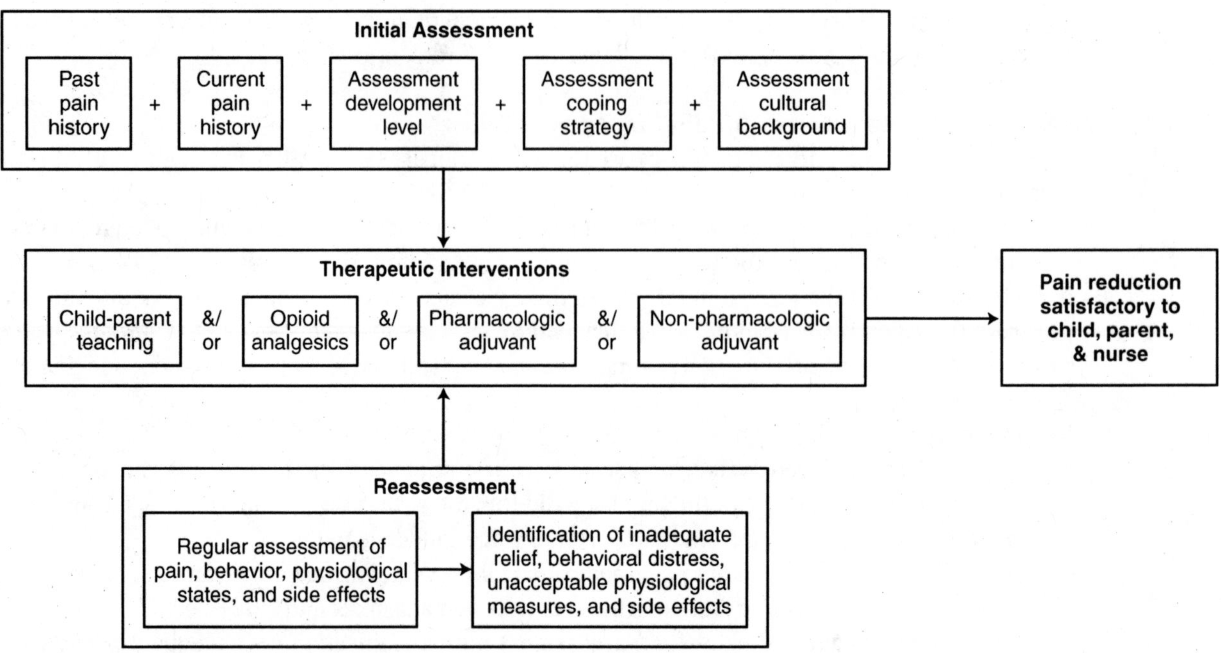

FIGURE 3-7 | Huth and Moore theory of acute pain management in infants and children.

Huth, M. M., & Moore, S. M. (1998). Prescriptive theory of acute pain management in infants and children. Journal of Society of Pediatric Nursing, 3(1), 23–32.

ments of developmental level, coping strategies, plus cultural backgrounds leads to choice of appropriate therapeutic intervention."

(2) "Therapeutic interventions, consisting of child–parent teaching and/or opioid analgesics, pharmacologic and nonpharmacologic adjuvants, contribute to pain reduction that is satisfactory to child, parent, and nurse."

(3) "Reassessment consisting of regular assessment of pain by child or parent report, assessment of behavioral and physiological states, and side effects leads to identification of inadequate pain relief, behavioral distress, unacceptable physiological measures, and side effects, which contributes to a choice of appropriate therapeutic interventions." (Huth & Moore, 1998, p. 26)

3. Relevance to pain management nurses
   a. The potential of this middle-range theory is to assist nurses in managing clinical pain and to expand the knowledge and research base in children's pain.
   b. It has the potential to "assist nurses to assure that infants and children suffer less and avoid the consequences of unmanaged pain" (Huth & Moore, 1998, p. 28).

Summary

Nursing theories exist to help explain nursing and nursing's relationship with the person, environment, and health. "Utilization of nursing models and their theories are a means of organizing the reasoning process for critical thinking in professional nursing practice" (Alligood & Marriner-Tomey, 2006, p. 3). Different views of various theorists have been presented to help pain management nurses to view pain and their role effectively and to develop strategies to manage pain based on scientific, humanistic, and holistic views. Nursing incorporates many paradigms, including the scientific medical model, holism, and self-transcendence (Sarter, 1988). There is a shift in nursing paradigms—perhaps not as revolutionary as some would think—but it is important to reevaluate the values and structures that shape the discipline (Newman, 1996). Many pain management nurses are on the forefront of new paradigms that view people in their situation holistically and do not compartmentalize the individual. Such nurses use many modalities to help people maximize their health potential despite pain. The reader is encouraged to read the theorists' original works and any further developments to appreciate each theory fully. Middle-range theories signify a growth of knowledge development in nursing. "Middle range theories offer valuable organizing frameworks to phenomena being researched by interdisciplinary teams. Hospitals seeking magnet status are required to articulate some nursing theoretic perspective that guides nursing practice in the facility. The quality of the practice environment is important for the quality of care and the retention of nurses. Theory-guided practice elevates the work of nurses leading to fulfillment and satisfaction and provide a satisfying professional model of practice." (Smith, 2008, p. 9).

References

Ackley, B. J., & Ladwig, G. B. (2006). *Nursing diagnosis book: A guide to planning care* (7th ed.). St. Louis: Mosby Elsevier.

Acute Pain Management Guideline Panel. (1992a). *Acute care management: Operative or medical procedures and trauma.* Clinical Practice Guideline. (AHCPR Publication No. 92-0032.) Rockville, MD: Agency for Health Policy and Research, Public Health Service, U.S. Department of Health and Human Services.

Acute Pain Management Guideline Panel. (1992b). *Acute care pain management in infants, children and adolescents: Operative and medical procedures. Quick reference for clinicians.* (AHCPR Publication No. 92-0020). Rockville, MD: Agency for Health Care Policy and Research, Public Health Service, U.S. Department of Health and Human Services.

Alligood, M., & Marriner-Tomey, A. (2006). *Nursing theory: Utilization and application* (3rd ed.). St. Louis: Mosby/Elsevier.

American Nurses Association. (2005). *Standards of nursing practice.* Kansas City, MO: Author.

Black, J., & Matassarin-Jacob, E. (1993). *Luckmann & Sorensen's medical–surgical nursing: A psychophysiologic approach* (4th ed., pp. 1–23). Philadelphia: W. B. Saunders.

Donaldson, S. K., & Crowley, D. M. (1978). The discipline of nursing. *Nursing Outlook, 26,* 113–113–120.

Erikson, E. (1963). *Childhood and society* (2nd ed.). New York: W. W. Norton.

Fawcett, J. (1997). The structural hierarchy of nursing knowledge: Components and their definitions. In I. King & J. Fawcett (Eds.), *The language of nursing theory and metatheory* (pp. 11–18). Indianapolis, IN: Sigma Theta Tau International Center Nursing Press.

Fawcett, J. (2000). *Analysis and evaluation of contemporary nursing knowledge: Nursing models and theories.* Philadelphia: F. A. Davis.

Fitzpatrick, J. (1997). Nursing theory and metatheory. In I. King & J. Fawcett (Eds.), *The language of nursing theory and metatheory* (pp. 36–40). Indianapolis, IN: Sigma Theta Tau International Center Nursing Press.

Fitzpatrick, J., & Whall, A. (Eds.). (1989). *Conceptual models of nursing: Analysis and application* (2nd ed.). Norwalk, CT: Appleton & Lange.

Gablik, S. (1991). *The reenchantment of art.* New York: Thames & Hudson.

Good, M., & Moore, S. M. (1996). Clinical practice guidelines as a new source of middle-range theory: Focus on acute pain. *Nursing Outlook, 44*(2), 74–79.

Hall, L. (1955). Quality of nursing care. *Public Health News: New Jersey State Department of Health, 36,* 212–215.

Henderson, V. (1960). *Basic principles of nursing care.* Geneva: International Council of Nurses.

Henderson, V. (1964). The nature of nursing. *American Journal of Nursing, 64,* 62–68.

Henderson, V., & Nite, G. (1978). *The principles and practice of nursing.* New York: Macmillan.

Huth, M. M., & Moore, S. M. (1998). Prescriptive theory of acute pain management in infants and children. *Journal of Society of Pediatric Nursing, 3*(1), 23–32.

International Council of Nurses. (2006). *Nurses' role in providing care to dying patients and their families.* Retrieved August 28, 2008, from http://www.icn.ch/pscare00.htm.

Johnson, M., Bulechak, G., Dochterman, J., Maas, M., & Morrhead, S., (2001). *Nursing diagnoses. Outcomes & interventions: NANDA International, NOC, and NIC linkages.* St. Louis: Mosby.

Johnson, M., Maas, M., & Moorhead, S. (Eds.), (2000). *Nursing outcomes classification (NOC)* (2nd ed.). St. Louis: Mosby.

Kim, H. (1997). Terminology in structuring and developing nursing knowledge. In I. King & J. Fawcett (Eds.), *The language of nursing theory and metatheory* (pp. 27–35). Indianapolis, IN: Sigma Theta Tau International Center Nursing Press.

King, I. (1981). *A theory for nursing: Systems, concepts, process.* New York: John Wiley.

King, I. (1989). King's general systems framework and theory. In J. Riehl-Sisca (Ed.), *Conceptual models for nursing practice* (3rd ed., pp. 149–158). Norwalk, CT: Appleton & Lange.

King, I. (1997). Knowledge development for nursing: A process. In I. King & J. Fawcett (Eds.), *The language of nursing theory and metatheory* (pp. 19–26). Indianapolis, IN: Sigma Theta Tau International Center Nursing Press.

Kramer, M. (1997). *Terminology in nursing: Definitions and comments.* Indianapolis, IN: Sigma Theta Tau International Center Nursing Press.

Kuhn, T. (1970). *The structure of scientific revolutions* (2nd ed.). Chicago: University of Chicago Press.

Kuhn, T. (1977). *The essential tension.* Chicago: University of Chicago Press.

Leininger, M. (1988). Leininger's theory of nursing: Cultural care diversity and universality. *Nursing Science Quarterly, 1,* 152–160.

Leininger, M. (1991). *Culture care diversity and universality: A theory of nursing.* New York: National League for Nursing.

Leininger, M. (1995). Madeleine M. Leininger: Cultural care diversity and universality theory. In C. McQuiston & A. Webb (Eds.), *Foundations of nursing theory* (pp. 371–402). Thousand Oaks, CA: Sage Publications.

Lutjens, L. (1995). Martha Rogers: The science of unitary human beings. In C. McQuiston & A. Webb (Eds.), *Foundations of nursing theory* (pp. 3–38). Thousand Oaks, CA: Sage Publications.

Maslow, A. (1970). *Motivation and personality.* New York: Harper & Row.

McEwen, M., & Wills, E. M. (2006). *Theoretical basis for nursing.* Philadelphia: Lippincott, Williams & Wilkins.

Newman, M. (1996). Prevailing paradigms in nursing. In J. Kenney (Ed.), *Philosophical and theoretical perspectives for advanced practice nurses* (pp. 302–307). Boston: Jones & Bartlett.

Nightingale, F. (1992). *Notes on nursing: What it is, and what it is not.* Philadelphia: J. B. Lippincott. (Original work published 1859)

North American Nursing Diagnosis Association International. (2003). *NANDA International nursing diagnoses: Definitions and classifications, 2003–2004.* Philadelphia: Author.

Orem, D. (1985). *Nursing: Concept of practice* (3rd ed.). New York: McGraw-Hill.

Orem, D. (1991). *Nursing: Concept of practice* (4th ed.). St. Louis: Mosby.

Parse, R. R. (1987). *Nursing science: Major paradigm theories and critiques.* Philadelphia: W. B. Saunders.

Piaget, J. (1969). *The theory of stages in cognitive development.* New York: McGraw-Hill.

Rogers, M. (1970). *An introduction to the theoretical basis of nursing.* Philadelphia: F. A. Davis.

Rogers, M. (1990). Nursing: Science of unitary, irreducible, human beings—Update 1990. In E. Barrett (Ed.), *Vision of Roger's science-based nursing* (Publication No. 15-2285, pp. 5–11). New York: National League for Nursing.

Roy, C., & Andrews, H. (1991). *The Roy adaptation model: The definitive statement.* Norwalk, CT: Appleton & Lange.

Sarter, B. (1988). Philosophic sources of nursing theory. *Nursing Science Quarterly, 1,* 52–59.

Silva, M. (1997). Philosophy, theory and research in nursing: A linguistic journey to nursing practice. In I. King & J. Fawcett (Eds.), *The language of nursing theory and metatheory* (pp. 51–60). Indianapolis, IN: Sigma Theta Tau International Center Nursing Press.

Smith, M. C. (2008). Disciplinary perspectives linked to middle range theory. In M. J. Smith and P. R Liehr (Eds.), *Middle range theory for nursing* (2nd ed., pp. 1–9). New York: Springer.

Smith, M. J., & Liehr, P. R. (2008). *Middle range theory for nursing* (2nd ed.). New York: Springer.

Waldman, A. (1997). Preparing for the NCLEX examination. In A. Stein & J. Miller (Eds.), *NCLEX-RN review* (3rd ed., pp. 1–12). Albany, NY: Delmar Publishers.

Walker, L., & Avant, K. (1988). *Strategies for theory construction in nursing* (2nd ed.). Norwalk, CT: Appleton & Lange.

Watson, J. (1979). *Nursing: The philosophy and science of caring.* Boston: Little, Brown.

Watson, J. (1981). Nursing's scientific quest. *Nursing Outlook, 29,* 413–416.

Watson, J. (1985). *Nursing: Human science and human care—A theory of nursing* (1st ed.). Norwalk, CT: Appleton-Century-Crofts.

Watson, J. (1988). *Nursing: Human science and human care—A theory of nursing* (2nd ed.). New York: National League for Nursing.

Watson, J., & Foster, R. (2003). The attending nurse caring model: Integrating theory, evidence and advanced care–healing therapeutics for transforming professional nursing practice. *Journal of Clinical Nursing, 12,* 360–365.

Yura, H., & Walsh, M. (1983). *The nursing process: Assessing, planning, implementing, evaluation* (4th ed.). New York: Appleton-Century-Crofts.

Websites

The two listed websites will provide links and information regarding grand theorists and middle-range theories. Most grand theorists have their own website.

Clayton State University Department of Nursing, Nursing theory link page
http://www.healthsci.clayton.edu/eichelberger/nursing.htm
Hahn School of Nursing and Health Sciences, San Diego, CA. nursing theory page
http://www.sandiego.edu/academics/nursing/theory

Suggested Readings

Frick-Helms, S. (1994). Comparison of theories of human growth and development. In C. Betz, M. Hunsberger, & S. Wright (Eds.), *Family-centered nursing care of children* (4th ed., pp. 74–76). Philadelphia: W. B. Saunders.

Good, M. (2004). Pain: A balance between analgesia and side effects. In S. Peterson & T. Bredow, *Middle range theories: Application to nursing research* (pp. 59–77). Philadelphia: Lippincott, Williams & Wilkins.

Good, M. (1998). A middle-range theory of acute pain management: Use in research. *Nursing Outlook, 45,* 120–124.

Marriner-Tomey, A. M., & Allingood, M. R. (2006). *Nursing theorists and their work* (6th ed.). St. Louis: Mosby.

Nightingale, F. (1949). Sick nursing and health nursing. In I. Hampton (Ed.), *Nursing of the sick* (pp. 24–43). New York: McGraw-Hill. (Original work published 1893)

North American Nursing Diagnosis Association. (1994). *Taxonomy 1 revised: 1990 with official nursing diagnosis.* St. Louis: North American Nursing Diagnosis Association.

Parker, M. E. (2006). *Nursing theories and nursing practice.* Philadelphia: F. A. Davis.

Peterson, S. J., & Bredow, T. S. (2004). *Middle range theories: Application to nursing research.* Philadelphia: Lippincott, Williams & Wilkins.

Selanders, L. (1995). Florence Nightingale: An environmental adaptation theory. In C. McQuiston & A. Webb (Eds.), *Foundations of nursing theory* (pp. 417–458). Thousand Oaks, CA: Sage Publications.

chapter

4

Theories of Pain

Connie Luedtke, MA, RN-BC
Pamela J. Nelson, PhD, RN-BC

Objectives

After studying this chapter, the reader should be able to:

1. Describe the evolution of theories about pain experiences.
   A. Understand that pain involves more than sensory experience.
   B. Review theories that address complexity of pain experience, including suffering.
2. Differentiate specificity theory from pattern theory.
3. Describe four behavioral theories of pain.
4. Describe the basic components and limitations of the gate-control theory of pain.
5. Identify new theories of pain proposed in the past decade.
6. Identify the theoretical perspective that best fits a current practice and describe its limitations.

I. Specificity Theory

A. The hypothesis that pain is related to specific anatomical structures and physiological functions replaced unproven, long-standing beliefs about pain, such as the following:
   1. Pain as a punishment for wrongdoing (ancient beliefs).
   2. Pain as an emotion—that pain was an emotion experienced in the heart, not a sensation experienced in the brain (Aristotelian).

B. Descartes first described pain in physical terms in 1664 (Melzack & Wall, 1983).
   1. The example described involved putting your foot in fire, resulting in the opening of a pore that pulls a thread, which rings a bell inside your head. As the bell swings back, it pulls the thread, which reflexively removes your foot from the fire before you have a chance to respond emotionally (Melzack & Wall, 1983).
   2. This example was consistent with people's experiences and could not be disputed with available and acceptable scientific methods.
   3. It was deduced logically that pain is a physical (not emotional) phenomenon traveling a specific anatomical path.

C. Johannes Müller, Max von Frey, and others in the 20th century detailed the elaborate anatomy and physiology of pain (Melzack & Wall, 1983).
   1. Müller described that sensory nerves responded to external stimuli (light, sound, taste, smell, and touch or feeling) and carried the encoded messages to specific areas of the brain.
   2. von Frey proved there were different kinds of sensory end organs, as opposed to the one type proposed by Müller, detailing the receptors that account for touch, warmth, cold, and pain.
   3. Other scientists (e.g., Angelo Ruffini, Charles Scott Sherrington, Peter O. Bishop, John D. Sinclair, Jerzey E. Rose, and Vernon B. Mountcastle) expanded on the propositions of Müller and von Frey with findings that thermal, mechanical, and chemical stimuli activated sensory nerves when a threshold was reached. These action potentials, in turn, transmitted information through specific peripheral and central pathways. In the case of pain, free nerve endings stimulated A delta (Aδ) and C fibers to transmit pain messages via an anterolateral (spinothalamic tract) pathway to pain centers in the thalamus (Melzack & Wall, 1983).

D. Specificity theory had a high level of utility because treatments (e.g., analgesics) were designed to block the generation (nonsteroidal antiinflammatory drugs) and transmission (opioids) of pain messages.

E. Challenging specificity theory
   1. Specificity theory does not explain all types of pain sensations (e.g., phantom limb pain and allodynia).
   2. Excessive noxious stimuli can be applied to the pain receptors without pain being perceived (e.g., the *walking wounded* soldiers who deny pain and refuse medication).
   3. Pain tolerance varies greatly among individuals and within the same individual at different times. This variation disputes the *hard-wired,* fixed, unidirectional system proposed by the specificity theory.
   4. Pain fibers can be cut or burned by nerve ablation, and pain persists or returns.

II. Pattern Theory

A. Pattern theory was articulated to account for the abnormal pain states (e.g., allodynia, hyperalgesia, and phantom limb sensation) not explained by specificity theory (Melzack & Wall, 1983).
   1. Pattern theory emphasizes the importance of stimulus intensity and central summation in the experience of pain and acknowledged variations within and among individuals in response to the same stimulus, which is painful when a crucial threshold is exceeded.
      a. At the end of the 19th century, Goldscheider first articulated the theory of how summation of stimuli in the central nervous system (e.g., dorsal horn) accounted for neuropathic pain syndromes (Melzack & Wall, 1965).
      b. By 1960, Livingston and Noordenbos described how this central summation in pathological states was due to a repatterning of the central nervous system, such as the development of

self-exciting, reverberating loops of neurons (Melzack & Wall, 1983). These abnormal loops were shown to affect adjacent sensory, motor, and autonomic nerves, accounting for spasticity, abnormal sweating, and increasing distribution of pain noted in some cases.

2. Pattern theory posits that all nerve endings are the same and that it is the pattern and intensity of the stimulus (not nerve ending type) that accounts for the pain experience.
3. Nerve types were described to be large or small, with a balance of fibers. An imbalance that favors the small fibers results in pain.
4. Research support and the utility of this theory were limited until more recent years, when concepts of primary and secondary sensitization, neuroplasticity, and up-regulation and down-regulation of spinal nerves have been supportive of the premise of this theory (Wall, 1999).

B. Challenging pattern theory
1. Physiological evidence reveals a high degree of receptor and fiber specialization or nerve differentiation that refutes a core premise of pattern theory.
2. Although pattern theory provides an explanation for neuropathic pain, it is not consistent with all types of pain experiences.

III. Psychosocial Theories of Pain

A. Psychological theories of pain
1. The psychological perspective views pain as an emotion or as the manifestation of an emotional state.
   a. The hypothesis that pain is an emotional state dates back more than 2 millennia to Aristotle.
   b. In 1894, Henry R. Marshall challenged specificity and pattern theory with his explanation of pain as an affect, not a physiological phenomenon (Holzman & Turk, 1986).
   c. Whether chronic pain is an antecedent or consequence of depression has been debated (Baker & Merskey, 1967; Blumer & Heilbron, 1981; Brown, 1990; Engel, 1959; Gatchel, Polatin, & Mayer, 1995; Magni, Moreschi, Rigatti-Luchini, & Merskey, 1994; Merskey & Boyd, 1978; Turk & Salovey, 1984; Woodforde & Merskey, 1967).
      (1) Extensive research has failed to find a consistent psychological profile of the *pain-prone patient.*
      (2) Prospective and longitudinal studies consistently find greater support for the conclusion that pain precedes, rather than follows, the development of depression (Breslau, Davis, Schultz, & Peterson, 1994; Brown, 1990; Cairns, Adkins, & Scott, 1996; Magni et al., 1994).
      (3) Chronic pain and depression may be related to a common pathophysiology involving the endogenous opiate system (Cowen, 1993; Kline et al., 1977; Krittayaphong, Light, Golden, Finkel, & Sheps, 1996; Tejedor-Real, Mico, Malsonado, Roques, & Gilbert-Rahola, 1995). Rome and Rome (2000) suggest that pain can be a limbically (involving the limbic portion of the brain responsible for our emotions) augmented syndrome, accounting for the emotional, physical, and behavioral features that often accompany chronic pain disorders regardless of the site of pain.
   d. Pain perception and tolerance relate to psychological factors, such as prior experiences, including social modeling, culture, attentional focus, suggestions by others, anxiety, and perceived meaning or cause of the pain (Turk & Nash, 1996; Turk & Rudy, 1986, 1992).
2. Pain may be a manifestation of some mental illnesses.
   a. Pain may be a hallucination in some individuals with schizophrenia or endogenous depression (Merskey & Spear, 1967).
   b. Pain may arise from some hysterical, fictitious, or hypochondriacal conditions (Ochoa, 1995).
   c. High stress levels compounded by distorted thinking and poor coping have been associated with chronic back pain (Melzack, 1999b; Turner, Clancy, & Vitaliano, 1987), which may be secondary to hormonal changes associated with prolonged stress (Lariviere & Melzack, 2000).

   d. Generally, these notions are believed to be true despite the limited research to support this perspective. The incidence of pain as a manifestation of mental illness is believed to be relatively rare (American Psychiatric Association, 1994).
3. Pain is the result of muscle tension, which is secondary to emotions.
   a. Physiological evidence supports that excessive or prolonged muscle tension can result in pain because of the buildup of waste products at the nerve endings.
   b. Sarno (1991) coined the term *tension myositis syndrome* to describe that most chronic pain problems result from tension (defined as repressed, unexpressed emotions) and an incorrect behavioral response. Treatment must include proper *conditioning* of the mind and body while gaining the insights needed to stop repressed emotions from causing further damage.
   c. Travell and Simons (1983) explained how muscles that are strained (by physical, psychological, or environmental stressors) can form *trigger points,* which are hypersensitive, knotted muscles associated with referred or regional pain when stimulated. These trigger points may be the source of acute or chronic pain and are treated (initially) by numbing and stretching the involved muscles (called myofascial release).
   d. Research to date neither clearly supports nor refutes these claims.
4. Although both perspectives can be supported or rejected, contemporary research supports that in some cases the emotional states accompanying pain are a consequence of noxious stimuli rather than the cause of pain. In contrast, in cases of chronic pain it is suggested that patients can experience physiological pain augmented by the limbic system, the system that modulates emotions (Rome & Rome, 2000).

B. Behavioral theories of pain
1. Pavlov (1927) viewed pain as a learned phenomenon with the context and meaning determining the perception and response. He showed that the meaning and response pattern to painful stimuli could be changed through *operant conditioning.*
2. Pilowsky and Spence (1976) described chronic pain syndrome as being one of abnormal illness behavior. The behaviors and limited functioning seem to be out of proportion to documented organic findings. This perspective suggests that chronic pain behaviors may be learned by social modeling and reinforcement, secondary gains, and deficient social skills.
3. Fordyce and associates (1973) described their method of looking beyond the physiological and psychological processes of pain to describe the observable, measurable, and potentially changeable *pain behaviors.* Rather than treating pain directly, the operant approach helps patients improve function and reduce or stop use of analgesics.
   a. Behaviors such as the verbal and nonverbal expressions of pain, drug intake, and limited activity continue to be displayed as long as positive reinforcement for those behaviors is received or perceived. If these behaviors are not reinforced (or are punished), they will be extinguished.
   b. The operant approach requires a well-controlled clinical setting, where pain and wellness behaviors can be evaluated carefully, monitored, and reinforced selectively. There is a deliberate attempt to respond neutrally to patients' thoughts and feelings surrounding their pain because attending to these thoughts and feelings would reinforce pain behavior.
   c. The conceptual basis and techniques of an operant conditioning treatment program are outlined in Fordyce's (1976) landmark book. Outcome data support the premise of this theory and the effectiveness (the ability to decrease medication use and improve function) of related therapies. The validity of many research projects supporting this form of therapy has been questioned because of methodological and sampling weaknesses (Portenoy & Kanner, 1996).
4. Turk and associates (Turk, 2003; Turk, Meichenbaum, & Genest, 1983) described a cognitive-behavioral framework for understanding and treating pain.
   a. The cognitive-behavioral framework views pain as a complex multidimensional experience. It was developed to improve the understanding and treatment of chronic pain and to address some shortcomings of the operant conditioning model (e.g., improving the application of behavioral changes beyond the treatment environment).

(1) In contrast to the behavioral model, the cognitive-behavioral model assumes the patient, not the professional, is the expert in managing personal pain through self-initiated techniques (not a fabricated clinical environment and reward system).
(2) The cognitive-behavioral model appears to be more compassionate than the operant model (by taking into account the patient's reports of pain and goals), while tapping into the patient's inner strengths, teaching the individual how to think, feel, and function better.

b. Therapy based on this cognitive-behavioral theory focuses on teaching the patient to monitor thoughts, feelings, and actions while learning and using self-initiated skills to reduce pain, improve function, enhance wellness behaviors, and reduce use of unnecessary medications or health care services.
(1) Thoughts, feelings, and attitudes must be examined for their relationship to pain and targeted behaviors (e.g., unrealistic expectations or emotional stress leading to increased pain levels).
(2) Behaviors must be recognized and monitored, with positive reinforcement (e.g., improved functioning with or without improved comfort).
(3) The patient determines which desirable behaviors must be added or increased and which self-defeating or unhelpful behaviors need to be decreased or eliminated.
(4) The patient becomes a behavioral engineer, changing personal behavior based on individualized goals, with internal and external rewards systems reinforcing behavior change.

c. Cognitive-behavioral theory has a growing body of research supporting its premises and the effectiveness and cost-effectiveness of related therapies (Caudill, Schnable, Zuttermeister, Benson, & Friedman, 1991; Gatchel & Okifui, 2006; Johansson, Dahl, Jannert, Melin, & Andersson, 1998; Johnson, Rice, Fuller, & Endress, 1978; Leibing, Pfingsten, Bartmann, Rueger, & Schuessler, 1999; Lorig, Mazonson, & Holman, 1993; Morley, Eccleston, & Williams, 1999; Thorn, 2004).

d. Recent scientific evidence using a nonrandomized two-group research design has demonstrated effectiveness of a pain rehabilitation program in improving functioning for opioid users undergoing medication withdrawal, as well as for nonopioid users (Townsend, et al., 2008).

IV. Gate-Control Theory of Pain

A. Melzack and Wall's (1965) gate-control theory defines pain as a complex perceptual experience influenced by physiological and psychological factors unique to the individual. This theory resulted from a critique and rearticulation of existing theories and data.
1. Elements of specificity theory were retained with descriptions of specialized receptors, fibers, and other components of the sensory system.
2. Elements of pattern theory were retained, such as the substantia gelatinosa in the dorsal horn, where sensitization and windup occur, accounting for pathological pain states (Davies & Lodge, 1987).
3. Components of psychosocial theories were retained because affect, motivation, perception, and the central control of the mind all contribute to the pain experience.

B. Propositions of the original theory (Melzack & Wall, 1965)
1. Small diameter (Aδ and C) fibers carry messages of pain to the dorsal horn of the spinal cord.
2. A neural mechanism in the dorsal horn of the spinal cord acts like a gate, which can increase (facilitate) or decrease (inhibit) the flow of nerve impulses from peripheral fibers to the central nervous system. This gating mechanism is located in the substantia gelatinosa.
3. Large-diameter (A beta) fibers (which transmit thermal or touch messages) can close the gate, reducing the transmission of pain messages.
4. The gating mechanism is influenced by the relative amount of input from small and large fibers entering the spine from parallel peripheral pathways.

5. Intense nonpainful stimuli could be perceived as pain if the gates are opened.
6. This gating mechanism is influenced by nerve impulses descending from the brain.
   a. An influence is exerted by *central control processes* of the brain (e.g., evaluating pain in terms of past experience) on the gating mechanism and discriminative and motivational systems.
   b. A specialized system, termed the *central intensity monitor* (parts of the motivational–affective, limbic, and reticular structures), modulates the gating system directly and indirectly through the central control processes of the brain.
7. When noxious stimuli entering the spinal cord exceed a crucial level, *T cells* (also termed the *action system*) responsible for the subjective experience and objective behavior of pain are activated. These T cells are believed to be the link between the mind and the body.
   a. Direct links are made from the (1) motivational–affective and (2) sensory–discriminatory systems, both of which link to the (3) central control processes.
   b. All three systems interact with one another and project to the motor system, determining the action to be taken.
   c. From the motivational perspective (Van Damme, Crobmez, & Eccleston, 2008), people with chronic pain are motivated to remove obstacles that keep them from attaining their goals or they adjust their goals to make them more easily obtainable. Knowing how and when to make each of these choices is equated with the successful ability to cope with chronic pain.

C. The following propositions have been added (Melzack & Wall, 1983, 1996) based on extensive new research and discoveries related to the original theory:
   1. Emphasis was added to the importance of the substantia gelatinosa in the establishment of an excitatory or inhibitory environment in the dorsal horn of the spine.
   2. The conceptualization of the gating mechanism was revised to imply that the gating mechanism could be presynaptic, postsynaptic, or both.
   3. The descending inhibitory gate-control system was strengthened because of evidence that unconscious central control processes and conscious motivational–affective systems had a greater influence over the perception of pain intensity than originally was suspected.
   4. The bidirectional nature of the perceptual, motivational, affective, and cognitive systems was detailed further as antecedents of the behavioral response to pain.
   5. Because extensive anatomical investigation has failed to find a single T cell structure, Melzack and Wall (1983) concluded that the action system is a complex, dynamic process of interactions among a multilayered neuromatrix, rather than a single localized structure.

D. Support and extension of the gate-control theory
   1. The gate-control theory has gained considerable recognition, with volumes of research and new clinical approaches supporting its validity and utility.
   2. Nonpharmacologic treatments (e.g., cold, heat, transcutaneous electrical nerve stimulation, and massage) exert their effect by stimulation of large *inhibitory* peripheral fibers, resulting in endorphin production and release. This common mechanism would account for the similar potency of various techniques described by Malone and Strube (1988).
   3. Segmental pain facilitation (opening the *gate*) has been shown to increase pain intensity and duration (Bennett, 1999).
      a. Peripheral nerve sensitization
         (1) Alterations in peripheral nerve threshold produce a state of hyperexcitability secondary to changes in ion channels (Waxman, Bib-Hajj, Cummins, & Black, 1999).
         (2) α-Adrenergic receptor activation (Perl, 1999) and chemical mediators of inflammation and pain (Watkins, Maier, & Goehler, 1995) produce peripheral sensitization.
      b. Windup and neuroplasticity
         (1) With repeated moderate-to-severe pain, *N*-methyl-D-aspartate receptors are activated, which produces a windup effect, changing intracellular calcium ion concentration and creating a synaptic buildup of excitatory amino acids. Pain intensity, duration, and geographical distribution become greater than expected for a given stimulus (Bennett, 1999; Coderre, Katz, Vaccarino, & Melzack, 1993).

(2) If moderate-to-severe pain persists for more than 24 hours, additional changes in the structure and function of the spinal segment of the nervous system occur. These changes are termed ***neuroplasticity*** and include further changes in ion channels, damage to pain inhibition systems, and protein synthesis that stimulates pain fiber growth, resulting in more intense, widespread pain (Arnstein, 1997; Coderre et al., 1993). Price and Staud (2005) suggest that fibromyalgia syndrome may be associated with neuroplastic changes. Dworkin and Fields (2005) postulate that fibromyalgia is a neuropathic pain condition.

c. Successive stage model of pain processing

(1) Developed by Wade, Dougherty, Archer, and Price (1996) and supported empirically by Rainville, Carrier, Hofbauer, Bushnell, and Duncan (1999), the successive stage model of pain processing describes how pain is processed cognitively (perception of pain intensity) and then influences pain affect (mood), which in turn governs subsequent behavioral responses.

(2) The central control concept of this theory may be inadequate given empirical evidence supporting that affect (particularly anger, fear, anxiety, and depression) or behavior (inactivity-induced deconditioning) can influence pain perception. The relationships among sensory, cognitive, affective, and behavioral domains of pain are probably bidirectional, not unidirectional as described (Novy, Nelson, Francis, & Turk, 1995). Rome and Rome (2000) suggest that pain and emotions influence one another through the limbic system.

4. Descending pain modulation system has been mapped and shown to exert an inhibitory effect (closing pain gates) at the dorsal horn.
   a. Hughes and associates (1975) and Pert and Snyder (1973) first described the discovery of opiate receptor sites in the brain.
   b. In 1976, two investigators, working independently, found opioid-like substances (endorphins) produced by central nervous system (enkephalin) interneurons (Hughes et al., 1975; Simanton & Snyder, 1976; Snyder, 1980). More than 20 varieties of endorphins are classified into three families: endorphins, enkephalins, and dynorphins (Fishman & Carr, 1992; Yaksh & Noveihed, 1985).
5. In relation to central control of pain, strong empirical evidence has clarified the relationship between cognitive patterns and the pain experience.
   a. Learned helplessness (Flor & Turk, 1988; Hill, Niven, & Knussen, 1995; Jensen, Turner, & Romano, 1991; LeSage, Slimmer, Lopez, & Ellor, 1989; Smith, Christensen, Peck, & Ward, 1994) and catastrophizing (Geisser, Robinson, Keefe, & Weiner, 1994; Jensen, Romano, Turner, Good, & Wald, 1999; Sullivan, Stnish, Waite, Sullivan, & Tripp, 1998) are associated with poor clinical outcomes. Imaging studies have demonstrated activation of pain centers in the brain when a person focuses on symptoms or catastrophizes about pain (Chen, 2001; Graceley et al., 2004).
   b. Strong beliefs in personal ability (self-efficacy) to manage pain, cope, and function, as well as acceptance of pain, have been associated with desired clinical outcomes (Anderson, Dowds, Pelletz, & Edwards, 1995; Arnstein, Caudill, Mandle, Norris, & Beasley, 1999; Estlander, Vanharanta, Moneta, & Kaivanto, 1994).
   c. Conflicting research reports raise questions about whether or not perceived *locus of control* accounts for individual differences in the perception of and response to pain (Bates & Rankin-Hill, 1994; Gallagher et al., 1995; Gustafsson & Gaston-Johansson, 1996; May, Reed, Schwoerer, & Potter, 1997; Scharff, Turk, & Marcus, 1995; Toomey, Seveille, Mann, Abashian, & Wingfield, 1995).
   d. The efficacy of distraction techniques, relaxation, imagery, cognitive restructuring, placebo effect, and other cognitive strategies capable of diminishing pain awareness supports that cognitive centers exert an effect on pain perception (Bruehl, Carlson, & McCibbin, 1993). Solicitous responses from significant others have been found to contribute to increased

symptoms and poorer patient outcomes for patients with chronic pain and fatigue (Newton-John & Williams, 2006; Schmaling, Smith, & Buchwald, 2000).

6. The action system, which directly links pain intensity to pain behavior, generally is supported with operant and cognitive-behavioral models (described in other sections), further delineating how psychosocial factors contribute to pain behavior.
   a. Physiological and psychosocial evidence supports that when nociceptive input reaches a crucial level it elicits the same *pain response* (e.g., muscle tension and flexion, adrenal release, and vocalization) regardless of age, sex, or race (Melzack & Wall, 1996).
   b. Population-based research supports that pain intensity is linked directly to behavioral response.
      (1) Large studies using multinational samples have found a consistent relationship between pain intensity and extent of disability (Cleeland, 1984; Serlin, Mendoza, Nakamura, Edwards, & Cleeland, 1995).
      (2) Mild or minimal pain intensity does not interfere with the individual's ability to "carry out daily activities," whereas moderate pain results in "extensive diminution in an individual's capacity," and severe pain "precludes . . . most activities of daily living" (American Medical Association, 1993).
      (3) In cases of chronic pain, pain intensity ratings do not necessarily correspond to functioning and quality of life; adaptive coping skills can be learned to improve functioning despite higher levels of pain (Hooten, Townsend, Sletten, Bruce, & Rome, 2007).

E. Multiple redundant systems (multiple gate control versus single gate control)
   1. Multiple parallel nerve pathways, neurotransmitters, and inflammatory neuroactive substrates are involved in the generation, transmission, and modification of pain signals (Dubner & Gold, 1999; Urban & Gebhart, 1999).
   2. The role of the serotonin and norepinephrine systems in modulating pain has been described and is the basis for administering antidepressant medications to inhibit noxious stimuli and produce analgesia (Max, 1994; Max et al., 1987; Yaksh, 1979). Recent studies have indicated shared mechanisms in depression and chronic pain for central hyperexcitability (Klauenberg et al., 2008).
   3. Silent nociceptors are dormant until peripheral sensitization occurs. The nociceptors are *turned on* by prostaglandins, bradykinins, serotonin, histamine, adenosine triphosphate, interleukins, tumor necrosis factor, and other cytokines (Kress & Reeh, 1996; Schaible & Grubb, 1993).
   4. Sympathetic fibers similarly sprout in the dorsal horn as the result of peripheral nerve injury or sensitization (Devor, Janig, & Michaelis, 1994), resulting in a rewiring of the dorsal horn and peripheral nerve sensitivity to adrenergic agonists.

F. Melzack's current thinking: the neuromatrix model of pain
   1. Rather than a linear model, Melzack (Godfrey, 2005; Lariviere & Melzack, 2000; Melzack, 1999a, 2001) supports the view that pain arises from complex, dynamic neuromatrices with parallel and redundant neurological and neurochemical systems within the brain that are not limited to activity in a discrete sensory cortex. Information from these multiple neural systems within the brain is integrated, producing the pain experience.
   2. The synaptic architecture is determined genetically at birth but changes constantly thereafter, based on sensory, chemical, cognitive, affective, behavioral, and perhaps spiritual experiences.
   3. Abnormal patterns of impulse generation (e.g., the absence of input after an amputation) or significant change in physical activity patterns may produce pathological pain states.
   4. Findings from brain-imaging studies have supported the neuromatrix model of pain. Evidence from brain-imaging studies in the last decade have advanced our understanding of where and how pain is processed in the central nervous system (Mersky, Loeser, & Dubner, 2005; Chen, 2001).
   5. The neuromatrix model contributes to our understanding of the psychological complexities because it integrates findings from brain-imaging studies, effects of stress on pain, and research on cognitive-behavioral factors (Keefe, Dixon, & Pryor, 2005).
   6. The connection of neuroscience of pain to human suffering is limited. Perhaps this is an area of future research appropriate for nurses to study.

G. Wall's most recent thinking, before his death in 2001
   1. Similar to Melzack, Wall (1999) discounted components of the gate-control theory of pain that promoted a specific nociceptive transmission system in favor of viewing pain as a drive or a need state (similar to hunger).
   2. The sensory system (viewed as the same system that controls motor function) is highly plastic, constantly changing based on physical, psychological, and social experiences.
   3. Pain is experienced as a signal for action. It demands that the person experiencing the pain or social contacts in the environment take action. Pain persists as long as the need is unmet. When appropriate actions are taken, pain awareness diminishes.

H. Challenging the gate-control theory
   1. The greatest strength of the theory is the exquisite articulation of the neuroanatomy and physiology of pain. This focus also is its greatest limitation.
      a. Although Melzack and Wall (1983) posited that affect, motivation, cognition, and behavior affect the perception of pain, the focus of the theory is a tiny zone of the spinal cord. Others described how the physical, psychological, behavioral, cognitive, cultural, and spiritual dimensions (Caudill, 1995; McCaffery & Pasero, 1999; Turk et al., 1983) fit into the context of the gate-control theory.
      b. Evidence that suggests a more broadly focused, multisystem model, which includes physiological evidence that endorphins are found in different parts of the brain, midbrain, spine, gastrointestinal tract, genitourinary tract, and musculoskeletal systems, is needed (Yaksh & Noveihed, 1985).
   2. The gate-control theory does not have a clear explanation for the role of the autonomic nervous system (sympathetic, parasympathetic) on the inhibition or facilitation of pain perception.
      a. Evidence shows that 20% of pain (unmyelinated C) fibers transmit their messages to the sympathetic chain rather than the dorsal horn (Ferrante, 1994).
      b. Research suggests activation of the sympathetic nervous system (e.g., a stress response) occurs with acute pain (Cahill, 1989; Houldin, Lev, Prystowsky, Redei, & Lowery, 1991; Stein, Price, & Gazzaniga, 1989; Wells-Federman et al., 1995).
   3. Complementary therapies are not explained by the gate-control theory but have demonstrated effectiveness (Caserta, 1992; Diers, 1972; Geisser et al., 1994) (see the chapter on Integrative Therapies Used in Pain Management Nursing).
      a. One explanation is the *placebo effect,* the nonspecific healing factor associated with being on the receiving end of another person's intent to help.
      b. Another explanation, based on Albert Einstein's theory ($E = MC^2$) that mass and energy are interchangeable, is that electromagnetic energy waves generated by topically applied magnets or certain interpersonal interactions can effect a change in the structure and function (mass) of the pain system.
      c. Many therapies are based on *theories* that have not been accepted by mainstream scientists or have not withstood the test of scientific investigations of multiple studies using rigorous methodologies. We may ponder whether current therapies satisfy our curiosity about pain and are sufficient to guide nursing practice or if a better explanation exists for the universal yet individual phenomenon of pain.
      d. New approaches to pain treatment, such as the role of healing in the mind–body connection (Sternberg, 2000) and the focus on spirituality and suffering, show potential significance to nursing practice and research.
      e. Addressing pain-related fear and avoidance (Asmundson, Norton, & Norton, 1999) and the relationship of emotional regulation processes and pain (Keefe, Lumley, Anderson, Lynch, & Carson, 2001) is another frontier that nurses are incorporating into their nursing practice. The nursing profession can assist in relieving the moral crisis of unrelieved pain by providing a caring relationship to people in pain and their family members. In the context of the nurse–patient relationship, by being present with, not just doing for, the patient, the nurse shows compassion and respect for the patient's pain experience (Ferrell, 2005).

References

American Medical Association. (1993). *Guide to the evaluation of permanent impairment* (4th ed.). Chicago: Author.

American Psychiatric Association. (1994). *Diagnostic and statistical manual of mental disorders* (4th ed.). Washington, DC: Author.

Anderson, K. O., Dowds, B. N., Pelletz, R. E., & Edwards, W. T. (1995). Development and initial validation of a scale to measure self efficacy beliefs in patients with chronic pain. *Pain, 63,* 77–84.

Arnstein, P. M. (1997). The neuroplastic phenomenon: A physiologic link between chronic pain and learning. *Journal of Neuroscience Nursing, 29,* 179–186.

Arnstein, P. M., Caudill, M., Mandle, C. L., Norris, A., & Beasley, R. (1999). Self-efficacy as a mediator of the relationship between pain intensity, disability and depression in chronic pain patients. *Pain, 80,* 483–491.

Asmundson, G. J. G., Norton, P. J., & Norton, G. R. (1999). Beyond pain: The role of fear and avoidance in chronicity. *Clinical Psychology Review, 19*(1), 97–119.

Baker, J. W., & Merskey, H. (1967). Pain in general practice. *Journal of Psychosomatic Research, 10,* 383–387.

Bates, M. S., & Rankin-Hill, L. (1994). Control, culture and chronic pain. *Social Science and Medicine, 39,* 629–645.

Bennett, R. M. (1999). Emerging concepts in the neurobiology of chronic pain: Evidence of abnormal sensory processing in fibromyalgia. *Mayo Clinic Proceedings, 74,* 385–398.

Blumer, D., & Heilbron, M. (1981). Chronic pain as a variant of depressive disease: The pain-prone disorder. *Journal of Nervous and Mental Diseases, 170,* 381–406.

Breslau, N., Davis, G. C., Schultz, L. R., & Peterson, E. L. (1994). Migraine and major depression: A longitudinal study. *Headache, 34,* 387–393.

Brown, G. K. (1990). A causal analysis of chronic pain and depression. *Journal of Abnormal Psychology, 99,* 127–137.

Bruehl, S., Carlson, C. R., & McCibbin, J. A. (1993). Two brief interventions for acute pain. *Pain, 54,* 29–36.

Cahill, C. A. (1989). Beta-endorphin levels during pregnancy and labor: A role in pain modulation? *Nursing Research, 38,* 200–203.

Cairns, D. M., Adkins, R. H., & Scott, M. D. (1996). Pain and depression in acute traumatic spinal cord injury: Origins of chronic problematic pain? *Archives of Physical Medicine and Rehabilitation, 77,* 329–335.

Caserta, J. E. (1992). A nursing presence. *Home Healthcare Nurse, 10,* 7–8.

Caudill, M. A. (1995). *Managing pain before it manages you.* New York: Guilford Press.

Caudill, M. A., Schnable, R., Zuttermeister, P., Benson, H., & Friedman, R. (1991). Decreased clinic use by chronic pain patients: Response to behavioral medicine intervention. *Clinical Journal of Pain, 7,* 305–310.

Chen, A. C. N. (2001). New perspectives in EEG/MEG brain mapping and PET/fMRI neuroimaging of human pain. *International Journal of Psychophysiology, 42,* 147–159.

Cleeland, C. S. (1984). The impact of pain on patients with cancer. *Cancer, 54,* 2635–2641.

Coderre, T. J., Katz, J., Vaccarino, A. L., & Melzack, R. (1993). Contribution of central neuroplasticity to pathologic pain: Review of clinical and experimental evidence. *Pain, 52,* 259–285.

Cowen, P. J. (1993). Serotonin receptor subtypes in depression: Evidence from studies in neuroendocrine regulation. *Clinical Neuropharmacology, 16*(Suppl. 3), S16–S18.

Davies, S. N., & Lodge, D. (1987). Evidence for involvement of *N*-methylaspartate receptors in "windup" of class 2 neurons in the dorsal horn. *Brain Research, 424,* 402–406.

Devor, M., Janig, W., & Michaelis, M. (1994). Modulation of activity in dorsal horn ganglion neurons by sympathetic activation in nerve-injured rats. *Journal of Neurophysiology, 71,* 38–47.

Diers, D. (1972). The effect of nursing interaction on patients in pain. *Nursing Research, 21,* 419–428.

Dubner, R., & Gold, M. (1999). The neurobiology of pain. *Proceedings of the National Academy of Sciences of the United States of America, 96,* 7627–7630.

Dworkin, R. H., & Fields, H. L. (2005). Fibromyalgia from the perspective of neuropathic pain. *Journal of Rheumatology, 32*(Suppl. 75), 1–5.

Engel, G. L. (1959). "Psychogenic" pain and the pain-prone patient. *American Journal of Medicine, 26,* 899–918.

Estlander, A. M., Vanharanta, H., Moneta, G., & Kaivanto, K. (1994). Anthropometric variables, self-efficacy beliefs and pain and disability ratings on the isokinetic performance of low back pain patients. *Spine, 19,* 941–947.

Ferrante, F. M. (1994). Pain neuroanatomy. In *Comprehensive review of pain management* (pp. 59–132 [unedited syllabus]). Chicago: American Society of Regional Anesthesia.

Ferrell, B. (2005). Ethical perspectives on pain and suffering. *Pain Management Nursing, 6*(3), 83–90.

Fishman, S. M., & Carr, D. B. (1992). Basic mechanisms of pain. *Hospital Practice, 27,* 63–76.

Flor, H., & Turk, D. C. (1988). Chronic pain and rheumatoid arthritis: Predicting pain and disability from cognitive variables. *Journal of Behavioral Medicine, 11,* 251–265.

Fordyce, W. E. (1976). *Behavioral methods for chronic pain and illness.* St. Louis: C. V. Mosby.

Fordyce, W. E., Fowler, R., Lehmann, J., DeLateur, B., Sand. P., & Trieschmann, R. (1973). Operant conditioning in the treatment of chronic pain. *Archives of Physical Medicine and Rehabilitation, 54,* 399–408.

Gallagher, R. M., Williams, R. A., Skelly, J., Haugh, L. D., Rauh, V., Milhous, R., & Frymoyer, J. (1995). Workers compensation and return to work in low back pain. *Pain, 61,* 229–307.

Gatchel, R. J., & Okifui, A. (2006). Evidence-based scientific data documenting the treatment and cost-effectiveness of comprehensive pain programs for chronic nonmalignant pain. *Journal of Pain, 7*(11), 779–793.

Gatchel, R. J., Polatin, P. B., & Mayer, T. G. (1995). The dominant role of psychosocial risk factors in the development of chronic low back pain disability. *Spine, 20,* 2702–2709.

Geisser, M. E., Robinson, M. E., Keefe, F. J., & Weiner, M. L. (1994). Catastrophizing, depression and the sensory, affective and evaluative aspects of chronic pain. *Pain, 59,* 79–83.

Godfrey, H. (2005). Understanding Pain, Part I: Physiology of pain. *British Journal of Nursing, 14*(16), 846–852.

Graceley, R. H., Geiser, M. E., Giesecke, T., Grant, M. A. B., Petzkey, F., Williams, D. A., & Clauw, D. J. (2004). Pain catastrophizing and neuro responses to pain among persons with fibromyalgia. *Brain, 127,* 835–843.

Gustafsson, M., & Gaston-Johansson, F. (1996). Pain intensity and health locus of control: A comparison of patients with fibromyalgia syndrome and rheumatoid arthritis. *Patient Education and Counselling, 29,* 179–188.

Hill, A., Niven, C. A., & Knussen, C. (1995). The role of coping in adjustment to phantom limb pain. *Pain, 62,* 79–86.

Holzman, A. D., & Turk, D. C. (1986). *Pain management: A handbook of psychological treatment approaches.* New York: Pergamon Press.

Hooten, W. M., Townsend, C. O., Sletten, C. D., Bruce, B. K., & Rome, J. D. (2007). Treatment outcomes after multidisciplinary pain rehabilitation with analgesic medication withdrawal for patients with fibromyalgia. *Pain Medicine, 8*(1), 8–16.

Houldin, A. D., Lev, E., Prystowsky, M. B., Redei, E., & Lowery, B. J. (1991). Psychoneuro-immunology: A review of literature. *Holistic Nursing Practice, 5,* 10–21.

Hughes, J., Smith, T. W., Kosterlitz, H. W., Fothergill, L. A., Morgan, B. A., & Morris, H. R. (1975). Identification of two related pentapeptides from the brain with potent opiate agonist activity. *Nature, 258,* 577–579.

Jensen, M. P., Romano, J. M., Turner, J. A., Good, A. B., & Wald, L. H. (1999). Patient beliefs predict patient functioning: Further support for a cognitive-behavioral model of chronic pain. *Pain, 81,* 95–104.

Jensen, M. P., Turner, J. A., & Romano, J. M. (1991). Self-efficacy and outcome expectancies: Relationship to chronic pain coping strategies and adjustment. *Pain, 44,* 263–269.

Johansson, C., Dahl, J., Jannert, M., Melin, L., & Andersson, G. (1998). Effects of a cognitive-behavioral pain management program. *Behavior Research and Therapy, 36,* 915–930.

Johnson, J. E., Rice, V. H., Fuller, S. S., & Endress, M. P. (1978). Sensory information, instruction in a coping strategy and recovery from surgery. *Research in Nursing and Health, 1,* 4–17.

Keefe, F. J., Dixon, K. E., & Pryor, R. W. (2005). Psychological contributions to the understanding and treatment of pain. In H. Merseky, J. D. Loeser, & R. Dubner (Eds.). *The paths of pain, 1975–2005* (pp. 403–420). Seattle: IASP Press.

Keefe, F. J., Lumley, M., Anderson, T., Lynch, T., & Carson, K. L. (2001). Pain and emotion: New research directions. *Journal of Clinical Psychology, 57*(4), 587–607.

Klauenberg, S., Maier, C., Assion, H. J., Hoffmann, A., Krumova, E. K., Magerl, W., Scherens, A., Treede, R. D., & Juckel, G. (2008). Depression and changed pain perception: Hints for a central disinhibition mechanism. *Pain, 140*(2), 332–343.

Kline, N. S., Li, C. H., Lehman, H. L., Lajta, A., Laski, E., & Cooper, T. (1977). Beta-endorphin-induced changes in schizophrenics and depressed patients. *Archives of General Psychiatry, 34,* 1111–1113.

Kress, M., & Reeh, P. W. (1996). Chemical excitation and sensitization in nociceptors. In C. Belmonte & F. Cervero (Eds.), *Neurobiology of nociceptors* (pp. 258–297). Oxford: Oxford University Press.

Krittayaphong, R., Light, K. C., Golden, R. N., Finkel, J. B., & Sheps, D. S. (1996). Relationship among depression scores, endorphin and angina pectoris during exercise in patients with coronary artery disease. *Clinical Journal of Pain, 12,* 126–133.

Lariviere, W. R., & Melzack, R. (2000). The role of corticotropin-releasing factor in pain and analgesia. *Pain, 84,* 1–12.

Leibing, E., Pfingsten, M., Bartmann, U., Rueger, U., & Schuessler, G. (1999). Cognitive-behavioral treatment in unselected rheumatoid arthritis outpatients. *Clinical Journal of Pain, 15,* 58–66.

LeSage, J., Slimmer, L. W., Lopez, M., & Ellor, J. R. (1989). Learned helplessness. *Journal of Gerontological Nursing, 15,* 8–15.

Lorig, K. R., Mazonson, P. D., & Holman, H. R. (1993). Evidence suggesting that health education for self management in patients with chronic arthritis has sustained health benefits while reducing health care costs. *Arthritis and Rheumatism, 36,* 439–446.

Magni, G., Moreschi, C., Rigatti-Luchini, S., & Merskey, H. (1994). Prospective study on the relationship between depressive symptoms and chronic musculoskeletal pain. *Pain, 56,* 289–297.

Malone, M. D., & Strube, M. J. (1988). Meta-analysis of non-medical treatments for chronic pain. *Pain, 34,* 231–244.

Max, M. B. (1994). Treatment of post-herpetic neuralgia: Antidepressants. *Annals of Neurology, 35*(Suppl.), S50–S53.

Max, M. B., Culnane, M., Schafer, S. C., Gracely, R. H., Walther, D. J., Smoller, B., & Dubner, R. (1987). Amitriptyline relieves diabetic neuropathy pain in patients with normal and depressed mood. *Neurology, 37,* 589–596.

May, D. R., Reed, K., Schwoerer, C. E., & Potter, P. (1997). Employee reactions to ergonomic job training: The moderating health effects of health locus of control and self efficacy. *Journal of Occupational Health Psychology, 2,* 11–24.

McCaffery, M., & Pasero, C. (1999). *Pain: Clinical manual* (2nd ed.). St. Louis: Mosby.

Melzack, R. (1999a). From the gate to the neuromatrix. *Pain* (Suppl.), S121–S126.

Melzack, R. (1999b). Pain and stress: A new perspective. In R. J. Gatchel & D. C. Turk (Eds.), *Psychosocial factors in pain* (pp. 89–106). New York: Guilford Press.

Melzack, R. (2001). Pain and the neuromatrix in the brain. *Journal of Dental Education, 65*(12), 1378–1382.

Melzack, R., & Wall, P. D. (1965). Pain mechanisms: A new theory. *Science, 150,* 971–979.

Melzack, R., & Wall, P. D. (1983). *The challenge of pain.* New York: Basic Books.

Melzack, R., & Wall, P. D. (1996). *The challenge of pain* (2nd ed.). New York: Penguin Books.

Merskey, H., & Boyd, D. (1978). Emotional adjustment and chronic pain. *Pain, 5,* 173–178.

Merskey, H., & Spear, F. G. (1967). The concept of pain. *Journal of Psychosomatic Research, 11,* 59–67.

Mersky, H., Loeser, J. D., & Dubner, R. (2005). *The paths of pain, 1975–2005.* Seattle: IASP Press.

Morley, S., Eccleston, C., & Williams, A. (1999). Systematic review and meta-analysis of randomized control trials of cognitive behavior therapy and behavior therapy for chronic pain patients, excluding headaches. *Pain, 80,* 1–13.

Newton-John, T. R., & Williams, A. C. (2006). Chronic pain couples: perceived marital interactions and pain behaviours. *Pain, 123,* 53–63.

Novy, D. M., Nelson, D. V., Francis, D. J., & Turk, D. C. (1995). Perspectives of chronic pain: An evaluative comparison of restrictive and comprehensive models. *Psychological Bulletin, 188,* 238–247.

Ochoa, J. L. (1995). Reflex sympathetic dystrophy: A common clinical avenue for somatoform expression. *Neurologic Clinics, 13,* 361–363.

Pavlov, I. P. (1927). *Conditioned reflexes.* Oxford: Humphrey Milford.

Perl, E. R. (1999). Causalgia, pathological pain and adrenergic receptors. *Proceedings of the National Academy of Sciences of the United States of America, 96,* 7664–7667.

Pert, C. B., & Snyder, S. H. (1973). Opiate receptor: Its demonstration in nervous tissue. *Science, 179,* 1011–1014.

Pilowsky, I., & Spence, N. D. (1976). Pain, anger and illness behaviour. *Journal of Psychosomatic Research, 20,* 411–416.

Portenoy, R. K., & Kanner, R. M. (1996). *Pain management: Theory and practice.* Philadelphia: F. A. Davis.

Price, D. D., & Staud, R. (2005). Neurobiology of fibromyalgia syndrome. *Journal of Rheumatology, 32*(Suppl. 75), 22–28.

Rainville, P., Carrier, B., Hofbauer, R. K., Bushnell, M. C., & Duncan, G. H. (1999). Dissociation of sensory and affective dimensions of pain using hypnotic modulation. *Pain, 82,* 159–171.

Rome, H., & Rome, J. (2000). Limbically augmented pain syndrome (LAPS): Kindling, corticolimbic sensitization, and the convergence of affective and sensory symptoms in chronic pain disorders. *Pain Medicine, 1*(1), 7–23.

Sarno, J. E. (1991). *Healing back pain.* New York: Warner Books.

Schaible, H. G., & Grubb, B. D. (1993). Afferent and spinal mechanisms of joint pain. *Pain, 55,* 5–54.

Scharff, L., Turk, D. C., & Marcus, D. A. (1995). The relationship of health locus of control and psychosocial–behavioral response in chronic headache. *Headache, 35,* 527–533.

Schmaling, K. B., Smith, W. R., & Buchwald, D. S. (2000). Significant other responses are associated with fatigue and functional status among patients with chronic fatigue syndrome. *Psychosomatic Medicine, 62,* 444–450.

Serlin, R. C., Mendoza, T. R., Nakamura, Y., Edwards, K. R., & Cleeland, C. S. (1995). When is cancer pain mild, moderate or severe? Grading pain severity by its interference with function. *Pain, 61,* 277–284.

Simanton, R., & Snyder, S. H. (1976). Morphine-like peptides in mammalian brain: Isolation, structure, elucidation and interactions with the opiate receptor. *Proceedings of the National Academy of Sciences of the United States of America, 73,* 2515–2519.

Smith, T. W., Christensen, A. J., Peck, J. R., & Ward, J. R. (1994). Cognitive distortion, helplessness and depressed mood in rheumatoid arthritis: A four-year longitudinal analysis. *Health Psychology, 13,* 213–217.

Snyder, S. (1980). Brain peptides as neurotransmitters. *Science, 209,* 976–983.

Stein, B. E., Price, D. D., & Gazzaniga, M. S. (1989). Pain perception in a man with a total corpus callosum transection. *Pain, 38,* 51–56.

Sternberg, E. (2000). *The balance within: The science connecting health and emotions.* New York: W. H. Freeman.

Sullivan, M. J., Stnish, W., Waite, H., Sullivan, M., & Tripp, D. A. (1998). Catastrophizing, pain and disability in patients with soft-tissue injuries. *Pain, 77,* 253–260.

Tejedor-Real, P., Mico, J. A., Malsonado, R., Roques, B. P., & Gilbert-Rahola, J. (1995). Implications of endogenous opioid system in the learned helplessness model of depression. *Pharmacology, Biochemistry and Behavior, 52,* 145–152.

Thorn, B. E. (2004). *Cognitive therapy for chronic pain: A step-by-step guide.* New York: Guilford Press.

Toomey, T. C., Seveille, J. L., Mann, J. D., Abashian, S. W., & Wingfield, M. S. (1995). Relationship of learned resourcefulness to measures of pain description, psychopathology, and health behavior in a sample of chronic pain patients. *Clinical Journal of Pain, 11,* 259–266.

Townsend, C., Kerkvliet, J., Bruce, B., Rome, J., Hooten, W. M., Luedtke, C., & Hodgson, J. (2008). A longitudinal study of the efficacy of a comprehensive pain rehabilitation program with opioid withdrawal: Comparison of treatment outcomes based on opioid use status at admission. *Pain, 140*(1), 177–189.

Travell, J. G., & Simons, D. G. (1983). *Myofacial pain and dysfunction: The trigger point manual* (Vols. 1–2). Baltimore: Williams & Wilkins.

Turk, D. C. (2003). Cognitive-behavioral approach to the treatment of chronic pain patients. *Regional Anesthesia and Pain Medicine, 28*(6), 573–579.

Turk, D. C., & Nash, J. M. (1996). Psychological issues in chronic pain. In R. K. Portenoy & R. M. Kanner (Eds.), *Pain management: Theory and practice.* Philadelphia: F. A. Davis.

Turk, D. C., & Rudy, T. E. (1986). Assessment of cognitive factors in chronic pain: A worthwhile enterprise? *Journal of Consulting and Clinical Psychology, 54,* 760–768.

Turk, D. C., & Rudy, T. E. (1992). Cognitive factors and persistent pain: A glimpse into Pandora's box. *Cognitive Theory Research, 16,* 99–122.

Turk, D. C., & Salovey, P. (1984). Chronic pain as a variant of depressive disease: A critical reappraisal. *Journal of Mental and Nervous Diseases, 172,* 398–404.

Turk, D. C., Meichenbaum, D., & Genest, M. (1983). *Pain and behavioral medicine.* New York: Guilford Press.

Turner, J. A., Clancy, S., & Vitaliano, P. P. (1987). Relationships of stress, appraisal and coping to chronic low back pain. *Behavioral Research and Therapy, 25,* 281–288.

Urban, M. O., & Gebhart, G. F. (1999). Supraspinal contributions to hyperalgesia. *Proceedings of the National Academy of Sciences of the United States of America, 96,* 7687–7692.

Van Damme, S., Crombez, G., & Eccleston, C. (2008). Coping with pain: A motivational perspective. *Pain, 139,* 1–4.

Wade, J. B., Dougherty, L. M., Archer, C. R., & Price, D. D. (1996). Assessing the stages of pain processing: A multivariate analytical approach. *Pain, 68,* 157–167.

Wall, P. D. (1999). *Pain: The science of suffering.* London: Weidenfeld & Nicholson.

Watkins, L. R., Maier, S. F., & Goehler, L. E. (1995). Immune activation: The role of pro-inflammatory cytokines in inflammation, illness responses and pathological pain states. *Pain, 63,* 289–302.

Waxman, S. G., Bib-Hajj, S., Cummins, T. R., & Black, J. A. (1999). Sodium channels and pain. *Proceedings of the National Academy of Sciences of the United States of America, 96,* 7635–7639.

Wells-Federman, C. L., Stuart, E. M., Deckro, J. P., Mandle, C. L., Blaim, M., & Medich, C. (1995). The mind–body connection: The psychophysiology of many traditional nursing interventions. *Clinical Nurse Specialist, 9,* 59–64.

Woodforde, J. M., & Merskey, H. (1967). Personality traits of patients with chronic pain. *Journal of Psychosomatic Research, 16,* 167–172.

Yaksh, T. L. (1979). Direct evidence that spinal serotonin and noradrenaline terminals mediate the spinal antinociceptive effects of morphine in the periaqueductal grey. *Brain Research, 160,* 180–185.

Yaksh, T. L., & Noveihed, R. (1985). The physiology and pharmacology of spinal opiates. *Annual Review of Pharmacology and Toxicology, 25,* 433–462.

chapter

5

Neurophysiology of Pain

Rosemary C. Polomano, PhD, RN, FAAN

Part One: Anatomy and Physiology of Pain

Objectives

After studying this chapter, the reader should be able to:

1. Discuss nociceptive pain mechanisms.
2. Distinguish the predominant characteristics of Aδ and C fibers.
3. Describe the pain pathways in the peripheral and central nervous system and the mechanisms involved in afferent nociceptive pain transmission, transduction, perception, and modulation.
4. Explain the role of neurotransmitters in mediating the pain response and known sites of receptors.

"Pain is 'normal' (nociceptive) when it results from the activity of healthy nociceptive afferents aroused by intense stimuli assuming the baseline sensitivity of the sensory system." (Devor, 1994)

I. Physiological Sources of Pain (Table 5-1) (Besson, 1999; Katz & Rothenberg, 2005)

A. Nociceptive
   1. Ongoing activation of nociceptor (free nerve endings capable of sensing pain) primary afferent neurons occurs in response to noxious stimuli.
   2. Pain is often consistent with the degree of tissue injury.
   3. Subtypes
      a. *Somatic:* Originating from nociceptive activation in the skin, subcutaneous tissue, bones, muscles, and blood vessels; typically well localized; and described as sharp, aching, or throbbing
      b. *Visceral:* Originating from nociceptor activation in the organs, linings of the organs, and body cavities; described as more diffuse gnawing or cramping

B. Neuropathic (non-nociceptive, pathological pain) (Treede et al., 2008)
   1. Pain is believed to be sustained by aberrant somatosensory processing in the peripheral nervous system or central nervous system (CNS).
   2. Pain can result from injury to or dysfunction of the peripheral nervous system or CNS.
   3. Such pain involves more than one mechanism and may result from abnormal peripheral nerve function and neural processing of impulses from abnormal neuronal receptor and mediator activity.
   4. Subtypes of neuropathic pain
      a. "Central generator": Deafferentation pain (e.g., central pain or phantom pain) or sympathetically maintained pain
      b. "Peripheral generator": Originating in the nerve root, plexus, or nerve (e.g., polyneuropathies or mononeuropathies)

II. Peripheral Nervous System: Components of Nociceptive Pain Messaging—Both Nociceptive and Primary Afferent Fibers (Katz & Rothenberg, 2005; Meyer, Ringkamp, Campbell, & Raja, 2006; Zhang & Bao, 2006)

A. Nociceptors
   1. Free nerve endings in the afferent peripheral nervous system are located in the muscle, fascia and blood vessels, knee joint, viscera, and dura.
   2. Nociceptors respond differentially to intense, potentially harmful stimuli of a thermal, chemical, or mechanical nature.

Table 5-1 Physiological Sources of Pain

Nociceptive Pain
Somatic Pain
• Complaints: constant, achy • Location: well localized in skin, subcutaneous tissues; less well localized in bone, muscle, blood vessels, connective tissues • Examples: incision pain, bone fractures, bony metastases, degenerative joint or spinal disease, osteoarthritis, rheumatoid arthritis, peripheral vascular disease, chronic stasis ulcers
Visceral Pain
• Complaints: cramping, splitting • Location: originates in internal organs or body cavity linings; poorly localized, diffuse, deep • Examples: chest or abdominal tubes, drains; bladder distention or spasms; intestinal distention; pericarditis; constipation; organ metastases; spastic bowel; inflammatory bowel disease; hiatal hernia; chronic hepatitis
Neuropathic Pain (nonnociceptive pain)
• Complaints: shooting, burning, electric shock–like, sharp, numb, motor weakness • Location: originates in injury to peripheral nerve, spinal cord, brain; poorly localized

3. Nociceptor subtypes respond to mechanical stimuli (mechanical nociceptors), mechanical and thermal stimuli (mechanothermal nociceptors), and mechanical, thermal, and chemical stimuli (polymodal nociceptors).
4. Nociceptors are associated with specific afferent nerve fiber (neuron) types (Aguggia, 2003).
   a. A fiber nociceptors are thought to evoke pricking pain, sharpness, and perhaps aching pain.
   b. C fibers thought to evoke a burning pain sensation.
5. Types of nociceptive pain
   a. First pain
      (1) Transmitted by A delta (Aδ) fibers
      (2) Fast pain: rapidly transmitting input to the somatosensory cortex
      (3) Sharp and pricking quality
   b. Second pain
      (1) Transmitted by C fibers
      (2) Slow pain
      (3) Dull, aching, or burning quality
      (4) May be long-lasting, even after painful stimuli subside
6. Specific nociceptor characteristics (Alvarez & Fyffe, 2000)
   a. *Sensitization* is an increased sensitivity of the receptor from neurochemicals and after repeated activation by noxious stimuli.
   b. Stimulus intensity is communicated through firing frequency (i.e., frequency increases as stimulus increases).
   c. Repeated stimulation can expand the receptive field (an area of the body surface over which a single sensory receptor, or its afferent nerve fiber, is capable of sensing stimuli).
   d. When sensitized, these nerve fibers are capable of responding to new forms of stimulation.
7. Variations between categories of nociceptors show complexity (Cho et al., 2006; Julius & Basbaum, 2001; Zhang & Bao, 2006).
   a. Nociceptors activating Aδ fibers
      (1) Mechanosensitive
         (a) Mechanosensitive nociceptors are receptive to mechanical stress or damage.
         (b) This is a major class of nociceptors in the skin dealing with mechanical pressure.
         (c) Pressure may be caused by distention, pressure, irritation, or infection.
         (d) The stimulus threshold remains stable through a range of intensities.
      (2) Mechanothermal
         (a) Mechanothermal is a major class of nociceptors in the skin healing with thermal stressors.
         (b) From 20% to 50% of Aδ fibers are in this category (Burgess & Perl, 1973).
      (3) Low-threshold mechanothermal (first pain)
         (a) This class responds to rapidly increasing heat stimuli.
         (b) It responds to heat in the 45°C to 47°C range.
         (c) Some nociceptors are activated by cold in the range of 0°C to 14°C; all are activated by temperature less than 0°C (Simone & Kajander, 1997).
         (d) These nociceptors are activated by intense mechanical stimulation.
      (4) High-threshold mechanoreceptor (Meyer & Campbell, 1981)
         (a) This class responds only after repeated stimuli.
         (b) The initial usual heat threshold is 50°C to 53°C.
         (c) These nociceptors develop sensitization to heat.
         (d) The threshold is lowered for heat with repeated exposure to stimuli.
      (5) Mechanoinsensitive (about 50% of Aδ nociceptors) (Meyer, Davis, Cohen, Treede, & Campbell, 1991)
         (a) Some may be insensitive to any mechanical stimulus.
         (b) Some may respond when pressure is greater than 600 kPa (60 g/mm^2).
      (6) Cold receptors, which respond to intense cold (Meyer et al., 2006)

b. Nociceptors activating Aβ fibers
   (1) Low-threshold mechanical stimulation (mechanoreceptors) occurs through fine touch or tactile stimuli.
c. Nociceptors activating C fibers (90% of afferent C fibers are nociceptive) (Fields, 1987)
   (1) Polymodal nociceptors are activated by cold, heat, pressure, and chemicals (Meyer, Ringkamp, Campbell, & Raja, 2006).
      (a) Heat activation occurs in the range of 38°C to 51°C by low and high rates of heating (McCormack, Prather, & Chapleo, 1998).
      (b) These nociceptors may develop ongoing discharge after sensitization.
      (c) Cold activation occurs in the range of −18°C to 14°C (Simone & Kajander, 1997).
      (d) Mechanical activation may not be changed by heat and chemical activity.
   (2) Mechanoinsensitive (about 30% of C fibers) (Meyer, Campbell, & Raja, 1988; Meyer et al., 1991)
      (a) Nociceptors may be insensitive or may respond to pressure.
      (b) They may be more responsive after inflammation.
      (c) They may be chemospecific (responding to specific chemical stimuli).
      (d) These nociceptors respond to intense heat or cold.
   (3) Evidence suggests subsets of receptors within nerve endings of the cutaneous receptive fields are capable of generating action potentials independent of heat and mechanical stimuli (Olausson, 1998).
d. Silent or sleeping nociceptors
   (1) Silent nociceptors are contained in the skin and deep tissues.
   (2) They are normally unresponsive to noxious mechanical and thermal stimuli but can be activated (responsive) by the onset of inflammation to the surrounding tissue, by mechanical stimulation during inflammation, and after tissue injury in the presence of inflammation and chemical sensitization.
   (3) When activated, silent nociceptors may discharge vigorously in response to nominal stimuli of pressure or temperature.
   (4) Many visceral nociceptors are silent nociceptors.
e. Other nociceptors
   (1) Articular nociceptors
      (a) Articular nociceptors are found in joints. Joint nerves contain about twice as many unmyelinated afferent axons as myelinated ones.
      (b) The ratio of nociceptors connected to unmyelinated versus myelinated neurons is about 2:1.
      (c) Group III axons are small myelinated afferents in joints and muscles.
      (d) Group IV axons are small unmyelinated afferents in joints and muscles.
      (e) Articular nociceptors respond to excess joint rotation that is noxious.
      (f) They can be sensitized by inflammation, causing response to even slight joint movements not in the noxious range.
   (2) Muscle nociceptors
      (a) Polymodal responsiveness of nociceptors is connected to group III and IV axons.
      (b) Some nociceptors connected to group IV are possibly activated more during ischemia.

Note: A growing body of evidence from experimental models has provided more specific details about the types and roles of nociceptors.

8. Nociceptors are sensitized or activated by chemicals released in response to tissue injury (Yaksh & Luo, 2007).
   a. Kinin
      (1) Bradykinin is a biologically active polypeptide triggered by the activation of the clotting cascade. It acts on specific bradykinin receptors.

(2) Kinin evokes a response in both A and C nociceptors, activating these free nerve endings, and plays a role in inflammatory pain and hyperalgesia.

b. Lipidic acids, such as cyclooxygenase (COX) products (e.g., prostaglandin E_2 and thromboxane A_2)

(1) Cell membranes are composed of phospholipids, and when cell membranes are damaged, the phospholipase enzyme breaks down the phospholipids to arachidonic acid; the enzyme, COX, breaks down arachidonic acid to prostaglandins.

(2) Prostaglandins sensitize nociceptors; they directly act on C fibers and facilitate their excitability.

c. Amines

(1) Histamine is released from mast cells.

(2) Serotonin (5-HT) is released from platelets.

(3) Both are produced in response to various stimuli such as tissue trauma and chemically medicated tissue damage.

d. Primary afferent peptides

(1) Calcitonin gene–related peptide and substance P are found in the peripheral terminals of C fibers.

(2) Both are released from responses to noxious stimuli and produce local cutaneous vasodilation, plasma extravasation, and sensitization in the skin region innervated by the stimulated sensory nerves.

e. Hydrogen (H^+) and potassium (K^+) ions present in injured tissues directly stimulate C fibers and lead to the local release of various vasodilatory peptides.

f. Cytokines, comprising interleukins or tumor necrosis factor, are powerful sensitizers of C fiber terminals and are part of the inflammatory and infection involving mast cells.

B. Transduction of nociceptive messaging

1. Transduction begins with activation of nociceptors in the peripheral nervous system in response to noxious stimuli.
2. Conversion of stimulus energy into an electrical impulse is made possible by the action potential in neuronal membranes.
3. Sodium (Na^+) and calcium channels open, causing depolarization of the nerve endings and release of an electrical signal.

C. Transmission of nociceptive messaging along the neuron

1. Nociceptive impulses initiated by activation are transmitted to the dorsal horn of the spinal cord.
2. Common neuronal membrane channels are involved in transmission.

a. Active and passive Na^+ and K^+ channels are typically involved.

b. Electrical membrane potential (action potential) transmits impulses.

c. Transduction initiates rapid exchange of electrolytes across neuronal membranes (i.e., impulse transmission), causing depolarization.

d. Not all impulses result in neurotransmitter release at the synapse in the dorsal horn.

e. Resting membrane potential reset occurs through active and passive electrolyte channel activity (repolarization).

f. The refractory period occurs when membrane potential goes below the resting potential, and it may not be stimulated for a period, limiting how many action potentials may be produced.

(1) The absolute refractory period is when no stimulus will create a response, no matter how strong.

(2) The relative refractory period is a much lower resting potential; therefore, a higher stimulus is needed.

D. Specific types and characteristics of afferent pain fibers

1. Aδ fibers

a. Small and thinly myelinated

b. Diameter: 2 to 5 micrometers

c. Conduction velocity: more than 10 and less than 40 meters/sec (Yaksh & Luo, 2007)

In Brief

Mechanical, thermal, or chemical stimuli activate nociceptors, which in turn stimulate primary afferent fibers. The intensity of stimuli may be strong enough to damage tissues and cause the release of neurochemical mediators (e.g., K^+, substance P, bradykinin, prostaglandin, histamine, and 5-HT), which sensitize or activate nociceptors. When nociceptors are activated, they transform the energy of the stimulus (transduction), causing the neuron to respond. This energy transformation generates an influx of Na^+ and an efflux of K^+ across the neuronal membrane. This ion exchange results in an action potential along the neuronal membrane of afferent fibers, terminating in the dorsal horn of the spinal cord (transmission).

d. Widely distributed in the body
   (1) Skin and subcutaneous tissue
   (2) Corneas
   (3) Teeth (intradental and periodontal)
   (4) Joint capsules
   (5) Mucous membranes of the mouth, nose, sinuses, and anus
   (6) Viscera
   (7) Respiratory system: J receptors (juxtapulmonary capillary receptors) in the lung interstitium near the capillaries connect to some C fibers
   (8) Digestive tract
   (9) Muscles, tendons, and fasciae
   (10) Bone periosteum
   (11) Urogenital system (kidneys and organs of reproduction)
   (12) Solid abdominal organs (liver, spleen, and pancreas)
   (13) Brain meninges and scalp
   (14) Cardiac muscle
   (15) Walls of blood vessels

e. Capable of localization of nociceptive stimuli

2. C fibers
   a. Small and unmyelinated
   b. Diameter: 0.3 to 3 micrometers
   c. Conduction velocity: approximately less than 2 m/sec (Yaksh & Luo, 2007)
   d. Widely distributed
   e. Potentially diffuse localization of nociceptive stimuli; diffuse receptive fields
3. Aβ fibers
   a. Large and myelinated
   b. Conduction velocity: more than 40 to 50 m/sec (Yaksh & Luo, 2007)
   c. Fine touch and proprioception fibers
4. Receptive fields
   a. A receptive field is the area monitored by a single nerve. The smaller receptive fields produce more precise localization of pain, whereas larger receptive fields produce less precise pain sensations.
   b. Receptive fields can overlap.
   c. Receptive fields for Aδ fibers can have a cluster of many small, separate nociceptive fields.
   d. Receptive fields for C fibers usually comprise one continuous, receptive field per fiber.
5. Transient receptor potential vanilloid 1 (TRPV1) (Cui et al., 2006)
   a. TRPV1 is expressed in primary sensory afferents. The best known vanilloid is capsaicin.
      (1) TRPV1 is extracted from capsicum chili peppers. Capsaicin specifically activates fine afferent nerve fibers involved in pain transmission and neurogenic inflammation.

b. A ligand-gated nonselective cation channel believed to be an important integrator of various pain stimuli, such as endogenous lipids, capsaicin, heat, and low pH.
c. TRPV1 plays a role in the acute detection of noxious heat.
d. Activation of TRPV1 results in release of neurotransmitters from peripheral and central nerve terminals in the brain, resulting in pain and inflammation (Roberts & Connor, 2006).
e. Activation of the antinociceptive descending pathway via TRPV1 receptor stimulation in the periaqueductal gray offers promise as a novel strategy for providing analgesia.

E. Dorsal root ganglion (DRG)
1. The anatomical location is outside of but close to the dorsal region of the CNS bilaterally (not present above the level of spinal nerves).
2. DRG contains cell bodies of somatic and visceral sensory nerves (except from cranial nerves, as mentioned later).
3. The soma is bulbous end of the neuron which contains the nucleus and acts as the cell's central control. The soma for sympathetic nerve fibers are located in the DRG.
4. Mu (μ) receptors are present, along with evidence for kappa (κ), delta (δ), and epsilon (ϵ) receptors.
5. Primary afferent cell bodies may have synaptic connections with other fiber-type cell bodies in the DRG.
6. Most nociceptive fibers enter the spinal cord through the dorsal root after passing through the DRG.
7. A few may enter the cord via the ventral root.

F. Sensory ganglia contain cell bodies from cranial nerves V, VII, IX, and X, which include nociceptive inputs.

G. Tract of Lissauer (Coggeshall, Chung, Chung, & Langford, 1981)
1. The tract is located in the dorsal root entry zone of spinal nerves (area in the white matter between the edge of spinal cord where afferent fibers enter and the beginning of the dorsal horn gray matter in which they synapse).
2. It is made up of approximately 80% primary afferent fibers; approximately 20% are axons from gray matter cells in the spine.
3. Nociceptive fibers mainly enter the medial aspect of the tract, where input is shared up and down one or two segments (variable), then enter into and synapse in the dorsal horn.

III. Central Nervous System: Spinal Cord and Brain (Hudson, 2000; Westlund High, 2008; Woolf & Slater, 2006; Yaksh, 1993, 2007)

A. Dorsal horn (Fig. 5-1) (Woolf & Slater, 2006)
1. The dorsal horn is the inner, butterfly-shaped gray matter of spinal cord.
2. Primary afferents project into the dorsal horn.
3. Gray matter is organized by 10 Rexed (based on histological appearance) laminae, I through X.
   a. Laminae I through VI are referred to as the dorsal horn.
   b. Laminae VII through IX are referred to as the ventral horn.
   c. Lamina X surrounds the central canal.
   d. Laminae I, II, V, and X have significant nociceptive input and possible afferent inhibitory inputs (Siddall & Cousins, 1998; Yaksh & Luo, 2007).
   e. Lamina I
      (1) Lamina I is the anatomical region in the marginal layer.
      (2) Input comes from cutaneous C, Aδ, and Aβ fibers.
      (3) Lamina I has muscle and visceral nociceptive afferents (Aδ and C).
      (4) Most are nociceptive-specific cells.
   f. Lamina II
      (1) Lamina II is the anatomical region substantia gelatinosa.
      (2) Input comes from cutaneous C, Aδ, and Aβ fibers.
      (3) Input comes from visceral C fibers.
      (4) This category is subdivided into laminae IIo (outer) and IIi (inner).

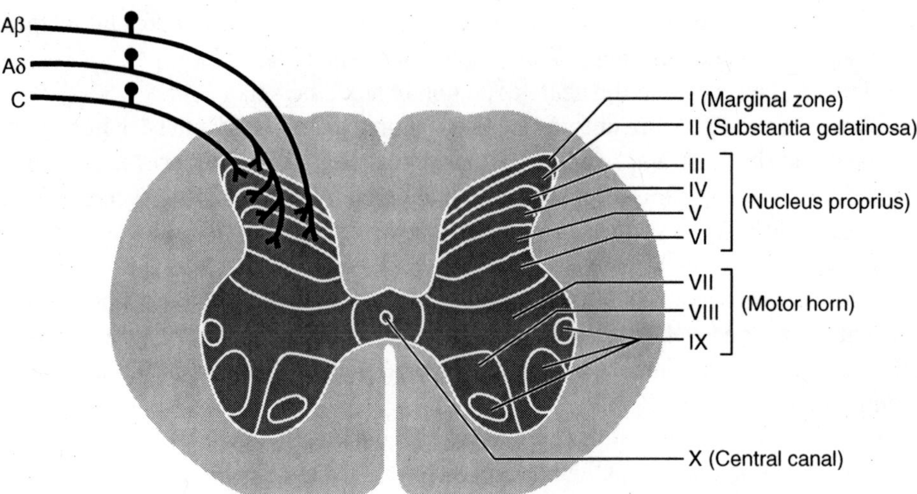

FIGURE 5-1 | Dorsal horn.

From *Pain Management*, volume 1 by Waldman, 2006. Copyright Elsevier Health Services. Used with permission.

g. Laminae III through VI
   (1) The anatomical region is the nucleus proprius.
   (2) Input comes from Aδ and Aβ fibers.
   (3) Input comes from muscle and visceral nociceptive afferents (Aδ and C fibers).
h. Lamina X
   (1) For lamina X, the anatomical region is central canal.
   (2) Input comes from Aδ fibers.
   (3) Input comes from visceral nociceptive afferents.
i. Laminae VII through IX lie in the motor horn.

Note: Lamina VIII is known to have some nociceptive input, but the overall significance is not clear because it seems to originate from scattered areas and is defined poorly.

4. Spinal neurons
   a. Spinal interneurons
      (1) Most neurons in the dorsal horn are spinal neurons.
      (2) These neurons contain many of the neuroactive substances involved in excitatory and inhibitory mechanisms with pain, and they are classified as neurotransmitters or modulators of pain.
      (3) Many interconnections of mixed fiber types exist between laminae (e.g., Aβ fibers have collaterals to laminae III, IV, and V and may play a role in referred pain patterns).
5. Neurotransmitter and modulators in the dorsal horn (peptides and amino acids) (Basbaum, 1985; Besse, Lombard, Zakac, Roques, & Besson, 1990; Carlton, Westlund, Zhang, Sorkin, & Willis, 1990; Otsuka, Konishi, Yanagisawa, Tsunoo, & Tagagi, 1982; Siddall & Cousins, 1998; Yaksh, 1997)
   a. Excitatory substances
      (1) Substance P is found most densely in laminae I and II but is also found in sympathetic ganglia, probably from primary afferent terminals.
      (2) Glutamate and aspartate, amino acids, are found in laminae I through III.
      (3) Cholecystokinin is found mostly in lamina II.
      (4) Calcitonin gene–related peptide is released from the spinal terminals of primary afferent neurons by high-intensity mechanical and thermal stimuli, as well as by the injection of local irritants (Garry & Hargreaves, 1992).
      (5) Vasoactive intestinal polypeptide is found most densely in lamina I.
      (6) Nitric oxide is involved in presynaptic transmission leading to postsynaptic excitation.

b. Inhibitory substances
   (1) Dynorphin, an endogenous opiate, works mainly on κ-receptors. Dynorphin A has a distinct action from other endogenous opioid peptides, exerting a significant neuronal excitatory and neurotoxic effect mediated not by the opioid receptors but by the bradykinin receptor (Lai, Luo, Chen, & Porreca, 2008).
   (2) Enkephalin, an endogenous opiate, is found in laminae I through III. It works mainly on δ-receptors.
   (3) β-Endorphin, an endogenous opiate, acts mainly on μ and δ-receptors.
   (4) Norepinephrine is found in laminae I, II, IV, V, VI, and X.
   (5) 5-HT is found in laminae I through III.
   (6) Somatostatin is found mostly in lamina II (less in lamina I). It inhibits nociceptors.
   (7) γ-Aminobutyric acid (GABA) is found mostly in laminae I and II.
   (8) While inhibitory, glycine acts as a coagonist at the glycine site of *N*-methyl-D-aspartate (NMDA) receptors to potentiate nociceptive transmission (Zhou, Zhang, Chen, & Pan, 2008).

6. The following are examples of receptor types present on presynaptic neurons, which modulate incoming afferent input (Siddall & Cousins, 1998):
   a. Opiate (μ, κ, and δ) receptors (75% of dorsal horn population) (Besse et al., 1990; Yaksh, 1997)
      (1) μ_1-Receptors are involved primarily with analgesia.
      (2) κ-Receptors are involved primarily with analgesic activity in the spinal cord.
      (3) δ-Receptors not only may have analgesic activity but also may produce euphoria.
   b. $GABA_B$
   c. Serotonin receptors ($5\text{-}HT_2$, $5\text{-}HT_3$)
   d. α_2-Adrenoreceptors
   e. Neurokinin-1 (NK-1)

7. The following are examples of receptor types present on postsynaptic neurons. These receptors provide opportunities to modulate the response of the second-order neuron to the incoming afferent input (Siddall & Cousins, 1998).
   a. Opiate (μ, κ, and δ) receptors (25% of dorsal horn population) (Besse et al., 1990; Yaksh, 1997)
   b. Glutamate receptors (Bleakman, Alt, & Nisenbaum, 2006)
      (1) Glutamate receptors include ionotropic NMDA receptors, kainate receptors (non-NMDA ionotropic) and α-amino-3-hydroxy-5-methyl-4-isoxazolepropionic acid (AMPA) receptors to which excitatory amino acids such as glutamate bind.
      (2) Metabotropic (mGlu1 to mGlu8) receptors
      (3) Both of these receptor groups play an important role in chronic pain states.
   c. Neurokinin
   d. $GABA_A$ (inhibitory)
   e. Serotonin receptors ($5\text{-}HT_{1B}$)
   f. Adenosine
   g. α_2-Adrenoreceptors (inhibitory)

8. Dorsal horn second-order neurons
   a. Three types are present in variable quantities.
      (1) Projection neurons relay messages to higher brain centers.
      (2) Excitatory neurons relay messages to projection neurons, various other interneurons, and motor spinal reflex neurons.
      (3) Inhibitory neurons can reduce afferent inputs to higher centers of the brain.
   b. Spinal cord gray matter is divided by Rexed into 10 laminae.
      (1) The first 6 make up the dorsal horn, receive all afferent neural activity, and represent the principle site for modulation of pain.
      (2) Second-order neurons either are nociceptive specific or have a wide dynamic range.

c. The following are characteristics of lamina I second-order neurons (lamina I is also called the *marginal zone*):
   (1) Most are nociceptive specific (also called ***high-threshold neurons***).
   (2) Projection neurons (ascending tract to thalamus) predominate.
   (3) Some local interneuron connections occur within the lamina.
   (4) A few are wide dynamic range neurons (i.e., respond to noxious and nonnoxious stimuli).
d. The following are characteristics of lamina II second-order neurons (lamina II is also called the *substantia gelatinosa* because of its appearance).
   (1) Some projection neurons ascend to the brain stem and thalamus.
   (2) Many local interneuron connections are made.
      (a) Some travel up or down a couple of segments within lamina II and synapse again.
      (b) Most synapse with other lamina II cells in the same segment.
      (c) Some connect to fibers from laminae I, III, IV, and V that penetrate into lamina II.
e. Lamina III second-order neurons are mainly projection neurons.
f. The following are characteristics of lamina V second-order neurons:
   (1) Projection neurons are mainly to the thalamus.
   (2) More are wide dynamic range neurons (compared with lamina I).
      (a) Convergent input is received from Aβ, Aδ, and C afferents.
      (b) Cutaneous receptive fields overlap.
      (c) High and low stimulus thresholds are found.
      (d) Convergence of somatic and viscera stimuli occurs.
      (e) These are responsible for ***windup*** states, characterized by a progressive increase in action potential from dorsal horn neurons elicited from a repeated low-frequency C fiber or nociceptor stimuli (Dostrovsky & Craig, 2006).
      (f) Some dendrites extend into laminae I and II.
   (3) Receptive fields are larger (compared with lamina I).
g. The following are characteristics of lamina X second-order neurons:
   (1) Projection neurons are mainly to the brain stem and reticular formation.
   (2) These neurons represent mostly small nociceptive fields.

B. Elements of ascending inhibitory inputs (not part of descending opiate system)
   1. Activation of mechanoreceptors causes activation of dorsal horn inhibitory neurons.
   2. Release of inhibitory amino acid neurotransmitters and peptides by dorsal horn interneurons is caused by activation of nociceptors in the dorsal horn.

C. Ascending nociceptive pathways (Fig. 5-2)
   1. The spinothalamic tract (STT) relays sensory information from the spinal cord to the thalamus, the main site for sensory information integration. Axons cross the dorsal and ventral commissures of the spinal cord, reaching to the contralateral side. Two locations exist where axons are concentrated: the middle of the lateral funiculus (lateral STT) and the middle of the anterior ventral funiculus (the anterior STT) (Craig, Zhang, & Blomqvist, 2002). In the spinal cord in the

In Brief

Where the primary afferent fibers terminate in the dorsal horn at the presynaptic junction, there is a release of neuropeptides, such as substance P, somatostatin, and vasoactive intestinal polypeptide, and a large quantity of other neurochemicals, many of which act as neurotransmitters. Some of these chemicals, including substance P, bind with receptors on secondary neurons, creating an action potential. Opiate receptors also are located in the dorsal horn on the end of the afferent pain fibers. Endogenous opiates bind to these receptors, resulting in the inhibition of the release of neurotransmitters (such as substance P), which can stop the nociceptive impulse from being communicated to the next order neuron.

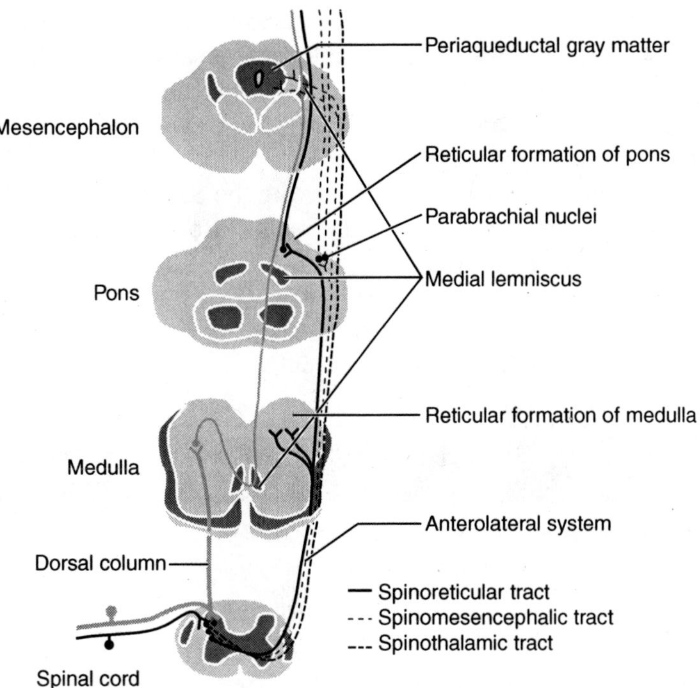

FIGURE 5-2 Projections of spinal neurons. The brain stem projections of spinal neurons into the medulla and mesencephalon. Third-order projections arising from the medullary and mesencephalic neurons project into the intralaminar and ventrobasal thalamus.

anterior white commissure, these tracts ascend in the white matter in the ventrolateral and lateral funiculus.

a. The lateral STT (the ***neospinothalamic tract***) projects to the ventroposterolateral nucleus of the thalamus and then to the somatosensory cortex for location, density, and duration of pain.
   (1) It is primarily composed of nociceptive neurons from laminae I and V and less so from lamina IV, most terminating in the ventroposterolateral nucleus of the thalamus.
   (2) A few lamina I neurons project into nucleus submedius of the thalamus, while a few lamina I neurons project into medial thalamus.
   (3) Individual variability does exist regarding the exact location and extent of this SST (Dostrovsky & Craig, 2006).
b. The medial STT (the ***paleospinothalamic tract***), which also includes input from the spinoreticular tract and spinomesencephalic tract, projects to the medial thalamus, with projections to the reticular formation, pons, midbrain, periaqueductal gray, hypothalamus, various other thalamic nuclei, and other areas of the brain.
   (1) It is primarily composed of nociceptive neurons from deeper laminae.
   (2) Most distal neurons to the brain lie in the outermost part of the tract, while the more proximal neurons, such as those from the cervical area, are in the innermost area of the tract.

2. The trigeminothalamic tract from the face and head has two parts similar to the STT:
   a. The neotrigeminothalamic tract to ventroposteromedial thalamic nucleus
   b. The paleotrigeminothalamic tract to medial thalamic nuclei
3. Spinoreticular pathways
   a. Projection axons from the spinal cord provide innervation to regions of the brain stem.
   b. The spinoreticular pathway contains cells from cervical areas and less so from laminae I, V, VII, VIII, and X, many with wide dynamic range characteristics.
   c. It has the most direct connection to the reticular formation from the spinal cord.

d. It connects with multiple nuclei, including areas in the medulla and pons.
e. The spinoreticular pathway is responsible for arousal and autonomic responses to pain.

4. Spinomesencephalic tract
   a. Most cells originate in laminae I and V.
   b. This tract is primarily nociceptive specific.
   c. It follows through the medulla and pons with the STT and spinoreticular tract. Then, at the level of the mesencephalon, it turns and connects to the subnucleus lateralis of the periaqueductal gray and other nuclei.
5. Ventral STT
   a. The ventral STT is composed of cells from laminae I and IV through VII.
   b. It seems to play an indirect role in nociception.

In Brief

The STT neurons are combined in the portion of the spinal cord called the anterolateral quadrant. These ascending neurons continue to transmit the nociceptive messages through to the thalamus and midbrain.

D. Centers in the brain receiving nociceptive input
1. Hypothalamus
   a. The hypothalamus integrates autonomic arousal and neuroendocrine responses.
   b. It relates to emotional responses.
   c. It is a strong activator of motivational inputs.
2. Thalamus
   a. The thalamus has two sections:
      (1) *Paleothalamus:* Medial and intralaminar nuclei
         (a) The paleothalamus is not organized somatotopically.
         (b) It has diffuse connections throughout the brain.
      (2) *Neothalamus:* Ventrobasal area
         (a) The neothalamus is somatotopically arranged.
         (b) It communicates with cerebral cortex areas, the primary somatosensory cortex (SI) and the secondary somatosensory cortex (SII).
   b. The thalamus controls relay messaging to higher centers of the brain.
   c. It provides cutaneous awareness for localization and discrimination.
   d. It may play a role in motor control and increased cortical activity.
3. Cerebral cortex: SI and SII, cortical modulation of pain (Ohara, Vit, & Jasmin, 2005)
   a. Somatotopically arranged cells in SI help with fine sensory discrimination.
   b. SII is not somatotopically arranged but receives information from SI.
4. Limbic system
   a. The limbic system generates purposeful, goal-directed behavior.
   b. It affects mood states.
   c. It generates incentive and motivational reactions.
5. Reticular formation (in the brain stem)
   a. Reticular formation mediates motor, autonomic, and sensory functions.
   b. It triggers arousal and alertness.
   c. It adds to emotive responses, including aversive drive (pain behaviors).
   d. It is composed of many nuclei, including the raphe magnus (part of descending analgesic system).
   e. The presence of ϵ-opioid receptors is probable.
6. Tectum (at back of midbrain): enhanced reflexes and learned behavior patterns (Nowak & Handford, 1994)

In Brief

From the thalamus, fibers transmit nociceptive messages to the somatosensory cortex, the parietal lobe, the frontal lobe, and the limbic system. At this level of processing, the individual perceives the painful sensation. Stimulation of the limbic system in the area of the anterior cingulate gyrus may produce the emotional reaction to pain. As pain management nurses, we must familiarize ourselves with the inner workings of the brain and pain perception. The future of pain research lies in the brain.

E. Descending modulation of pain (Bonica, 1990; Fields, 1987; Siddall & Cousins, 1998)
   1. Periaqueductal gray
      a. The periaqueductal gray receives input from multiple brain centers:
         (1) Locus coeruleus (in the pons): sends noradrenergic input to the periaqueductal gray
         (2) Limbic system
         (3) Cortex (frontal and insular areas)
         (4) Other cerebral cognitive centers
         (5) Thalamus
         (6) Hypothalamus (major contributor): sends β-endorphin axons
      b. The periaqueductal gray consists of multiple neuron types with various neurotransmitters that exert inhibitory antinociceptive effects:
         (1) Enkephalin
         (2) Dynorphin
         (3) 5-HT
         (4) Neurotensin
      c. The periaqueductal gray contains receptors for many transmitters:
         (1) Enkephalin
         (2) β-Endorphin
         (3) Substance P: produces analgesia if injected into periaqueductal gray
   2. Nucleus raphe dorsalis and mesencephalic reticular formation
      a. These consist of multiple neuron types with various neurotransmitters:
         (1) Enkephalin
         (2) Dynorphin
         (3) 5-HT
         (4) Neurotensin
      b. They project axons to nucleus raphe magnus and nucleus gigantocellularis.
      c. They contribute to serotoninergic input by way of dorsolateral funiculus to all dorsal horn laminae: most densely in laminae I, II, V, and IX.
   3. Medulla (primarily the rostroventral medulla)
      a. The medulla receives multiple inputs from the periaqueductal gray.
      b. It contains as many nuclei as the nucleus raphe magnus and nucleus magnocellularis.
      c. Most neurons from here release 5-HT and norepinephrine.
      d. Some neurons from here release enkephalin, substance P, and other peptides (substance P in the periphery activates nociceptors).
      e. The medulla may have some dynorphin-producing neurons.
      f. Some neurons may make 5-HT and enkephalin.
      g. The medulla is thought to have *on-cells* and *off-cells,* giving bidirectional control over nociceptive inputs.
         (1) Brain centers or pathways descend to the spinal cord and modulate pain.
         (2) Off-cells inhibit transmission of pain-related information to the brain.
         (3) On-cells facilitate transmission of pain-related signals to the brain.

4. Pons
   a. Neurons release primarily norepinephrine and 5-HT.
   b. Synapses are mostly in laminae I, II, IV, V, and X.
5. Descending modulation control
   a. Noradrenergic tract (norepinephrine tract) (Ruda, Bennett, & Dubner, 1986)
      (1) The locus coeruleus provides the main source of noradrenergic input to the periaqueductal gray.
      (2) The noradrenergic tract passes down the dorsolateral, ventrolateral, and ventral funiculi.
      (3) Termination occurs in all laminae but densely in laminae I, II, IV, V, VI, and X.
      (4) The noradrenergic tract seems to have crucial role in opiate-induced analgesia.
   b. Hypothalamospinal tract
      (1) The hypothalamospinal tract starts from hypothalamic nuclei, including the medial and paraventricular.
      (2) Major synapses are to laminae I and X.
      (3) Minor synapses are to laminae II, III, and V.
      (4) Primary chemistries of neurons include vasopressin and oxytocin.
      (5) Minor neuronal chemistry input includes enkephalin.
   c. Periaqueductal gray to spinal projections
      (1) Projections bypass nuclei in the medulla.
      (2) Chemistry is primarily 5-HT and noradrenergic.
      (3) Projections descend by way of the dorsolateral funiculus.
      (4) Main synapses are in laminae I, II, V, and X.
6. Dorsal horn cells
   a. Dorsal horn neurons may contain endogenous opiates and other substances (Xie, Woods, Traynor, & Ko, 2008).
      (1) Enkephalin-releasing cells (endogenous opiate or endorphin)
         (a) These cells are most densely found postsynaptically in laminae I, II, and V.
         (b) Some are also found postsynaptically in laminae VII and X.
      (2) Dynorphin-releasing cells (Iadarola, Brady, Draisci, & Dubner, 1988)
         (a) These cells are most dense in laminae I and V.
         (b) They may provide a presynaptic input to primary afferents.
         (c) Inflammation over time causes increased amounts of dynorphin in laminae I, II, V, and VI on the ipsilateral side.
      (3) Neurotensin-releasing cells (an endogenous peptide found to decrease pain when released into the periaqueductal gray)
         (a) Cell bodies dominate in laminae II and III.
         (b) Terminals are found in laminae I through III.
         (c) These cells may activate other inhibitory neurons.
      (4) GABA-releasing cells (a pain-inhibiting neurotransmitter)
         (a) These cells are mainly found in laminae I and II.
         (b) They provide presynaptic control of small primary afferents.
         (c) They may act as inhibitory interneurons to second-order nociceptors.
      (5) Substance P and other peptides
      (6) 5-HT
         (a) 5-HT comes from descending neurons in the dorsal horn.
         (b) It mainly has a postsynaptic effect on STT projection cells.
         (c) It causes inhibition of laminae I and V neurons.
         (d) It causes excitation of lamina VI neurons.
      (7) Norepinephrine cells
         (a) Norepinephrine cells are found primarily in laminae I, II, IV, V, VI, and X.
         (b) They act primarily on STT and trigeminothalamic tract neurons (Ruda et al., 1986).

(8) Specific opioid receptor types
   (a) μ_1 and μ_2 (μ = Mu)
   (b) δ_1 and δ_2 (δ = Delta)
   (c) κ_1, κ_2, and κ_3 (κ = Kappa)
   (d) σ-Receptors are present, but their role in nociception is unclear (σ = Sigma)
   (e) β-Endorphin (β = Beta)
   (f) Probable other receptors (not yet defined clearly)

b. Receptors are found on some central terminals of primary afferents.
   (1) About 33% of thalamic projection cells in lamina I have enkephalin input.
   (2) About 50% of thalamic projection cells in lamina V have enkephalin input.

c. There is some evidence for a postsynaptic local negative feedback loop activated by arriving afferent impulses.

d. Some dorsal horn interneurons contain endogenous opiates.

7. Endogenous endorphin release may be altered secondary to many factors.
   a. Factors that may increase endorphin release are as follows:
      (1) Pain
      (2) Acupuncture
      (3) Exercise
      (4) Sexual response
      (5) Short-term stress
   b. Factors that may decrease endorphin release are as follows:
      (1) Prolonged stress
      (2) Anxiety in acute and chronic pain
      (3) Depression in chronic pain
      (4) Suffering or severe distress caused by loss
      (5) Alcohol use in excess
      (6) Prolonged pain

F. Other factors affecting pain perception and processing (Fillingim, 2005)
   1. Age (Cole, Farrell, Gibson, & Egan, 2008; Gibson & Farrell, 2004)
   2. Gender (Gazerani, Andersen, & Arendt-Nielsen, 2005; Vallerand & Polomano, 2000)
   3. Genetics (Edwards, 2006; Russell, 2007; Zhang, 2006)
   4. Race, ethnicity, and culture (Cintron & Morrison, 2006; Zatzick & Dimsdale, 1990)

Note: Common wisdom held that a neuron released one type of neurotransmitter, which had a specific action and responded to one type of transmitter. It now seems that some neurons may respond to multiple transmitters, that they may create and release many transmitters, and that when released a neurotransmitter may have a role in multiple actions at the same time.

In Brief

Midbrain activation by nociceptive input causes fibers with descending projections to the dorsal horn of the spinal cord to modulate pain through descending pathway activation. This system often works to decrease the amount of pain and can explain why some individuals in the face of devastating and painful injuries may not feel pain. It is also explains the basis for why nonpharmacological approaches such as visual imagery, distraction, hypnosis, and relaxation reduce pain. 5-HT is released in the brain by specific neurons, particularly within the nucleus raphe magnus, and binds to the next neuron of the descending analgesic tract (which can be activated). It is then released back into the synaptic cleft, where the original 5-HT reuptake occurs. Neurons that play a role in the descending analgesic system in the medulla and pons release norepinephrine in the same manner. When the reuptake of norepinephrine and 5-HT is inhibited, the descending analgesic system is enhanced, resulting in improved inhibition of the transmission of nociceptive messages within the dorsal horn.

References

Aguggia, M. (2003). Neurophysiology of pain. *Neurological Sciences, 24* (Suppl. 2), S57–S60.

Alvarez, F. J., & Fyffe, R. E. (2000). Nociceptors for the 21st century. *Current Review of Pain, 4,* 451–458.

Basbaum, A. I. (1985). Functional analysis of the cytochemistry of the spinal dorsal horn. In H. L. Fields, R. Dubner, & F. Cevero (Eds.), *Advances in pain research and therapy* (pp. 149–175). New York: Raven Press.

Besse, D., Lombard, M. C., Zakac, J. M., Roques, B. P., & Besson, J. M. (1990). Pre- and postsynaptic distribution of μ, δ, and κ opioid receptors in the superficial layers of the cervical dorsal horn of the rat spinal cord. *Brain Research, 521,* 15–22.

Besson, J. M. (1999). The neurobiology of pain. *Lancet, 353,* 1610–1615.

Bleakman, D., Alt, A., & Nisenbaum, E. S. (2006). Glutamate receptors and pain. *Seminars in Cell Developmental Biology, 17,* 592–604.

Bonica, J. J. (1990). Anatomic and physiologic basis of nociception and pain. In J. Bonica (Ed.), *The management of pain* (2nd ed., pp. 28–94). Philadelphia: Lea & Febiger.

Burgess, P. R., & Perl, E. R. (1973). Cutaneous mechanoreceptors and nociceptors. In A. Iggo (Ed.), *Handbook of sensory physiology: Vol. 2. Somatosensory system* (pp. 29–78). Berlin: Springer-Verlag.

Carlton, S. M., Westlund, K. N., Zhang, D., Sorkin, L. S., & Willis, W. D. (1990). Calcitonin gene–related peptide containing primary afferent fibers synapse on primate spinothalamic tract cells. *Neuroscience Letters, 109,* 76–81.

Cho, H., Koo, J. Y., Kim, S., Park, S. P., Yang, Y., & Oh, U. (2006). A novel mechanosensitive channel identified in sensory neurons. *European Journal of Neuroscience, 23,* 2543–2550.

Cintron, A., & Morrison, R. S. (2006). Pain and ethnicity in the United States: A systematic review. *Journal of Palliative Medicine, 9,* 1454–1473.

Coggeshall, R. E., Chung, K., Chung, J. M., & Langford, L. A. (1981). Primary afferent axons in the tract of Lissauer in the monkey. *Journal of Comparative Neurology, 196,* 431–442.

Cole, L. J., Farrell, M. J., Gibson, S. J., & Egan, G. F. (2008). Age-related differences in pain sensitivity and regional brain activity evoked by noxious pressure. *Neurobiology of Aging,* in press.

Craig, A. D., Zhang, E. T., & Blomqvist, A. (2002). Association of spinothalamic lamina I neurons and their ascending axons with calbindin immunoreactivity in monkey and human. *Pain, 97,* 105–115.

Cui, M., Honore, P., Zhong, C., Gauvin, D., Mikusa, J., Hernandez, G., Chandran, P., Gomtsyan, A., Brown, B., Bayburt, E.K., Marsh, K., Bianchi, B., McDonald, H., Niforators, W., Neelands, T.R., Moreland, R.B., Decker, M.W., Lee, C.H., Sullivan, J.P., & Faltynek, C.R. (2006). TRPV1 receptors in the CNS play a key role in broad-spectrum analgesia of TRPV1 antagonists. *Journal of Neuroscience, 26,* 9385–9393Devor, M. (1994). The pathophysiology of damaged nerves. In P. D. Wall & R. Melzak (Eds.), *Textbook of pain* (3rd ed., pp. 79–100). New York: Churchill Livingstone.

Dostrovsky, J. O., & Craig, A. D. (2006). Ascending projection systems. In S. B. McMahon & Koltzenberg, M. (Eds.), *Textbook of pain* (5th ed., pp. 187–204). Philadelphia: Elsevier Churchill Livingstone.

Edwards, R. R. (2006). Genetic predictors of acute and chronic pain. *Current Rheumatology Reports, 8,* 411–417.

Fields, H. (1987). *Pain.* New York: McGraw-Hill.

Fillingim, R. B. (2005). Individual differences in pain responses. *Current Rheumatology Reports, 7,* 342–347.

Garry, M. G., & Hargreaves, K. M. (1992). Enhanced release of immunoreactive CGRP and substance P from spinal dorsal horn slices occurs during carrageenan inflammation. *Brain Research, 582,* 139–142.

Gazerani, P., Andersen, O. K., & Arendt-Nielsen, L. (2005). A human experimental capsaicin model for trigeminal sensitization: Gender-specific differences. *Pain, 118,* 155–163.

Gibson, S. J., & Farrell, M. (2004). A review of age differences in the neurophysiology of nociception and the perceptual experience of pain. *Clinical Journal of Pain, 20,* 227–239.

Hudson, A. J. (2000). Pain perception and response: Central nervous system mechanisms. *Canadian Journal of Neurological Science, 27,* 2–16.

Iadarola, M. J., Brady, L. S., Draisci, G., & Dubner, R. (1988). Enhancement of dynorphin gene expression in spinal cord following experimental inflammation: Stimulus specificity, behavioral parameters and opioid receptor binding. *Pain, 35,* 313–326.

Julius, D., & Basbaum, A. I. (2001). Molecular mechanisms of nociception. *Nature, 413,* 203–210.

Katz, W. A., & Rothenberg, R. (2005). Section 3: The nature of pain: pathophysiology. *Journal of Clinical Rheumatology, 11*(2 Suppl.), S11–S15.

Lai, J., Luo, M. C., Chen, Q., & Porreca, F. (2008). Pronociceptive actions of dynorphin via bradykinin receptors. *Neuroscience Letters, 437,* 175–179.

McCormack, K., Prather, P., & Chapleo, C. (1998). Some new insights into the effects of opioids in phasic and tonic nociceptive tests. *Pain, 78,* 79–98.

Meyer, R. A., & Campbell, J. N. (1981). Myelinated nociceptive afferents account for the hyperalgesia that follows a burn to the hand. *Science, 213,* 1527–1529.

Meyer, R. A., Campbell, J. N., & Raja, S. N. (1988). Antidromic nerve stimulation in monkey does not sensitize unmyelinated nociceptors to heat. *Brain Research, 441,* 168–172.

Meyer, R. A., Davis, K. D., Cohen, R. H., Treede, R. D., & Campbell, J. N. (1991). Mechanically insensitive afferents (MIAs) in cutaneous nerves of monkey. *Brain Research, 561,* 252–261.

Meyer, R. A., Ringkamp, M., Campbell, J. N., & Raja, S. N. (2006). Peripheral mechanisms of cutaneous nociception. In S. B. McMahon & M. Koltzenberg (Eds.), *Textbook of pain* (5th ed., pp. 11–57). Philadelphia: Elsevier Churchill Livingstone.

Nowak, T. J., & Handford, A. G. (1994). *Essentials of pathophysiology: Concepts and applications for health care professionals* (pp. 609–629). Dubuque, IA: Wm. C. Brown Publishers.

Ohara, P. T., Vit, J. P., & Jasmin, L. (2005). Cortical modulation of pain. *Cell and Molecular Life Science, 62,* 44–52.

Olausson, B. (1998). Recordings of polymodal single c-fiber nociceptive afferents following mechanical and argon-laser heat stimulation of human skin. *Experimental Brain Research, 122,* 44–54.

Otsuka, M., Konishi, S., Yanagisawa, M., Tsunoo, A., & Tagagi, H. (1982). Rose of substance P as a sensory transmitter in spinal cord and sympathetic ganglia. *Ciba Foundation Symposium, 91,* 13–34.

Roberts, L. A., & Connor, M. (2006). TRPV1 antagonists as a potential treatment for hyperalgesia. *Recent Patents in CNS Drug Discovery, 1,* 65–76.

Ruda, M. A., Bennett, G. J., & Dubner, R. (1986). Neurochemistry and neural circuitry in the dorsal horn. *Progress in Brain Research, 66,* 219–268.

Russell, M. B. (2007). Genetics in primary headaches. *Journal of Headache Pain, 8,* 190–195.

Siddall, P. J., & Cousins, M. J. (1998). Introduction to pain mechanisms: Implications for neural blockade. In M. J. Cousins & P. O. Bridenbaugh (Eds.), *Neural blockade in clinical anesthesia and management of pain* (3rd ed., pp. 675–699). Philadelphia: Lippincott-Raven.

Simone, D. A., & Kajander, K. C. (1997). Responses of cutaneous A-fiber nociceptors to noxious cold. *Journal of Neurophysiology, 77,* 2049–2060.

Treede, R. D., Jensen, T. S., Campbell, J. N., Cruccu, G., Dostrovsky, J. O., Griffin, J. W., Hansson, P., Hughes, R., Nurmikko, T., & Serra, J. (2008). Neuropathic pain: Redefinition and a grading system for clinical and research purposes. *Neurology, 70,* 1630–1635.

Vallerand, A. H., & Polomano, R. C. (2000). The relationship of gender to pain. *Pain Management Nursing, 1*(3 Suppl. 1), 8–15.

Westlund High, K. N. (2008). Pain pathways: Peripheral, spinal, ascending and descending pathways. In H. T. Benzon, J. P. Rathmell, C. L. Wu, D. C. Turk, & C. F. Argoff (Eds.), *Raj's practical management of pain* (4th ed., pp. 199–134). Philadelphia: Mosby Elsevier.

Woolf, C. J., & Slater, M. W. (2006). Plasticity and pain: Role of the dorsal horn. In S. B. McMahon & M. Koltzenberg (Eds.), *Textbook of pain* (5th ed., pp. 91–106). Philadelphia: Elsevier Churchill Livingstone.

Xie, H., Woods, J. H., Traynor, J. R., & Ko, M. C. (2008). The spinal antinociceptive effects of endomorphins in rats: Behavioral and G protein functional studies. *Anesthesia & Analgesia, 106,* 1873–1881.

Yaksh, T. L. (1993). New horizons in our understanding of the spinal physiology and pharmacology of pain processing. *Seminars in Oncology, 20*(Suppl. 1), 6–18.

Yaksh, T. L. (1997). Pharmacology and mechanisms of opioid analgesic activity. *Acta Anaesthesiologica Scandinavica, 41*(Suppl. 2), 94–111.

Yaksh, T. L. (2007). Dynamics of the pain processing system. In S. D. Waldman (Ed.), *Pain management* (Vol. 1, pp. 21–32). Philadelphia: Saunders, Elsevier.

Yaksh, T. L., & Luo, D. (2007). Anatomy of the pain processing system. In S. D. Waldman (Ed.), *Pain management* (Vol. 1, pp. 11–20). Philadelphia: Saunders, Elsevier.

Zatzick, D. F., & Dimsdale, J. E. (1990). Cultural variations in response to painful stimuli. *Psychosomatic Medicine, 52,* 544–557.

Zhang, X., & Bao, L. (2006). The development and modulation of nociceptive circuitry. *Current Opinion in Neurobiology, 16,* 460–466.

Zhou, H. Y., Zhang, H. M., Chen, S. R., & Pan, H. L. (2008). Increased C-fiber nociceptive input potentiates inhibitory glycinergic transmission in the spinal dorsal horn. *Pharmacology Experimental Therapeutics, 324,* 1000–1010.

Suggested Readings

Green, B. G. (2004). Temperature perception and nociception. *Journal of Neurobiology, 61,* 13–29.

Miaskowski, C. (2004). Recent advances in understanding pain mechanisms provide future directions for pain management. *Oncology Nursing Forum, 31*(4 Suppl.), 25–35.

Paice, J. A. (1991). Unraveling the mystery of pain. *Oncology Nursing Forum, 18,* 843–849.

Renn, C. L., & Dorsey, S. G. (2005). The physiology and processing of pain: A review. *AACN Clinical Issues, 16,* 277–290; quiz, 413–415.

Schnitzler, A., & Ploner, M. (2000). Neurophysiology and functional neuroanatomy of pain perception. *Journal of Clinical Neurophysiology, 17,* 592–603.

Part Two: Pathophysiology of Pain

Objectives

After studying this chapter, the reader should be able to:

1. Describe the changes in the peripheral and central nervous systems in response to injury and how mechanisms of pain transduction, transmission, modulation, and perception are affected.
2. Explain the mechanisms for central sensitization.
3. Discuss the mechanisms and manifestations of central pain syndromes.

IV. Pathophysiological Pain

A. Pathophysiological pain, in contrast to physiological sources of pain, results from a change in baseline somatosensory sensitivity (Devor, 1994).

1. This section addresses the pathophysiology of pain and the somatosensory sensitivity of the nociceptive system and disruptions in pain transduction and transmission that lead to alterations in peripheral and central processing and ***pathophysiological pain states*** (Devor, 1994).
   a. Pathophysiological pain can be caused by a specific disease (e.g., diabetes or cancer) or painful condition (e.g., low back pain, headache syndromes, postherpetic neuralgia, phantom limb pain, or fibromyalgia).
   b. When there is tissue or nerve damage in an area, there may be increased sensitivity around and extending beyond the site of injury.
      (1) This increased sensitivity, or hyperalgesia, may serve as an adaptive process to remind an individual to protect the injured area.
      (2) If it persists after healing has taken place, it can become chronic and associated with changes in the nervous system and how pain is perceived and processed.
2. Peripheral sensitization is defined as an increased sensitivity of nociceptors.
   a. After tissue injury and inflammatory response, nociceptor thresholds are lowered and pain hypersensitivity often occurs. The reduction in pain thresholds and an increase in the responsiveness of the peripheral terminals of high-threshold nociceptor neurons can lead to nociceptors firing with *increased frequency* to both nonnoxious and noxious stimuli.

b. COX also plays an important role in both peripheral and central sensitizations.
   (1) COX-2 is among the enzymes that are produced with inflammation.
   (2) COX-2 converts arachidonic acid to prostaglandins, which in turn increase the sensitivity of peripheral nociceptor terminals.
c. Nociceptors may fire in response to stimuli that *previously were insufficient* to elicit a response (Wang, Ehnert, Brenner, & Woolf, 2006). There is an enhanced transmission of nociceptive inputs to the brain associated with the loss of discriminatory processing of nonnoxious and noxious stimuli (Romanelli & Esposito, 2004).

3. Damaged peripheral nerve axons can produce *ectopic* nerve impulses or paroxysmal firing.
   a. Afferent neurons can transmit signals, but they produce impulses that are initiated from abnormal sites or processes (e.g., not originating from the transduction of a nociceptive stimulus acting on the nociceptor).
   b. Ectopic firing of nerve cells can occur when nerve fibers such as Aβ touch fibers that typically do not transmit pain; these fibers then become responsive to pain.
   c. This sensitization occurs when DRG cells also become hypersensitive to nerve pain impulses.
      (1) This is further complicated by windup in the dorsal horn cell bodies through sprouting of Aβ mechanical and touch fibers into the superficial areas of the dorsal horn.
      (2) Activation of glutamate-specific postsynaptic NMDA receptors, which are located in the dorsal horn, increases painful inputs.
      (3) Ectopic firing of injured nerves often observed with neuropathic pain syndromes can produce electric shock-like pain or stabbing pain.
4. The central processing circuits of the nervous system develop an increased gain, including the formation of spontaneous impulses. This is called *central sensitization.*
   a. Central sensitization refers to an increased sensibility of somatosensory neurons in the dorsal horn of the spinal cord to pain and occurs after intense peripheral noxious input from tissue injury or nerve damage (Ji, Kohno, Moore, & Woolf, 2003).
   b. The CNS becomes overresponsive to sensory input, and pain may be experienced in areas that are not generating painful stimuli.
      (1) This process occurs from repeated C fiber inputs from tissue or nerve damage that leads to the release of glutamate, an excitatory amino acid, in the dorsal horn, which acts on NMDA receptors to produce this sensitization.
   c. Pain prevention strategies and effective pain control are critical to preventing early mechanisms for central sensitization.
5. Windup, or physiological responses of spinal neurons, is increased with repeated stimulation of C fibers.
   a. Windup, like central sensitization and hyperalgesia, is induced by C fiber inputs and is attenuated by NMDA and neurokinin-1 (NK-1) receptor antagonists.
      (1) These inputs create many problems, including the sprouting of wide dynamic range neurons and induction of glutamate-dependent NMDA receptors.
      (2) Windup, however, is different from central sensitization; it can be short-lasting, whereas central sensitization and hyperalgesia persist over time.
   b. The synaptic processes that produce windup are capable of causing central sensitization, but the reverse is not true (Woolf, 1996).
6. Neuroplasticity normally refers to an intricate group of processes that allow neurons in the brain to compensate for injury and adjust their responses to new situations or changes in their environment (Katz & Rothenberg, 2005).
   a. Brain-derived neurotrophic factor (BDNF) is a well-known regulator of synaptic plasticity and is involved in descending pain pathway facilitation.
   b. Following peripheral nerve injury, there are dynamic changes that occur in the capabilities for descending pain pathways to modulate pain (Danziger, Weil-Fugazza, Le Bars, & Bouhassira, 2001).

(1) After tissue injury, BDNF and neurotrophic tyrosine kinase receptor (TrkB) signaling in the brain stem is rapidly activated (Ren & Dubner, 2007).

(2) Animal models demonstrate that with persistent pain transmission is facilitated. Functional, chemical, and structural plasticity of neurons can contribute to adaptive mechanisms in reducing pain and to maladaptive mechanisms in enhancing pain.

c. Genetic makeup and variability among individuals may play important roles in the synthesis and function of proteins affecting the plasticity of the CNS (Gjerstad, 2007). This may explain interpatient differences in pain responses and help readers understand the development of many persistent pain conditions.

7. Primary and secondary hyperalgesia

a. Primary hyperalgesia occurs at the site of tissue injury. Sensitized primary afferent nociceptors are partially responsible for increased response to stimuli such as heat.

b. Secondary hyperalgesia is experienced in the surrounding uninjured tissue areas and is thought to be more related to central sensitization rather than to peripheral sensitization.

(1) The presence of inflammatory mediators in the tissues may cause the recruitment of large and small fibers outside of the injured area to be sensitized.

(2) This is called secondary hyperalgesia, and it can extend 10 to 20 cm beyond the injured area. There is strong evidence that secondary hyperalgesia is most likely due to central sensitization (Guilbaud, Kayser, Attal, & Benoist, 1992).

(3) Secondary hyperalgesia is characterized by hyperalgesia to mechanical stimuli but not heat stimuli (Campbell & Meyer, 2006).

(a) This mechanical hyperalgesia is similar to hyperalgesia commonly noted in patients with neuropathic pain.

(b) Mechanical hyperalgesia can be in response to stimuli from light-stroking (i.e., allodynia) and can punctate stimuli (Campbell & Meyer, 2006).

8. Opioid-induced hyperalgesia (OIH): broadly defined, is a state of nociceptive sensitization caused by exposure to opioids (Chu, Angst, & Clark, 2008; DuPen, Shen, & Ersek, 2007; Mitra, 2008).

a. It is a state characterized by a paradoxical response in which patients actually become more sensitive to certain painful stimuli and have increased pain with exposure to opioid therapy.

b. Furthermore, opioid hyperalgesia can occur in the treatment of both acute and chronic pain.

(1) The exact mechanism for this phenomenon is not clearly understood, but it is believed to be related to neuroplastic changes in the peripheral nervous system and CNS that lead to sensitization of pronociceptive pathways (Chu et al., 2008).

(2) This may explain why opioids tend to lose their effectiveness in certain patients over time.

V. Peripheral Sensitization

A. Peripheral sensitization occurs with increased sensitivity of nociceptors and greater spontaneous activity of afferents, resulting in hyperalgesia and pain.

1. Injured tissues release several activating substances from mast cells, white blood cells, and damaged tissues.

a. These chemicals are often referred to as the "inflammatory soup," which contains substances such as bradykinin, 5-HT, and prostaglandin E_2 (Katz & Gold, 2006).

b. These pain inflammatory mediators can directly affect nociceptors or may sensitize them to touch (allodynia) or movement. This may even occur in areas distant from the inflammatory field.

c. Tissue injury promotes the likelihood of a peripheral stimulus activating a pain neuron, and the injury increases the receptive fields of the pain neurons.

2. Mechanisms for inflammatory pain are complex and have important implications for understanding symptoms that patients experience (Kidd & Urban, 2001).

B. Exposure of the nociceptor to chemicals derived from the process of inflammation can cause alterations in nociceptor activity.
   1. Chemicals derived from the inflammatory response can act to sensitize or activate nociceptors *in the area of injury*. Sites of action for neurochemicals involved in mediating pain vary; some have specific actions in the periphery, and others act on receptors in the dorsal horn.
      a. Sensitization of primary afferent nociceptors may occur directly through stimulation from heat, mechanical, or chemical stimulation; or indirectly through other inflammatory mediators.
      b. Nociceptors fire in response to stimuli of lesser strength than usual.
      c. Nociceptors may generate more frequent impulses than usual to suprathreshold stimuli.
      d. Nociceptors may fire from stimuli that do not typically cause pain (allodynia), such as light touch (Devor, 1991).
      e. Afterdischarge can occur following repeated or intense stimuli (e.g., the neuron continues to fire after the stimulus is removed).
      f. Nociceptor sensitization occurs within an area of about 5 to 10 mm of the injury site (Campbell, Meyer, & Raja, 1984).
      g. Ongoing pain without a clear explanation for hyperalgesia is common (Basbaum et al., 2006).
   2. *Silent nociceptors* can become responsive; they may discharge with normal movement and show changes in their receptive field size (Siddall & Cousins, 1998).
      a. Silent nociceptors do not respond to nociceptive stimuli until sensitization has occurred.
   3. Some neurochemicals derived from the inflammatory response may directly activate nociceptors even in the absence of any other stimuli.
   4. 5-HT acts differently in the peripheral nervous system and CNS.
      a. Peripherally, it has a hyperalgesic effect, participating with other neurochemicals to exert a pronociceptive effect.
      b. Centrally, its action in the CNS is antinociceptive by facilitating descending pathway pain modulation (Sommer, 2006).
   5. The second messenger system mediated by cyclic adenosine monophosphate (cAMP) has a major role in the development of primary afferent hyperalgesia (Levine & Taiwo, 1994).

C. Sensitization may occur as a result of chemical toxins (e.g., interleukin-1) released from bacteria.

D. Peripheral sensitization, if maladaptive, may represent failure of an inflammatory response feedback loop (Strausbaugh et al., 1999).

VI. Ectopic Nerve Impulses

A. Damaged or injured peripheral nerve axons may produce ectopic impulses through several mechanisms (Devor, 1994).

B. Mechanisms for ectopic firing of damaged nerves vary, as illustrated by individuals with the same type of pain exhibiting different symptoms to express the pain.
   1. Mechanisms contributing to ectopic discharge in nerves along the length of the peripheral afferent neuron distal to the cell body are as follows:
      a. Damaged nerves sprout and cause collateral sprouting of nearby undamaged intact neurons. Sprouts can cause neuromas, which are often the site of ectopic impulse generation and mechanosensitivity (e.g., seen in diabetic neuropathy and amputation).
         (1) Neuromas may be trapped in scar tissue, causing ongoing activations (often referred to as *neuromas in continuity*).
         (2) Neuromas may be extremely small and difficult to detect by palpation.
         (3) Neuromas typically form after limb amputations.
         (4) Neuromas form where nerve sheaths are breached.
         (5) Neuromas form on both myelinated and unmyelinated nerve fibers.

(a) The rate of spontaneous discharge from neuromas on myelinated neurons increases with warming and is suppressed by cooling.

(b) The rate of spontaneous discharge from neuromas on unmyelinated neurons increases with cooling and is suppressed by heat. (This may be the basis for cold intolerance often observed in amputees.)

(6) Neuromas may initiate impulses with mechanical stimulus or spontaneously.

b. When myelinated nerves are damaged, the myelin sheath retreats, exposing a longer length of neuronal membrane than originally present.

(1) This results in demyelinated areas along myelinated nerves.

(2) This can be caused by diabetes, chemotherapeutic or neurotoxic drugs, trauma, progressive neurological disease, and heavy metal toxicity.

(a) Demyelinated areas exhibit spontaneous impulse discharge.

(b) Demyelinated areas are hyperexcitable to mechanical stimuli.

(c) Demyelinated areas show ongoing rhythmical after discharge following stimulation.

c. Constricted nerves develop mechanosensitive hot spots.

d. Up-regulation of α-adrenergic receptors (increased numbers) may occur in a damaged neuron's membrane; few α-adrenergic receptors are found on the normal afferent nociceptive neuron, which may partially explain the mechanisms for complex regional pain syndrome.

(1) Adrenergic receptors may fire when exposed to norepinephrine from sympathetic nerve fiber activity or from circulating epinephrine.

(2) They may bring the threshold of the nociceptive afferent nerve closer to firing, enhancing hyperalgesia to thermal and mechanical stimuli.

e. An imbalance in Na^+ channels may be evident in the damaged neuron's membrane.

(1) The number of Na^+ channels per unit length along the neuronal membrane increases as neurons attempt to use the usual replacement channels that are unable to reach the distal areas of innervation.

(2) The number of channels per unit length along the neuronal membrane may increase as the neuron sends more than the usual replacement components in an effort to repair the damaged neuron.

(3) Passive influx of Na^+ through an increased number of channels may initiate impulses without a stimulus.

f. Up-regulation and increased numbers of stretch-activated receptors in the damaged neuron's membrane result in impulse generation with light pressure (e.g., allodynia in an amputation residual limb [stump] area).

g. Crossed afterdischarge may develop in which ongoing stimulation of an afferent causes a self-sustained discharge in an adjacent afferent that is not itself being directly stimulated. This is chemically mediated and may play a role in the development of lancinating pain, as in trigeminal neuralgia.

h. Ephaptic communication or cross-talk of C fibers in the injured zones can occur.

(1) This is an *electrical* transmission event whereby a transected neuron can short-circuit the insulation of a neighboring undamaged neuron.

(2) This results in inducing an electrical impulse on that other neuron, increasing the number of pain messages to the CNS.

i. Collateral neuronal sprouting may occur.

(1) Neurons sharing a common border with a damaged nerve may send sprouts into the damaged nerve's territory, perhaps secondary to nerve growth factor, and become exposed to chemicals of sensitization.

(2) Intact neurons within the area of damaged nerves may send sprouts into the damaged

nerve's area, also likely secondary to nerve growth factor, and become exposed to chemicals of sensitization.

j. Antidromic impulses (impulses in axon conduction opposite to the normal) occur when ectopic impulses are initiated midaxon or from the DRG.
    (1) For example, the impulse may run toward the periphery and toward the CNS.
    (2) These impulses may stimulate the release of neurochemicals in the periphery, such as substance P, causing local vasodilation that leads to warmth, redness, and edema, often called *neurogenic inflammation.*
    (3) This may play a role in the trophic changes seen in complex regional pain syndrome II (see the chapter on Persistent Pain Management).
k. A crushed nerve may cause less disruption than a cut nerve because sprouts from crushed nerves are more likely to come into contact with Schwann cells (myelin-producing cells) than are sprouts on a cut nerve. The Schwann cells provide a source of nerve growth factor that helps the damaged nerve to recover (Wall, 1991).

2. Ectopic mechanisms in DRG cell bodies can occur.
    a. These cells have inherent normal rhythmical discharges, but the magnitude of discharge can be enhanced in nerve damage states, causing sensitization.
    b. Mechanical pressure on the DRG (e.g., as from a herniated disk) may increase neuronal discharge.
    c. Sympathetic nerve activity can cause innervation of the DRG, activating primary afferent nociceptive neurons. This mechanism is due to noradrenergic sprouting in the DRG after peripheral nerve damage.
    d. DRG cells may develop ephaptic coupling after herpes zoster infection, which is possibly involved in mechanisms causing postherpetic neuralgia (Devor, 1991).
    e. DRG cells developing crossed afterdischarge play a role in hyperalgesia after nerve injury and can spread abnormal messaging across a dermatome.

Note: Ongoing peripheral ectopic input can maintain central sensitization.

VII. Central Sensitization

A. Central sensitization plays a crucial role in the pathogenesis of chronic pain (Dubner, 1997; Woolf, 2007). Central sensitization is a complex condition that is defined by an increase in the excitability of neurons within the CNS so that normal sensory inputs cause abnormal sensing and responses to painful and other stimuli.
    1. The central processing circuits of the nervous system are disrupted, including the development of spontaneous impulses.
    2. Some aspects of central sensitization can persist after peripheral inputs cease; however, peripheral and central neural mechanisms are involved in causing central sensitization, and it can be a long-lasting problem.

B. There are distinctions for the initial sensitization versus ongoing central sensitization in which the initial central sensitization is the result of an afferent barrage that can be short lived and ongoing central sensitization is sustained by peripheral inputs caused by severe tissue injury (Coderre & Katz, 1997).
    1. There are new insights to the mechanisms of central sensitization and how it is responsible for *secondary hyperalgesia* (the extension of tenderness or increase pain sensitivity outside of an area of injury) and *tactile allodynia* (pain in response to light touch).
    2. Central sensitization is an important factor for both inflammatory and neuropathic pain (Woolf, 2007).
    3. Central pain can be caused by mechanisms that are independent of peripheral inputs.

C. The process by which acute, unrelieved pain leads to central sensitization, and subsequently chronic pain syndromes, is outlined by Carr and Goudas (1999).

1. Acute tissue injury produces a cascade of events that involve the release of neurotransmitters; electrophysiological, intracellular stress; and structural and neuropsychological responses.
2. Even brief intervals of acute pain are capable of inducing long-term neuronal remodeling and sensitization ("plasticity"), chronic pain, and lasting psychological distress (Carr & Goudas, 1999).

D. Dorsal horn mechanisms play a role in central sensitization (these mechanisms are strongly linked to ongoing peripheral input).

1. Sprouting of nerve endings into adjacent laminae after peripheral nerve damage results in activation of central pain pathways by neurons communicating nonnociceptive information as light touch (e.g., sprouting of Aβ fibers from lamina III into laminae I and II has been observed) (Woolf, Shortland, & Coggeshall, 1992).
2. Unmasked latent synapses within the dorsal horn that can be active only in a state of sensitization result in activation of central pain pathways by neurons communicating nonnociceptive information as light touch or in recruitment of additional second-order nociceptive neurons, increasing the number of pain signals going to the brain.
3. Chemical sensitization occurs when nitric oxide and COX-2, which are released from second-order neurons after intense stimulation, diffuse into primary afferents and cause increased release of glutamate.
   a. Glutamate excites NMDA receptors and further activates second-order neurons. This positive feedback loop contributes to pain sensitization.
   b. Glutamate also plays a major role in central sensitization, which produces hyperexcitability (reduction in the threshold for action potential firing) (DeLeo, 2006).
4. Dorsal horn neurons whose receptive fields are adjacent to injury sites may expand their receptive fields following tissue damage so that they react to stimuli elicited within the damaged area itself (McMahon & Wall, 1984).
5. Wide dynamic range neurons, which usually discriminate between nociceptive and nonnociceptive stimuli, when sensitized, may signal pain with light tactile stimuli *(allodynia)* (Siddall & Cousins, 1998).
6. Prolonged activation of the non-NMDA receptors (i.e., AMPA and neurokinin receptors) on second-order neurons prime NMDA receptors into a state of activation.
7. Sustained activation of NMDA receptors leads to changes in the CNS, playing an important role in chronic pain states.
   a. ***Windup*** is the progressive increase in the magnitude of response to C fiber activity by dorsal horn neurons to repetitive activation of these fibers.
   b. ***Central sensitization*** occurs where nociceptive neurons in the dorsal horns of the spinal cord become sensitized by peripheral tissue damage or inflammation, leading to an increased sensibility of the dorsal horn to stimuli.
   c. ***Long-term potentiation*** is a concept that a cellular ***memory*** for pain may lead to future increased responses to nociceptive stimuli.
   d. ***Facilitation*** is the development of a state in which, because of the repeated stimulation of a neuron, the impulse threshold is reduced and intensity of the response is increased.
   e. Receptive field alterations in the periphery are orchestrated from the dorsal horn.
   f. Oncogene induction can cause long-term changes in a cell's responsiveness to stimuli.
8. Hyperalgesia (an exaggerated response to painful stimuli that are typically painful) may be evident in different ways, probably depending on the source of the peripheral input. Patients with neuropathic pain generally experience cutaneous hypersensitivity, increased pain from thermal or mechanical stimuli.
9. Other cutaneous manifestations associated with neuropathic pain may include painful numbness, redness, swelling, or warmth in the injured area.
   a. Some may have sensitivity to heat and find relief with cold, while others may seek comfort with the warmth and experience pain from exposure to cold.
   b. Some improve with Aβ fiber blocks, some with C fiber blocks, and others with sympathetic nerve blocks (Schwartzman, Grothusen, Kiefer, & Rohr, 2001).

E. Changes may occur in the spinal cord, resulting in central pain. (Some of these changes may be independent of peripheral inputs.)
   1. If contralateral ascending spinal pathways for pain (i.e., spinothalamic, spinoreticular, and spinomesencephalic) are surgically or chemically severed in an effort to treat pain, this may result in pain messages being carried by a latent ipsilateral (same side) pathway that eventually takes over.
      a. This explains why immediate pain relief may occur for some time after such a procedure before pain returns (Noordenbos & Wall, 1981).
      b. This includes the results of neuroablative procedures such as neurectomy, cordotomy, and rhizotomy (Loeser, 2006; Overton, Kornbluth, Saulino, Holding, & Freedman, 2008).
   2. Trauma to the spinal cord at any level for any cause (ischemic, transection, neoplastic, hemorrhagic, compression, radiation, or surgery) on or near the cord can cause damage to any part of the spinothalamic, spinoreticulothalamic, or spinomesencephalic pathways. Epidemiology and taxonomy for pain associated with spinal cord injuries are outlined in the report on the International Spinal Cord Injury Pain Basic Data Set (Widerström-Noga et al., 2008).
   3. Disease processes may injure the cord directly, such as with myelitis or multiple sclerosis.
F. Changes may occur in supraspinal CNS neurons. (Some of these changes may be independent of peripheral inputs.)
   1. Possible direct causes of changes to supraspinal CNS neurons that may lead to central pain are as follows:
      a. Strokes or other ischemic injury to the thalamus or other areas of the brain
      b. Surgical or traumatic lesions
      c. Malignancy invasion
      d. Radiation damage
   2. The role of supraspinal structures may change with central sensitization or CNS injury.
      a. Thalamus (Siddall & Cousins, 1998)
         (1) With acute pain, a positron emission tomography (PET scan) shows increased thalamic activity, but with chronic or cancer pain, decreased thalamic activity is shown.
         (2) Regional blood flow changes with neuropathic pain.
         (3) The patient develops spontaneous neuronal hyperactivity.
         (4) Somatotopic organization is altered.
      b. Cortex (Flor et al., 1995; Jensen, 1996)
         (1) Neuronal sprouting occurs.
         (2) Intracortical connections are unmasked.
         (3) Gene expression changes after peripheral nerve injury (Devor, 1994).
         (4) Regional blood flow increases.
      c. The cingulate cortex shows activation and increased regional blood flow.
      d. The right gyrus cinguli is activated in some neuropathic pain states.

Summary

Mounting evidence supports a biological, genetic, and environmental basis to explain individual variations in inflammation and neuropathic pain responses (Buffington, 2001; Limer, Nicholl, Thomson, & McBeth, 2008; Max & Stewart, 2008). While assessing pain, listening to what the patient is telling you can give you clues into the etiology of pain. We can take note of the words of Bowsher (1991) who wrote about what he believed to be the lowest common denominator of all symptoms for central pain: It is burning in nature, often with a paradoxical burning pain caused by a cold stimulus, and is made worse by light touch or the rubbing of clothing. We are learning about the neuromechanisms that cause painful conditions, and increasing our understanding of variations that previously we referred to as "pain of unknown etiology" help elevate our clinical practice. Evidence is accumulating that nutritional factors may play a role in pain; for example, soy may suppress neuropathic hypersensitivity (Shir, Sheth, Campbell, Raja, & Seltzer, 2001; Valsecchi et al., 2008). We can look forward to increasing our options for pain relief as neuroscience continue to explore the territories of pain mechanisms and pain perception.

Helpful Distinctions

Referred pain seems to have components of central sensitization, such as the expansion of receptive fields after inflammatory injuries in areas such as the colon, joints, bladder, and esophagus. This is possible because a large percentage of spinal neurons (possibly 90%) receive convergent input from visceral and somatic afferents.

Sympathetic mediated pain occurs when sympathetic afferents play a role in the peripheral inputs that maintain pain.

Sympathetic independent pain describes a pain syndrome in which sympathetic afferents do not play a significant role in the maintenance of pain but pain apparently is supported by other peripheral inputs, such as collateral sprouting in the dorsal horn and ephaptic connections.

Phantom limb pain is mediated by nerves that are severed by the removal of a body part but continue to generate sensory input to the CNS. There are some central features to phantom limb pain as well, which would explain pain *memories* that are felt in the phantom body part that existed before amputation or avulsion of the actual body part (Flor, 2008). This syndrome can develop and be expressed when nonlimb areas of the body, in which pain was felt, are removed by surgery or avulsion, including teeth, breasts, stomach areas removed because of ulcers, special sense organs, the uterus (may feel labor pains or cramps), the rectum, the bladder, and the cornea (Coderre & Katz, 1997). Amputees can be pain-free for years and then suddenly have their old pain return after a peripheral stimulus to the stump site, which implies the presence of quiescent central sensitized neuronal pathways for pain (Noordenbos & Wall, 1981).

References

Basbaum, A. I., Bushnell, M. C., Campbell, J. N., Chaplan, S.R., Mantyh, P.W., Porreca, F., Price, D.D., Urban, L., Vierck, C.J., & Zubieta, J.K. (2006). Measurement and new technologies: Rapporteur report. In J. N. Campbell, A. I. Basbaum, A. Dray, R. Dubner, R. H. Dworkin, & C. N. Sang (Eds.), *Emerging strategies for the treatment of neuropathic pain* (pp. 361–381). Seattle: IASP Press.

Bowsher, D. (1991). Neurogenic pain syndromes and their management. *British Medical Bulletin, 47,* 644–666.

Buffington, C. A. (2001). Visceral pain in humans: Lessons from animals. *Current Pain and Headache Report, 5*(1), 44–51.

Campbell, J. N., & Meyer, R. A. (2006). Mechanisms of neuropathic pain. *Neuron. 52,* 77–92.

Campbell, J. N., Meyer, R. A., & Raja, S. N. (1984). Hyperalgesia: New insights. *Pain, 2*(Suppl.), S3.

Carr, D. B., & Goudas, L. C. (1999). Acute pain. *Lancet, 353,* 2051–2058.

Chu, L. F., Angst, M. S., & Clark, D. (2008). Opioid-induced hyperalgesia in humans: Molecular mechanisms and clinical considerations. *Clinical Journal of Pain, 24,* 479–496.

Coderre, T. J., & Katz, J. (1997). Peripheral and central hyperexcitability: Differential signs and symptoms in persistent pain. *Behavior and Brain Sciences, 20,* 404–419.

Danziger, N., Weil-Fugazza, J., Le Bars, D., & Bouhassira, D. (2001). Stage-dependent changes in the modulation of spinal nociceptive neuronal activity during the course of inflammation. *European Journal of Neuroscience, 13,* 230–240.

DeLeo, J. A. (2006). Basic science of pain. *Journal of Bone and Joint Surgery, 88*(Suppl. 2), 58–62.

Devor, M. (1991). Neuropathic pain and injured nerve: Peripheral mechanisms. *British Medical Bulletin, 47,* 619–630.

Devor, M. (1994). The pathophysiology of damaged nerves. In P. D. Wall & R. Melzak (Eds.), *Textbook of pain* (3rd ed., pp. 79–100). New York: Churchill Livingstone.

Dubner, R. (1997). Neural basis of persistent pain: Sensory specialization, sensory modulation, and neuronal plasticity. In T. S. Jensen, J. A. Turner, & Z. Wiesenfeld-Hallin, (Eds.), *Proceedings of the 8th World Congress on Pain, Progress in Pain Research and Management* (pp. 243–257). Seattle: IASP Press.

DuPen, A., Shen, D., & Ersek, M. (2007). Mechanisms of opioid-induced tolerance and hyperalgesia. *Pain Management Nursing, 8,* 113–121.

Flor, H. (2008). Maladaptive plasticity, memory for pain and phantom limb pain: Review and suggestions for new therapies. *Expert Review of Neurotherapeutics, 8,* 809–818.

Flor, H., Elbert, T., Knecht, S., Wienbruch, C., Pantev, C., Birbaumer, N., Larbig, W., & Taub, E. (1995). Phantom-limb pain as a perceptual correlate of cortical reorganization following arm amputation. *Nature, 375,* 482–484.

Gjerstad, J. (2007). Genetic susceptibility and development of chronic non-malignant back pain. *Reviews in Neuroscience, 18,* 83–91.

Guilbaud, G., Kayser, V., Attal, N., & Benoist, J. M. (1992). Evidence for a central contribution to secondary hyperalgesia. In W. D. Willis (Ed.), *Hyperalgesia and allodynia* (pp. 187–201). New York: Raven Press.

Jensen, T. S. (1996). Mechanisms of neuropathic pain. In J. N. Campbell (Ed.), *Pain 1996: An updated review* (pp. 77–86). Seattle: IASP Press.

Ji, R. R., Kohno, T., Moore, K. A., & Woolf, C. J. (2003). Central sensitization and LTP: Do pain and memory share similar mechanisms? *Trends in Neuroscience, 26,* 696–705.

Katz, E. J., & Gold, M. S. (2006). Inflammatory hyperalgesia: A role for the C-fiber sensory neuron cell body? *Journal of Pain, 7,* 170–178.

Katz, W. A., & Rothenberg, R. (2005). Section 3: The nature of pain: pathophysiology. *Journal of Clinical Rheumatology, 11*(2 Suppl.), S11–S15.

Kidd, B. L., & Urban, L. A. (2001). Mechanisms of inflammatory pain. *British Journal of Anaesthesia, 87,* 3–11.

Levine, J., & Taiwo, Y. (1994). Inflammatory pain. In P. D. Wall & R. Melzak (Eds.), *Textbook of pain* (3rd ed., pp. 45–56). New York: Churchill Livingstone.

Limer, K. L., Nicholl, B. I., Thomson, W., & McBeth, J. (2008). Exploring the genetic susceptibility of chronic widespread pain: The tender points in genetic association studies. *Rheumatology (Oxford), 47,* 572–577.

Loeser, J. D. (2006). Other surgical interventions. *Pain Practice, 6,* 58–62.

Max, M. B., & Stewart, W. F. (2008). The molecular epidemiology of pain: A new discipline for drug discovery. *Nature Review and Drug Discovery, 7,* 647–658.

McMahon, S. B., & Wall, P. D. (1984). Receptive fields of rat lamina I projection cells move to incorporate a nearby region of injury. *Pain, 19,* 235–247.

Mitra, S. (2008). Opioid-induced hyperalgesia: Pathophysiology and clinical implications. *Journal of Opioid Management, 4,* 123–130.

Noordenbos, W., & Wall, P. D. (1981). Implications of the failure of nerve resection and graft to cure chronic pain produced by nerve lesions. *Journal of Neurology, Neurosurgery and Psychiatry, 44,* 1068–1073.

Overton, E. A., Kornbluth, I. D., Saulino, M. F., Holding, M. Y., & Freedman, M. K. (2008). Interventions in chronic pain management. Interventional approaches to chronic pain management. *Archives of Physical Medicine Rehabilitation, 89*(3 Suppl. 1), S61–S64.

Ren, K., & Dubner, R. (2007). Pain facilitation and activity-dependent plasticity in pain modulatory circuitry: Role of BDNF–TrkB signaling and NMDA receptors. *Molecular Neurobiology, 35,* 224–235.

Romanelli, P., & Esposito, V. (2004). The functional anatomy of neuropathic pain. *Neurosurgery Clinics of North America, 15,* 257–268.

Schwartzman, R. J., Grothusen, J., Kiefer, T. R., & Rohr, P. (2001). Neuropathic central pain: Epidemiology, etiology, and treatment options. *Archives of Neurology, 58,* 1547–1550.

Shir, Y., Sheth, R., Campbell, J. N., Raja, S. N., & Seltzer, Z. (2001). Soy-containing diet suppresses chronic neuropathic sensory disorders in rats. *Anesthesia and Analgesia, 92,* 1029–1034.

Siddall, P. J., & Cousins, M. J. (1998). Introduction to pain mechanisms: Implications for neural blockade. In M. J. Cousins & P. O. Bridenbaugh (Eds.), *Neural blockade in clinical anesthesia and management of pain* (3rd ed., pp. 675–699). Philadelphia: Lippincott-Raven.

Sommer, C. (2006). Is serotonin hyperalgesic or analgesic? *Current Pain and Headache Reports, 10,* 101–106.

Strausbaugh, H. J., Green, P. G., Lo, E., Tangemann, K., Reichling, D. B., Rosen, S. D., & Levine, J. D. (1999). Painful stimulation suppresses joint inflammation by inducing shedding of L-selectin from neutrophils. *Nature Medicine, 5,* 1057–1061.

Valsecchi, A. E., Franchi, S., Panerai, A. E., Sacerdote, P., Trovato, A. E., & Colleoni, M. (2008). Genistein, a natural phytoestrogen from soy, relieves neuropathic pain following chronic constriction sciatic nerve injury in mice: Anti-inflammatory and antioxidant activity. *Journal of Neurochemistry, 107,* 230–240.

Wall, P. D. (1991). Neuropathic pain and injured nerve: Central mechanisms. *British Medical Bulletin, 47,* 631–643.

Wang, H., Ehnert, C., Brenner, G. J., & Woolf, C. J. (2006). Bradykinin and peripheral sensitization. *Biological Chemistry, 387,* 11–14.

Widerström-Noga, E., Biering-Sørensen, F., Bryce, T., Cardenas, D. D., Finnerup, N. B., Jensen, M. P., Richards, J. S., & Siddall, P. J. (2008). The International Spinal Cord Injury Pain Basic Data Set. *Spinal Cord,* Dec, 46,12, 818–823

Woolf, C. J. (1996). Windup and central sensitization are not equivalent. *Pain, 66*(2–3), 105–108.

Woolf, C. J. (2007). Central sensitization: Uncovering the relation between pain and plasticity. *Anesthesiology, 106*(4), 864–867.

Woolf, C. J., Shortland, P., & Coggeshall, R. E. (1992). Peripheral nerve injury triggers central sprouting of myelinated afferents. *Nature, 355,* 75–77.

Suggested Readings

Gregg, J. M. (1990). Studies of traumatic neuralgias in maxillofacial region: Surgical pathology and neural mechanisms. *Journal of Oral Maxillofacial Surgery, 48,* 228–237.

McMahon, S. B., Bennett, D. L., & Bevan, S. (2006). Inflammatory medicators and modulators of pain. In S. B. McMahon & M. Koltzenberg (Eds.), *Textbook of pain* (5th ed., pp. 49–72). New York: Elsevier Churchill Livingstone.

Melzack, R., Coderre, T. J., Katz, J., & Vaccarino, A. L. (2001). Central neuroplasticity and pathological pain. *American New York Academy of Science, 933,* 157–174.

Treede, R. D., Jensen, T. S., Campbell, J. N., Cruccu, G., Dostrovsky, J. O., Griffin, J. W., Hansson, P., Hughes, R., Nurmikko, T., & Serra, J. (2008). Neuropathic pain: Redefinition and a grading system for clinical and research purposes. *Neurology, 70,* 1630–1635.

chapter

6

Research Utilization in Pain Management Nursing

Patricia Bruckenthal, PhD, RN, ANP-C

Objectives

After studying this chapter, the reader should be able to:

1. Describe the importance of research to the practice of pain management nursing.
2. Evaluate research findings to facilitate clinical decision making in pain management.
3. Apply strategies to promote a culture of evidence-based practice in pain management in the work settings.

Nurses involved in pain management are continually challenged to provide the best care to patients. Research focused on pain management can provide guidance for clinically sound decision making regarding many aspects of care, including pain assessment and successful intervention. Nurses must have a basic understanding of the research process to generate or use research findings to improve patient outcomes. While some nurses are involved in the discovery of new scientific findings, others must evaluate the data and apply relevant findings to practice. Nurses play an important role in the advancement of knowledge and providing best practices in pain management.

I. **Understanding Research Utilization**
   A. Historical perspectives
      1. Evidence-based practice (EBP)
         a. *Evidence-based practice* is the use of current best evidence in making decisions about patient care that incorporates a systematic approach for and critical appraisal of the most relevant evidence to answer a clinical question, the nurse's clinical experience, and the patient's preferences and values (Sackett, Straus, Richardson, Rosenberg, & Hayes, 2000).
      2. EBP to provide empirical support
         a. In 1972, Archie Cochrane challenged payment for health care unless supported by empirical evidence.
         b. He proposed that randomized, controlled trials (RCTs) provided strongest evidence on which to base proactive care.
         c. In 1992, the Cochrane Center launched in Oxford, England.
         d. In 1994, the Cochrane Collaboration was founded to develop, maintain, and update systematic reviews of clinical trials and make these accessible to the public (Melnyk & Fineout-Overholt, 2005).
      3. Research utilization
         a. *Research utilization* is the use of research findings in practice to improve care.
            (1) *Conceptual utilization* is the use of findings to enhance understanding of a problem or issue in nursing.
            (2) *Instrumental utilization* is the direct application of knowledge gained to change practice, which includes adoption of nursing intervention, new procedures, clinical protocols, and guidelines, and to support appropriateness of current practice.
      4. Research utilization models (examples) (Beyea & Nicoll, 1997)
         a. Western Interstate Commission for Higher Education (mid-1970s)
         b. Conduct and Utilization of Research in Nursing (1975)
         c. Nursing Child Assessment Satellite Training (1976)
         d. Stetler-Marram Model (1976, revised 1994 and 2001)
         e. Dracup-Breu Model (1977)
         f. Iowa Model (1994)
      5. Knowledge related to research utilization
         a. Basic research concepts
         b. Tables of evidence
         c. Criteria to determine usability of a credible research study
         d. Inferential statistics
         e. Substantive area under consideration
      6. Steps in EBP (Dicenso, Cullum, Ciliska, & Guyatt, 2004)
         a. Identify a problem or clinical question.
         b. Systematically search appropriate research.
         c. Critically review and appraise the quality and applicability of findings.
         d. Implement a plan to incorporate findings into practice.
         e. Implement the practice change.
         f. Evaluate the outcomes of research-based practice.

II. Impact of Research Utilization on Pain Management Nursing

A. Contributions to practice
   1. Research utilization builds professionalism that defines parameters of practice.
   2. It provides accountability to patients, health care agencies, and third-party payers.
   3. It demonstrates the efficacy of nursing in the changing health care arena.
   4. Research utilization promotes critical thinking and reflective practice.
   5. It expands knowledge related to pain management nursing.
   6. It validates the efforts of researchers.
   7. It improves patient outcomes.

B. Guideline development (examples)
   1. The use of "as needed" range orders for opioid analgesics (Gordon et al., 2004)
   2. *Principles of Analgesic Use in the Treatment of Acute Pain and Cancer Pain* (American Pain Society [APS], 2003)
   3. *Pain Management in the Long-Term Care Setting: Clinical Practice Guidelines* (American Medical Directors Association, 2003)
   4. "The management of persistent pain in older persons" (American Geriatrics Society, 2002)
   5. "An interdisciplinary expert consensus statement on assessment of pain in older persons" (Hadjistavropoulos et al., 2007)
   6. *Evidence-Based Practice Guideline: Acute Pain Management in Older Adults* (Herr, Bjoro, Steffensmeier, & Rakel, 2006)
   7. *Guideline for the Management of Pain in Osteoarthritis, Rheumatoid Arthritis, and Juvenile Chronic Arthritis,* Clinical Practice Guideline No. 2 (APS, 2002)
   8. "Diagnosis and treatment of low back pain: A joint clinical practice guideline from the American College of Physicians and the American Pain Society" (American College of Physicians & American Pain Society, 2007)
   9. *Guideline for the Management of Fibromyalgia Syndrome Pain in Adults and Children* (APS, 2005)

III. Evaluating Research for Clinical Decision Making

A. *Evaluation* is careful, critical appraisal of the strengths and limitations of a piece of research.

B. Purposes
   1. Evaluation should advance an area of knowledge by informing the researchers of ways to improve the study.
   2. It facilitates decision making about how or if the findings should be incorporated into nurses' practice.

C. Elements of a research critique for a quantitative study (Gillis & Jackson, 2002) (for a quantitative research definition, see IV. Generating Evidence: The Research Process).
   1. *Substantive and theoretical dimensions* determine whether the study was important in terms of the significance of the problem studied, the soundness of the conceptualizations, and the creativity and appropriateness of the theoretical framework.
      a. Critique problem statements and the hypothesis.
         (1) The purpose and problem statement are clearly articulated.
         (2) The potential contribution to nursing is stated.
         (3) Research questions or hypotheses are clearly stated.
         (4) Concepts and variables clearly are defined.
      b. Critique research literature reviews.
         (1) Classic and current literature is synthesized relevant to the research question.
         (2) Gaps in knowledge are identified.
         (3) The rational for how the current study will extend previous research is provided.
      c. Critique theoretical and conceptual frameworks.
         (1) The framework provides a rationale for the study.

2. *Methodological dimensions* analyze how the researcher chose to address the research question or test the research hypotheses.
   a. Critique the research design.
      (1) The study design is specified.
      (2) Evidence of a pilot study conducted.
      (3) The design is appropriate to the research purpose and question.
      (4) Design control of the extraneous variable is explicated.
   b. Critique the sampling plan.
      (1) The type of sampling is described.
      (2) The population to whom results will be generalized is described.
      (3) The demographic characteristics of the sample are described.
      (4) The inclusion and exclusion criteria are described.
      (5) The sample size is appropriate to meet assumptions of statistical tests (e.g., power analysis).
   c. Critique the methods and measurement issues.
      (1) The methods are appropriate to meet the study purpose and to answer questions.
      (2) Evidence of reliable and valid data collection procedures is given.
      (3) Data collection instruments are described in sufficient detail.
   d. Critique the data collection procedures.
      (1) Techniques to ensure consistency in data collection are described.
      (2) The procedure to keep conditions same for all participants is described.
      (3) Strategies to limit errors in data collection, recording, and analysis are described.
   e. Critique the quantitative data analyses.
      (1) Data analysis procedures are described.
      (2) Statistical techniques are appropriate for the study methodology.
      (3) Statistical tests answer the research questions.
3. *Interpretative dimensions* allow the researcher to review the findings, seek to understand what they mean in relation to the research hypothesis and the theoretical framework, and discuss the implications of the findings for the nursing profession.
   a. Critique the interpretation of the findings.
      (1) Findings are presented clearly and correctly.
      (2) A statement identifies whether or not findings support the hypothesis or answer the research question.
      (3) Tables and graphs are clearly labeled and congruent with results described in the text.
      (4) Findings are unbiased.
   b. Critique the nursing implications.
      (1) Important implications to practice, education, or research are identified.
      (2) The relationship to advancement of nursing knowledge is described.
      (3) Newly emerging research questions are identified.
   c. Critique the conclusions.
      (1) Clinical and statistical findings are discussed.
      (2) Alternative explanations are offered.
      (3) Major strengths and limitations are identified.
      (4) The major contribution to nursing knowledge development is described.
4. *Ethical dimensions* address the ethical aspects of conducting the study.
   a. Critique that the human subjects rights have been adhered to.
   b. All people involved with conduct of the study have gone through human subjects training. As an example, see http://hhs.gov/ohrp/humansubjects/guidance/belmont.htm.
5. *Presentational and stylistic dimensions* address the presentation of a research report.
   a. Critique that all research components are addressed and in sufficient detail.
   b. Critique the grammar and writing style.

D. Additional elements of a research critique for a qualitative study (Lincoln & Guba, 1985)

1. Qualitative research is an approach to understanding the phenomenon of interest that limits the disruption of the natural context of the phenomena, is committed to the participants' viewpoint, acknowledges the participation of the researcher, and is committed to the belief in multiple realities.
   a. Trustworthiness
      (1) *Credibility* methods have the goal of increasing the possibility that the research will produce credible results. The researcher can look at the use of various data sources or can verify the interpretation of the data with participants during and at the completion of the study.
      (2) *Transferability* is the ability of others to use the results or the ability of the results to be transferred to another context because there is a thorough description of the phenomena.
      (3) *Confirmation* assures the reader that the findings, conclusions, and recommendations are supported by the data.
      (4) *Dependability* enables someone else to follow logically the process and procedures that the researcher used in the study. Dependability is confirmed by having two researchers examine the process and the product of the research independently.

E. Hierarchy of evidence (Table 6-1)
   1. Evaluating the "strength of evidence" provides a mechanism to guide clinicians in evaluating research for health care decision making.
   2. Grading the strength of a body of evidence incorporates three domains.
      a. *Quality:* The extent to which a study's design, conduct, and analysis has minimized selection, measurement, and confounding biases
      b. *Quantity:* The number of studies that have evaluated the question, sample size across studies, and magnitude of treatment effects
      c. *Consistency:* Whether investigators with both similar and dissimilar study designs report similar findings (Agency for Healthcare Research and Quality, 2002)

F. Searchable databases (examples)
   1. Cumulative Index of Nursing and Allied Health Literature (CINAHL), http://www.cinahl.com
   2. Cochrane Database of Systematic Reviews, http://www.cochrane.org
   3. EMBASE, http://www.embase.com
   4. Medline, http://www.ncbi.nlm.gov
   5. PsycINFO, http://www.apa.org/psychinfo

Table 6-1 Hierarchy of Evidence

Level 1	Evidence from a systematic review or meta-analysis of all relevant Random Clinical Trials (RCTs) or evidence-based clinical practice guidelines based on systematic reviews of RCTs
Level 2	Evidence obtained from at least one well-designed RCT
Level 3	Evidence obtained from well-designed controlled trials without randomization
Level 4	Evidence from well-designed case-control and cohort studies
Level 5	Evidence from systematic reviews of descriptive and qualitative studies
Level 6	Evidence from a single descriptive or qualitative study
Level 7	Evidence from the opinion of authorities, reports of expert committees, or both

From Geyett, G., & Rennie, D. (2002). *Users' guide to the medical literature.* Chicago, IL: American Medical Association Press.
Harris, R. P., Helfand, M., Woolf, S. H., Lohr, K.N., Mulrow, C.D., Teutsch, S.M., & Atkins, D.. (2001). Current methods of the U.S. Preventative Health Task Force: A review of the process. *American Journal of Preventative Medicine, 20,* 21–35.{.)

IV. Generating Evidence: The Research Process

A. *Nursing research* involves a systematic process that leads to the generation of new knowledge, refinement of knowledge, or extension of knowledge that contributes to the discipline of nursing and in particular to pain management nursing.

1. Purposes of nursing research (Burns & Grove, 2006)
    a. *Describe:* Depict the characteristics of individuals, groups, situation, and health states.
    b. *Explore:* Investigate the dimensions of a phenomenon.
    c. *Explain:* Attempt to understand the underpinnings of phenomena and their interrelationships.
    d. *Predict and control:* Forecast how combinations of variables will operate in different circumstances involving different groups of individuals.
2. Limitations of the research process
    a. Every study has limitations based on the design and sampling techniques that were selected.
    b. Moral and ethical constraints, protection of human subjects, and institutional review boards also impose limitations.
    c. The complexity of humans can be considered a limitation.
    d. Measurement and data collection difficulties are possible.
    e. Obstacles prevent complete control in the research environment, such as extraneous variables.

B. Steps in the research process

1. Identify the sources of research problems in pain management nursing.
    a. Experiences in the clinical setting
    b. Nursing literature
    c. Theories and conceptual frameworks
    d. External sources (e.g., government agencies and task forces)
2. Narrow the topic by generating a list of researchable questions.
3. Evaluate research problems.
    a. Identify the significance of the problem and its relevance to pain management nursing.
    b. Assess the ability to research the problem and its relevance to pain management nursing.
        (1) Does the problem have empirical reality or an objective focus (evidence rooted in an understandable, predictable, or controllable clinical world and gathered through data collection by using the senses to generate knowledge)?
        (2) Does it employ defined concepts?
        (3) Is it able to capture the phenomena being studied?
    c. Determine the feasibility of the research by considering the following factors:
        (1) What is the time (e.g., the project will be completed in the allotted time frame) and timing (e.g., the subjects will be available during the period the study takes place)?
        (2) Does it have empirical reality or an objective focus?
        (3) Does it employ defined concepts?
        (4) Is it able to capture the phenomena being studied?
        (5) What is the availability of financial resources, including funding?
        (6) What is the experience of the researcher?
        (7) What are the ethical considerations related to working with human subjects?
4. State the research problem.
    a. Delineate the problem. The statement of the research problem guides the development of the study and must be presented clearly.
        (1) Research problems become refined further by reviewing the literature to discover what research has been conducted on the topic, focusing on research designs and sampling techniques.
        (2) The research purpose is generated from the problem. Because the problem identifies a gap within nursing knowledge in a selected area, the purpose clarifies the knowledge that will be produced from the specific investigation (Burns & Grove, 2006).

(3) In a quantitative study, the purpose statements should indicate the independent and dependent variables of the study population. In a qualitative study, the purpose is to identify the phenomenon of interest and the study population (Burns & Grove, 2006; Polit & Hungler, 2007).

b. Ask the research question. From the research problem, the purpose of the study and research question is generated.
   (1) Many research studies contain a statement of purpose and several more specific research questions.
   (2) The question directs the methodology.

5. Research the hypothesis.
   a. Characteristics of a hypothesis
      (1) The hypothesis must be empirically testable and inferred from measured or observed phenomena.
      (2) It translates problem statements into predictions of expected outcomes.
      (3) It is not used in descriptive research because descriptive research describes phenomena instead of explaining them.
      (4) *Hypotheses are never proven;* they are supported only.
   b. Purpose of hypotheses
      (1) Hypotheses are a means of generating knowledge through the testing of theoretical statements or relationships that have been identified in previous research, proposed by theorists, or observed in practice.
   c. Characteristics of workable hypotheses
      (1) Testable
         (a) Hypotheses have measurable variables.
         (b) They predict a relationship between at least two variables.
         (c) They are statistically testable.
      (2) Justifiable
         (a) Specific instances are observed, collated, and combined into a general statement.
         (b) Deductive reasoning moves from the general to the specific or from a general premise to a particular conclusion.

6. Review the literature.
   a. Purposes
      (1) Literature is a source for research ideas.
      (2) Using it, the researcher can understand the current state of the science for a particular phenomenon.
      (3) It documents the prevalence and significance of the research problem.
      (4) A literature review provides the conceptual framework or theory to guide the study design and data interpretation.
      (5) It supports the choice of variables for the study.
      (6) A review can be used to identify studies to determine previous methods, research instruments, and samples.
   b. Scope of the literature review
      (1) Types of sources
         (a) A primary source is a description written by the person who conducted the study.
         (b) A secondary source is a description of a study prepared by someone other than an original researcher. It is less desirable than a primary source.
   c. Locating relevant literature for a research review
      (1) Electronic literature searches (e.g., CINAHL, Medline, PubMed, Ovid)
      (2) Journal resources
         (a) *Pain Management Nursing*
         (b) *Advances in Nursing Science*
         (c) *Journal of Advanced Nursing*

(d) *Journal of Nursing Scholarship*
(e) *Journal of Pain and Symptom Management*
(f) *Nursing Research*
(g) *Oncology Nursing Forum*
(h) *Pain*
(i) *Clinical Journal of Pain*
(j) *Research in Nursing and Health*

C. Quantitative research
1. *Quantitative research* involves the systematic collection of numerical information under conditions of considerable control and the analysis of the data. It involves the manipulation of such data through statistical procedures for the purpose of describing phenomena or assessing the magnitude and reliability of relationships among them (Polit & Hungler, 2007).
2. Types of quantitative research designs
a. *Descriptive study designs:* Studies focus on the accurate portrayal of the characteristics of people, situations, or groups and the frequency with which certain phenomena occur. A summary includes mean and standard deviation. No manipulation of the variables occurs.
(1) *Typical descriptive study design:* This research design examines the characteristics of a specific group.
(a) Example: a chronic low back pain population study to obtain characteristics of lifestyles, sleep habits, health habits, and work setting
(2) *Comparative descriptive design:* This research design examines and describes differences in variables between two or more groups.
(a) Example: taking the aforementioned example study and comparing these same characteristics in the fibromyalgia population
(3) *Time-dimensional designs:* These designs examine sequences and patterns of change, growth, or trends across time.
(a) Longitudinal designs examine changes in the same subjects over an extended period.
(i) Example: long-term effects of opioid therapy
(b) Cross-sectional designs are used to examine groups of subjects in various stages of development simultaneously.
(i) Example: long-term effects of opioid therapy in patients with history of chemical abuse and patients with no history of chemical abuse
(4) *Case-study design:* This design involves an intensive exploration of a single unit of study, which may be a person, family, group, community, or institution.
b. *Correlational studies:* These research investigations explore the interrelationships among variables of interest without any active intervention on the part of the researcher.
(1) Example: the relationship between gender and pain rating during a dental procedure
c. *Quasi-experimental study designs:* The purpose of these designs is to examine causality. This design can threaten validity because the subjects cannot be assigned randomly to treatment conditions, although the researcher does manipulate the independent variable and exercises certain controls to enhance the internal validity of the results.
(1) Nonequivalent control group pretest–posttest design
(2) One-group pretest–posttest design (preexperimental)
(3) Nonequivalent or untreated control group posttest only design (preexperimental; no randomization and pretest weakens the results)
d. *Experimental study designs:* These studies examine causality by controlling the independent variable and randomly assigning subjects to different conditions. This involves the essential elements of random sampling, researcher-controlled manipulation of the independent variable, and control of the experimental situation, including a control group. The key components are manipulation, control, and randomization.
(1) Example: randomly assigning postoperative patients to receive morphine patient–controlled analgesia with continuous infusion or without continuous infusion

(2) Randomized clinical trials evaluate innovative treatment using a before–after only design.
 (a) Example: randomly selecting patients for the clinical trial of intranasal sumatriptan

(3) Double-blind studies are useful when data are collected by observation. Double-blind techniques remove observer biases because neither the subject nor the observer knows the group assigned to a given subject. This blinding prevents the researcher bias from entering the data and affecting the study results.

e. Additional research designs
 (1) *Evaluation research:* This form of applied research identifies how well a program, policy, procedure, or practice is working.
  (a) Example: end-of-life consultation service and its impact on quality of life
 (2) *Needs assessment:* This research is similar to evaluation, representing an effort to provide a decision maker or policymaker with information for action. Data are collected to estimate the needs of a group, community, or organization and thus to assist in a planning process.
 (3) *Methodological research:* Controlled investigations explore ways of obtaining, organizing, and analyzing data. These studies address the development, validation, and evaluation of research tools or techniques.

D. Qualitative research
 1. *Qualitative research* is a systematic, interactive, subjective approach used to describe life experiences and give them meaning (Burns & Grove, 2006).
 2. Characteristics of qualitative research
  a. Its purpose is to describe or generate theories so that they may be used to develop hypotheses or study phenomena about which little is known.
  b. It has a purposeful sample: participants are selected because they have characteristics in common.
  c. The researcher is involved closely with the participants.
  d. It involves inductive data analysis.
  e. It uses a narrative approach to reporting the findings.
 3. Types of qualitative studies
  a. *Grounded theory* is an approach to data collection with the purpose of developing theories about the phenomena under study.
  b. *Ethnography* focuses on the culture of people.
   (1) An *emic approach* is the investigation of behaviors from within the culture.
   (2) An *etic approach* is the investigation of behaviors from outside the culture by examining similarities and differences across culture.
  c. *Phenomenology* considers the lived experience of people (e.g., study the phenomenon of pain flare in the chronic pain population).
  d. *Historical research* is focused on looking for patterns and relationships from the past in a systematic way to evaluate past occurrences.
  e. *Philosophical research* seeks to clarify meanings, make values manifest, identify ethics, and study the nature of knowledge.
  f. *Content analysis* provides a systematic means of measuring the frequency, order, or intensity of occurrence of words, phrases, or sentences because of their theoretical importance.
  g. *Narrative inquiry* is the lens through which a study takes form (Stevens, 1998). This is often used in a marginalized and vulnerable population. The results of this method can be used to affect social policy.

V. Applying Evidence to Clinical Practice

A. *Knowledge use* is the process of disseminating and using research-generated information to influence or change existing practices.
 1. Clinical relevance

a. Determine whether a significant problem will be solved by applying a new intervention or a change in practice.

2. Scientific merit
    a. Critique each study to assess whether the findings and conclusions are accurate and generalizable. Can this study influence clinical practice?
    b. Replication studies have been done and resulted in the same findings.
    c. Studies have been conducted in a clinical setting.
3. Implementation potential
    a. Transferability asks, Should the selected innovation be attempted in the new clinical setting?
    b. Feasibility considers the availability of resources and staff, organizational climate, availability of external resources, and potential for clinical evaluation. Nurses will have control over the implementation of the innovation.
    c. Consider the cost-benefit ratio of implementing or not implementing the innovation to the client, organization, and profession.

B. Process for a research usage project (Gillis & Jackson, 2002)
1. Select a relevant clinical problem.
    a. Problem-focused triggers
    b. Knowledge-focused triggers
2. Review and critique the research literature.
    a. Use guidelines (previously described).
    b. Use an organizing framework (create a grid) to summarize findings.
3. Determine the transferability and feasibility of the studies to the setting.
    a. Utility to nursing practice
    b. Applicability to nursing practice
    c. Scientific merit
    d. Client safety and preference
    e. Sufficient resources for implementation
4. Develop the research-based protocol.
5. Establish outcome indicators.
6. Plan and develop educational sessions to introduce the new protocol.
    a. Involve stakeholders in the process.
    b. Use an established planned change model or diffusion of innovations model.
    c. Obtain feedback on the change process.
7. Evaluate the protocol based on the outcome indicators.
    a. Identify barriers to implementation.
    b. Identify factors to enhance implementation process.
8. Revise as needed.
9. Disseminate the evaluation of the protocol to other nursing professionals.
    a. Institutionwide
    b. Professional and clinical journals
    c. Scientific meeting presentations and posters

VI. Creating a Culture for Research Utilization and EBP in Pain Management

A. Identifying barriers to using nursing research in practice
1. Research characteristics
    a. Lack of extensive knowledge based on valid, reliable, and generalizable study results
    b. Dearth of reported replication studies
2. Organizational characteristics
    a. Lack of resources
    b. Lack of rewards for research
    c. Resistance to change
    d. Lack of institutional commitment for research

3. Nursing profession characteristics
    a. Lack of time for clinical nurses to perform steps in the research utilization process
    b. Lack of skills in critical appraisal
    c. Shortage of appropriate role models
    d. Lack of autonomy or control over the practice

B. Strategies for improving research use
1. Adopt a reflective inquiring approach.
2. Read research articles.
3. Attend professional conferences.
4. Learn to expect evidence that a procedure or practice is effective.
5. Attend a journal club.
6. Participate as a team member in a research study or utilization project.
7. Replicate a study.
8. Use findings in the literature to change practice.
9. Compare and contrast mythical concepts to concepts well grounded in the research.
    a. Example: when colleagues say meperidine is the only opioid that works on bone pain, suggest that they find the research that supports their statement.
10. Collaborate with academic nurse educators, researchers, and clinicians.
    a. Encourage nursing students to engage in critical appraisal of research literature.
    b. Clinicians have clinical knowledge and clinical questions.
    c. Collaboration enhances the research process and usage.
    d. It can be helpful to collaborate with "seasoned" researchers to enhance chances for research funding from granting mechanisms.
    e. Collaboration can facilitate research for bedside nurses because time and workload constraints inhibit full participation in research process.
11. Facilitate EBP in organizations.
    a. Set institutional goals to use research findings to promote excellence.
    b. Enhance job descriptions to include EBP in performance appraisals.
    c. Offer incentives for research utilization (e.g., prizes, books, or conference registration).
    d. Allot time, funds, and resources to support nursing research at all levels of nursing practice.

C. Fostering mentorship
1. Mentoring is crucial in integrating nursing research at all levels. Mentoring in pain management nursing helps define, document, and improve health outcomes.
2. The following attributes apply to the relationship with a mentor (Stewart & Krueger, 1996):
    a. Career development relationship
    b. Teaching and learning process
    c. Knowledge or competence differential among participants (Stewart & Krueger, 1996)
3. There are two types of mentors.
    a. Academic researcher
    b. Clinical-based researcher (crucial in integrating nursing research at all levels)

References

Agency for Healthcare Research and Quality. (2002). *Systems to rate the strength of scientific evidence.* Retrieved December 14, 2008, from http://www.ahrq.gov/clinic/tp/strengthtp.htm.

American College of Physicians & American Pain Society. (2007). Diagnosis and treatment of low back pain: A joint clinical practice guideline from the American College of Physicians and the American Pain Society. *Annals of Internal Medicine, 147*(7), 478–491.

American Geriatrics Society. (2002). The management of persistent pain in older persons: AGS Panel on Persistent Pain in Older Persons. *Journal of the American Geriatric Society, 50,* S205–S224.

American Medical Directors Association. (2003). *Pain management in the long-term care setting: Clinical practice guidelines.* Columbia, MD: Author.

American Pain Society. (2002). *Guideline for the management of pain in osteoarthritis, rheumatoid arthritis, and juvenile chronic arthritis.* Clinical Practice Guideline No. 2. Glenview, IL: Author.

American Pain Society. (2005). *Guideline for the management of fibromyalgia syndrome pain in adults and children* (Vol. 4). Glenview, IL: Author.

American Pain Society (Ed.). (2003). *Principles of analgesic use in the treatment of acute pain and cancer pain* (5th ed.). Glenview, IL: Author.

Beyea, S. C., & Nicoll, L. H. (1997). Research utilization models help disseminate research findings and ultimately improve patient outcomes. *AORN Journal, 65*(3), 640–642.

Burns, N., & Grove, S. (2006). *The practice of nursing research: Conduct, critiques, utilization* (6th ed.). Philadelphia: W. B. Saunders.

Dicenso, A., Cullum, N., Ciliska, D., & Guyatt, G. (2004). *Evidence-based nursing: a guide to clinical practice.* Philadelphia: Elsevier.

Geyett, G., & Rennie, D. (2002). *Users' guide to the medical literature.* Chicago, IL: American Medical Association Press.

Gillis, A., & Jackson, W. (2002). *Research for nurses methods and interpretation.* Philadelphia: F. A. Davis.

Gordon, D. B., Dahl, J., Phillips, P., Frandsen, J., Cowley, C., Foster, R. L., Fine, P.G., Miaskowski, C., Fishman, S., & Finley, R.S.. (2004). The use of "as-needed" range orders for opioid analgesics in the management of acute pain: A consensus statement of the American Society for Pain Management Nursing and the American Pain Society. *Pain Management Nursing, 5*(2), 53–58.

Hadjistavropoulos, T., Herr, K., Turk, D. C., Fine, P. G., Dworkin, R. H., Helme, R., Jackson, K., Parmelee, P.A., Rudy, T.E., Lynn Beattie, B., Chibnall, J.T. Craig, K.D., Ferrell, B.R., Ferrell, B., Fillingim, R. B., Gagliese, L., Gallagher, R., Gibson, S.J., Harrison, E.L., Katz, B., Keefe, F.J., Lieber, S.J., Lussier, D., Schmader, K.E., Tait, R.D., Weiner, D.K., & Williams, J. (2007). An interdisciplinary expert consensus statement on assessment of pain in older persons. *Clinical Journal of Pain, 23*(1 Suppl.), S1–S43.

Harris, R. P., Helfand, M., Woolf, S. H., Lohr, K.N., Mulrow, C.D., Teutsch, S.M., & Atkins, D. (2001). Current methods of the U.S. Preventative Health Task Force: A review of the process. *American Journal of Preventative Medicine, 20,* 21–35.

Herr, K., Bjoro, K., Steffensmeier, J., & Rakel, B. (2006). *Evidence-based practice guideline: Acute pain management in older adults.* Iowa City: University of Iowa, Geriatric Nursing Research Intervention Center.

Lincoln, Y. S., & Guba, E. G. (1985). *Naturalistic inquiry.* Beverly Hills, CA: Sage.

Melnyk, B. M., & Fineout-Overholt, E. (2005). *Evidence-based practice in nursing and health care: A guide to practice.* Philadelphia: Lippincott Williams & Wilkins.

Polit, D., & Hungler, B. (2007). *Nursing research: Principles and methods* (8th ed.). Philadelphia: Lippincott.

Sackett, D. L., Straus, S. E., Richardson, W. S., Rosenberg, W., & Hayes, R. B. (2000). *Evidence-based medicine: How to practice and teach EBM.* Edinburgh: Churchill Livingston.

Stevens, P. E. (1998). The experiences of lesbians of color in health care encounters: Narrative insights for improving access and quality. *Journal of Lesbian Studies, 2*(1), 77–94.

Stewart, B. M., & Krueger, L. E. (1996). An evolutionary concept analysis of mentoring in nursing. *Journal of Professional Nursing, 12*(5), 311–321.

chapter

7

Benefits of Proper Pain Management

Diana L. Ruzicka, RN-BC, MSN, CNS

Objectives

After studying this chapter, the reader should be able to:

1. Discuss the economic impact of managing and treating patients with pain.
2. Discuss the benefits of appropriate pain management.
3. Describe the concept of quality of life and its impact on physiological, psychological, social, and spiritual well-being.
4. Identify measures to reduce morbidity and mortality in patients with acute, persistent (chronic), and cancer pain.

I. Costs of Uncontrolled Pain

A. Acute pain

1. Inadequate management of pain creates a financial burden on the health care system and society (Dahl, Berry, Stevenson, Gordon, & Ward, 1998; Turk, 1996).
2. Intravenous patient-controlled analgesia (PCA) may result in cost savings because it reduces amount of nursing time on analgesia-related activities by 20%, and nursing costs with intravenous PCA are lower than with other conventional therapies (Wasylak, Abbott, English, & Jeans, 1990).
3. Pain is the leading cause of emergency department visits and hospitalization in patients with sickle cell disease (Platt et al., 1991).
   a. A study of 50 patients with frequent emergency department admissions with sickle cell disease was conducted. The patients were switched from intramuscular meperidine to intravenous morphine or hydromorphone and then were switched to oral controlled-release morphine as soon as pain was controlled. Admissions decreased by 44%, length of stay decreased by 25%, and emergency department visits decreased by 67% (McCaffery & Pasero, 1999).
   b. Identifying modifiable psychosocial variables, such as stress, coping behavior, social support, personality factors, and mental status, associated with use of health care services could aid in the development of psychological interventions aimed at decreasing emergency department visits and other health care costs (Reese & Smith, 1997).

B. Cancer and human immunodeficiency virus (HIV) pain

1. Unscheduled cancer pain admissions are costly.
2. Unscheduled hospital admissions for the treatment of cancer pain cost $4.7 million annually (Larsen, 1996).
3. Of the 1,166 total admissions recorded during a 6-month period at the University of Texas M. D. Anderson Cancer Center, 14% of admissions were for pain.
   a. The mean length of stay was 10.5 days, and the mean patient charge per admission was $19,000.
4. Poorly treated pain in patients with HIV or acquired immunodeficiency syndrome (AIDS) creates an economic burden on patients, families, and society (Carr, 1994).
   a. Diagnostic algorithms are needed to establish efficient cost-effective care in patients with HIV or AIDS (Carr, 1994).

C. Persistent (nonmalignant) pain

1. It is estimated that greater than 50 million Americans suffer from some form of pain. This pain has a significant impact economically (Turk & Okifuji, 1998).
2. Common pain conditions that affect both men and women (e.g., arthritis, back pain, headache, and other musculoskeletal pain) cost $61.2 billion annually due to lost income, decreased productivity, and medical expenses.
   a. This cost is much higher as the preceding estimate does not include lost productive time costs associated with other pain conditions (e.g., dental pain, cancer pain, gastrointestinal pain, neuropathy, or pain associated with menstruation), pain-induced disability that leads to continuous absence of 1 week or more, secondary costs for hiring and training replacement workers, or chronic lost productivity due to chronic pain, which an employee may underestimate over time (Stewart, Ricci, Chee, Morganstein, & Lipton, 2003).
   b. Of the total workforce, 13% experienced a loss in productive time during a 2-week period due to common pain conditions—headache (5.4%), back pain (3.2%), arteritis (2%), and other musculoskeletal pain (2%)—losing a mean of 4.6 hours/week (Stewart et al., 2003).
   c. The majority (76.6%) of the lost productive time was explained by reduced performance while at work, not by work absence (e.g., lost concentration, repeated a job, worked more slowly than usual, felt fatigued at work, and did nothing at work on days when not feeling well). Only 1.1% of the workforce was absent from work 1 or more days per week because of the four pain conditions (Stewart et al., 2003).

3. Headache pain costs $19.6 billion annually in the United States; $4.2 billion is due to absenteeism, and $15.4 billion is due to lost productivity at work (Stewart et al., 2003).
4. Osteoarthritis affects more than 50 million older Americans and is the most common arthritic condition (Beach, 2007).
   a. Arthritis pain costs $10.3 billion annually in the United States; $1.6 billion is due to absenteeism and $8.7 billion is due to lost productivity at work (Stewart et al., 2003).
5. Back pain costs $19.8 billion annually in the United States; $6 billion is due to absenteeism and $13.8 billion is due to lost productivity at work (Stewart et al., 2003).
   a. Other musculoskeletal pains cost $11.6 billion annually in the United States; $2.6 billion is due to absenteeism and $9 billion is due to lost productivity at work (Stewart et al., 2003).
6. Approximately 6 million patients suffer from fibromyalgia (Sprott, 2003).
   a. One prospective study showed that patients with fibromyalgia have more than $2,000 per year in medical costs, have approximately 10 outpatient clinic visits per year, and have one hospitalization every 3 years (Wolfe et al., 1990).
   b. Another prospective study showed that total annual costs for fibromyalgia patients were close to $6,000, compared with $2,500 for typical patients. For every dollar spent on fibromyalgia-specific claims, the employer spent $57 to $143 on additional direct and indirect costs (Robinson et al., 2003).
7. A study of 15 primary care centers in 14 countries revealed that 22% of primary care patients report persistent pain, with a wide prevalence rate among facilities ranging from 5.5% to 33% (Gureje, Von Korff, Simon, & Gater, 1998).
8. Benefits of appropriate pain relief may include increase in level of functioning, reduction or elimination of pain complaint, and positive and hopeful attitude (American Chronic Pain Association, 2008).
9. Considerable controversy exists about the use of opioids for the treatment of chronic pain of noncancer origin.
   a. Many physicians feel that chronic pain is inadequately treated and that opioids can play an important role in the treatment of all types of chronic pain.
   b. Others caution against the widespread use of opioids, noting problems with hyperalgesia (increased pain sensitivity), tolerance, loss of benefit with time, and escalating usage with decreasing function in many individuals (American Chronic Pain Association, 2008).
10. Multidisciplinary pain centers, which involve multiple disciplines of health care providers in the physical, psychosocial, and behavioral issues in chronic pain, are important in the treatment of individuals with chronic pain (Turk & Okifuji, 1998). Multidisciplinary pain centers have been shown to decrease health care use.
    a. Pain clinic visits decreased by 30% in the first years after treatment (Turk & Okifuji, 1998).
    b. Return to work occurred at a higher rate in those patients who completed treatment at a multidisciplinary pain center (Shealy & Cady, 1998; Turk & Okifuji, 1998).
       (1) Follow-up data was provided at 6 months and 2 years from 800 patients, with 600 followed up at more than 2 years and 200 at 2 months and 6 months showing that 35% returned to work (Shealy & Cady, 1998).
       (2) Hospital and medication expenses decreased (Shealy & Cady, 1998). Fewer than 55 patients had additional surgical procedures after treatment.
          (a) Total medical expenses decreased by 80% to 85%, and medication expenses decreased by 85%
          (b) Of patients treated, 62% to 90% did not seek additional treatment 3 to 12 months after completion at a multidisciplinary pain center (Turk & Okifuji, 1998).
       (3) The status of 201 chronic pain patients 13 years after treatment in a pain management center showed no increase in risk of mortality; half the patients were gainfully employed. Before admission to pain clinic, 88% were unemployed (i.e., away from full-time work for more than 1 month), with a median unemployment period of 24.5 months (Maruta, Malinchoc, Offord, & Colligan, 1997).

c. Costs can be reduced by establishing an ambulatory pain rehabilitation program. Costs to third parties for pain rehabilitation were $321,000 in 1985 for inpatient treatment compared with $61,000 in 1987 for outpatient treatment. The average cost per inpatient treatment in 1985 was $22,848 compared with $7,640 for outpatient treatment in 1987.
   (1) Success rates as determined by return to work were relatively similar (13 of 25 in 1985 and 11 of 25 in 1987) (Cicala & Wright, 1989).
   (2) A cost-benefit analysis of a multidisciplinary chronic pain program indicated a reduction in posttreatment outpatient visits, a decrease in inpatient length of hospital stay by 3 days, and a decrease in health care dollars of nearly $500,000 during a 5-year period for pain treatment for the 30 patients in the study (Kee, Middaugh, & Pawlick, 1997).

d. Medical expenditure savings were estimated as follows:
   (1) A decrease occurred in the number of additional surgeries (17.5% less); the follow-up interval was 2 years (Turk & Okifuji, 1998).
   (2) Medical costs were reduced in the year after surgery by 58% (Turk & Okifuji, 1998).
   (3) Costs savings were estimated at $626,091,051 for an estimated 4,140 individuals treated at multidisciplinary pain centers in 1 year (Turk & Okifuji, 1998).

II. Benefits of Managing Pain

A. Benefits and outcomes of managing pain are well documented. Table 7-1 summarizes these benefits.

B. Approximately 50% of patients with acute or persistent noncancer pain receive inadequate care, and as many as 90% of people with pain associated with cancer or other terminal illnesses are untreated (Ferrell, 2005).

C. Acute pain

1. Preemptive analgesia may reduce both acute and chronic pain by reducing the peripheral sensitization from the injury and the central sensitization with its subsequent windup (Malchow & Black, 2008; Perkins & Kehlet, 2000; Rueben, 2007).
   a. Intraoperative ketorolac, at 60 mg, was injected locally into the underlying sphincter muscle in a group of patients undergoing hemorrhoidectomy, who were given ketorolac, 30 mg intramuscularly, postoperatively every 6 hours and a 5-day supply of oral ketorolac. This regimen provided pain control comparable to opioid therapy and had a higher satisfaction rating. There was no associated urinary retention or bleeding (O'Donovan, Ferrara, Larach, & Williams, 1994).
   b. Premedication with oral dextromethorphan (*N*-methyl-D-aspartate receptor antagonist), at 45 mg, in 12 patients undergoing tonsillectomy resulted in lower pain scores at rest and on swallowing throughout 7 days and in less postoperative analgesia compared with the control group. The group that was premedicated with 30 mg of dextromethorphan had lower pain scores than the control group when at rest but not on swallowing (Kawamata, Omote, Kawamata, & Namiki, 1998).
   c. Preemptive analgesia may modify the pain perceived after a tissue injury by administering an analgesic before the precipitating noxious stimulus.

2. Epidural analgesia administered before an amputation has been shown to decrease phantom limb pain (Grass, 1993).
   a. Intraoperative plus postoperative epidural analgesia decreased the incidence of post-thoracotomy pain syndrome from 67% to 33% at 6 months when compared with just postoperative epidural analgesia in a prospective, randomized, single-blind study (Obata et al., 1999).

3. More than 60% of surgery is now performed in an ambulatory care setting. Despite improved analgesics and sophisticated drug delivery systems, surveys indicate that more than 80% of patients experience moderate to severe pain postoperatively (Shang & Gan, 2003).
   a. In a sample of 250 adults who had undergone surgical procedures in the United States, 80% experienced acute pain after surgery; 86% of these patients reported it was moderate, severe, or extreme pain, with more patients experiencing pain after discharge than before discharge (Apfelbaum, Chen, Mehta, Gan, & Tong, 2003).

Table 7-1 Outcomes and Measures of Effectiveness and Benefits of Pain Management
Mortality
Morbidity
Major
Myocardial infarction
Pneumonia
Pulmonary embolism
Minor
Nausea
Vomiting
Readmission
Patient satisfaction
Quality of life
Economic (cost) analysis (length of stay, readmission, increased emergency room visits, lost wages or absenteeism, reduced performance on days at work, etc.)
Type of analysis
Cost identification or cost minimization
Cost-effectiveness
Cost-utility
Cost-benefit
Type of cost and benefit
Direct medical
Direct nonmedical
Indirect morbidity and mortality
Intangible
Perspective for analysis
Societal
Patient
Payer
Provider

Adapted from Fleisher, L.A., Mantha, S., Roizen, M.F. (1998). Medical technology assessment: an overview. *Anesthesia and Analgesia,* 87(6), 1271–1282.

4. Although intravenous PCA had been the "gold standard" for acute pain management, there are now more analgesic options and compelling data to support the combination of analgesics or multimodal therapy, the timing of analgesic interventions, and the use of newer drug delivery systems (Polomano, Rathmell, Krenzischek, & Dunwoody, 2008).
   a. A meta-analysis of the randomized, controlled trials comparing postoperative epidural and intravenous PCA with opioids in adults (n = 299) published between 1966 and 2004 revealed that epidural analgesia, regardless of analgesic agent, epidural regimen, and type and time of pain assessment, provided superior postoperative analgesia compared to intravenous PCA (Wu et al., 2005).

b. Regional anesthesia, when compared to general anesthesia, decreased the odds of deep venous thrombosis by 44%, pulmonary embolism by 55%, transfusion by 50%, pneumonia by 39%, respiratory depression by 59%, myocardial infarction by 33%, and renal failure by 43% in various surgical patients included in a review of 142 trials of 9,553 subjects (Schug, 1999). Epidural analgesia decreased length of stay, which resulted in decreased costs.
c. General anesthesia combined with epidural anesthesia and analgesia in patients undergoing major peripheral vascular surgery decreased the intensive care unit (ICU) stay by 1.8 days and the total hospital stay by 2.5 days when compared to patients receiving general anesthesia with postoperative parenteral, oral, or both types of opioids (Tuman et al., 1991).
d. Epidural analgesia in patients undergoing total esophagectomy decreased the ICU stay by 2 days and the total hospital stay by 7 days when compared to patients receiving intravenous morphine. This resulted in a savings of Canadian $12,770 per patient (Smedstad, Beattie, Blair, & Buckley, 1992).
e. Epidural analgesia with morphine and bupivacaine shortened the time to fulfill discharge criteria by 35 hours, thus potentially saving $1,200 per patient as compared with the use of epidural or PCA morphine in a prospective, randomized, controlled clinical trial of 54 patients undergoing colon surgery. However, other factors prevented timely hospital discharge in this study (Liu et al., 1995).
f. Local anesthetics infiltrated into the surgical area may decrease the need for pain medication postoperatively.
    (1) Mastectomy patients who had a paravertebral block intraoperatively had pain control 23 hours because of the sensory block. This resulted in a cost savings of $800 per outpatient (Weltz, Greengrass, & Lyerly, 1995).
    (2) A suprascapular nerve block before general anesthesia for pain relief in arthroscopic shoulder surgery resulted in a 51% reduction in demand and a 31% reduction in consumption of morphine delivered by PCA.
        (a) There was a greater than 5-fold reduction in the incidence of nausea, as well as reduced visual analogue and verbal pain scores.
        (b) The length of hospital stay was reduced by 24%.
        (c) At home, there was a 40% reduction of analgesic consumption and reduction in verbal pain scored at rest on abduction (Ritchie et al., 1997).
    (3) Ilioinguinal hypogastric nerve block (as opposed to general anesthesia or spinal anesthesia) was the most cost-effective anesthetic technique for outpatients undergoing unilateral inguinal herniorrhaphy with respect to speed of recovery (133 ± 68 minutes for nerve block versus 171 ± 40 minutes for general anesthesia versus 280 ± 83 minutes for spinal anesthesia), patient comfort (15 ± 14 mm versus 39 ± 28 mm versus 34 ± 32 mm, respectively), and associated incremental costs ($132.73 ± $33.80 versus $172.67 ± $29.83 versus $164 ± $31.03, respectively) (Song, Greilich, White, Watcha, & Tongier, 2000).
    (4) Local anesthesia with sedation for anorectal surgery in the ambulatory setting was more cost-effective than spinal or general anesthetic techniques ($69 ± $20 versus $104 ± $18 versus $145 ± $25, respectively) due to lower intraoperative and recovery costs. The local anesthesia and spinal group required less pain medication (19% versus 19% versus 45%, respectively) and more patients in local anesthesia group were highly satisfied with the care they received (68% versus 58% versus 39%, respectively) (Li et al., 2000).
    (5) The use of combined analgesic therapy, such as the addition of a nonsteroidal anti-inflammatory drug (NSAID) to a Percocet®-morphine regimen, shortened the length of stay (4.2 to 3 days) and lowered visual analogue scale scores (average of 5.3 to 3.8) in craniotomy patients (Rahimi et al., 2006).
    (6) The infiltration of botulinum toxin in the chest wall musculature following mastectomy significantly reduced postoperative spasm, pain intensity scores (1 ± 1 versus 3 ± 2, with botulinum toxin injections or no injections, respectively), and length of stay in

hours (26 ± 8 hours versus 37 ± 19 hours), thus facilitating tissue expander reconstruction. Patients were able to tolerate a greater volume during expansion, thereby decreasing the number of expansion sessions (Layeeque et al., 2004).

5. Educating the patient and family is the hallmark of achieving optimal pain management in patients with sickle cell disease.
   a. Psychological (education, imagery), behavioral (relaxation exercises, biofeedback), and physical (massage, hydration, physical therapy) strategies are geared toward producing pain relief, reducing stress, and increasing function.
   b. These modalities, when integrated into treatment plans, should be culturally sensitive and tailored to the individual patient (American Pain Society [APS], 1999).

D. Cancer pain
1. It is currently estimated that there are nearly 9 million people with a history of cancer in the United States and an estimated 1.3 million people will be diagnosed in 2002 alone, of whom 60% will survive at least 5 years after diagnosis (Ferrell et al., 2001; Miaskowski & Dibble, 1995; National Institutes of Health State-of-the-Science Statement, 2002).
   a. Of patients in the early and intermediate stages of cancer, 30% to 45% experience moderate-to-severe pain; 75% of patients are in the advanced stage of cancer experience pain (Pargeon & Hailey, 1999).
   b. Older people are a primary age group for cancer and its associated pain, and responses to pain may be modified by various psychosocial factors. Generational and cultural variations exist in attitudes to pain (All & Huycke, 1999) (see the chapter on Historical and Cultural Influences on Pain Perceptions and Barriers to Treatment).
   c. The two largest ethnic minority groups with cancer in the United States are African Americans and Hispanics.
      (1) In a study of 108 African-American and Hispanic patients with cancer, physicians underestimated pain for 64% of the Hispanic patients and 74% of the African American patients.
      (2) Although there are improvements in analgesic prescribing practices, inadequate pain assessment remains a barrier to optimal pain management (Anderson et al., 2000).
   d. Of 126 oncology patients interviewed 48 hours after admission to an Australian hospital, 47.6% experienced moderate to severe pain in the previous 24 hours but had only received 40.4% of available analgesic. In addition, 41% held strong beliefs about the potential for addiction to narcotics, and these reported higher current pain, worst pain intensity, and higher-than-average pain intensity in the previous 24 hours (Cohen et al., 2007).
2. Pain can be managed better by educating health care providers on the recommended guidelines for the treatment of cancer pain and involving patients and families as active participants in the management of pain. A comprehensive assessment of pain is needed to recognize various syndromes and identify the cause and pathophysiology of the pain (Portenoy, 1997).
3. Opioids are the most cost-effective because they are effective in managing most cancer pain (Agency for Health Care Policy and Research, 1994; Levy, 1994).
   a. Opioid therapy can relieve pain adequately in more than 75% of patients with cancer pain (Portenoy, 1997).
4. NSAIDs have been shown to be effective in some specific cancer pain syndromes, including pain from bone metastasis and soft tissue infiltration.
   a. The peripheral mechanisms of NSAIDs are similar to the effect of infiltrating the area with local anesthetic.
   b. NSAIDs weaken effect of peripheral nociceptors, afferent nociceptor activity, and C fiber-mediated central sensitization.
   c. A central effect has been suggested (Mercadante et al., 1999).
5. Corticosteroids are used to treat cancer pain by decreasing the inflammation at the site of injury (e.g., bone metastasis, epidural cord compression, bowel obstruction, cerebral edema secondary to brain tumor, and neuropathic pain) (Perin, 2000).

6. Continuous subcutaneous infusion of opioid for pain control resulted in a cost savings because less skill is needed than with other interventional therapies (Poniatowski, 1991).

E. HIV or AIDS pain
1. Pain often is undertreated in patients with HIV or AIDS, and the treatment is complicated by polypharmacy (various antiretroviral agents) and drug-drug interactions.
2. A comprehensive pain assessment should be done to determine the type of pain and what other prescribed medications are being taken to prevent medication interactions (Breitbart, Kaim, & Rosenfield, 1999; McCaffery & Pasero, 1999).
3. At all stages of HIV or AIDS in children, pain is important.
   a. Pain related to procedures is worse than disease-related pain for many children.
   b. An eutectic mixture of local anesthetics has been shown to decrease procedure-related pain in children undergoing venipuncture, lumbar puncture, and central catheter placement (Czarnecki, Dollfas, & Strafford, 1994).
   c. Behavioral methods, such as guided imagery and relaxation techniques, often are used to give children a sense of control over their pain symptoms (Czarnecki et al., 1994).

F. Persistent (chronic nonmalignant) pain
1. People suffering with chronic pain felt less confident in their ability to care for themselves compared to the public (61% versus 73%, respectively; $p < 0.05$) (McCarberg, Nicholson, Todd, Palmer, & Penles, 2008).
2. Significantly more chronic pain respondents reported experiencing pain during sports activities (72%), yard work (60%), walking (54%), household chores (50%), lifting heavy objects (47%), sitting extended periods (43%), and shopping (41%) than the acute pain respondents ($p < 0.05$) (McCarberg et al., 2008).
3. Acute and chronic pain suffers reported trouble falling asleep and staying asleep at least 29% of the time for acute and at least 38% for chronic pain patients (McCarberg et al., 2008).
4. Participants with chronic pain conditions reported more sleep disruptions and loss of quality of sleep compared with the public ($p < 0.05$) (McCarberg et al., 2008).
5. Ethnic differences exist in the prevalence and severity of persistent pain, with African Americans suffering more pain from cancer, arthritis and other debilitating diseases (Creamer, Lethbridge-Cejku, & Hochberg, 1999; Moore & Brodsgaard, 1999; Payne, Medina, & Hampton, 2003) (see chapter on Disparities in Pain Management).
6. Benefits for the patient, institutions, and health professionals include the following:
   a. Patients have the right to and health care organizations have the obligation to support pain management because unrelieved pain has adverse physical and psychological effects (Joint Commission, 2008).
   b. Health care organizations plan, support, and coordinate activities and resources to ensure that pain is recognized and addressed appropriately. Health care organizations educate all relevant providers about assessing and managing pain (Joint Commission, 2008).
7. Health care professionals assess for pain and educate patients and families, when appropriate, about their role in pain management and the potential limitations and side effects of pain treatment. The patient is educated to understand pain, the risk for pain, the importance of effective pain management, the pain assessment process, and the method for pain management (Joint Commission, 2008).
8. Patients are assessed based on clinical presentation, services sought, and in accordance with the care services provided.
   a. A comprehensive pain assessment is conducted as appropriate for the patient's condition and the scope of care, treatment, and services.
   b. Regular assessment and follow-up occur according to the criteria developed by the hospital. The assessment methods are appropriate to the patient's age, abilities, or both.
   c. When pain is identified, the patient is treated by the hospital or referred for treatment (Joint Commission, 2008).

d. Each patient's physiologic status, mental status and pain level are monitored immediately after procedures, administration of moderate or deep sedation or anesthesia, or both (Joint Commission, 2008).

9. The hospital collects data on the perception of care, treatment, and services of patients, including the effectiveness of pain management (Joint Commission, 2008).

III. Quality of Life (Figure 7-1)

A. Acute pain

1. Quality improvement guidelines to improve treatment outcomes of acute pain have been developed by the APS (1995) (see the chapter on Quality Evaluation and Improvement).
2. The core of these guidelines centers on assessment and appropriate management of pain to improve quality of life and patient comfort.
3. Patients are more likely to be satisfied if the management of pain is individualized to their needs and side effects are titrated against efficacy (Borsook, LeBel, & McPeck, 1996).
4. Quality of life is affected adversely by moderate and greater levels of pain intensity.
5. The severity of postoperative pain in patients undergoing elective total hip or knee replacement correlated with a decrease in both the physical and the mental components of quality of life in the immediate postoperative period (within 2 weeks of surgery) as measured by the 12-Item Short-Form Health Survey (Wu et al., 2003).

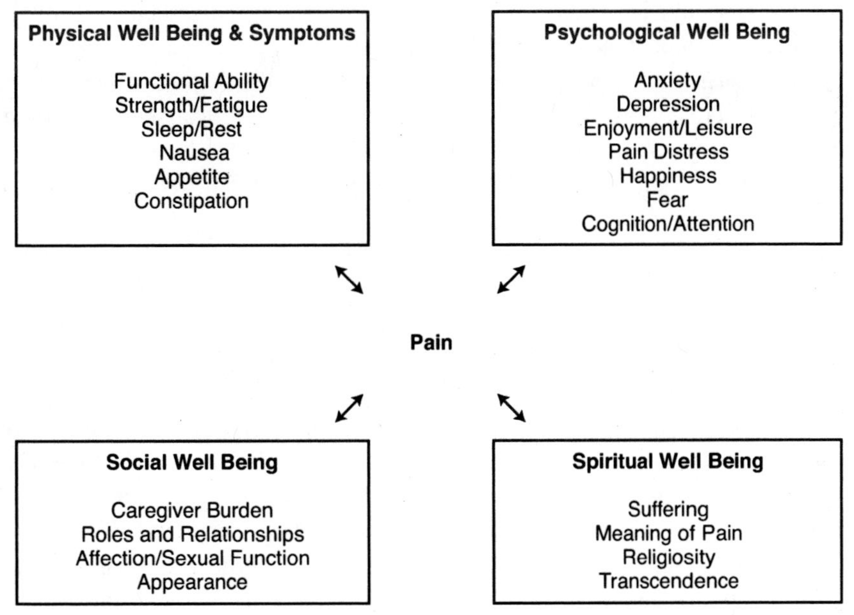

References

Ferrell BR, Wisdom C, Wenzl C, Schneider C. (1989). "Quality of Life as an Outcome Variable in the Management of Cancer Pain." *Cancer*, 63: 2321–2327.

Ferrell BR, Wisdom C, Wenzl C, Brown J. (1989). "Effects of Controlled-Release Morphine on Quality of Life for Cancer Pain." *Oncology Nursing Forum*, 6(4): 521–526.

Padilla G, Ferrell BR, Grant M, Rhiner M. (1990). "Defining the Content Domain of Quality of Life for Cancer Patients with Pain." *Cancer Nursing*, 13(2): 108–115.

Ferrell BR, Grant M, Padilla G, Vemuri S, Rhiner M. (1991). "The Experience of Pain and Perceptions of Quality of Life: Validation of a Conceptual Model." *The Hospice Journal*, 7(3): 9–24.

Ersek M, Ferrell BR. (1994). "Providing Relief from Cancer Pain by Assisting in the Search for Meaning." *Journal of Palliative Care*, 10: 15-22.

Ferrell BR, Dean GE. (1995). "The Meaning of Cancer Pain." *Seminars in Oncology Nursing, 11(1): 17–22.*

Ferrell BR. (1995). "The Impact of Pain on Quality of Life: A Decade of Research." *Nursing Clinics of North America*, 30(4): 609–624.

Juarez G, Ferrell BR, Borneman T. (1998). "Perceptions of Quality of Life in Hispanic Patients with Cancer." *Cancer Practice*, 6(6): 318–324.

Figure 7-1 | Quality of life model.

Betty Ferrell PhD., FAAN and Marcia Grant DNSc, FAAN, City of Hope Medical Center, with permission.

B. Sickle cell pain
   1. Pain management should be aggressive to decrease pain and enable patients to obtain functional ability.
      a. A study of 25 children ages 6 to 16 with sickle cell disease compared with children without the disease showed that children affected by sickle cell pain had seven times increased risk of not attending school and that pain was highly disruptive of social and recreational activities (Fuggle, Shand, Gill, & Davies, 1996).
C. Cancer and HIV pain
   1. Pain can affect adversely the quality of life. It is important to identify high-risk patients.
      a. A study of 133 patients with pancreatic cancer showed that there was a significant correlation between pain and depressive symptoms among patients who experienced pain. Patients with moderate or greater pain had significantly impaired functional activity and poorer quality-of-life scores (Kelsen et al., 1995).
   2. The conceptual model of pain and quality of life initially described by B. R. Ferrell (1995) identifies four dimensions affected by pain (Ferrell, 2005; Ferrell & Coyle, 2002).
      a. *Physical well-being:* Pain leads to lack of sleep, fatigue, and associated symptoms such as nausea or severe gastrointestinal distress from pain or pain medications. Dyspnea, delirium, agitation, and anorexia are possible (Ferrell & Coyle, 2002).
      b. *Psychological well-being:* Anxiety, depression, and fear of future pain occur. Sadness, loneliness, hopelessness, and anger are also common.
      c. *Social concerns:* Pain affects family caregivers and others surrounding the patient by increasing caregiver burden, interfering with sexuality, and greatly impacting role and relationships. For many, pain becomes a family experience.
      d. *Spiritual well-being:* Pain may be viewed as a spiritual crisis as patients experience hopelessness or a sense of abandonment, and undertreated pain causes the person to question the meaning of life and in some situations consider assisted suicide.
   3. Undertreatment of pain has resulted in some patients being labeled as "drug seeking" (McCaffery, Grimm, Pasero, Ferrell, & Uman, 2005).
   4. Helping family members cope can increase their effectiveness as caregivers and can improve the quality of life of patients (Warner, 1992).
   5. Palliative care for the terminally ill focuses on symptom control and pain management. When pain is controlled, other symptoms of terminal illness can be addressed (McCabe, 1997; McMillan, 1996).
      a. Pain can serve as a constant reminder of the progressive nature of the disease. Patients with cancer worry about pain and dying without pain relief. The fear of an inability to cope with the symptoms and the pain of an incurable disease may cause patients to have intense feelings of helplessness and hopelessness (All & Huycke, 1999; Portenoy, 1997).
      b. Dying in America continues to be associated with needless suffering. Pain and other symptoms are poorly assessed and managed. The End of Life Nursing Education Consortium program provides a comprehensive curriculum that can be taught to nurses at various levels in an effort to improve pain and symptom management at the end of life (Paice et al., 2006).
   6. A structured pain education program for patients and their families provides support and improves pain management and quality of life (Ferrell, Ferrell, Ann, & Tran, 1994).
   7. Cognitive-behavioral and psychological interventions can help improve quality of life by giving patients a sense of control and improving their coping skills (Pargeon & Hailey, 1999).
   8. Patients with HIV or AIDS often report hopelessness and suicidal ideation. Children with HIV or AIDS with poorly managed pain are prevented from enjoying life (Carr, 1994).
D. Persistent (chronic nonmalignant) pain
   1. Assessment and management of chronic pain can improve the quality of life. Factors that need to be assessed include the following:
      a. Individual's coping methods and meaning of pain.
      b. Gender and culture.

c. Pain history, present medications, and analgesics that have been used in the past (Luggen, 1998).

2. A comprehensive approach to chronic pain can improve (Gatchel & Turk, 1996) self-care abilities and functional status, as well as coping skills to manage pain.
3. How pain is managed may profoundly affect the quality of life in elderly patients with chronic pain (Closs, 1994).
   a. Mobility and function may be improved (B. R. Ferrell, 1995).
   b. Decreased depression and improved socialization occur (B. R. Ferrell, 1995).
   c. Sleep may be improved (B. R. Ferrell, 1995).
   d. Managing pain can create improvement in functional status, sleep, relationships, and amount of time exercising, which can all positively affect quality of life.
4. Consequences of persistent pain among older people include depression, anxiety, decreased socialization, sleep disturbance, impaired ambulation, and increased health care utilization and costs (American Geriatrics Society [AGS] Panel on Persistent Pain in Older Adults, 2002).
   a. Conditions known to be potentially worsened by the presence of pain include gait disturbances, slow rehabilitation, and adverse effects from multiple drug prescriptions (AGS Panel on Persistent Pain in Older Adults, 2002).
   b. In Europe, 66% of older patients with postherpetic neuralgia and allodynia, who were unable to tolerate systemic treatment, claimed that a lidocaine 5% plasters was superior to systemic treatment; 78% claimed it had improved their quality of life (Meier, Wasner, & Faust, 2003).
   c. Pain management training and education may reduce pain and increase patient satisfaction in the geriatric population, as evidenced by chronic pain treatment outcome studies (Cutler, Fishbain, Rosomoff, & Rosomoff, 1994).
5. In a study of 15 primary care centers in 14 countries, patients with persistent pain were more likely to have an anxiety or depressive disorder, experience significant activity limitations, and have unfavorable health perceptions.
   a. The relationship between disability and persistent pain was inconsistent across centers, indicating a need for further investigation into the role of culture in shaping response (Gureje et al., 1998).

IV. Morbidity and Mortality

A. Acute pain

1. Unrelieved pain evokes a stress response characterized by tachycardia, increased myocardial oxygen consumption, hypercoagulability, immunosuppression, and persistent catabolism (Jacobi et al., 2002).
   a. Pain is associated with reduced natural killer cell counts, indicating an impaired immune response, which can delay or inhibit healing (APS, 2003) (see the chapter on Immunity and Pain).
   b. Pain causes catabolism, which can lead to poor healing, weakness, and muscle breakdown (APS, 2003).
   c. Studies demonstrate an increased incidence of thromboembolic events associated with inadequate pain control due to stress hormone effects and decreased mobility (APS, 2003).
      (1) Deep venous thrombosis was almost four times more likely following general anesthesia than with regional anesthesia techniques in patients with traumatic femoral neck fractures undergoing operative repair (Sorenson & Pace, 1992).
      (2) In a study of 80 patients undergoing major peripheral vascular surgery, venous thrombosis of a coronary artery, deep vein complications, or vascular complications developed in 11 patients receiving general anesthesia with postoperative parenteral, oral, or both types of opioids and in only 1 receiving general anesthesia with epidural anesthesia and analgesia (Tuman et al., 1991).
   d. Pain can impair effective respiration through localized guarding of muscles around the area of pain and a generalized muscle rigidity or spasm that restricts movement of the chest wall

and diaphragm (APS, 2003; Jacobi et al., 2002). Studies demonstrate a decreased incidence of pulmonary complications associated with improved pain control (Wu et al., 2006).

   e. In a meta-analysis of 48 randomized, controlled, clinical trials, when compared to systemic opioids, epidural opioids decreased the incidence of atelectasis; when compared to systemic opioids, epidural local anesthetic decreased the incidence of pulmonary infection and pulmonary complications overall (Ballatyne et al., 1998).

2. Pain can decrease gastrointestinal motility (APS, 2003). Studies demonstrate that improved analgesia is associated with earlier return of gastrointestinal function.
   a. Thoracic epidural analgesia with a local anesthetic-based regimen, when compared with systemic opioid analgesia after general surgery, is associated with significantly earlier return of gastrointestinal function after abdominal surgery in seven randomized trials (Schug, 1999).
   b. The use of epidural local anesthetic, as compared to epidural opioids for postoperative analgesia, is associated with earlier return of gastrointestinal motility after abdominal surgery in four randomized clinical trials (Schug, 1999).
3. Improved analgesia is associated with less agitation, sedation, and mechanical ventilation in the ICU (Malchow & Black, 2008).
4. Pain increases salt and water retention and increases blood pressure (APS, 2003).
5. Poor pain control can cause anxiety, depression, and sleep deprivation (APS, 2003).
6. Poor pain control can lead to the development of posttraumatic stress disorder (PTSD) (Malchow & Black, 2008).
   a. Greater levels of early postinjury emotional distress and physical pain were associated with an increased risk (23%) of symptoms consistent with a PTSD diagnosis in a representative sample of 2,931 injured trauma survivors age 18 to 84 recruited from 9,983 in-patients at 69 hospitals across the United States (Zatzick et al., 2007).
   b. Perioperative low-dose intravenous ketamine may decrease the prevalence of PTSD.
      (1) Soldiers injured in Operation Iraqi Freedom or Operation Enduring Freedom receiving perioperative ketamine had a lower incidence of PTSD than soldiers receiving no ketamine during their surgeries despite having larger burns, having a higher injury severity score, undergoing more operations, and spending more time in the ICU (McGhee, Maani, Garza, Gaylord, & Black, 2008).
7. Poor pain control can lead to the development of chronic pain.
   a. Acute pain can evolve directly into chronic pain, possibly as a reflection of acute pain-induced changes in the central nervous system (neuronal plasticity) (APS, 2008, APS, 2003).
   b. The intensity of acute postoperative pain is a predictor of chronic pain.
      (1) Chronic pain is common after amputation, inguinal hernia surgery, breast surgery, gallbladder surgery, and lung surgery.
      (2) The type of nerve injury may explain the increase in both acute and chronic pain, but other psychological or physiological factors may heighten pain sensitivity (Perkins & Kehlet, 2000).
   c. Patients with serious illnesses who had a high level of pain during hospitalization were at risk for continuous pain 6 months after discharge.
      (1) Of the patients reporting level 4 pain (defined as moderately severe pain occurring most of the time or extremely severe pain occurring half of the time) and level 5 pain (defined as moderately severe pain occurring most or all of the time or extremely severe pain occurring at least half of the time), 39.7% reported level 4 or 5 pain 2 to 6 months later (Desbiens et al., 1997).
8. In a review of 142 trials of 9,553 subjects, when compared with general anesthesia, regional anesthesia reduced overall mortality by approximately 30%. Deaths were most commonly (75%) due to pulmonary embolism, cardiac event, stroke, or infection (Schug, 1999).
   a. In a 5% nationally random sample of Medicare beneficiaries from 1997 to 2001 undergoing various surgical procedures, the presence of epidural analgesia was associated with a signifi-

cantly lower odds of death at 7 and 30 days after surgery; however, no difference was seen among the groups with regard to overall major morbidity, with the exception of an increase in pneumonia at 30 days in the epidural group (Wu et al., 2004).

B. Sickle cell pain
  1. Inadequate treatment of painful events may last 1 week.
  2. Vasoocclusive events (painful crisis), which result in hospitalizations more than three times per year, are associated with an increase in the death rate of patients 20 years and older. Repeated vaso-occlusive crisis may lead to organ or tissue damage and chronic pain (McCaffery & Pasero, 1999).
  3. Chronic pain states can be severely debilitating, physically and psychologically. Chronic pain often is associated with bone changes, such as avascular necrosis or vertebral collapse, or with chronic recurrent leg ulcers.

C. Cancer and HIV pain
  1. Each year, approximately 1.2 million patients are diagnosed with cancer and more than 500,000 die from cancer (Miaskowski et al., 2005).
  2. Pain is present in 20% to 75% of adult patients at the time of cancer diagnosis, in 17% to 57% of patients in active cancer treatment, and in 23% to 100% of patients in advanced and terminal stages of cancer (Miaskowski et al., 2005).
  3. Pain is present in 62% of children at the time of cancer diagnosis, in 25% to 85% of children receiving active treatment, and in 62% to 90% of children at the end of life (Miaskowski et al., 2005).
  4. Unrelieved pain impairs patients' ability to function; results in anxiety, depression, and other mood disturbances; and impairs quality of life (Miaskowski et al., 2005).
     a. Participation in a support group by patients with cancer pain may have a positive impact on their survival (Rustoen & Wikland, 1998).
     b. Management of symptoms and pain is a focus of palliative care and is important in increasing hope and decreasing thoughts of suicide (Beckwith & Cole, 1998).
     c. New pain in immunoincompetent HIV-infected people may signify life-threatening disease.

V. Treatment Outcomes

A. Computer tomography-guided radiofrequency ablation of the spinothalamic tract or trigeminal tract nucleus in the upper cervical region of the spinal cord provided initial pain relief (from 8.5 ± 0.8 to 1.2 ± 1.06) and 6-month follow-up (2.3 ± 0.6) and improvement in sleep (3.25 to 7 hours and then 4.8 hours, respectively) (Raslan, 2008).

B. For many children, treatment-related pain may be more painful than the disease itself.
  1. In children, infections tend to recur and are painful and prolonged. Encephalopathy can cause allodynia and spasticity with severe developmental delays (Czarnecki et al., 1994).

C. Persistent (chronic) nonmalignant pain
  1. Several distinct types of pain exist: nociceptive, inflammatory, neuropathic, and functional.
     a. Identification of the mechanisms responsible for production of distinct pain syndromes and pharmacological tools that act specifically on these mechanisms are key to preventing persistent pain syndromes (Woolf, 2004).
     b. Secondary interventions that promote a return to activity through rehabilitation are needed (Gatchel & Turk, 1996).

D. Psychological interventions and assessing barriers to recovery may be needed to prevent the development of chronic pain.
  1. Follow-up and maintenance may be important for long-term outcomes. Strategies to prevent relapse are needed (Linton & Bradley, 1996).
  2. Identifying risk factors and general screening for risk are important in an attempt to isolate patients who are likely to develop chronic pain problems.
  3. Pain prevention can occur in patients with acute musculoskeletal pain through the following:
     a. Addressing pain behaviors that reinforce pain.
     b. Counseling on the issues of fear and avoidance of movement.

4. The interaction among pain, depression, and functional ability is not fully understood.
    a. A study of 74 elderly (60 to 95 years old) African Americans living in Detroit found that pain interference was significantly related to physical functioning and frequency of aerobic exercise, indicating that pain interference influences participation in these health behaviors.
        (1) Depression was found to account for 28% of the relationship between pain and exercise frequency. Depression was not a mediator between the pain and the physical functioning variable (Patil, Johnson, & Lichtenberg, 2008).
    b. Chronic pain is associated with feelings of depression, which may lead to suicidal ideation (Hitchcock, Ferrell, & McCaffery, 1994).
        (1) Approximately 30% of patients with fibromyalgia are diagnosed as having concurrent depression or anxiety disorders. Patients with fibromyalgia also display high lifetime rates of migraine, irritable bowel syndrome, chronic fatigue, and panic disorder (Hudson, Goldenberg, Pope, Keck, & Schlesinger, 1992).

References

Agency for Health Care Policy and Research. (1994). *Management of cancer pain.* Clinical Practice Guideline. (AHCPR Publication No. 94-0592.) Rockville, MD: U.S. Department of Health and Human Services.

All, A. C., & Huycke, L. I. (1999). Pain, cancer, and older adults. *Geriatric Nursing, 20,* 241–246.

American Chronic Pain Association. (2008). *ACPA chronic pain medication supplement.* Retrieved August 4, 2008, from http://www.theacpa.org/documents/.

American Geriatrics Society Panel on Persistent Pain in Older Adults. (2002). The management of persistent pain in older persons: Clinical practice guideline. *Journal of the American Geriatrics Society,* 50(6 Suppl.), S205–S224.

American Pain Society. (1995). Quality improvement guidelines for the treatment of acute pain and cancer pain. *Journal of the American Medical Association, 274,* 1874–1880.

American Pain Society. (1999). *Guidelines for the management of acute and chronic pain in sickle cell disease.* Glenview, IL: Author.

American Pain Society. (2003). *Principles of analgesic use in the treatment of acute pain and cancer pain* (5th ed.). Glenview, IL: Author.

American Pain Society. (2008). *Principles of analgesic use in the treatment of acute pain and cancer pain* (6th ed.). Glenview, IL: Author.

Anderson, K. O., Mendoza, T. R., Valero, V., Richman, S. R., Russel, C., Hurley, J., DeLeon, C., Washington, P., Palos, G., Payne, R., & Cleeland, C. S. (2000). Minority cancer patients and their providers: Pain management attitudes and practice. *Cancer, 88,* 1929–1938.

Apfelbaum, J. L., Chen, C., Mehta, S. S., Gan, T. J., & Tong, J. (2003). Postoperative pain experience: results from a national survey suggest postoperative pain continues to be under managed. *Anesthesia & Analgesia, 97*(2), 534–540.

Ballantyne, J. D., Carr, D. B., deFerrati, S., Suaree, T., Lau, J., Chalmers, T. C., Angellilo, I. F., & Mosteller, F. (1998). The comparative effects of postoperative analgesic therapies on pulmonary outcomes: Cumulative meta-analyses of randomized, controlled trials. *Anesthesia & Analgesia, 86,* 598–610.

Beach, P. (2007). *Osteoarthritis: Evidence-based nursing monographs.* Retrieved July 31, 2008, from http://www.nursingconsult.com/das/ebnm/view/100994197-2.

Beckwith, S. K., & Cole, B. E. (1998). Hospice, cancer pain management, and symptoms control. In R. S. Weiner (Ed.), *Pain management* (Vol. 2, pp. 703–720). Boca Raton, FL: St. Lucia Press.

Borsook, D., LeBel, A. A., & McPeck, B. (Eds.). (1996). *The Massachusetts General Hospital handbook of pain management.* Boston: Little, Brown.

Breitbart, W., Kaim, M., & Rosenfield, B. (1999). Clinician's perceptions of barriers to pain management in AIDS. *Journal of Pain and Symptom Management, 18,* 203–212.

Carr, D. B. (Ed.). (1994). *Pain in HIV/AIDS.* Washington, DC: Robert G. Addison, France, USA Pain Association.

Cicala, R. S., & Wright, H. (1989). Outpatient treatment of patients with chronic pain: An analysis of cost savings. *Clinical Journal of Pain, 5,* 223–226.

Closs, S. J. (1994). Pain in elderly patients: A neglected phenomenon? *Journal of Advanced Nursing, 19,* 1072–1081.

Cohen, E., Botti, M., Hanna, B., Leach, S., Boyd, S., & Robbins, J. (2007). Pain beliefs and pain management of oncology patients. *Cancer Nursing, 31*(2), E1–E8.

Creamer, P., Lethbridge-Cejku, M., & Hochberg, M. C. (1999). Determinants of pain severity in knee osteoarthritis: Effect of demographic and psychosocial variables using three pain measures. *Journal of Rheumatology, 26,* 1785–1792.

Cutler, R. B., Fishbain, D. A., Rosomoff, R. S., & Rosomoff, H. L. (1994). Outcomes in treatment of pain in geriatric and younger age groups. *Archives of Physical Medicine and Rehabilitation, 75,* 457–464.

Czarnecki, L., Dollfas, C., & Strafford, M. (1994). Children with pain and HIV/AIDS. In D. B. Carrr (Ed.), *Pain in HIV/AIDS* (pp. 48–54). Washington, DC: Robert G. Addison, France, USA Pain Association.

Dahl, J., Berry, P., Stevenson, K. M., Gordon, D., & Ward, S. (1998). Institutionalizing pain management: Making pain assessment and treatment an integral part of the nation's health care system. *APS Bulletin, 8,* 19–20.

Desbiens, N. A., Wu, A. W., Alzola, C., Mueller-Rizap, N., Wenger, N. S., Connors, A. F., Lynn, J., & Phillips, R. S. (1997). Pain during hospitalization is associated with continuous pain six months later in survivors of serious illness. *American Journal of Medicine, 102,* 269–276.

Ferrell, B. (2005). Ethical perspectives on pain and suffering. *Pain Management Nursing, 6*(3), 83–90.

Ferrell, B. R. (1995). Pain evaluation and management in the nursing home. *Annals of Internal Medicine, 123,* 681–687.

Ferrell, B. R. (1995). The impact of pain on quality of life. *Nursing Clinics of North America, 30,* 609–624.

Ferrell, B. R., & Coyle, N. (2002). An overview of palliative nursing care. *American Journal of Nursing, 7*(4), 163–168.

Ferrell, B. R., Ferrell, B. A., Ann, C., & Tran, K. (1994). Pain management for elderly patients with cancer at home. *Cancer, 74*(7 Suppl.), 2139–2146.

Ferrell, B. R., Novy, D., Sullivan, M. D., Banja, J., Dubois, M. Y., & Gitlin, M. (2001). Ethical dilemmas in pain management. *Journal of Pain, 2,* 171–180.

Fuggle, P., Shand, P. A., Gill, L. J., & Davies, S. C. (1996). Pain, quality of life, and coping in sickle cell disease. *Archives of Disease in Childhood, 75,* 1999–2003.

Gatchel, R. J., & Turk, D. C. (Eds.). (1996). *Psychological approaches to pain management.* New York: Guilford Press.

Grass, J. A. (1993). Surgical outcome: Regional anesthesia and analgesia versus general anesthesia. *Anesthesiology Review, 20,* 117–125.

Gureje, O., Von Korff, M., Simon, G., & Gater, R. (1998). Persistent pain and well-bring: A World Health Organization study in primary care. *Journal of the American Medical Association, 280*(2), 147–151.

Hitchcock, L. S., Ferrell, B. F., & McCaffery, M. (1994). The experience of chronic nonmalignant pain. *Journal of Pain and Symptom Management, 9,* 312–318.

Hudson, J., Goldenberg, D., Pope, H., Keck, P., & Schlesinger, L. (1992). Comorbidity of fibromyalgia with medical and psychiatric disorders. *American Journal of Medicine, 92,* 363–367.

Jacobi, J., Fraser, G. L., Coursin, D. B., Riker, R. R., Fontaine, D., Wittbrodt, E. T., Chalfin, D. B., Masica, M. F., Bjerke, H. S., Coplin, W. M., Crippen, D. W., Fuchs, B. D., Kelleher, R. M., Marik, P. E., Nasraway, S. A., Murray, M. J., Peruzzi, W. T., & Lum, P. D. (2002). Clinical practice guidelines for the sustained use of sedatives and analgesics in the critically ill adult. *Critical Care Medicine, 30*(1), 119–141.

Joint Commission. (2008). *Comprehensive accreditation manual for hospitals.* Oakbrook Terrace, IL; Author.

Kawamata, R., Omote, K., Kawamata, M., & Namiki, A. (1998). Premedication with oral dextromethorphan reduces postoperative pain after tonsillectomy. *Anesthesia & Analgesia, 86,* 594–597.

Kee, W. G., Middaugh, S., & Pawlick, K. (1997). Cost benefit analysis of a multidisciplinary chronic pain program. *American Journal of Pain Management, 7,* 59–62.

Kelsen, D. P., Portenoy, R. K., Thaler, H. T., Niedzwieck, D., Passik, S. D., Tao, Y., Banks, W., Brennan, M. L., & Foley, K. M. (1995). Pain and depression in patients with newly diagnosed pancreatic cancer. *Journal of Clinical Oncology, 13,* 748–755.

Larsen, M. M. (1996). Unscheduled cancer pain admissions costly: Close to $5 million a year at M. D. Anderson. *Oncology News International, 5,* 3.

Layeeque, R., Hochberg, J., Siegel, E., Kunkel, K., Kepple, J., Henry-Tillman, R., Dunlap, M., Seibert, J., & Klimberg, V. S. (2004). Botulinum toxin infiltration for pain control after mastectomy and expander reconstruction. *Annals of Surgery, 240*(4), 608–614.

Levy, M. H. (1994). Pharmacologic management of cancer pain. *Seminars in Oncology, 21,* 718–739.

Li, S. S., Coloma, M., White, P., Watcha, M., Chiu, J. W., Li, H., & Huber, P. J. (2000). Comparison of the costs and recovery profiles of three anesthetic techniques for ambulatory anorectal surgery. *Anesthesiology, 93*(5), 1225–1230.

Linton, S. J., & Bradley, L. A. (1996). Strategies for the prevention of chronic pain. In A. J. Gatchel & D. C. Turk (Eds.), *Psychological approaches to pain management* (pp. 438–457). New York: Guilford Press.

Liu, S. S., Carpenter, R. L., Mackey, D. C., Thirlby, R. C., Rupp, S. M., Shine, T. S. J., Feinglass, N. G., Metzger, P. P., Flumer, J. T., & Smith, S. L. (1995). Effects of perioperative analgesia technique on rate of recovery after colon surgery. *Anesthesiology, 83,* 757–765.

Luggen, A. S. (1998). Healthy people 2000 chronic pain in older adults: A quality of life issue. *Journal of Gerontological Nursing, 24,* 48–54.

Malchow, R. J., & Black, I. H. (2008). The evolution of pain management in critically ill trauma patients: emerging concepts from the global war on terrorism. *Critical Care Medicine, 36*(7 Suppl.), S346–S357.

Maruta, T., Malinchoc, M., Offord, K. P., & Colligan, R. C. (1997). Status of patients with chronic pain 13 years after treatment in a pain management center. *Pain, 74,* 199–204.

McCabe, M. J. (1997). Ethical issues in pain management. *Hospice Journal, 12,* 25–32.

McCaffery, M., & Pasero, C. (1999). *Pain: Clinical Manual* (2nd ed.). St. Louis: Mosby.

McCaffery, M., Grimm, M. A., Pasero, C., Ferrell, B., & Uman, G. (2005). On the meaning of "drug seeking." *Pain Management Nursing, 6*(4), 122–136.

McCarberg, G., Nicholson, B., Todd, K., Palmer, T., & Penles, L. (2008). The impact of pain on quality of life and the unmet needs of pain management: Results from pain sufferers and physicians participating in an internet survey. *American Journal of Therapeutics, 15*(4), 312–320.

McGhee, L. L., Maani, C. V., Garza, T. H., Gaylord, K. M., & Black, I. H. (2008). The correlation between ketamine and posttraumatic stress disorder in burned service members. *Trauma, 64*(2 Suppl.), S195–S199.

McMillan, S. C. (1996). Pain and pain relief experienced by hospice patients with cancer. *Cancer Nursing, 19,* 298–307.

Meier, T., Wasner, G., & Faust, M. (2003). Efficacy of lidocaine patch 5% in the treatment of focal peripheral neuropathic pain syndromes: A randomized, double blind, placebo-controlled study. *Pain, 106*(1–2), 151–158.

Mercandante, S., Casuccio, A., Angello, A., Pumo, S., Kargar, J., & Garofalo, S. (1999). Analgesics effects of non-steroidal anti-inflammatory drugs in cancer pain due to somatic or visceral mechanisms. *Journal of Pain and Symptom Management, 5,* 351–356.

Miaskowski, C., & Dibble, S. L. (1995). The problem of pain in outpatients with breast cancer. *Oncology Nursing Forum, 22,* 791–797.

Miaskowski, C., Cleary, J., Burney, R., Coyne, P., Finley, R., Foster, R., Grossman, S., Janjan, N., Ray, J., Syrjala, K., Weisman, S., & Zahrbock, C. (2005). *Guideline for the management of cancer pain in adults and children* (No. 3). Glenview, IL: American Pain Society.

Moore, R., & Brodsgaard, I. (1999). Cross-cultural investigations of pain. In P. R. Croft, S. J. Linton, L. LeResche, & M. Von Korff (Eds.), *Epidemiology of pain* (pp. 63–80). Seattle: IASP Press.

National Institutes of Health State-of-the-Science Statement. (2002). *Symptom management in cancer pain, depression and fatigue.* Retrieved August 13, 2008, from http:/consensus.nih.gov/2002/2002CancerPainDepressionFatigue/.

Obata, H., Saito, S., Fujita, N., Fuse, Y., Ishizaki, K., & Goto, F. (1999). Epidural block with mepivacaine before surgery reduces long-term post-thoracotomy pain. *Canadian Journal of Anaesthesia, 46,* 1127–1132.

O'Donovan, S., Ferrara, A., Larach, S., & Williams, P. (1994). Intraoperative use of Toradol facilitates outpatient hemorrhoidectomy. *Diseases of the Colon and Rectum, 37,* 793–799.

Paice, J. A., Ferrell, B. R., Virani, R., Grant, M., Malloy, P., & Rhome, A. (2006). Graduate nursing education regarding end-of-life care. *Nursing Outlook, 54*(1), 46–52.

Pargeon, K. L., & Hailey, B. J. (1999). Barriers to effective cancer pain management: A review of the literature. *Journal of Pain and Symptom Management, 18,* 358–368.

Patil, S. K., Johnson, A. Sc., & Lichtenberg, P. (2008). The relation of pain and depression with various health-promoting behaviors in African American elders. *Rehabilitation Psychology, 53*(1), 85–92.

Payne, R., Medina, E., & Hampton, J. W. (2003). Quality of life concerns in patients with breast cancer: Evidence for disparity of outcomes and experiences in pain management and palliative care among African-American women. *Cancer, 97,* 311–317.

Perin, M. L. (2000). Corticosteroids for cancer pain. *American Journal of Nursing, 100,* 15–16.

Perkins, F. M., & Kehlet, H. (2000). Chronic pain as an outcome of surgery: A review of predictive factors. *Anesthesiology, 93*(4), 1123–1133.

Platt, O. S., Thorington, B. D., Brambilla, D. J., Milner, P. F., Rosse, W. F., Vichinsky, E., & Kinney, T. R. (1991). Pain in sickle-cell disease: Rates and risk factors. *New England Journal of Medicine, 325,* 11–16.

Polomano, R., Rathmell, J., Krenzischek, D., & Dunwoody, C. (2008). Emerging trends and new approaches to acute pain management. *Pain Management Nursing, 9*(Suppl. 1), S33–S41.

Poniatowski, B. C. (1991). Continuous subcutaneous infusion for pain control. *Journal of Intravenous Nursing, 14,* 30–35.

Portenoy, R. K. (1997). *Contemporary diagnosis and management of pain in oncologic and AIDS patients.* Newtown, PA: Handbooks in Health Care.

Rahimi, S. Y., Vender, J. R., Macomson, S. D., French, A. B. S., Smith, J. R., & Alleyne, C. H. (2006). Postoperative pain management after craniotomy: Evaluation and cost analysis. *Neurosurgery, 59*(4), 852–857.

Raslan, A. M. (2008). Percutaneous computed tomography–guided radiofrequency ablation of upper spinal cord pain pathways for cancer-related pain. *Operative Neurosurgery, 62*(3 Suppl. 1), 226–234.

Reese, F. L., & Smith, W. R. (1997). Psychosocial determinants of health care utilization in sickle cell disease patients. *Annals of Behavioral Medicine, 19,* 171–178.

Ritchie, E. D., Tong, D., Chung, F., Norris, A. M., Miniaci, A., & Vairavanathan, S. D. (1997). Suprascapular nerve block for postoperative pain relief in arthroscopic shoulder surgery: A new modality. *Anesthesia & Analgesia, 84*(6), 1306–1312.

Robinson, R., Birnbaum, H., Morley, M., Sisitsky, S. Greenberg, P., & Claxton, A. (2003). Economic cost and epidemiological characteristics of patients with fibromyalgia claims. *Journal of Rheumatology, 30,* 1318–1325.

Rustoen, T., & Wikland, I. (1998). Nursing intervention to increase hope and quality of life in newly diagnosed cancer patients. *Cancer Nursing, 21,* 235–245.

Schug, S. A. (1999). Is regional anesthesia better than general anesthesia? In *Syllabus of the 24th Annual Meeting of the American Society of Regional Anesthesia* (pp. 62–64). Philadelphia: American Society of Regional Anesthesia.

Shang, A., & Gan, T. (2003). Optimising postoperative pain management in the ambulatory patient. *Drugs, 63*(9), 855–867.

Shealy, C. N., & Cady, R. (1998). Multidisciplinary pain clinics. In R. J. Weiner (Ed.), *Pain management* (pp. 35–44). Boca Raton, FL: St. Lucia Press.

Smedstad, K. G., Beattie, W. S., Blair, W. S., & Buckley, D. N. (1992). Postoperative pain relief and hospital stay after total esophagectomy. *Clinical Journal of Pain, 8*(2), 149–153.

Song, D., Greilich, N. B., White, P. F., Watcha, M. F., & Tongier, W. K. (2000). Recovery profiles and costs of anesthesia for outpatient unilaterial inguinal herniorrhaphy. *Anesthesia & Analgesia, 91*(4), 876–881.

Sorenson, R. M., & Pace, N. L. (1992). Anesthetic techniques during surgical repair of femoral neck fractures: A meta-analysis. *Anesthesiology, 77,* 1095–1104.

Sprott, H. (2003). What can rehabilitation interventions achieve in patients with primary fibromyalgia? *Current Opinions in Rheumatology, 15,* 145–150.

Stewart, W., Ricci, J., Chee, E., Morganstein, D., & Lipton, R. (2003). Lost productive time and cost due to common pain conditions in the U.S. workforce. *Journal of the American Medical Association, 290*(18), 2443–2454.

Tuman, K. J., McCarthy, R. J., March, R. J., DeLaria, G. A., Patel, R. V., & Ivankovich, A. D. (1991). Effects of epidural anesthesia and analgesia on coagulation and outcome after major vascular surgery. *Anesthesia & Analgesia, 73,* 696–704.

Turk, D. C. (1996). Biopsychosocial perspective on chronic pain. In R. J. Gatchel & D. C. Turk (Eds.), *Psychological approaches to pain management* (pp. 3–32). New York: Guilford Press.

Turk, D. C., & Okifuji, A. (1998). Interdisciplinary approach to pain management: Philosophy, operations, and efficacy. In M. A. Ashburn & L. J. Rice (Eds.), *The management of pain* (pp. 235–248). New York: Churchill Livingstone.

Warner, T. E. (1992). Involvement of families in pain control of terminally ill patients. *Hospice Journal, 8,* 155–170.

Wasylak, R. J., Abbott, F. V., English, M. J., & Jeans, M. E. (1990). Reduction of postoperative morbidity following patients controlled morphine. *Canadian Journal of Anesthesia, 27,* 726–731.

Weltz, C. R., Greengrass, R. A., & Lyerly, H. K. (1995). Ambulatory surgical management of breast carcinoma using paravertebral block. *Annals of Surgery, 222,* 19–21.

Wolfe, F., Smythe, H., Yunus, M., Bennett, R., Bombardier, C., Goldeberg, D., Tugwell, P., Campbell, S., Abeles, M., Clark, P., Fam, A., Farber, S., Fiechtner, J., Franklin, C., Gatter, R., Hamaty, D., Lessard, J., Lichtbroun, A., Masi, A., McCkain, G., Reynolds, W., Romano, T., Russell, I., & Sheon, R. (1990). The American College of Rheumatology 1990 criteria for the classification of fibromyalgia: Report of the Multicenter Criteria Committee. *Arthritis & Rheumatism, 33,* 160–172.

Woolf, C. J. (2004). Pain: Moving from symptom control toward mechanism-specific pharmacologic management. *Annals of Internal Medicine, 140*(6), 441–451.

Wu, C., Cohen, S. R., Richman, J. M., Rowlingson, A. J., Courpas, G. E., Cheung, K., Lin, E. E., & Liu, S. S. (2005). Efficacy of postoperative patient-controlled and continuous infusion epidural analgesia versus intravenous patient-controlled analgesia with opioids: A meta-analysis. *Anesthesiology, 103,* 1079–1088.

Wu, C., Hurley, R. W., Anderson, G. F., Herbert, R., Rowlingson, A. J., & Fleisher, L. A. (2004). Effect of postoperative epidural analgesia on morbidity and mortality following surgery in Medicare patients. *Regional Anesthesia & Pain Medicine, 29,* 525–533.

Wu, C., Naqibuddin, M., Rowlingson, A. J., Steven, A., Jermyn, R. M., & Fleisher, L. A. (2003). The effect of pain on health-related quality of life in the immediate postoperative period. *Anesthesia & Analgesia, 97,* 1078–1085.

Wu, C., Sapirstein, A., Herbert, R., Rowlingson, A. J., Michaels, R. K., Petrovic, M. A., & Fleisher, L. A. (2006). Effect of postoperative epidural analgesia on morbidity and mortality after lung resection in Medicare patients. *Journal of Clinical Anesthesia, 18,* 515–520.

Zatzick, D. F., Rivara, F. P., Nathens, A. B., Jurkovich, G. J., Wang, J., Fan, M., Russo, J., Salkever, D. S., & Mackenzie, E. J. (2007). A nationwide U.S. study of post-traumatic stress after hospitalization for physical injury. *Psychological Medicine, 37,* 1469–1480.

Suggested Readings

Ferrell, B. R., & Coyle, N. (2007). *Textbook of palliative nursing.* New York: Oxford University Press.

Moore, C. M., Cross, M. H., Desborough, J. P., Burrin, J. M., MacDonald, I. A., & Hall, G. M. (1995). Hormonal effects of thoracic extradural analgesia for cardiac surgery. *British Journal of Anaesthesia, 75,* 387–393.

St. Marie, B., & Arnold, S. (Eds.). (2002). *When your pain flares up: Easy, proven techniques for managing chronic pain.* Minneapolis: Fairview Press.

Warfield, C. A., & Bajwa, Z. H. (2004). *Principles & practice of pain management* (2nd ed.). New York: McGraw-Hill.

Wu, C. L., & Fleisher, L. A. (2000). Outcomes research in regional anesthesia and analgesia. *Regional Anesthesia & Pain Medicine, 91,* 1232–1242.

section

2

Advocating for Patients in Pain

chapter

8

Historical and Cultural Influences on Pain Perceptions and Barriers to Treatment

Christina L. Clyde, MS, RN-BC
Kathleen Anne Kwiatkowski, BA, RN, L.Ac

Objectives

After studying this chapter, the reader should be able to:

1. **Describe the evolution of pain concepts, cause, and treatment from primitive societies to the present.**
2. **Define cultural concepts examining the effects of culture on the expression and treatment of pain.**
3. **Examine cultural perspectives related to pain among several select populations.**
4. **Discuss communication barriers and strategies to enhance pain assessment and treatment.**
5. **Identify cultural barriers and disparities among populations.**

The French surgeon Daetigus wrote: "Were we to imagine ourselves suspended in timeless space over an abyss out of which the sounds of revolving earth rose to our ears, we would hear naught but an elemental roar of pain uttered as with one voice by suffering mankind" (Bonica, 1990). Pain is considered one of the greatest factors to shape the course of human events, for it affects all humans (Bonica, 1990).

Beliefs regarding pain and its treatment are influenced by historical events that are unique to any given culture. Examination of these events may give some insight into current cultural beliefs and the treatment of pain today.

Part One: Evolution of Pain: A Historical Perspective

I. **Early Societies (BC, AD)**
   A. Pain treatment was influenced primarily by magic and religious undercurrents.
   B. Treatment modalities
      1. Ritual activity, charms, tattoos, herbs, chants, and incantations were used to ward off demons (Warfield, 1988).
      2. Administration of medicine was assigned to a sorceress, priestess, or shaman.
      3. Physical therapies were common (Bonica, 1990).
         a. Methods of physical therapies
            (1) Pressure, friction, and application of heat and cold were used in alleviating pain.
            (2) Oil, stones, massage, and laying of hands over the affected area were used.
   C. Mesopotamian and early Hebrew civilizations (AD) (Raj, 1995)
      1. Mesopotamians
         a. Mesopotamians introduced drugs (e.g., opium) and surgical procedures such as bloodletting and burr holes as pain therapies.
         b. They developed a multidisciplinary approach to pain management.
         c. The team of practitioners may have included a shaman, priest, physician, and exorcist.
      2. Early Hebrews
         a. Early Hebrews considered pain and suffering as punishment from God.
         b. This belief was based on biblical interpretation.
   D. Egyptians
      1. Egyptians considered pain to be a result of spirits of the dead entering living bodies by way of the ears and nares (Bonica, 1990).
      2. They promoted treatment and practices based primarily on purging the body of such influences (Warfield, 1988).
      3. They used medicinal herbs to induce vomiting, sweating, urinating, and sneezing.
      4. Egyptians performed surgery such as trephining (drilling of the skull) for treatment of headaches.
      5. They introduced the application of an electrotherapy technique.
         a. The process involved the placement of an electric fish from the Nile River over the wound.
         b. The practice was similar to modern-day transcutaneous electrical nerve stimulation therapy.
   E. Ancient Indians
      1. Buddhist philosophy held that pain was brought on by a frustration of desires (Keele, 1957).
         a. Ancient Indians placed great significance on the relationship between emotion and pain.
      2. Hindus believed that pain originated and was experienced in the heart (Warfield, 1988).
      3. Treatment and modalities
         a. Ancient Indians encouraged the practice of chanting as a diversional activity in relief of pain.
            (1) The practice compared with modern-day relaxation techniques and biofeedback (Warfield, 1988).

F. Ancient China
 1. Medical practice was influenced by two important figures: Emperor Shen Nung and Emperor Huang Ti in 2800 to 2500 BC, respectively. These practices of medicine are used in China today (Bonica, 1990).
  a. Shen Nung (Raj, 1995)
   (1) The emperor assisted in the vast expansion of Chinese pharmacopoeia by introducing the willow plant.
    (a) The willow contains salicylic acid.
    (b) This was used in treatment of rheumatic pain.
   (2) Siberian wort was also used.
    (a) Siberian wort is antispasmodic.
    (b) It offered relief for back pain sufferers.
  b. Huang Ti
   (1) Huang Ti developed the theories and practice of acupuncture.
   (2) Concepts and practice (Bonica, 1990)
    (a) Two opposing forces—yin (negative, feminine, passive) and yang (positive, masculine, active)—are instrumental in maintaining balance and vital energy (chi) within the body. Illness, stress, and pain cause disruption to these forces.
    (b) The practice works to correct physical imbalances in the body brought on by stress, pain, and illness by the placement of small needles along a network of meridians (composed of 14 channels), which connect to each organ; the practice alters organ function.

G. Ancient Greeks
 1. Ancient Greeks expanded their pharmacopoeia with opium derivatives and began significant use of topical medicine applied locally to wounds to reduce pain, dry secretions, and hasten healing (Raj, 1995).
 2. Philosophers explored the origin and nature of sensory data and the sense organs (Bonica, 1990).
  a. Aristotle (Warfield, 1988)
   (1) Aristotle believed that pain originated in the heart and began with increased sensitivity to touch.
   (2) He distinguished the five senses as seeing, hearing, tasting, smelling, and touching.
  b. Hippocrates (Warfield, 1988)
   (1) Hippocrates believed pain was exhibited as a manifestation of disequilibrium of humors and classified patients in categories.
    (a) Blood: heart ailments
    (b) Phlegm: respiratory ailments
    (c) Yellow or black bile: gastrointestinal ailments

H. Romans (AD 1st century)
 1. Roman philosophers Celsus and Galen influenced Roman thought regarding pain management.
  a. Celsus
   (1) Celsus was the first to document the use of analgesic pills (Raj, 1995).
  b. Galen
   (1) Galen classified dispositions based on the Greek theory of humors as phlegmatic, sanguine, choleric, and melancholic (Raj, 1995).
   (2) He classified nerves as sensory and motor (Bonica, 1990).

I. Middle Ages
 1. Major epidemics plagued the population.
 2. Many people became disillusioned with the deficits of medical thought and knowledge.
 3. At this time, Christianity was on the rise; consequently, religious beliefs, not reason, strongly influenced the practice of medicine (Raj, 1995).

J. Renaissance
   1. Universities promoted advances in chemistry (alchemy), physics, and anatomy and physiology (Bonica, 1990).
   2. Paracelsus (physician, early to mid-1500s)
      a. Paracelsus is thought to be the first to make ether (Raj, 1995).
      b. He combined ether and alcohol to create laudanum, allowing greater potency as an analgesic (Clendening, 1933).
      c. He advocated physical therapies, such as massage, exercise, and electrotherapy.

II. 16th to Early 19th Centuries (Cousins & Phillips, 1986)

A. Refrigeration anesthesia (application of cold) was used before surgery in 1646.
   1. Compression anesthesia (use of tourniquets to numb area) was first used in the late 16th century.

B. Progress in pain management developed slowly until the mid-19th century, when major advances took place in three important fields.
   1. Administration of opiates and hypnotics
   2. Inhalation of analgesic and anesthetic gases
   3. Administration of local anesthetics by various means

C. Morphine was isolated from opium in 1803 (Warfield, 1988).
   1. A dosage scale was established in 1817 (Raj, 1995).

D. Ether was recognized by 1846 as an effective general anesthetic (Warfield, 1988).

E. Chloroform was introduced as an alternative to ether in childbirth as the need arose to avoid ether side effects.

III. Late 19th Century

A. Silas Weir Mitchell studied patients from the Civil War.
   1. He acknowledged symptoms from wounds to peripheral nerves.
   2. He termed this "causalgia" (University of Illinois, Department of Neurology, 2008).

B. Cocaine was recognized as effective local anesthetic agent in 1884 (Cousins & Phillips, 1986).

C. Radiotherapy
   1. Wilhelm Röntgen was instrumental in providing roentgen rays as a new modality to alleviate pain in 1895 (Clendening, 1960).

D. Aspirin was introduced as an analgesic in 1899 (Warfield, 1988).

E. Surgery
   1. Key contributors in the development of surgical procedures in pain therapy include the following (Raj, 1995):
      a. Hersley of England developed surgery for trigeminal neuralgia.
      b. Robert Abbe introduced posterior rhizotomy in 1896.
      c. William G. Spiller and Charles H. Frazier performed neurectomy and cordotomy.
      d. Professor Della G. Ruggi proposed sympathectomy in treatment of visceral pain.

F. Physical therapy
   1. Physical measures reemerged in pain management.
   2. Techniques included light therapy, electrotherapy, hydrotherapy, thermotherapy, and mechanotherapy (Krusen, 1940, as cited in Raj, 1995).

G. Neurophysiology discoveries (see the chapter on Theories of Pain)

IV. 20th Century

A. Progress in the field of pain at the cellular and tissue level in specific body areas was the work of leading pain pioneers.

B. Rene Leriche, French surgeon
   1. Leriche developed periarterial sympathectomies after observing vasomotor changes in limbs and studied phantom limb pain in 1916 during World War I (Zimmermann, M., 2006).

C. William K. Livingston, American surgeon
   1. Livingston studied phantom limb pain and developed ganglionectomies and novocaine blocks to treat patients during World War II (Livingston & Fields, 1998).
D. Ronald Melzack, Canadian psychologist, and Patrick Wall, British physiologist
   1. Melzack and Wall published a paper introducing the gate-control theory to pain.
   2. Their paper, "Pain mechanisms: A new theory" (Melzack & Wall, 1965) has been described as "the most influential ever written in the field of pain" (see the chapter on Theories of Pain).
E. John C. Liebeskind, American psychologist
   1. Liebeskind published findings that stimulus-produced analgesia was blocked by the opiate antagonist, naloxone, in 1972 (Terman, 1999).
F. Hans Kosterlitz, British biologist, and associates
   1. Kosterlitz and associates discovered enkephalin, the first known opioid produced in the human body, in 1977 (Nash, 2008).
G. John Bonica, American anesthesiologist
   1. Bonica was the first physician to address chronic pain complicated by psychological problems and drug abuse from injured veterans who are home from World War II.
   2. He believed chronic pain was best managed by a team of interdisciplinary specialists (Raj, 1995).
H. Evolution of pain centers (Raj, 1995)
   1. Post-World War II (1944-1948)
      a. Pain clinics were established by anesthesiologists, initially known as *nerve block clinics,* secondary to the method or technique preferred in treating pain.
      b. The 1950 to 1960 decade was an era of continued growth of nerve block clinics.
   2. In 1960, Bonica developed the first multidisciplinary pain center at the University of Washington. This served as a prototype for the development of many clinics in the United States and abroad.
   3. In 1979, selective spinal analgesia was discovered (Cousins, Mather, Glynn, Wilson, & Graham, 1979).
I. Hospice (see the chapter on Palliative Care)
   1. Cicely Saunders is credited with founding of the modern hospice movement, which developed out of her work with patients in the late 1940s.
   2. St. Christopher's Hospice was opened in London in 1967 as a teaching and research institution dedicated to the emotional, physical, and spiritual needs of the dying.
   3. Saunders promoted substituting pain medication "on demand" for the "time-based" dose regimes used in hospitals (De Boulay, 1984).
      a. Saunders advocated for the use of Brompton's mixture or cocktail for hospice patients as a pain suppressant.
         (1) Primary ingredients included morphine, cocaine, ethyl alcohol, and chlorpromazine.
         (2) Variations in replacing agents in the mixture were based on patient needs (De Boulay, 1984).
J. Organization of pain societies
   1. The International Association for the Study of Pain (IASP) was established in 1974.
      a. Journal: *Pain*
      b. There are 55 IASP chapters on six continents and 6,708 members.
      c. IASP holds a World Congress on Pain every 3 years (IASP, 2008).
   2. The American Society of Regional Anesthesia was established in 1976.
      a. Journal: *Regional Anesthesia and Pain Medicine*
   3. The American Pain Society (APS) was established in 1977.
      a. Journal: *Pain Forum Quarterly*
      b. There are 3,550 members representing 30 fields.
      c. APS holds yearly scientific meetings (American Pain Society, 2008).
   4. The American Academy of Pain Medicine was formed in 1983.

5. The American Society of Pain Management Nurses (ASPMN) was established in 1990. It was later renamed the American Society for Pain Management Nursing.
   a. Journal: *Pain Management Nursing*
   b. ASPMN meets annually (ASPMN, 2008).
   c. First pain management certification examination in 2005 in a partnership venture between the American Nurses Credentialing Center (ANCC) and ASPMN.
6. The American Association of Cancer Pain Initiative was established in 1998.

K. Policies and legislation (see chapter on Social, Political and Ethical Forces Influencing Nursing Practice)

Part Two: Current Cultural Viewpoints

I. Cultural Concepts

A. It is important to define terminology accurately to fully understand how these concepts interrelate and to ensure the same point of reference.

1. *Culture* is the beliefs, values, and practices shared by a group or community of people. This *learned* behavior is passed down from one generation to the next (Weber, 1996).
2. The term *race* is often used interchangeably with *ethnicity. Race* is defined as a shared biological origin (Shire, 2002). Race classifies major groups of people according to ancestry, physical characteristics, and heredity (Tan, Jensen, Thornby, & Anderson, 2005).
3. *Ethnicity* is the circumstance of belonging to a particular ethnic group, sharing characteristics such as common geographical origin, race, language, religion, tradition, values, symbols, literature, folklore, music, food, settlement patterns, and employment patterns (Spector, 1985).
4. *Ethnocentrism* is the belief that one's own culture is better or superior to all others, believing that one's own way of acting, thinking, and behaving is the best way (Leininger, 1995).
5. *Stereotyping* is an assumption about an individual or group based on some common information related to ethnic background (Weber, 1996). It is an ending point; no attempt is made to find out more information about the individual or group (Galanti, 1991).
6. *Generalization* refers to traits that are common to a group, considered a beginning point; however, further information must be obtained before any conclusions can be made about a particular individual (Galanti, 1991).
7. *Acculturation* is a process by which an individual or group takes on the behaviors, values, and lifeways of the dominant culture (Leininger, 1995).
8. *Assimilation* is the incorporation of select characteristics or features of another culture by an individual or group without taking on the total attributes of the particular culture (Leininger, 1995).
9. *Cultural humility* is a commitment and active engagement in a lifelong process that one enters into with others, including oneself. This process includes self-evaluation and humility to balance the dynamics that exist between practitioner-patient communication by using patient-focused care, as well as developing advocacy partnerships with the communities served. For further information on ground work in this area, refer to http://www.ampainsoc.org/advocacy/ethnoracial.htm (American Pain Society, 2009)
   a. For example, an African-American nurse caring for a Hispanic woman just after surgery attributes the patient's moans to the "overexpression of pain," which she believes is related to a cultural response rather than the pain itself. The nurse had undergone cultural training in nursing school and considered herself knowledgeable. Cultural humility is more than completing a series of training classes; it involves self-evaluation and an openness to engage in a dialogue that is focused on the patient, with the interaction being directed more by the patient than by the health care provider (Tervalon & Murray-Garcia, 1998).
10. *Cultural diversity* encompasses the cultural differences that exist between people, including language, dress, traditions, social organization, beliefs about morality and religion, and their interaction with the environment.

B. Nursing perspective
   1. The quality of care is influenced greatly by nurses' perceptions of the patient's physical and mental state.
      a. Conflicting perceptions can lead to miscommunication, distrust, poor compliance, and inappropriate treatment (Molzahn & Northcott, 1989).
      b. Nurses must respect and support the cultural uniqueness of their patients to provide effective care.
   2. Traditional cultural values may not be consistent within ethnic groups.
      a. Factors such as assimilation, acculturation, age, sex, and individual variation all can contribute to these differences.
      b. Care should be taken to avoid presumptions about an individual based on cultural background. A cultural assessment should be completed to determine individual health beliefs and practices.
   3. Nurses' cultural backgrounds and beliefs may affect the treatment of pain.
      a. Assessment of pain is complicated and influenced by the interaction between the nurse and the patient.
      b. Each party has its own set of values, experiences, meanings, and expectations (Walker, Tan, & George, 1995).
   4. Examination of personal cultural beliefs related to health and illness and associated behaviors is crucial to providing effective care to culturally diverse populations. Health care providers must be cognizant of their own cultural and ethnic biases before caring for patients (Smith, Curci, & Silverman, 2002).
   5. Nurses can play an important role in the treatment of pain for diverse groups by providing culturally sensitive education materials regarding pain medication administration and side-effect treatment (Cope, 2000).

C. Pain and cultural influences
   1. Culture influences the expression and perception of pain and whether an individual is likely to communicate that pain to others, including health care providers (Honeyman & Jacobs, 1996).
   2. Beliefs and attitudes affect how someone interprets, perceives, and responds to injury or illness.
      a. These beliefs and attitudes reflect the cultural and social background of the individual (Yates, Dewar, & Fentiman, 1995).
      b. Culture influences illness beliefs, behaviors, health care practices, ability to seek treatment, and response and receptivity to treatment (Lasch, 2000).
   3. Pain may have a personal meaning to an individual as influenced by cultural background.
      a. For example, some Jewish patients may be more concerned with the underlying disease causing the pain and with the long-term effects than with the pain itself (Garro, 1990).
      b. Sensations, emotions, beliefs, and thoughts are part of the pain experience (Davidhizar, Dowd, & Giger, 1997).
   4. Pain usually results in an affective response, which is expressed differently based on cultural background. Pain expression can be divided into two categories: stoic or emotive (Davidhizar et al., 1997).
      a. Stoic patients generally are silent regarding their pain; they have a "grin and bear it" attitude.
      b. Emotive patients are verbally expressive and may display such pain behaviors as moaning and crying.
   5. An understanding of potential patterns regarding pain responses in various cultural groups is essential for the effective treatment of pain; however, cultural awareness should be used with a complete individual pain assessment (Davidhizar et al., 1997).
   6. Patients who are cared for by health care providers with the same cultural background are seen as more participatory. This improved communication can lead to increased patient involvement, satisfaction with their caregiver, and improved health outcomes (Shire, 2002).

D. Gender, race, and pain (see the chapter on Gender/Sex Differences in Pain and Analgesia)
   1. Weisse, Sorum, Sanders, and Syat (2001) examined gender and race as determinants of decisions regarding pain management and found that there may be differences in the treatment styles of male and female physicians.
      a. Male physicians may identify with those of the same gender or race.
      b. Female physicians identified with disadvantaged patient groups.
   2. Many cultures have defined gender-specific roles.
      a. Women may be the family caretakers, and men may be the decision makers of the family or community.
   3. Gender differences in pain responses exist; however, it is unlikely that these differences can be related solely to cultural background.
      a. Some studies have found that women report more intense pain than men (Affleck et al., 1999; Unruh, Ritchie, & Merskey, 1999) and may show an increased sensitivity to pain (Edwards et al., 1999).
      b. These variations may have an impact on nursing response to the treatment of pain.

E. Influences of pain care
   1. Components of patient and health care provider interaction may be influenced by ethnicity and culture. This interaction consists of four elements:
      a. Pain experience
      b. Expression of pain
      c. Assessment of pain
      d. Decision to treat the pain (Todd, 2001)

F. Genetics and pain
   1. Subpopulations within ethnic groups may exhibit genetic variations that predict slow or rapid medication metabolism, atypical responses, and sensitivities to pain medications (Sakauye, 2005) (see the chapter on Overview of Pharmacology).

G. Cultural barriers and disparities in the management of pain (see the chapter on Disparities in Pain Management)
   1. Disparities exist in the treatment of minority populations, specifically those of African-American and Hispanic ethnicities (Ezenwa, et al., 2006).
   2. Two studies involving the treatment of cancer pain in these two groups examined the pain treatment of socioeconomically disadvantaged patients and the attitudes of the health care providers treating these patients.
      a. Barriers to treatment of pain were identified as the following:
         (1) Physician and patient discrepancy with regard to the severity of pain experienced by the patients and the effect of their pain on sleep
         (2) Inadequate pain assessment
         (3) Communication problems related to language differences between the health care provider and the patient
         (4) Inadequate staff knowledge
         (5) Reluctance of the patient to report pain
      b. In addition, lack of financial resources and access to care affect pain assessment and treatment (Cope, 2000).
   3. Substantial ethnic disparities for various health-related measures exist in the literature, including health status, services, and quality of care, in the literature.
      a. Lower socioeconomic status may account for some of these disparities; however, subtle forms of racism among health care providers may account for some of these findings.
      b. The meaning and behaviors associated with pain are influenced by the cultural background of the patient and the health care provider.
         (1) When the "backgrounds" of the patient and health care provider differ, pain may be more difficult to communicate.

(2) Ethnic stereotypes may impair pain assessment, and conscious or subconscious racism may contribute to the undertreatment of pain (Todd, 2001).

H. Clinical examples of cultural influences on pain management
1. Ethnic minority patients and those with low socioeconomic status are less likely to accept an epidural for the management of postoperative pain when compared to those of non minority backgrounds and higher socioeconomic status (Ochroch, Troxel, Frogel, & Farrar, 2007).
2. Hispanic patients with cancer pain, particularly those of lower socioeconomic status, are often undertreated.
   a. Factors that may contribute to this are Hispanic concerns about addiction, fewer resources, greater difficulty accessing care, difficulty filling prescriptions, and language and cultural differences between clinicians and patients.
   b. A qualitative study also found that because Hispanics felt marginalized due to their immigrant status, they endured pain and did not complain about perceived unfair treatment (Im, Guevara, & Chee, 2007).
3. Racial or ethnic differences in the behavioral response to pain may also be related to the meaning of pain for specific cultural groups. For example, pain that interferes with work and the ability to maintain employment may be particularly difficult for minorities who are in a lower income bracket (Riley et al., 2002).
4. Western civilization tends to provide more attentive and compassionate care to those who display a stoic rather than an expressive attitude toward pain because in the Western culture stoicism is valued (i.e., "no pain, no gain").The treatment of pain may be affected by a mismatch between the health care provider's and the patient's cultural backgrounds (Weissman, Gordan, & Bidar-Sielaff, 2004).

I. Cultural assessment
1. Purpose (Leininger, 1995) (see the chapter on Nursing Theories: Support of Pain Management Nursing)
   a. To discover individual health patterns and meanings
   b. To provide a basis for nursing decisions and actions
   c. To identify potential areas of conflict
2. The following are components of an abbreviated cultural assessment (Andrews & Boyle, 1999):
   a. Family and kinship systems
      (1) Is the family nuclear or extended?
      (2) What is the role or status of individual family members?
   b. Social life
      (1) What is the daily routine of the group?
      (2) Are there special nutritional patterns?
   c. Language and traditions
      (1) What language or dialect is spoken?
      (2) What are the patterns of verbal and nonverbal communication?
      (3) How does the use of personal space relate to communication?
      (4) What are the major cultural traditions?
   d. Religion
      (1) What are the religious beliefs and practices?
      (2) How do religious beliefs and practices relate to health practices?
   e. Health beliefs and practices
      (1) What is the attitude regarding health and illness?
      (2) Who makes decisions about health care?
      (3) Are folk remedies, rituals, or healers used?
3. In addition to the preceding cultural assessment, pointed questions about pain beliefs can help guide treatment (Lasch, 2000).
   a. What do you call your pain?
   b. Why do you think you have this pain, and what does it mean?
   c. How long does the pain last?

d. How bad is your pain?
e. How does your pain interfere with your life (sleep, activity, etc.)?
f. What treatments have you tried, and what do you think will work?
g. Who do you talk to about your pain (family or friend)?
h. Who helps you with your pain?

4. Cultural competence (Weissman et al., 2004)
   a. Be aware of your cultural and family values.
   b. Consider personal biases about those whose values may be different than your own.
   c. Accept cultural differences.
   d. Strive to understand the dynamics of the differences.
   e. Adapt to diversity.
5. Communication
   a. Definition and relationship to pain
      (1) *Communication* is a transactional process whereby two or more people engage in the creation of meaning. It involves generating and receiving messages. The most important factor is not the message sent but how the message was perceived. The goals of communication between two cultures are to decrease uncertainty and to establish a trusting relationship (Nance, 1995).
      (2) Pain expression is influenced by the ability to communicate effectively verbally and nonverbally. Individuals who can articulate their pain and are able to request analgesia are more successful in receiving appropriate pain treatment; individuals who cannot may suffer (Waddie, 1996). Nurses' interpretations of pain expression affect the treatment of pain.
      (3) Cultural or religious deterrents may be associated with the verbal or nonverbal expression of pain. Pain admission may be associated with shame or weakness of character, or pain may be thought of as a punishment for wrongdoings. Visual assessment of pain behaviors, such as grimacing, agitation, guarding, or lying, still may be the only clue nurses have in patients experiencing pain (Moddeman, 1995).
   b. Communication characteristics, such as tone of voice, personal space, eye contact, touch, and time orientation, may be influenced by cultural background. These differences may impede communication between the patient and the caregiver (Lipson, Dibble, & Minarik, 1996).

J. Facilitating communication (Kavanagh & Kennedy, 1992)
   1. *Promote a feeling of acceptance.* This gives the patient an opportunity to express concerns to the caregiver without fear of judgment.
   2. *Strive for a trusting relationship.* Do not be resentful if this is not achieved. Cultural differences may lead to misunderstandings or mistrust.
   3. *Understand the meaning of caring within the context of the cultural group.* Attitudes and behaviors regarding caring may differ among cultural groups.
   4. *Understand the patient's desire to please and the motivation that may cause noncompliance.* The patient's cultural beliefs may prevent the individual from participating in the health care provider's plan of care.
   5. *Avoid stereotyping.* Individual differences within cultural groups are affected by many factors, including age, sex, acculturation, and assimilation.
   6. *Understand the patient's goals and expectations.*
   7. *Respect health beliefs, practices, and folk remedies.* Do not discredit practices unless they are known to be harmful.
   8. *Be prepared to accommodate family.* Include them in the treatment process.
   9. *Show respect toward family members.* It is especially important to respect the primary decision maker. This may be an individual other than the patient.
   10. *Be aware that physical or eye contact may be inappropriate.* It may have an unintended meaning, which may inhibit effective communication.
   11. *Overcome communication barriers.*

a. An interpreter may be used to communicate when language is a barrier; however, be aware that the interpreter's perceptions and attitudes may influence the translation.
   (1) For example, if the interpreter believes that pain medication can lead to addiction, the interpreter may pass this belief to the patient, making the patient resistant to taking the medication (Buchanan, Voigtman, & Mills, 1997).
   (2) In some cultures, it may not be appropriate to have interpreters who are of the opposite sex.
b. The use of visual aids, such as a visual analogue scale, or written material in the patient's native language may be helpful to communicate pain and assess its treatment (see Appendix 8-1).
c. Patient-controlled analgesia may minimize some problems associated with communication between health care providers and patients regarding pain treatment because it allows the patient to administer pain medication without having to communicate the need for it (Lee, Gin, & Oh, 1997).

II. Portrait of Race and Hispanic Origin in the United States (Greico & Cassidy, 2001)

A. The 2000 U.S. Census Bureau report revised the questions on race and Hispanic origin to more clearly define the country's expanding diversity (U.S. Census Bureau, 2000).
   1. The federal government regards race and Hispanic origin as two separate concepts.
      a. All Census 2000 respondents were asked to answer two self-identification questions.
         (1) Are you Spanish, Hispanic, or Latino?
         (2) What race do you consider yourself to be?
B. The Census 2000 question on race differed from the Census 1990 question because, for the first time, respondents were given the option of selecting one or more races to indicate their racial affiliation. This acknowledges the complexity of the racial diversity within the populations in the United States (Shire, 2002).
   1. Nearly 98% of respondents reported only one race; the remaining 2% chose two or more.
   2. Six categories of race were identified; results from the total percentage of the population are as follows:
      a. White (75%)
      b. Black or African American (12.3%)
      c. Asian (3.6%)
      d. American Indian or Alaska Native (0.9%)
      e. Native Hawaiian or other Pacific Islander (0.1%)
      f. "Some other race"
         (1) Respondents had to select one of two categories: Hispanic/Latino or non-Hispanic/Latino.
         (2) Most respondents in this category reported they were Hispanic or Latino (12.5%).
C. Census 2000 further defines each race as follows (U.S. Census Bureau, 2000):
   1. African American or Black: origins in Black racial groups of Africa
   2. American Indian or Alaska Native: origins in original peoples of North, South, or Central America who maintain tribal affiliation
   3. Asian: origins in original peoples of the Far East, Southeast Asia, or Indian subcontinent
   4. Hispanic or Latino: origins in Cuba, Mexico, Puerto Rico, or South or Central America
   5. Native Hawaiian or other Pacific Islander: origins in original peoples of Hawaii, Guam, Samoa, or other Pacific Islands
   6. White: origins in Europe, the Middle East, or North Africa

III. Health Beliefs Regarding Pain in Select Cultural Groups

A. The meaning, expression, and treatment of pain are influenced by cultural background.
   1. Providing effective pain relief requires two-way communication between those experiencing pain and those treating pain.

2. Pain assessment, pain management strategies, education, and patient expectations regarding pain relief need to be addressed to institute an individual plan of care for each patient.
3. Interaction with patients from diverse cultural backgrounds presents a challenge to health care professionals, not only because communication may be an issue secondary to language differences but also because cultural barriers may exist between the patient and the health care provider (Table 8-1).

B. It is especially important for pain management nurses to understand the health beliefs, traditions, and healing practices of a given culture.
1. These unique cultural perspectives should be considered in guiding the treatment of pain. Incorporating the patient's beliefs into the treatment plan is essential for success.
2. Cultural variables such as communication, gender, modesty, diet, objects, social organization, religion, space, and time must be taken into account. All these factors influence the healing process (Spector, 2009).

C. The following section provides examples of unique characteristics, communication styles, and nursing considerations for select cultural groups found in the United States as defined by the U.S. Census Bureau (2000). The degree of acculturation and assimilation, age, sex, and individual differences must be taken into account when interacting with patients from differing cultural backgrounds. Characteristics of these groups are generalizations only; individual variables must be taken into account to avoid stereotyping.
1. African American or Black: origins in Black racial groups of Africa; 12.3% of the total U.S. population (Greico & Cassidy, 2001).
a. Unique cultural perspectives (Lipson & Dibble, 2005).
(1) There is strong religious affiliation; laying of hands and prayer are used to treat illness (Spector, 2009).
(2) Prayer, religion, and church provide support during stressful times (Tan et al., 2005).
(3) African Americans may use faith healers, herbalists, or both to treat illness.
(4) Home remedies such as poultices and food practices are often used to treat or prevent illness (Spector, 2009).
(5) There is a family-oriented support system, often matriarchal in structure (Spector, 2009).

Table 8-1 Cultural and Communication Considerations

Language	Can patient communicate with providers effectively? When using interpreters, consider the gender and age of the patient and the interpreter.
Eye or physical contact	Direct eye or physical contact may be considered disrespectful in some cultures.
Personal space	Be aware of personal space issues. Close personal space may be reserved for family members only.
Speech style	Tone and pace of speech may be culturally specific. Silence may indicate respect or lack of understanding.
Nonverbal communication	Watch for nonverbal cues that may indicate lack of understanding. This also may be important in pain assessment (e.g., grimacing or immobility).
Spiritual or religious beliefs	Beliefs may be important to the healing process. Allow time for personal spiritual practices such as praying or rituals.
Health beliefs	Are there cultural disparities between the practitioner's and the patient's health beliefs?
Familial relationships	Who are the decision makers, caretakers, or both? Include them in the treatment process.

From Clyde, C. L., & Kwiatkowski, K. (2002). Cultural perspective and pain. In B. J. St. Marie (Ed.) *Core Curriculum for Pain Management Nursing*. Philadelphia: Elsevier Press.

(6) Fear of addiction comes with use of pain medication.
(7) The use of numerical, pictorial, and word pain rating scales is beneficial in assessing pain.
(8) African Americans report less control over their pain and use more external coping strategies (Tan et al., 2005).
(9) They experience higher levels of depression and disability with chronic pain when compared to White Americans (Tan et al., 2005).
(10) African Americans may be skeptical of procedures (Lipson & Dibble, 2005).

b. Communication (Lipson & Dibble, 2005)
(1) English is the primary language, including nonstandard vernacular Black English.
(2) Tone is often loud and animated.
(3) Direct eye contact may vary; it generally indicates respect.
(4) Close personal space is acceptable.
(5) Silence may indicate distrust.
(6) African Americans generally have an open and expressive pain style.

c. Nursing considerations
(1) Allow extended family presence when possible because it provides physical and emotional support.
(2) Dispel myths surrounding addiction and the use of pain medication.
(3) Assess pain frequently; use the pain scales.
(4) Allow home remedies and food.
(5) Encourage spiritual support.
(6) Establish a trusting relationship with the patient and family.

2. American Indian or Alaska Native: origins in original peoples of North, South, or Central America who maintain tribal affiliation; 0.9% of the total U.S. population (Greico & Cassidy, 2001); more than 550 recognized tribes in the United States; 200 tribes are not federally recognized (Lipson & Dibble, 2005)

a. Unique cultural perspectives (Spector, 1985)
(1) Individuals believe illness may be caused by evil spirits in nature.
(2) There is a strong relationship between nature and humans.
(3) Optimism is important to the healing process (Cornelison, 2001).
(4) Individuals may use spiritual healers to realign the body if they are not in harmony with life; use of prayer, ceremony, and spiritual rituals are important in the treatment process.
(5) Home remedies such as herbs and roots may be used to treat illness.
(6) Female family members are caretakers; kinship roles may extend to friends. The spokesperson, for example, may be child or family friend.
(7) Pain is related directly to a past or future event and is described as a cause-and-effect relationship.
(8) Pain is often undertreated due to stereotypes about this population, i.e., substance abusers and those who are able to manage pain stoically (Lipson & Dibble, 2005).

b. Communication (Lipson & Dibble, 2005)
(1) English is usually spoken, along with more than 100 indigenous dialects.
(2) Individuals appreciate a soft tone of voice in health care setting.
(3) Interpreters should be mature; ask the patient about gender preference.
(4) Avoiding eye contact indicates respect.
(5) Individuals value adequate personal space, especially when meeting for the first time (2 to 3 feet).
(6) Nonverbal communication is important; silence is respected (Andrews & Boyle, 1999).
(7) Listening is an important cultural skill.
(8) Explain the necessity for touch during a physical examination.

(9) The patient may be unwilling to express pain and may use general terms of not feeling "right or good."
(10) The patient will not ask for pain relief measures repeatedly.

c. Nursing considerations
   (1) Provide a quiet environment and ample time for verbalization.
   (2) Ask direct questions regarding pain.
   (3) Pay attention to nonverbal cues.
   (4) Respect spiritual and ritual practices.

3. Asian: origins of original peoples of the Far East, Southeast Asia, or Indian subcontinent; 3.6% of total U.S. population (Greico & Cassidy, 2001); three groups presented: Chinese, South Asian, and Hmong
   a. Chinese
      (1) Unique cultural perspectives (Lipson & Dibble, 2005)
         (a) Chinese people believe illness is caused by an imbalance of yin and yang in the body.
         (b) Yin (cold) and yang (hot) foods are used to treat imbalances in the body.
         (c) The patient avoids discussion of death (Cornelison, 2001).
         (d) Depending on religious affiliation, Chinese people pray alone or in church. It is common for families to honor their ancestors.
         (e) Chinese people traditionally use of acupuncture, acupressure, and herbs to treat pain and illness.
         (f) Family is placed above individual and society; extended families are common.
         (g) Stoicism is valued. Chinese people believe pain should be endured, which may lead to avoidance or taking less of pain medication (Lai et al., 2003).
            (i) The patient may request less pain medicine or stop its use prematurely because of fear of side effects (Lee et al., 1997).
            (ii) The patient may avoid procedures (e.g., blood draw) and surgery.
      (2) Communication (Lipson & Dibble, 2005)
         (a) The primary languages are Cantonese and Mandarin.
         (b) Individuals often use a loud tone of voice.
         (c) The patient may choose to use close family members as interpreters when possible; nonfamily interpreters should be fluent in the patient's dialect.
         (d) Avoidance of eye contact and silence may signify respect.
         (e) Respect personal space; individuals prefer a distance of 4 to 5 feet.
         (f) Privacy and modesty are important, especially for women.
         (g) The use of touch is uncommon among nonfamily members. Touching the head of an older person is considered disrespectful.
         (h) The patient may not ask questions because this may be viewed as disrespectful.
         (i) Pain complaints may be reported to the family or physician rather than the nurse (Walker et al., 1995).
         (j) The patient may not verbalize pain complaints.
         (k) The patient may be reluctant to discuss problems or complaints in the presence of others, which is related to a cultural belief of "losing face" (Man, Chu, Chen, Ma, & Gin, 2007).
      (3) Nursing considerations
         (a) Offer pain medication; patients may not ask for it.
         (b) Assess nonverbal pain cues, such as grimacing or lying still.
         (c) Respect illness and pain therapies, such as food remedies and acupuncture.
         (d) Explain the need to touch for health care purposes.
   b. South Asian: includes Indians, Pakistanis, Sri Lankan, Nepalese, and East Africans
      (1) Unique cultural perspectives (Lipson et al., 1996)
         (a) South Asians believe that illness results from bad actions.

(b) Prayer and ritualistic acts (chanting, use of charms) are thought to relieve suffering.
(c) Traditional medicine (Ayurvedic) is important in treatment of pain.
(d) Home remedies are used to manage acute muscular or joint pain before medical treatment is sought.
(e) Common home remedies (East Indian) include mustard paste or herbal leaf poultice and oils applied to painful areas, as well as warmed turmeric paste to applied joints (Lipson & Dibble, 2005).
(f) Extended family is important and may live in same household. Daughters usually move in with the husband's family.
(g) The patient may prefer intramuscular injections for pain (Lipson & Dibble, 2005).
(h) Patients are generally able to understand and use numerical pain scales.
(i) Cultural values of privacy and modesty may affect disclosure and physical pain assessment.

(2) Communication (Lipson & Dibble, 2005)
(a) Many different languages and dialects are spoken depending on origin; however, most are fluent in English.
(b) A soft-spoken tone of voice is used to communicate; loudness may indicate disrespect or is considered impolite.
(c) South Asians prefer older, same-sex interpreters within the family.
(d) Direct eye contact may be considered rude. Men and women who are not related do not sustain direct eye contact.
(e) Silence usually indicates approval, acceptance, or tolerance.
(f) Close personal space or contact is reserved for family members. Unrelated men and women maintain an approximate 3-foot distance.
(g) South Asians prefer word descriptors for pain.

(3) Nursing considerations
(a) Respect modesty and personal space. Explain the need for touch related to physical assessment.
(b) Methods of distraction, positioning, reassurance, and mild analgesics, antispasmodics, and sedatives may be used to manage pain (Walker et al., 1995).
(c) Allow time for prayer.
(d) Assess pain through direct, open-ended questions, word descriptor scales.

c. Hmong: distinct ethnic group originating in Southeastern Asia who migrated to parts of southern China, Laos, Vietnam, Burma, and Thailand; U.S. Census reports 186,301 Hmong in United States (Greico & Cassidy, 2001)

(1) Unique cultural perspectives (Lipson & Dibble, 2005)
(a) The cause of sickness may be attributed to spirits in nature.
(b) Christian Hmong request to see their ministers when hospitalized.
(c) Traditional Hmong may participate in spiritual ceremonies conducted by a shaman (ceremonies are usually conducted at home); herbal remedies and foods are important in the healing process.
(d) Home remedies, such as cupping, coining, and pinching, may be used over painful areas. These cause ecchymotic spots that are intended to release evil spirits or toxins from the body.
(e) The family is involved with the care and treatment of the sick, especially in times of crisis. Decisions are made collectively by the family, usually male members (O'Connor, 1995).
(f) Traditionally, women are caretakers of the sick.
(g) The patient may not adhere to dosage instructions (may increase an analgesic dose if pain relief is inadequate).
(h) The patient may fear invasive procedures, such as surgery, nerve blocks, and epidural catheter placement for pain relief.

(2) Communication (Lipson & Dibble, 2005)
  (a) Many Hmong elders speak only Hmong. There are two dialects: White and Green (sometimes referred to as Blue).
  (b) Use a moderate tone of voice when speaking.
  (c) Hmong prefer a same-sex family member for an interpreter. Many English words have no Hmong equivalent, which may lead to confusion. The interpreter must be given a full sentence, paragraph, or thought to translate.
  (d) Prolonged direct eye contact or no eye contact is considered impolite.
  (e) Moderate personal space is acceptable.
  (f) Hmong usually communicate indirectly.
  (g) Saying "yes" may not mean an affirmative answer.
  (h) Hmong are polite: they may not disagree or say "no" publicly. Hmong respect authority: they may not admit to not understanding the meaning of a conversation.
  (i) Hmong prefer no public display of affection or touching.
  (j) Most older Hmong are not literate in their own language or in English; they may have trouble interpreting numbered or written pain assessment tools.
  (k) Pain expression tends to be stoic, but the patient will request pain medication if its availability is known.

(3) Nursing considerations
  (a) Use a moderate tone of voice.
  (b) Explain procedures and benefits of pain therapies to the patient and, more importantly, to the family.
  (c) Have the patient and family repeat instructions to ensure understanding.
  (d) Do not use pain scales; use illustrated or diagrammatic scales to assess pain, or ask if pain is mild, moderate, or severe.
  (e) Assess pain and pain relief measures frequently.
  (f) Teach pain-relieving techniques, such as positioning, application of heat or cold, and distraction, to the patient and assigned caretaker.

4. Hispanic or Latino: origins in Cuba, Mexico, Puerto Rico, or South or Central America; 12.5% of the total U.S. population (Greico & Cassidy, 2001)
   a. Unique cultural perspectives
      (1) Illness may be viewed as the will of God or as being caused by living a bad life (Lipson & Dibble, 2005).
      (2) Depending on the country of origin, some may use folk healers or spiritualists to treat illness. Folk or home remedies may be used by traditionalists and are passed down from one generation to the next.
      (3) Hispanics and Latinos have strong spiritual or religious ties; they believe in folk medicine and prayer for healing (Lipson et al., 1996).
      (4) Strong family ties often extend to non-blood-related family members (Julia, 1996).
      (5) Women may have been raised in a culture of *familism,* a cultural belief where the importance of family comes before everything, including personal needs. Women are less likely to report pain until it becomes intolerable so that they do not disrupt family life (Im et al., 2007).
      (6) Men are often stoic in response to pain because of traditional gender roles for males known as *machism,* where the expression of pain is viewed as a weakness (Im et al., 2007).
      (7) Pain may be viewed as a consequence of immoral behavior, a punishment, a duty, fate, or an obligation (Duggleby, 2003).
      (8) Hispanics and Latinos prefer an oral or intravenous route for analgesia.
      (9) Hispanics and Latinos have a fear of addiction and are concerned about tolerance (Im et al., 2007).

(10) Pain is managed by creating balance between a person and the environment (Duggleby, 2003).
(11) Strategies used to decrease pain include prayer, distraction, massage, herbs and teas, heat and cold, ointments, care and advice from families, and promises (Duggleby, 2003).

b. Communication (Lipson et al., 1996)
(1) Language is Spanish, with different dialects depending on region.
(2) A moderate tone of voice is used in daily conversation; individuals may be louder with family members.
(3) Hispanics and Latinos prefer same-sex interpreters.
(4) They may avoid direct eye contact as sign of respect.
(5) Close personal space is accepted.
(6) Silence may indicate a lack of understanding or disagreement.
(7) Touch is usually reserved for family and close friends.
(8) Hispanics and Latinos prefer word descriptor pain scales and open-ended questions to assess pain (Duggleby, 2003).
(9) Display of pain may differ in various Hispanic ethnic groups; the patient may be stoic or expressive.

c. Nursing considerations
(1) Expect and encourage family support and involvement.
(2) Discuss patient's addiction fears.
(3) Respect and allow time for spiritual needs.
(4) Assess pain frequently using open-ended questions, and pay attention to nonverbal cues.

5. Native Hawaiian (Lipson & Dibble, 2005) or other Pacific Islander: origins in original peoples of Hawaii, Guam, Samoa, or other Pacific Islands; 0.1% of the total U.S. population (Greico & Cassidy, 2001)

a. Unique cultural perspectives
(1) *Native Hawaiian* (uppercase "N") refers to all people of Hawaiian ancestry, regardless of blood measure. Those who have 50% or more Hawaiian blood are referred to as *native Hawaiians* (lowercase "n"). The difference between the two determines eligibility for such things as land ownership and health care benefits.
(2) Historically, spirituality is based on maintaining balance and harmony; Hawaiians believe the disruption of balance leads to illness and misfortune.
(3) Hawaiians may use traditional healers; spirituality plays an important role in healing modalities including massage.
(4) Older Hawaiians may use traditional medicines and herbs to treat illness.
(5) Many treat illness and symptoms using over-the-counter medicines.
(6) Family includes extended family; those related by blood, marriage, or adoption; and friends. Hawaiians believe that the family is more important than the individual.
(7) The family spokesperson is usually the eldest family member (Hawaiians prefer a male spokesperson if available).
(8) Hawaiians understand pain rating scales but usually underreport pain. They will accept pain medication.

b. Communication
(1) Hawaiian is the official language; however, English is most commonly spoken.
(2) Hawaiians prefer soft tones and nod to show that they are listening.
(3) Use direct eye contact when communicating.
(4) Accepted personal space between nonfamily members is 18 to 20 inches.
(5) Silence may indicate agreement or acceptance even if communication is not fully understood.

(6) A handshake or touching a shoulder is within acceptable limits; touching the head is unacceptable (the head is thought to be the source of power or knowledge).
(7) Pain expression is usually stoic. Hawaiians will not complain of pain.

c. Nursing considerations
(1) Assess pain by encouraging the patient to use word descriptors and assess nonverbal cues.
(2) Have the patient and family repeat instructions to ensure understanding.
(3) Use a moderate tone of voice to communicate.

6. White: origins in Europe, the Middle East, and North Africa; 75% of the total U.S. population; includes those who indicated their race as White and wrote in entries such as Irish, Italian, German, Polish, or Arab (Greico & Cassidy, 2001); Three groups presented: Arab, Irish, and Italian

a. Arab: More than 1.24 million people reported Arab ancestry (Greico & Cassidy, 2001).
(1) Unique cultural perspectives (Lipson & Dibble, 2005)
(a) Illness may be caused by bad luck, stress, loss, germs, imbalance of hot and cold or dry and moist, and sudden fears. It may also be caused by the evil eye, punishment from God for sins.
(b) The predominant religion is Islam. It is broader than Christianity and considered a way of life (Julia, 1996).
(c) Prayer is an important daily ritual.
(d) Arabs may use folk remedies to treat illness or pain, such as herbal teas and poultices, camphor oil, and hot chicken soup.
(e) Family is the central focus and takes precedence over the individual. This includes extended family, usually patriarchal (Cornelison, 2001).
(f) Pain is feared; it is less frightening if the patient understands the source and prognosis.
(g) Arabs describe pain using metaphors (e.g., fire, iron, knives, or rocks).
(h) Pain may be seen as a punishment; suffering may be viewed as atonement.
(i) Arabs believe injections are more effective than pills.
(2) Communication (Lipson & Dibble, 2005)
(a) Arabic is the spoken language, with many dialects and variation based on the country of origin.
(b) Most Arab professionals are fluent in English.
(c) Use a loud voice to signify the importance of a message, silence may mean respect or that the patient did not understand the message.
(d) Same-sex interpreters are preferred; use only same-sex family members as interpreters when translating sensitive issues (be aware that the message may be edited by family).
(e) Women may avoid eye contact when communicating with men.
(f) Close personal space is preferred for family members and trusted people of the same gender.
(g) Arabs prefer to have a terminal illness or poor prognosis discussed with the family, not the patient.
(h) Arabs have an expressive pain style, especially around family members.
(3) Nursing considerations
(a) Have the patient define the pain descriptors used.
(b) To decrease anxiety, offer an explanation of procedures, the cause of pain, and treatment options.
(c) Respect spiritual practices.
(d) Incorporate the family into the plan of care.

b. Irish: More than 33 million people reported Irish ancestry (Greico & Cassidy, 2001).
(1) Unique cultural perspectives (Lipson & Dibble, 2005)
(a) The Irish believe that physical illness is God's will; it may be related to sin or guilt.

(b) Many spiritual healing practices come from the Catholic faith, (e.g., prayer). Priests may be called to deliver sacrament of the sick.
(c) The Irish use home and folk remedies to treat illness before seeking medical care (e.g., willow bark tea for pain).
(d) Families are mostly nuclear, with a strong sense of family obligation to the extended family.
(e) The decision maker is usually the male head of household in the past, but recently women have had a more important role.
(f) Irish men are not as compliant with medications; taking medications is perceived as weakness.
(g) Pain is viewed as part of life.

(2) Communication
(a) English is the common language of the Irish.
(b) Tone in ordinary conversation is quiet and relaxed.
(c) Direct eye contact is acceptable; the patient may perceive someone who does not make direct eye contact as untrustworthy. The patient may avoid eye contact to disguise emotion.
(d) Comfortable personal space is greater than that of other Northern European Americans.
(e) Engaging in touch during conversation is not usually done, even with family members.
(f) Irish men tend to be stoic and reluctant to take pain medications; women are more expressive.

(3) Nursing considerations
(a) For important decisions, quietly ascertain who the decision maker of the family is and include that person in the plan of care.
(b) Explain to the patient the importance and benefits of taking pain medication.
(c) Assess pain frequently, and pay attention to nonverbal cues.

c. Italians: More than 15.7 million people identified their ancestry as Italian (Greico & Cassidy, 2001).

(1) Unique cultural perspectives (Lipson & Dibble, 2005)
(a) Older Italians may attribute illness to God's will, fate, the evil eye, genetics, or other causes such as guilt and anxiety.
(b) The majority of Italians are Catholic. Families may contact a Catholic priest when a family member is very ill to receive forgiveness of sins through confession and the sacrament of the sick, which is thought to give spiritual strength for healing or preparation for death.
(c) The use of folk or home remedies comes mostly from plants and may include lemon juice, olive oil, vinegar, and garlic.
(d) The traditional Italian American family consists of mother, father, and children. Parents and the eldest son are the most respected.
(e) Italians prefer a non-oral route for medications and may self-medicate or stop treatment early if symptoms subside.
(f) Pain is viewed as an evil and is a frightening experience to be avoided, considered to deprive one of life.
(g) Patients may describe pain as loss of energy or depression.

(2) Communication
(a) Italian is the official language with many dialects; some other languages spoken in regions of Italy are French, German, Ladino, Slovene, and Albanian.
(b) Tone of voice among family members may be loud.
(c) Italians prefer an educated family member as an interpreter; the family interpreter may not divulge all information to the patient to protect that individual.

(d) Use direct eye contact to show a sincere interest in conversation; avoiding eye contact considered very impolite.
(e) Italians are comfortable with close personal space.
(f) Italians have an expressive pain style, both verbal and nonverbal.

(3) Nursing considerations
(a) Allow time for prayer, and address spiritual needs.
(b) Incorporate the family into the plan of care.
(c) Explain the rationale for pain medications and procedures.
(d) Assess depressive symptoms that may be related to pain.

Summary

Pain assessment and treatment continue to be challenges despite the efforts to improve the management of pain over the last decade. Individual variability, as well as cultural factors, including health beliefs and practices, must be taken into account when treating patients whose culture may differ from those of the health care providers involved in their care. The nurse cannot use a broad brush to paint all individuals the same color based on ethnicity or race. The degree of acculturation, assimilation, education, occupation, socioeconomic status, and community cultural ties can affect responses to pain and illness.

Cultural barriers to pain management include communication problems related to language; inadequate staff knowledge regarding cultural influences, which may affect the presentation, assessment, and treatment of pain; lack of financial resources; and access to care (Cope, 2000). Respecting cultural values should be incorporated into the care of patients experiencing illness and pain; however, personal bias and differences between provider and patient values and beliefs may interfere. Thus, another barrier to care is the patient's diversity (Cornelison, 2001).

One important goal of Healthy People 2010 is the elimination of health disparities associated with race and ethnicity (Riley et al., 2002). Despite all the attention to the crisis of inadequate pain management, the literature suggests that disparities continue in minority populations, especially those of African American and Hispanic ethnicity. Subtle forms of racism and stereotyping may exist. Understanding personal attitudes or biases is an important first step in overcoming cultural barriers. Educational efforts to address pain undertreatment related to race and ethnicity should include not only assessment of pain in diverse cultural groups but also suggestions for treatment options, including analgesic choices that would be appropriate for the type and severity of the pain the patient is experiencing (Todd, 2001).

Weissman et al. (2004) proposes four steps to cultural competence: Listen to the patient's pain description, and then (1) explain your perception, (2) acknowledge the differences and similarities, (3) recommend treatment options, and (4) negotiate agreement. The goals of culturally competent care are to incorporate the specific cultural health beliefs and practices of the individual and family into the care (Duggleby, 2003), to find common words to describe pain, and to develop pain management strategies that are culturally acceptable (Sakauye, 2005).

References

Affleck, G., Tennen, H., Keefe, F. J., Lefebvre, J. C., Kashikar-Zuck, S., Wright, K., Starr, K., & Caldwell, D. S. (1999). Everyday life with osteoarthritis or rheumatoid arthritis: Independent effects of disease and gender on daily pain, mood, and coping. *Pain, 83,* 601–609.

American Pain Society. (2008). American Pain Society: Research, Education, Treatment, Advocacy. Retrieved December 14, 2008, from http://www. ampainsoc.org.

American Pain Society. (2004) Racial and Ethnic Identifiers in Pain Management: The Importance to Research, Clinical Practice, and Public Health Policy. Advocacy: Pain Care Coalition. Retrieved May 15, 2009, from http://www.ampainsoc.org/advocacy/ethnoracial.htm.

Andrews, M. M., & Boyle, J. S. (1999). *Transcultural concepts in nursing care* (3rd ed.). Philadelphia: Lippincott Williams & Wilkins.

Bonica, J. J. (1990). *The history of pain concepts and therapies: The management of pain* (2nd ed., Vol. 1). Philadelphia: Lea & Febiger.

Buchanan, L., Voigtman, J., & Mills, H. (1997). Implementing the agency for health care policy and research pain management pediatric guidelines in a multicultural practice setting. *Journal of Nursing Quality Care, 11,* 23–35.

Clendening, L. (1933). *Behind the doctor.* New York: Alfred A. Knopf.

Clendening, L. (1960). *Source book of medical history.* Mineola, NY: Dover.

Clyde, C. L., & Kwiatkowski, K. (2002). Cultural perspective and pain. In B. J. St. Marie (Ed.) *Core Curriculum for Pain Management Nursing.* Philadelphia: Elsevier Press.

Cope, D. (2000). Cultural and educational issues in pain management. *Clinical Journal of Oncology Nursing, 4*(5), 237–241.

Cornelison, A. H. (2001). Cultural barriers to compassionate care: Patient's and health professional's perspectives. *Bioethics Forum, 17*(1), 7–14.

Cousins, M., & Phillips, G. (1986). *Acute pain management.* New York: Churchill Livingstone.

Cousins, M. J., Mather, L. E., Glynn, C. J., Wilson, P. R., & Graham, J. R. (1979). Selective spinal analgesia. *Lancet, 1,* 1141–1142.

Davidhizar, R., Dowd, S., & Giger, J. N. (1997). Cultural differences in pain management. *Radiologic Technology, 68,* 345–348.

De Boulay, S. (1984). *Cicely Saunders: Founder of the modern hospice movement.* London: Hodder and Stoughton.

Duggleby, W. (2003). Helping Hispanic/Latino home health patients manage their pain. *Home Health Care Nurse, 21*(3), 174–179.

Edwards, R. R., Fillingim, R. B., Yamauchi, S., Sigurdsson, A., Bunting, S., Mohorn, S. G., & Maixner, W. (1999). Effects of gender and acute dental pain on thermal pain responses. *Clinical Journal of Pain, 15,* 233–237.

Ezenwa, M. O., Ameringer, S., Ward, S. E., & Serlin, R. C. (2006). Racial and ethnic disparities in pain management in the United States. *Journal of Nursing Scholarship, third quarter,* 225–233.

Galanti, G. (1991). Basic concepts. In *Caring for patients from different cultures* (pp. 1–14). Philadelphia: University of Pennsylvania Press.

Garro, L. (1990). Culture, pain, and cancer. *Journal of Palliative Care, 6,* 34–44.

Grieco, E. M., & Cassidy, R. C. (2001). Overview of race and Hispanic origin: census 2000 brief, United States census 2000. Washington, DC: US Department of Commerce, US Census Bureau: 2001. Retrieved from http://www.census.gov/prod/2001pubs/c2kbr01-1.pdf on May 15, 2009.

Honeyman, P. T., & Jacobs, E. A. (1996). Effects of back pain on Australian Aboriginals. *Spine, 21,* 841–843.

Im, E. O., Guevara, E., & Chee, W. (2007). The pain experience of Hispanic patients with cancer in the United States. *Oncology Nursing Forum, 34*(4), 861–868.

International Association for the Study of Pain. (2008). *Welcome to IASP.* Retrieved December 14, 2008, from http://www.iasp-pain.org//AM/Template.cfm?Section=Home.

Julia, M. C. (1996). *Multicultural awareness in the health care professions.* Needham Heights, MA: Allyn & Bacon.

Kavanagh, K. H., & Kennedy, P. H. (1992). Communication, intervention, and diversity. In *Promoting cultural diversity* (pp. 31–82). Newbury Park, CA: Sage.

Keele, K. D. (1957). *Anatomies of pain.* Springfield, IL: Charles C. Thomas.

Lai, Y. H., Dalton, J. A., Belyea, M., Chen, M. L., Tsai, L. Y., & Chen, S. C. (2003). Development and testing of the pain opioid analgesics belief scale in Taiwanese cancer patients. *Journal of Pain and Symptom Management, 25*(4), 376–385.

Lasch, K. E. (2000). Culture, pain, and culturally sensitive pain care. *Pain Management Nursing, 1*(3 Suppl. 1), 16–22.

Lee, A., Gin, T., & Oh, T. E. (1997). Opioid requirements and response in Asians. *Anaesthesia and Intensive Care, 25,* 665–670.

Leininger, M. (1995). Transcultural nursing perspectives: Basic concepts and culture care incidents. In *Transcultural nursing: Concepts, theories, research and practice* (2nd ed., pp. 57–92). New York: McGraw-Hill.

Lipson, J. G., & Dibble, S. L. (Eds.). (2005). *Culture and clinical care.* San Francisco: UCSF Nursing Press.

Lipson, J. G., Dibble, S. L., & Minarik, P. A. (1996). *Culture and nursing care: A pocket guide.* San Francisco: UCSF Nursing Press.

Livingston, W. K., & Fields, H. (1998). *Pain and suffering.* Washington, DC: IASP Press.

Man, A. K. Y., Chu, M. C., Chen, P. P., Ma, M., & Gin, T. (2007). Clinical experience with a chronic pain management program in Hong Kong Chinese patients. *Hong Kong Medicine Journal, 13*(5), 372–378.

Melzack, R., & Wall, P. D. (1965). Pain mechanisms: A new theory. *Science, 150,* 971–979.

Moddeman, G. R. (1995). Barriers to pain management in elderly surgical patients. *AORN Journal, 61,* 1073–1075.

Molzahn, A. E., & Northcott, H. C. (1989). The social basis of discrepancies in health/illness perceptions. *Journal of Advanced Nursing, 14,* 132–140.

Nance, T. A. (1995). Intercultural communication: Finding common ground. *Journal of Obstetric, Gynecologic, and Neonatal Nursing, 24,* 249–255.

Nash, M. (2008). *Hans Kosterlitz and the enkephalins.* Retrieved December 14, 2008, from http://opioids.com/endogenous/index.html.

Ochroch, E. A., Troxel, A. B., Frogel, J. K., & Farrar, J. T. (2007). The influence of race and socioeconomic factors on patient acceptance of perioperative epidural analgesia. *Anesthesia & Analgesia, 105*(6), 1787–1792.

O'Connor, B. B. (1995). *Healing traditions: Alternative medicine and the health professions (studies in health, illness, and caregiving).* Philadelphia: University of Pennsylvania Press.

Raj, P. P. (1995). Tutorial #19: History of pain medicine. *Pain Digest, 5,* 198–205.

Riley, J. L., Wade, J. B., Myers, C. D., Sheffield, D., Papas, R. K., & Price, D. D. (2002). Racial/ethnic differences in the experience of chronic pain. *Pain, 100,* 291–298.

Sakauye, K. (2005). Cultural influences on pain management in the elderly. *Comprehensive Therapy, 31*(1), 78–82.

Shire, N. (2002). Effects of race, ethnicity, gender, culture, literacy, and social marketing on public health. *Journal of Gender Specific Medicine, 5*(2), 48–54.

Smith, R., Curci, M., & Silverman, A. (2002). Pain management: The global connection. *Nursing Management* (June), 27–29.

Spector, R. E. (1985). Culture health and illness. In *Cultural diversity in health and illness* (2nd ed., (pp. 57–77). Norwalk, CT: Appleton-Century-Crofts.

Spector, R. E. (2009). *Cultural diversity in health and illness* (7th ed.). Upper Saddle River, NJ: Pearson Education.

Tan, G., Jensen, M., Thornby, J., & Anderson, K. O. (2005). Ethnicity, control appraisal, coping, and adjustment to chronic pain among Black and White Americans. *Pain Medicine, 6*(1), 18–28.

Terman, G. W. (1999). *John C. Liebeskind (1935–1997): A tribute.* Retrieved December 14, 2008, from http://www.pubmedcentral.nih.gov/articlerender.fcgi?artid=33592.

Tervalon, M., & Murray-Garcia, J. (1998). Cultural humility versus cultural competence: A critical distinction in defining physician training outcomes in multicultural education. *Journal of Health Care for the Poor and Underserved, 9*(2), 117–125.

Todd, K. H. (2001). Influence of ethnicity on emergency department pain management. *Emergency Medicine, 13,* 274–278.

U.S. Census Bureau. (2000). *Your gateway to Census 2000.* Retrieved December 13, 2008, from http://www.census.gov/main/www/cen2000.html.

University of Illinois, Department of Neurology. (2008). *Dr. Silas Weir Mitchell.* Retrieved December 14, 2008, from http://www.uic.edu/depts/mcne/founders/page0062.html.

Unruh, A. M., Ritchie, J., & Merskey, H. (1999). Does gender affect appraisal of pain and pain coping strategies? *Clinical Journal of Pain, 15,* 31–40.

Waddie, N. A. (1996). Language and pain expression. *Journal of Advanced Nursing, 23,* 868–872.

Walker, A. C., Tan, L., & George, S. (1995). Impact of culture on pain management: An Australian perspective. *Holistic Nursing Practice, 9,* 48–57.

Warfield, C. A. (1988). A history of pain relief. *Hospital Practice, 23,* 121–122.

Weber, S. E. (1996). Cultural aspects of pain in childbearing women. *Journal of Obstetric, Gynecologic, and Neonatal Nursing, 25,* 67–72.

Weisse, C. S., Sorum, P. C., Sanders, K. N., & Syat, B. L. (2001). Do gender and race affect decisions about pain management? *Journal of General Internal Medicine, 16,* 211–217.

Weissman, D. E., Gordan, D., & Bidar-Sielaff, S. (2004). Cultural aspects of pain management. *Journal of Palliative Medicine, 7*(5), 715–716.

Yates, P., Dewar, A., & Fentiman, B. (1995). Pain: The views of elderly people living in long-term residential care settings. *Journal of Advanced Nursing, 21,* 667–674.

Zimmermann, M. (2006). Historical evolution of pain concepts. In Oh (Ed.), *The nociceptive membrane.* Boston: Elsevier Press.

appendix

8-1

Translations of 0–10 Pain Rating Scales

English

Please point to the number that best describes your pain.

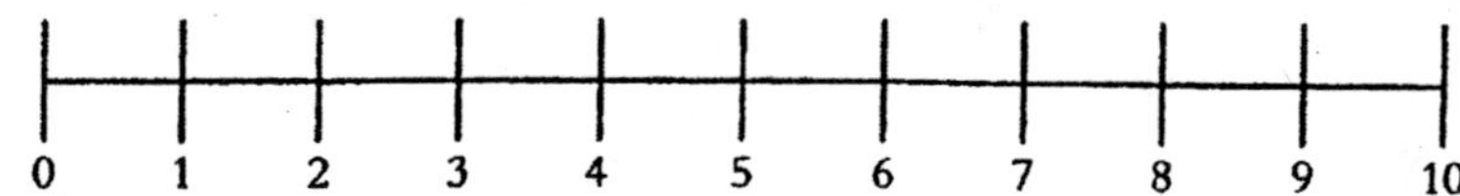

No pain — Terrible pain

Chinese*

請指出那個數字反映你痛的程度

Please point to the number that best describes your pain.

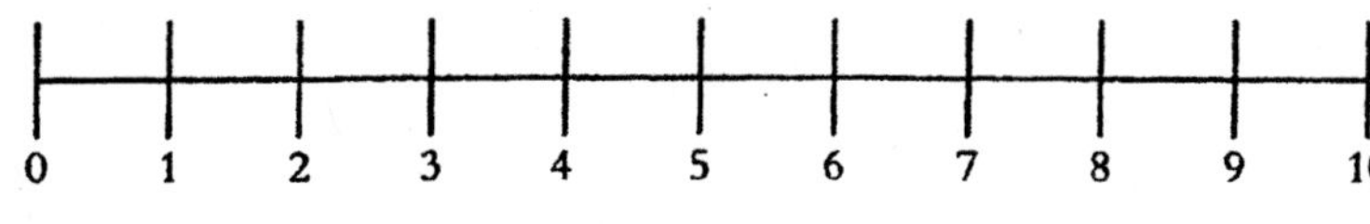

無痛 No pain — **劇痛** Terrible pain

French†

S'il vous plait, indiquez le chiffre qui décrit le mieux votre douleur.

Please point to the number that best describes your pain.

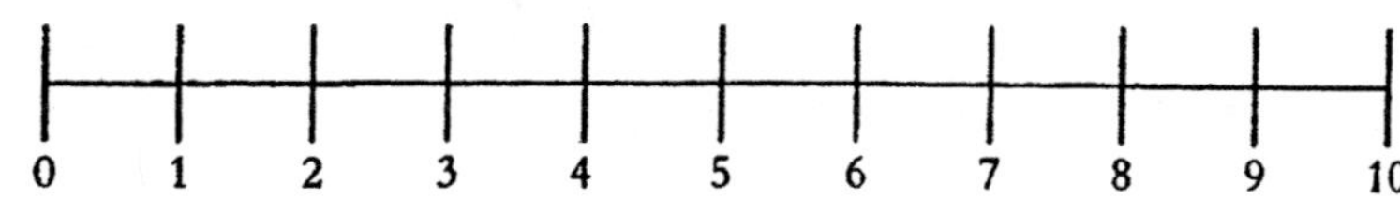

Pas de douleur No pain — **Douleur intense** Terrible pain

Note: Most of the translations of the pain rating scales were done by volunteers. No back and forth translations have been done, so the reader is advised that errors may occur. These scales have been used extensively, however, by the facilities that submitted them.

* Pain Management Committee, St. Francis Medical Center, Honolulu, HI.

From *Pain Clinical Manual* 2nd edition by Margo McCaffery and Chris Pasero, pages 68-73. Copyright Elsevier, 1999. Reprinted by permission.

Hebrew†

בבקשה תשימו אצבע על המספר מאפס עד עשר:
שמראה לנו כמה חזק הכאב

Please point to the number that best describes your pain.

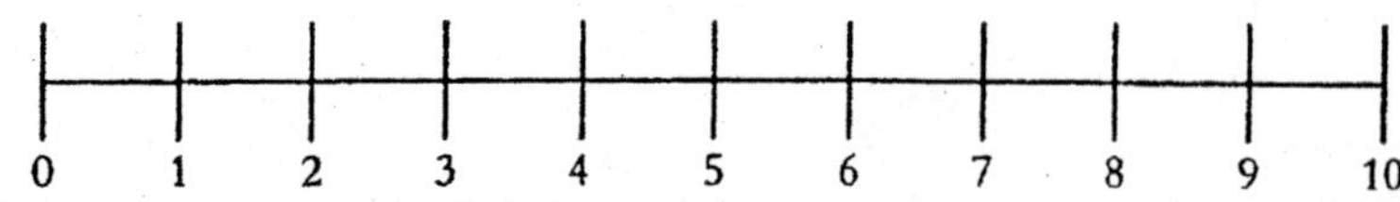

בלי כאב — כאב חזק

No pain — Terrible pain

Ilocano* (Spoken in the Philippines)

Paki tudo ti numero nga mangipakita ti kinasakitna.

Please point to the number that best describes your pain.

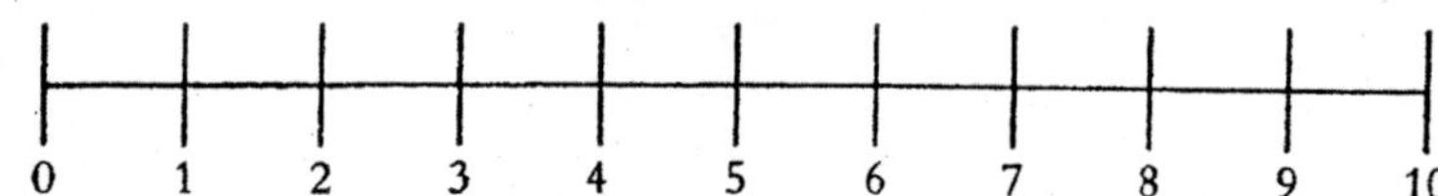

Awan sakit na — **Nakasaksakit unay**

No pain — Terrible pain

Italian†

Segna il numero che indica il level del dolore.

Please point to the number that best describes your pain.

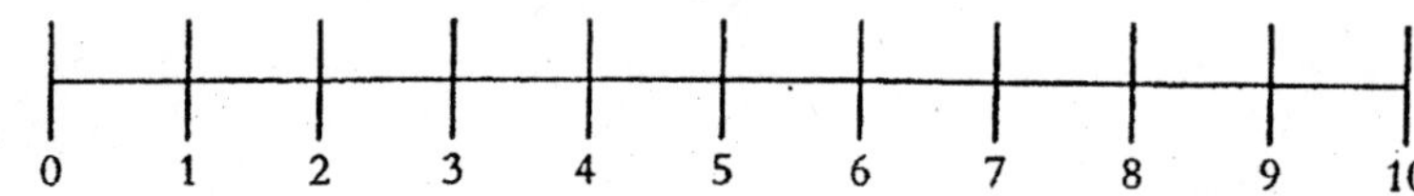

Nessun dolore — **Dolore insuportable**

No pain — Terrible pain

Japanese†

痛みの強さの度合を0～10までの階段で示して下さい。

Please point to the number that best describes your pain.

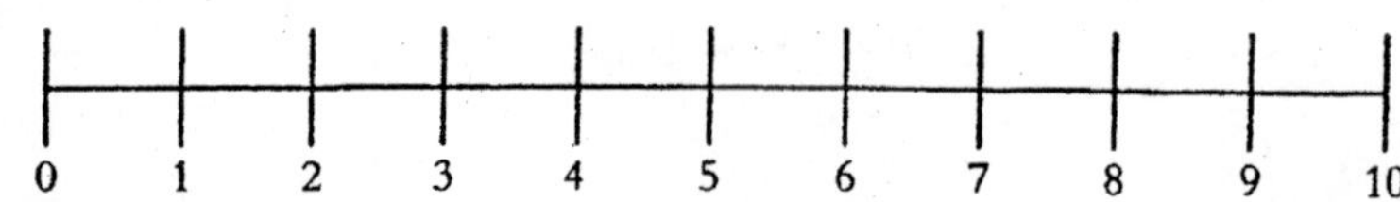

ゼロ　全く痛みがない — 激痛 敫痛

No pain — Terrible pain

* Pain Management Committee, St. Francis Medical Center, Honolulu, HI.

† Compiled by Josephine Musto, RN, MS, ONC, Nursing Care Manager, Pain Management Service, and members of Nursing Department, Saint Vincent's Hospital and Medical Center, New York, NY.

Korean

현재 통증의 강도를 가장 잘 나타내는 번호에 표시하십시오.

Please point to the number that best describes your pain.

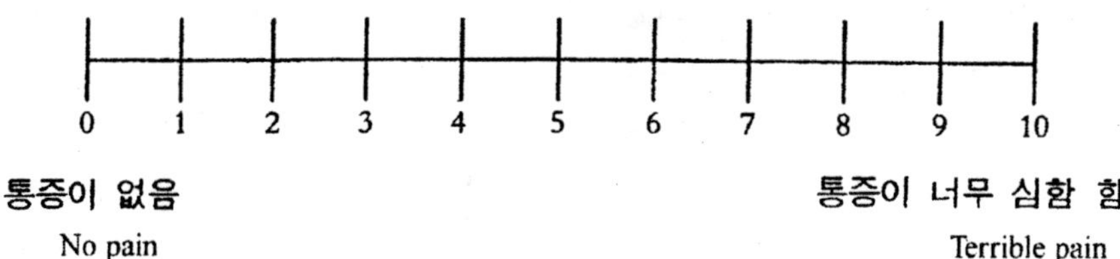

통증이 없음　　　　　　　　　　통증이 너무 심함 함

No pain　　　　　　　　　　Terrible pain

Pakistan†

برائے مہربانی اپنے درد کی شدت بتانے کے لیے نیچے لکھے ہوئے نمبروں میں سے کسی ایک کی طرف اپنی انگلی سے اشارہ کریں۔

Please point to the number that best describes your pain.

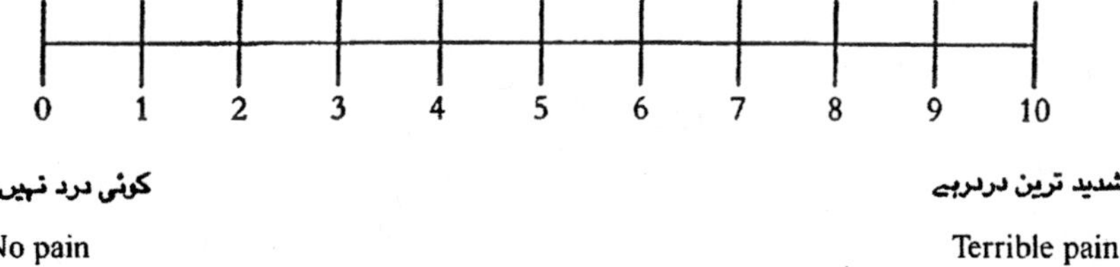

کوئی درد نہیں ہے　　　　　　　　　　شدید ترین دردہے

No pain　　　　　　　　　　Terrible pain

Polish†

Proszę wskazać numer, który najlepiej określa jak silny jest ten ból

Please point to the number that best describes your pain.

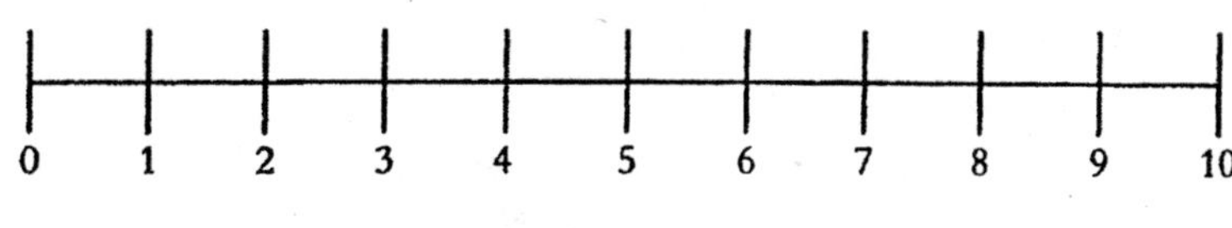

Nie mam bólu　　　　　　　　　　**Straszny ból**

No pain　　　　　　　　　　Terrible pain

Russian†

Выбирите число, которое указывает вашу боль по десятибальной системе.

Please point to the number that best describes your pain.

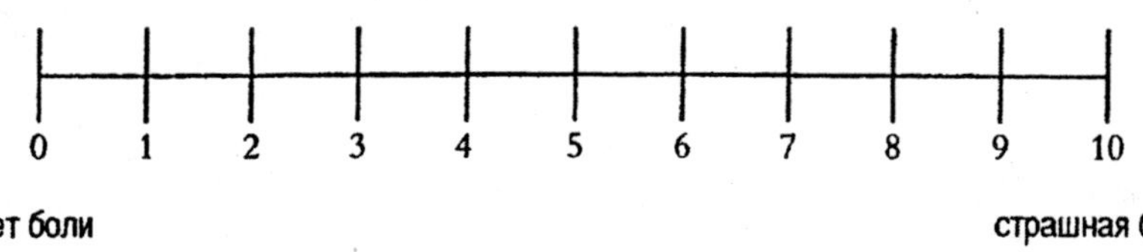

нет боли　　　　　　　　　　**страшная боль**

No pain　　　　　　　　　　Terrible pain

† Compiled by Josephine Musto, RN, MS, ONC, Nursing Care Manager, Pain Management Service, and members of Nursing Department, Saint Vincent's Hospital and Medical Center, New York, NY.

Samoan*

Fa'amolemole ta'u mai le numera e fa'amatala ai le itu-aiga tiga o loo e lagonaina

Please point to the number that best describes your pain.

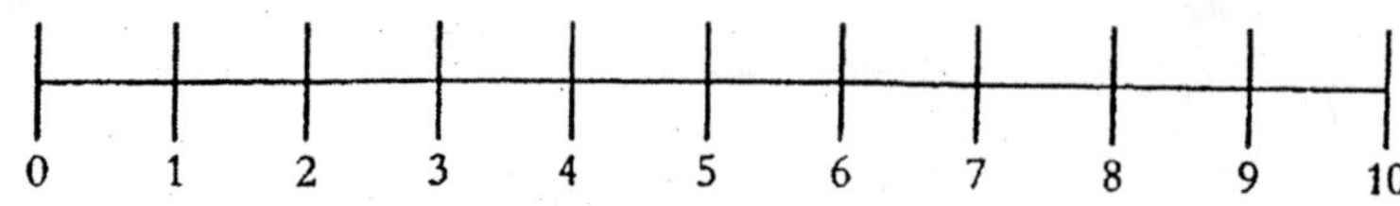

Le tiga — No pain

Tiga tele — Terrible pain

Spanish†

Por favor senale al numero que mejor describe su dolor. (Mas grande el numero mayor su dolor.)

Please point to the number that best describes your pain.

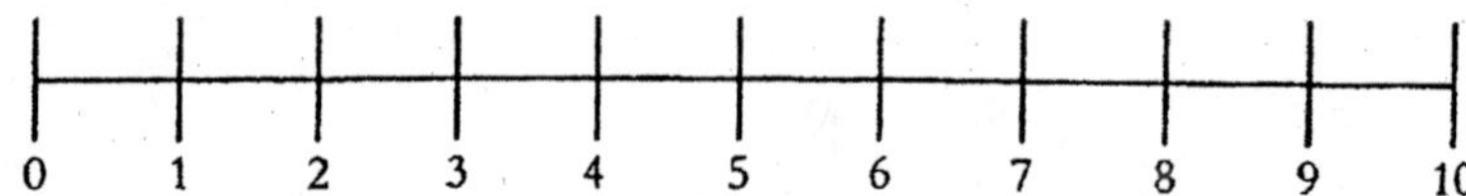

No tiene dolor — No pain

Tiene un terrible dolor — Terrible pain

Tagalog† (Spoken in the Philippines)

Ituro po ninyo ang numerong nagpapaliwanag kung gaano kasakit.

Please point to the number that best describes your pain.

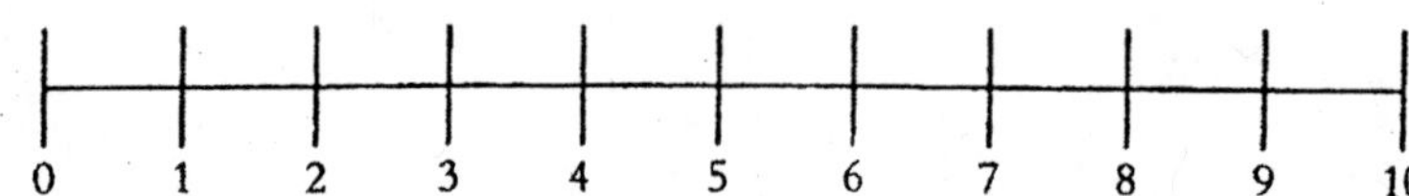

Walang masakit — No pain

Napakasakit — Terrible pain

Tongan† (Spoken in Tonga, an Island in the South Pacific)

I he ngaahi fika koena, fakailongai mai ai e tuunga ho falangaaki.

Please point to the number that best describes your pain.

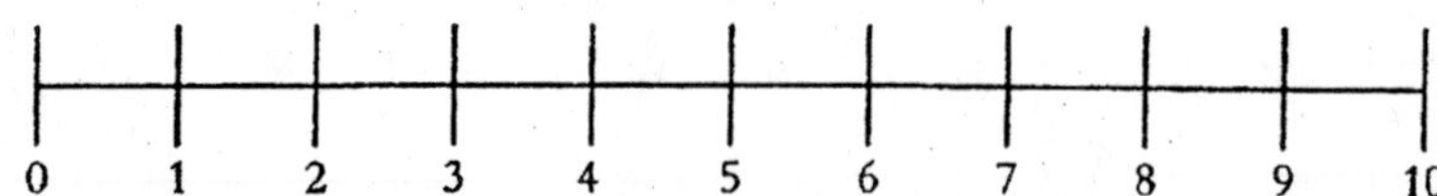

Ikai ha felangaaki — No pain

Ikai matuuaki'e langa — Terrible pain

† Compiled by Josephine Musto, RN, MS, ONC, Nursing Care Manager, Pain Management Service, and members of Nursing Department, Saint Vincent's Hospital and Medical Center, New York, NY.

* Pain Management Committee, St. Francis Medical Center, Honolulu, HI.

† Compiled by Josephine Musto, RN, MS, ONC, Nursing Care Manager, Pain Management Service, and members of Nursing Department, Saint Vincent's Hospital and Medical Center, New York, NY.

Vietnamese

Xin chỉ số mô tả đúng nhất sự đau nhức của quý vị

Please point to the number that best describes your pain.

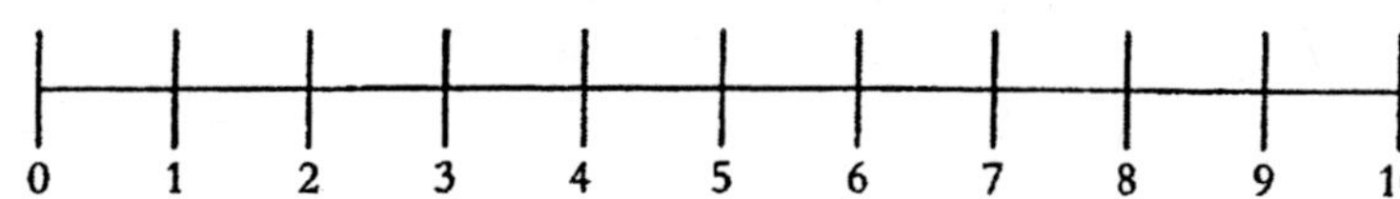

Không đau — No pain

Đau rất nhiều — Terrible pain

[†] Compiled by Josephine Musto, RN, MS, ONC, Nursing Care Manager, Pain Management Service, and members of Nursing Department, Saint Vincent's Hospital and Medical Center, New York, NY.

chapter

9

Epidemiology of Pain

Karen P. Hall, MSHSA, RN-BC, NE-BC
Barbara St. Marie, ANP, GNP, RN-BC, PhD Candidate

Objectives

After studying this chapter, the reader should be able to:

1. Discuss the significance of epidemiology as a foundational component of pain management practice.
2. Cite general studies of pain prevalence in various populations.
3. Describe how results of epidemiological studies are used to improve care.

Epidemiology offers the field of pain management a broad view of the impact of pain on our society. It is through epidemiology that programs can develop, groups are studied, and the statistical figures that are attained can be used to influence social policy. Throughout this text, we read about health disparities regarding pain management, we see the impact of uncontrolled pain, and we see proclamations of the benefit of pain management on the biological, social, and psychological domains of humanity. Understanding epidemiology is more than just knowing the prevalence of particular pain syndromes; it is a plan for delivery, a tool used to redesign access to care, and a measurement of outcome, and it is systematic in the investigation. Epidemiological figures historically have facilitated the development of programs (e.g., eliminating certain diseases in the world, reducing perinatal mortality, and studying groups at risk for heart disease, acquired immunodeficiency syndrome, and cancer). Historically, pain has had limited research using methods of epidemiology. Nurses have been on the forefront of the specialty of pain management in recent years as information has been unveiling related to pain epidemiology. We are challenged, as nurses, to continue growing in our knowledge of the area of epidemiology and to forward the information obtained through this form of study to appropriate groups to facilitate change, to redesign care delivery, and to promote access that will reduce and eventually eliminate disparities in pain management.

I. Pain Epidemiology: Historical Perspective

A. Epidemiology is "the study of the distribution and determinants of health-related states or events in a specified population and the application of this study to the control of health problems" (Last, 1988).

B. Epidemiology is the study of the following:
   1. Causes of disease.
   2. Natural history of disease and predictors of outcome.
   3. Impact of disease on groups of people, society, or both.
   4. Where disease occurs.
   5. How disease is transmitted.

C. International Association for the Study of Pain (IASP)
   1. The IASP developed a task force in 1994 to focus on improving epidemiological studies relevant to pain. Members of this task force represented different aspects of epidemiological sciences.
   2. The IASP published *Epidemiology of Pain* in 1999 (Crombie, Croft, Linton, LeResche, & Von Korff, 1999).
   3. The IASP continues to build on its epidemiological work (Carlton, 2005).

II. Epidemiological Study and Pain Management

A. Uses of epidemiological work (Carlton, 2005)
   1. Epidemiology measures burden in our society.
      a. Knowing the incidence of common pain syndromes helps us understand the burden to our society.
   2. Epidemiology is used in determining etiology.
   3. It determines natural history and identifies predictors of outcome.
   4. Communication is used to affect interventional management and policy.

B. Uses of epidemiological work for pain management
   1. Plan an approach for improving the delivery of pain management.
   2. Determine access to pain management services.
   3. Ascertain patient satisfaction with the delivery of care.
   4. Establish the outcomes of a pain management service.
   5. Develop a systematic investigation of pain patients to establish valid diagnostic groups.
   6. Uncover the cause of pain so that preventive measures can be developed.
      a. Primary prevention focuses on stopping a pain condition from ever occurring.
      b. Secondary prevention focuses on early detection of disease with the aim of intervening to reduce subsequent ill health.

c. Tertiary prevention seeks to minimize the impairments and disabilities that could arise from incurable disease and to promote the patient's adjustment to the chronic condition.

7. Identify factors that contribute to the susceptibility to pain and disability caused by pain (Crombie et al., 1999).

C. Techniques of epidemiology

1. Studies must have the following:
   a. Well-defined purpose.
   b. Defined plan.
   c. Appropriate study design.
   d. Appropriate analysis.
   e. Valid interpretation of findings.
2. Prevalence studies
   a. Are measured at a single point in time or over a long period.
   b. Show how the frequency of pain can vary across different body sites and how pain affects the lives of individuals and their families.
3. Cohort studies follow patients over time to determine how pain changes.
4. Case-control studies compare characteristics of patients who have pain with a suitable control group.
5. Statistical measurement helps us to understand the strength of association between risk factors and certain pain problems (Carlton, 2005).
   a. Measurements include odds ratios, relative risks, and confidence intervals.
   b. Date includes age, gender and other demographics.
   c. Lifestyle measurements can be included, such as chemical use, weight, exercise frequency, sleep, injury, and genetics.
   d. Psychological, social, and cultural information can also be used.

III. Pain Prevalence per Population

A. Pain prevalence and ethnicity

1. A 2006 study in the United States of 11,021 people age 51 and older.
   a. Higher pain prevalence was reported in the non-Hispanic Blacks (28%) and Hispanics (33%) than in the non-Hispanic Whites (27%).
   b. One-fourth of non-Hispanic Blacks and Hispanics reported predominantly having severe pain, compared with 17% of non-Hispanic Whites (Reyes-Gibby, Aday, Todd, Cleeland, & Anderson, 2006).
2. Sickle cell pain
   a. Pain in a sickle cell epidemiology study (Smith, 2005)
      (1) The purpose of the study was to build predictive models for patient behavior in response to pain.
      (2) The study had 226 participants.
      (3) Based on patient diaries, 56% of participants had some pain; 26% had pain every day. In addition, 30% had severe pain (chronic pain syndrome) and 13% had pain 5% of days or less.
      (4) Health care usage did not accurately reflect pain.
      (5) Patients with a hemoglobin SS genotype had pain more frequently than SC patients.
      (6) Painful sites were thigh, shoulder, and knee.
      (7) Of those studied, 28% reported depression; 31% reported alcohol abuse.
   b. Sickle cell disease is associated with long-standing controversy about analgesic addiction (Lusher, Elander, Bevan, Telfer, & Burton, 2006).
      (1) There is evidence to the contrary that sickle cell disease and analgesic dependency are correlated. It has been shown that disputes about analgesics are associated with pseudoaddiction (Lusher et al., 2006).

B. Pain prevalence in children
   1. Headache
      a. In a study of 9,000 schoolchildren, prevalence of headache in those at least 7 years old ranged from 37% to 51%. In those at least 15 years old, prevalence rose to 57% to 82%.
      b. "Frequent" headaches were reported in 2.5% of children at least 7 years old and 15% of those at least 15 years old.
      c. Before puberty, headaches are more frequent in boys; after puberty, they are more frequent in girls (Lewis, 2002).
   2. Myofascial and musculoskeletal pain
      a. In children 9 to 12 years of age, 57 per 100,000 reported myofascial pain (Mikkelsson, Sourander, Piha, & Salminen, 1997).
      b. Of children and adolescents, 0.2% to 12% reported pain with opening their jaw (Crombie et al., 1999).
      c. Causes of musculoskeletal pain in order of highest to lowest occurrence are trauma, mechanical or overuse, and osteochondrosis.
      d. Chronic knee pain was defined as more than 3 months in an epidemiological study (Vahasarja, 1995).
         (1) All ages: girls at 12.6%, boys at 11.3%
         (2) Age 9 to 10: girls at 3.1%, boys at 4.8%
         (3) Age 14 to 15: girls at 19.8%, boys at 16.8%
   3. Postoperative pain
      a. A study of 84 children following tonsillectomy showed that parents administered less analgesic than prescribed and that children suffered from undertreatment of pain.
      b. Of parents, 77% stated that the pain relief was adequate, but 56% of the children had difficulty taking oral fluids because of complaints of pain (Sutters & Miaskowski, 1997).

C. Pain prevalence in the elderly (see the chapter on Gerontology Pain Management)
   1. Pain in cognitively impaired nursing home patients (Ferrell, Ferrell, & Rivera, 1995)
      a. Of 325 subjects randomly selected, 62% reported pain complaints during the interview and pain questionnaire.
      b. Of those studied, 38% denied any painful problems or could not give meaningful responses to the questionnaire.
      c. Location of pain
         (1) Back: 67.1%
         (2) Knee: 58.2%
         (3) Foot or ankle: 52.2%
         (4) Shoulder: 47.8%
         (5) Neck: 45.5%
      d. Etiology of pain
         (1) Arthritis: 70%
         (2) Old fracture, including prosthetic related: 13%
         (3) Neuropathy: 10%
      e. Interventions
         (1) Of those studied, 81% had acetaminophen ordered.
         (2) In the study, 13% were actively taking nonsteroidal anti-inflammatory drugs.
         (3) Orders for opioid analgesics had been placed by 34%.
         (4) In the preceding 6 months, 25% received physical therapy consultation.
         (5) Of those studied, 6% stated they had been to a pain management clinic at one time.
         (6) Untreated pain results in impaired mobility, depression, and diminishes quality of life.
   2. "Persistent Pain in Nursing Home Residents" (research letter to the editor) (Teno, Weitzen, Wetle, & Mor, 2001)
      a. Since 1998, information on frequency of pain (none, daily, or less than daily) and severity of pain (mild, moderate, or excruciating at times) has been collected on nursing home residents.

b. Analysis of a national repository of a minimum data set representing nursing home residents in all 50 states found the following:
(1) Persistent pain was defined as daily moderate or excruciating pain at a second assessment, 60 to 180 days later.
(2) For two assessments, 14.7% of nursing home residents were in persistent pain.
(3) Of residents, 41.2% in pain at first assessment were in severe pain 60–180 days later.
(4) These data were reported by nursing home staff, not the residents.

3. "Pain in the Oldest–Old During Hospitalization and Up to One Year Later" (Desbiens, Mueller-Rizner, Connors, Hamel, & Wenger, 1997)
   a. A prospective cohort study was conducted at four teaching hospitals; 1,266 patients were at least 80 years of age in the Hospitalized Elderly Longitudinal Project.
   b. Hospital interviews were obtained from 49.1% of the patients due to inability to communicate, failed cognitive screen, refusal, discharge or death, coma, or intubation. Surrogate interviews were available for 72.7% of the patients.
   c. Post-hospitalization, 83.7% survived 2 months; 68.4% survived 12 months.
   d. In the study, 45.8% complained of pain, and 19.0% reported extremely severe pain of any frequency or moderately severe pain occurring at least half the time (similar to prevalence of pain reports of hospitalized patients, with these studies having been conducted in 1987, 1992, and 1996).
   e. Patients with depressed mood were at higher risk for pain during hospitalization.

D. Pain prevalence in the patient with cancer (IASP, 2008)
   1. Prevalence of pain at the time of cancer diagnosis and early in the course of disease is estimated at 50%.
   2. In advanced stages, the pain prevalence increases to 75%.
   3. In cancer survivors, a meta-analysis found pain prevalence to be 33%.
   4. Types of tumors
      a. Pancreatic: 72% to 85%
      b. Head and neck: 67% to 91%
      c. Prostate: 56% to 94%
      d. Genitourinary: 58% to 90%
      e. Breast: 40% to 89%
      f. Uterine: 30% to 90%

E. Pain prevalence in the hospice patient with nonmalignant terminal disease (Zeppetella, O'Doherty, & Collins, 2001)
   1. A prospective survey was made of prevalence and characteristics of breakthrough pain in patients with ***nonmalignant terminal disease*** admitted to hospice.
   2. Breakthrough pain was classified as somatic, visceral, neuropathic, or mixed etiology.
   3. Of the patients who were studied, 66% had reasonable control of background pain, while 34% reported severe or excruciating pain.
   4. The mean daily episodes of breakthrough pain was five; 54% occurred suddenly, 56% of pain was unpredictable, 60% was severe or excruciating, and 73% of all pain lasted less than 30 minutes.
      a. Prior to hospice admission, 33% were prescribed mild analgesics for their breakthrough pain.
      b. Of the patients, 30% took opioids for moderate pain.
      c. Another 33% took opioids for severe pain.
   5. Patient satisfaction
      a. Of patients with background pain without breakthrough pain, 75% were satisfied.
      b. Of patients with breakthrough pain, 41% were satisfied.

F. Pain prevalence in hospice patients with malignant terminal disease (Zeppetella, O'Doherty, & Collins, 2000)
   1. A prospective survey sought prevalence and characteristics of breakthrough pain.
   2. Breakthrough pain was classified as somatic, visceral, neuropathic, and mixed.

3. Reports from patients of duration of persistent pain were for days (10%), weeks (55%), and months (35%), with 89% of patients reporting breakthrough pain.
4. The mean of daily episodes of breakthrough pain was seven.
   a. Approximately 50% occurred suddenly.
   b. Another 17% resulted from end-of-dose failure of scheduled analgesics.
   c. In addition, 50% were unpredictable.
   d. For pain episodes, 73% lasted 30 minutes or less.
   e. Neuropathic breakthrough pain was brief, with 91% lasting 30 minutes or less.
   f. Of somatic pain, 60% lasted 30 minutes or less.
   g. Of visceral pain, 62% lasted 30 minutes or less.
5. Treatments
   a. The following treatments were reported to relieve pain the best: analgesics (57%) and lying still (32%).
   b. Of patients studied, 34% were prescribed nonopioid analgesics.
   c. The study found that 23% were prescribed weak opioids.
   d. Another 64% were prescribed strong opioid.
   e. Finally, 43% were not prescribed "rescue" medications.
6. Patient satisfaction
   a. Of patients with chronic pain without breakthrough pain, 78% were satisfied.
   b. Of patients with breakthrough pain, 25% were satisfied. Dissatisfied patients have significantly more occurrences of breakthrough pains.

G. Pain prevalence and gender (IASP, 2007) (see the chapter on Gender/Sex Differences in Pain and Analgesia)
1. Chronic pain: Prevalence rates are higher for women than for men for most common chronic pain conditions.
2. Female-to-male ratios
   a. Headache, neck, shoulder, knee, and back pain average around 1.5:1 (American Psychiatric Association, 2000, p. 501; IASP, 2007).
   b. Orofacial pain is 2:1.
   c. Migraine headache is 2.5:1.
   d. Fibromyalgia is 4:1.
3. Depression and comorbid features are risk factors for common pain conditions.
4. Women experience more physical symptoms than men.

Summary

Epidemiological studies are needed in the field of pain management, in particular regarding issues of nursing care. Advocacy begins with having a correct representation of the populations we work with. Epidemiological studies help get us closer to the truth.

References

American Psychiatric Association. (2000). *Diagnostic and statistical manual of mental disorders* (4th ed., text rev.) (DSM-IV-TR). Arlington, VA: Author.

Carlton, J. E. (2005). *Core curriculum for professional education in pain.* Seattle: IASP Press.

Crombie, I., Croft, P., Linton, S., LeResche, L., & Von Korff, M. (1999). *Epidemiology of pain.* London: IASP Press.

Desbiens, N. A., Mueller-Rizner, N., Connors, A. F., Hamel, M. B., & Wenger, N. S. (1997). Pain in the oldest–old during hospitalization and up to one year later. *Journal of the American Geriatrics Society, 45*(10), 1167–1172.

Ferrell, B. A., Ferrell, B. R., & Rivera, L. (1995). Pain in cognitively impaired nursing home patients. *Journal of Pain and Symptom Management, 10*(8), 591–598.

International Association for the Study of Pain. (2007). *Global year against pain in women.* Retrieved December 17, 2008, from http://www.iasp-pain.org/AM/Template.cfm?Section=Resources2&Template=/CM/ContentDisplay.cfm&ContentID=4469.

International Association for the Study of Pain. (2008). *Global year against cancer pain.* Retrieved December 17, 2008, from http://www.iasp-pain.org/AM/Template.cfm?Section=Resources3&Template=/CM/ContentDisplay.cfm&ContentID=7395.

Last, J. M. (1988). A dictionary of epidemiology. *International Journal of Epidemiology, 25*(5), 1098-1101.

Lewis, D. W. (2002). *Headaches in children and adolescents: American Family Physician.* Retrieved October 18, 2008, from http://www.aafp.org/afp/20020215/625.html.

Lusher, J., Elander, J., Bevan, D., Telfer, P., & Burton, B. (2006). Analgesic addiction and pseudoaddiction in painful chronic illness. *Clinical Journal of Pain, 22*(3), 316–324.

Mikkelsson, M., Sourander, A., Piha, J., & Salminen, J. J. (1997). Psychiatric symptoms in preadolescents with musculoskeletal pain and fibromyalgia. *Pediatrics, 100,* 220–227.

Reyes-Gibby, C. C., Aday, L. A., Todd, K. H., Cleeland, C. S., & Anderson, K. O. (2006). Pain in aging community–dwelling adults in the United States: Non-Hispanics Whites, non-Hispanic Blacks, and Hispanics. *Journal of Pain, 8,* 75–84.

Smith, W. (2005). *Pain in sickle cell epidemiology study.* Retrieved December 17, 2008, from http://www.nhlbi.nih.gov/meetings/scd/2005-11minutes.htm.

Sutters, K. A., & Miaskowski, C. (1997). Inadequate pain management and associated morbidity in children at home after tonsillectomy. *Journal of Pediatric Nursing, 12,* 178–185.

Teno, J. M., Weitzen, S., Wetle, T., & Mor, V. (2001). Persistent pain in nursing home residents. [Research letter]. *Journal of the American Medical Association, 285*(16), 2081.

Vahasarja, V. (1995). Prevalence of chronic knee pain in children and adolescents in northern Finland. *Acta Paediatrica, 84,* 803–805.

Zeppetella, G., O'Doherty, C. A., & Collins, S. (2000). Prevalence and characteristics of breakthrough pain in cancer patients admitted to a hospice. *Journal of Pain and Symptom Management, 20*(2), 87–92.

Zeppetella, G., O'Doherty, C. A., & Collins, S. (2001). Prevalence and characteristics of breakthrough pain in patients with non-malignant terminal disease admitted to a hospice. *Palliative Medicine, 15,* 243–246.

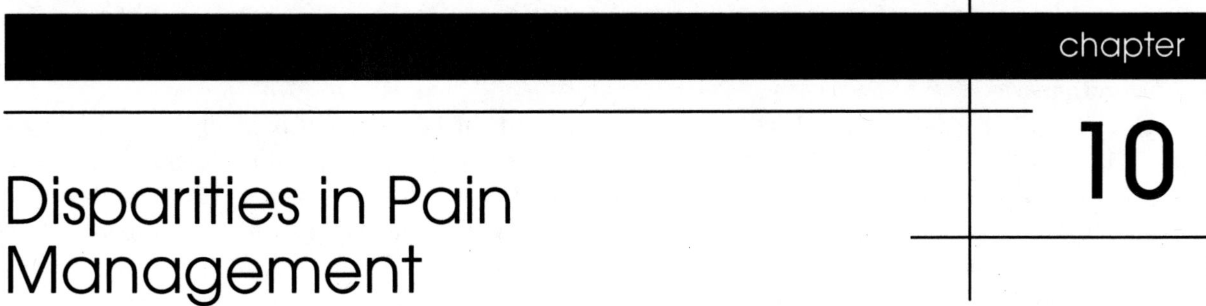

chapter

10

Disparities in Pain Management

Helen N. Turner, DNP, RN-BC, PCNS-BC

Objectives

After studying this chapter, the reader should be able to:

1. Explain at least five causes of health disparities affecting pain management.
2. Identify patient populations at high risk for inadequate pain care secondary to disparities.
3. Describe at least five personal and professional activities to decrease disparities in pain management.

I. Definitions

A. Disparities are defined as follows by Healthy People 2010 and the Institute of Medicine.
   1. Healthy People 2010: "Population-specific differences in the presence of disease, health outcomes, or access to health care" and "unequal burden in disease morbidity and mortality rates experienced by ethnic/racial groups as compared to the dominant group" (U.S. Department of Health and Human Services [USDHHS], 2000)
   2. Institute of Medicine: "Differences in the quality of health care that are not due to access-related factors or clinical needs, preferences or appropriateness of intervention" (Smedley, Stith, & Nelson, 2003)

II. Disparities in Health Care

A. Major causes
   1. The Institute of Medicine delineates two sources of disparities:
      a. Health care systems, including legal and regulatory climate
      b. Discrimination (e.g., biases, stereotyping, clinical communication, and decision making) (Smedley et al., 2003)
   2. Disparities are caused by treatment decisions, differences in income, differences in education, sociocultural factors, and failure by the medical profession (Lebovits, 2005).

B. Prevalence
   1. Fourteen percent of the U.S. population is without health insurance.
      a. Health insurance facilitates access to health care systems.
   2. Of the U.S. population, 68% of people live in medically underserved areas (Sullivan & Eagel, 2005).

C. Results of disparity in health care
   1. Those who suffer disparity in general have poorer health, are diagnosed later, are sicker when hospitalized, and die earlier (USDHHS, 2008).
   2. African Americans and Asians have a higher risk of death than Caucasians after injury (Arthur, Hedges, Newgard, Diggs, & Mullins, 2008).
   3. Patients who are Asian, older, female, or married tend to receive less aggressive cardiac care (Blomkalns et al., 2005; Diercks & Miller, 2008; Gnavi et al., 2007).
   4. African Americans and Hispanics receive less surgery for liver cancer (Sloane, Chen, & Howell, 2006; Sonnenday, Dimick, Schulick, & Choti, 2007).
   5. African Americans have greater numbers of emergency department visits for acute asthma (Ginde, Espinola, & Camargo, 2008).
   6. African Americans more often diagnosed with schizophrenia than Caucasians; contributing factors may include higher rates of substance abuse, cultural mistrust being interpreted as paranoia, misdiagnosis, methods used for diagnosis, provider influence or bias, and care setting (DeCoux Hampton, 2007).
   7. Women of color are less likely to have access to reproductive health care (Webb, 2004).
   8. African-Americans with severe sepsis are less likely to receive intensive care unit care than Caucasians (Barnato, Alexander, Linde-Zwirble, & Angus, 2008).
   9. Uninsured and African-American females less likely to be hospitalized for traumatic brain injury (Selassie, Pickelsimer, Frazier, & Ferguson, 2004).
   10. African Americans, Hispanics, and Asians less likely to receive invasive cardiovascular procedures (Kressin & Petersen, 2001).
   11. Less educated (below ninth grade) and African-American patients have lower rates of cardiac catheterizations (Schecter et al., 1996).
   12. This is a global issue, not just one in the United States.
       a. In Sweden, men received more treatment than women for dermatological conditions (Nyberg, Osika, & Evengard, 2008).
       b. In Jerusalem, Israel, Jewish residents received better diabetes care than Arab patients (Tirosh, Calderon-Margalit, Mazar, & Stern, 2008).

c. In Torino, Italy, statins are prescribed less based on age (older) and sex (female) for secondary prevention of ischemic heart disease (Gnavi et al., 2007).
d. In Canada, females and Asians receive less aggressive cardiac treatment (Diercks & Miller, 2008).
e. In South Africa, racial differences account for infant mortality rates (Burgard & Treiman, 2006).
f. In Glasgow, Scotland, women are less often prescribed statins and angiotensin-converting enzyme inhibitors after stroke (McInnes, McAlpine, & Walters, 2007).

III. Disparities in Pain Management

A. Population segments
1. Pain management differs among population segments. Those at particular risk are children, the elderly, people with a history of chemical dependency, the mentally ill, women, racial and ethnic minorities, and those with a socioeconomic disadvantage, language barriers, geographical remoteness, poor health literacy, specific types of pain-related conditions (acute, chronic nonmalignant, cancer, and experimental), and specific comorbidities (Green et al., 2003; Green, Todd, Lebovits, & Francis, 2006; Sullivan & Eagel, 2005).

B. Sociodemographics
1. Gender: female
   a. Women are more likely to receive fewer opioids and more often receive sedatives rather than analgesics (Green & Wheeler, 2003; Paulson, Dekker, & Aguilar-Gaxiola, 2007).
2. Race and ethnicity (Ezenwa, Ameringer, Ward, & Serlin, 2006; Green et al., 2003; Green et al., 2006; Paulson et al., 2007).
   a. Hispanics with long-bone fractures are twice as likely as non-Hispanics to *not* receive pain medication in a large, urban, level 1 trauma center; if they did receive medication, the doses were generally lower (Todd, Samaroo, & Hoffman, 1993).
   b. African Americans with long-bone fractures are less likely to receive analgesics in the emergency department than Caucasians, and risk of receiving no analgesics was 66% higher for African Americans than for Caucasians (Todd, Deaton, D'Adamo, & Goe, 2000).
   c. African Americans and other people of color in Medicaid managed care plans had one-third less odds of receiving a COX-2 prescription than Caucasians (Shaya & Blume, 2005).
   d. Hispanic ethnicity predicts limited access to care for chronic pain (Nguyen, Ugarte, Fuller, Haas, & Portenoy, 2005).
3. Age: the extremes
   a. Children are undertreated due to the challenges of assessing and communicating pain (Yaffa Zisk, 2003; Yaffa Zisk, Grey, MacLaren, & Kain, 2007).
   b. Regardless of setting, older patients are more likely to die in moderate to severe pain (SUPPORT Principle Investigators, 1995).
4. Socioeconomic disadvantage (Bernheim, Ross, Krumholz, & Bradley, 2008; Poleshuck & Green, 2008)
   a. Socioeconomic disadvantage includes factors of neighborhood socioeconomic status, education, and income.
   b. Socioeconomic disadvantage is consistently associated with increased risk for pain. In one study, the authors address the challenges of defining the socioeconomic disadvantaged (Poleshuck & Green, 2008).
5. Patient or family education level (Poleshuck & Green, 2008)
   a. Lower level of education is generally associated with lower income, decreased access to care, and possibly decreased quality of care (Bernheim et al., 2008; Field, 2008).
   b. Education has a greater association with health than does income (Poleshuck & Green, 2008).

C. Location
1. Those in rural areas have less access to care and specialty care than do those in urban areas

(Baicker, Chandra, & Skinner, 2005; Green et al., 2006; Nelson Bolin, Phillips, & Hawes, 2006; Tollefson & Usher, 2006).

2. Distance limits access to specialists, especially pain specialists who tend to practice in urban areas (Green et al., 2006).
3. People from lower-income neighborhoods have less access to health care generally and to pain care specifically.
    a. Pharmacies in some low-income areas not stocking adequate opioids (Green, Ndao-Brumblay, West, & Washington, 2005; Morrison, Wallenstein, Natale, Senzel, & Huang, 2000).
    b. Pharmacies in the state of Washington had adequate opioid supplies regardless of location and economic status (Mayer, Kirlin, Rehm, & Loeser, 2008).
4. Homeless people (Kushel & Miaskowski, 2006)
    a. The homeless have limited access to basic health care.
    b. Care is often poorly coordinated with inconsistent providers.
    c. There is a lack of data; however, the homeless are more generally ill and have increased premature death rates.
5. Health care setting affects quality and consistency of pain management.
    a. In the emergency department, delivery of analgesia is often delayed, ineffective, or both based on race, ethnicity, and gender (Arendts & Fry, 2006; Epps, Jowers Ware, & Packard, 2008; Heins et al., 2006; Pletcher, Kertesz, Kohn, & Gonzales, 2008; Quazi, Eberhart, Jacoby, & Heller, 2008; Rupp & Delaney, 2004; Todd et al., 1993).
    b. Nursing home residents experience significant amounts of moderate to severe pain (Cadogan, 2004; Green et al., 2003; Nelson Bolin et al., 2006).
    c. Despite improvements, many patients receive inadequate analgesia at the end of life (Brunnhuber, Nash, Meier, Weissman, & Woodcock, 2008; Harris, 2007; Rabow & Dibble, 2005).

D. Special populations
1. *Chronic pain:* It is unclear whether undertreatment in this population is solely based on undertreatment or is confounded by differences in coping and psychological responses (Green 2003; Watkins, Wollan, Melton, & Yawn, 2006).
2. *Cognitive impairment:* This population tends to be undertreated because of assessment and communication challenges (Cadogan, 2004; Jowers Ware, Epps, Herr, & Packard, 2006).
3. *Mental illness:* Pain involves both physical and psychological elements and is confounded by mental illness, often resulting in undertreatment (Gureje et al., 2008; Hughes, Nosek, & Robinson-Whelen, 2007; Ohayon, 2006).
    a. Mental illness often complicates history taking, assessment, treatment, compliance, and follow-through (Broyles, Colbert, Tate, Swigart, & Happ, 2008; Fishbain, 2005).
4. *Chemical dependency:* This population is often poorly treated due to inadequate provider knowledge related to pain and addiction treatment, as well as to providers' fears of repercussions from authorities and regulators and personal biases (American Society for Pain Management Nursing, 2002; Fosnocht, Swanson, & Barton, 2005; Morgan, 2006; Paulson et al., 2007; Rupp & Delaney, 2004; Sullivan & Eagel, 2005).
5. *Immigrants or culture:* Difficulty in assessment and history taking, delays or lack of treatment seeking, cultural norms dictating pain response, and providers lacking knowledge of cultural variability in pain response are common (Sobralske & Katz, 2005).
6. *Incarcerated:* Prison medical care is often substandard (Moore & Elkavich, 2008).
    a. Barriers to pain management identified by health care providers included concern for misuse diversion and patient credibility (Lin & Mathew, 2005).
    b. Similar to nonincarcerated minorities, there is a high incidence of uncontrolled cancer pain and severe chronic pain (Lin & Mathew, 2005).
    c. Prison policies prohibiting inmates from carrying medications (Lin & Mathew, 2005).
    d. There is a higher percentage of minorities in prisons (Bonney, Clarke, Simmons, Rose, & Rich, 2008).

7. *Workers' compensation* (Chibnall, Tait, Andresen, & Hadler, 2005; Scherzer, Rugulies, & Krause, 2005; Tait & Chibnall, 2001)
   a. Treatment is often inadequate (Chibnall et al., 2005).
   b. Negative provider attitudes or outright refusal to accept workers' compensation cases is seen (Chibnall et al., 2005; Scherzer et al., 2005).
   c. Those in low-wage jobs experience a higher burden of illness, injury, and disability; this burden falls on workers who are disadvantaged in society (female and minorities) (Scherzer et al., 2005).
   d. Underreporting of work-related injuries occurs due to punitive attitudes of managers, inadequate compensated time off, inadequate treatment, and failure to address workplace hazards (Scherzer et al., 2005).
   e. The adversarial nature of the workers' compensation process is an issue (Chibnall et al., 2005).

IV. Barriers Contributing to Disparities in Pain Management

A. Patient family
   1. Age, sex, socioeconomic status, and educational level can be barriers.
   2. Race and ethnicity can influence where patients seek care and the quality of care received (Iwashyna, Curlin, & Christakis, 2002; Kahn et al., 1994).
   3. Communication between patients and health care providers and concerns about risk of addiction, abuse, or diversion can be problems (Sullivan & Eagel, 2005).
   4. The disease process can cause disparities.
   5. Anxiety, grief, and anger can be barriers.
   6. Misconceptions, concerns, biases, and beliefs often contribute to disparities.

B. Health care providers
   1. Attitudes and beliefs could create disparities.
      a. Some physicians underestimate pain in African-American patients (Staton et al., 2007).
      b. Physicians' and nurses' ethnic, cultural, and gender biases and knowledge influence treatment (Berger, 2008; Clarke et al., 1996; Ferrell, McGuire, & Donovan, 1993; Fosnocht et al., 2005; Hamers, Abu-Saad, van den Hout, & Halfens, 1998; Layman Young, Horton, & Davidhizar, 2006; Manworren & Hayes, 2000; McCaffery, & Ferrell, 1997; Tamayo-Sarver et al., 2003; Weisse, Sorum, & Dominguez, 2003).
      c. Clinical management decisions are influenced by patients' socioeconomic status. The population in one article consisted entirely of Medicaid patients, so they had insurance coverage (Bernheim et al., 2008).
   2. Providers' who had personal experience with pain tended to be more empathetic in the management of pain (Abu-Saad & Hamers, 1997; Banja, 2006; Fuller, 1996; Griffin, Polit, & Byrne, 2007; Horbury, Henderson, & Bromley, 2005; Wilson, 2007).
   3. Lack of training in pain medicine or addiction medicine can be a barrier (Fosnocht et al., 2005; Paulson et al., 2007; Sullivan & Eagel, 2005).
   4. Lack of priority may be given to pain care.
   5. Accountability to provide pain management may be lacking.
   6. Time restrictions may be placed on providers in clinical settings.

C. Health care systems
   1. Access (Green et al., 2006; Kahn et al., 1994)
      a. Pharmacies may not be stocking sufficient medications to treat severe pain adequately (Green, et al., 2005; Morrison et al., 2000).
      b. Medication decisions may be based on potential for abuse rather than effectiveness (Flugsrud-Breckenridge, Gervitz, Paul, & Gould, 2007).
   2. Society
      a. The war on drugs and diversion prevention can create barriers (Joranson, Elliott, & Lipman, 2003).

3. Insurance
    a. Ethnicity and insurance were found to be significant determinants of whether or not an epidural was used for labor analgesia in a sample of more than 2,300 women.
        (1) Women who had Medicaid insurance were almost twice as likely not to receive an epidural when compared to privately insured and noninsured women.
        (2) Women who had Medicaid insurance were more likely to be younger, less educated and mostly African American.
        (3) Hispanic ethnicity was also strongly associated with nonuse of epidural procedures, which may be related to lack of resources such as insurance, education, and ability to navigate the health care system (Atherton DeCarolis Feeg, & Fouad Lel-Adham, 2004).

V. Ethical Implications

A. Pain relief was declared a basic human right by the World Health Organization (Green et al., 2006).

B. The American Nurses Association (ANA) and American Medical Association (AMA) codes of ethics (AMA, 2002; ANA, 2001) outline ethical practices, including those related to pain care.
   1. Autonomy
      a. Self-determination is respecting the choices and wishes of people who have the capacity to decide and protecting those who do not have this capacity.
   2. Nonmaleficence
      a. Do no harm.
      b. We know untreated pain results in harm.
   3. Beneficence
      a. Care should benefit patients and protect their interests.
   4. Justice
      a. Justice is "fair, equitable, and appropriate distribution in society of a privilege, benefit, or service" (Lebovits, 2005, p. 3).

VI. Legislation or Policies Addressing Disparities in Pain Management

A. Health care reform (American Pain Foundation, 2008)
   1. The National Pain Care Policy Act of 2008 (HR 2994) calls for a congressional finding for improved pain care research, education, access, and care. These are national health care priorities requiring appropriate funding.
   2. The Veterans Pain Care Act is part of the Veterans Health Care Policy Enhancement Act of 2008 (HR 6445) and addresses assessment and management of pain (acute and chronic), standardization of pain care, pain research, pain education of health care providers and patients, and performance accountability for veterans' pain care.
   3. The Military Pain Care Act of 2008 is part of the FY09 National Defense Authorization Act and directs the U.S. secretary of defense to plan a pain care initiative in all health care facilities of the military.

B. Advocacy groups
   1. Pain and Policy Studies Group, University of Wisconsin, Paul P. Carbone Comprehensive Cancer Center, World Health Organization Collaborating Center for Policy and Communications in Cancer Care (2008).
      a. Through research, education, and communication, the focus is on identifying and addressing barriers to appropriate use of opioids, especially in chronic pain and palliative care.
         (1) State report cards on pain policy
         (2) Collaboration with the U.S. Drug Enforcement Administration
      b. The mission includes balancing international, national, and state policies to assure access to pain medications while minimizing diversion and abuse and to support communication around the globe to improve access to information about pain relief, palliative care, and policy.

2. Center for Practical Bioethics Balancing Pain Policy (2008)
   a. The center works with pain policy groups, state medical boards, and attorneys general to educate, advocate, and influence pain policy nationally.

VII. Pain Management Disparities in Current Literature and Media

A. There is a need for increased coverage of disparities in the popular media (television, Internet, and printed press) to increase public awareness.

B. Research activities may result in low-socioeconomic-status participants to be missed in traditional pain studies that recruit by phone or in a medical setting.

C. The following are pain management organizations that address education, advocacy, and disparities in pain care:
   1. American Society for Pain Management Nursing
   2. American Pain Society
   3. American Pain Foundation
   4. American Academy of Pain Medicine
   5. International Association for the Study of Pain
   6. Alliance of State Pain Initiatives
   7. American Chronic Pain Association
   8. The Pain Relief Foundation
   9. Mayday Fund
   10. National Foundation for the Treatment of Pain

D. Governmental organizations addressing disparities include the following:
   1. Agency for Healthcare Research and Quality
   2. National Guideline Clearinghouse
   3. National Institutes of Health
   4. National Library of Medicine
   5. U.S. Drug Enforcement Administration
   6. U.S. Food and Drug Administration
   7. Veterans Health Administration Office of Quality and Performance, clinical practice guidelines

VIII. What We Can Do?

A. Increase awareness of disparities and populations at greatest risk (Green, Tait, & Gallagher, 2005; Paulson et al., 2007; Sullivan & Eagel, 2005).

B. Participate in ongoing research and monitoring of pain management disparities (American Pain Society, 2004; Green et al., 2006; Sullivan & Eagel, 2005).

C. Address disparities through health care education and continuing education (Green et al., 2006; Paulson et al., 2007).

D. Promote cultural competence and social justice (Green et al., 2006).

E. Encourage and inspire minority students to pursue careers in pain management (Green et al., 2006).

F. Develop and advocate for policy and legislation directed at removing barriers to pain management (APS, 2004; Green, Tait, et al., 2005; Green et al., 2006; Taylor, Gostin, & Pagonis, 2008).
   1. Education to address prescribing fears needs more attention (Passik, 2006; Rich, 2006; Rowe, 2006).
   2. Access is needed to appropriate pain care and medications (Lin, Crawford, & Salmon, 2005; von Gunten, 2006).

G. Work with third-party payers and pharmacy organizations to improve access to care and treatment (Paulson et al., 2007).

H. Improve communication between patients and providers (Carcaise-Edinboro & Bradley, 2008; Kalauokalani, Franks, Wright Oliver, Meyers, & Kravitz, 2007).

I. Advocate for patient and family involvement in pain management care (McNeill, Reynolds, & Ney, 2007; Walker, Signal, Russell, Smiler, & Tuhiwai-Ruru, 2008).

J. Advocate for comprehensive multidisciplinary pain management at hospital, local, state, and national levels (APS, 2004; Paulson et al., 2007).
   1. Close working relationships should be developed with addiction specialists (Paulson et al., 2007).

K. "Still, an insightful clinician will always need to avoid ethnic or racial stereotypes, eschew the notion of cultural uniformity, and assess and manage each patient as an individual" (Rollman, 2005, p. 4).

L. "Our greatest opportunities for reducing health disparities are in empowering individuals to make informed health care decisions and in promoting communitywide safety, education, and access to health care" (USDHHS, 2000, p. 16).

References

Abu-Saad, H., & Hamers, J. P. H. (1997). Decision-making and paediatric pain: A review. *Journal of Advanced Nursing, 26,* 946–952.

American Medical Association Council on Ethical and Judicial Affairs. (2002). *Code of medical ethics.* Chicago: AMA Press, p. 269.

American Nurses Association. (2001). *Code of ethics for nurses with interpretive statements.* Silver Spring, MD: American Nurses Publishing.

American Pain Foundation. (2008). Retrieved October 1, 2008, from http://www.painfoundation.org/page.asp?file=Action/intro.htm.

American Pain Society. (2004). *Position statement. Racial and ethnic identifiers in pain management: The importance to research, clinical practice, and public health policy.* Retrieved October 6, 2008, from http://www.ampainsoc.org/advocacy/ethnoracial.htm.

American Society for Pain Management Nursing. (2002). *Position statement. Pain management in patients with addictive disease.* Retrieved October 6, 2008, from http://www.aspmn.org/Organization/documents/addictions_9pt.pdf.

Arendts, G., & Fry, M. (2006). Factors associated with delay to opioid analgesia in emergency departments. *Journal of Pain, 7*(9), 682–686.

Arthur, M., Hedges, J. R., Newgard, C. D., Diggs, B. S., & Mullins, R. J. (2008). Racial disparities in mortality among adults hospitalized after injury. *Medical Care, 46*(2), 192–199.

Atherton, M. J., DeCarolis Feeg, V., & Fouad Lel-Adham, A. (2004). Race, ethnicity, and insurance as determinants of epidural use: Analysis of a national sample survey. *Nursing Economics, 22*(1), 6–13.

Baicker, K., Chandra, A., & Skinner, J. S. (2005). Geographic variation and the problem of measuring racial disparities in health care. *Perspectives in Biology and Medicine, 48*(Suppl. 1), S42–S53.

Banja, J. D. (2006). Empathy in the physician's pain practice: Benefits, barriers, and recommendations. *Pain Medicine, 7*(3), 265–275.

Barnato, A. E., Alexander, S. L., Linde-Zwirble, W. T., & Angus, D. C. (2008). Racial variation in the incidence, care, and outcomes of severe sepsis. *American Journal of Respiratory Critical Care Medicine, 117,* 279–284.

Berger, J. T. (2008). The influence of physicians' demographic characteristics and their patients' demographic characteristics on physician practice: Implications for education and research. *Academic Medicine, 83*(1), 100–105.

Bernheim, S. M., Ross, J. S., Krumholz, H. M., & Bradley, E. H. (2008). Influence of patients' socioeconomic status on clinical management decisions: A qualitative study. *Annals of Family Medicine, 6*(1), 53–59.

Blomkalns, A. L., Chen, A. Y., Hochman, J. S., Peterson, E. D., Trynosky, K., Diercks, D. B, Brogan, G.X., Jr., Boden, W.E., Roe, M.T., Ohman, E.M., Gibler, W.B., & Newby, L.K. (2005). Gender disparities in the diagnosis and treatment of non–ST-segment elevation acute coronary syndromes: Large-scale observations from the CRUSADE (can rapid risk stratification of unstable angina patients suppress adverse outcomes with early implementation of the American College of Cardiology/American Heart Association Guidelines) national quality improvement initiative. *Journal of the American College of Cardiology, 45*(6), 832–837.

Bonney, L. E., Clarke, J. G., Simmons, E. M., Rose, J. S., & Rich, J. D. (2008). Racial/ethnic sexual health disparities among incarcerated women. *Journal of the National Medical Association, 100,* 553–558.

Broyles, L. M., Colbert, A. M., Tate, J., A., Swigart, V. A., & Happ, M. B. (2008). Clinicians' evaluation and management of mental health, substance abuse, and chronic pain conditions in the intensive care unit. *Critical Care Medicine, 36,* 87–93.

Brunnhuber, K., Nash, S., Meier, D. E., Weissman, D. E., & Woodcock, J. (2008). *Putting evidence into practice: Palliative care.* Retrieved October 8, 2008, from http://www.unitedhealthfoundation.org/download/EndofLife.pdf.

Burgard, S. A., & Treiman, D. J. (2006). Trends and racial differences in infant mortality in South Africa. *Social Science and Medicine, 62,* 1126–1137.

Cadogan, M. (2004). Exploring the great barrier myth: another look at obstacles to effective pain management. *Journal of American Medical Directors Association, 5*(2), 133–134.

Carcaise-Edinboro, P., & Bradley, C. J. (2008). Influence of patient–provider communication on colorectal cancer screening. *Medical Care, 46,* 738–745.

Center for Practical Bioethics Balancing Pain Policy. (2008). Retrieved October 1, 2008, from http://www.practicalbioethics.org/cpb.aspx?pgID=978.

Chibnall, J. T., Tait, R. C., Andresen, E. M., & Hadler, N. M. (2005). Race and socioeconomic differences in post-settlement outcomes for African American and Caucasian Workers' Compensation claimants with low back injuries. *Pain, 114,* 462–472.

Clarke, E. B., French, B., Bilodeau, M. L., Capasso, V. C., Edwards, A., & Empoliti, J. (1996). Pain management knowledge, attitudes and clinical practice: The impact of nurses' characteristics and education. *Journal of Pain and Symptom Management, 11,* 18–31.

DeCoux Hampton, M. (2007). The role of treatment setting and high acuity in the overdiagnosis of schizophrenia in African Americans. *Archives of Psychiatric Nursing, 21*(6), 327–335.

Diercks, D. B., & Miller, C. D. (2008). Disparities in the care of chest pain. *Canadian Medical Association Journal, 179,* 631–632.

Epps, C. D., Jowers Ware, L., & Packard, A. (2008). Ethnic wait time differences in analgesic administration in the emergency department. *Pain Management Nursing, 9*(1), 26–32.

Ezenwa, M. O., Ameringer, S., Ward, S. E., & Serlin, R. C. (2006). Racial and ethnic disparities in pain management in the United States. *Journal of Nursing Scholarship, 38*(3), 225–233.

Ferrell, B. R., McGuire, D. B., & Donovan, M. I. (1993). Knowledge and beliefs regarding pain in a sample of nursing faculty. *Journal of Professional Nursing, 9,* 79–88.

Field, D. (2008). Disparities in pain management: An expert interview with Carmen R. Green, M. D. *Medscape Neurology and Neurosurgery.* Retrieved October 6, 2008, from http://www.medscape.com/viewarticle/581003? src=mp&spon=17&uac=123889FT.

Fishbain, D. A. (2005). Polypharmacy treatment approaches to the psychiatric and somatic comorbidities found in patients with chronic pain. *American Journal of Physical Medicine and Rehabilitation, 84*(Suppl.), S56–S63.

Flugsrud-Breckenridge, M. R., Gervitz, C., Paul, D., & Gould, H. J., III. (2007). Medication of abuse in pain management. *Current Opinion in Anaesthesiology, 20,* 319–324.

Fosnocht, D. E., Swanson, E. R., & Barton, E. D. (2005). Changing attitudes about pain and pain control in emergency medicine. *Emergency Medicine Clinics of North America, 23,* 297–306.

Fuller, B. (1996). Meanings of discomfort and fussy-irritable in infant pain assessment. *Journal of Pediatric Health Care, 10,* 255–263.

Ginde, A. A., Espinola, J. A., & Camargo, C. A. (2008). Improved overall trends but persistent racial disparities in emergency department visits for acute asthma, 1993–2005. *Journal of Allergy and Clinical Immunology, 122,* 313–318.

Gnavi, R., Migliardi, A., Demaria, M., Petrelli, A., Caprioglio, A., & Costa, G. (2007). Statins prescribing for the secondary prevention of ischaemic heart disease in Torino, Italy: A case of ageism and social inequalities. *European Journal of Public Health, 17*(5), 492–496.

Green, C. R., Anderson, K. O., Baker, T. A., Campbell, L. C., Decker, S., Fillingim, Todd, K.H., & Vallerand, A.H. (2003). The unequal burden of pain: Confronting racial and ethnic disparities in pain. *Pain Medicine, 4*(3), 277–294.

Green, C. R., Ndao-Brumblay, S. K., West, B., & Washington, T. (2005). Differences in prescription opioid analgesic availability: Comparing minority and White pharmacies across Michigan. *Journal of Pain, 6*(10), 689–699.

Green, C. R., Tait, R. C., & Gallagher, R. M. (2005). The unequal burden of pain: Disparities and differences. *Pain Medicine, 6*(1), 1–2.

Green, C. R., Todd, K. H., Lebovits, A., & Francis, M. (2006). Disparities in pain: Ethical issues. *Pain Medicine, 7*(6), 530–533.

Green, C. R., & Wheeler, J. R. (2003). Physician variability in the management of acute postoperative and cancer pain: A quantitative analysis of the Michigan experience. *Pain Medicine, 4,* 8–20.

Griffin, R. A., Polit, D. F., & Byrne, M. W. (2007). Stereotyping and nurses' recommendations for treating pain in hospitalized children. *Research in Nursing & Health, 30,* 655–666.

Gureje, O., Von Korff, M., Kola, L., Demyttenaere, K., He, Y., Posada-Villa, J., Lepine, J. P., Angermeyer, M. C., Levinson, D., Alonso, J., de Girolamo, G., Iwata, N., Karam, A., Guimaraes Borges, G. L., de Graaf, R., Browne, M. O., Stein, D. J., Haro, J. M., Bromet, E. J., Kessler, R. C., & Alonso, J. (2008). The relation between multiple pains and mental disorders: Results from the World Mental Health surveys. *Pain, 135,* 82–91.

Hamers, J. P. H., Abu-Saad, H., van den Hout, M. A., & Halfens, R. J. G. (1998). Are children given insufficient pain-relieving medication postoperatively? *Journal of Advanced Nursing, 27,* 37–44.

Harris, D. (2007). Forget me not: Palliative care for people with dementia. *Postgraduate Medical Journal, 83,* 362–266.

Heins, J. K., Heins, A., Grammas, M., Costello, M., Huang, K., & Mishra, S. (2006). Disparities in analgesia and opioid prescribing practices for patients with musculoskeletal pain in the emergency department. *Journal of Emergency Nursing, 32*(3), 219–224.

Horbury, C., Henderson, A., & Bromley, R. (2005). Influences of patient behavior on clinical nurses' pain assessment: Implications for continuing education. *Journal of Continuing Education in Nursing, 36*(1), 18–24.

Hughes, R. B., Nosek, M. A., & Robinson-Whelen, S. (2007). Correlates of depression in rural women with physical disabilities. *Journal of Obstetric, Gynecologic, and Neonatal Nursing, 36,* 105–114.

Iwashyna, T. J., Curlin, F. A., & Christakis, N. A. (2002). Racial, ethnic, and affluence differences in elderly patients' use of teaching hospitals. *Journal of General Internal Medicine, 17,* 696–703.

Joranson, D. E., Elliott, D., & Lipman, A. G. (2003). Pain and the pharmacist. *Pain Medicine, 4*(2), 190–194.

Jowers Ware, L., Epps, C. D., Herr, K., & Packard, A. (2006). Evaluation of the Revised Faces Pain Scale, Verbal Descriptor Scale, and Iowa Pain Thermometer in older minority adults. *Pain Management Nursing, 7*(3), 117–125.

Kahn, K. L., Pearson, M. L., Harrison, E. R., Desmond, K. A., Rogers, W. H., Rubenstein, L. V., Brook, R. H., & Keeler, E. B., et al. (1994). Health care for Black and poor hospitalized Medicare patients. *Journal of the American Medical Association, 271,* 1169–1174.

Kalauokalani, D., Franks, P., Wright Oliver, J., Meyers, F. J., & Kravitz, R. L. (2007). Can patient coaching reduce racial/ethnic disparities in cancer pain control? Secondary analysis of a randomized controlled trial. *Pain Medicine, 8*(1), 17–24.

Kressin, N. R., & Petersen, L. A. (2001). Racial differences in the use of invasive cardiovascular procedures: Review of the literature and prescription for future research. *Annals of Internal Medicine, 135,* 352–366.

Kushel, M. B., & Miaskowski, C. (2006). End-of-life care for homeless patients: "She says she is there to help me in any situation." *Journal of the American Medical Association, 296,* 2959–2966.

Layman Young, J., Horton, F. M., & Davidhizar, R. (2006). Nursing attitudes and beliefs in pain assessment and management. *Journal of Advanced Nursing, 53,* 412–421.

Lebovits, A. (2005). The ethical implications of racial disparities in pain: Are some of us more equal? *Pain Medicine, 6*(1), 3–4.

Lin, J. T., & Mathew, P. (2005). Cancer pain management in prisons: A survey of primary care practitioners and inmates. *Journal of Pain and Symptom Management, 29,* 466–473.

Lin, S., Crawford, S. Y., & Salmon, C. J. (2005). Potential access and revealed access to pain management medications. *Social Science & Medicine, 60,* 1881–1891.

Manworren, R. C. B., & Hayes, J. S. (2000). Pediatric nurses' knowledge and attitudes survey regarding pain. *Pediatric Nursing, 26,* 610–614.

Mayer, J. D., Kirlin, B., Rehm, C., & Loeser, J. D. (2008). Opioid availability in outpatient pharmacies in Washington State. *Clinical Journal of Pain, 24*(2), 120–123.

McCaffery, M., & Ferrell, B. R. (1997). Nurses' knowledge of pain assessment and management: How much progress have we made? *Journal of Pain and Symptom Management, 14*(3), 175–188.

McInnes, C., McAlpine, C., & Walters, M. (2007). Effect of gender on stroke management in Glasgow. *Age and Ageing, 37*(2), 220–222.

McNeill, J. A., Reynolds, J., & Ney, M. L. (2007). Unequal quality of cancer pain management: Disparity in perceived control and proposed solutions. *Oncology Nursing Forum, 34*(6), 1121–1128.

Moore, L. D., & Elkavich, A. (2008). Who's using and who's doing time: Incarceration, the war on drugs, and public health. *American Journal of Public Health, 98,* 782–786.

Morgan, B. D. (2006). Knowing how to play the game: Hospitalized substance abusers' strategies for obtaining pain relief. *Pain Management Nursing, 7*(1), 31–41.

Morrison, R. S., Wallenstein, S., Natale, D. K., Senzel, R. S., & Huang, L. (2000). "We don't carry that": Failure of pharmacies in predominantly non-White neighborhoods to stock opioids analgesics. *New England Journal of Medicine, 342,* 1023–1026.

Nelson Bolin, J., Phillips, C. D., & Hawes, C. (2006). Urban and rural differences in end-of-life pain and treatment status on admission to a nursing facility. *American Journal of Hospice and Palliative Medicine, 23*(1), 51–57.

Nguyen, M., Ugarte, C., Fuller, I., Hass, B., & Portenoy, R. K. (2005). Access to care for chronic pain: Racial and ethnic differences. *Journal of Pain, 6*(5), 301–314.

Nyberg, F., Osika, I., & Evengard, B. (2008). "The laundry bag project": Unequal distribution of dermatological healthcare resources for male and female psoriatic patients in Sweden. *International Journal of Dermatology, 47,* 144–149.

Ohayon, M. M. (2006). Interlacing sleep, pain, mental disorders and organic diseases. *Journal of Psychiatric Research, 40,* 677–679.

University of Wisconsin Pain and Policy Studies Group, University of Wisconsin Paul P. Carbone Comprehensive Cancer Center, & World Health Organization Collaborating Center for Policy and Communications in Cancer Care. (2008). Retrieved October 1, 2008, from http://www.painpolicy.wisc.edu/.

Passik, S. D. (2006). Pain management misstatements: Ceiling effects, red and yellow flags. *Pain Medicine, 7*(1), 76–77.

Paulson, M. R., Dekker, A. H., & Aguilar-Gaxiola, S. (2007). Eliminating disparities in pain management. *Journal of American Osteopathic Association, 107*(Supplement 5), ES17–ES20.

Pletcher, M. J., Kertesz, S. G., Kohn, M. A., Gonzales, R. (2008). Trends in opioid prescribing by race/ethnicity for patients seeking care in U.S. emergency departments. *Journal of the American Medical Association, 299,* 70–78.

Poleshuck, E. L., & Green, C. R. (2008). Socioeconomic disadvantage and pain. *Pain, 136,* 235–238.

Quazi, S., Eberhart, M., Jacoby, J., & Heller, M. (2008). Are racial disparities in ED analgesia improving? Evidence from a national database. *American Journal of Emergency Medicine, 26,* 462–464.

Rabow, M. W., & Dibble, S. (2005). The unequal burden of pain: Disparities and differences (continuation) ethnic differences in pain among outpatients with terminal and end-stage chronic illness. *Pain Medicine, 6*(3), 235–241.

Rich, B. A. (2006). Of smoke, mirrors, and passive–aggressive behaviors. *Pain Medicine, 7*(1), 78–79.

Rollman, G. B. (2005). The need for ecological validity in studies of pain and ethnicity. *Pain, 113,* 3–4.

Rowe, W. (2006). Pain, the DEA, and the impact on patients. *Pain Medicine, 7*(1), 86.

Rupp, T., & Delaney, K. A. (2004). Inadequate analgesia in emergency medicine. *Annals of Emergency Medicine, 43*(4), 494–503.

Schecter, A. D., Goldschmidt-Clermont, P. J., McKee, G., Hoffeld, D., Myers, M., Velez, R., Duran, J., Schulman, S. P., Chandra, N. G., & Ford, D. E. (1996). Influence of gender, race, and education on patient preferences and receipt of cardiac catheterizations among coronary care unit patients. *American Journal of Cardiology, 78,* 996–1001.

Scherzer, T., Rugulies, R., & Krause, N. (2005). Work-related pain and injury and barriers to workers' compensation among Las Vegas hotel room cleaners. *American Journal of Public Health, 95*(3), 483–488.

Selassie, A. W., Pickelsimer, E. E., Frazier, L., Ferguson, P. L. (2004). The effect of insurance status, race, and gender on ED disposition of persons with traumatic brain injury. *American Journal of Emergency Medicine, 22,* 465–473.

Shaya, F. R., & Blume, S. (2005). Prescriptions for cyclooxygenase-2 inhibitors and other nonsteroidal anti-inflammatory agents in a Medicaid managed care population: African Americans versus Caucasians. *Pain Medicine, 6*(1), 11–17.

Sloane, D., Chen, H., & Howell, C. (2006). Racial disparity in primary hepatocellular carcinoma: Tumor stage at presentation, surgical treatment and survival. *Journal of the National Medical Association, 98*(12):1934–1939.

Smedley, B., Stith, A., & Nelson, A. (2003). *Unequal treatment: Confronting racial and ethnic disparities in health care.* Washington, DC: National Academies Press.

Sobralske, M., & Katz, J. (2005). Culturally competent care of patients with acute chest pain. *Journal of the American Academy of Nurse Practitioners, 17,* 342–349.

Sonnenday, C. J., Dimick, J. B., Schulick, R. D., & Choti, M. A. (2007). Racial and geographic disparities in the utilization of surgical therapy for hepatocellular carcinoma. *Journal of Gastrointestinal Surgery, 11,* 1636–1646.

Staton, L. J., Panda, M., Chen, I., Genao, I., Kurz, J., Pasanen, M., Mechaber, A., Memon, M., O'Rourke, J., Wood, J., Rosenberg, E., Faselis, C., Carey, T., Calleson, D., & Cykert, S. (2007). When race matters: Disagreement in pain perception between patients and the physicians in primary care. *Journal of the National Medical Association, 99,* 532–538.

Sullivan, L. W., & Eagel, B. A. (2005). Leveling the playing field: Recognizing and rectifying disparities in management of pain. *Pain Medicine, 6*(1), 5–10.

SUPPORT Principle Investigators. (1995). A controlled trial to improve care for seriously ill hospitalized patients: The study to understand prognoses and preferences for outcomes and risks of treatments (SUPPORT). *Journal of the American Medical Association, 274,* 1591–1598.

Tait, R. C., & Chibnall, J. T. (2001). Work injury management of refractory low back pain: Relations with ethnicity, legal representation, and diagnosis. *Pain, 91,* 47–56.

Tamayo-Sarver, J. H., Dawson, N. V., Hinze, S. W., Cydulka, R. K., Wigton, R. S., Albert, J. M., Ibrahim, S. A., & Baker, D. W. (2003). The effect of race/ethnicity and desirable social characteristics on physicians' decision to prescribe opioid analgesics. *Academy of Emergency Medicine, 10*(11), 1239–1248.

Taylor, A. L., Gostin, L. O., & Pagonis, K. A. (2008). Ensuring effective pain treatment. *Journal of the American Medical Association, 299,* 89–91.

Tirosh, A., Calderon-Margalit, R., Mazar, M., & Stern, Z. (2008). Differences in quality of diabetes care between Jews and Arabs in Jerusalem. *American Journal of Medical Quality, 23*(1):60–65.

Todd, K. H., Deaton, C., D'Adamo, A. P., & Goe, L. (2000). Ethnicity and analgesic practice. *Annals of Emergency Medicine, 35*(1), 11–16.

Todd, K. H., Samaroo, N., & Hoffman, J. R. (1993). Ethnicity as a risk factor for inadequate emergency department analgesia. *Journal of the American Medical Association, 269,* 1537–1539.

Tollefson, J., & Usher, K. (2006). Short report chronic pain in the rural arena. *Australian Journal of Rural Health, 14,* 134–135.

U.S. Department of Health and Human Services. (2000). *Healthy people 2010: National health promotion and disease prevention objectives.* Retrieved May 1, 2008, from http://www.healthypeople.gov/Document/pdf/uih/2010uih.pdf.

U.S. Department of Health and Human Services, Agency for Healthcare Research and Quality. (2008). *National healthcare disparities report 2007.* Rockville, MD: Author.

von Gunten, C. F. (2006). Who makes the rules? *Journal of Palliative Medicine, 9*(1), 2–3.

Walker, T., Signal, L., Russell, M., Smiler, K., & Tuhiwai-Ruru, R. (2008). The road we travel: Maori experience of cancer. *New Zealand Medical Journal, 121*(1279), 27–35.

Watkins, E., Wollan, P. C., Melton, J., & Yawn, B. P. (2006). Silent pain sufferers. *Mayo Clinic Proceedings, 81*(2), 167–171.

Webb, R. (2004). *Reproductive health disparities for women of color.* Washington, DC National Association of Social Workers, Office of Human Rights and International Affairs, pp. 1–5.

Weisse, C. S., Sorum, P. C., & Dominguez, R. E. (2003). The influence of gender and race on physicians' pain management decisions. *Journal of Pain, 4*(9), 505–510.

Wilson, B. (2007). Nurses' knowledge of pain. *Journal of Clinical Nursing, 16,* 1012–1020.

Yaffa Zisk, R. (2003). Our youngest patients' pain: from disbelief to belief? *Pain Management Nursing, 4*(1), 40–51.

Yaffa Zisk, R., Grey, M., MacLaren, J. E., Kain, Z. N. (2007). Exploring sociodemographic and personality characteristic predictors of parental pain perceptions. *Anesthesiology and Analgesia, 104,* 790–798.

chapter

11

Pain Initiatives

Nancy Kowal, MS, APRN, BC
Jerri Patterson, RN, MSN, APN, BC

Objectives

After studying this chapter, the reader should be able to:

1. Describe the beginning of the pain initiatives.
2. Understand the national transition of the American Alliance of State Pain Initiatives.
3. Examine the effect of the national state initiatives on pain management as a public health problem.
4. Identify state initiatives' historical contributions.
5. Discuss the influence of pain initiatives on professional organizations and their contributions.
6. Discuss the influence of state pain initiatives on the national pain management action.

I. Goals of State Pain Initiatives (PIs)

A. Focus on cancer pain at all stages of the disease.
B. Discuss the initiation of pain management education to change practice.
C. Identify the creation of pain management standards, guidelines, and programs designed for health care professionals.

II. History of the Cancer Pain Initiatives (CPIs)

A. CPIs began in 1986 (Alliance of State Pain Initiatives, 2008).
B. They focused on the state licensure process for health care professionals.
C. They addressed the geographical and demographical diversity of each state.
D. The purpose was to design programs in each state based on its unique strengths and characteristics.
E. The Alliance of State Pain Initiatives identified state barriers, licensure issues, and regulatory problems.

III. Initial construct

A. Pain was identified as a major public health problem despite the advances in pain management science and medical care (Dahl, 1993, 1998).
   1. Pain providers and innovators supported the concept that pain was not managed well in the 1980s.
   2. Charles Cleeland's work with cancer pain, along with that of his colleagues, defined pain barriers and care deficits in practice (Cleeland et al., 1994; Joranson & Gilson, 1997).
   3. Quality initiatives validated these concerns and ranked fear of pain as the number one concern, even over death, in 2000 (Daut & Cleeland, 1982).
B. The national status of pain as a public health problem was staggering.
   1. The prevalence of pain in the United States affected greater than 50 million Americans.
   2. More than 25 million experienced acute pain as a result of surgery or injuries (Greene, 1993).
   3. One-third of patients with cancer indicated that upon diagnosis they had been in pain, and two-thirds with advanced disease experienced moderate to severe pain.
   4. The facts supported the concept that most pain can be relieved. The reality of practice did not manage pain well.

IV. Pain Management Obstacles Identified Through These Initiatives

A. Pain management education was deemed inadequate.
B. There was exaggerated fear of opioids, addiction, and side effects.
C. Communication and education by health care providers to patients were lacking.
D. There was a low priority for pain management in the health care systems.
E. Licensure, laws, and regulations did not support effective pain care.
F. Pain costs exceeded $100 million annually for chronic pain alone (Dahl, 1993; Greene, 1993; Ward et al., 1993).

V. Definition of Initiative

A. PIs created a driving vision for change. They were defined as follows:
   1. The power or ability existed to begin and follow an action plan.
   2. The state CPIs set in motion a blueprint containing a series of action to create positive change in pain management.
   3. Goals were defined with a common outcome: improved pain management.
B. State CPIs met annually.
   1. The meetings provided the opportunity to share expertise and resources while building collaborative relationships.

VI. Innovators

A. The first state PI was in Madison, Wisconsin, in 1986.
   1. The Wisconsin CPI endorsed the World Health Organization pain focus.

2. The Wisconsin CPI detailed this in the planning and research clinical practice guideline: *Management of Pain* (Dahl, Bennett, Bromley, Joranson, 2002).
3. Wisconsin created attention through innovation in cancer pain management (Dahl, Joranson, Engber, & Dosch, 1988).
4. Other states that were concerned with the same issues stepped forward to model their CPIs using Wisconsin's template.

B. Wisconsin's basic principles included the following:
   1. Pain treatment exists but is underused.
   2. Education on pain did not change practice.
   3. Cancer pain must address attitudes and behaviors of health care professionals (Dahl, 1993, 1998; Greene, 1993; Ward et al., 1993).

VII. Transition from CPIs to State PIs

A. From 2001 to 2003, the Alliance of State Pain Initiatives (2008) worked with 10 state PIs to gain a broader focus.
   1. The goal was to promote positive changes in pain management practices at an institutional level.
   2. Each state initiative recruited 15 to 25 long-term care facilities, home health agencies, or community programs committed to the following:
      a. Assessment of the structures in place at each facility to support pain assessment and management
      b. Formation of a quality improvement pain team
      c. Evaluation of team activities
      d. Team development of a quality assurance plan and assessment of the impact of quality improvement initiatives on the system's structure and the patients' expression of pain
   3. Outcomes included the following:
      a. A significant decrease occurred in the percentage of moderate and severe pain.
      b. There was a decreased report of pain in the last 24 hours.
      c. Structural elements necessary for affective pain management increased.
      d. The Robert Wood Johnson Grant provided support for Michigan, North Carolina, Connecticut, Delaware, New Mexico, and Virginia.
      e. Project on Death in America was created. The project is now closed, but it focused on understanding and transforming the culture and experience of death and bereavement. It supported Arizona and Iowa (http://www.soros.org/initiatives/pdia) initiatives.
         (1) The American Cancer Society supported this program in Massachusetts and Vermont.

B. State PIs were recognized as facilitating organization to effect change.
   1. State PI work was expanded to address all pain areas:
      a. Acute
      b. Chronic noncancer
      c. Cancer pain (Dahl et al., 2003; Gordon, 1996; Gordon, Dahl, & Stevenson, 2000; Gordon et al., 1999; Weissman, Griffie, Muchka, & Matson, 2000).

VIII. American Alliance of Cancer Pain Initiatives (AACPI)

A. In 1996, the leaders of 44 CPIs created AACPI, a national network of state-based PIs.

B. The goal was to link all CPIs, combine resources, and improve pain management.

C. Steps to achieve goals were as follows:
   1. Create a national communicative network with list serves, newsletters, websites, pain standards, and educational programs.
   2. Provide a consultative process for development of resources and programs to improve state and national vision for cancer pain issues (Dahl, 1993, 1998).
   3. Define shared goals.
   4. Develop priorities.
   5. Facilitate change.

6. Create strong partnerships with maximal impact and sustained movement through common goals (Ward et al., 1993; Dahl, 1993, 1996, 1998; Dahl et al., 1988).

IX. Facilitation of State PIs with Other Organizations

A. During the state PI movement, other organizations made pain management a priority in their programs.
B. These partnerships facilitated the state PI work.
C. Specific organizations in action included the following:
   1. The Oncology Nursing Society published a position paper that guides the education of nurses and presents a core curriculum on pain (Spross, McGuire, & Schmitt, 1991).
   2. The society's pain management interest groups became involved in state PIs.
   3. Publication of a curricular guideline for cancer pain began in 1992 (Jacox et al., 1994).
   4. Collaboration occurred with the American Pain Society, University of Wisconsin Cancer Pain Initiative, Agency for Health Care Policy and Research, American Pain Foundation, National Cancer Institute's Cancer Information Service, and American Cancer Society.
D. The American Society of Pain Management Nursing, from 1998 to 2008, published position papers:
   1. "Procedural sedation in emergency care setting"
   2. "Pain management at the end of life"
   3. "Neonatal circumcision pain relief"
   4. "Pain management in patients with addictive disease"
   5. "Registered nurse management and monitoring of analgesia by catheter techniques"
   6. "Authorized and unauthorized ('PCA by proxy') dosing of analgesic infusion pumps" (statement endorsed by the Oncology Nursing Society and the Hospice and Palliative Nurses Association)
   7. "Pain assessment in the nonverbal patient"
   8. "Balancing pain relief and abuse"
   9. National All Schedules Rx Electronic Reporting Act
   10. Letter to the U.S. Drug Enforcement Administration, docket DEA-261
   11. *ASPMN Health Policy Guiding Principles*
   12. "Assisted suicide"
   13. "Use of placebos in pain management"
   14. "Joint statement: The use of as needed range orders for opioid analgesics in the management of acute pain"
E. The American Pain Foundation was a national extension to focus on data collection and legislative action.

X. Professional Education on Pain Management

A. The Wisconsin CPI developed the Cancer Pain Role Model Program (Dahl, 1999).
B. From 1990 to 2000, Cancer Pain Role Model conferences were held in 31 states.
C. Creation of an acute pain model of education incorporated academic training for health care professionals.
   1. Educational materials were developed.
   2. Standards for various pain management areas were created.
   3. Statewide seminars, conferences, and workshops were sponsored.
   4. Pain report cards via the Policy & Studies Group at the University of Wisconsin were developed, with results released in 2007. The report card grades the state on quality of laws, regulations, and other public policies that affect pain management (http://www.aspi.wisc.edu/newsletter).

XI. PIs in Action

A. Arizona PI
   1. The Arizona PI was established in 1991.

2. It trained greater than 500 health care professionals on cancer pain.
3. It held a "Train the Trainers" workshop modeled after American Alliance of Cancer Pain Initiatives institutional change projects and the City of Hope Pain Resource Training (Berry & Dahl, 2000).
4. The goal was to improve pain management competence.
5. Pain team leaders were recruited in facilities to lead pain management efforts.

B. Alaska PI
1. Development began of pain news monthly online to broaden pain knowledge.
2. Greater than 600 health care professionals received pain news.

C. Southern California PI
1. The Southern California PI has been a role model for PIs since 1993.
2. Programs have been sponsored on cancer pain management, palliative care, and American Medical Association education on end-of-life care.
3. The Southern California PI recognized pain champions.
4. It developed a pocket card devoted to principles of cancer pain management and given to health care professionals in Southern California.

D. New Jersey PI
1. The New Jersey PI created best practices in a pain management course.

E. Virginia PI
1. Successful advocacy occurred for legislative proposals to improve state law, (i.e., access to hospice, health maintenance organizations, insurance companies, and cancer reimbursement).
2. Access was provided to pain management experts and oncologists for a 5-year state palliative study to create a cancer control plan for Virginia.

F. Massachusetts PI
1. The Massachusetts PI obtained a governor's proclamation declaring pain management awareness month.
2. Pain education pocket tools were created and distributed nationally.
3. Power over Pain Action Network (2008) lectures take place statewide.
4. In 2007 and 2008, approval was given to the pain policy for the Massachusetts Medical Society.
5. The PI has been drafting pain policies for nursing, pharmacy, and dentistry pending approval.
6. Pain management education was developed in the geriatric population.
7. Pain workshops have been held at Massachusetts General Hospital.
8. The PI has been placing stories about pain and pain management in media markets.

G. Maryland PI
1. In 2002, House Bill 423 created the Maryland State Advisory Council on Pain Management.
2. Council was activated in 2004.
3. A website resource list has been developed.
4. The PI created a treatment model for pain management with a video teaching tool.
5. It completed a pain survey on its website (American Pain Foundation, 2002).
6. The governor has proclaimed a pain awareness month.

H. Idaho PI
1. In April 2008, the Idaho PI expanded and energized membership at a successful educational seminar "A New Surge Against Pain."

I. Washington State PI
1. The Washington State PI collaborated with the Alaska PI, Western Pain Society, and Washington Academy of Pain Management to foster dialogue among health care professionals, licensing boards, and regulatory bodies to balance pain issues.
2. Five areas of concern include the following:
   a. Clinical practice guidelines.
   b. Health care professional education.
   c. Laws and regulation.

d. Consumer protection.
e. Prescription monitoring.

J. Montana PI
   1. The Montana Board of Medicine disseminated the Federation of State Medical Boards book, *Responsible Opioid Prescribing: A Physician's Guide* by Scott Fishman (Fishman, 2007).

K. West Virginia PI
   1. The West Virginia PI provided free "Pain Management 101" training in four regions statewide.

L. Connecticut PI
   1. Education was provided to health care professionals on a new state electronic prescription monitoring program to promote understanding about its use.

XI. PI Endpoints

A. Promote public awareness of pain.
B. Collect data on the outcomes of the individual states' State Pain Initiatives.
C. Fund pain research by grants and legislation for treatment options (Berry & Dahl, 2000; Dahl & Gordon, 2002; Gordon et al., 2000; Jansen, 2008; Shorten, Carr, Harmon, Puig, & Browne, 2006; Weir, 2005; Weissman et al., 2000).
D. Review state report cards on pain, and create change in the areas needed.
E. Foster standards, guidelines, and skill sets with schools, enhancing clinical practice and treatment (American Society for Pain Management Nursing, 2002; Cherkin, Deyo, & Berg, 1991; Ferrell et al., 1993; Max, 1990; McCaffery, Ferrell, O'Neil-Page, Lester, & Ferrell, 1990; Shorten et al., 2006; Weissman, Dahl, & Beasley, 1993).
F. Provide public awareness of pain management issues via print, radio, and television forums.
G. Maintain regulatory and licensure scrutiny regarding pain management issues.
H. Promote model pain policies and guidelines state by state (Ashburn, Love, & Pace 1994; Ballantyne et al., 1993; Dahl, 2005; Federation of State Medical Boards of the United States, 1999; Harold Rogers Drug Prescription Monitoring Program, 2008; Marcario, 2005; Office of Diversion Control, 2008; Substance Abuse & Mental Health Services Administration, 2008; University of Wisconsin Pain and Policy Studies Group, 2000, 2003).
I. Support improved clinical outcomes with quality pain management, especially for the millions living with severe and chronic pain (Harold Rogers Drug Prescription Monitoring Program, 2008; National All Schedules Prescription Electronic Reporting Act, 2005).
J. Support core curriculum training on pain management in medicine, nursing, pharmacy, and dentistry schools (Cherkin et al., 1991; Ferrell et al., 1993; McCaffery et al., 1990; Shorten et al., 2006).
K. Evaluate various clinical practice areas treating acute, chronic, and cancer pain.

XII. Innovation in Key Health Care Settings

A. Press Gainey scores and Centers for Medicare and Medicaid Services ratings are used to evaluate acute pain management effectiveness and reimbursement action.
B. Acute pain evaluation and its relevance to hospital readmissions are key to positive clinical outcomes (Berry & Dahl, 2000; Dahl, 1999; Dahl & Gordon, 2002; Joint Commission, 2008).
C. A Joint Commission evaluation is used relative to pain and hospital licensure issues.
D. Long-term care pain scores are positive in 40% of these patients in a diverse population with cognitive and chronic pain issues.
E. Data in specific populations are used to create assessment and treatment protocols based on research data (Ballantyne et al., 1993; Cleeland et al., 1994; Jamison et al., 1997; McNeill, Sherwood, Starck, & Thompson 1998).
F. Treatment of acute pain should be improved to decrease chronic pain problems (American Pain Society Committee on Quality Assurance Standards, 1991; American Pain Society Quality of Care Committee, 1995; U.S. Pharmacopeia Quality Review, 2004; Warfield & Kahn, 1995).

XIII. Future for PIs

A. Create a process to universalize up-to-date pain management across the country.
B. Enhance research in multimodal pain management approaches.
C. Create state PIs that continue to grow, influence social policies on behalf of pain management, and support the state's pain management programs.

References

Alliance of State Pain Initiatives. (2008). State Pain Initiatives. Retrieved December 7, 2008, from http://www.aspi.wisc.edu/.

American Pain Foundation. (2004). *New survey shows one in three Marylanders suffer with serious pain.* Retrieved December 15, 2008, from http://www.painfoundation.org/downloads/md_survey_release.pdf.

American Pain Society Committee on Quality Assurance Standards. (1991). Quality assurance standards for pain relief of acute and cancer pain. In: M. Bond, J. Charlton, & C. Woolf (Eds.), *Proceedings from the VI World Congress on Pain* (pp. 186–189). Amsterdam: Elsevier.

American Pain Society Quality of Care Committee. (1995). Quality improvement guidelines for the treatment of acute and cancer pain. *Journal of the American Medical Association, 274,* 1874–1880.

American Society of Pain Management Nursing. (2002). *ASPMN position statement: Pain management in patients with addictive disease.* Retrieved June 4, 2003, from http://www.aspmn.org/html/addiction.htm.

Ashburn, M. A., Love, G., & Pace, N. L. (1994). Respiratory-related critical events with intravenous patient-controlled analgesia. *Clinical Journal of Pain, 10,* 52–56.

Ballantyne, J. C., Carr, D. B., Chalmers, T. C., Dear, K. B., Angelillo, I. F., & Mosteller, F. (1993). Postoperative patient-controlled analgesia: Meta-analyses of initial randomized control trials. *Journal of Clinical Anesthesia, 5,* 182–193.

Berry, P. H., & Dahl, J. L. (2000). The new JCAHO pain standards: Implications for pain management nurses. *Pain Management Nursing, 11,* 3–12.

Cherkin, D., Deyo, R. A., & Berg, A. O. (1991). Evaluation of a physician education intervention to improve primary care for low back pain: Impact on patients. *Spine, 16,* 1173–1178.

Cleeland, C. S., Gonin, R., Hatfield, A. K., Edmonson, J. H., Blum, R. H., Stewart, J. A., & Pandya, K. J. (1994). Pain and its treatment in outpatients with metastatic cancer. *New England Journal of Medicine, 330,* 592–596.

Dahl, J. L. (1993). State cancer pain initiatives. *Journal of Pain and Symptom Management, 8,* 372–375.

Dahl, J. L. (1996). The state cancer pain initiative form a national organization: The American Alliance of *Cancer Pain* Initiatives. *APS Bulletin, 6,* 3.

Dahl, J. L. (1998). State cancer pain initiatives: A decade of progress. *Cancer Prevention International, 3,* 157–164.

Dahl, J. L. (1999). New JCAHO standards focus on pain control. *Oncology Issues, 14,* 27–28.

Dahl, J. L. (2005). How to reduce fears or legal/regulatory scrutiny in managing pain in cancer patients. *Journal of Supportive Oncology, 3,* 384–388.

Dahl, J. L., Bennett, M. E., Bromley, M. D., Joranson, D. E. (2002). Success of the State Pain Initiatives. Cancer Pain, May/June, *10,* 1, S9–S13.

Dahl, J. L., & Gordon, D. B. (2002). Joint Commission pain standards: A progress report. *APS Bulletin, 12*(6), 1, 11–12.

Dahl, J. L., Gordon, D., Ward, S., Skemp, M., Wochos, S., & Schurr, M. (2003). Institutionalizing pain management: The post-operative management quality improvement project. *Journal of Pain, 4,* 361–371.

Dahl, J. L., Joranson, D. E., Engber, D., & Dosch, J. (1988). The cancer pain problem: Wisconsin's response. *Journal of Pain and Symptom Management, 3,* s1–s20.

Daut, R. I., & Cleeland, C. S. (1982). The prevalence and severity of pain in cancer. *Cancer, 50,* 1913–1918.

Federation of State Medical Boards of the United States. (2004). *Model policy for the use of controlled substances for the treatment of pain: Guidance document.* Retrieved December 15, 2008, from http://www.fsmb.org/fsmb_search_results.asp.

Fishman, S. M. (2007). *Responsible opioid prescribing: A physician's guide.* Federation of State Medical Boards. Washington, DC: Waterford Life Science.

Ferrell, B. R., Grant, M., Ritchey, K. J., Ropchan, R., & Rivera, L. M. (1993). The pain resource nurse training program: A unique approach to pain management. *Journal of Pain and Symptom Management, 9,* 549–556.

Gordon, D. B. (1996). Critical pathways: A road to institutionalizing pain management. *Journal of Pain Symptom Management, 11,* 252–259.

Gordon, D. B., Dahl, J. L., & Stevenson, K. (2000). *Building an institutional commitment to pain management: The Wisconsin Resource Manual.* Madison, Wisconsin: The Resource Center of the American Alliance of Cancer Pain Initiatives, University of Wisconsin-Madison.

Gordon, D. A., Stewart, J. A., Dahl, J. L., & Stevenson, K., (1999). Institutionalizing pain management. *Journal of Pharmaceutical Care in Pain and Symptom Control, 7,* 3–16.

Greene, P. E. (1993). America responds to cancer pain: A survey of state initiative. *Cancer Practice, 1,* 65–73.

Harold Rogers Drug Prescription Monitoring Program. *Bureau of Justice Assistance.* Retrieved December 15, 2008, from http://www.ojp.usdoj.gov/BJA/grant/prescripdrugs.html.

Jacox, A. K., Carr, D. B., Payne, R., Berde, C. B., Breibart, W. Cain, J. M., Chapman, C. R., Cleeland, C. S., Ferrell, B. T., Finley, R. S., Hester, N. O., Stratton Hill, C., Leak, W. D., Lipman, A. G., Logan, C. L., McGarvey, C. L., Miaskowski, C. A., Mulder, D. S., Paice, J. A., Shapiro, B. S., Silberstein, E. B., Smith, R. S., Stover, J., Tsou, C. V., Vecchiarelli, L., & Weissman, D. E. (1994). *Management of cancer pain.* Clinical Practice Guideline No. 9. (AHCPR Publication No. 94–0592.) Rockville, MD: Agency for Healthcare Policy and Research, Public Health Service, U.S. Department of Health and Human Services.

Jamison, R. N., Ross, M. J., Hoopman, P., Griffin, F., Levy, J., Daly, M., & Scaffer, J. L. (1997). Assessment of postoperative pain management: Patient satisfaction and perceived helpfulness. *Clinical Journal of Pain, 13,* 229–236.

Jansen, M. (2008). *Managing pain in the older adult.* New York: Springer.

Joint Commission. (2008). The Joint Commission Names Five New Members to the Board of Commissioners. Retrieved December 15, 2008, from http://www.jointcommission.org/NewsRoom/NewsReleases/nr_11_24_08a.htm.

Joranson, D. E., & Gilson, A. M. (1997). State intractable pain policy: Current status. *APS Bulletin, 7,* 7–9.

Marcario, A. (2005). Systematic literature review of the economics of intravenous patient-controlled analgesia. *Pharmacy and Therapeutics, 30,* 392–399.

Max, M. D. (1990). Improving outcomes of analgesic treatment: Is education enough? *Annals of Internal Medicine, 113,* 885–889.

McCaffery, M., Ferrell, B., O'Neil-Page, E., Lester, M., & Ferrell, B. (1990). Nurses knowledge or opioid analgesic drugs and psychological dependence. *Cancer Nursing, 13,* 21–27.

McNeill, J. A., Sherwood, G. D., Starck, P. L., & Thompson, C. J. (1998). Assessing clinical outcomes: patient satisfaction with pain management. *Journal of Pain and Symptom Management, 16,* 29–40.

National All Schedules Prescription Electronic Reporting Act of 2005. (2005). *A review of implementation of existing state controlled substance monitoring programs.* Retrieved December 15, 2008, from http://www.nasper.org/articles.htm.

Office of Diversion Control, U.S. Department of Justice. (2008). *A closer look at state prescription monitoring programs: Questions and answers.* Retrieved January 2, 2008, from http://www.deadviersion.usdoj.gov/faq/rx_monitor.htm.

Power Over Pain Action Network. (2008). *American Pain Foundation.* Retrieved December 15, 2008, from http://www.painfoundation.org/poweroverpain/default.asp.

Shorten, G., Carr, D. B., Harmon, D., Puig, M., & Browne, J. (2006). *Postoperative pain management: An evidence-based guide to practice.* Philadelphia: Saunders.

Substance Abuse & Mental Health Services Administration. (2008). *SAMHSA.* Retrieved December 15, 2008, from http://www.samhsa.gov/index.aspx.

Spross, J. A., McGuire, D. B., & Schmitt, R. M. (1991). Oncology Nursing Society position paper on cancer pain. *Oncology Nursing Forum, 17,* 595–614, 751–760, 943–955.

University of Wisconsin Pain and Policy Studies Group. (2000). *A guide to evaluation: Achieving balance in federal and state pain policy.* Madison, WI: University of Wisconsin-Madison.

University of Wisconsin Pain and Policy Studies Group. (2003). *Database of state laws, regulations and other official governmental policies.* Retrieved June 4, 2003, from http://wwwlmedsch.wisc.edu/painpolicy/matrix.htm.

U.S. Pharmacopeia Quality Review. (2004). *Patient Controlled Analgesia Pumps.* Retrieved July 12, 2005, from http://www.usp.org/pdf/EN/patientSafety/qr812004–09–01.pdf.

Ward, S. E., Goldberg, N., Miller-McCauley, V., Mueller, C., Nolan, A., Pawlik-Plank, D., et al. (1993). Patient-related barriers to management of cancer pain. *Pain, 52,* 319–324.

Warfield, C. A., & Kahn, C. H. (1995). Acute pain management: Programs in U.S. hospitals and experiences and attitudes among U.S. adults. *Anesthesiology, 83,* 1090–1094.

Weir, V. L. (2005). Best-practice protocols: Preventing adverse drug events. *Nurse Management, 36,* 24–30.

Weissman, D. E., Dahl, J. L., & Beasley, J. W. (1993). The cancer pain role model program of the Wisconsin Cancer Pain Initiative. *Journal of Pain and Symptom Management, 8,* 29–35.

Weissman, D. E., Griffie, J., Muchka, S., & Matson, S. (2000). Building an institutional commitment to pain management in long-term care facilities. *Journal of Pain and Symptom Management, 20,* 35–42.

Suggested Readings

American Medical Directors Association. (2003). *Pain management in the long-term care setting.* Clinical Practice Guideline. Columbia, MD: Author.

American Society of Addiction Medicine. (1998). Public policy statement on the rights and responsibilities of physicians in the use of opioids for the treatment of pain. *Journal of Addictive Diseases, 17,* 131–133.

Apfelbaum, J. L., Chen, C., Mehta, S. S., & Gan, T. J. (2003). Postoperative pain experience: Results from a national survey suggest postoperative pain continues to be undermanaged. *Anesthesia & Analgesia, 97,* 534–540.

Carr, D. B., Jacox, A., Chapman, C. R., Ferrell, B., Fields, H.L., Heidrich III, G.,et al. (1992). *Acute pain management: Operative or medical procedures and trauma.* Clinical Practice Guideline No. 1. (AHCPR Publication No. 92–0032.) Rockville, MD: Agency for Health Care Policy and Research, Public Health Service, U.S. Department of Health and Human Services.

Clark, M. E., Gironda, R. J., & Young, R. W. (2003). Development and validation of the Pain Outcomes Questionnaire-VA. *Journal of Rehabilitation Research & Development, 40,* 381–395.

Ersek, M., & Wilson, S. A. (2003). The challenges and opportunities in providing end-of-life care in nursing homes. *Journal of Palliative Medicine, 6,* 45–57.

Feldt, K. S., Tyden, M. D., & Miles, S. (1998). Treatment of pain in cognitively impaired compared with cognitively intact older patients with hip-fracture. *Journal of the American Geriatric Society, 46,* 1079–1085.

Ferrell, B. A., & Ferrell, B. R. (1991). Pain management at home. *Geriatric Home Care, 7,* 765–775.

Fries, B. E., Simon, S. E., Morris, J. N., Flodstrom, C., & Bookstein, F. L. (2001). Pain in U.S. nursing homes: validating a pain scale for the minimum data set. *Gerontologist, 41,* 173–175.

Gallagher, R. (2004). Opioids in chronic pain management: Navigating the clinical and regulatory challenges. *Family Practice, 53,* S23–S32.

Gan, T. J., Lubarsky, D. A., Flood, E. M., Thanh, T., Mauskopf, J., Mayne, T., & Chen, C. (2004). Patient preferences for acute pain treatment. *British Journal of Anaesthesia, 92,* 681–688.

Gibson, R. (1998). The Robert Wood Johnson Foundation grant-making strategies to improve end-of-life care. *Journal of Palliative Medicine, 1,* 415–417.

Herr, K. (2002). Chronic pain challenges and assessment strategies. *Journal of Gerontological Nursing, 28,* 20–27.

Herr, K. (2002). Pain assessment in cognitively impaired older adults: New strategies and care observation help pinpoint unspoken pain. *American Journal of Nursing, 102*(12), 65–66, 68.

Horgas, A. L., & Tsai, P. F. (1998). Analgesic drug prescription and use in cognitively impaired nursing home residents. *Nursing Research, 47,* 235–242.

Idvall, E., Hamrin, E., Sjostrom, B., & Unosson, M. (2002). Patient and nurse assessment of quality of care in postoperative pain management. *Quality and Safety in Health Care, 11,* 327–334.

Joranson, D. E., Gilson, A. M., Ryan, K. M., Maurer, M. A., Nischik, J. A., & Nelson, J. M. (2000). *Achieving balance in federal and state pain policy: A guide to evaluation.* Madison, WI: Pain and Policy Studies Group, University of Wisconsin Comprehensive Cancer Center.

Landi, F., Onder, G., Cesari, M., Gambassi, G., Steel, K., Russo, A., et al. (2001). Pain management in frail, community-living elderly patients. *Archives of Internal Medicine, 161,* 2721–2724.

McCaffery, M., & Ferrell, B. R. (1992). Does the gender gap affect your pain control decisions? *Nursing, 22,* 48–51.

Moyers, B. *On our own terms: Moyers on dying in America. Leadership guide.* Retrieved December 15, 2008, from http://www.pbs.org/wnet/onourownterms.

Ross, M. M., & Crook, J. (1998). Elderly recipient of home nursing services: Pain disability and functional competence. *Journal of Advanced Nursing, 27,* 1117–1126.

Skinner, M. (1997). Aspects of the problems in treating chronic pain: Florida pain management guidelines. *Journal of the Florida Medical Association, 84,* 85–86.

Vincente, K. J., Kada-Bekhaled, K., Hillet, G., Cassano, A., & Orser, B. A. (2003). Programming errors contribute to death from patient-controlled analgesia: Case report and estimate of probability. *Canadian Journal of Anesthesia, 50,* 328–332.

Weiner, D. K., & Rudy, T. E. (2002). Attitudinal barriers to effective treatment of persistent pain in older persons. *Journal of the American Geriatric Society, 50,* 2035–2040.

Weissman, D. E., Griffie, J., Muchka, S., & Matson, S. (2001). Improving pain management in long-term care facilities. *Palliative Medicine, 4,* 567–573.

Won, A., Lapane, K., Vallow, S., Schein, J., Morris, J., & Lipsitz, L. (2004). Persistent nonmalignant pain and analgesic prescribing patterns in elderly nursing home residents. *Journal of the American Geriatrics Society, 52,* 867–874.

World Health Organization. (1990). *Cancer pain relief and palliative care: Report of a WHO Expert Committee.* WHO Technical Report Series, No. 804. Geneva: Author.

World Health Organization. (2002). *National cancer control programmes: Policies and managerial guidelines.* Retrieved December, 15, 2008, from http://www.who.int/cancer/nccp/en.

chapter

12

Social, Political, and Ethical Forces Influencing Nursing Practice

Micke A. Brown, BSN, RN
Pamela Bennett, BSN, RN

Objectives

After studying this chapter, the reader should be able to:

1. Describe how patient rights to pain care affect nursing care priorities.
2. Explain the key elements of medical ethics as they are relevant to pain management nursing practice.
3. Discuss the sociopolitical pressures on prescribing and pain practice that may impede access to effective pain care.
4. Acknowledge the legal and regulatory influences on pain practice and engage in social change activities that positively enhance and help eliminate negative policies.
5. Comprehend the role of the nurse as a patient advocate and demonstrate effective advocacy skills within the sphere of influence of that practice setting.

I. Patient Rights and Social Justice

A. Pain management as a fundamental human right
   1. The American Association of Colleges of Nursing has made explicit the values that form the cornerstone of professional nursing: altruism, autonomy, human dignity, integrity, and social justice (Murphy, Canales, Norton, & DeFilippis, 2005).
   2. A critical first step is for society to recognize pain management as a human right (Fishman, 2007).
   3. Many of the world's nations have written constitutions enumerating the right of their citizens to receive adequate health care. No nations articulate a right to pain relief. Pain is an international problem that requires an international solution.
      a. The World Health Organization, as the ultimate health agency of the United Nations, holds a critical role in any solution. It has been involved with pain in three overlapping areas: promotion and dissemination of guidelines on pain management, advocacy of improved access to opioid analgesics, and national programs of palliative care and pain relief.
      b. Much work and continuing vigilance are required to make the transition from the current assertion that pain management is a fundamental human right to a future in which appropriate pain management is a global reality (Brennan, Carr, & Cousins, 2007).
      c. Pain management is the subject of many initiatives within the disciplines of medicine, ethics, and law. Unreasonable failure to treat pain is viewed worldwide as poor medicine, unethical practice, and an abrogation of a fundamental human right (Brennan et al., 2007).
   4. Ethical tenant of autonomy
      a. Patients have a right to receive optimal pain relief and be involved in their pain management treatment plan.
      b. Patients have a right to be informed of pain management treatments, benefits and risks of procedures, alternative pain management modalities, and expected outcomes (Ferrell, 1994).
      c. "Patients have the right to appropriate assessment and management of their pain" (Joint Commission, 2001).
         (1) This significantly raises the profile of pain in all populations and settings.
         (2) This raises in priority a major symptom of why people seek health care for help: pain is too often underappreciated and undertreated.
         (3) It is the foundation for all other standards that address pain (Quinn, 2003).
      d. The Agency for Healthcare Research and Quality (1992, 1994) guidelines reinforce that pain management is every patient's right.

II. Discrimination and Disparity Issues Impede Equal Access to Pain Care (see the Chapter on Disparities in Pain Management)

A. In the current U.S. health care system, both good health and a higher quality of health care are more likely to be experienced by those who have access to money, power, and privilege. And for those without this access, health disparities are an everyday part of their lives (Murphy et al., 2005).

B. The treatment of pain must be afforded to all those who are capable of feeling and experiencing pain. Health care providers must rely on contemporary neuroscientific knowledge to compel and sustain a philosophy and ethics of pain care. This must be available and provided to all people across their life span (Niebroj, Jadamus-Niebroj, & Giordano, 2008).

C. The variations on health and cost outcome among people of various races and ethnicities have not been the object of pharmacoeconomists, outcome researchers, and pain researchers (Lafleur, Said, McAdam-Marx, Jackson, & Mortazavi 2007).
   1. Lack of disparity and pain outcomes research may be due to various factors:
      a. Limited availability of race and ethnicity data in secondary data sets
      b. Lack of priority for public and private funding organizations to support this type of research
      c. Potential biases of researchers and funding organizations
   2. Eradicating health disparities and increasing health-related quality of life are the overall goals of Healthy People 2010 (Erlen, 2003).

   a. Human suffering is the most significant consequence of racial disparity, and a cost estimate is difficult to attain (Harrison & Falco, 2005).
   b. The challenge to the nursing profession is to develop strategies to refuse to give in to the dominance of economic interests over the need to prevent harm (Heggen & Wellard, 2004).
3. The American Nurses Association (ANA) is committed to working toward the eradication of discrimination and racism in the profession of nursing, in the education of nurses, in the practice of nursing, and in the organizations in which nurses' work. The ANA is further committed to working toward egalitarianism and the promotion of justice in access and delivery of health care to all people (ANA, 1998).

D. The Genetic Discrimination Act focuses on the potential impact on pain patients and their pain treatment.
   1. This became Public Law No. 110–233 on May 21, 2008.
   2. This amends the Employee Retirement Income Security Act of 1974, Public Health Service Act, and Internal Revenue Code to prohibit a group health plan from adjusting premium or contribution amounts for a group on the basis of genetic information.
   3. There is a need for revising the Health Insurance Portability and Accountability Act of 1996 (HIPAA) privacy regulations to
      a. Treat genetic information as health information.
      b. Prohibit the use or disclosure by a group health plan, health insurance coverage, or Medicare supplemental policy of genetic information about an individual for underwriting purposes.
   4. HIPAA prohibits discrimination against an employee, individual, or member because of genetic information.
   5. As genome science uncovers more genetic links to pain conditions and individual response to medication therapies that drive pharmacotherapy selection, HIPAA has potential to affect patients and their pain treatment in a comprehensive manner. The bill details are at http://www.govtrack.us/congress/bill.xpd?bill=h110-493&tab=summary.
      a. Nurses, as patient advocates, need to apply ethical standards of conduct and moral imperative to safeguard patients while "taking care" of them in the context of genetic health information (Giarelli, 2003).

III. Ethical Dimensions: Influence on Practice

A. Ethics is concerned with right and wrong. Agreeing on what is right can be challenging; however, this understanding is essential to the delivery of skilled professional health care.
   1. Ethics is relevant to clinical, practice-based issues and influences all areas of the professional nursing role.
   2. To apply ethics effectively, nurses must develop reasoning skills and understand the concepts and principles that assist ethical analysis (Chaloner, 2007).

B. The core principles of pain management nursing are based on tenets of medical ethics. Seven of the values that commonly apply are as follows:
   1. *Autonomy:* A patient has the right to self-determination regarding health care. The patient has the right to refuse or choose treatment ***(voluntas aegroti suprema lex)***.
      a. Patients must be allowed to "self-determine when they need analgesia to guarantee . . . autonomy" (Greipp, 1992, p. 51).
      b. The patient's report of pain is an important part of autonomy and should be believed.
      c. The autonomy of vulnerable populations is violated easily (Borneman & Ferrell, 1996).
      d. Individuals have the right to make decisions that determine the course of their lives (doctrine of informed consent) (Henkelman, 1994).
      e. "Persons would be free to choose and act without controlling constraints imposed by others" (Faden & Beauchamp, 1986, p. 8).
      f. "A patient has the right to be involved in decisions regarding pain management interventions, so health care providers are obliged to provide the information necessary to guide an informed decision" (Henkelman, 1994, pp. 48A–48B).

g. "The kind of pain management and side effects that are acceptable to patients varies directly with their present and future goals, and their unique view of themselves and the world" (Cain & Hammes, 1994, p. 162).
h. Involvement includes teaching the patient about pain, pain management techniques, and availability of management options.
i. Discussion with patients about the cultural and religious meanings of pain to them provides insight toward appropriate interventions (Taylor & Ersek, 1995).

2. *Beneficence:* Beneficence is commitment to do good and avoid harm (Thompson, 1996). A practitioner should act in the best interest of the patient *(salus aegroti suprema lex)*.
   a. "The question as to whom one's beneficence should be directed is open and assumes an obligation to weigh and balance benefits against harms, against alternative benefits, and against alternative harms" (Faden & Beauchamp, 1986, p. 13).
   b. "The duty to benefit another or to achieve good ends . . . can be problematic when there is a question of what is . . . 'good' . . ." (Henkelman, 1994, p. 48B).
   c. "The duty to benefit through relief of pain is by itself adequate to support the use of increasing doses (of opioids) to alleviate pain, even if there might be life shortening and expected side effects" (Cain & Hammes, 1994, p. 161).
3. *Dignity:* The patient (and the person treating the patient) has the right to dignity, the state of being worthy of esteem and respect for the individual as a unique and important person.
   a. "The nurse who provides pain management uses personal and professional codes of ethics to guide pain management practice that is characterized by respect for human dignity" (American Society for Pain Management Nursing [ASPMN], 1996, p. 116).
   b. "An attitude of respecting and seeking the patient's perspective and advocating for that outcome is a basic ethical duty" (Cain & Hammes, 1994, p. 163).
   c. Dignity is a highly abstract, vague concept that is difficult to measure within the context of general nursing, yet it is a central phenomenon to nursing.
      (1) Respect, autonomy, empowerment, and communication have been identified as being the defining attributes of dignity.
      (2) This concept analysis is important for areas in which the maintenance of dignity may be unintentionally overlooked. This can occur in facilities where patients may have to wait for hospital rooms in a corridor, which does not lend itself to upholding dignity, privacy, and confidentiality.
      (3) Patients' dignity should be maintained at all times, and health care workers need to recognize their own dignity to promote dignity in others (Griffin-Heslin, 2005).
   d. Respect is the act of esteeming another. This is demonstrated by word and deed. It is fostered by attending to the whole person and by involving the patient and family in decision making, providing family-centered care, bearing witness, and adopting a broader perspective marked by cultural humility.
      (1) By creating processes that ensure everyone's views are heard, health care professional, as well as patients and their families, are supported.
      (2) One process, known as "council process," shifts dialogue from telling to discovering, from judging to inquiring. It neutralizes conjecture, fosters the acceptance of moral conflict, and protects the integrity of health care professionals and their organizations (Rushton, 2007).
4. *Fidelity:* Fidelity is responsibility to keep one's promises (Taylor & Ersek, 1995).
   a. Health care providers have a responsibility to provide appropriate follow-up care and support of the patient.
   b. The patient has the responsibility for keeping appointments, implementing the treatment plan, and reporting side effects and outcome of the plan to the health care provider.
5. *Justice:* Fairness, impartial treatment, and high quality of care are necessary for all patients, regardless of race, ethnicity, or diagnosis. This includes fair distribution of health care resources (Borneman & Ferrell, 1996; Faden & Beauchamp, 1986; Thompson, 1996).

a. "Efforts to relieve pain must be ongoing and extended to all clients in order to be just" (Greipp, 1992, p. 51).
b. The patient's financial and social situation should be considered when choosing methods of pain relief (Taylor & Ersek, 1995).
c. The least expensive and least invasive (but effective) interventions should be chosen whenever possible (Taylor & Ersek, 1995).

6. *Nonmaleficence:* "First, do no harm" *(primum non nocere).*
   a. Nurses must work with patients and physicians to achieve safe and effective analgesia (Greipp, 1992).
   b. When life-supportive treatments are withdrawn, the patient must be kept comfortable so as to minimize pain and suffering (Morray, 1995).
7. *Veracity:* Veracity is the duty to tell the truth and to avoid lies and deception (Taylor & Ersek, 1995). Truthfulness and honesty are the concepts of informed consent. Since the Nuremberg trials and Tuskegee Syphilis Study, this ethical tenet has been applied to clinical practice and in clinical research.
   a. This ethical tenet requires honest, open communication so that patients and families are able to participate in decision making (Taylor & Ersek, 1995).
   b. "Veracity is essential in the nurse–patient relationship," unless the patient requests that the truth be withheld (Thompson, 1996, p. 63).
   c. The patient is entitled to know potential complications and risks related to treatment choices, including the choice of no treatment.
   d. The patient is entitled to know about any conflict of interest that may exist between health care providers and services offered (e.g., who owns the pain service).
   e. The administration of placebos violates the principle of veracity (Borneman & Ferrell, 1996).

C. The field of feminist ethics can be applied to pain management to understand the perspective of both the patient and the nurse. Three concepts derived from feminist ethics are applied to the care of people in pain: relationship, compassion, and respect (Ferrell, 2005).

IV. ANA *Code for Nurses* (2001) (Table 12-1)

A. "The nurse promotes, advocates for, and strives to protect the health, safety, and rights of the patient" (ANA, 2001). Pain management nurses are on the front line in the care of patients most vulnerable due to pain and its undertreatment. Pain management nurses are duty bound both ethically and morally to protect the patient's right to appropriate pain assessment and treatment.
B. Creating a caring environment is a cornerstone for effective pain management nursing
   1. Continued assessment of the values of the patient, family, and nurse is essential (Taylor & Ersek, 1995).
   2. "Understanding what pain means to a patient can provide insight regarding how to intervene" (Taylor & Ersek, 1995).
   3. Caring implies a commitment to all the bioethical principles (Thompson, 1996). Caring is a willingness to respect the patient's informed choices based on the patient's values and beliefs.
   4. Ethics committees play a vital role in ensuring institutional commitment to pain management (Ferrell, 1997).

V. Greipp's Model of Ethical Decision Making (Fig. 12-1)

A. Greipp's model of ethical decision making was designed as an ethical framework to illustrate an overall conception of the interaction between nurse and patient in the management of pain (Greipp, 1992).
B. This model is based on general systems theory and is consistent with Madeleine Leininger's transcultural caring theory.
C. There are learned psychosociocultural variable that may negatively affect decisions made by nurses and patients.

Table 12-1 ANA *Code for Nurses*
1. The nurse, in all professional relationships, practices with compassion and respect for the inherent dignity, worth, and uniqueness of every individual, unrestricted by considerations of social or economic status, personal attributes, or the nature of health problems.
2. The nurse's primary commitment is to the patient, whether an individual, family, group, or community.
3. The nurse promotes, advocates for, and strives to protect the health, safety, and rights of the patient.
4. The nurse is responsible and accountable for individual nursing practice and determines the appropriate delegation of tasks consistent with the nurse's obligation to provide optimum patient care.
5. The nurse owes the same duties to self as others, including the responsibility to preserve integrity and safety, to maintain competence, and to continue personal and professional growth.
6. The nurse participates in establishing, maintaining, and improving health care environments and conditions of employment conducive to the provision of quality health care and consistent with the values of the profession through individual and collective action.
7. The nurse participates in the advancement of the profession through contributions to practice, education, administration, and knowledge development.
8. The nurse collaborates with other health professionals and the public in promoting community, national, and international efforts to meet health needs.
9. The profession of nursing, as represented by associations and their members, is responsible for articulating nursing values, for maintaining the integrity of the profession and its practice, and for shaping social policy.

From American Nurses Association. (2001). *Code for nurses, with interpretive statement.* Retrieved December 3, 2008, from http://www.nursingworld.org/MainMenuCategories/ThePracticeofProfessionalNursing/EthicsStandards/CodeofEthics/AboutTheCode.aspx. Courtesy American Medical Association.

D. Learned psychosociocultural variables acquired by nurses are their belief system, culture and personal experiences, professional experiences, education, and ethics. These variables potentially inhibit practice.
   1. A person with a chemical dependency history may not receive opioids for pain because of the nurse's belief that opioids are not as effective in this group of individuals.
   2. A nurse who believes that a certain amount of pain builds character may have little tolerance for patients who freely express pain and demand analgesics.

E. Learned psychosociocultural variables acquired by patients include their belief system, culture, education, and personal experiences.
   1. A patient who believes that a request for pain medication will annoy the nurse may suffer in silence.
   2. A patient who believes a display of emotions will result in better pain management will act out to gain more attention.

VI. Other Organizations' View of Pain Management

A. American Academy of Pain Medicine
   1. Pain management nursing practice mirrors the precepts reflected in the ethics charter of the American Academy of Pain Medicine. It states that it is the ethical imperative to provide relief from pain and that all physicians look to improve the following areas:
      a. Assess the pain sufferer as a whole person, including all relevant biological, social, psychological, and spiritual dimensions pertaining to etiology and impact of pain.
      b. Treat the person in pain with competence and compassion.

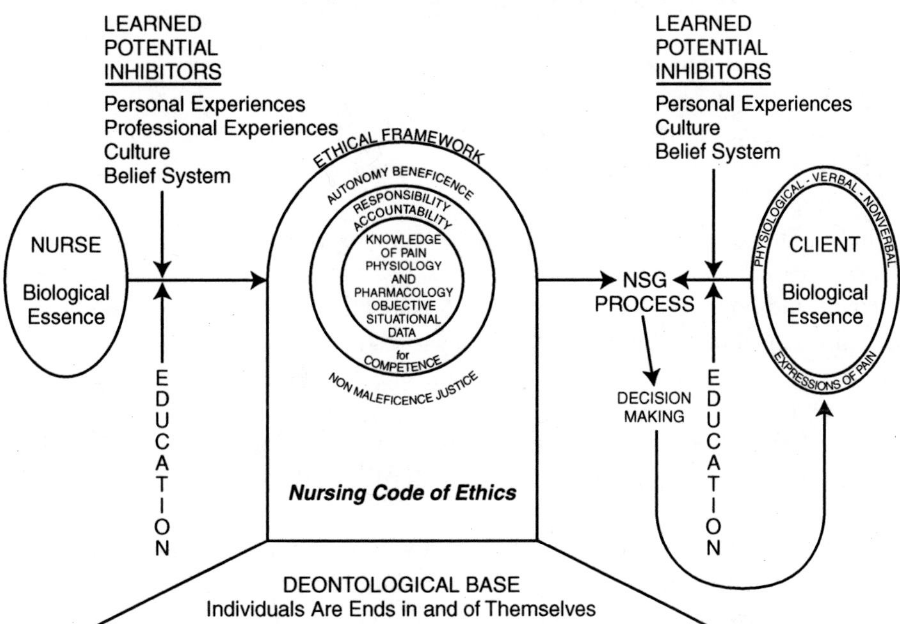

Figure 12-1 | Greipp's model of ethical decision making in the management of clients' pain.

From *Advances in Nursing Science*, 16, by M.E. Greipp, 1992. Reprinted by permission of Wolters Kluwer Health. Permission conveyed through Rightslink.

c. Educate professional colleagues, patients, the public, and policymakers on the principles and methods of pain medicine.
d. Support and/or participate in basic and clinical pain research.
e. Advocate assurance of access to pain care and its continuous improvement (American Academy of Pain Medicine Council on Ethics, 2005).

B. Oncology Nursing Society (ONS) and International Society of Nurses in Cancer Care
1. The ONS issued a position statement on cancer pain (ONS, 1991, updated 2006), and the International Society of Nurses in Cancer Care (1999) developed a position statement on cancer pain.
2. In a survey of oncology nurses, the undertreatment of pain was identified as the number one ethical issue to be addressed (Ersek, Scanlon, Glass, Ferrell, & Steeves, 1995).
3. In 2008, the ONS Ethics Advisory Council ranked pain management issues third (Hansen, 2008). The first two priorities were nurse responsibility in addressing treatment limitation and transition to palliative care.

C. The Joint Commission, formerly known as the Joint Commission on Accreditation of Healthcare Organizations, developed standards for pain management to support the individual's right to pain assessment and treatment (see the chapter on Quality Evaluation and Improvement).
1. "Effective pain management is a crucial component of good health care, and treating pain is the responsibility of all caregivers. The Joint Commission encourages patients to ask the right questions so that they can find relief" (Joint Commission, 2008).
2. This education campaign coincided with September as pain awareness month.

D. The American Pain Society (APS) has several position statements (APS, 2008), some in collaboration with the American Academy of Pain Medicine. Topics include opioids, chronic pain, and end-of-life issues. These support ethical tenets for the treatment of pain by the health care professional and society.

E. Primary care providers need an ethical framework to adopt the principles of palliative care, as well as to guide efforts to relieve persistent pain.
1. Accept all patient pain reports as valid.
2. Negotiate treatment goals early in care.

3. Avoid harming patients.
4. Improve the overall health and quality of life of the patient.

VII. Advocating for Pain Management

A. Clinical practice guidelines

1. Clinical guidelines provide a sustainable set of directions for the decision-making process.
2. There is constant change in knowledge, parameters of practice, and economic, political, and social milieu.
3. Guidelines must be part of a progressive learning process. New information supersedes old, and relative values of particular techniques, technologies, and procedures are reappraised, reaffirmed, and revised to be resonant with those of the participant communities.
4. Guidelines must be dynamic and part of a paradigm of change.
5. For change to be affective, it must be preceded by learning (see the chapter on the Pain Management Nurse as a Change Agent).
6. Incorporation of knowledge of the phenomenon (pain) and bringing forward new information using experience and wisdom must occur (Giordano, 2007).

B. Placebo use

1. ASPMN holds the position that placebos should not be used by any route of administration in the assessment or management of pain in any individual regardless of age or diagnosis. ASPMN supports the use of placebos only in institutional review board (IRB)–approved clinical trials (ASPMN, 2004). Placebo use for the assessment or treatment of pain, including the evaluation of response to pain treatments, constitutes fraud and deception.
2. Placebo use in this manner is associated with substandard assessment and treatment of pain. Therefore, the ASPMN adamantly opposes the use of placebos.
3. Professionals are urged to refuse to administer placebos, and institutions are advised to establish policies that prohibit their use outside the context of an IRB-approved research study.
   a. A *placebo* is "a form of medical therapy, or an intervention designed to simulate medical therapy, that is believed to be without specific activity for the condition being treated, and that is used either for its symbolic effect or to eliminate observer bias in a controlled experiment" (Brody, 1982, p. 113).
   b. The *placebo effect* is "the change in the patient's condition that is attributable to the symbolic import of the healing intervention rather than to the intervention's specific pharmacologic or physiologic effects" (Brody, 1982, p. 113).
   c. Placebo responses in the literature vary from 15% to 58% (Turner, Deyo, Loeser, Von Korff, & Fordyce, 1994) and from 0% to 100% (Wall, 1992).
   d. Many factors influence placebo responses, including the therapeutic relationship between patient and health care provider. "The placebo response is well documented, and therapeutic trials have shown that an inert pill, given as an apparent active therapy, is more effective than no treatment at all" (Bradley, Daroff, Fenichel, & Marsden, 2000, pp. 861–866). Both this effect and the beneficial influence of the therapeutic relationship may be explained, for example, by release of endorphins; another possibility is that patients report a positive response to please a physician and thereby continue that support. Part of the art of medicine is to encourage the patient's positive belief in the efficacy of a recommended treatment, and the physician can take advantage of this response, whatever its mechanism.
   e. Pain relief from a placebo proves nothing (McCaffery & Pasero, 1999).
4. Arguments against placebos
   a. The Agency for Health Care Policy and Research guidelines for cancer pain state "placebos should not be used in the management of cancer pain" (Jacox et al., 1994, p. 17).
   b. Placebo use violates the American Medical Association's *Code of Medical Ethics* (Opinion E-8.083, revised November 2006; see Guidelines on Placebo Use in Clinical Practice at http://www.ama-assn.org/ama/pub/physician-resources/medical-ethics/code-medical-ethics/opinion 8083.shtml) and the ANA's *Code for Nurses* (2001).

Table 12-2 Placebo Use in Clinical Practice

A placebo is a substance provided to a patient that the physician believes has no specific pharmacological effect on the condition being treated. In the clinical setting, the use of a placebo without the patient's knowledge may undermine trust, compromise the patient–physician relationship, and result in medical harm to the patient.

Physicians may use placebos for diagnosis or treatment only if the patient is informed of and agrees to its use. A placebo may still be effective if the patient knows it will be used but cannot identify it and does not know the precise timing of its use. A physician should enlist the patient's cooperation by explaining that a better understanding of the medical condition could be achieved by evaluating the effects of different medications, including the placebo. The physician need neither identify the placebo nor seek specific consent before its administration. In this way, the physician respects the patient's autonomy and fosters a trusting relationship, while the patient still may benefit from the placebo effect.

A placebo must not be given merely to mollify a difficult patient, because doing so serves the convenience of the physician more than it promotes the patient's welfare. Physicians can avoid using a placebo yet produce a placebo-like effect through the skillful use of reassurance and encouragement. In this way, the physician builds respect and trust, promotes the patient–physician relationship, and improves health outcomes.

From American Medical Association. (2006). *Code of medical ethics*. Retrieved December 3, 2008, from http://www0.ama-assn.org/apps/pf_new/pf_online?f_n=browse&doc=policyfiles/HnE/E-8.083.HTM&&s_t=&st_p=&nth=1&prev_pol=policyfiles/HnE/E-7.05.HTM&nxt_pol=policyfiles/HnE/E-8.01.HTM.Courtesy American Medical Association.

c. Use of placebos violates patient's rights according to the Joint Commission (Fox, 1994).
d. Nurses, as moral agents, have an ethical obligation to avoid the use of placebos and to establish institutional policies to preclude their use in pain management (McCaffery, Ferrell, & Turner, 1996, p. 1592).
    (1) "Use of placebos to assess and treat pain is one of the most unfortunate examples of the continuing ignorance about pain management, the under-treatment of pain, and the violation of patients' rights" (McCaffery et al., 1996, p. 1587).
    (2) A survey conducted by Ferrell and McCaffery (1996) found that only 8% of respondents worked in institutions that had a policy regarding placebo use.
    (3) All hospitals and health care agencies need a written policy that addresses unethical placebo use (McCaffery & Ferrell, 1997).
    (4) Nurses may use this policy to communicate their concerns with the physician who prescribes a placebo and to explain why they refuse to administer a placebo even with a written order (McCaffery & Ferrell, 1997).
        (a) Fidelity and veracity principles are violated unless informed consent takes place.
        (b) Placebo use violates the rights of all patients who receive them outside the context of an approved clinical trial in which the patient has given informed consent to participate (McCaffery & Ferrell, 1997, pp. 9–10).
        (c) A positive placebo response cannot be predicted in an individual, and a placebo may be effective at one time and not another (McCaffery & Ferrell, 1997, p. 9).
        (d) Placebos are not without side effects. Placebos may include drowsiness, headaches, nervousness, nausea, constipation, or insomnia (Brody, 1982; Turner et al., 1994).
            (i) Placebos have been found to alter laboratory results and other physiological measurements (Brody, 1982).
            (ii) Nonspecific influences of treatments may produce adverse effects called *nocebo effects* (Turner et al., 1994).
            (iii) The learning process or conditioning can occur as a result of a negative association with treatments in the past (Turner et al., 1994).
e. The APS analgesic guidelines state, "Do not use placebos to assess the nature of pain" (APS, 2003, p. 37) and "the deceptive use of placebos and the misinterpretation of the placebo response to discredit the patient's pain report are unethical and should be avoided" (APS, 2003, p. 37).

(1) This was revised in 2005 and stated that "the deceptive use of placebos and [consequent] misinterpretation of placebo response to discredit the patient's pain are unethical" (Sullivan & Ferrell, 2005).

(2) It also includes a section suggesting that exceptions could be made in the administration of placebos outside of IRB-approved clinical trials.

(a) Such an exception involves the use of an "N-of-1 trial" (meaning "number of one trial"). N-of-1 trials evaluate the effectiveness of a procedure or treatment in a single person rather than in a larger cohort of subjects. In short, N-of-1 trials are thought to evaluate the individual's potential for benefiting from active treatment. If a patient responds to a placebo with pain relief, active treatment may be denied (Sullivan & Ferrell, 2005).

f. The ASPMN's position is that an N-of-1 trial has too many limitations to be used for the purpose of denying active treatment—especially because N-of-1 trials are performed without the oversight of an IRB.

(1) Nurses should be aware of the difference in the positions taken by the APS and the ASPMN and carefully consider what they will do if asked to administer a placebo.

(2) ASPMN hopes that nurses will refuse to participate or endorse placebo use outside of an IRB-approved trial.

(3) Hospitals and clinics should establish policies that specify this and that optimal pain control requires individualized treatment plans using interventions known to be effective.

g. The American Osteopathic Association position statement is against use of placebos for pain management in end-of-life care.

(1) Exquisite management of end-of-life pain is a medical imperative.

(2) Use of a placebo in place of known effective pain medication for determining whether the patient is really in pain is under no circumstances appropriate.

(3) Use of placebos does not meet the accepted criteria to diagnose substance abuse.

(4) There is no medical justification for the use of placebos to assess or treat patients in pain at end of life (Nichols et al., 2005).

h. The use of placebos in pain management has areas of agreement among organizations.

(1) Placebos cannot be used to diagnose malingering or psychogenic pain.

(2) A placebo response provides no information about the cause of pain or its severity.

(3) A placebo should not be given, even when there is a written order for it, unless its use is part of an IRB-approved trial.

(4) Placebos should not be used without informed consent (McCaffery & Arnstein, 2006).

i. Placebo use is justified only in a research situation (approved clinical trials) for which informed consent was obtained from participants (Fox, 1994; McCaffery & Pasero, 1999).

(1) There is a paradox when a placebo is used in clinical research particularly for patients with pain.

(2) First, the use of placebo-controlled trials in the face of proven effective treatments violates the health care professional's therapeutic obligation to offer optimal medical care to patients. Second, testing new treatments against a placebo when proven effective treatments exist lacks scientific and clinical merit.

(3) Allowing subjects to enroll in a trial in which a placebo is used (and not disclosed) would imply that a proportion of enrollees receive medical attention that is considered inferior by the expert community (Freedman, Glass, & Weijer, 1996).

j. Placebos often are given to difficult patients as punishment, to prove a patient wrong, or to patients who did not obtain relief from standard treatment (McCaffery & Ferrell, 1997).

k. In addition to ethical issues associated with placebos, there is the danger of precipitating withdrawal symptoms in opioid-tolerant patients when a placebo or a reduced dose of an opioid is substituted for the usual opioid.

5. Arguments for placebos are arguments about the impact of placebo effect rather than about the use of a placebo.

a. The placebo response can be used therapeutically without deception (Brody, 1982).
   (1) Health care providers "can use nondeceptive means to promote a positive placebo response in their patients" (Brody, 1982, p. 112).
b. Every clinical encounter provides a placebo effect.
   (1) The expectation is of comfort and the caring relationship between the patient and the nurse.
   (2) The patient's expectation is that treatment will relieve symptoms (Turner et al., 1994). For example, "This pill will really help," when said before administration of a drug or treatment, can enhance the response.
   (3) The learning process or conditioning is a result of positive association with effective treatments in the past (Turner et al., 1994).
c. In medical research, the placebo effect is an important methodological tool.
   (1) A placebo is given to participants in clinical trials, with the intention of mimicking an experimental intervention. The nocebo effect, on the other hand, is the phenomenon whereby a patient who believes that a treatment will cause harm actually does experience adverse effects.
   (2) The placebo effect strongly influences the way the results of clinical trials are interpreted.
   (3) Placebo responses vary with the choice of study design, the choice of primary outcome measure, the characteristics of the patients, and the cultural setting in which the trial is conducted (Antonaci et al., 2007).
   (4) The placebo effects in published trials of acute migraine medications are highly variable and often substantial. This variability in placebo response means that active control equivalence trials or the use of historical controls will not provide adequate proof of the safety or efficacy of new drugs and will not differentiate between drugs that are active versus placebo but of unknown efficacy relative to each other.
   (5) The potential for approval of ineffective drugs, the inability to compare results of studies performed in different locations, and poor characterization of the tolerability and safety profiles of new drugs represent a greater danger to migraineurs than does the limited-duration use of a placebo in carefully monitored clinical trials of consenting subjects. These observations support the view that the inclusion of a placebo group remains of major scientific and ethical importance in trials of migraine medications (Loder, Goldstein, & Biondi, 2005).
   (6) Placebo control use in clinical research is contentious in areas where effective treatments already exist. Determination of appropriate standards for placebo use is especially difficult in areas such as pain treatment and psychiatry, in which substantial placebo responses can occur.
      (a) Debates are characterized by three common themes:
         (i) Whether the state of existing treatments forbids placebo use
         (ii) Whether the nature of the condition being treated and the level of additional risk permit placebo control use
         (iii) Whether methodological concerns are sufficient to justify placebo use (Nagasako & Kalauokalani, 2005)

VIII. Assisted Suicide, Euthanasia, and Double Effect

A. Compassionate care
   1. In accordance with our commitment to compassionate care for all individuals, ASPMN supports the position statements by the American Nurses' Association (ANA) on active euthanasia and assisted suicide (ASPMN, 2003).
   2. The ANA believes that the nurse should not participate in assisted suicide. Such an act is in violation of the *Code for Nurses* and the ethical traditions of the profession. Nurses, individually and collectively, have an obligation to provide comprehensive and compassionate end-of-life care, which

includes promoting comfort, relieving pain, and at times, foregoing life-sustaining treatments (ANA, 2004).

B. Physician-assisted suicide and euthanasia
   1. An increased interest in physician-assisted suicide and euthanasia seems to be related to the prevalence of inadequate pain management (Shapiro, 1994).
   2. The philosophical principle of preference utilitarianism (a morally right action as that which produces the most favorable consequences for the people involved; Singer 1993) and the concept of "nurses as healer praxis" (ethically caring: What I do to you will ultimately affect me) do not support the role of nurses in euthanasia (McCabe, 2007a; McCabe, 2007b).

C. End-of-life care (see the chapter on Palliative Care)
   1. There are seven major legal <u>myths</u> regarding end-of-life care (Meisel, Snyder, & Quill, 2000).
      a. Foregoing life-sustaining treatment for patients without decision-making capacity requires evidence that this was the patient's actual wish.
      b. Withholding or withdrawing of artificial fluids and nutrition from terminally ill or permanently unconscious patients is illegal.
      c. Risk management personnel must be consulted before life-sustaining medical treatment may be terminated.
      d. Advanced directives must comply with specific forms, are not transferable between states, and govern all future treatment decisions; oral advance directives are unenforceable.
      e. If a physician or nurse prescribes or administers high doses of medication to relieve pain or other discomfort in a terminally ill patient, resulting in death, that physician or nurse will be criminally prosecuted.
      f. When a terminally ill patient's suffering is overwhelming despite palliative care and the patient requests a hastened death, there are no legally permissible options to ease suffering.
      g. The 1997 U.S. Supreme Court decisions outlawed physician-assisted suicide.

D. Double effect
   1. The issue of double effect is a concern of nurses. Pain management nurses should understand the concept of double effect to provide ethically sound end-of-life pain care.
   2. *Principle of double effect:* An intended treatment may have deleterious side effects (Cain & Hammes, 1994).
      a. "The intent of treatment must be clearly focused on the good or beneficial (and medically appropriate) outcome" (Cain & Hammes, 1994, p. 161).
      b. To be beneficent, nurses must seek actively to relieve clients' pain (Greipp, 1992).
         (1) The doctrine of double effect is derived from the principle of nonmaleficence. Administration of high doses of opioids required for pain relief not only may relieve the pain but also may hasten death (Taylor & Ersek, 1995).
         (2) Controlling the pain of patients at the end of life can be challenging both clinically and ethically. One ethical obstacle arises when analgesia has the potential to hasten the death of the patient, thus invoking the principle of double effect to resolve such dilemmas.
         (3) Pain management can be administered effectively from a Jewish perspective in most clinical scenarios (Rabbi Weiss, 2007).

E. Physician-assisted suicide
   1. The U.S. Supreme Court's 6-3 decision in *Gonzales v. Oregon* (Oregon's physician-assisted suicide law) from both the majority opinion and the major dissent in Oregon provides an opportunity to assess the dangers inherent in allowing a political agenda that polarizes the sanctity of life against quality patient care at the end of life and minimizes professional ethical obligations (Hilliard, 2007; Kapp, 2006).
      a. Oregon Death with Dignity Law of 1997 allows terminally ill Oregonians to end their lives through the voluntary self-administration of lethal medications. This is expressly prescribed by a physician for that purpose.

b. Patients who meet certain criteria can request a prescription for lethal medication from a licensed Oregon physician.
   (1) The physician must be a doctor of medicine or doctor of osteopathy licensed to practice medicine by the Board of Medical Examiners for the state of Oregon.
   (2) The physician must also be willing to participate in the act. Physicians are not required to provide prescriptions to patients, and participation is voluntary.
   (3) In addition, some health care systems (for example, a Catholic hospital or the Veterans Health Administration) have prohibitions against practicing the act that physicians must abide by as terms of their employment.
   (4) A patient must be
      (a) 18 years of age or older.
      (b) A resident of Oregon.
      (c) Capable of making and communicating personal health care decisions.
      (d) Diagnosed with a terminal illness that will lead to death within 6 months.
   (5) It is up to the attending physician to determine whether these criteria have been met.
   (6) It is up to the physician to determine the prescription. To date, most patients have received a prescription for an oral dosage of a barbiturate.

2. Nurses must not participate in assisted suicide by helping the patient self-administer a lethal dose of medication nor bear witness to this activity; these activities are considered unethical.
3. The implications and ramifications of the U.S. Supreme Court's decision to uphold the Oregon Death with Dignity Act, as well as three crucial cases, Terri Schiavo, Karen Quinlan, and Nancy Cruzan, directly affect nursing practice and emphasize the ethical obligation of pain management nurses to advocate for patients at the end of life (Ball, 2006).

IX. Palliative Sedation (see the chapter on Palliative Care)

A. Intractable symptom management
   1. Terminal illnesses can cause distressing symptoms, such as severe pain, mental confusion, muscle spasms, feelings of suffocation, and agitation.
   2. Despite skilled palliative care, these symptoms may not respond to standard interventions.
   3. After all other means to provide comfort and relief to a dying patient have been tried and are unsuccessful, doctors and patients can consider palliative sedation.

B. Definition of palliative sedation
   1. Palliative sedation is the use of sedative medications to relieve extreme suffering by making the patient unaware and unconscious (as in a deep sleep) while the disease takes its course, eventually leading to death.
   2. The sedative medication is gradually titrated until the patient is comfortable and able to relax.
   3. Palliative sedation is not intended to hasten death or shorten life (Brender, 2005).
   4. Double effect (described earlier)
      a. The doctrine of double effect, the traditional justification for palliative sedation, permits physicians to provide high doses of opioids and sedatives to relieve suffering, provided that the intention is not to cause the patient's death and that certain other conditions are met.
      b. Such high doses are permissible even if the risk of hastening death is foreseen. The patient or family should agree with plans for palliative sedation.
      c. Because intention plays a key role in this doctrine, clinicians must understand and document which actions are consistent with an intention to relieve symptoms rather than to hasten death (Bernard & Rubenfeld, 2005).
      d. End-of-life sedation remains a controversial and ill-defined clinical practice; its applications vary considerably. Doctors and nurses are more in favor of palliative sedation when physical suffering is refractory to treatment and they are confronted with a patient's existential suffering (Blondeau, Roy, Dumont, Godin, & Martineau, 2005; Howland, 2005).

5. The attending physician needs to explain to patients and family, as well as to the medical and nursing staff, the details of care and the justification for palliative sedation.
    a. Because cases involving palliative sedation are emotionally stressful, the patient, family, and health care workers can all benefit from talking about the complex medical, ethical, and emotional issues they raise (Bernard & Rubenfeld, 2005).

C. The U.S. Supreme Court in its decisions regarding physician-assisted suicide fundamentally sanctioned palliative sedation, yet it remains a controversial intervention (*Washington v. Glucksberg*, 1997).
    1. Suffering is a "dynamic and transforming process" that offers the opportunity for healing at the end of life. As such, "the ethical arguments for the use of palliative sedation for existential suffering may not satisfy the requirements for proportionality, nonmaleficence, and intent" (Shaver & Rousseau, 2005).
    2. There may become a societal "obligation to die" that would endanger the rights of vulnerable populations, including the disabled and the frail elder. A truly autonomous choice relating to how one dies is impossible, especially for vulnerable populations (Hallenbeck, 2000).

D. The National Hospice and Palliative Care Organization and the American Academy of Hospice and Palliative Medicine support the use of palliative sedation to treat unrelieved suffering.
    1. The Veterans Health Administration had no formal statement or policy on sedative therapy.
    2. The National Ethics Committee of the Veterans Health Administration developed a creditable and well-written summary of palliative sedation, supporting its use as an ethically appropriate therapy of last resort for patients experiencing severe, unremitting, refractory clinical symptoms at the end of life.
    3. This is a recommended policy guide for veterans care facilities across the nation (National Ethics Committee, 2007).

X. Medical Futility and Pain Management Nursing Care

A. Medical futility is described as proposed therapy that should not be performed because available data have shown that it will not improve the patient's medical condition.
    1. Medical futility remains ethically controversial for several reasons. Some health care providers claim that a treatment is futile without knowing the relevant outcome data.
    2. There is, unfortunately, no consensus as to the statistical threshold for a treatment to be considered futile.
    3. It is important for nurses to help patients determine whether medical interventions are futile and their goals of care and end-of-life care decisions while maintaining quality pain and palliative care (Poncy, 2006).
    4. Nurses rate prolonging the dying process with inappropriate measures as their most disturbing ethical issue and protecting patients' rights to be of great concern (Johnstone, DaCosta, & Turale, 2002). Paradoxically, ethical codes assume nurses have the autonomy to uphold patients' health care choices (Seal, 2007).

B. Critical care nursing and medical teams are inadequately prepared to deliver palliative care for the critically ill geriatric patient.
    1. Nursing and medical providers caring for the frail elderly within an intensive care unit often reveal feelings of concern for overtreatment of patients when hope for improvement has diminished.
    2. Decline of critically ill elders regularly results in conflicts and disagreements surrounding care directives among patient, family, nursing, and specialty service teams.
    3. Nursing and medical providers caring for the critically ill elderly population who waiver between aggressive verses palliative care measures may be troubled by ethical dilemmas of "doing more harm than good."
    4. Collaborative, interdisciplinary practice in the face of such dilemmas offers an interactive and practical approach that promotes clinical excellence and improves quality of care for the critically ill (Dawson, 2008).
    5. Pain management nurses can serve as clinical advisors and patient advocates to guide ethical, respectful care.

C. Medical futility is brought to the clinical experience when
   1. The patients' wishes are impossible to realize.
   2. Decision making was performed by others regardless of whether the patients' wishes were known.
D. Nurses' view of medical futility
   1. Many nurses want to respect the wishes of dying patients. However, they questioned how patients die in intensive care units and are therefore faced with ethical dilemmas.
   2. At the same time, many nurses realize that respecting patients' wishes about end-of-life care in an intensive care unit is difficult and that being unable to respect these wishes is often unavoidable (Kinoshita, 2007).
   3. If nurses are to be effective patient advocates at end of life, they need to do the following:
      a. Develop clear criteria within which nursing assessments of patient status can be framed.
      b. Develop specialized skills to manage the nonmedical needs of dying people.
      c. Develop organizational and political skills to negotiate changing clinical practice and workplace relations (Sorensen & Iedema, 2007).
   4. The combined role for pain and palliative care nursing is positioned to fulfill this need.
E. Case law regarding medical futility
   1. Such cases, as in the Case Law Example box, tend to be the product of a severe breakdown of trust in the relationship between the clinicians and the patient's family. The deficiency is exacerbated when the communication must occur across the gaps created by language, class, and culture.
      a. Clinicians may justify their efforts to override the requests of family members by claiming that the continued use of life support is causing the patient unwarranted pain and suffering or is contributing to an undignified death.
      b. Health care is not an unlimited resource, and physicians have an ethical obligation to ensure that it is distributed fairly. Motivations may include financial considerations and concern about excessive expense, and this may seem to be an ethically legitimate reason to refuse continued treatment to patients.
      c. Clinicians may justify their refusal to treat on the basis of their right to refuse to participate in medical interventions that they believe violate their moral integrity.
   2. Texas Advance Directives Act (Table 12-3)
      a. The principal advantage of the act is that it provides a path for resolving intractable dilemmas in situations in which clinicians may feel compelled to do whatever patients and families demand.
      b. This statute incorporates a due-process standard by insisting that all allegations of futility go forward only after they have been reviewed and approved by the hospital ethics committee.
      c. In such situations, the ethics committee is acting, under Texas law, as a surrogate judge and jury, with the statutory power to authorize clinicians to take actions against the wishes of a patient and family, with protection against civil and criminal liability (Truog, 2007).

Case Law Example

Emilio Gonzales was an 18-month-old boy who had Leigh's disease, a progressive and fatal neurometabolic disorder. He had been on life support in the intensive care unit of an Austin Texas Hospital for 5 months. National attention was focused on a mother's struggle to prevent the Children's Hospital from withdrawing life support from her infant son. The hospital had invoked the Texas Advance Directives Act, which authorized it to withdraw life support if an ethics committee had determined that further life support was medically inappropriate and provided the hospital gave the family 10 days' notice and attempted to transfer Emilio to an alternative provider (*Washington Post*, 2007).

Table 12-3 Key Provisions for Resolving Futility Cases under the Texas Advance Directives Act

- The physician's refusal to comply with the patient's or surrogate's request for treatment must be reviewed by a hospital-appointed medical or ethics committee in which the attending physician does not participate.
- The family must be given 48 hours' notice and be invited to participate in the consultation process.
- The ethics consultation committee must provide a written report detailing its findings to the family and must include this report in the medical record.
- If the ethics consultation process fails to resolve the dispute, the hospital, working with the family, must make reasonable efforts to transfer the patient's care to another physician or institution willing to provide the treatment requested by the family.
- If after 10 days (measured from the time the family receives the written summary from the ethics consultation committee) no such provider can be found, the hospital and physician may unilaterally withhold or withdraw therapy that has been determined to be futile.
- The patient or surrogate may request a court-ordered time extension, which should be granted only if the judge determines that there is a reasonable likelihood of finding a willing provider of the disputed treatment.
- If the family does not seek an extension or the judge fails to grant one, futile treatment may be unilaterally withdrawn by the treatment team with immunity from civil and criminal prosecution.

From *Annals of Intern Med*, 2003, by R. L. Fine, & T. W. Mayo. Permission conveyed by Copyright Clearance Center.

3. Therefore, this type of law may serve a useful purpose in the following situations:
   a. Patients are subjected to unwarranted pain and suffering.
   b. Clinicians have defensible claims that family or advocate demands compromise their moral integrity (Truog, 2007).

XI. Sociopolitical Pressures

A. Numerous sociopolitical pressures may affect a patient's ability to receive appropriate and effective pain care. In addition, various factors may influence the ability of nurses to provide needed care. Nurses need to be aware of these pressures and understand the potential impact on patient care.
   1. Economic factors
      a. Conflict of interest from pharmaceutical marketing practices that may surround a nurse practitioner's prescribing choices may be reduced by the use of relevant guidelines (Crigger, 2005).
      b. As the business of pain management has escalated, hospitals, home care agencies, and physicians may have become owners of pain management services. Potential problem arise when owners make decisions about treatments that cause conflict between what is in the patient's best interest and what is in the owner's financial interest (Whedon & Ferrell, 1991).
      c. Nurses need to be aware of economic incentives related to interventional pain medicine (Schofferman, 2006).
      d. Nurses play various roles in patient care. It is important for nurses to recognize those roles to ensure that unacceptable ethical boundaries are not crossed (Sullivan & Main, 2007).
      e. Lack of adequate insurance coverage produces barriers for patients in obtaining appropriate pain management (Cain & Hammes, 1994).
      f. Lack of access to optimal pain control can be limiting (Ferrell, et.al., 2002).
      g. Improper use of technological interventions can be an issue (Taylor & Ersek, 1995).
         (1) Reimbursement biases mean that intravenous infusions via an infusion pump ($3,000 per month) are covered by insurance companies, but oral analgesics ($100 per month) are not (Whedon & Ferrell, 1991).

(2) A conflict of interest can arise between the patient's best interest and the personal financial interest of the health care provider (Whedon & Ferrell, 1991).
(3) Use of technology is inappropriate when it decreases quality of life, when it diverts resources inappropriately, or when complications outweigh probable benefits (Ferrell & Rhiner, 1991; Whedon & Ferrell, 1991).
(4) Technology may affect the patient and family adversely through significant physical, financial, and psychological burdens, including their ability to use technological equipment safely (Ferrell & Rhiner, 1991; Taylor & Ersek, 1995; Whedon & Ferrell, 1991).

2. Practitioner attitudes are important. Nurses need to understand how their own fears, bias, and lack of knowledge, as well as those of their peers, can greatly affect appropriate and effective patient care.
   a. Opiophobia and fear of addiction (Davis & Walsh, 2004; Ferrell & Rhiner, 1991; Greipp, 1992; Martino, 1998; Popenhagen, 2006; Rhodin, 2006)
   b. Fear of investigation and censure for prescribing opioids because of laws and regulations aimed at prevention of drug abuse (Dahl, 2005; Federation of State Medical Boards of the United States House of Delegates, May 1998) or prevention of the hastening of death (Gilson & Joranson, 2006; Taylor & Ersek, 1995)
   c. Fear of prescribing at the end of life (Quill & Meier, 2006; Trehan, 2007) (see the earlier discussion and the chapter on Palliative Care)
   d. Psychological barriers of the clinician (Passik, Byers, & Kirsh, 2007)
   e. Clinician bias
      (1) Race and ethnicity (Burgess, van Ryn, Crowley-Matoka, & Malat, 2006; Maze & Martino, 2005) (see the chapter on Disparities in Pain Management)
      (2) Gender (Criste, 2003; Werner, Isaksen, & Malterud, 2004) (see the chapter on Gender or Sex Differences in Pain and Analgesia)
      (3) Age (Zwakhalen, Hamers, Peijnenburg, & Berger, 2007)
   f. Bias in research
      (1) Importance of minimizing bias in research (Merskey & Teasell, 2007) (see the chapter on Research Utilization in Pain Management Nursing)

XII. Public Health Implications

A. The public health problem of pain that is undertreated or not treated is well documented (see the chapter on Disparities in Pain Management).
B. There is a second growing public health problem of prescription drug abuse.
   1. Nurses have a responsibility to assist in the prevention of misuse, abuse, and diversion of prescription medications.
   2. Nurses also have a responsibility to ensure those with the disease of chemical dependency have access to appropriate pain management care.
C. There is a need for a comprehensive public policy to address pain management with its existing barriers to care (Dilcher, 2004).
D. Public health surrounding chronic pain and healthy communities are affected by legal, ethical, and policy concerns (Johnson & Todd, 2007).
E. Ethical, societal, and regulatory barriers face opioid prescribers (Reddy, 2006).
F. The United Nations' *Single Convention on Narcotic Drugs* seeks to ensure balance between access to opioid analgesics while discouraging drug trafficking on the international stage; therefore, it affects global availability on opioid analgesics (Taylor, 2007).
G. Legal parameters exist for the medical use of controlled substances and are established by international treaties, federal and state laws, and regulations (Gilson & Joranson, 2006).
H. International drug control treaties
   1. Treaties ensure the availability of controlled substances for medical purposes.
   2. They prevent illegal drug diversion (Gilson & Joranson, 2006).

I. Federal controlled substances policies: the U.S. Drug Enforcement Administration (DEA) and the Controlled Substances Act (http://www.usdoj.gov/dea/pubs/csa.html)
   1. Policies acknowledge that controlled substances are necessary for public health and that their availability for medical and scientific purposes must be ensured.
   2. Policies recognize that prescribing narcotics for intractable pain is a legitimate medical practice (Gilson & Joranson, 2006).
   3. The U.S. DEA asserts that controlled substances should be prescribed, dispensed, or administered for legitimate reasons.

J. State laws or regulations
   1. The Project on Legal Constraints on Access to Effective Pain Relief, conducted by the American Society of Law, Medicine and Ethics, proposes the following pain relief act for adoption by state legislatures.
      a. "Neither disciplinary action nor state criminal prosecution shall be brought against health care provider for the prescription, dispensing, or administration of medical treatment for the therapeutic purpose of relieving intractable pain (when that provider) can demonstrate by reference to an accepted guideline that his or her practice substantially complied with that guideline" (Hyman, 1996).
   2. The U.S. DEA publishes controlled substance manuals for ***midlevel*** practitioners, such as nurse practitioners. State boards of nursing may be contacted for specific questions (Gilson & Joranson, 2006).
      a. To obtain an informational outline of the Controlled Substances Act, see the following website: http://www.deadiversion.usdoj.gov/pubs/manuals/pract/index.html (Rannazzisi & Caverly, 2006).
      b. The Federation of State Medical Boards is providing to registrants of numerous states the following resource. It also can be ordered from the Federation of State Medical Boards website at http://www.fsmb.org/Pain/default.html.
         (1) *Responsible Opioid Prescribing* offers physicians effective strategies for reducing the risk of addiction, abuse, and diversion of opioids that they prescribe for their patients in pain. Written by pain medicine specialist Scott M. Fishman (2008), this concise handbook translates the Federation of State Medical Board's "Model policy for the use of controlled substances for the treatment of pain" (2005) into pragmatic steps for risk reduction and improved patient care, including the following:
            (a) Patient evaluation, including risk assessment
            (b) Treatment plans that incorporate functional goals
            (c) Informed consent and prescribing agreements
            (d) Periodic review and monitoring of patients
            (e) Referral and patient management
            (f) Documentation
            (g) Compliance with state and federal law

K. Opioid prescribing
   1. The risks and benefits of chronic opioid therapy need to be carefully considered before initiation of therapy and in relation to ongoing therapy. Patient selection is critical (Ballantyne, 2006).
   2. The role of trust between the clinician and the patient has significant value in the therapeutic relationship (Miller, 2007; Morse, 1991).
   3. The role of ethics surrounding the use of opioids in patients with pain following spinal cord injury is illustrated in the literature using case studies (Richards, Kezar, & Ness, 2007).
   4. Subjective factors influence the prescribing practices of advanced practice nurses for patients with chronic pain (Fontana, 2008).
   5. Physicians underprescribe, nurses give less than is prescribed, and patients often take less medication than is prescribed (Greipp, 1992; Lisson, 1987; Taylor & Ersek, 1995; Taylor, Ferrell, Grant, & Cheyney, 1993).
   6. The counterproductive philosophy of underprescribing is perpetuated by three principles (Martino, 1998).

a. *"Just Say No" campaign slogan:* Drug addiction and abuse harm individuals and society and have created an opiophobia.
b. *"Grin and bear it" philosophy:* Pain happens.
   (1) Pain builds character.
   (2) Society rewards practitioners who uphold this principle (by choosing to underprescribe) with substance control laws, rules, and regulations.
c. *Avoidance of risks:* This ensures no harm is done (internal reward) and secures for practitioners income, power, prestige, and status (external rewards).

7. The American Academy of Pain Medicine, American Pain Society, and American Society of Addiction Medicine (2004) published a consensus document titled "Public policy statement on the rights and responsibilities of health care professionals in the use of opioids for the treatment of pain."
   a. Recommendations
      (1) Health care professionals who prescribe opioids for the treatment of pain should use clear and reasonable medical judgment to establish that a pain state exists and to determine whether opioids are an indicated component of treatment. Opioids should be prescribed in a lawful and clinically sound manner. Patients should be followed at reasonable intervals for ongoing medical management to confirm as nearly as is reasonable that the medications are used as prescribed, to ensure that the goals of treatment are met, and to revise therapy as indicated. Such initial decision making and ongoing management should be appropriately documented.
      (2) Health care professionals who are practicing medicine in good faith and who use reasonable medical judgment regarding the prescription of opioids for the treatment of pain should not be held responsible for the willful and deceptive behavior of patients who successfully obtain opioids for nonmedical purposes. It is an appropriate role of the U.S. DEA, pharmacy boards, and other regulatory agencies to inform physicians of the behavior of such patients when it is detected.
      (3) Interventions to correct the clinical care practices of health care professionals who consistently fail to recognize addictive disorders, medication misuse, or medication diversion in their patients or fail to evaluate and treat pain are appropriate. Interventions may include education, licensing sanction, legal sanction, or a combination of these as indicated after careful and appropriate review of records and other available information.
      (4) For the purpose of performing regulatory, legal, quality assurance, and other clinical case reviews, it should be recognized that judgment can only be made properly with full and detailed understanding of a particular clinical case regarding the following:
         (a) The medical appropriateness of the prescription of opioids for pain in a specific context
         (b) The selection of a particular opioid drug or drugs
         (c) The determination of indicated opioid dosage and interval of medication administration,
      (5) Regulatory, legal, quality assurance, and other reviews of clinical cases involving the use of opioids for the treatment of pain should be performed when they are indicated by reviewers with a requisite level of understanding of pain medicine and addiction medicine.
      (6) Appropriate education in addiction medicine and pain medicine should be provided as part of the core curriculum at all medical and other provider training schools.
      (7) Legal actions, licensing actions, or both against health care professionals who are proven to be knowingly complicit in the diversion of scheduled drugs or other illegal prescribing activities are appropriate.

8. Legal and regulatory issues related to opioid prescribing
   a. It is vital to obtain valid informed consent and agreement for treatment with controlled substances (Bolen, 2006b; Jacobson & Mann, 2004; Lowe, 2004).

b. Prescribers should educate patients about the risks and benefits of opioid analgesics (Bloodworth, 2006).
c. Case rulings and implications for prescribers of opioids include both inappropriate prescribing and undertreatment of pain (Bolen, 2006a; Brushwood, 2007a, 2007b; Johnson, 2005; Reidenberg & Willis, 2007; Reynolds, 2006; Shapiro, 1994).
d. Prescribers need to be aware of the state of flux in the current regulatory and legal environment and to continue to monitor current and future trends to ensure appropriate practice (Chan & Fishman, 2006).
e. Prescription monitoring programs study the impact on patient care (Fishman, Papazian, Gonzales, Riches, & Gilson, 2004).
f. The Federation of State Medical Boards of the United States published "Model policy for the use of controlled substances for the treatment of pain," which can be used a prescription guideline for advanced practice nurses (Federation of State Medical Boards of the United States, 2005).
g. Findings of a survey of state medical board members' beliefs about pain, addiction, and diversion and abuse demonstrate that medical regulators believe criminal investigations and prosecutions of physicians for their prescribing practices have increased (Gilson, Maurer, & Joranson, 2007).
h. Balance between pain management and drug law enforcement is critical (Joranson & Portenoy, 2005; Lawrence, 2005).
i. Adequate documentation may decrease U.S. DEA action (Jung & Reidenberg, 2006; Rannazzisi, 2007).

L. Addictive disease, misuse, abuse, and diversion of prescription medications
1. "ASPMN position statement: Pain management in patients with addictive disease" (ASPMN, 2004)
a. Patients with addictive disease have the right to be treated with respect and to receive the same quality of pain management as all other patients. Providing this care addresses the potential for increased drug use or relapse associated with unrelieved pain. Nurses are in an ideal position to advocate and intervene for these patients across all treatment settings.
b. Specific recommendations are provided for all patients with addictive disease, patients who are actively using, patients in recovery, and patients on methadone maintenance treatment.
2. Patient selection and monitoring are critical when assessing the appropriateness for opioid therapy (Ballantyne, 2006; Ineck & Rule, 2006).
3. There are complex ethical issues in caring for the patient with chronic pain and substance use disorders. The nurse needs to understand these issues to be able to provide appropriate care (Geppert, 2004).
4. It is important for nurses to become educated on the impact of prescription drug abuse on public health. In addition, it is important for nurses to know the role they can play in educating others about prescription drug abuse. Nurses working with other health care professionals, patients, law enforcement, regulators, legislators, payers, and the media can affect this growing public health problem (Manchikanti, 2007; Passik, Heit, & Kirsh, 2006).
5. Nurses need to be aware of aberrant drug related behavior (Todd, 2005).

XIII. Legal and Regulatory Influences: General

A. Accountability and culpability
1. A legal distinction exists between the regulatory authority of guidelines and that of regulations. Guidelines are developed by nationally recognized organizations or specialty societies or are contained in authoritative textbooks or articles. Guidelines have no force of law and are merely suggestions for safe conduct. Regulations are a *rule or order of law* issued by executive authority of government (Hyman, 1996).
2. Community practice standards are a consideration in culpability.
3. Institutional leadership is required to establish safe pain management policies, protocols, and orders and to ensure staff competency and accountability.

B. Liability issues in pain management
   1. *Liability resulting from improper pain management:* Improper pain management is the failure to adhere to good and accepted practice. Lawsuits have focused on the responsibility of health care providers to ensure the proper administration of pain medications and doses.
      a. In the *Estate of Henry Janes v. Hillhaven Corp.*, the jury awarded $15 million in damages to the family of a patient whose dying days were made intolerable by the decision of a nurse and her employer, a nursing home, to withhold or reduce pain medication ordered by the patient's physician. The nurse assessed the patient as "being addicted to morphine" and, without the consent of the physician, instituted her own "pain management plan" by substituting analgesics and a mild tranquilizer (Shapiro, 1994).
      b. Liability is emerging for the undertreatment of pain (Vaglienti & Grinberg, 2004).
      c. Elder abuse and undertreatment of pain are cited in the literature (McIntire, 2004; Rich, 2004; Tucker, 2004).
   2. *Health care provider liability to third parties:* A health care provider's legal duty may extend to the driving public when administering drugs or treatment that can induce drowsiness or compromise judgment.
      a. In *Wilschinsky v. Medina,* the New Mexico Supreme Court ruled that a physician was liable when an individual was injured by an automobile driven by the physician's patient. The patient, already receiving an oxycodone–acetaminophen drug, was administered meperidine by a physician for complaints of a debilitating migraine. After the meperidine, the patient developed nausea, and the physician administered a second drug to combat the symptoms. Approximately 1 hour later, when the patient was driving home, she struck and injured another individual (Shapiro, 1994).
      b. Driving while on chronic opioid analgesic therapy case reports and recommendations are found in the literature (Fishbain, Lewis, Cole, Rosomoff, & Rosomoff, 2007).
   3. Nurses who are involved in outpatient pain management treatment or interventional pain management should ensure they do the following:
      a. Explain and document information provided regarding the benefits, risks, and side effects associated with medications (i.e., impairment of mental alertness or dexterity).
      b. Provide verbal and written instructions to the patient and family members regarding potential adverse complications of invasive pain management procedures and when to seek medical attention.
      c. Document patient instructions and patient understanding.
      d. Arrange for alternative transportation if the patient is without a driver.
   4. *Pain control versus euthanasia:* Health care providers who administer lethal doses of medication deliberately are at risk for prosecution. Many states have laws imposing criminal sanctions for aiding, assisting, causing, or promoting suicide (Shapiro, 1994).
   5. *Liability for risks and side effects of prescription drugs:* The manufacturer of pain management devices can be liable if it provides substandard directions or instructions for safe product use or warns health care providers inadequately about potential or known side effects or dangers. In cases in which manufacturer warnings are adequate but the health care provider fails to follow the directions or convey them to the patient, the health care provider may be held liable (Shapiro, 1994).

C. Negligence and malpractice consideration for pain management nurses
   1. Definitions
      a. *Negligence* is the failure to do something that a "reasonable" nurse would do or is doing something that a "reasonable" nurse would not do in the same situation (Cushing, 1998).
      b. *Malpractice* is any professional misconduct or unreasonable lack of skill in carrying out professional duties (Cushing, 1998).
      c. A *standard of care* consists of safe and accepted nursing care practices. The standard of care is assessed by policies and guidelines written by nationally recognized organizations or specialty societies and formal training, as outlined in hospital policies or contained in authoritative textbooks and articles.

2. Elements of negligence and malpractice
   a. *Duty* is established when a professional patient–nurse relationship exists.
      (1) The pain management nurse is in charge of the patient.
      (2) The primary care nurse monitors the patient alone or in conjunction with the pain management nurse.
   b. *Breach of duty* is failure of the pain management nurse to exercise reasonable care. Examples include, but are not limited to, the following:
      (1) Failure to implement appropriate pain management policies, procedures, and protocols
      (2) Failure to provide appropriate pain management education for staff
      (3) Failure to report changes in a patient's condition
      (4) Negligent administration of opioids
      (5) Failure to monitor an epidural site for signs of infection (Kuc, 1997)
   c. *Causation* occurs when injury to the patient was proximately caused by the negligent conduct of the nurse.
      (1) For example, allowing an epidural patient with known right leg numbness to ambulate unassisted resulted in the patient's falling and fracturing a hip or injuring a knee.
   d. *Damages* occur when the patient suffered a compensable injury.
      (1) Using the fractured hip example, damages include the risk of unnecessary anesthesia and surgery for hip arthroplasty, rehabilitation, pain and suffering, and the potential need for future hip surgery.

D. Documentation
   1. Nurses have a responsibility to thoroughly document the patient's history, assessments, plan of care, interventions, patient and family education and their understanding of the teachings of adverse events, outcomes, and other relevant information. Nurses also have a responsibility to document relevant communications about the patient to other health care practitioner team members. Documentation should be timely and in accordance with state laws and policies and procedures of the employer.

XIV. Nursing Practice Issues

A. Nurses need to systematically assess pain and offer pain medications to nursing home residents to overcome barriers to effective pain management (Jones et al., 2005).
B. Ethical and legal considerations exist for the clinical nurse specialists in treating patients with pain (O'Malley, 2005).
C. It is vital to obtain valid informed consent and agreement for treatment with controlled substances (Bolen, 2006b; Jacobson & Mann, 2004; Lowe, 2004).
D. There is a role for opioid treatment agreements.
   1. A statement of support for opioid agreements by the American Academy of Pain Management can be found at http://www.aapainmanage.org/literature/Articles/OpioidAgreements.Pdf.
   2. Communication of opioid agreements with all providers and pharmacists is helpful in addressing clinical challenges (Fishman, Bandman, Edwards, & Borsook, 1999; Gallagher, 2004; Gudin, 2007).
E. Urine drug testing in clinical practice can be a valuable tool if the appropriate test is used.
   1. The pain management nurse can be well positioned to establish expectations of urine toxicology screenings.
   2. The pain management nurse understands the ethical considerations of interpretation of the urine toxicology results.
   3. Practical guidelines are available in the literature (Gourlay & Heit, 2005; Gourlay, Caplan, & Heit, 2006; Hammett-Stabler & Webster, 2008; Moeller, Lee, & Kissack, 2008; Swope, Amero, Kujawski, Miller, & St. Marie, 2009).
      a. Tufts Health Care Institute (2005) has information on opioid risk management. See http://www.thci.org/opioid for a PowerPoint presentation.

b. The International Association for Pain and Chemical Dependency is an international organization dedicated to promoting appropriate and effective treatment for all patients with pain, including individuals with substance abuse, mental health, or other cooccurring problems that may make treatment more challenging. See http://www.iapcd.org/index.php?option=com_frontpage&Itemid=1 for more information on guidelines and educational opportunities.

XV. Advocacy

A. Role of nurses as advocates (patient and nurse)
   1. Advocacy is core to nursing practice and is a cornerstone to excellence in patient care. Nurses have not only an obligation but also a privilege to serve as an advocate for their patients who, often because of their age, medical condition, or mental health, are unable to advocate for themselves.
   2. Due to the respect that nurses enjoy within the broader community, they can serve as a powerful and effective advocate voice with policymakers and the press.

B. Patient advocacy
   1. Pain management delivery equipment is not a substitute for being with patients and acknowledging their pain and suffering (Whedon & Ferrell, 1991).
   2. Nurses have an obligation to explore all pain management options within the scope of their nursing practice, including pharmacological and nonpharmacological methods, holistic and spiritual support, technological advances, and noninvasive treatment.
   3. Patients who may not be able to communicate their pain management needs adequately are infants, children, mentally impaired patients, speech-impaired or hearing-impaired patients, intubated patients, and semicomatose patients.
   4. When patients are unable to express their need for pain relief, it is imperative that the nurse be especially observant.
   5. Advocacy is a vital nursing issue comprising valuing, apprising, and interceding. These concepts should be understood as they can affect patient care either positively or negatively (Baldwin, 2003).
   6. Advocacy themes include protection, communication or giving voice, doing, and comfort and caring (Boyle, 2005).
   7. Three core attributes of the concept of patient advocacy identified are
      a. Safeguarding patients' autonomy.
      b. Acting on behalf of patients.
      c. Championing social justice in the provision of health care (Bu & Jezewski, 2007).

C. Preparing nurses for advocacy
   1. Nursing advocacy appears to integrate aspects of individuality and professionalism and experiences of empowering, exceptional care. Advocacy occurs over time and is described as a process of analyzing, counseling, responding, and shielding and whistle-blowing activities in clinical nursing practice (Vaartio & Leino-Kilpi, 2005).
      a. Nurses should strongly advocate for patients' choices (Altun & Ersoy, 2003).
      b. The concept and application of nursing advocacy are complex and require further study (MacDonald, 2007; Vaartio & Leino-Kilpi, 2005).
      c. Nurses can affect professional practice through their advocacy efforts (Stevens, 1999).
      d. Nurses can affect professional practice through their leadership examples (Murphy & Roberts, 2008).
   2. Advocacy is an ethical response of nurses for patients who are vulnerable or socially isolated (Erlen, 2006; Holley, 2007).
   3. A "Sphere of nursing advocacy model" may be useful in guiding research or for teaching nursing advocacy (Hanks, 2005).
      a. Research in nursing advocacy is expanding into different models, including facilitating the use of complementary therapies (Kubsch, Sternard, Hovarter, & Matzke, 2004).
   4. Nurse advocacy plays an important role in a multidisciplinary team due to the limited time physicians spend with patients (McGrath, Holewa, & McGrath, 2006).

a. Advocacy is an essential skill for case managers (Tahan, 2005).
b. The role of the nurse as an advocate in end-of-life care is essential (Thacker, 2008).

5. When prepared, nurses can play a vital role in advocating for regulatory or legislative change in larger health care systems.
   a. Legislative advocacy skills can be easily learned, and proficiency can be developed.
   b. Critical components include an interest, time, energy, and patience (Abood, 2007).
   c. Clinicians should consider participating in an informed manner in policy advocacy (Altilio, 2006; Spenceley, Reutter, & Allen, 2006).
   d. The University of Wisconsin Pain and Policy Studies Group (http://www.painpolicy.wisc.edu/) has done significant policy research and produced report cards for state policies, laws, and regulations (see the chapter on Pain Initiatives). Pain advocates often use this information to assist and direct them in their policy advocacy work (Gilson, Joranson, & Maurer, 2007; Gilson, Joranson, Maurer, Ryan, & Garthwaite, 2005; Gilson, Maurer, & Joranson, 2005).
   e. Nurses should recognize that pain is political (Rich, 2005).
   f. Nursing is one of the top respected professions.

D. Websites to help facilitate involvement in advocacy
   1. Advocacy competencies (Counselors for Social Justice, 2004–2007), http://counselorsforsocialjustice.com/advocacycompetencies.html
   2. The American Organization of Nurse Executives (2005) vision for 2020, http://www.aone.org/aone/advocacy/npec.html

E. Nurses and the media
   1. Nurses with good media credibility are often a source of "go to" information for the media.
      a. Nurses have been ranked number one in the Gallup polls for honesty and ethics of the professions, with 84% of respondents ranking nurses high or very high (Saad, 2008).
      b. Nurses have topped Gallup's Honesty and Ethics ranking every year but one since they were added to the list in 1999. The year that was an exception is 2001, when firefighters were added to the list.
   2. Nurses can learn media advocacy skills and effectively deploy them to educate larger audiences on pain management and other health issues affecting patient care, access to care, or both.
   3. Opportunities to advocate in the media are most commonly found with print, radio, and television forums.
   4. Proficiency in media requires preparation; i.e., background information on issues and other resources for media work can be found online.
      a. ASPMN's website has information about advocacy occurring from the organization. This can be found at http://www.aspmn.org/Public/advocacy.htm.
      b. The American Pain Foundation Power Over Pain Action Manual can be found at http://www.painfoundation.org/poweroverpain/default.asp?file=Media/mediaguide.htm&menu=2.
      c. The Purdue Pharma Pain Advocacy Community Non-Branded Program has a website with an advocacy resource titled "In the Face of Pain Advocacy Toolkit." It can be found on http://www.inthefaceofpain.com.

Summary

Taking care of peoples' pain, one patient at a time is an important endeavor. However, pain management nurses must also serve society by working to impact social policy, giving voice to the marginalized, and ensuring that pain management is available to everyone everyday.

References

Abood, S. (2007). Influencing health care in the legislative arena. *Online Journal of Issues in Nursing, 12*(1), 3.

Agency for Healthcare Research and Quality. (1992). *Acute pain management (critical guide): Operative medical procedures.* Clinical Practice Guideline. (AHRQ Publication No. 92-0032.) Rockville, MD: Author.

Agency for Healthcare Research and Quality. (1994). *Cancer pain management guidelines.* Publication No. 94-0592. Rockville, MD: Author.

Altilio, T. (2006). Pain and symptom management clinical, policy, and political perspectives. *Journal of Psychosocial Oncology, 24*(1), 65–79.

Altun, I. & Ersoy, N. (2003). Undertaking the role of patient advocate: A longitudinal study of nursing students. *Nursing Ethics, 10*(5), 462–471.

American Academy of Pain Medicine, American Pain Society, & American Society of Addiction Medicine. (2004). Public policy statement on the rights and responsibilities of health care professionals in the use of opioids for the treatment of pain: A consensus document from the American Academy of Pain Medicine, the American Pain Society, and the American Society of Addiction Medicine. *Pain Medicine, 5*(3), 301–302.

American Academy of Pain Medicine Council on Ethics. (2005). Ethics charter from American Academy of Pain Medicine. *Pain Medicine, 6*(3), 203–212.

American Medical Association. (2006). *Code of medical ethics.* Retrieved December 3, 2008, from http://www0.ama-assn.org/apps/pf_new/pf_online?f_n=browse&doc=policyfiles/HnE/E-8.083.HTM&&s_t=&st_p=&nth=1&prev_pol=policyfiles/HnE/E-7.05.HTM&nxt_pol=policyfiles/HnE/E-8.01.HTM&.

American Nurses Association. (1998). *Discrimination and racism in health care.* Retrieved December 3, 2008, from http://www.nursingworld.org/MainMenuCategories/HealthcareandPolicyIssues/ANAPositionStatements/EthicsandHumanRights.aspx.

American Nurses Association. (2001). *Code for nurses, with interpretive statement.* Retrieved December 3, 2008, from http://www.nursingworld.org/MainMenuCategories/ThePracticeofProfessionalNursing/EthicsStandards/CodeofEthics/AboutTheCode.aspx.

American Nurses Association. (2004). *Assisted suicide.* Retrieved December 3, 2008, from http://www.nursingworld.org/MainMenuCategories/HealthcareandPolicyIssues/ANAPositionStatements/EthicsandHumanRights.aspx.

American Organization of Nurse Executives. (2005). *Vision 2020 for nursing.* Retrieved December 3, 2008, from http://www.aone.org/aone/advocacy/npec.html.

American Pain Foundation. (2006). *Power over pain action manual.* Retrieved December 3, 2008, from http://www.painfoundation.org/poweroverpain/default.asp?file=Media/mediaguide.htm&menu=2.

American Pain Society. (2003). *Principles of analgesic use in the treatment of acute pain and cancer pain* (5th ed.). Glenview, IL: Author.

American Pain Society (2008).

American Pain Society & American Academy of Pain Medicine. (1996). *The use of opioids for the treatment of chronic pain.* Retrieved November 30, 2008, from http://www.ampainsoc.org/advocacy/opioids.htm.

American Society for Pain Management Nursing. (1996). *Standards of clinical nursing practice for pain management.* Pensacola, FL: Author.

American Society for Pain Management Nursing. (2003). *Nursing position statements on assisted suicide: End of life issues–placebo use.* Retrieved December 3, 2008, from http://www.aspmn.org/ORGANIZATION/position_papers.htm.

American Society for Pain Management Nursing. (2004). ASPMN position statement: Pain management in patients with addictive disease. *Journal of Vascular Nursing, 22*(3), 99–101.

Antonaci, F., Chimento, P., Bono, G., Antonaci, F., Chimento, P., Sances, G., & Diener, H. C. (2007). Lessons from placebo effects in migraine treatment. *Journal of Headache and Pain, 8*(1), 63–66.

Baldwin, M. A. (2003). Patient advocacy: a concept analysis. *Nursing Standard, 17*(21), 33–39, 5–11.

Ball, S. C. (2006). Nurse–patient advocacy and the right to die. *Journal of Psychosocial Nursing and Mental Health Services, 44*(12), 36–42.

Ballantyne, J. C. (2006). Opioids for chronic nonterminal pain. *Southern Medical Journal, 99*(11), 1245–1255.

Bernard, L., & Rubenfeld, G. (2005). Palliative sedation in dying patients: "We turn to it when everything else hasn't worked." *Journal of the American Medical Association, 294,* 1810–1816.

Blondeau, D., Roy, L., Dumont, S., Godin, G., & Martineau, I. (2005). Physicians' and pharmacists' attitudes toward the use of sedation at the end of life: Influence of prognosis and type of suffering. *Journal of Palliative Care, 21*(4), 238–245.

Bloodworth, D. (2006). Opioids in the treatment of chronic pain: Legal framework and therapeutic indications and limitations. *Physical Medicine & Rehabilitation Clinics of North America, 17*(2), 355–379.

Bolen, J. (2006a). The Fourth Circuit Court of Appeals' decision in *United States v. Hurwitz:* An important victory for pain management professionals and those living with pain. *Journal of Opioid Management, 2*(5), 262–267.

Bolen, J. (2006b). Getting informed consent and agreement for treatment right: A legal perspective on key obligations for practitioners who use controlled substances to treat chronic pain. *Journal of Opioid Management, 2*(4), 193–200.

Borneman, T., & Ferrell, B. R. (1996). Ethical issues in pain management. *Clinics in Geriatric Medicine, 12,* 615–627.

Boyle, H. J. (2005). Patient advocacy in the perioperative setting. *American Peri-Operative Registered Nurses Journal, 82*(2), 250–262.

Bradley, W. G., Daroff, R. B., Fenichel, G. M., & Marsden, C. D. (2000). Management of neurological disease. In W. G. Bradley, R. B. Darroff, G. M. Fenichel, & C. D. Marsden (Eds.), *Neurology in clinical practice: Principles of diagnosis and management* (Vol. 1, 3rd ed., pp. 861–866). Boston: Butterworth-Heinemann. Brender, E. (2005). Palliative care. *Journal of the American Medical Association, 294,* 1850.

Brennan, F., Carr, D. B., & Cousins, M. (2007). Pain management: A fundamental human right [review article]. *Anesthesia & Analgesia, 105*(1), 205–221.

Brody, H. (1982). The lie that heals: The ethics of giving placebos. *Annals of Internal Medicine, 97,* 112–118.

Brushwood, D. B. (2007a). The "general recognition and acceptance" standard of objectivity for good faith in prescribing: Legal and medical implications. *Journal of Pain & Palliative Care Pharmacotherapy, 21*(2), 35–38.

Brushwood, D. B. (2007b). Patient perspectives on criminal prosecutions of pain management practitioners: Lessons from the Fisher-Miller case. *Journal of Pain & Palliative Care Pharmacotherapy, 21*(3), 73–78.

Bu, X., & Jezewski, M. (2007). Developing a mid-range theory of patient advocacy through concept analysis. *Journal of Advanced Nursing, 57*(1), 101–110.

Burgess, D. J., van Ryn, M., Crowley-Matoka, M., & Malat, J. (2006). Understanding the provider contribution to race/ethnicity disparities in pain treatment: Insights from dual process models of stereotyping. *Pain Medicine, 7*(2), 119–134.

Cain, J. M., & Hammes, B. L. (1994). Ethics and pain management: Respecting patient wishes. *Journal of Pain and Symptom Management, 9,* 160–165.

Chaloner, C. (2007). An introduction to ethics in nursing. *Nursing Standard, 21*(32), 42–46.

Chan, K. T., & Fishman, S. M. (2006). Legal aspects of chronic opioid therapy. *Current Pain & Headache Reports, 10*(6), 426–430.

Counselors for Social Justice. (2004–2007). *Advocacy competencies: Task force on advocacy competencies.* Retrieved December 3, 2008, from http://counselorsforsocialjustice.com/advocacycompetencies.html.

Crigger, N. J. (2005). Pharmaceutical promotions and conflict of interest in nurse practitioner's decision making: The undiscovered country. *Journal of the American Academy of Nurse Practitioners, 17*(6), 207–212.

Criste, A. (2003). Do nurse anesthetists demonstrate gender bias in treating pain? A national survey using a standardized pain model. *American Association of Nurse Anesthetists Journal, 71*(3), 206–209.

Cushing, M. (1998). *Nursing jurisprudence: Establishing the standard of care.* Norwalk, CT: Appleton & Lange.

Dahl, J. L. (2005). How to reduce fears of legal/regulatory scrutiny in managing pain in cancer patients. *Journal of Supportive Oncology, 3*(5), 384–388.

Davis, M. P., & Walsh, D. (2004). Epidemiology of cancer pain and factors influencing poor pain control. *American Journal of Hospice & Palliative Care, 21*(2), 137–142.

Dawson, K. A. (2008). Palliative care for critically ill older adults: Dimensions of nursing advocacy. *Critical Care Nursing Quarterly, 31*(1), 19–23.

U.S. Drug Enforcement Administration. (2002). *DEA and Controlled Substances Act.* Retrieved December 14, 2008, from http://www.usdoj.gov/dea/pubs/csa.html.

Dilcher, A. J. (2004). Damned if they do, damned if they don't: The need for a comprehensive public policy to address the inadequate management of pain. *Annals of Health Law, 13*(1), 81–144.

Erlen, J. A. (2003). When all do not have the same: Health disparities. *Orthopaedic Nursing, 22*(2), 151–154.

Erlen, J. A. (2006). Who speaks for the vulnerable? *Orthopaedic Nursing, 25*(2), 133–136.

Ersek, M., Scanlon, C., Glass, E., Ferrell, B. R., & Steeves, R. (1995). Priority ethical issues in oncology nursing: Current approaches and future directions. *Oncology Nursing Forum, 22,* 803–807.

Faden, R. R., & Beauchamp, T. L. (1986). *A history and theory of informed consent.* Oxford Press, New York.

Federation of State Medical Boards of the United States. (1998). *House of Delegates, May 1998.* Retrieved December 15, 2008, from http://www.fsmb.org/grpol_pain_policy_resource_center.html.

Federation of State Medical Boards of the United States. (2005). Model policy for the use of controlled substances for the treatment of pain. *Journal of Pain & Palliative Care Pharmacotherapy, 19*(2), 73–78.

Ferrell, B.A., Casarett, D., Epplin, J., Fine, P., Gloth III, M., Herr, K., Katz, P., Keefe, F., Koo, J.S., O'Grady, M., Szwabo, P., Vallerand, & A.H., Weiner, D. (2002). The Management of Persistent Pain in Older Persons: AGS Panel on Persistent Pain in Older Persons. Journal of the American Geriatric Society, 50, S205-224.

Ferrell, B. R. (1994). Ethical and professional issues in pain technology: A challenge to supportive care. *Supportive Care in Cancer, 2,* 21–26.

Ferrell, B. R. (1997). The role of ethics committees in responding to the moral outrage of unrelieved pain. *Bioethics Forum, 13,* 11–16.

Ferrell, B. R. (2005). Ethical perspectives on pain and suffering. *Pain Management Nursing, 6*(3), 83–90.

Ferrell, B. R., & McCaffery, M. (1996). Current placebo practice and policy. *ASPMN Pathways, winter,* 12–14.

Ferrell, B. R., & Rhiner, M. (1991). High-tech comfort: Ethical issues in cancer pain management for the 1990s. *Journal of Clinical Ethics, 2,* 108–112.

Fine, R. L., & Mayo, T. W. (2003). Resolution of futility by due process: Early experience with the Texas advance directives. *Annals of Internal Medicine, 138,* 743–746.

Fishbain, D. A., Lewis, J. E., Cole, B., Rosomoff, R. S., & Rosomoff, H. L. (2007). Medicolegal rounds: Medicolegal issues and alleged breaches of standards of medical care in a patient motor vehicle accident allegedly related to chronic opioid analgesic therapy. *Journal of Opioid Management, 3*(1), 16–20.

Fishman, S. M. (2007). Recognizing pain management as a human right: A first step. *Anesthesia & Analgesia, 105*(1), 8–9.

Fishman, S. M. (2008). *Responsible opioid prescribing: A physician's guide.* Washington, DC: Waterford Life Sciences.

Fishman, S. M., Bandman, T. B., Edwards, A., & Borsook, D. (1999). The trilateral opioid contract bridging the pain clinic and the primary care physician through the opioid contract. *Journal of Pain and Symptom Management, 24*(3), 335–344.

Fishman, S. M., Papazian, J. S. Gonzalez, S., Riches, P. S., & Gilson, A. (2004). Regulating opioid prescribing through prescription monitoring programs: Balancing drug diversion and treatment of pain. *Pain Medicine, 5*(3), 309–324.

Fontana, J. S. (2008). The social and political forces affecting prescribing practices for chronic pain. *Journal of Professional Nursing, 24*(1), 30–35.

Fox, A. E. (1994). Confronting the use of placebos for pain. *American Journal of Nursing, 94,* 42–46.

Freedman, B., Glass, K. C., & Weijer, C. (1996). Placebo orthodoxy in clinical research: Placebo orthodoxy in clinical research. II. Ethical, legal, and regulatory myths. *Journal of Law, Medicine & Ethics, 24,* 252–259.

Gallagher, R. (2004). *Opioids in chronic pain management: Navigating the clinical and regulatory challenges.* Retrieved December 3, 2008, from http://findarticles.com/p/articles/mi_m0689/is_10_53/ai_n6249281/pg_5.

Geppert, C. M. A. (2004). To help and not to harm: Ethical issues in the treatment of chronic pain in patients with substance use disorders. *Advances in Psychosomatic Medicine.* 25, 151–171.

Giarelli, E. (2003). Safeguarding being: A bioethical principle for genetic nursing care. *Nursing Ethics, 10*(3), 255–268.

Gilson, A. M., & Joranson, D. E. (2006). *Continuing concerns about DEA's "prescription series" proposal.* Retrieved June 6, 2007, from http://www.painpolicy.wisc.edu/DEA/Rx_series.pdf.

Gilson, A. M., Joranson, D. E., & Maurer, M. A. (2007). Improving state pain policies: Recent progress and continuing opportunities. *CA: A Cancer Journal for Clinicians, 57*(6), 341–353.

Gilson, A. M., Joranson, D. E., Maurer, M. A., Ryan, K. M., & Garthwaite, J. P. (2005). Progress to achieve balanced state policy relevant to pain management and palliative care: 2000–2003. *Journal of Pain & Palliative Care Pharmacotherapy, 19*(1), 13–26.

Gilson, A. M., Maurer, M. A., & Joranson, D. E. (2005). State policy affecting pain management: Recent improvements and the positive impact of regulatory health policies. *Health Policy, 74*(2), 192–204.

Gilson, A. M., Maurer, M. A., & Joranson, D. E. (2007). State medical board members' beliefs about pain, addiction, and diversion and abuse: A changing regulatory environment. *Journal of Pain, 8*(9), 682–691.

Giordano, J. (2007). Techniques, technology and tekne: The ethical use of guidelines in the practice of interventional pain management. *Pain Physician, 10*(1), 1–5.

Gourlay, D. L., & Heit, H. A. (2005). Universal precautions in pain medicine: The treatment of chronic pain with or without the disease of addiction. *Medscape Neurology & Neurosurgery, 7*(1), and *Pain Medicine, 6*(2).

Gourlay, D. L., Caplan, Y. L., & Heit, H. A. (2006). *Urine drug testing in clinical practice: Dispelling the myths & designing strategies* (3rd ed.). Stamford, CT: California Academy of Family Physicians in cooperation with PharmaCom Group.

Greipp, M. E. (1992). Undermedication for pain: An ethical model. *Advances in Nursing Science, 15,* 44–53.

Griffin-Heslin, V. L. (2005). An analysis of the concept dignity. *Accident & Emergency Nursing, 13*(4), 251–257.

Gudin, J. (2007). Opioid agreement or patient-centric action plan? *American Journal of Medicine, 120*(9), 19.

Hallenbeck, J. L. (2000). Terminal sedation: Ethical implications in different situations. *Journal of Palliative Medicine, 3,* 313–320.

Hammett-Stabler, C. A., & Webster, L. R. (2008). A clinical guide to urine drug testing: Augmenting pain management and enhancing patient care. Piscataway, NJ: University of Medicine and Dentistry of New Jersey, Center for Continuing and Outreach Education.

Hanks, R. G. (2005). Sphere of nursing advocacy model. *Nursing Forum, 40*(3), 75–78.

Hansen, A. (2008). *Ethics SIG quality improvement and needs assessment survey results.* Oncology Nursing Society Ethics Special Interest Group Newsletter. Retrieved December 3, 2008, from http://onsopcontent.ons.org/Publications/SIGNewsletters/eth/eth19.1.html#story5.

Harrison, E., & Falco, S. M. (2005). Health disparity and the nurse advocate: Reaching out to alleviate suffering. *Advances in Nursing Science, 28*(3), 252–264.

Heggen, K., & Wellard, S. (2004). Increased unintended patient harm in nursing practice as a consequence of the dominance of economic discourses. *International Journal of Nursing Studies, 41*(3), 293–298.

Henkelman, W. L. (1994). Inadequate pain management: Ethical considerations. *Nursing Management, 21,* 48A–48D.

Hilliard, B. (2007). The politics of palliative care and the ethical boundaries of medicine: *Gonzales v. Oregon* as a cautionary tale. *Journal of Law, Medicine & Ethics, 35*(1), 158–174. Holley, U. A. (2007). Social isolation: A practical guide for nurses assisting clients with chronic illness. *Rehabilitation Nursing, 32*(2), 51–56.

Howland, J. (2005). Questions about palliative sedation: An act of mercy or mercy killing? *Ethics & Medics, 30*(8), 1–2.

Hyman, C. S. (1996). Pain management and disciplinary action: How medical boards can remove barriers to effective treatment. *Journal of Law, Medicine & Ethics, 24*(4), 338–343.

Ineck, J. R., & Rule, A. M. (2006). Opioid analgesics in the substance abuser: Pros and cons. *Journal of Pain & Palliative Care Pharmacotherapy, 20*(3), 39–41.

International Society of Nurses in Cancer Care. (1999). Cancer pain position statement. *International Cancer Nursing News, 11,* 4.

Jacobson, P. L., & Mann, J. D. (2004). The valid informed consent-treatment contract in chronic non-cancer pain: Its role in reducing barriers to effective pain management. *Comprehensive Therapy, 30*(2), 101–104.

Jacox, A., Carr, D. B., Payne, R., Berde, C. B., Breitbart, W., Cain, J. M., Chapman, C.R., Cleeland, C.S., Ferrell, B.T., Finley, R.S., Hester, N.O., Stratton Hill, C., Leak, W.D., Lipman, A.G., Logan, C.L., McGarvey, C.L., Miaskowski, C.A., Mulder, D.S., Paice, J.A., Shapiro, B.S., Silberstein, E.B., Smith, R.S., Stover, J., Tsou, C.V., Vecchiarelli, L., & Weissman, D.E. (1994). *Management of cancer pain.* Clinical Practice Guideline No. 9. (AHCPR Publication No. 94-0592.) Rockville, MD: U.S. Public Health Service.

Johnson, S. H. (2005). Legal issues in the use of controlled substances in pain management. *Medical Ethics, 12*(1), 4, 12.

Johnson, S. H., & Todd, K. (2007). Chronic pain and healthy communities: Legal, ethical, and policy issues in improving the public's health. Proceedings of the Public's Health and the Law in the 21st Century: Fifth Annual Partnership Conference. *Journal of Law, Medicine & Ethics, 35*(4), 69–71.

Johnstone, M. J., DaCosta, C., & Turale, S. (2002). *Registered nurses' experiences of ethical issues in nursing practice.* Final Report to the Nurse Board of Vieloria. Melbourne, Australia: Royal Melbourne Institute of Technology University.

Joint Commission. (2008). *Speak up campaign.* Retrieved December 3, 2008, from http://www.jointcommission.org/NR/rdonlyres/C581F557-BD6C-4139-8C5B-149214C0AE27/0/painmanagementbrochure.pdf.

Joint Commission. *Pain standards for 2001.* Retrieved May 17, 2009, from http://www.jointcommission.org/NewsRoom/health_care_issues.htm#9.

Jones, K. R., Fink, R. M., Clark, L., Hutt, E., Vojir, C.P., & Mellis, B. K. (2005). Nursing home resident barriers to effective pain management: Why nursing home residents may not seek pain medication. *Journal of the American Medical Directors Association, 6*(1), 10–17.

Joranson, D. E., & Portenoy, R. K. (2005). Pain medicine and drug law enforcement: An important step toward balance. *Journal of Pain & Palliative Care Pharmacotherapy, 19*(1), 3–5.

Jung, B., & Reidenberg, M. M. (2006). The risk of action by the Drug Enforcement Administration against physicians prescribing opioids for pain. *Pain Medicine, 7*(4), 353–357.

Kapp, M. B. (2006). The U.S. Supreme Court decision on assisted suicide and the prescription of pain medication: Limit the celebration. *Journal of Opioid Management, 2*(2), 73–74.

Kinoshita, S. (2007). Respecting the wishes of patients in intensive care units. *Nursing Ethics, 14*(5), 651–664.

Kubsch, S. M., Sternard, M. J., Hovarter, R., & Matzke, V. (2004). A holistic model of advocacy: Factors that influence its use. *Complementary Therapies in Nursing & Midwifery, 10*(1), 37–45.

Kuc, J. A. (1997). Liability issues related to epidural analgesia. *Journal of Legal Nurse Consulting, 8,* 2, 7–11.

Lafleur, J., Said, Q., McAdam-Marx, C., Jackson, K., & Mortazavi, M. (2007). Problems in studying the association between race and pain in outcomes research. *Journal of Pain & Palliative Care Pharmacotherapy, 21*(3), 57–62.

Lawrence, L. L. (2005). Legal issues in pain management: Striking the balance. *Emergency Medicine Clinics of North America, 23*(2), 573–584.

Lisson, E. L. (1987). Ethical issues related to pain control. *Nursing Clinics of North America, 22,* 649–659.

Loder, E., Goldstein, R., & Biondi, D. (2005). Placebo effects in oral triptan trials: The scientific and ethical rationale for continued use of placebo controls. *Cephalalgia, 25*(2), 124–131.

Lowe, N. K. (2004). Context and process of informed consent for pharmacologic strategies in labor pain care [see comment]. *Journal of Midwifery & Women's Health, 49*(3), 250–259.

MacDonald, H. (2007). Relational ethics and advocacy in nursing: Literature review. *Journal of Advanced Nursing, 57*(2), 119–126.

Manchikanti, L. (2007). National drug control policy and prescription drug abuse: Facts and fallacies. *Pain Physician, 10*(3), 399–424.

Martino, A. M. (1998). In search of a new ethic for treating patients with chronic pain: What can medical boards do? *Journal of Law, Medicine & Ethics, 26,* 332–349.

Maze, C. D., & Martino, A. M. (2005). Registered nurses' personal rights vs. professional responsibility in caring for members of underserved and disenfranchised populations. *Journal of Clinical Nursing, 14*(5), 546–554.

McCabe, H. (2007a). Nursing involvement in euthanasia: How sound is the philosophical support. *Nursing Philosophy, 8*(3), 167–175.

McCabe, H. (2007b). Nursing involvement in euthanasia: A "nursing-as-healing-praxis" approach. *Nursing Philosophy, 8*(3), 176–186.

McCaffery, M., & Arnstein, P. (2006). The debate over placebos in pain management: The ASPMN disagrees with a recent placebo position statement. *American Journal of Nursing, 106*(2), 62–65.

McCaffery, M., & Ferrell, B. R. (1997). Pain and placebos: Ethical and professional issues. *Orthopaedic Nursing, 16,* 5–11.

McCaffery, M., & Pasero, C. (1999). *Pain: clinical manual* (2nd ed., p. 492). St. Louis: Mosby.

McCaffery, M., Ferrell, B. R., & Turner, M. (1996). Ethical issues in the use of placebos in cancer pain management. *Oncology Nursing Forum, 23,* 1587–1593.

McGrath, P., Holewa, H., & McGrath, Z. (2006). Nursing advocacy in an Australian multidisciplinary context: Findings on medico-centrism. *Scandinavian Journal of Caring Sciences, 20*(4), 394–402.

McIntire, T. (2004). Grandma's pain: How elder abuse litigation led to a regulatory revolution in the duty to provide palliative care. *Tennessee Medicine, 97*(12), 549–551, 554.

Meisel, A., Snyder, D., & Quill, T. (2000). American College of Physicians–American Society of Internal Medicine End-of-Life Care Consensus Panel: Seven legal barriers to end-of-life care; myths, realities, and grains of truth. *Journal of the American Medical Association, 284,* 2495–2501.

Merskey, H., & Teasell, R. W. (2007). Problems with insurance-based research on chronic pain. *Medical Clinics of North America, 91*(1), 31–43.

Miller, J. (2007). The other side of trust in health care: Prescribing drugs with the potential for abuse. *Bioethics, 21*(1), 51–60.

Moeller, K. E., Lee, K. C., & Kissack, J. C. (2008). Urine drug screening: Practical guide for clinicians. *Mayo Clinic Proceedings, 83*(1), 66–76.

Morray, B. (1995). Pain medication for the patient following treatment withdrawal. *Dimensions in Critical Care Nursing, 14*(2), 92–98.

Morse, J. M. (1991). Negotiating commitment and involvement in the nurse–patient relationship. *Journal of Advanced Nursing, 16,* 455–468.

Murphy, N., & Roberts, D. (2008). Nurse leaders as stewards at the point of service. *Nursing Ethics, 15*(2), 243–253.

Murphy, N., Canales, M. K., Norton, S. A., & DeFilippis, J. (2005). Striving for congruence: The interconnection between values, practice, and political action. *Policy, Politics, & Nursing Practice, 6*(1), 20–29.

Nagasako, E. M., & Kalauokalani, D. A. (2005). Ethical aspects of placebo groups in pain trials: Lessons from psychiatry. *Neurology, 65*(12 Suppl. 4), S59–S65.

National Ethics Committee, Veterans Health Administration. (2006). The ethics of palliative sedation as a therapy of last resort. *American Journal of Hospice & Palliative Care, 23*(6), 483–491.

Nichols, K. J., Galluzzi, K. E., Bates, B., Husted, B. A., Leleszi, J. P., Simon, K., Lavery, D., & Cass, C. (2005). AOA's position against use of placebos for pain management in end-of-life care. *Journal of the American Osteopathic Association, 105*(3 Suppl. 1), S2–S5.

Niebroj, L. T., Jadamus-Niebroj, D., & Giordano, J. (2008). Toward a moral grounding of pain medicine: Consideration of neuroscience, reverence, beneficence, and autonomy. *Pain Physician, 11*(1), 7–12.

O'Malley, P. (2005). The undertreatment of pain: Ethical and legal implications for the clinical nurse specialist. *Clinical Nurse Specialist, 19*(5), 236–237.

Oncology Nursing Society. (1991). *Oncology Nursing Society position paper on cancer pain.* Pittsburgh: Oncology Nursing Society Press.

Passik, S. D., Byers, K., & Kirsh, K. L. (2007). Empathy and the failure to treat pain. *Palliative & Supportive Care, 5*(2), 167–172.

Passik, S. D., Heit, H., & Kirsh, K. L. (2006). Reality and responsibility: A commentary on the treatment of pain and suffering in a drug-using society. *Journal of Opioid Management, 2*(3), 123–127.

Poncy, M. (2006). *Ethics and futile care.* Program and abstracts of the National Conference of Gerontological Nurse Practitioners 25th Annual Meeting, September 27–October 1, Ponte Vedra Beach, Florida.

Popenhagen, M. P. (2006). Collaborative practice: Undertreatment of pain and fears of addiction in pediatric chronic pain patients–How do we stop the problem? *Journal for Specialists in Pediatric Nursing, 11*(1), 61–67.

Quill, T. E., & Meier, D. E. (2006). The big chill: Inserting the DEA into end-of-life care. *New England Journal of Medicine, 354*(1), 1–3.

Quinn, T. E. (2003). JCAHO pain standards: Impact on practice. *Pain Relief Connection, 2,* 3–4.

Rabbi Weiss, R. B. (2007). Pain management at the end of life and the principle of double effect: A Jewish perspective. *Cancer Investigation, 25*(4), 274–277.

Rannazzisi, J. T. (2007). The DEA's balancing act to ensure public health and safety. *Clinical Pharmacology & Therapeutics, 81*(6), 805–806.

Rannazzisi, J. T., & Caverly, M. W. (2006). Practitioners manual: An informational outline of the controlled substances act. Retrieved December 3, 2008, from http://www.deadiversion.usdoj.gov/pubs/manuals/pract/index.html.

Reddy, B. S. (2006). The epidemic of unrelieved chronic pain: The ethical, societal, and regulatory barriers facing opioid prescribing physicians. *Journal of Legal Medicine, 27*(4), 427–442.

Reidenberg, M. M., & Willis, O. (2007). Prosecution of physicians for prescribing opioids to patients. *Clinical Pharmacology & Therapeutics, 81*(6), 903–906.

Reynolds, S. (2006). Science at the mercy of the mob: Dr. Hurwitz's legal problems in perspective. *Journal of Opioid Management, 2*(6), 312–313.

Rhodin, A. (2006). The rise of opiophobia: Is history a barrier to prescribing? *Journal of Pain & Palliative Care Pharmacotherapy, 20*(3), 31–32.

Rich, B. A. (2004). Thinking the unthinkable: The clinician as perpetrator of elder abuse in patients in pain. *Journal of Pain & Palliative Care Pharmacotherapy, 18*(3), 63–74.

Rich, B. A. (2005). The politics of pain: Rhetoric or reform. *DePaul Journal of Health Care Law, 8*(3), 519–558.

Richards, J. S., Kezar, L. B., & Ness, T. J. (2007). Ethics in pain management of persons with spinal cord injury. *Topics in Spinal Cord Injury, 13*(3), 95-107.

Rushton, C. H. (2007). Respect in critical care: A foundational ethical principle. *American Association of Critical-Care Nursing Advanced Critical Care, 18*(2), 149–156.

Saad, L. (2008). *Nurses shine, bankers slump in ethics ratings: Gallup Poll.* Retrieved January 5, 2009, from http://www.gallup.com/poll/112264/Nurses-Shine-While-Bankers-Slump-Ethics-Ratings.aspx.

Schofferman, J. (2006). Interventional pain medicine: Financial success and ethical practice–An oxymoron. *Pain Medicine, 7*(5), 457–460.

Seal, M. (2007). Patient advocacy and advance care planning in the acute hospital setting. *Australian Journal of Advanced Nursing, 24*(4), 29–36.

Shapiro, R. S. (1994). Liability issues in the management of pain. *Journal of Pain and Symptom Management, 9,* 146–152.

Shaver, W. A., & Rousseau, P. C. (2005). *A challenge to the ethical validity of palliative sedation.* Abstract 318. Program and abstracts of the American Academy of Hospice and Palliative Medicine/Hospice and Palliative Nurses Association Annual Assembly, January 19–23, New Orleans, Louisiana.

Sorensen, R., & Iedema, R. (2007). Advocacy at end-of-life research design: An ethnographic study of an ICU. *International Journal of Nursing Studies, 44*(8), 1343–1353.

Spenceley, S. M., Reutter, L., & Allen, M. N. (2006). The road less traveled: Nursing advocacy at the policy level. *Policy, Politics, & Nursing Practice, 7*(3), 180–194.

Stevens, C. (1999). *The Professional Advocacy Initiative: Making it happen, Arizona Nurse.* Retrieved December 5, 2008, from http://findarticles.com/p/articles/mi_qa3928/is_199903/ai_n8828977.

Sullivan, M. J. L., & Ferrell, B. R. (2005). Ethical challenges in the management of chronic nonmalignant pain: Negotiating through the cloud of doubt. *Journal of Pain, 6*(1), 2–9.

Sullivan, M. J. L., & Main, C. (2007). Service, advocacy and adjudication: Balancing the ethical challenges of multiple stakeholder agendas in the rehabilitation of chronic pain. *Disability & Rehabilitation, 29*(20–21), 1596–1603.

Swope, E., Amero, L., Kujawski, T., Miller, K., & St. Marie, B. J. (2009). *American Society for Pain Management Nursing: Urine drug testing self-directed learning module.* Lenexa, Kansas: American Society for Pain Management Nurses.

Tahan, H. A. (2005). Essentials of advocacy in case management. *Lippincott's Case Management, 10*(3), 136–140.

Taylor, A. L. (2007). Addressing the global tragedy of needless pain: Rethinking the United Nations Single Convention on Narcotic Drugs. *Journal of Law, Medicine & Ethics, 35*(4), 556–570, 511.

Taylor, E. J., & Ersek, M. (1995). Ethical and spiritual dimensions of cancer pain management. In D. B. McGuire, C. H. Yarbro, & B. R. Ferrell (Eds.), *Cancer pain management* (2nd ed., pp. 41–60). Boston: Jones & Bartlett.

Taylor, E. J., Ferrell, B. R., Grant, M., & Cheyney, L. (1993). Managing cancer pain at home: The decisions and ethical conflicts of patients, family caregivers, and homecare nurses. *Oncology Nursing Forum, 20,* 919–927.

Thacker, K. S. (2008). Nurses' advocacy behaviors in end-of-life nursing care. *Nursing Ethics, 15*(2), 174–185.

Thompson, M. H. (1996). Ethics committees: Their share in the advocacy role. *Seminars in Perioperative Nursing, 5,* 62–67.

Todd, K. H. (2005). Chronic pain and aberrant drug-related behavior in the emergency department. *Journal of Law, Medicine & Ethics, 33*(4), 761–769.

Trehan, A. B. (2007). Fear of prescribing: How the DEA is infringing on patients' right to palliative care. *University of Miami Law Review, 61,* 961–995.

Truog, R. D. (2007). Tackling medical futility in Texas. *New England Journal of Medicine, 357*(1), 1–3.

Tucker, K. L. (2004). The debate on elder abuse for undertreated pain. *Pain Medicine, 5*(2), 214–228.

Tufts Health Care Institute. (2005). *Opioid risk management: THCI conference presentations.* Retrieved December 5, 2008, from http://www.thci.org/opioid/.

Turner, J. A., Deyo, R. A., Loeser, J. D., Von Korff, M., & Fordyce, W. E. (1994). The importance of placebo effects in pain treatment and research. *Journal of the American Medical Association, 271,* 1609–1614.

Vaartio, H., & Leino-Kilpi, H. (2005). Nursing advocacy: A review of the empirical research 1990–2003. *International Journal of Nursing Studies, 42*(6), 705–714.

Vaglienti, C. S., & Grinberg, M. (2004). Emerging liability for the undertreatment of pain. *Journal of Nursing Law, 9*(3), 7–17.

Wall, P. D. (1992). The placebo effect: An unpopular topic. *Pain, 51,* 1–3.

Washington v. Glucksberg. (1997). No. 117 Supreme Court 2258. Retrieved December 5, 2008, from http://www.oyez.org/cases/1990-1999/1996/1996_96_110/.

Washington Post. (2007). Case puts Texas futile-treatment law under a microscope. Retrieved December 15, 2008, from http://www.washingtonpost.com/wp-dyn/content/article/2007/04/10/AR2007041001620_pf.html.

Werner, A., Isaksen, L. W., & Malterud, K. (2004). "I am not the kind of woman who complains of everything": Illness stories on self and shame in women with chronic pain. *Social Science & Medicine, 59*(5), 1035–1045.

Whedon, M., & Ferrell, B. R. (1991). Professional and ethical considerations in the use of high-tech pain management. *Oncology Nursing Forum, 18,* 1135–1143.

Zwakhalen, S. M., Hamers, J. P., Peijnenburg, R. H., & Berger, M. P. (2007). Nursing staff knowledge and beliefs about pain in elderly nursing home residents with dementia. *Pain Research & Management, 12*(3), 177–184.

Suggested Readings

Disparity Impact

Cintron, A., & Morrison, R. S. (2006). Pain and ethnicity in the United States: A systematic review. *Journal of Palliative Medicine, 9*(6), 1454–1473.

Ezenwa, M. O., Ameringer, S., Ward, S. E., & Serlin, R. C. (2006). Racial and ethnic disparities in pain management in the United States [see comment]. *Journal of Nursing Scholarship, 38*(3), 225–233.

Gaskin, D. J., & Frick, K. D. (2008). Race and ethnic disparities in valuing health. *Medical Decision Making, 28*(1), 12–20.

Green, C. R., Anderson, K. O., Baker, T. A., Campbell, L. C., Decker, S., Fillingim, R. B., Kalauokalani, D. A., Lasch, K. E., Myers, C., Tait, R. C., Todd, K. H., & Vallerand, A. H. (2003). The unequal burden of pain: Confronting racial and ethnic disparities in pain. *Pain Medicine, 4*(3), 277–294.

Green, C. R., Ndao-Brumblay, S. K., West, B., & Washington, T. (2005). Differences in prescription opioid analgesic availability: Comparing minority and White pharmacies across Michigan. *Journal of Pain, 6,* 689–699.

Green, C. R., Tait, R. C., & Gallagher, R. M. (2005). The unequal burden of pain: Disparities and differences. *Pain Medicine, 6*(1–2), 689–699.

Green, C. R., Todd, K. H., Lebovits, A., & Francis, M. (2006). Disparities in pain: Ethical issues. *Pain Medicine, 7*(6), 530–533.

Heins, A., Grammas, M., Heins, J. K., Costello, M. W., Huang, K., & Mishra, S. (2006). Determinants of variation in analgesic and opioid prescribing practice in an emergency department. *Journal of Opioid Management, 2*(6), 335–340.

Heins, J. K., Heins, A., Grammas, M., Costello, M., Huang, K., & Mishra, S. (2006). Disparities in analgesia and opioid prescribing practices for patients with musculoskeletal pain in the emergency department. *Journal of Emergency Nursing, 32*(3), 219–224.

Malloy, D. C., & Hadjistavropoulos, T. (2004). The problem of pain management among persons with dementia, personhood, and the ontology of relationships. *Nursing Philosophy, 5*(2), 147–159.

McNeill, J. A., Reynolds, J., & Ney, M. L. (2007). Unequal quality of cancer pain management: Disparity in perceived control and proposed solutions. *Oncology Nursing Forum Online, 34*(6), 1121–1128.

Paulson, M., III, & Dekker, A. H. (2005). Healthcare disparities in pain management. *Journal of the American Osteopathic Association, 105*(6 Suppl. 3), S14–S17.

Paulson, M. R., Dekker, A. H., & Aguilar-Gaxiola, S. (2007). Eliminating disparities in pain management. *Journal of the American Osteopathic Association, 107*(9 Suppl. 5), ES17–ES20.

United Nations. (1961). *Single Convention on Narcotic Drugs.* Retrieved December 13, 2008, from http://www.incb.org/incb/convention_1961.html.

Vaartio, H., Leino-Kilpi, H., Salanterä, S., & Suominen, T. (2006). Nursing advocacy: How is it defined by patients and nurses, what does it involve and how is it experienced? *Scandinavian Journal of Caring Sciences,* 20(3), 282–292.

Genetic Discrimination Act

Genetic Discrimination Act. (2008). Public Law No. 110-233. Retrieved May 17, 2009, from http://www.govtrack.us/congress/bill.xpd?bill=h110-493&tab=summary.

Ethical Dimensions: Influence on Practice

Carr, E. (1997). Myths and fears about pain relieving drugs. *Nursing Time, 93,* 50–51.

Chaloner, C. (2007). Ethics in nursing: The way forward. *Nursing Standard, 21*(38), 40–41.

Ersek, M. (1999). Enhancing effective pain management by addressing patient barriers to analgesic use. *Journal of Hospice and Palliative Nursing, 1,* 87–96.

Federation of State Medical Boards of the United States. (2007). Retrieved December 12, 2008, from http://www.fsmb.org/Pain/default.html

Hofland, S. L. (1992). Elder beliefs: Blocks to pain management. *Journal of Gerontological Nursing, 18,* 19–24.

Murphy, T. F. (2008). The ethics of responding to pain and suffering. *Cancer Treatment & Research, 140,* 117–135.

Oncology Nursing Society. (1999). *Cancer pain management.* Retrieved May 17, 2009, from http://www.ons.org/publications/positions/CancerPainManagement.shtml.

U.S. Department of Health and Human Services. (1996). *The summary of HIPPA privacy rule.* Retrieved December 16, 2008, from http://www.hhs.gov/ocr/privacysummary.pdf.

Placebo Use

Sullivan, M., Paice, J. A., & Benedetti, F. (2004). Placebos and treatment of pain. *Pain Medicine, 5*(3), 325–328.

Sullivan, M., Terman, G.W., Peck, B., Correll, D.J., Rich, B., Crawford Clark, W., Latta, K., Lebovits, A., & Gebhart, G. (2005). APS position statement on the use of placebos in pain management.

Journal of Pain, 6(4), 215–217.

Clinical Research: Ethical Challenges

Behi, R., & Nolan, M. (1995). Ethical issues in research. *British Journal of Nursing, 4,* 712–717.

Cahana, A. (2005). Ethical and epistemological problems when applying evidence-based medicine to pain management. *Pain Practice, 5*(4), 298–302.

International Association for the Study of Pain. (1982). *Ethical guidelines for pain research in humans.* Retrieved May 17, 2009, from http://www.iasp-pain.org/AM/Template.cfm?Section=Ethics1&Template=/CM/HTMLDisplay.cfm&ContentID=1953#humans.

Levine, R. J. (1986). *Ethics and regulation of clinical research* (2nd ed.). Baltimore, MD: Urban & Schwarzenberg.

Oberle, K., & Allen, M. (2006). Ethical considerations for nurses in clinical trials. *Nursing Ethics, 13*(2), 180–186.

Weymuller, E. A. (1996). A consideration of ethical issues in the design of clinical trials. *American Journal of Otolaryngology, 17,* 2–11.

Wilkes, L., Cert, R., & Beale, B. (2005). Role conflict: Appropriateness of a nurse researcher's actions in the clinical field. *Nurse Researcher, 12*(4), 57–70.

Informed Consent (Clinical Trials)

Berry, D. L., Dodd, M. J., Hinds, P. S., & Ferrell, B. R. (1996). Informed consent: Process and clinical issues. *Oncology Nursing Forum, 23,* 507–512.

Cantini, F., & Ells, C. (2007). The role of the clinical trial nurse in the informed consent process. *Canadian Journal of Nursing Research, 39*(2), 126–144.

Goodwin, J. A. (2004). Patient advocacy: Witnessing informed consent for research in acute care. *MEDSURG Nursing, 13*(4), 227–231.

End-of-Life Challenges

American Nurses Association. (2003). *Position statement: Pain management and control of distressing symptoms in dying patient.* Retrieved May 17, 2009, from http://www.nursingworld.org/MainMenuCategories/HealthcareandPolicyIssues/ANAPositionStatements/EthicsandHumanRights.aspx.

Oncology Nursing Society & Association of Oncology. (2003). *Social work: Joint position on end-of-life care.* Retrieved May 17, 2009, from http://www.ons.org/publications/positions/EndOflifeCare.shtml.

Assisted Suicide, Euthanasia, Double Effect

Oregon Death with Dignity Act. (1997). Retrieved May 17, 2009, from http://www.oregon.gov/DHS/ph/pas/faqs.shtml#whocan.

Singer, P. (1993). *Practical ethics* (pp. 108–109, 232–234). Cambridge University Press.

Medical Futility

Bernat, J. L. (2005). Medical futility: Definition, determination, and disputes in critical care. *Neurocrit Care, 2,* 198–205.

Texas Advance Directive Act. (1999). Retrieved May 17, 2009, from http://tlo2.tlc.state.tx.us/statutes/docs/HS/content/htm/hs.002.00.000166.00.htm.

Nursing Practice Issues

American Academy of Pain Management. (1996). *Statement of support: Prescribing issue on opioid agreements & contracts.* Retrieved May 17, 2009, from http://www.aapainmanage.org/literature/Articles/OpioidAgreements.pdf.

section

3

Clinical Practice of Pain Management Nursing

chapter

13

Pain Assessment

Yvonne D'Arcy, MS, CRNP, CNS

Objectives

After studying this chapter, the reader should be able to:

1. Identify the key elements of pain assessment for all patients.
2. Identify tools for assessing pain for acute, chronic, cancer, and pediatric patients and for patients unable to self-report pain.
3. Understand the multidimensional features of pain assessment.
4. Identify patients in special populations who need different types of pain assessment tools.

Pain assessment is the foundation of good pain management and sets the stage for care planning, implementation, and evaluation. Self-report of pain intensity is the most dependable method of pain assessment (American Pain Society, 2003). The patient's report of pain is subjective and includes both the sensory component and the psychological, cultural, and emotional elements of the experience (Ackley, Ladwig, Swan, & Tucker, 2008; D'Arcy, 2007). The Joint Commission (2000) states that each patient has the right to have pain assessed and reassessed at regular intervals. Ongoing assessment and documentation provide direction for a pain management plan of care; adjustments are based on the patient's response (Ackley et al., 2008; Berry, Covington, Dahl, Katz, & Miaskowski, 2006).

I. Components of Pain Assessment (Ackley et al., 2008; D'Arcy, 2007; St. Marie, 2002)

A. Location
1. Ask the patient to identify the location of the pain.
2. Ask the patient to point to the location of the pain if possible.
3. Use pictures so that the patient can point to the location of the pain.
4. Use body diagrams on which the patient can draw the location of the pain.
5. Ask the patient if the pain radiates, and have the patient point to the body location of the radiation.

B. Description
1. Have the patient describe the pain in his or her own words.
2. Supply the patient with a group of verbal pain descriptors such as those on the McGill Pain Questionnaire, or use the Verbal Descriptor Scale for a patient who is unable to describe the pain.
3. Assess the patient for the presence of a neuropathic pain component by identifying and documenting descriptors such as burning, shooting, shocklike, painful numbness, and tingling.

C. Intensity
1. For basic pain assessment in patients who can self-report pain, use a Numeric Pain Intensity Scale.
2. Use tools to rate pain intensity that are reliable and valid for the population being assessed.
3. Use the same assessment tool to assess pain over the continuum: current pain level, best pain level, and worst pain level.

D. Duration
1. Ask the patient when the pain first started.
2. Determine how long it lasts.
3. Identify when the pain is worse.
4. Identify when the pain is better.

E. Alleviating and relieving factors
1. Ask the patient what makes the pain better.
2. Ask the patient what makes the pain worse.
3. Determine what medications or treatments have helped to make the pain better.
4. Ask the patient what home remedies, over-the-counter medications, complementary methods, or use of other substances such as alcohol have been tried to treat the pain.

F. Associative factors
1. Ask if the patient has been nauseated or has vomited because of the pain.
2. Is the patient constipated?
3. Is the patient sedated, delirious, confused, or depressed?
4. Is the patient having difficulty sleeping?

G. Pain goal
1. Have the patient set a numerical pain goal that he or she thinks is reasonable to achieve.
2. Develop a plan of care that uses the pain goal as an outcome.

H. Functional goal
1. Function may be a better measure of pain relief for chronic pain patients.
2. Pain is dynamic and will increase with activity (Dahl & Kehlet, 2006).
3. Ask the patient how the pain interferes with daily living, self-care, walking, etc.
4. Ask the patient to keep a pain diary that records changes or improvements in ability to function.

II. Pertinent Medical History

A. Past pain experiences
B. Current or past chemical use, illicit or prescription substance abuse, or history of substance abuse disorder
C. Medical history
D. Surgical history
E. Psychiatric history
F. Medication history
G. Laboratory findings
H. Imaging results, such as computerized axial tomography (CT) scans or magnetic resonance imaging scans (MRIs)
I. Other pertinent workup, such as EMG

III. Barriers to Assessment (D'Arcy, 2008)

A. Language
B. Culture
C. Physical condition
D. Psychological condition
E. Behavioral issues
F. Developmental level
G. Cognitive ability
H. Level of consciousness
I. Verbal or nonverbal
J. Nursing bias
K. Nursing knowledge deficits about assessment

IV. Acute Pain Assessment Tools

A. The goal of acute pain management is to alleviate pain or reduce pain to a level that is acceptable to the patient (Dochterman & Bulechek, 2004).
B. Assessing acute pain requires the use of pain assessment tools that are quick and easy to use and can provide usable data for pain assessment and reassessment.
   1. Qualities needed for acute assessment tools
      a. The tools are simple and easy to use.
      b. They allow for quick assessment and reassessment.
      c. They provide for easy documentation.
      d. They are understandable for patients of different cultures or languages.
      e. These tools are most commonly used for acute pain, procedural pain assessment (Ackely et al., 2008), perianesthesia pain assessment (Krenzischek & Wilson, 2003), and postoperative pain assessment.
C. Unidimensional assessment tools
   1. A systematic review of 164 articles on pain assessment found that single-item ratings of pain intensity are reliable and valid measures of pain intensity (Jensen, 2003).
      a. These tools measure one element of the pain experience: intensity.
      b. They are designed for a quick and easy assessment that can also determine how effective pain medications and interventions have been.
   2. A decrease of two points on the pain intensity rating has been found to be clinically significant (Farrar, Young, Lamoreaux, Werth, & Poole, 2001).
   3. The *Visual Analog Scale (VAS)* is one of the simplest scales to use. It consists of a 100-mm line that the patient marks to indicate pain intensity. The line is measured from the beginning to the mark, and the pain intensity is determined. A mark at the 30-mm line would translate into a 3 out of 10 for pain intensity, or 3/10: mild pain. This tool was originally designed for use in research studies. Administration is visual.

a. Advantages
   (1) Response is quick.
   (2) The scale is simple to use.
   (3) It is easy to score.
   (4) It is easy to compare results with previous ratings.
   (5) The scale is easy to translate.
   (6) It is considered one of the best tools for assessing variations in pain intensity and a reliable tool for research (Carlsson, 1983).
   (7) The scale has a high degree of sensitivity.
b. Disadvantages
   (1) Some older adult patients have difficulty marking on the line and place the mark above or below the 100-mm line (D'Arcy, 2003; Herr & Mobily, 1993).
   (2) It is difficult to use with very young or very old patients with impairment.
   (3) Reproducibility is poor with patents with cognitive dysfunction, postoperative patients, or patients with dementia.
   (4) The 100-mm line is often variable.
   (5) The results do not qualify as interval-level scores for purposes of statistical procedures (Carlsson, 1983).
c. Clinical application
   (1) The VAS is validated for use with
      (a) Patients with chronic pain.
      (b) Patients with rheumatic disease.
      (c) Children older than 5 years of age.
   (2) Using the absolute VAS, the patient is asked the present level of pain intensity.
   (3) For estimates in change of pain intensity, the comparative VAS can be used.

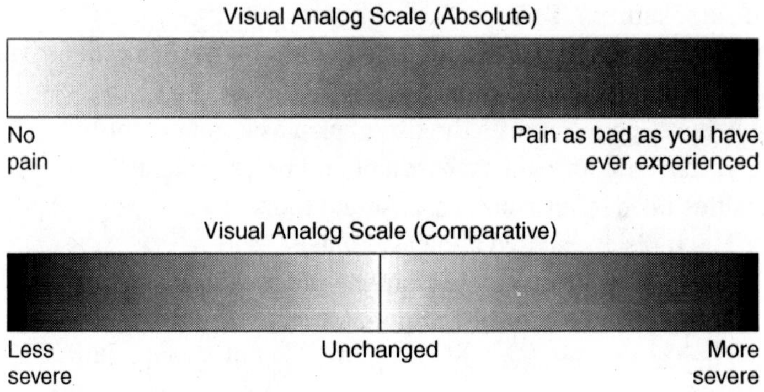

Visual Analog Scale (Absolute)

No pain — Pain as bad as you have ever experienced

Visual Analog Scale (Comparative)

Less severe — Unchanged — More severe

4. The *Verbal Descriptor Scale (VDS)* uses verbal descriptors to describe pain.
   a. This scale uses six phrases: ***no pain, mild pain, moderate pain, severe pain, very severe pain,*** and ***worst pain possible.*** The patient is instructed to pick a word that represents the closest level of pain intensity (D'Arcy, 2007). Administration is verbal or visual.
   b. Advantages
      (1) Some patients prefer to use words rather than numbers to describe their pain.
      (2) Response is quick.
      (3) The scale is simple.
      (4) It is easy to score.
      (5) Although normally used for cognitively intact patients, Feldt, Ryden, and Miles (1998) found a 73% completion rate with the VDS in cognitively impaired patients.
   c. Disadvantages
      (1) The patient must be able to understand the meaning of the words.
      (2) The VDS is difficult for very young and very old patients.
      (3) The English form with translations alters the reliability of scale.

(4) It is less sensitive for changes in pain.
(5) The VDS measures an ordinal scale, making statistical use meaningless.

d. Clinical application
   (1) The VDS has been validated for use with
      (a) Patients with chronic pain.
      (b) Patients with acute pain.

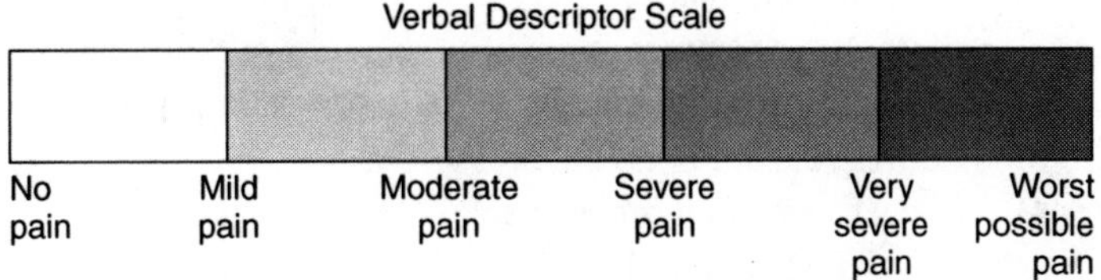

5. A *Numeric Pain Intensity (NPI) Scale* can be used for patients who can self-report pain.
   a. Advantages
      (1) Response is quick.
      (2) The scale is simple to use.
      (3) It is easy to score.
      (4) It is easy to make comparative pain ratings
      (5) The NPI can provide a method for consistency of pain assessments.
      (6) It can be translated into other languages.
      (7) It detects treatment effects.
   b. Disadvantages
      (1) The NPI cannot be used with nonverbal patients or cognitively impaired patients.
      (2) Older patients may have difficulty finding a number for pain.
      (3) Reliability decreases with visual or auditory impairment.
      (4) Patients in severe pain may have difficulty using a numerical rating.
   c. Clinical application
      (1) This tool has been validated for use with
         (a) Patients with chronic pain.
         (b) Patients with rheumatic disease.
         (c) Patients with postoperative pain.
         (d) Patients with cancer pain.
         (e) Trauma patients.

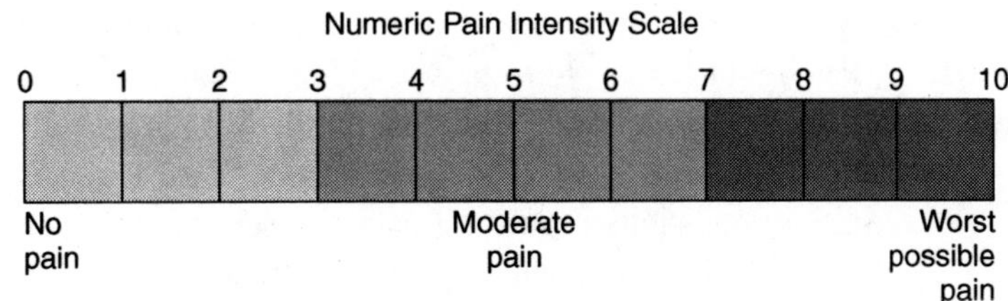

V. Tools for chronic, persistent pain assessment

A. Persistent pain assessment requires the use of tools that assess more than just the intensity of pain.

B. The degree of functionality for patients with chronic pain may provide more of an indication of pain relief than a numerical rating (Ackely et al., 2008; D'Arcy, 2007; Pasero & McCaffery, 2004).

C. Tools to assess patients with persistent pain are used in primary care, in chronic pain programs, and for hospitalized patients who have persistent pain.

D. *Multidimensional pain scales* are used to measure more than one component of the pain experience. They measure not only the intensity but also the nature and location of the pain and may include a section that assesses for mood, medication efficacy, and impact of pain on activity and sleep (Marin, Cyhan, & Miklos, 2006; Tang & Crane, 2006). Such scales are most commonly used for patients with persistent pain. They can be used as a self-report or in a research setting as an interview.

1. The *McGill Pain Questionnaire* is used to measure experimentally induced pain, postprocedural pain, and pain resulting from numerous medical and surgical conditions.
   a. Description
      (1) The questionnaire has multiple questions regarding pain.
      (2) It is available in two forms.
         (a) The short form measures sensory and affective dimensions of pain, along with pain intensity.
         (b) The long form measures location of pain, pattern of pain over time, sensory and affective dimensions of pain, and pain intensity.
      (3) Administration is verbal and visual.
      (4) It has three chief measures:
         (a) Pain rating index
         (b) Number of words chosen from a standard list of descriptive terms
         (c) Present pain intensity
   b. Advantages
      (1) Many research studies support its reliability and validity (Chok, 1998; Graham, Bond, Gerkovich, & Cook, 1980; McDonald & Weiskopf, 2001; MacIntye, Hopkins, & Harris, 1995; Melzack, 1975, 1987; Mystakidou et al., 2002; Wilkie, Savedra, Holzemer, Tesler, & Paul, 1990).
      (2) The short form takes 2 to 3 minutes and provides basically the same information as the long form.
      (3) The questionnaire measures sensory, affective, and evaluative experiences of pain.
      (4) It can discriminate among changes in the pain experience.
   c. Disadvantages
      (1) The long form takes 30 minutes to complete.
      (2) Scoring and weighting the descriptors are difficult.
      (3) Difficulty arises in translating the verbal descriptor section into words that indicate syndromes (Gracely & Dubner, 1987; Graham et al., 1980).
      (4) It does not include impaired or remaining function, pain complaints, or interventions that have been tried.
   d. Clinical application
      (1) The questionnaire is validated in many patient populations.
      (2) It has been translated into numerous languages.
      (3) It has been validated for children older than 12 years of age.
2. The *Brief Pain Inventory* (BPI) was originally developed to assess pain in patients with cancer but has reliability and validity in patients with chronic nonmalignant pain (Daut, Cleeland, & Flannery, 1983; Raiche, Osborne, Jensen, & Cardenas, 2006; Tan, Jensen, Thornby, & Shanti, 2004; Tittle, McMillan, & Hagan, 2003; Williams, Smith, & Fehnel, 2006).
   a. Description
      (1) Multiple questions regarding pain provide information on pain, how it interferes with patient function, and whether pain medications are effective.
      (2) Administration is both verbal and visual.
      (3) The inventory can be used as self-report or interview.
   b. Advantages
      (1) It includes a body diagram.
      (2) It addresses the multidimensionality of pain.
      (3) The inventory assesses location, intensity, and pattern.
      (4) Many studies support its reliability and validity when translated into other languages (Ger, Ho, Sun, Wang, & Cleeland, 1999; Klepstad et al., 2002; Mystakidou et al., 2001; Radbruch et al., 1999).
   c. Disadvantages
      (1) The inventory requires cognitive skills to complete (Cleeland & Ryan, 1994).
      (2) The patient must be able to correlate pain experience through various scales.

d. Clinical application
   (1) The inventory is validated in
      (a) Patients with cancer pain.
      (b) Patients with arthritis pain.
   (2) It has been translated into various languages.

3. The *West Haven-Yale Multidimensional Pain Inventory* has three parts.
   a. Description (Kerns, Turk, & Rudy, 1985)
      (1) The inventory uses 12 scales.
      (2) It examines the impact and meaning of pain on the patient's life.
      (3) It evaluates the physical, emotional, cognitive, and behavioral responses that occur with pain.
      (4) The inventory evaluates pain location, intensity, and quality, as well as the chronology of the pain experience and treatment.
      (5) It examines the extent to which the patient participates in common daily activities.
   b. Advantages
      (1) The inventory is brief.
      (2) It has clarity of design.
      (3) It uses contemporary psychological theory.
      (4) There is a multidimensional focus.
      (5) The inventory has strong psychometric properties.
      (6) The inventory's hallmark is its ability to measure the patient's perspective of self-control and problem-solving abilities.
   c. Disadvantages
      (1) At 52 items, the inventory is long.
      (2) The generalizability of results of this tool has yet to be determined.
   d. Clinical application
      (1) The inventory can be applied to chronic pain patients in clinical settings.

4. The *Pain Outcomes Questionnaire* was developed by the U.S. Department of Veterans Affairs to assess pain in chronic pain patients (Clark, Gironda, & Young, 2003).
   a. Advantages
      (1) The questionnaire was developed over 5 years at multiple sites.
      (2) It uses self-report.
      (3) It is a comprehensive tool.
      (4) The questionnaire is efficient.
   b. Disadvantages
      (1) It has not been replicated.
   c. Clinical application
      (1) The questionnaire is reliable and valid when used to evaluate the effectiveness of treatment for veterans experiencing chronic noncancer pain.

5. Other multidimensional pain assessment tools for chronic pain include the following:
   a. Dartmouth Pain Questionnaire
   b. Minnesota Multiphasic Personality Inventory (MMPI)
   c. State-Trait Anxiety Inventory
   d. UAB Pain Behavior Scale

6. Another way to assess pain quickly in patients with chronic pain is to use a set of structured questions for interview such as those in the *Brief Pain Impact Questionnaire* (*BPIQ*).
   a. Advantages
      (1) The BPIQ is quick and easy.
      (2) It covers the main elements of pain assessment.
      (3) It highlights the impact of pain on the individual.
      (4) The BPIQ addresses the use of alcohol.
   b. Disadvantages
      (1) It cannot be scored objectively.

(2) It cannot be used for comparison.
(3) The BPIQ needs more reliability and validity testing.

c. Clinical application
(1) The BPIQ is applicable to patients with chronic pain conditions.

VI. Assessing Pain Using an Interview

A. Using one of the multidimensional tools or the BPIQ as an interview can provide additional information and provide a venue for answering patient questions.

B. Setting the stage for the interview
1. Review the chart.
2. Establish the environment, for example, courtesy, interest, and desire to help.

C. Approach to the present pain situation
1. Greet the patient, for example, Mr., Mrs., or Ms., unless talking with an adolescent or child.
2. Be alert to the individual's comfort, for example, improve the patient's position and attempt to create comfort, realizing your purpose does not end there.
3. Ask an opening question: "Can you tell me about your headaches?"
4. Follow the patient's lead; people in pain may or may not have complicated psychosocial behavior.
   a. *Facilitation:* Use action, posture, eye contact, and words to encourage the patient to say more.
   b. *Reflection:* Repetition of the patient's words encourages the patient to give more detail.
   c. *Clarification:* If the patient's words or demeanor is ambivalent, ask "Can you tell me what you mean?"
   d. *Empathic responses:* Respond to the patient in a manner that shows understanding and acceptance. This allows the patient to feel more secure.

Brief Pain Impact Questionnaire

- *How strong is your pain, right now? Is it worse or average over the past week?*
- *How many days over the past week have you been unable to do what you would like to do because of your pain?*
- *Over the past week, how often has pain interfered with your ability to take care of yourself, for example, bathing, eating, dressing and going to the toilet?*
- *Over the past week, how often has pain interfered with your ability to take care of your home-related chores, such as grocery shopping, preparing meals, paying bills, and driving?*
- *How often do you participate in pleasurable activities such as hobbies, socializing with friends, and travel? Over the past week, how often has pain interfered with these activities?*
- *How often do you do some type of exercise? Over the past week, how often has pain interfered with your ability to exercise?*
- *Does pain interfere with your ability to think clearly?*
- *Does pain interfere with your appetite? Have you lost weight?*
- *Does pain interfere with your sleep? How often over the last week?*
- *Has pain interfered with your energy, mood, personality, or relationships with other people?*
- *Over the past week, have you taken pain medications?*
- *Has your use of alcohol or other drugs ever caused a problem for you or those close to you?*
- *How would you rate your health at the present time?*

From Weiner, D. K., Herr, K., & Rudy, T. (2002). *Persistent pain in older adults: An interdisciplinary guide for treatment.* New York: Springer. Reprinted by permission of the authors.

e. *Confrontation:* When observing clues of anger, anxiety, and depression, confronting these behaviors may help bring certain feelings forward for discussion.
f. *Interpretation:* You may infer something in the conversation. This inference (if correct) can show empathy and increase understanding.

D. General demeanor
1. Patients observe nonverbal behaviors as they are being interviewed.
2. Appear calm and unhurried, even with limited time.
3. Avoid condescending behaviors, stereotyping, or making sport of the patient.

E. Obtaining more data
1. Encourage a chronological account by asking "What then?" or "What happened next?"
2. Use direct questions: "How would you describe your pain?" "Where do you feel it? Show me." "Does the pain travel?"
3. Make sure direct questions do not lead the answer.
4. Use language that is appropriate and understandable to the patient.

F. Sensitive topics
1. Mentor with a skilled practitioner
2. Alcohol and drugs
   a. Ask "How much alcohol do you drink?" rather than "Do you drink alcohol?"
   b. Use CAGE questions (Barker & Whitfield, 1991).
      (1) "Have family members or friends ever *criticized* your drinking?"
      (2) "Has their criticism annoyed you?"
      (3) "Have you ever felt guilty about your drinking?"
      (4) "Have you ever had a drink in the morning as an eye opener?"
3. Physical violence
   a. Observe for domination of an interview by the person accompanying the patient or if that person refuses to leave the room or appears unusually anxious or concerned.
   b. Observe for bruises, especially on the breast or abdomen.
   c. If the patient seems embarrassed by talking about it, an opening question may be, "Many women tell me that someone at home is abusing or hurting them. How is it for you?"
4. Sexual history
   a. This is best discussed late in the interview.
   b. The patient may not be comfortable discussing sexual history on the first encounter.
   c. Begin by saying, "I'd like to ask you questions about your sexual health. May I go ahead?"
   d. If the answer is yes, proceed.
   e. Do not make assumptions about sexual preference, marital status, or attitudes toward pregnancy or contraception.

G. Closing
1. Ask "Is there anything else we should talk about?" or "Have we omitted anything?"
2. Clarify for the patient what to do next or what to expect.
3. Write down instructions.

H. Talking with parents
1. Conduct interviews of children with the parents or caregiver present.
2. Observe parent and child interaction.
3. Sensitive topics may need to be discussed with the parents only.
4. Questions directed to the parents are similar to those given previously; however, be aware that their answers reflect their assumptions, perceptions, biases, and needs.
5. Refer to the infant or child by name.
6. Use open-ended questions rather than direct questions.

I. Talking with children (see the chapter on Pediatric Pain Management)
1. Children 5 years or older may be interviewed with or without the parent present.
2. Children 5 years or older are able to portray their history and describe more accurately the severity of their pain than are their parents.

3. Start with open-ended questions.
    a. "Your mother says you have a stomachache; what can you tell me about it?"
    b. "Does it worry you?"
    c. "What helps make your stomachache go away?"
    d. "What do you think causes it?"
    e. "Can you show me where it hurts?"
    f. "Is it like a pinprick, or does it ache?"

J. Talking with adolescents
1. Adolescents may appear laconic or disdainful.
2. The conversation may be sustained if genuine interest is shown by the interviewer.
3. Focus the conversation on the adolescent rather than the problem, such as informal questions about friends, school, hobbies, and family.
4. Confidential conversation is appropriate at this age, based not on keeping secrets but rather on mutual respect.
5. The adolescent needs to be involved in the process if sensitive topics are discussed and are to be discussed with the parents.
6. Communication skills
    a. Reflection is avoided with cognitively immature adolescents because it is confusing.
    b. Silence rarely is successful.
    c. Confrontation may cause anxiety and avoidance in adolescents.
    d. Adolescents may find discussing feelings with adults difficult.
7. The environment should be friendly and informal.

K. Talking with aging patients
1. Hearing and vision may be impaired, and response may be slower.
2. Give older patients extra time to respond to questions.
3. Determine priorities and goals.
4. Learn how crises in the past have been handled, if appropriate.
5. Learn how older patients function in their daily lives.
6. Home safety is important and may need evaluation.
7. Include the family in the evaluation.

VII. Pediatric Pain Assessment Tools

A. The *FACES Scale* consists of six faces that range from smiling to tearful. It can be used for younger children and cognitively impaired older adults (Ackley et al., 2008; Wong & DiVito-Thomas, 2006). To use the scale, the patient is asked to point to the picture that best represents the pain being experienced (Fig. 13-1).
1. Advantages
    a. The scale is simple and easy to use.
    b. It is easy to score.
    c. It requires no reading or verbal skills.
    d. It has no cultural or gender influence.
2. Disadvantages
    a. Sometimes this scale is seen as measuring mood rather than pain.
    b. Sad or crying faces are not universal.
3. Clinical application
    a. The FACES scale is reliable and valid for use with younger children, Asian children, and cognitively impaired older adults (Ackley et al., 2008; Wong & DeVito Thomas, 2006).
4. *Bieri FACES,* a variation of the standard FACES scale, contains seven faces derived from a series of children's facial representations of pain intensity (Fig. 13-2) (Bieri, Reeve, Champion, Addicoat, & Ziegler, 1990).
    a. Advantages
        (1) This scale was developed using children's representation of pain intensity.
        (2) It has good test–retest reliability.

0
No hurt
1
Hurts little bit
2
Hurts little more
3
Hurts even more
4
Hurts whole lot
5
Hurts worst

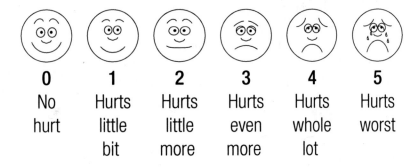

Explain to the person that each face is for a person who feels happy because he has no pain (hurt) or sad because he has some or a lot of pain.
Face 0 is very happy because he doesn't hurt at all.
Face 1 hurts just a little bit.
Face 2 hurts a little more.
Face 3 hurts even more.
Face 4 hurts a whole lot.
Face 5 hurts as much as you can imagine, although you don't have to be crying to feel this bad.

Figure 13-1 | Wong-Baker FACES Pain Rating Scale.

FACES Pain Rating Scale from Hockenberry MJ, Wilson D, Winkelstein ML: *Wong's Essentials of Pediatric Nursing*, ed. 7, St. Louis, 2005, p. 1259. Used with permission. Copyright Mosby.

(3) This is a rapid assessment with little respondent burden (Patrician, 2004).
(4) This scale gives a more stylized representation.
(5) It has no gender bias.

b. Disadvantages
(1) This scale can be focused on affective state rather than pain intensity.

c. Clinical application
(1) Children of all races can use this scale to assess pain intensity.

B. *CRIES* measures the psychological elements of crying, requires oxygen, increased vital signs, expression, and sleeplessness. It was developed for measuring pain in neonates (Merkel & Malviya, 2000).

1. Advantages
   a. This assessment is quick.
   b. It is easy to score.
   c. It provides a consistent method of assessment.
2. Disadvantages
   a. It measures pain and distress.
   b. It relies on observation.
   c. Scoring is based on numerical equivalents.
3. Clinical application
   a. This assessment is designed for neonates.

C. *FLACC* is designed to measure pain in infants and children from 2 months to 7 years of age (Voepel-Lewis, Merkel, Tait, Trzcinka, & Maliviya, 2002). It uses the elements of faces, legs, activity, cry, and consolability. A numerical score is derived. This score has a positive correlation with NPI results (Voepel-Lewis, Malviya, et al., 2002).

1. Advantages
   a. The method is quick and easy to use.
   b. Scoring is easy.

Faces Pain Scale – Revised (FPS-R)

From ***Pediatric Pain Sourcebook***, **www.painsourcebook.ca**
Version: 7 Aug 2007 CL von Baeyer

In the following instructions, say "hurt" or "pain," whichever seems right for a particular child.

"These faces show how much something can hurt. This face *[point to left-most face]* shows no pain. The faces show more and more pain *[point to each from left to right]* up to this one *[point to right-most face]* – it shows very much pain. Point to the face that shows how much you hurt [right now]."

Score the chosen face 0, 2, 4, 6, 8, or 10, counting left to right, so '0' = 'no pain' and '10' = 'very much pain.' Do not use words like 'happy' and 'sad'. This scale is intended to measure how children feel inside, not how their face looks.

Sources. Hicks CL, von Baeyer CL, Spafford P, van Korlaar I, Goodenough B. The Faces Pain Scale – Revised: Toward a common metric in pediatric pain measurement. ***Pain*** 2001;93:173-183. Bieri D, Reeve R, Champion GD, Addicoat L, Ziegler J. The Faces Pain Scale for the self-assessment of the severity of pain experienced by children: Development, initial validation and preliminary investigation for ratio scale properties. ***Pain*** 1990;41:139-150.

Fold here

0 2 4 6 8 10

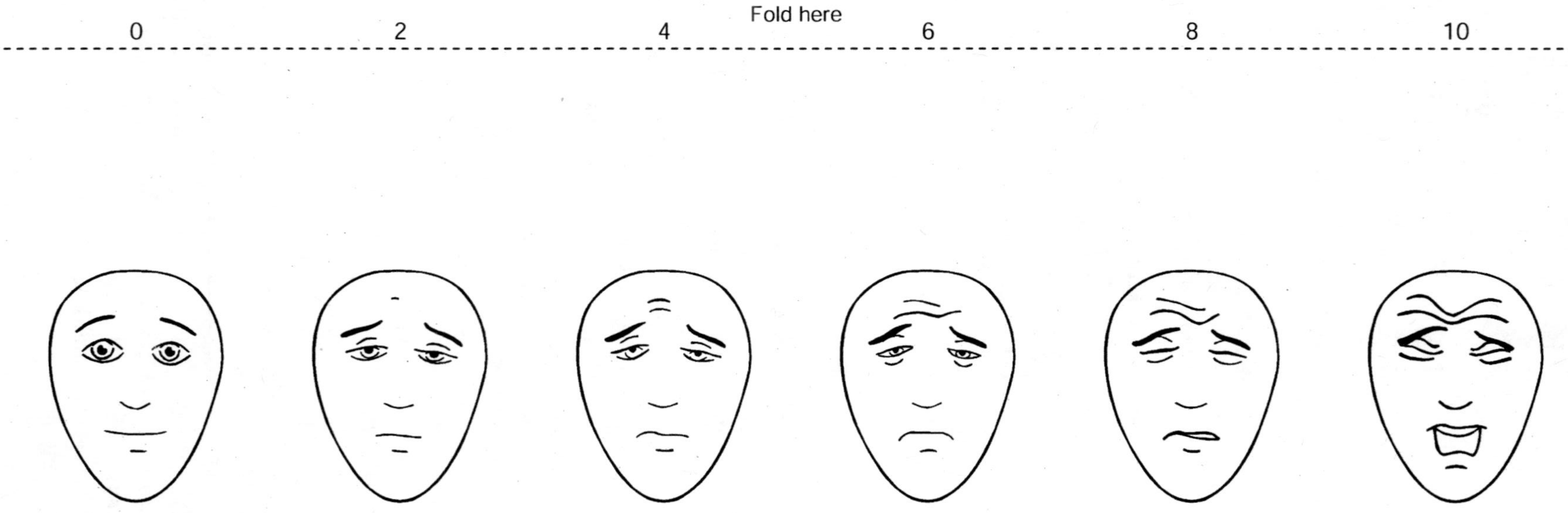

Figure 13-2 | FACES Pain Scale. Numbers 0 to 6, left to right.

Bieri D, Reeve RA, Champion GD, Addicoat L, Ziegler JB. The Faces Pain Scale from *Pain* 190 May, 41(2). Used with permission from IASP.

c. There are no ethnic or cultural differences.
d. It provides a consistent method for pain assessment.

2. Disadvantages
a. The method relies on the observation of care providers.
b. Correlating a numerical rating to a pain level is difficult.

3. Clinical application
a. This method can be applied to children who are 2 months to 7 years old.
b. It can be used effectively with children who have a cognitive impairment (Voepel-Lewis, Malviya, et al., 2002).

VIII. Pain Assessment in Specialty Populations: Nonverbal and Older Patients with Dementia, Critically Ill Intubated Patients, and Patients with Substance Abuse Disorders

A. The Joint Commission mandates that all patients have their pain assessed. This includes patients who cannot self-report pain.

B. The rule of thumb for using a behavioral pain assessment scale is to attempt a self-report whenever possible, assume pain is present for patients who have a painful condition but cannot self-report pain (Ackely et al., 2008), and use the best tool available for assessing pain in this population.

C. The behavioral scales are not all fully developed but do provide a means of assessing difficult-to-assess nonverbal populations.

D. The *Checklist of Nonverbal Pain Indicators (CNPI)* provides a list of six behaviors that indicate pain in nonverbal patients: vocalizations, facial grimacing, bracing, rubbing, restlessness, and vocal complaints (Feldt, Ryden, & Miles, 1998). Trials took place with verbal and nonverbal patient cohorts (Feldt, 2000). These behaviors were expanded by the American Geriatrics Society (2002).

1. Advantages
a. CNPI identifies behaviors that indicate pain.
b. It can be used as a screening tool to identify patients who are in pain.

2. Disadvantages
a. It relies on observation.
b. No numerical equivalent is possible.
c. Potential inconsistencies are related to observer variation.

3. Clinical application
a. CNPI is designed for use with older, cognitively impaired adults in acute care (Herr, Bjoro, & Decker, 2006).
b. It provides reliable, valid determination of behaviors that indicate pain through test comparison of behaviors in verbal, cognitively intact patients compared to nonverbal, cognitively impaired patients.

E. *Pain Assessment in Advanced Dementia (PAINAD)* was developed by the U.S. Department of Veterans Affairs for patients who have dementia and are nonverbal (Hutchinson, Tucker, Kim, & Gilder, 2006; Lane et al., 2003; Warden, Hurley, & Volicer, 2003). It uses the elements of breathing, negative vocalization, facial expression, body language, and consolability.

1. Advantages
a. PAINAD provides a systematic assessment of some elements that have been determined to indicate pain.
b. It can be used to screen demented patients for pain behaviors.
c. One study determined the psychometric properties of a German version of this tool. This study demonstrated good reliability and asserts this is a valid tool to measure pain (Schuler et al., 2007).

2. Disadvantages
a. PAINAD is less comprehensive than needed to assess pain (Herr, Coyne, et al., 2006).
b. It relies on caregivers' assessment of pain intensity (Herr, Coyne, et al., 2006).

3. Clinical application
a. This assessment is used for nonverbal patients with dementia or Alzheimer's disease.
b. PAINAD is developing reliability and validity for use with demented, nonverbal patients.

F. The *Payen Behavioral Pain Scale* is designed for critically ill patients who are intubated. It contains a three-point assessment with elements that fit the patients population: facial expression, upper limb movement, and compliance with ventilation (Payen et al., 2001).
  1. Advantages
     a. The pain rating correlates with NPI for observed activity (Aissaoui, 2005; Payen et al., 2001; Purdum & D'Arcy, 2005).
     b. It gives a specific measurement of ventilator compliance.
     c. This scale provides a method for pain assessment with ventilated patients.
     d. Correlation is seen in all levels of sedation.
     e. Replication studies have consistent, similar findings.
  2. Disadvantages
     a. The scale relies on observation for rating.
     b. Sedation is being used.
  3. Clinical application
     a. This scale is reliable and valid for assessing pain in critically ill intubated patients (Li, Puntillo, & Miaskowski, 2008).

G. The *Critical-Care Pain Observation Tool (CPOT) in Adult Patients* is designed to assess pain in critically ill adult patients. It uses four behaviors: facial expression, body movement, muscle tension, and compliance with the ventilator, for those patients who are ventilated, or vocalization, for extubated patients.
  1. Advantages
     a. CPOT provides an organized assessment for the critically ill adult patients.
     b. It provides discriminate validity with sedated patients (Gelinas & Johnston, 2007; Gelinas, Fillion, Puntillo, Viens, & Fortier, 2006; Li et al., 2008).
     c. This tool provides for an assessment in both ventilated and nonventilated patients.
  2. Disadvantages
     a. The tool relies on observations.
     b. Sedation is used, and patients with ventilation support are being assessed.
  3. Clinical application
     a. CPOT applies to adult critically ill patients, both ventilated and nonventilated.
     b. It is reliable and valid for assessing pain in critically ill patients who are intubated and who can self-report pain.

H. The *Opioid Risk Tool (ORT)* is used to assess the risk of opioid use when prescribing opioids for pain. It consists of a short list of questions related to family history of substance abuse, personal history of substance abuse, age, history of any preadolescent sexual abuse, any psychological disease, and depression. A score of greater than 8 is highly predictive for the development of aberrant behavior with opioid use.
  1. Advantages
     a. ORT is quick and easy to use.
     b. Quick scoring is possible.
     c. It is a quick screen for patients who, despite their pain, may develop aberrant behaviors with long-term opioid use.
  2. Disadvantages
     a. The tool relies on patient response.
     b. It does not address the full extent of the pain experience.
  3. Clinical application
     a. Adult patients who are being considered for long-term opioid therapy can use ORT.
     b. There is a high degree of specificity and sensitivity in both male and female patients (Webster & Webster, 2005).

I. The *Screener and Opioid Assessment for Patients with Pain (SOAPP-R)*—is used when patients are being considered for long-term opioid therapy for chronic pain. It consists of 24 questions related to substance abuse history, medication-related behaviors, antisocial behaviors, doctor–patient relationships, and personal care and lifestyle issues (Butler, Budmna, Fernandez, & Jamison, 2004). Each question has a point value. A score above 18 indicates a high risk for abuse.

1. Advantages
    a. This is a quick screen for patients who may need to be more closely monitored during opioid therapy.
    b. It helps to identify patients who will have a low risk of difficulty with opioid therapy.
2. Disadvantages
    a. It relies on patients to make a truthful report.
    b. It does not address the full scope of the pain experience.
3. Clinical application
    a. This screen is applicable to chronic pain patients who are being given opioids for pain relief.

J. *Neuropathic pain scales* are used to differentiate and measure pain intensity for pain that is neuropathic rather than nociceptive in nature. Such scales are used to measure the intensity of neuropathic pain. In the most common scale, there are 11 items using 0 to 10 rating scales (Galer & Jensen, 1997).

1. Advantages
    a. Two items measure the global dimensions of pain intensity and pain unpleasantness.
    b. Eight items assess specific components of neuropathic pain: sharp, hot, dull, cold, sensitive, itchy, deep, and surface pain.
    c. One item addresses the fluctuation of pain from constant with intermittent increases, to intermittent, to constant with fluctuation.
    d. Higher scores are indicative of a pain that is more neuropathic (Bennett, Smith, Torrance, & Lee, 2006).
    e. The scale can measure the effects of treatments (Galer & Jensen, 1997).
2. Disadvantages
    a. Data collected from chronic pain clinic patients do not reflect the total experience of the larger patient population with neuropathic pain.
    b. The validation study is not a randomized, double-blind construct.
    c. Not all types of neuropathic pain complaints are covered in the 11 items of the scale.
3. Clinical application
    a. This scale is used to assess pain intensity in chronic pain patients who have a neuropathic pain syndrome.

K. The *Leeds Assessment of Neuropathic Symptoms and Signs* is a self-administered assessment tool to determine whether pain is neuropathic (Weingarten et al., 2007).

1. Advantages
    a. This assessment is easy to use.
    b. It is in a self-administered survey format.
2. Disadvantages
    a. Specificity and sensitivity: less sensitive when used in population studies.
    b. It is best suited as a screening tool rather than an assessment tool (Weingarten et al., 2007).
3. Clinical application
    a. This assessment is used to screen pain for a neuropathic component in chronic pain patients of all types.

References

Ackley, B., Ladwig, G., Swan, B. A., & Tucker, S. J. (2008). *Evidence-based nursing care guidelines.* St. Louis: Mosby Elsevier.

Aissaoui, Y., et al. (2005). Validation of behavioral pain scale in critically ill, sedated and mechanically ventilated patients. *Anesthesia & Analgesia, 101*(5), 1470–1476.

American Geriatrics Society. (2002). The management of persistent pain in older persons: The American Geriatrics Society Panel on Persistent Pain in Older Persons. *Journal of the American Geriatrics Society, 50*(6), 205–224.

American Pain Society. (2003). *Principles of analgesic use in the treatment of acute and cancer pain* (5th ed.). Glenview, IL: Author.

Barker, L. R., & Whitfield, C. L. (1991). Alcoholism. In L. R. Barker, J. R. Burtage, & P. D. Zieve (Eds.), *Principles of ambulatory medicine* (3rd ed., p. 211). Baltimore: Williams & Wilkins.

Bennett, M. I., Smith, B. H., Torrance, N., & Lee, A. J. (2006). Can pain be more or less neuropathic? Comparison of symptom assessment tools with ratings of certainty by clinicians. *Pain, 122*(3), 289–294.

Berry, P. H., Covington, E., Dahl, J., Katz, J., & Miaskowski, C. (2006). *Pain: Current understanding of assessment, management, and treatments.* Reston, VA: National Pharmaceutical Council & the Joint Commission.

Bieri, D., Reeve, R. A., Champion, G. D., Addicoat, L., & Ziegler, J. B. (1990). The FACES pain scale for the self-assessment of the severity of pain experienced by children: Development, initial validation, and preliminary investigation for ratio scale properties. *Pain, 41*(2), 139–150.

Butler, S., Budmna, S. H., Fernandez, K., & Jamison, R. N. (2004). Validation of a screener and opioid assessment measure for patients with chronic pain. *Pain, 112,* 65–75.

Carlsson, A. M. (1983). Assessment of chronic pain. I. Aspects of reliability and validity of the visual analog scale. *Pain, 16,* 87–101.

Chok, B. (1998). An overview of the Visual Analogue Scale and the McGill Pain Questionnaire. *Physiotherapy Singapore, 1*(3), 88–93.

Clark, M. E., Gironda, R. J., & Young, R. W. (2003). Development and validation of the Pain Outcomes Questionnaire-VA. *Journal of Rehabilitation Research and Development, 40*(5), 381–395.

Cleeland, C., & Ryan, K. M. (1994). Pain assessment: Global use of the Brief Pain Inventory. *Annals of the Academy of Medicine, 23,* 129–138.

Dahl, J. B., & Kehlet, H. (2006). Postoperative pain and its management. In S. B. McMahon & M. Kolzenburg (Eds.), *Wall & Melzack's textbook of pain* (5th ed.). Philadelphia: Churchill Livingstone.

D'Arcy, Y. M. (2003). Pain assessment. In P. Iyer (Ed.), *Medical–legal aspects of pain and suffering.* Tucson, AZ: Lawyers and Judges Publishing.

D'Arcy, Y. (2007). *Pain management: Evidence-based tools and techniques for nursing professionals.* Marblehead, MA: HcPro.

D'Arcy, Y. (2008). Nursing 2008 pain management survey report. *Nursing 2008, 38*(6), 42–49.

Daut, R. L., Cleeland, C. S., & Flannery, R. (1983). Development of the Wisconsin Brief Pain Questionnaire to assess pain in cancer or other diseases. *Pain, 17,* 197–210.

Dochterman, J. M., & Bulechek, G. M. (Eds.). (2004). *Nursing interventions classification* (4th ed.). St. Louis: Mosby.

Farrar, J. T., Young, J. P., Lamoreaux, L., Werth, J. L., & Poole, R. M. (2001). Clinical importance of changes in chronic pain intensity measured on an 11 point numerical pain rating scale. *Pain, 94,* 149–158.

Feldt, K. S. (2000). The Checklist of Non-Verbal Pain Indicators (CNPI). *Pain Management Nursing, 1*(1), 13–21.

Feldt, K. S., Ryden, M. B., & Miles, S. (1998). Treatment of pain in cognitively impaired compared with cognitively intact older patients with hip fractures. *Journal of the American Geriatrics Society, 46,* 1079–1085.

Galer, B., & Jensen, M. (1997). Development and preliminary validation of a pain measure specific to neuropathic pain: The Neuropathic Pain Scale. *Neurology, 48*(2), 332–338.

Gelinas, C., & Johnston, C. (2007). Pain assessment in the critically ill ventilated adult: Validation of the critical-care pain observation tool and physiologic indicators. *Clinical Journal of Pain, 23*(6), 497–505.

Gelinas, C., Fillion, L., Puntillo, K., Viens, C., & Fortier, M. (2006). Validation of the Critical Care Pain Observation Tool in adult patients. *American Journal of Critical Care, 15*(4), 420–427.

Ger, L., Ho, S., Sun, W., Wang, M., & Cleeland, C. (1999). Validation of the Brief Pain Inventory in a Taiwanese population. *Journal of Pain and Symptom Management, 18*(5), 316–322.

Gracely, R. H., & Dubner, R. (1987). Reliability and validity of verbal descriptor scales of painfulness. *Pain, 29,* 175–185.

Graham, C., Bond, S., Gerkovich, M., & Cook, M. (1980). Use of the McGill Pain Questionnaire in the assessment of cancer pain: Replicability and consistency. *Pain, 8,* 377–387.

Herr, K. A., & Mobily, P. (1993). Comparison of selected pain assessment tools for use with the elderly. *Applied Nursing Research, 6*(1), 39–46.

Herr, K., Bjoro, K., & Decker, S. (2006). Tools for assessment of pain in nonverbal older adults with dementia: A state-of-the-science review. *Journal of Pain and Symptom Management, 31*(2), 170–192.

Herr, K., Coyne, P., Key, T., Manworren, R., McCaffery, M., Merkel, S., Perlosi-Kelly, J., & Wild, L. (2006). Pain assessment in the nonverbal patient: Position statement with clinical practice recommendations. *Pain Management Nursing, 7*(2), 44–52.

Hutchinson, R. W., Tucker, W. F., Kim, S., & Gilder, R. (2006). Evaluation of a behavioral assessment tool for the individual unable to self-report pain. *American Journal of Hospice & Palliative Medicine, 23*(4), 328–331.

Jensen, M. P. (2003). The validity and reliability of pain measures in adults with cancer. *Journal of Pain, 4*(1), 2–21.

Joint Commission. (2000). *Pain assessment and management: An organizational approach.* Oakbrook Terrace, IL: Author.

Kerns, R. D., Turk, D., & Rudy, T. E. (1985). The West Haven-Yale Multidimensional Pain Inventory (WHYMPI). *Pain, 23,* 345–356.

Klepstad, P., Loge, J. H., Borchgrevink, P. C., Mendoza, T. R., Cleeland, C., & Kaasa, S. (2002). The Norwegian Brief Pain Inventory Questionnaire: Translation and validation in cancer pain patients. *Journal of Pain and Symptom Management, 24*(5), 517–525.

Krenzischeck, D. A., & Wilson, L. (2003). An introduction to the ASPAN pain and comfort clinical guideline. *Journal of Perianesthesia Nursing, 18*(4), 228–236.Lane, P., Kuntupis, M., MacDonald, S., McCarthy, P., Panke, J. A., Warden, V., & Volicer, L. (2003). A pain assessment tool for people with advanced Alzheimer's and other progressive dementias. *Home Healthcare Nurse, 21*(1), 32–37.

Li, D., Puntillo, K., & Miaskowski, C. (2008). A review of objective pain measures for use with critical care adult patients unable to self-report. *Journal of Pain, 9*(1), 2–10.

Marin, R., Cyhan, T., & Miklos, W. (2006). Sleep disturbance in patients with chronic low back pain. *American Journal of Physical Medicine and Rehabilitation, 85*(5), 430–435.

McDonald, D. D., & Weiskopf, C. S. A. (2001). Adult patients' postoperative pain descriptions and responses to the Short Form McGill Pain Questionnaire. *Clinical Nursing Research, 10*(4), 442–452.

MacIntyre, D. L., Hopkins, P. M., & Harris, S. R. (1995). Evaluation of pain and functional activity in patellofemoral pain syndrome: Reliability and validity of two assessment tools. *Physiotherapy of Canada, 47*(3), 164–170.

Melzack, R. (1975). The McGill Pain Questionnaire: Major properties and scoring methods. *Pain, 1,* 277–299.

Melzack, R. (1987). The Short Form McGill Pain Questionnaire. *Pain, 30,* 191–197.

Merkel, S., & Malviya, S. (2000). Pediatric pain, tools and assessment. *Journal of Perianesthesia Nursing, 15*(6), 386–391.

Mystakidou, K., Mendoza, T., Tsilika, E., Befon, S., Parpa, G., Bellos, G., Vlahos, L., & Leeland, C. (2001). Greek Brief Pain Inventory: Validation and utility in cancer pain. *Oncology, 60*(1), 35–42.

Mystakidou, K., Parpa, E., Tsilika, E., Kalaidopoulou, O., Georgaki, S., Galanos, A., & Vlahos, L. (2002). Greek McGill Pain Questionnaire: Validation and utility in cancer patients. *Journal of Pain and Symptom Management, 24*(4), 370–387.

Pasero, C., & McCaffery, M. (2004). Pain control: Comfort-function goals. *American Journal of Nursing, 104*(9), 77–78.

Patrician, P. (2004). Single-item graphic representational scales. *Nursing Research, 53*(5), 347–352.

Payen, J. F., Bru, O., Bosson, J.L., Lagrasta, A., Novel, E., Deschaux, I., Lavagne, P., & Jacquot, C. (2001). Assessing pain in critically ill sedated patients by using a behavioral pain scale. *Critical Care Medicine, 29*(12), 1–11. Purdum, A., & D'Arcy, Y. (2005). *A comparison of two behavioral pain scales with intubated intensive care (ICU) patients.* San Antonio, TX: American Pain Society.

Radbruch, L., Liock, G., Kiencke, P., Lindena, G., Sabatowski, R., Grond, S., Lehmann, A., & Cleeland, C. (1999). Validation of the German version of the Brief Pain Inventory. *Journal of Pain and Symptom Management, 18*(3), 180–187.

Raiche, K. A., Osborne, T. L., Jensen, M. P., & Cardenas, D. (2006). The reliability and validity of pain interference measures in persons with spinal cord injury. *Journal of Pain, 7*(3), 179–186.

Schuler, M. S., Becker, S., Kaspar, R., Nikolaus, T., Kruse, A., & Basler, H. D. (2007). Psychometric properties of the German Pain Assessment in Advanced Dementia Scale (PAINAD-G) in nursing home residents. *Journal of the American Medical Directors Association, 8,* 388–395.

Tan, G., Jensen, M. P., Thornby, J. I., & Shanti, B. F. (2004). Validation of the Brief Pain Inventory for chronic non-malignant pain. *Journal of Pain and Symptom Management, 5*(2), 133–137.

Tang, N. K., & Crane, C. (2006). Suicidality in chronic pain: A review of the prevalence, risk factors and psychological links. *Psychological Medicine, 36*(5), 575–586.

Tittle, M. B., McMillan, S. C., & Hagan, S. (2003). Validating the Brief Pain Inventory for use with surgical patients with cancer. *Oncology Nursing Forum, 30*(2), 325–330.

Voepel-Lewis, T., Malviya, S., Tait, A., Merkel, S., Foster, R., Krane, E., & Davis, P. (2002). A comparison of the clinical utility of pain assessment tools for children with cognitive impairment. *Anesthesia & Analgesia, 106*(1), 72–78.

Voepel-Lewis, T., Merkel, S., Tait, A., Trzcinka, A., & Maliviya, S. (2002). The reliability and validity of the Faces, Legs, Activity, Cry, Consolability observational tool as a measure of pain in children with cognitive impairment. *Anesthesia & Analgesia, 95*(5), 1224–1229.

Warden, V., Hurley, A. C., & Volicer, L. (2003). Development and psychometric evaluation of the Pain Assessment in Advanced Dementia (PAINAD) scale. *Journal of the American Medical Directors Association, 4,* 9–15.

Webster, L. R., & Webster, R. M. (2005). Predicting aberrant behaviors in opioid treated patients: Preliminary validation of an opioid risk tool. *Pain Medicine, 6*(6), 432–442.

Weiner, D. K., Herr, K., & Rudy, T. (2002). *Persistent pain in older adults: An interdisciplinary guide for treatment.* New York: Springer.

Weingarten, T. N., Watson, J. C., Hooten, W. M., Wollan, P. C., Melton, L. J., Locketz, A. J., Wong, G. Y., & Yawn, B. P. (2007). Validation of the S-LANSS in the community setting. *Pain, 132*(1–2), 189–194.

Wilkie, D., Savedra, M., Holzemer, W., Tesler, M., & Paul, S. (1990). Use of the McGill Pain Questionnaire to measure pain: A meta-analysis. *Nursing Research, 39*(1), 36–41.

Williams, V. S. L., Smith, M. Y., & Fehnel, S. E. (2006). The validity and utility of the BPI interference measures for evaluating the impact of osteoarthritis pain. *Journal of Pain and Symptom Management, 31*(1), 48–57.

Wong, D., & DiVito-Thomas, P. (2006). The validity, reliability, and preference of the Wong-Baker FACES pain rating scale among Chinese, Japanese, and Thai children. Abstract retrieved May 17, 2009, from http://evolve.elsevier.com/productPages/s_97.html.

chapter 14

Overview of Pharmacology

Virginia L. Ghafoor, PharmD, RPh
Barbara St. Marie, ANP, GNP, RN-BC, PhD Candidate

Objectives

After studying this chapter, the reader should be able to:

1. Understand pharmacological differences in the actions of drugs used for analgesia.
2. Identify key pharmacokinetic principles affecting the physiological response to pain medication.
3. Determine drug selection based on route of administration and efficacy in pain relief.
4. Recognize appropriate drug doses, side effects, and interactions with other medications.
5. Establish monitoring parameters to evaluate outcomes associated with administration of pain medication.

I. Drug Pharmacology

A. α_2-Agonists (Appendix 14–1)
   1. Multiple activities occur via G protein–linked mechanisms, including inhibition of cyclic adenosine monophosphate formation and the opening of K^+ channels. α_2-agonists are used for treatment in pain, spasticity, and opioid withdrawal (Elliott, 2003).
   2. Clonidine
      a. Duraclon® (neuraxial, epidural treatment)
      b. Catapres-TTS® (transdermal patch)
      c. Catapres® (tablet form)
   3. Dexmedetomidine (Precedex®)
   4. Tizanidine (Zanaflex®)

B. Anticonvulsants (Appendix 14–2)
   1. Anticonvulsants inhibit sustained high-frequency neuronal firing by blocking sodium (Na^+) channels after an action potential, reducing excitability in sensitized C-nociceptors (Loughrey, 2003).
      a. Carbamazepine (Tegretol®)
      b. Lamotrigine (Lamictal®)
      c. Oxcarbazepine (Trileptal®)
      d. Phenytoin (Dilantin®)
   2. Anticonvulsants block Na^+ channels and increase synthesis and activity of γ-aminobutyric acid A ($GABA_A$), an inhibitory neurotransmitter in the brain (Silberstein, 1996).
      a. Topiramate (Topamax®)
      b. Valproic acid (Depakote®)
   3. Anticonvulsants bind to the $\alpha_2\delta$ subunit of the calcium channel to reduce neurotransmitter release (Dooley, Taylor, Donevan, & Feltner, 2007; Gajraj, 2007).
      a. Gabapentin (Neurontin®)
      b. Pregabalin (Lyrica®): schedule V controlled substance (U.S. Drug Enforcement Administration, 2005)
   4. Benzodiazepines (see E. Anxiolytics)
      a. Clonazepam (Klonopin®)
      b. Diazepam (Valium®)
      c. Lorazepam (Ativan®)

C. Antidepressants (Appendix 14–3)
   1. Tricyclic antidepressants inhibit presynaptic neuronal reuptake of norepinephrine and serotonin (5-hydroxytryptamine [5-HT]) at the descending tract (Sindrup, Otto, Finnerup, & Jensen, 2005).
      a. Amitriptyline (Elavil®)
      b. Amoxapine (Asendin®)
      c. Clomipramine (Anafranil®)
      d. Desipramine (Norpramin®)
      e. Doxepin (Sinequan®)
         (1) Topical cream (Prudoxin®, Zonalon®)
      f. Imipramine (Tofranil®)
      g. Maprotiline (Ludiomil®)
      h. Nortriptyline (Pamelor®)
      i. Protriptyline (Vivactil®)
      j. Trimipramine (Surmontil®)
   2. Selective serotonin reuptake inhibitors inhibit presynaptic neuronal reuptake of serotonin (Sindrup et al., 2005).
      a. Citalopram (Celexa®)
      b. Escitalopram (Lexapro®)
      c. Fluoxetine (Prozac®)
      d. Fluvoxamine (Luvox®)

e. Paroxetine (Paxil®, Paxil CR®)
f. Sertraline (Zoloft®)

3. The serotonin noradrenaline reuptake inhibitor inhibits the reuptake of serotonin and norepinephrine (Sindrup et al., 2005).
   a. Duloxetine (Cymbalta®)
   b. Venlafaxine (Effexor®, Effexor XR®)
4. Atypical antidepressants (Iosifescu, Alpert, & Fava, 2003)
   a. Bupropion (Wellbutrin®, Wellbutrin SR®) is a second-generation non-TCA. It inhibits the reuptake of norepinephrine and dopamine.
   b. Mirtazapine (Remeron®) is a tricyclic structural analogue with nonselective receptor activities. The main mechanism involves antagonist activity at central presynaptic α_2-adrenergic receptors, which enhances the activity of norepinephrine and serotonin (5-HT_2 and 5-HT_3). Mirtazapine is a potent antagonist of histamine H_1-receptors.
   c. Nefazodone (Serzone®) is chemically related to trazodone, with serotonin 5-HT_2 blockade but less α_1 blockade.
   d. Trazodone (Desyrel®) inhibits serotonin reuptake, blocks serotonin 5-HT_2, and is an antagonist at α_1-adrenergic receptors.

D. Antihistamines (Appendix 14–4)
1. H_1 antihistamines (first generation) bind to histamine, muscarinic, α-adrenergic, and serotonin receptors to reduce transmission of itch and pain from afferent C-type nerve fibers in the periphery (O'Donoghue & Tharp, 2005; Stander & Schmelz, 2006).
   a. Diphenhydramine and promethazine are most commonly used for treatment of opioid-induced itching, general pruritus, nausea, and vomiting.
   b. Hydroxyzine is most commonly used for anxiety, acute pain, opioid-induced itching, general pruritus, nausea, and vomiting.
   c. Other antihistamines are primarily used for allergic rhinitis.
      (1) Chlorpheniramine (Chlor-Trimeton®, various products)
      (2) Cyproheptadine (limited to generic products)
      (3) Diphenhydramine (Benadryl®, various products)
      (4) Hydroxyzine (Vistaril®, Atarax®, various products)
      (5) Promethazine (Phenergan®, various products)
      (6) Pyrilamine (various products)
2. H_2 antihistamines (second generation) have a slower dissociation rate from the histamine receptor, less central nervous system penetration, and minimal activity with nonhistamine receptors (O'Donoghue & Tharp, 2005).
   a. Cetirizine (Zyrtec®)
   b. Desloratadine (Clarinex®)
   c. Fexofenadine (Allegra®)
   d. Loratadine (Claritin®)

E. Anxiolytics (Appendix 14–5)
1. Benzodiazepines directly bind to the $GABA_A$ receptor–chloride (Cl^-) ion channel complex to modulate the binding of GABA (inhibitory neurotransmitter). The primary use is for anxiolytic, anticonvulsant, and antispasmodic activity (Bateson, 2004; Rudolph & Mehler, 2006).
   a. Alprazolam (Xanax®)
   b. Chlordiazepoxide (Librium®)
   c. Clonazepam (Klonopin®)
   d. Clorazepate (Tranxene®)
   e. Diazepam (Valium®)
   f. Lorazepam (Ativan®)
   g. Midazolam (Versed®)
   h. Oxazepam (Serax®)

2. Buspirone (BuSpar®) is a presynaptic serotonin 5-HT_{1A} agonist that decreases neuronal firing and reduces synthesis and release of serotonin. No interaction occurs with GABA receptors. It is primarily used for anxiety disorders.
3. Flumazenil (Romazicon®) is a benzodiazepine receptor antagonist used for complete or partial reversal of sedation.

F. Hypnotics (Appendix 14–6)
1. Benzodiazepines directly bind to the $GABA_A$ receptor–Cl^- ion channel complex to modulate the binding of GABA (inhibitory neurotransmitter) (Bateson, 2004; Rudolph & Mohler, 2006).
    a. Flurazepam (Dalmane®)
    b. Temazepam (Restoril®)
    c. Triazolam (Halcion®)
2. Nonbenzodiazepines are structurally unrelated to benzodiazepines but interact at the $GABA_A$ receptor-Cl^- ion channel complex. They are used for short-term management of insomnia (Ebert, Wafford, & Deacon, 2006; Ramakrishnan & Scheid, 2007).
    a. Eszopiclone (Lunesta®)
    b. Zaleplon (Sonata®)
    c. Zolpidem (Ambien®, Ambien CR®)
3. Ramelteon (Rozerem®) is a potent, selective agonist of melatonin receptors MT_1 and MT_2 within the suprachiasmic nucleus of the hypothalamus, an area responsible for determination of circadian rhythms and synchronization of the sleep-wake cycle (Ebert et al., 2006)

Box 14–1 Nursing Considerations While Caring for Patients Receiving Local Anesthetics

Local anesthetics agents are used in treating patients undergoing procedures (see chapter on Moderate Sedation/Analgesia), as well as patients with acute, persistent, and cancer pain states (see chapter on Cancer Pain Management). New formulations of these local anesthetics allow the delivery to be prolonged and to occur through various routes, i.e., intravenous, subcutaneous, intramuscular, intraarticular, perineural, intrapleural, epidural, intrathecal, and topical. These methods may be a single bolus injection or a continuous infusion of local anesthetic agent over some time.

Mechanisms of action against pain, which go beyond the descriptive blockade on page 239 of this chapter, are based on complex research and understanding of the neuromechanisms involved. Intravenous and oral preparations have been successfully used to treat neuropathic pain syndromes (Challapalli, Tremont-Lukats, McNicol, Lau, & Carr, 2005). Heavner (2007), in his review of the literature, found that Zhang, Li, and Munir (2004) had discovered systemic lidocaine in rats reduced sympathetic nerve sprouting in dorsal root ganglion associated with some neuropathic pain states. Takatori, Kuroda, and Hirose (2006) showed with local anesthetic agents that there is an inhibition of nerve growth factor-stimulating tyrosine kinase activity, which suppresses neurite outgrowth (i.e., projections from the neuron).

In clinical practice, we see the use of epinephrine with the local anesthetic agents. Epinephrine is sometimes used with local anesthetic to test an epidural catheter for placement. The epinephrine is used to determine whether the catheter tip is in an epidural vein; if it is, the heart rate will increase and the epidural catheter needs to be adjusted by the anesthesiologist. Epinephrine is a vasoconstrictor that can inhibit the absorption of local anesthetic agents into the circulation and can prolong the efficacy of the local anesthetic. An anesthesiologist or interventional pain physician well trained in its use can put these effects of the drug to good use. Side effects from the epinephrine may include tachycardia, hypertension, and cardiac arrest.

Reactions to local anesthetic agents can be evident to nurses in their monitoring process. There may be a *localized or systemic reaction* that is thought to be an allergic reaction. If the patient has a history of allergy to local anesthetic agents, the nurse can query the patient about what type of reaction occurred and what the local anesthetic agent was when the reaction occurred. Obtaining past

G. Induction anesthetics
   1. Ketamine (Ketalar®) binds to the phencyclidine receptor on the *N*-methyl-D-aspartate (NMDA) channel and noncompetitively inhibits glutamate activation (Okon, 2007).
      a. The NMDA receptor is a ligand-gated ion channel that is activated by glutamate.
      b. This channel is highly permeable to calcium.
   2. Propofol (Diprivan®) is an ultra-short-acting general anesthetic unrelated to benzodiazepines and barbiturates (Lundstrom, Zachrisson, & Furst, 2005).
      a. Mechanism of action is uncertain.
H. Local anesthetics
   1. Local anesthetics are injectable; they block conduction of nerve impulses by decreasing or preventing an increase in the permeability of excitable membranes to Na^+ (Heavner, 2007) (see Box 14–1).
      a. Bupivacaine (Marcaine®, Sensorcaine®)
      b. Levobupivacaine (Chirocaine®)
      c. Chloroprocaine (Nesacaine®)
      d. Etidocaine (Duranest®)
      e. Lidocaine (Xylocaine®): also used for topical application
      f. Mepivacaine (Carbocaine®)
      g. Prilocaine (Citanest®)
      h. Procaine (Novocaine®)

medical records will also facilitate this discovery. Local reactions may be rash or urticaria. Certain local anesthetics will have fewer allergic reactions than others. Nursing communication with the health care team, even with a minor reaction, is necessary to provide the best care to the patient. Another type of reaction is a *systemic reaction* that may result in cardiovascular or central nervous system reactions, or methemoglobinemia. Local anesthetic agents have a vasodilation effect; when plasma concentrations become high, toxicity can occur. Cardiovascular reactions could result in myocardial suppression, bradycardia, hypotension, and cardiovascular collapse. *Central nervous system* reactions may range from a reaction as minor as lightheadedness and dizziness, to difficulty focusing or tinnitus or circumoral numbness, to more severe reactions such as muscle twitching, convulsions, loss of consciousness, or even death. Such reactions may also involve transient neurological symptoms such as prolonged anesthesia and paresthesia.

Methemoglobinemia is more common in infants less than 6 months old than in adults. Methemoglobinemia results in anemia and tissue hypoxia.

Precautions against Toxicity

To assure optimal patient care, nurses should screen the patient for a past history of reaction to local anesthetics, renal or hepatic dysfunction, preexisting heart block or heart conditions, and history of respiratory acidosis. Toxicity may occur more often in pregnancy, in the very old or very young, and those with hypoxia. Toxicity usually occurs from inadvertent intravascular injection, excessive dose or rate of injection, delayed clearance of the drug, or injection into vascular tissue. Nurses should read the medication label and inform the physician if epinephrine is on the label of the local anesthetic agent. Close assessment of and monitoring by nursing staff can detect side effects early before they become toxic.

Challapalli, V., Tremont-Lukats, I. W., McNicol, E. D., Lau, J., & Carr, D. B. (2005). Systemic administration of local anesthetic agents to relieve neuropathic pain. *Cochrane Database of Systematic Reviews,* Issue 4. Retrieved May 24, 2009, from http://www.cochrane.org/reviews/en/ab003345.html

Heavner, J. T. (2007). Local anesthetics. *Current Opinion in Anaesthesiology, 20,* 336–342.

Takatori, M., Kuroda, Y., & Hirose, M. (2006). Local anesthetics suppress nerve growth factor-mediated neurite outgrowth by inhibition of tyrosine kinase activity of TrkA. *Anesthesia & Analgesia, 102,* 462–467.

Zhang, J. M., Li, H., & Munir, M. A. (2004). Decreasing sympathetic sprouting in pathologic sensory ganglia: A new mechanism for treating neuropathic pain using lidocaine. *Pain, 109,* 143–149.

i. Ropivacaine (Naropin®)
j. Tetracaine (Pontocaine®)
2. Topical use is limited to mucous membranes and skin. These forms are not suitable for injection because of irritating or ineffective properties. The mechanism of action is the same as with injectable local anesthetics (Heavner, 2007). Refer to Tables 14–1 and 14–2 for information on topical compounds for pain management. Examples of topical local anesthetics products are as follows:
 a. Benzocaine (Americaine®, Hurricaine® spray)
 b. Cocaine solution
 c. Dibucaine (Nupercainal®)
 d. Dyclonine (Dyclone®, Sucrets®)
 e. Pramoxine (Anusol®, ProctoFoam®, Tronothane®)
 f. Lidocaine or prilocaine (EMLA® cream)
 g. Lidocaine (Lidoderm® 5% patch)
3. Oral local anesthetic
 a. Mexiletine (Challapalli et al., 2005)

I. Muscle relaxants (Appendix 14–7) (Beebe, Barkin, & Barkin, 2005)
1. Baclofen (Lioresal®) activates $GABA_B$ receptors to reduce the release of neurotransmitters and amino acids. It acts specifically at the spinal end of the upper motor neurons to cause muscle relaxation.
2. Benzodiazepines (see E. Anxiolytics)
3. Carisoprodol (Soma®, Soma Compound®) is a centrally acting skeletal muscle relaxant. The precise mechanism of action is unknown. Benefits of this drug are most likely from the sedative side effects. Additive effects occur with other central nervous system depressants. Psychological dependence has been reported with long-term use. It is also metabolized to meprobamate, which has anxiolytic and sedative effects.
4. Chlorzoxazone (Parafon Forte®) is a centrally acting skeletal muscle relaxant. It acts on the spinal cord and subcortical levels by depressing polysynaptic reflexes.
5. Cyclobenzaprine (Flexeril®) is a centrally acting skeletal muscle relaxant pharmacologically related to tricyclic antidepressants. It reduces tonic somatic motor activity, influencing both α- and γ-motor neurons, and is a $5\text{-}HT_2$ receptor antagonist (Beebe et al., 2005).
6. Metaxalone (Skelaxin®) is a centrally acting muscle relaxant. Its mechanism of action is unknown.
7. Methocarbamol (Robaxin®) is a centrally acting skeletal muscle relaxant. The precise mechanism of action is unknown. Benefits of this drug are most likely from the sedative side effects.
8. Orphenadrine (Norflex®, Norgesic®) is a muscarinic H_1 receptor antagonist. It inhibits the norepinephrine transporter and is an NMDA receptor ion channel blocker (Beebe et al., 2005).
9. Tizanidine (Zanaflex®) (see A. α_2-Agonists)

J. Nonsteroidal antiinflammatory drugs (NSAIDs) (Appendix 14–8) (Herndon et al., 2008).
1. Cyclooxygenase (COX)–1 is a primary enzyme isoform that converts arachidonic acid to prostaglandins. Nonselective NSAIDs that inhibit COX-1 prevent formation of prostaglandin mediators that trigger inflammation. Under normal physiological conditions, prostaglandins regulate gastrointestinal cytoprotection, renal vasodilation, renal Na^+ and Cl^- reabsorption, platelet aggregation, fever, and uterine contraction. Inhibition of prostaglandin synthesis by NSAIDs produces gastrointestinal irritation, renal ischemia, electrolyte imbalances (Na^+ retention), increased bleeding, and fever reduction.
 a. Aspirin®
 b. Choline magnesium trisalicylate (Trilisate®)
 c. Diclofenac (Voltaren®, Arthrotec®)
  (1) Diclofenac Epolamine (Flector®) patch
  (2) Diclofenac Na^+ (Voltaren®) gel
 d. Diflunisal (Dolobid®)
 e. Etodolac (Lodine®)
 f. Fenoprofen (Nalfon®)

Table 14-1 Topical Compounds for Pain Management (Prescription Required)

U.S. Food and Drug Administration (FDA) Approved, Commercially Available	Off-Label Use, Pharmacy Compounded
Anticonvulsants	
• None	• Carbamazepine 2% • Gabapentin 6%
Antidepressants	
• Doxepin 5% cream (Prudoxin®, Zonalon®)	• Amitriptyline 2% • Nortriptyline
Local Anesthetics	

• Lidocaine
  • 2% solution for iontophoresis (Numby Stuff®)
  • 2% viscous solution for oral use
  • 2% cream, gel
  • 3% cream, lotion
  • 4% cream, solution
  • 5% patch, cream, ointment
  • 10% patch for iontophoresis (LidoSite® Topical System)
• Lidocaine or prilocaine 2.5%: EMLA®, various products
• Cetacaine®
  • 14% benzocaine
  • 2% tetracaine gel, solution, ointment, aerosol
	• Lidocaine
	  • 2%, 4%, 5% compounded in various products
	  • FDA warning on the risk of potentially fatal arrhythmias with compounded lidocaine products
	• Prilocaine, various products
	• Bupivacaine, various products
	• Tetracaine, various products

Nonsteroidal Anti-inflammatory Drugs (NSAIDs)	
• Diclofenac 1.5% transdermal patch (Flector®) • Diclofenac 1% gel (Voltaren®) • Diclofenac 3% gel (Solaraze®)	• Diclofenac • Ketoprofen 4%, 5%, 10% • Flurbiprofen 5% • Ibuprofen 2% • Indomethacin • Piroxicam 0.5%, 2%
NMDA Receptor Antagonists	
• None	• Ketamine 5%, 10%, 15%, 20% • Dextromethorphan • Amantadine
Opioids	
• Fentanyl, various products (see I. K. 1. c. for more information on Fentanyl)	• Hydromorphone • Morphine • Methadone
Other	
• None	• Baclofen 5% • Orphenadrine • Cyclobenzaprine 0.5%, 1%, 2% • Clonidine 0.2% • Guanethidine 1%, 2%

Table 14-2 Topical Compounds for Pain Management Over the Counter

Local Anesthetics
• Lidocaine 0.5% spray, gel, cream, ointment (Solarcaine®, various products)
• Lidocaine 2.5% spray (Bactine®)
• Benzocaine 6.3% liquid, gel (Anbesol®)
• Pramoxine 1% cream, ointment, aerosol, pads (Tucks®, ProctoFoam®, various products)
Salicylates
• Methyl salicylate 30% cream (Icy Hot®, Bengay Ultra Strength®, various products)
• Trolamine salicylate 10% cream (Aspercreme®, Sportscreme®, various products)
Counterirritants
• Menthol 16% ointment (Maximum Strength Flexall®, various products)
• Menthol 5% transdermal (Icy Hot Back Pain Relief®, various products)
• Menthol 1.3% and Camphor 1.3% ointment (Mentholatum®, various products)
Capsaicin
• 0.25%, 0.5%, 0.75% cream, lotion, gel (Zostrix®, Capsaicin®, various products)
• 0.75% roll-on (No Pain-HP®)

g. Flurbiprofen (Ansaid®)
h. Ibuprofen (Motrin®, Advil®)
i. Indomethacin (Indocin®, Indocin SR®)
j. Ketoprofen (Orudis®, Orudis KT®)
k. Ketorolac (Toradol®)
l. Meclofenamate (Meclomen®)
m. Mefenamic acid (Ponstel®)
n. Meloxicam (Mobic®)
o. Nabumetone (Relafen®)
p. Naproxen (Naprosyn®, Aleve®)
q. Piroxicam (Feldene®)
r. Salsalate (Disalcid®)
s. Sulindac (Clinoril®)
t. Tolmetin (Tolectin®)

2. Celecoxib (Celebrex®) is a selective COX-2 inhibitor (American Pain Society [APS], 2002). The COX-2 enzyme isoform is produced in tissues after injury occurs. The COX-2 enzyme is induced by inflammatory stimuli and cytokines (i.e., bacterial lipopolysaccharide, interleukins, and tumor necrosis factor). Selective NSAIDs that inhibit COX-2 reduce inflammation at the tissue site but exert no effect on COX-1.

K. Opioids (Appendices 14–9A through 14–9C)
1. Receptor agonists are exogenous opioids selective for μ-receptors that mimic endogenous endorphins and enkephalins to produce supraspinal or spinal analgesia (Table 14–3). Pure μ-agonists are strong opioids and typically require only a small percentage (10% to 20%) of the available receptors to be occupied to produce a maximum pharmacological response (Janicki & Parris, 2003).
   a. Alfentanil (Alfenta®)
   b. Codeine (various products)
   c. Fentanyl
      (1) Intravenous (Sublimaze®)
      (2) Oral transmucosal fentanyl citrate (OTFC; Actiq®) (Aronoff, Brennan, Pritchard, & Ginsberg, 2005)

Table 14-3 Opioid Receptor Agonists

Opioid Receptor	Endogenous Opioid	Exogenous Opioid	Antagonist
Mu (μ)	Enkephalin	Alfentanil	Naloxone
	β-Endorphin	Codeine	Pentazocine
		Fentanyl	Nalbuphine
		Hydrocodone	
		Hydromorphone	
		Levorphanol	
		Meperidine	
		Morphine	
		Methadone	
		Oxycodone	
		Oxymorphone	
		Propoxyphene	
		Remifentanil	
		Sufentanil	
Kappa (κ)	Dynorphin A	Levorphanol	Naloxone
		Pentazocine	
Delta (δ)	Enkephalin	Levorphanol	Naloxone
		Oxymorphone	

(3) Fentanyl buccal tablet (FBT, Fentora®) (Blick & Wagstaff, 2006)
(4) Transdermal (Duragesic®) (Skaer, 2004)
(5) Fentanyl iontophoretic transdermal system (ITS, Ionsys®) (Herndon, 2007)

d. Hydrocodone (various oral combinations with acetaminophen)
e. Hydromorphone (Dilaudid®)
f. Levorphanol (Levo-Dromoran®)
g. Meperidine (Demerol®, Pethidine®)
h. Methadone (Lugo, Satterfield, & Kern, 2005)
   (1) Intravenous (various products)
   (2) Oral solution (Methadose®, various products)
   (3) Oral tablets (Dolophine®, Methadose® discontinued)
   (4) Oral-dispersible 40-mg tablet restricted to maintenance programs (Methadose®, Methadone® diskette)
i. Morphine
   (1) Short-acting formulations (various products)
   (2) Long-acting oral formulations (MS Contin®, Oramorph®, Kadian®, Avinza®)
   (3) Extended-release liposomal suspension, epidural (DepoDur®) (Keck, Glennon, & Ginsberg, 2007)
   (4) Intraspinal preparations, preservative free (Duramorph®, Astramorph®)
j. Oxycodone (Oxycontin®, various oral combinations with acetaminophen)
k. Oxymorphone (Chamberlin, Cottle, Neville, & Tan, 2007)
   (1) Intravenous (Opana®, Numorphan® discontinued)
   (2) Oral immediate-release tablet (Opana®)
   (3) Oral extended-release tablet (Opana ER®)

l. Propoxyphene (Darvocet®, Darvon®) (Barkin, Barkin, & Barkin, 2006)
m. Remifentanil (Ultiva®)
n. Sufentanil (Sufenta®)

2. Partial agonists are exogenous opioids with mixed μ- and κ-receptor activity to produce spinal analgesia. These opioids require 75% to 100% receptor occupancy to produce a maximum response (Janicki & Parris, 2003).
   a. Buprenorphine (Buprenex®) is a partial μ-agonist and κ-antagonist (Heit & Gourlay, 2008).
   b. Butorphanol (Stadol®) is a partial μ-agonist and partial κ-agonist (Rozen, Ling, & Schade, 2005).
   c. Nalbuphine (Nubain®) is a μ-antagonist and κ-agonist (Rozen et al., 2005).
   d. Pentazocine (Talwin®) is a partial μ-agonist and partial κ-agonist (Rozen et al., 2005).
3. Antagonists competitively interact at opioid receptors to displace the opioid, producing reversal of analgesia, recovery from respiratory depression, relief of opioid-induced constipation, and treatment of opioid withdrawal.
   a. Nonselective for a receptor, central acting
      (1) Nalmefene (Revex®) is an intravenous form for opioid withdrawal treatment or overdose.
      (2) Naloxone (Narcan®) is for opioid overdose and opioid–induced constipation (off-label use) (Clarke, Dargan, & Jones, 2005).
      (3) Naltrexone comes in two forms:
         (a) Oral tablets (ReVia®) for opioid withdrawal treatment
         (b) Intravenous extended-release suspension (Vivitrol®) for opioid overdose
   b. Selective for a μ-receptor, peripheral acting
      (1) Alvimopan (Entereg®) is for postoperative ileus (Kraft, 2007).
      (2) Methylnaltrexone (Relistor®) is for opioid-induced constipation in palliative care (DeHaven-Hudkins, DeHaven, Little, & Techner, 2007; Thomas et al., 2008).

L. Steroids (Appendices 14-10A through 14-10C)
   1. Glucocorticoid steroids bind to the glucocorticoid receptor in the cellular cytoplasm. Exogenous steroid binding activates the receptor by changing the transcription of target genes. This change results in multiple antiinflammatory actions, including blocking production and release of cytokines (e.g., interleukins and tumor necrosis factor) and inhibiting IgE dependent histamine release from basophils. Cortisol, the endogenous glucocorticoid, is suppressed with the administration of exogenous glucocorticoid steroids (Czock, Keller, Rasche, & Haussler, 2005).
      a. Betamethasone (Celestone®)
      b. Dexamethasone (Decadron®)
      c. Methylprednisolone (Medrol®)
      d. Prednisone (Deltasone®)
      e. Triamcinolone (Aristocort®, Kenalog®)
   2. Mineralocorticoid steroids bind to the mineralocorticoid receptors in the kidney, colon, salivary glands, sweat glands, and hippocampus. The endogenous analogue, aldosterone, is converted to cortisone, which interacts with mineralocorticoid receptors. This interaction results in multiple physiological functions, with the most predominant effects on electrolyte and water homeostasis in the body (Czock et al., 2005).
      a. Cortisone (Cortizone®, Cortone®)
      b. Fludrocortisone (Florinef®)
      c. Hydrocortisone (Cortef®, Hydrocortone®, Solu-Cortef®)

M. Serotonin agonists (Appendix 14–11)
   1. Agonists bind to serotonin 5-HT_{1B} and 5-HT_{1D} receptors located on the trigeminal nerve. This leads to inhibition of firing of serotoninergic neurons and reduction in the synthesis and release of serotonin, resulting in vasoconstriction of dural blood vessels (Ahn & Basbaum, 2005; Moskowitz, 2007).

   a. Almotriptan (Axert®)
   b. Eletriptan (Relpax®)
   c. Frovatriptan (Frova®)
   d. Naratriptan (Amerge®)
   e. Rizatriptan (Maxalt®)
   f. Sumatriptan (Imitrex®)
   g. Zolmitriptan (Zomig®)

N. Miscellaneous
   1. Acetaminophen (Tylenol®) inhibits prostaglandin synthetase in the central nervous system to produce pain relief and reduction of fever. It has weak peripheral antiinflammatory activity (Appendix 14–12A) (Barkin, 2001; Smith, 2003). It also reinforces descending inhibitory serotonergic pain pathways (Pickering et al., 2008).
   2. Tramadol (Ultram®) weakly binds to μ-opioid receptors and inhibits the reuptake of norepinephrine and serotonin (Appendix 14–12B).
   3. Ergot alkaloids, at therapeutic doses, produce peripheral vasoconstriction by stimulating α-adrenergic receptors. At high doses, they act as competitive α-adrenergic blocker. Vascular headaches are aborted through direct vasoconstriction of the dilated carotid artery producing the headache. Serotonin agonist activity also is induced by ergot alkaloids (Appendix 14–11) (Saper & Silberstein, 2006).
   4. Ethanol augments inhibitory effects (especially when combined with benzodiazepines) at the $GABA_A$ receptor/Cl^- ion channel complex and at low doses inhibits glutamate-activated NMDA receptors.
   5. Capsaicin induces release of substance P, the principal chemomediator of pain impulses from the periphery to the central nervous system, from peripheral sensory neurons. After repeated application, capsaicin depletes the neuron of substance P and prevents reaccumulation. Refer to Table 14–2 for products (Stanos, 2007).
   6. Tetrahydrocannabinol (THC) is a synthetic oral cannabinoid formulation designed to replicate naturally occurring cannabis (endocannabinoids). The endocannabinoid system consists of CB_1 and CB_2 receptors that are molecular targets of Δ^9-THC (stated delta 9 THC). CB_1 is found mainly in the brain and causes the psychological effects of THC. CB_2 is found in the immune system. Both receptors are activated by G protein-linked mechanisms to produce weak modulatory effects for neuronal transmission.
      a. Endocannabinoids and CB_1 receptor distributions are not always equal in their locations in the brain. However, adaptation occurs with either the endocannabinoids or the receptors to create an equal balance (Fride, 2005).
      b. Endocannabinoids play a role in brain plasticity, leading to long-term effects on movement and coordination, habit formation, and reward and addiction.
      c. Endocannabinoids may be found to play a role in most if not all brain function. This research is recent and complex.
         (1) Dronabinol (Marinol®) is FDA approved for treatment of chemotherapy-induced nausea, vomiting, or both and human immunodeficiency virus-induced anorexia.
         (2) Nabilone (Cesamet®) is FDA approved for refractory nausea, vomiting, or both secondary to chemotherapy (Hall, Christie, & Currow, 2005; McCarberg, 2007).

II. Pharmacokinetics and Pharmacodynamics

Nurses must have a thorough understanding of applied pharmacology as they administer and potentially intervene in any of these phases of drug administration (Box 14-2). Direct administration of medication incorporates an understanding of onset of action, steady-state plasma levels, duration, and elimination of the medications given (Table 14-4) (Gutierrez, 1999)

A. Absorption
   1. Absorption is passive diffusion of a drug molecule across a lipid membrane into the circulation. The rate and extent of absorption determines when a drug becomes available to exert its action,

Box 14-2 Drug Efficacy Definitions

Pharmaceutics

Drug formulation properties include dosage form, dissolution, disintegration, and route of administration.

Pharmacokinetics

Pharmacokinetics is the biological process by which a drug is transported to target site, detoxified, and excreted from the body. The abbreviation ADME represents absorption, distribution, metabolism (biotransformation), and elimination.

Pharmacodynamics

Pharmacodynamics is the effect of a drug at its site of action, including drug-receptor interactions, dose-response relationship, drug interactions, and physiological variation (age, gender, genetics).

influencing duration and intensity of drug action. Absorption allows distribution, metabolism, and excretion to occur.

a. Factors that influence drug absorption
   (1) *Solubility:* Water-soluble drugs are absorbed readily.
   (2) *Concentration:* High drug concentrations are absorbed more rapidly at the site of administration compared with lower concentrations.
   (3) *Gastric pH:* This pH affects the solubility of drugs. The stomach mucosa is a buffer system with a gradient that ranges from a pH of 1 to 2 on the luminal side to a pH of 6 to 7 on the epithelial cells. The pH of the drugs has an effect on gastric absorption.
   (4) *Gastric emptying rate:* This is the rate at which the stomach empties into the duodenum of the small intestine.
   (5) *Blood flow:* The amount of blood flow to the site of administration is a factor. Heat or massage at the site of administration increases blood flow and rate of absorption; vasoconstrictors and shock conditions decrease blood flow and rate of absorption.
   (6) *Surface area:* Rapid absorption occurs from the surface of the cell membrane, such as the pulmonary alveolar epithelium, intestinal mucosa, or layers of the skin.
   (7) Dosage form variations prevent
      (a) Decomposition of drugs by gastric secretion.
      (b) Dilution of the drug before it reaches the intestine.
      (c) Nausea and vomiting from stomach irritation.
      (d) Immediate release of a drug into the stomach.
b. *Bioavailability* is the percentage of active drug substances absorbed and available to tissues after administration. Absorption varies with different routes of administration (Roberts, Keir, & Hanks, 1998; Severijnen, Baat, Bakker, Tolboom, & Bongaerts, 2004).
   (1) *Gastric absorption* primarily occurs in the stomach and small intestine. The rate of gastric emptying can increase or decrease drug absorption. The gastric emptying rate can be increased by taking some medications on an empty stomach and drinking a lot of water to allow dissolution, rapid passage into the small intestine, and drug absorption into a large surface area. Upright body position assists this process.
   (2) The *small intestine* is highly vascular, has numerous villi, and creates a larger absorption area than the stomach. The intestinal fluids are alkaline, with a pH of 7 or 8. Increased intestinal motility decreases exposure of drugs to the small intestine and decreases absorption. Drug bioavailability (e.g., the amount that reaches systemic circulation) depends on the following:
      (a) Extent of first-pass metabolism in small intestine (e.g., mucosa and flora) and liver

Table 14-4 Mode of Analgesic Medication Administration

Intervention	Advantages	Disadvantages
Oral Nonopioid Analgesics Examples: Acetaminophen, aspirin, NSAIDs, antidepressants, anticonvulsants, serotonin agonists	1. Primary therapy for headache, inflammation, or neuropathic pain 2. Low risk of drug addiction 3. Additive analgesia when combined with opioids and other treatment modalities 4. Ease of administration	1. Ceiling dose limit because of major side effects 2. Most forms are for oral administration, which results in slower onset of action 3. Drug interactions with other medications
Oral Opioid Analgesics Examples: Fentanyl, hydrocodone, morphine, methadone, hydromorphone	1. For acute or chronic pain 2. No ceiling dose limit on single opioid medications unless adverse effects of excessive sedation or respiratory depression 3. Multiple routes of administration 4. Extended-release oral dose forms	1. Tolerance possible with long-term administration 2. Addiction in patients with a high risk of chemical dependency 3. Ceiling dose limit with opioid combinations containing acetaminophen 4. Constipation prophylaxis needed
Rectal	1. Alternative when no oral or intravenous routes access 2. Many suppository combinations	1. Not widely accepted by patients 2. Slow onset of action
Transdermal	1. For patients who cannot take medications orally 2. Continuous medication administration without the use of pumps or needles 3. Ease of administration	1. Restrictions on use for acute postoperative pain and in opioid-naïve patients 2. Slow onset of action with initial subcutaneous depot formation (i.e., fentanyl) 3. Side effects of respiratory depression and sedation may not be quickly reversed 4. Difficult to titrate dose 5. Additional short-acting medication required for breakthrough pain 6. Constipation prophylaxis with opioids
Subcutaneous	1. Rapid pain relief without intravenous access 2. Hydromorphone or morphine preferred 3. For PCA administration	1. Volume limitations for infusion (2–4 ml/hr) 2. Risk of induration and irritation at infusion site 3. Constipation prophylaxis with opioids
Intravenous	1. Rapid relief for severe pain 2. Bolus dosing, continuous infusion, and PCA modes	1. Skilled nursing and pharmacy support required 2. Infusion pump required for continuous and PCA modes 3. Constipation prophylaxis with opioids
Intraspinal	1. Useful for pain that is unresponsive to less invasive measures 2. Greater analgesia possible with local anesthetics	1. Tolerance may occur sooner than with oral administration 2. Risk of central nervous system infection 3. Pruritus and urinary retention more common than with oral and IV administration 4. Special expertise required from anesthesiologists 5. Careful monitoring needed at initiation of therapy and with dose adjustments 6. Skilled nursing and pharmacy support required 7. Infusion pump required for continuous and PCA administration

NSAID, nonsteroidal antiinflammatory drug; PCA, patient-controlled analgesia.

(b) Physical characteristics of the drug
(1) *Solid form:* Tablets need to disintegrate before being absorbed into the small intestine. Enteric-coated tablets and controlled- or sustained-release tablets delay drug dissolution and are slower to be absorbed. Capsule and powder forms are absorbed more rapidly.
(2) *Liquid form:* Liquids are absorbed more rapidly for gastrointestinal absorption than solid form.
(c) Capacity to absorb drugs (e.g., emesis, gastrectomy, and extensive intestine and bowel resection limit drug absorption); for example, roux-en-y gastric bypass decreases small intestine absorption of medications and nutrients (Miller & Smith, 2006; Severijnen et al., 2004)
(1) The procedure bypasses the duodenum and jejunum.
(2) Decreased intestinal length leads to reduced absorption of extended-release oral drug formulations.

c. *Sublingual (under the tongue) and buccal (between the teeth and the mucous membrane of the cheek)* (Reisfield & Wilson, 2007) absorption from the oral mucosa of the mouth delivers drug directly into the venous blood flow going to the superior vena cava. Drugs absorbed rapidly by this route have minimal first-pass metabolism by the liver. The sublingual mucosa is the most permeable region in the oral cavity, with a thickness of 100 to 200 μm (micrometers). In contrast, the buccal mucosa is 500 to 800 μm in thickness.
d. *Rectal absorption* delivers the drug into the superior, middle, and inferior rectal veins. Drugs absorbed into the middle and inferior rectal veins directly reach the systemic circulation without hepatic alteration. The superior rectal vein drains into the portal system and exposes the drug to first-pass metabolism. Extent of absorption depends on rectal content, localized irritation, and drug retention (Roberts et al., 1998).
e. The *intravenous route* depends on blood flow. The drug is administered directly into the systemic circulation, and the absorption process is not necessary. First-pass metabolism is circumvented with this route of administration. Intravenous administration should be slow to prevent adverse effects.
f. *Subcutaneous absorption* is slow. The drug is administered beneath the skin into the connective tissue or fat under the dermis. The drug solubility and vasoconstriction of blood vessels cause delays in drug absorption. With continuous drug administration, the rate of drug delivery into the systemic circulation is similar to an intravenous infusion. First-pass metabolism is circumvented with this route of administration.
g. The *intramuscular absorption* rate depends on blood flow and generally is more rapid with administration in the deltoid or vastus lateralis muscles. Drug absorption in the gluteus maximus is slower, especially in women because of increased subcutaneous fat. Absorption can be altered in obese or emaciated patients. Repeated injections can cause scar tissue, which also affects absorption. First-pass metabolism is circumvented with this route.
(1) The intramuscular route is not recommended for pain management because it is painful; absorption varies and can be unpredictable; and it delivers a large bolus of opioid in an infrequent schedule, creating peaks and valleys of blood levels.
(2) Typically, intramuscular orders are written as PRN (as needed) orders. With PRN orders, the patient has to
(a) Hurt first.
(b) Ask for pain medications.
(c) Receive the intramuscular administration.
(d) Wait for onset of action.
(e) Become sedated and sleep.
(f) Awaken in pain again to ask for more pain medications.
(3) Intramuscular and PRN orders set the patient up for pain because of delayed adminis-

tration, variable dosing, irritation of the injection site, variable absorption effects, and severe tissue damage (Small, 2004).

h. *Intraarterial absorption* depends on blood flow because the drug is injected directly into an artery. First-pass metabolism is circumvented with this route.
i. *Intraperitoneal absorption* uses the large surface area of the abdomen for administration of drugs that enter into the portal vein circulation. First-pass metabolism can occur with this route of administration.
j. *Pulmonary absorption* uses the large surface area of the pulmonary epithelium and mucous membranes. Entry into the systemic circulation is virtually instantaneous, and first-pass metabolism is circumvented.
k. *Cutaneous absorption* includes topical application of drugs to mucous membranes of the conjunctiva, nasopharynx, oropharynx, vagina, colon, urethra, and urinary bladder for local effects. Generally, there is minimal systemic absorption.
l. *Topical (skin) absorption* can be obtained from drugs formulated in ointments or transdermal patches. Normally, compounds are lipid-soluble compounds. The skin must be intact to prevent an increase in systemic absorption of potentially toxic chemicals. Massaging the skin enhances absorption because the capillaries become dilated and local blood flow increases (Stanos, 2007). Refer to Tables 14-1 and 14-2 for topical products.
    (1) *Transdermal (passive)* (Grond, Radbruch, & Lehmann, 2000) cutaneous permeation of drugs is primarily mediated by diffusion. Diffusion into the systemic circulation varies depending on the thickness of the lipophilic keratinous stratum corneum (i.e., formation of depot in subcutaneous fat tissue).
    (2) *Transdermal (iontophoresis)* (Herndon, 2007) iontophoretic delivery requires the creation of an external electrical current from positive and negative terminals. Through this mechanism, positively charged, ionizable drug is actively transported into the systemic circulation in a nonsaturable manner (i.e., it does not need to form a depot in the subcutaneous fat tissue).
m. *Intrathecal* refers to a drug injected directly into the spinal subarachnoid space, bypassing the blood-brain barrier (Ghafoor et al., 2007).
n. *Epidural* refers to a drug injected in the space outside the dura mater. For this route to be effective, it is necessary for the drug to diffuse through the dura mater. There also is some vascular uptake of drug, especially with initial administration (Rathmell, Lair, & Nauman, 2005).

B. Distribution
1. *Distribution* is transport of a drug in body fluids from the bloodstream to various tissues of the body and its site of action. *Volume of distribution* defines the drug concentration in the body.
2. Factors that affect drug distribution
    a. Alterations in cardiac output affect volume of fluid distribution.
    b. Regional permeability of the capillaries in muscle, skin, and organs varies for the drug's molecules. The drug distributes first to organs with the largest circulatory supply, such as the heart, kidney, liver, and brain, then redistributes to areas with less blood flow, such as muscle and fat.
    c. Drug accumulation occurs in tissues, especially fat-soluble drugs.
    d. Protein binding occurs, especially albumin and α_1-acid glycoprotein for basic drugs.
    e. Distribution varies with age, gender, and disease states.
    f. Obesity increases the volume of distribution if the drug is distributed in both lean and fat tissues (Casati & Putzu, 2005).
3. Barriers to drug distribution
    a. The blood-brain barrier allows for distribution of lipid-soluble drugs into the brain and cerebrospinal fluid.
    b. Drugs that are lipid insoluble cannot pass through the blood-brain barrier.

c. The placental barrier has membranous layers that separate the blood vessels of the mother and the fetus. The barrier is nonselective, allowing the passage of lipid-soluble and lipid-insoluble drugs, providing the fetus with little protection. Steroid, opioid, and anesthetic agents cross the placental barrier easily.

4. Body fluid distribution
   a. *Cerebrospinal fluid* distribution is restricted by the blood-brain barrier. Blood flow in the central nervous system is permeable to nonpolar, lipid-soluble drugs (e.g., fentanyl). Strongly ionized drugs normally are not permitted to enter the central nervous system from the systemic circulation.
   b. *Plasma protein binding* results in decreased drug availability for tissue distribution (e.g., only an unbound drug can cross tissue membranes). Competitive binding for plasma protein sites can displace other protein-bound drugs. The displaced protein-bound drugs continue to circulate in the bloodstream, remaining inactive and creating a drug reservoir or storage depot. Toxicity may result.
      (1) Caution needs to be used with combining drugs. For example, when warfarin (Coumadin®) is at a stable dose for a patient, and phenytoin is added to the medication regimen, it displaces warfarin. These drugs compete for the binding sites, releasing more free drug of warfarin and creating toxicity (hemorrhage).
      (2) If there is a low albumin level in the blood (as in hepatic damage or body cavity drainage), there is less albumin to bind with and more free drug available to travel to the point of action. Toxicity could result if the normal dosage is given.
   c. *Tissue binding* with fat tissue (adipose tissue) is more likely to occur with lipid-soluble drugs because adipose tissue has low blood flow and is a stable reservoir for drugs.

C. Metabolism (biotransformation)
1. The body eliminates a drug through transformation and excretion. *Drug metabolism* is the chemical reactions involved in the biotransformation of drugs to more water-soluble compounds or metabolites, which are ionized at a physiological pH (i.e., 7.0 to 7.4) and then excreted by the kidneys. Sites of drug metabolism include the liver, intestinal mucosa, kidneys, skin, and lungs (Sweeney & Bromilow, 2006).
   a. The liver is the primary organ for drug metabolism because of its dual blood supply from the hepatic artery (25% of blood flow) and portal vein (75% of blood flow). Gaps (called *fenestrae*) between the endothelial cell lining of hepatic sinusoids allow plasma to make contact with the microvilli of hepatocytes. The cytochrome P450 enzymes are located in the smooth endoplasmic reticulum cell structure inside the hepatocyte. These enzymes create the chemical alterations of drugs (Lee, 2003).
   b. Major factors that affect drug metabolism
      (1) Hormones
         (a) Hyperthyroidism increases metabolism.
         (b) Growth hormone deficiency decreases metabolism.
         (c) Estrogen and progesterone inhibit or induce metabolism.
      (2) Hepatic blood flow affected by severe cardiovascular dysfunction, starvation, or renal problems
         (a) Genetic polymorphism
         (b) Chronic liver disease (e.g., obstructive jaundice or hepatic disease and cirrhosis)
         (c) Age (Aubrun & Marmion, 2007; Delco et al., 2005)
2. Process for drug metabolism
   a. Phase I: Cytochrome P450 (CYP450) monooxygenase system (the name is derived from the enzymes' absorption peak at 450 nm; the "P" signifies red pigment) (Table 14–5) (McKindley & Glen, 2001; Sweeney & Bromilow, 2006).
      (1) First-pass hepatic effect
         (a) Oral medications pass through the portal vein into the liver before entering the general circulation.

Table 14-5 Cytochrome P450

Substrate		Inhibitor		Inducer	
Definition: Drug that is metabolized by the CYP450 enzyme		Definition: Drug that prevents the binding of the substrate to the CYP450 enzyme		Definition: Drug that increases the CYP450 enzyme metabolism of the substrate	
CYP1A2					
Acetaminophen	Imipramine	Amiodarone	Grapefruit juice	Insulin	Smoking
Amitriptyline	Naproxen	Cimetidine	Isoniazid	Omeprazole	Cruciferous vegetables
Caffeine	Ondansetron	Ciprofloxacin	Ketoconazole	Phenobarbital	Char-grilled meats
Cyclobenzaprine	Propranolol	Clarithromycin	Levofloxacin	Phenytoin	
Desipramine	Ropivacaine	Erythromycin	Norfloxacin	Rifampin	
Diazepam	Verapamil	Fluvoxamine	Paroxetine	Ritonavir	
Haloperidol	R-warfarin				
CYP3A4					
Alfentanil	Dronabinol	Cannabinoids	Indinavir	Carbamazepine	
Alprazolam	Fentanyl	Ciprofloxacin	Itraconazole	Dexamethasone	
Amitriptyline	Imipramine	Ciprofloxacin	Ketoconazole	Ethosuximide	
Bupivacaine	Lidocaine	Erythromycin	Propofol	Phenobarbital	
Cannabinoids	Midazolam	Fluconazole	Ritonavir	Phenytoin	
Carbamazepine	Prednisone	Fluoxetine	Verapamil	Primidone	
Cocaine	Ropivacaine	Fluvoxamine		Rifampin	
Codeine	Sertraline	Grapefruit juice		St. John's wort	
Dexamethasone	Trazodone				
Cyclobenzaprine	Temazepam				
Dextromethorphan					
Diazepam					
CYP2C9					
Amitriptyline	Ibuprofen	Amiodarone	Ketoconazole	Phenobarbital	
Diclofenac	Imipramine	Fluconazole	Paroxetine	Rifampin	
Fluoxetine	Phenytoin	Itraconazole	Ritonavir		
Glipizide	S-warfarin	Isoniazid	Sertraline		
			Trimethoprim		
CYP2C19					
Citalopram	Pantoprazole	Cimetidine	Omeprazole	Phenobarbital	
Diazepam	Phenytoin	Fluoxetine	Paroxetine	Rifampin	
Indomethacin	Propranolol	Fluvoxamine Ritonavir			
Omeprazole	Topiramate	Ketoconazole Ritonavir	Sertraline		

(continued)

Table 14-5 (*continued*)

Substrate		Inhibitor		Inducer
CYP2D6				
Amitriptyline	Meperidine	Amiodarone	Fluoxetine	Dexamethasone
Amphetamine	Metoclopramide	Celecoxib	Methadone	Carbamazepine
Codeine	Mexiletine	Cimetidine	Paroxetine	Phenobarbital
Cyclobenzaprine	Morphine	Citalopram	Ritonavir	Phenytoin
Desipramine	Nortriptyline	Cocaine	Sertraline	Rifampin
Dextromethorphan	Ondansetron	Desipramine		Tramadol
Doxepin	Oxycodone			
Fluoxetine	Paroxetine			
Haloperidol	Tramadol			
Hydrocodone	Trazodone			
Imipramine	Venlafaxine			
CYP2E1				
Acetaminophen	Methoxyflurane	Disulfiram	Acetone	Isoniazid
Alcohol	Ropivacaine		Alcohol	
Halothane	Sevoflurane		Fasting	
Isoflurane	Theophylline			Obesity

(b) When certain drugs are metabolized by the hepatic microsomal enzyme system, a small fraction of the drug is available for distribution to produce effect.

(c) In some cases, the first-pass hepatic effect results in complete elimination of the drug, resulting in less pharmacological effect.

(2) Phase I metabolism consists of three types of chemical reactions: oxidation, reduction, and hydrolysis. It is estimated that 90% of drug oxidation involves CYP1A2, CYP3A4, CYP2C9, CYP2C19, CYP2D6, and CYP2E1. The most significant CYP isoenzymes in terms of quantity are CYP3A4 and CYP2D6. CYP enzymes exist predominantly in the liver but also in extrahepatic tissues, including the brain, lungs, intestine, and kidneys. Any drug metabolized by these enzymes is called a substrate (see Table 14-5 for specific drug interactions) (Sweeney & Bromilow, 2006).

(a) *Enzyme inhibition:* The most common type of inhibition reaction is reversible at the CYP450 active site (Sikka, Magauran, Ulrich, & Shannon, 2005).

(i) Competitive inhibition occurs when an inhibitor drug prevents binding of the substrate drug to the active site on the enzyme. This type of inhibition can be overcome by giving more of the substrate drug, thus a reversible process.

(ii) Noncompetitive inhibition occurs when the inhibitor drug binds to another site on the enzyme to form an inactive complex. This type of inhibition cannot be overcome by adding more of the substrate drug.

(b) *Enzyme induction:* This adaptive response protects cells by increasing the detoxification activity of the liver enzymes, thereby decreasing the length of drug effect. For example, if an individual was taking diazepam, the addition of carbamazepine results in increased metabolism of diazepam and a shorter duration of action (Sikka et al., 2005). CYP2E1 is an alcohol-inducible enzyme with a significant role in the metabolism of acetaminophen. CYP2E1 catalyzes the oxidation of acetaminophen to produce the hepatotoxic metabolite N-acetyl-p-benzoquinoneimine. Long-term ethanol use induces CYP2E1 production and increases the production acetaminophen toxic metabolite (Lee, 2003).

(c) *Genetic polymorphism:* The distribution within a population for inheriting liver enzymatic activity is controlled at a single genetic locus. Significant genetic polymorphisms have been described for CYP2C9, CYP2C19, and CYP2D6 (Ingelman-Sundberg, Sim, Gomez, & Rodrigues-Antona, 2007; Sikka et al., 2005).

(i) CYP2C9 constitutes the majority of the CYP2C family. Two allelic variants have been found with a prevalence of 6% to 12% in white populations. Individuals homozygous for each genetic variant are poor metabolizers and require a lower dose of substrate (e.g., warfarin).

(ii) With CYP2C19, up to 20% of Asian Americans and African Americans are homozygous for a defective allele and classified as poor metabolizers. Only about 3% to 5% of Caucasians inherit this deficiency. Poor metabolizers have higher-than-normal plasma concentration of drug substrates from usual doses (e.g., benzodiazepines, proton pump inhibitors, and tricyclic antidepressants).

(iii) With CYP2D6, approximately 5% to 10% of the Caucasian population inherit an autosomal recessive allele on chromosome 22 for this enzyme deficiency and are poor metabolizers of CYP2D6 drug substrates. Only 1% to 4% of African Americans are reported as poor metabolizers. Poor metabolizers have higher plasma drug concentrations and prolonged elimination half-lives of CYP2D6 drug substrates when given at usual doses. Examples of medications include codeine (cannot convert codeine to morphine), paroxetine, venlafaxine, fluoxetine, desipramine, imipramine, nortriptyline, and oxycodone.

b. Phase II: Conjugation reactions are biosynthetic in nature and involve conjugation reactions. The metabolic process combines drugs or phase I metabolites to small endogenous substances. For conjugation reaction to occur, the drugs and metabolites combine with glucuronic acid, sulfate, glycine, or glutathione; this allows drugs and metabolites to be detoxified (Sweeney & Bromilow, 2006).

(1) Glucuronosyltransferases: Uridine diphosphate-glucuronosyltransferases (UGT) are the enzymes that produce glucuronidation reactions. For example, after morphine administration, morphine undergoes CYP450 enzyme metabolism, which produces three metabolites. Two of these metabolites undergo phase II conjugation with glucuronic acid to form the morphine-3-glucuronide (M3G) and morphine-6-glucuronide (M6G).

(a) UGT1A1 is involved in the glucuronidation of morphine, buprenorphine, and nalorphine.

(b) UGT1A3/1A4 is involved in the glucuronidation of tricyclic antidepressants (amitriptyline, doxepin, imipramine, desipramine, and nortriptyline) and lamotrigine.

(c) UGT2B7 is involved in the glucuronidation of benzodiazepines.

D. Elimination

1. *Elimination* is the process whereby drugs and active and inactive metabolites are excreted primarily through the kidneys. The kidneys receive 20% to 25% of the cardiac output and are sensitive to changes in the blood supply.
2. The *clearance* is the volume of blood that is cleared completely of the drug in a unit of time. The *elimination half-life* is the measure of time taken for half the drug in the body to be cleared by the kidney. Half-life depends on the volume of distribution and clearance of the drug. Elimination may occur through the liver, bile, feces, lungs, sweat, and salivary and mammary glands.
3. Elimination in the kidney occurs through passive glomerular filtration, active tubular secretion, and partial reabsorption.

a. Free drugs and water-soluble metabolites are filtered by the glomeruli.

b. Protein-bound drugs do not pass through the glomerular filtration system.
c. After filtration, lipid-soluble drugs are not excreted but instead are reabsorbed by the tubular nephron and reenter the systemic circulation.
d. Nonionized, water-soluble drugs go through the kidney, bypassing the glomerular filtration system, and go through hepatic metabolism before returning to the kidney for excretion.

4. *Hemodialysis:* Substances that normally are excreted by the kidney either completely or partially can be dialyzed out. Examples of these drugs are central nervous system depressants or stimulants and some nonnarcotic analgesics.
5. *Intestinal excretions:* After hepatic metabolism, the metabolite is secreted into the bile, to the duodenum, and eliminated with the feces.
6. Lung excretion
   a. Drugs administered into the respiratory system usually are eliminated by the same system.
   b. These drugs enter by inspiration and are eliminated through expiration.
   c. An example of excretion of a drug through the respiratory system is ethyl alcohol, in which a small amount is eliminated through expiration. The breath can be analyzed for alcohol content.
7. Sweat and salivary gland excretion
   a. Elimination and metabolites in sweat may be responsible for dermatitis and other skin reactions.
   b. When drugs are eliminated through the salivary gland, some patients may complain of tasting the drug.
8. Mammary gland excretion
   a. Breast milk is acidic, and opioids such as morphine sulfate and codeine sulfate are basic; these drugs achieve high concentration in the breast milk.
   b. Weak acids, such as barbiturates, are less concentrated in breast milk. For example, a nursing mother taking medications may give her infant a small amount of drug; however, because the infant has an undeveloped metabolizing system, there may be a cumulative effect.

III. Therapeutic Drug Monitoring (Sirot et al., 2006)

A. Drug levels[s1]
   1. Cmax: peak level of drug (i.e., maximum concentration)
   2. Cmin: trough level of drug (i.e., minimal concentration)
   3. Tmax: time to achieve maximum concentration of drug
   4. Tmin: time to achieve minimum concentration of drug
   5. Steady state: achieved when the plasma drug level remains constant and does not peak or trough significantly. The concentration at steady state (*Css*) depends on the drug elimination and frequency of administration. It takes approximately four drug half-lives to reach a 95% steady-state plasma concentration (see earlier text for a definition of elimination half-life).

B. Pharmacodynamics
   1. *Pharmacodynamics* is the response or effect of tissues to specific chemical agents at various sites in the body. The effects of a drug on the body may be in the form of increasing, decreasing, or replacing enzymes, hormones, or body metabolic functions.
   2. *Mechanism of action* is drug-induced alteration in function at the site of action.
   3. Drug-receptor interaction (Chudler & Bonica, 2001; Ferrante, 1996)
      a. A receptor is a reactive cellular site that binds with a drug to produce an effect.
      b. This is a lock-and-key effect creating a complementary relationship between a certain portion of the drug molecule and the receptor site of the cell.
      c. *Affinity* is the ability of the drug to bind at the receptor site.
      d. *Efficacy* is the ability of the drug to initiate biological activity in that drug-receptor interaction.
      e. An *agonist* produces the effect.
      f. An *antagonist* reverses the effect by competing with the agonist at the receptor.
         (1) *Competitive antagonism* involves an agent with the same affinity for the receptor as the agonist. This competition reduces the effect of the agonist at the receptor site (Box 14–3).

Box 14-3 Example of Opioid Receptor Antagonism

A patient received epidural morphine and develops pruritus. A lower dose of antagonist (0.05 mg of intravenous naloxone) reverses the pruritus, whereas a higher dose (0.4 mg of intravenous naloxone) of antagonist reverses the side effect and the analgesia.

(2) Nonreceptor interactions
   (a) Some drugs require no receptor site affinity to create action. These enter a cell or accumulate along a membrane, where they influence the chemical or physical function along the cell membrane.
   (b) For example, anesthetic agents are lipid-soluble drugs that have similar properties to the cell membranes. They interact with ion (or chemical) exchanges along the cell membranes. The electrochemical gradient between the internal and the external cell membranes regulates the ion flow, such as sodium, calcium, and potassium channels.

4. Drug-enzyme interaction
   a. A drug can produce its effect by interacting with a cellular enzyme.
   b. The enzyme produces a catalyst, and drugs can inhibit the action of specific enzymes, producing an altered response.
5. Nonspecific drug interaction
   a. Cell membranes are lipoproteins that regulate the flow of ions and metabolites and maintain electrochemical propensity between the interior and the exterior surfaces of the cell.
   b. For example, general anesthetics are lipid soluble.
6. Adverse drug reactions (Box 14-4) (Sirot et al., 2006)
   a. Exaggerated drug response
   b. Unwanted effect on an organ system different from that being treated
   c. Allergic or hypersensitivity reaction

Box 14-4 Adverse Drug Reaction Examples

Overdose or Toxicity

Example: High opioid dose results in respiratory depression.

Side Effect

Example: Constipation is caused by chronic opioid use.

Drug Interaction

Example: Torsades de pointes (QT_c prolongation) results from inhibition of haloperidol metabolism by CYP2D6 when methadone is started.

Allergic (Hypersensitivity or Immunological)

Example: Anaphylactic reactions involve an immune response created by antigen binding to immunoglobulin E (IgE) antibodies.

Pseudoallergic (Nonimmunological)

Example: Administration of morphine by intravenous or oral routes can cause nonimmunological degranulation of mast cells to release histamine in a dose-dependent fashion. Patients who are sensitive to changes in histamine levels may experience an itching or burning sensation, most commonly on the face, chest, and trunk.

Box 14-5 High-Risk Drugs for QT_c Prolongation

Amiodarone (Cordarone®, Pacerone®)
Chlorpromazine (Thorazine®)
Clarithromycin (Biaxin®)
Disopyramide (Norpace®)
Droperidol (Inapsine®)
Erythromycin
Haloperidol (Haldol®)
Methadone (Dolophine®)
Pentamidine (Pentam®)
Pimozide (Orap®)
Procainamide (Pronestyl®, Procan®)
Quinidine (Cardioquin®)
Sotalol (Betapace®)
Sparfloxacin (Zagam®)
Thioridazine (Mellaril®)

d. Idiosyncratic reaction
   (1) Drug interaction causing either increased or decreased response
e. Side effect
   (1) A dose-related predictable reaction to a drug is seen.
   (2) This has been observed with frequency in the population.
   (3) It is expected based on the pharmacological activity of the agent (Fincham, 1991).
f. Variables affecting adverse drug reactions
   (1) Patient variables
      (a) Elderly
      (b) Neonates
      (c) Genetic factors (e.g., CYP450 enzyme deficiencies)
   (2) Drug variables
      (a) Route of administration
      (b) Product formulation
      (c) Duration of therapy
   (3) Drug-induced diseases

7. *Toxic effects* result from excessive drug levels given to or taken by the patient.
8. Drug interaction
   a. Drug interaction is a change in magnitude or duration of a response to one drug in the presence of another drug. This change results in an increase or decrease in concentration of drug at the site of action (Boxes 14-4 and 14-5).
   b. Causes of drug interaction
      (1) Rapid or slow biotransformation or metabolism
      (2) Displacement of a drug from plasma protein
      (3) Poor gastrointestinal uptake of drug
      (4) Renal or hepatic impairment resulting in altered clearance of drug (Table 14-6) (Davis, 2007; Dean, 2004; Delco et al., 2005; Looi & Audisio, 2007)
      (5) Modifications in receptor or blocking receptor channels
      (6) Changes in electrolyte balance or body fluid pH
      (7) Changes in rate of protein synthesis
   c. Examples of drug interactions
      (1) *Additive effect:* Two drugs with similar pharmacological action are taken and produce a summed effect.

Table 14-6 Opioid Selection for Side Effect Reduction

Opioid Side Effect Profile	Opioid Selection for Side Effect Reduction
Confusion	Fentanyl
	Hydromorphone
	Oxycodone
Myoclonus	Hydromorphone
Sedation	Tramadol
Impaired Organ Function	**Opioid Selection for Side Effect Reduction**
Hepatic insufficiency	Hydromorphone
	Morphine
Renal insufficiency	Fentanyl
	Hydromorphone
	Methadone
	Oxycodone

(2) *Synergistic effect:* Two drugs with a combined effect greater than the sum of each drug acting alone, produce an increased effect.

(3) *Potentiation:* One drug increases the effect of a second drug (McKenry & Salerno, 1990).

C. Selection of analgesic medications (see also Table 14–6)

1. Pain assessment
2. Route of administration
   a. Patient factors to assess
      (1) Can the patient swallow medications by mouth?
      (2) Is the patient NPO (nothing by mouth) because of abdominal problems or risk of aspiration?
      (3) Does the patient have a colostomy or short bowel, which would decrease medication absorption from the gastrointestinal tract?
      (4) Does the patient have intravenous access?
   b. Mode of medication administration (Table 14–4)
3. Special populations (Box 14–6)

IV. Multimodal Analgesia

A. Multimodal analgesia uses a rational approach to analgesia with a combination of medications and non-medication (see the chapter on Quality Evaluation and Improvement). The American Society of Anesthesiologists Task Force on Acute Pain Management believe that opioids combined with an NSAID, COX-2 inhibitor (coxib), or acetaminophen have opioid "dose-sparing effect" (Ashburn et al., 2004, p. 1576). This task force recommends multimodal analgesia when not contraindicated by comorbidity and scheduling around-the-clock administration of NSAIDs, COX-2 inhibitors, or acetaminophen, in addition to consideration for regional blockade with local anesthetics (Ashburn et al., 2004, p. 1577).

Box 14-6 Special Population Drug Selection

Chemical dependency: see Chapter 26
Geriatrics: see Chapter 22
Moderate sedation: see Chapter 16
Pediatrics: see Chapter 20

B. Multimodal analgesia is rational combinations of analgesics with differing mechanisms of actions. It incorporates pharmacological and nonpharmacological interventions (see the chapters on Cancer Pain Management and Integrative Therapies Used in Pain Management Nursing).

C. Rational for using multimodal analgesic techniques
   1. Such techniques can reduce complications of side effects of opioid analgesia.
   2. Further studies are needed to correlate the use of multimodal analgesia in reducing chronic pain syndrome.

D. Postoperatively, there are abundant pain signals (see the chapter on Neurophysiology of Pain).
   1. These pain signs produce secondary inflammatory responses.
   2. This contributes to prolonged changes in peripheral and central nervous system.
   3. Amplification and prolongation of postoperative pain can result in the following:
      a. Peripheral sensitization
         (1) Results from inflammation at a surgical site
         (2) Results in a lower threshold to activate peripheral pain
      b. Central sensitization
         (1) Results from persistent exposure of the peripheral neurons to painful input
         (2) Results in an increase in excitability of spinal neurons
   4. Both peripheral and central sensitization contributes to spinal windup, which produces a hypersensitive state and a decrease in the pain threshold in injured and uninjured tissue.
   5. Prolonged central sensitization may lead to permanent alterations of the central nervous system.
      a. Changes such as death of inhibitory neurons
      b. Replacement with new afferent excitatory neurons
      c. Establishment of aberrant excitatory synaptic connections (see the chapter on Neurophysiology of Pain)

E. Treatment using multimodal analgesic techniques (see the chapter on Acute Pain Management)
   1. NSAIDs and acetaminophen
      a. These inhibit production of prostaglandins at spinal cord and periphery.
      b. They have an opioid-sparing effect.
      c. They should be administered around-the-clock postoperatively unless contraindicated.
      d. Acetaminophen mechanisms of action remains poorly defined. Speculation regarding COX-3 receptor activity and serotonergic mechanisms are referenced (Hersh, Lally, & Moore, 2005; Pickering et al., 2006).
      e. It is appropriate to administer an NSAID, a COX-2 inhibitor, or acetaminophen unless contraindicated by comorbidity (Ashburn et al., 2004; Carroll, Angst, & Clark, 2004).
   2. $\alpha_2\delta$-ligands (gabapentin and pregabalin)
      a. Gabapentin provides significant analgesia in experimental models of inflammatory pain (Carroll et al., 2004, p. 583).
      b. There are two clinical trials indicating a reduced postoperative pain when gabapentin is "administered preoperatively (1,200 mg) or postoperative (1,200 mg/day)" (Dirks et al., 2002, and Fassoulaki et al., 2002, as cited in Carroll et al., 2004, p. 583).
   3. Local anesthetic and regional analgesia
      a. Peripheral nerve blocks are shown to be opioid sparing, provide superior analgesia, and have greater patient satisfaction. Peripheral nerve blocks of local anesthetic agents can be administered via a single-shot injection or through placement of a catheter in or around a surgical or trauma site for continuous infusion. Studies of peripheral nerve blocks involving surgeries of the upper extremities show the effectiveness of nerve blocks in the axillary, supraclavicular, and interscalene regions (Carroll et al., 2004, p. 584). The literature also supports the use of peripheral nerve blocks in other locations such as intercostal, ilioinguinal, penile, interpleural, or plexus (Ashburn, 2004, p. 1576). The American Society of Anesthesiologists Task Force on Acute Pain Management recommends the use of peripheral nerve block when these can be applied and maintained safely (Ashburn et al., 2004, p. 1576).

b. The literature supports the use of epidural or intrathecal morphine or fentanyl. There is greater associated pruritus and urinary retention with the use of morphine by these routes as compared to systemic administration (Ashburn et al., 2004, p. 1576). The literature is insufficient to describe the side effect profiles of epidural or intrathecal hydromorphone or sufentanil. Local anesthetic agents such as bupivacaine, levobupivacaine, or ropivacaine may be added to the infusion for "selective neural blockade and augment[ed] opioid-mediated analgesia" (Mitra & Sinatra, 2004, p. 222).

4. Ketamine is an analgesic agent and general anesthetic agent that has many pharmacological effects.
   a. NMDA receptors have been linked to nociceptive signal transmission and opioid tolerance.
   b. Ketamine is an NMDA receptor antagonist.
   c. It is best understood as an adjuvant analgesic (Carroll et al., 2004, p. 582; Mitra & Sinatra, 2004, p. 221).
5. α_2-Adrenergic receptor agonists such as clonidine work at the peripheral, spinal, and brain stem sites. Mechanisms of why clonidine creates analgesia are unknown thus far, but it has been shown to potentiate the action of opioids and local anesthetics (Chong, Mungani, & Hill, 2003, p. 413).

V. Preemptive Analgesia

A. Preliminary principles of preemptive analgesia
   1. Analgesic intervention started before nociception is more effective than same intervention after nociception.
   2. The benefit of preemptive analgesia would outlast the duration of action of the analgesic agent used (Ong & Seymour, 2003, p. 159).
   3. Assumptions were that preemptive analgesia provided more effective analgesia, reduced postoperative analgesic requirements, and possibly prevented chronic pain syndromes.

B. Results of a critical analysis between 1981 and 2001 of 27 randomized, controlled trials published indicated the following.
   1. Animal studies show consistent efficacy of preemptive analgesia.
   2. Human studies show conflicting results.
      a. Methodological deficiencies were found with 19 studies.
      b. Analysis showed 4 studies were valid and showed positive preemptive effect.
         (1) One of the positive studies showed preemptive effect of a duration of 11.2 hours using dextromethorphan (Wu et al., 1999, as cited in Ong & Seymour, 2003, p. 171).
      c. Analysis found that 4 studies were valid and showed negative preemptive effect (Ong & Seymour, 2003, p. 169).

C. The validity of preemptive analgesia as a routine presurgical strategy requires further well-designed clinical trials (Ong & Seymour, 2003, p. 170).
   1. The American Society of Anesthesiologists Task Force on Acute Pain Management has found "insufficient literature to evaluate the efficacy of the preoperative initiation of treatment(s) either to reduce preexisting pain, or as part of a multimodal analgesic pain management program" (Ashburn, et al., 2004, p. 1575).
   2. Drs. Paul F. White, Henrik Kehlet, and Spencer Liu write on what is known about perioperative analgesia.
      a. "Postoperative administration of COX-2 inhibitors has consistently been demonstrated to have beneficial effects in improving analgesia, reducing opioid-related side effects, and improving the quality of patient recovery in the early and intermediate postoperative period. However, the potential for long-term clinical benefits remains to be confirmed by other investigative groups" (White, Kehlet, & Liu, 2009, p. 1366–1367)
      b. "There is no longer unequivocal evidence supporting the preemptive effect of NSAIDs and COX-2 inhibitors" (White, Kehlet, & Liu, 2009, p. 1367).
      c. "The ability of a multimodal preemptive analgesic regimen to prevent the development of chronic pain after major orthopedic surgery remains unproven" (White, Kehlet, & Liu, 2009, p. 1367).

Summary

The priorities in using the analgesics described in this chapter in a thoughtful manner are immediate pain control and maintaining pain control. The Acute Pain Management chapter describes goal setting with the patients and setting up goals of care that are intentional, are expedited without hesitancy, and are expected.

References

Ahn, A. H., & Basbaum, A. I. (2005). Where do triptans act in the treatment of migraine? *Pain, 115,* 1–4.

American Pain Society. (2008). Principles of Analgesic Use in the Treatment of Acute Pain and Cancer Pain. Glenville, IL: Author.

American Pain Society. (2002). *Guideline for the management of pain in osteoarthritis, rheumatoid arthritis, and juvenile chronic arthritis.* Glenville, IL: Author.

Aronoff, G. M., Brennan, M. J., Pritchard, D. D., & Ginsberg, B. (2005). Evidence-based oral transmucosal fentanyl citrate (OTFC) dosing guidelines. *Pain Medicine, 6*(4), 305–314.

Ashburn, M. A., Caplan, R. A., Carr, D. B., Connis, R. T., Ginsberg, B., Green, C. R., Lema, M.J., Nickinovich, D.G., & Rice, L.J. (2004). Practice guidelines for acute pain management in the perioperative setting: An updated report by the American Society of Anesthesiologists Task Force on Acute Pain Management. *Anesthesiology, 100*(6), 1573–1581.

Aubrun, F., & Marmion, F. (2007). The elderly patient and postoperative pain treatment. *Best Practice & Research Clinical Anaesthesiology, 21*(1), 109–127.

Barkin, R. L. (2001). Acetaminophen, aspirin or ibuprofen in combination analgesic product. *American Journal Therapeutics, 8,* 433–442.

Barkin, R. L., Barkin, S. J., & Barkin, D. S. (2006). Propoxyphene (dextropropoxyphene): A critical review of a weak opioid analgesic that should remain in antiquity. *American Journal Therapeutics, 13,* 534–542.

Bateson, A. N. (2004). The benzodiazepine site of the $GABA_A$ receptor: An old target with new potential. *Sleep Medicine, 5*(Suppl. 1), S9–S15.

Beebe, F. A., Barkin, R. L., & Barkin, S. (2005). A clinical and pharmacological review of skeletal muscle relaxants for musculoskeletal conditions. *American Journal Therapeutics, 12,* 151–171.

Blick, S. K., & Wagstaff, A. J. (2006). Fentanyl buccal tablet in breakthrough pain in opioid-tolerant patients with cancer. *Drugs, 66*(18), 2387–2393.

Bredgaard Sorensen, M., Strom, J., Sloth Madsen, P., Angelo, H. R., & Reiz, S. (1984). Haemodynamic, electrocardiographic cardiometabolic changes after overdose of propoxyphene: An experimental study in pentobarbitone-anaesthetized pigs. *Human Toxicology, 3*(Suppl.), 53S–59S.

Carroll, I. R., Angst, M. S., & Clark, J. D. (2004). Management of perioperative pain in patients chronically consuming opioids. *Regional Anesthesia and Pain Medicine, 29,* 576–591.

Casati, A., & Putzu, M. (2005). Anesthesia in the obese patient; pharmacokinetic considerations. *Journal of Clinical Anesthesia, 17,* 134–145.

Challapalli, V., Tremont-Lukats, I. W., McNicol, E. D., Lau, J., & Carr, D. B. (2005). Systemic administration of local anesthetic agents to relieve neuropathic pain. *Cochrane Database of Systematic Reviews,* Issue 4. Retrieved May 24, 2009 from http://www.cochrane.org/reviews/en/ab003345.html.

Chamberlin, K. W., Cottle, M., Neville, R., & Tan, J. (2007). Oral oxymorphone for pain management. *Annals of Pharmacotherapy, 41,* 1144–1152.

Chong, C. A., Mungani, R., & Hill, R. G. (2003). Atypical analgesic drugs and sympathetic blockers. In R. Melzack & P. D. Wall (Eds.), *Handbook of pain management: A clinical companion to Wall and Melzack's textbook of pain* (pp. 413–414). New York: Churchill Livingstone.

Chudler, E. H., & Bonica, J. A. (2001). Supraspinal mechanisms of pain and nociception. In Loesser, J. D. (Ed.), *Bonica's management of pain.* Philadelphia: Lippincott Williams & Wilkins.

Clarke, S. F. J., Dargan, P. I., & Jones, A. L. (2005). Naloxone in opioid poisoning: Walking the tightrope. *Emergency Medicine Journal, 22,* 612–616.

Czock, D., Keller, F., Rasche, F., & Haussler, U. (2005). Pharmacokinetics and pharmacodynamics of systemically administered glucocorticoids. *Clinical Pharmacokinetics, 44*(1), 61–98.

Davis, M. (2007). Cholestasis and endogenous opioids: Liver disease and exogenous opioid pharmacokinetics. *Clinical Pharmacokinetics, 46*(10), 825–850.

Dean, M. (2004). Opioid in renal failure and dialysis patients. *Journal of Pain and Symptom Management, 28,* 497–504.

DeHaven-Hudkins, D. L., DeHaven, R. N., Little, P. J., & Techner, L. M. (2008). The involvement of the mu opioid receptor in gastrointestinal pathophysiology: Therapeutic opportunities for antagonism at this receptor. *Pharmacology and Therapeutics, 117,* 162–187.

Delco, F., Tchambaz, L., Schlienger, R., Drewe, J., Krahenbuhl, S. (2005). Dose adjustment in patients with liver disease. *Drug Safety, 28*(6), 529–545. Dooley, D. J., Taylor, C. P., Donevan, S., & Feltner, D. (2007). Ca^{+2} channel $\alpha_2\delta$ ligands: Novel modulators of neurotransmission. *Trends in Pharmacological Sciences, 28*(2), 75–82.

Ebert, B., Wafford, K. A., & Deacon, S. (2006). Treating insomnia: Current and investigational pharmacological approaches. *Pharmacology and Therapeutics, 112,* 612–629.

Elliott, J. A. (2003). α-2 Agonists (bedside). In H. S. Smith (Ed.), *Drugs in pain* (pp. 201–222). Philadelphia: Hanley and Belfus.

Ferrante, F. M. (1996). Principles of opioid pharmacotherapy: Practical implications of basic mechanisms. *Journal of Pain and Symptom Management, 11,* 265–273.

Fincham, J. E. (1991). An overview of adverse drug reactions. *American Pharmacy, NS31,* 47–52.

Fride, E. (2005). Endocannabinoids in the central nervous system: From neuronal networks to behavior. *Current Drug Targets: CNS & Neurological Disorders, 4,* 633–742.

Gajraj, N. M. (2007). Pregabalin: Its pharmacology and use in pain management. *Anesthesia & Analgesia, 105,* 1805–1815.

Gazelle, G., & Fine, P. G. (2004). Methadone for pain No. 75. *Journal of Palliative Medicine, 7*(2), 303–304.

Ghafoor, V. L., Epshteyn, M., Carlson, G. H., Terhaar, D. M., Charry, O., and Phelps, P. K. (2007). Intrathecal drug therapy for long-term pain management. *American Journal of Health-System Pharmacy, 64,* 2447–2461.

Grond, S., Radbruch, L., & Lehmann, K. A. (2000). Clinical pharmacokinetics of transdermal opioids. *Clinical Pharmacokinetics, 38*(1), 59–89.

Gutierrez, K. (1999). Pharmaceutics and pharmacokinetics. In K. Gutierrez (Ed.), *Pharmacotherapeutics: Clinical decision-making in nursing* (pp. 41–60). Philadelphia: W. B. Saunders.

Hall, W., Christie, M., & Currow, D. (2005). Cannabinoids and cancer: Causation, remediation, and palliation. *Lancet Oncology, 6,* 35–42.

Heavner, J. D. (2007). Local anesthetics. *Current Opinion in Anaesthesiology, 20,* 336–342.

Heit, H. A., & Gourlay, D. L. (2008). Buprenorphine, new tricks with an old molecule for pain management. *Clinical Journal of Pain, 4*(2), 93–97.

Herndon, C. M. (2007). Iontophoretic drug delivery system: Focus on fentanyl. *Pharmacotherapy, 27*(5), 745–754.

Herndon, C. M., Hutchison, R.W., Hildegarde, J.B., Stacy, Z.A., Chen, J.T., Farnsworth, D.D., Dang, D., & Fermo, J.D. (2008). Management of chronic nonmalignant pain with nonsteroidal antiinflammatory drugs. *Pharmacotherapy, 28*(6), 788–805.

Ingelman-Sundberg, M., Sim, S. C., Gomez, A., & Rodrigues-Antona, C. (2007). Influence of cytochrome P450 polymorphisms on drug therapies: Pharmacogenetic, pharmacoepigenetic and clinical aspects. *Pharmacology and Therapeutics, 116,* 496–526.

Iosifescu, D. V., Alpert, J. E., & Fava, M. (2003). Antidepressants: Clinical management. In H. S. Smith (Ed.), *Drugs in pain* (pp. 223–239). Philadelphia: Hanley and Belfus.

Janicki, P. K., & Parris, W. C. (2003). Clinical pharmacology of opioids. In H. S. Smith (Ed.), *Drugs in pain* (pp. 97–118). Philadelphia: Hanley and Belfus.

Keck, S., Glennon, C., & Ginsberg, B. (2007). DepoDur extended release epidural morphine: Reshaping postoperative care—what perioperative nurses need to know. *Orthopaedic Nursing, 26*(2), 86–93.

Kraft, M. (2007). Emerging pharmacologic options for treating postoperative ileus. *American Journal of Health-System Pharmacy, 64*(Suppl. 13), S13–S20.

Krantz, M. J., Martin, J., Stimmel, B., Mehra, D., & Halgney, M. C. P. (2009). QT_c interval screening in methadone treatment. CSAT Consensus Guideline. *Annals of Internal Medicine, 150,* 1, 1–9.

Lee, W. M. (2003). Drug-induced hepatotoxicity. *New England Journal of Medicine, 349,* 474–485.

Looi, Y. C., & Audisio, R. A. (2007). A review of literature on post-operative pain in older cancer patients. *European Journal of Cancer, 43,* 2222–2230.

Loughrey, J. P. R. (2003). Anticonvulsant drugs in the treatment of chronic pain states. In H. S. Smith (Ed.), *Drugs in pain* (pp. 165–182). Philadelphia: Hanley and Belfus.

Lugo, R. A., Satterfield, K. L., & Kern, S. E. (2005). Pharmacokinetics of methadone. *Journal of Pain & Palliative Care Pharmacotherapy, 19*(4), 13–24.

Lundstrom, S., Zachrisson, U., & Furst, C. J. (2005). When nothing helps: Propofol as sedative and antiemetic in palliative cancer care. *Journal of Pain and Symptom Management, 30,* 570–77.

McCarberg, B. H. (2007). Cannabinoids: Their role in pain and palliation. *Journal of Pain and Palliative Care Pharmacotherapy, 21*(3), 19–28.

McKenry, L. M., & Salerno, E. (1990). Principles of drug action. In *Mosby's pharmacology in nursing* (20th ed.). St. Louis: Mosby-Year Book.

McKindley, D. M., & Glen, V. L. (2001). Basic pharmacokinetics, pharmacodynamics and important drug interactions. In K. I. Bland (Ed.), *The practice of general surgery.* Philadelphia: W. B. Saunders.

McNulty, J. P. (2007). Can levorphanol be used like methadone for intractable refractory pain? *Journal of Palliative Medicine, 10*(2), 293–296.

Miller, A. D., & Smith, K. S. (2006). Medication and nutrient administration considerations after bariatric surgery. *American Journal of Health-System Pharmacy, 63,* 1852–1857.

Mitra, S., & Sinatra, R. S. (2004). Perioperative management of acute pain in the opioid-dependent patient. *Anesthesiology, 101*(1), 212–227.

Moskowitz, M. A. (2007). Pathophysiology of headache: Past and present. *Headache, 47*(Suppl. 1), S58–S63.

Nickander, R. C., Smits, S. E., & Steinberg, M. I. (1977). Propoxyphene and norpropoxyphene: Pharmacologic and toxic effects in animals. *American Society for Pharmacology and Experimental Therapeutics, 200*(1), 245–253.

Nickander, R. C., Emmerson, J. L., Hynes, M. D., Steinberg, M. I., & Sullivan, H. R. (1984). Pharmacologic and toxic effects in animals of dextropropoxyphene and its major metabolite. *Human Toxicology, 3*(Suppl.), 13S–36S.

O'Donoghue, M., & Tharp, M. D. (2005). Antihistamines and their role as antipruritics. *Dermatologic Therapy, 18,* 333–340.

Okon, T. (2007). Ketamine: An introduction for the pan and palliative medicine physician. *Pain Physician, 10,* 493–500.

Ong, K. S., & Seymour, R. A. (2003). Evidence-Based medicine approach to pre-emptive analgesia. *American Journal of Pain Management, 13,* 158–172.

Pickering, G., Lorior, M. A., Libert, F., Eschalier, A., Beaune, P., & Dubray, D. (2006). Analgesic effect of acetaminophen in humans: First evidence of a central serotonergic mechanism. *Clinical Pharmacology and Therapeutics, 79,* 371–378.

Ramakrishnan, K., & Scheid, D. C. (2007). Treatment options for insomnia. *American Family Physician, 76,* 517–528.

Rathmell, J. P., Lair, T. R., & Nauman, B. (2005). The role of intrathecal drugs in the treatment of acute pain. *Anesthesia & Analgesia, 101,* S30–S43.

Reisfield, G. M., & Wilson, G. R. (2007). Rational use of sublingual opioids in palliative medicine. *Journal of Palliative Medicine, 10*(2), 465–475.

Roberts, C. J., Keir, S., & Hanks, G. (1998). The principles of drug use in palliative medicine. In D. Doyle, G. W. C. Hanks, & N. MacDonald (Eds.), *Oxford textbook of palliative medicine* (2nd ed., pp. 223–238). New York: Oxford University Press.

Rozen, D., Ling, C., & Schade, C. (2005). Coadministration of an opioid agonist and antagonist for pain control. *Pain Practice, 5*(1), 11–17.

Rudolph, U., & Mohler, H. (2006). GABA-based therapeutic approaches: $GABA_A$ receptor subtype functions. *Current Opinion in Pharmacology, 6,* 18–23.

Saper, J. R., & Silberstein, S. (2006). Pharmacology of dihydroergotamine and evidence for efficacy and safety in migraine. *Headache, 46*(Suppl. 4), S171–S181.

Severijnen, R., Baat, N., Bakker, H., Tolboom, J., & Bongaerts, G. (2004). Enteral drug absorption in patients with a short small bowel. *Clinical Pharmacokinetics, 43*(14), 951–962.

Sikka, R., Magauran, B., Ulrich, A., & Shannon, M. (2005). Bench to bedside: Pharmacogenomics, adverse drug interactions and the cytochrome P450 system. *Academic Emergency Medicine, 12*(12), 1227–1235.

Silberstein, S. D. (1996). Divalproex sodium in headache: Literature review and clinical guidelines. *Headache, 36,* 547–555.

Sindrup, S. H., Otto, M., Finnerup, N. B., & Jensen, T. S. (2005). Antidepressants in the treatment of neuropathic pain. *Basic and Clinical Pharmacology and Toxicology, 96,* 399–409.

Sirot, E. J., van der Velden, J.W., Rentsch, K., Eap, C.B., Baumann, P.(2006). Therapeutic drug monitoring and pharmacogenetic tests as tools in pharmacovigilance. *Drug Safety, 29*(9), 735–768.

Skaer, T. L. (2004). Practice guidelines for transdermal opioids in malignant pain. *Drugs, 64*(23), 2629–2638.

Sloth Madsen, P., Strom, J., Reiz, S., & Bredgaard Sorensen, M. (1984). Acute propoxyphene self-poisoning in 222 consecutive patients. *Acta Anaesthesiology Scandinavia, 6,* 661–665.

Small, S. P. (2004). Preventing sciatic nerve injury from intramuscular injections: Literature review. *Journal of Advanced Nursing, 47*(3), 287–296.

Smith, H. S. (2003). Acetaminophen (bench). In H. S. Smith (Ed.), *Drugs in pain* (pp. 223–239). Philadelphia: Hanley and Belfus.

Stander, S., & Schmelz, M. (2006). Chronic itch and pain: Similarities and differences. *European Journal of Pain, 10,* 473–478.

Stanos, S. P. (2007). Topical agents for the management of musculoskeletal pain. *Journal of Pain and Symptom Management, 33,* 342–355.

Sweeney, B. P., & Bromilow, J. (2006). Liver enzyme induction and inhibition: Implications for anaesthesia. *Anaesthesia, 61,* 159–177.

Thomas, J., Karver, S., Cooney, G. A., Slatkin, N. (2008). Methylnaltrexone for opioid-induced constipation in advanced illness. *New England Journal of Medicine, 358,* 2332–2343.

U.S. Drug Enforcement Administration. (2005). Schedules of controlled substances: Placement of pregabalin into schedule V. Final rule. *Federal Register, 70*(144), 43633–43635. Retrieved December 19, 2008, from http://www.ncbi.nlm.nih.gov/sites/entrez?Db=pubmed&Cmd=ShowDetailView&TermToSearch=16050051&log$=activity.

White, P.F., Kehlet, H., Liu, S. (2009). Perioperative analgesia: What do we still know? International Anesthesia Research Society, 108, 5, 1364–1367.

Suggested Readings

Hersh, E. V., Lally, E. T., & Moore, P. A. (2005). Update on cyclooxygenase inhibitors: Has a third COX isoform entered the fray? *Current Medical Research and Opinion, 21,* 1217–1226.

Institute for Clinical Systems Improvement. (2007). *Assessment and management of chronic pain* (2nd ed.). Retrieved June 10, 2009[s2], from http://www.icsi.org.

Jacox, A., Carr, D. B., Payne, R., Berde, C.B., Breibart, W. Cain, J.M., Chapman, C.R., Cleeland, C.S., Ferrell, B.T., Finley, R.S., Hester, N.O., Stratton Hill, C., Leak, W.D., Lipman, A.G., Logan, C.L., McGarvey, C.L., Miaskowski, C.A., Mulder, D.S., Paice, J.A., Shapiro, B.S., Silberstein, E.B., Smith, R.S., Stover, J., Tsou, C.V., Vecchiarelli, L., & Weissman, D.E. (1994). *Management of cancer pain.* Clinical Practice Guideline No. 9. (AHCPR Publication No. 94-0592.) Rockville, MD: Agency for Health Care Policy and Research, Public Health Service, U.S. Department of Health and Human Services.

Preskorn, S. H. (1997). Clinically relevant pharmacology of selective serotonin reuptake inhibitors. *Clinical Pharmacokinetics, 32*(Suppl. 1), 1–21.

appendix

14-1

α_2-Agonists (Adult Drug Doses)

Name	Route	Average Dose Range	Average Dose Interval	Maximal Daily Dose	Half-Life (hours)	Clinically Important Metabolites (Active)
Clonidine (Catapres®)	PO	0.1–0.2 mg	bid	2.4 mg/d	6–20	None
	Major side effects: Bradycardia, severe rebound hypertension, orthostatic hypotension, constipation, dry mouth, pruritus **Monitoring:** Blood pressure, heart rate, pulse **Dose adjustment:** Do not discontinue dose abruptly. Reduce dose gradually over 2–4 days to prevent severe rebound hypertension. Administer 4–6 hours before surgery. Reduce initial dose 50% to 75% for patients with creatinine clearance of less than 10 ml/min.					
(Catapres-TTS®)	TD	0.1-to 0.3-mg patch	Applied every 7 days			None
	Major side effects: Same as clonidine, dermatitis with patch **Monitoring:** Blood pressure, heart rate, pulse **Dose adjustment:** Therapeutic plasma levels are achieved 2–3 days after initial patch application. Patients need oral clonidine for 1–2 days during initial transition from oral clonidine to the transdermal therapeutic system (TTS) patch. Remove transdermal systems when attempting defibrillation or synchronized cardioversion because of electrical conductivity. Gradually reduce dose to prevent severe rebound hypertension.					
Dexmedetomidine (Precedex®)	IV	Loading infusion: 1 microgram/kg over 10 minutes Maintenance infusion: 0.2–0.7 microgram/kg/hr				
	Major side effects: Hypotension, bradycardia, atrial fibrillation, nausea **Monitoring:** Blood pressure, heart rate, pulse (monitor continuously) **Dose adjustment:** Administer only if skilled in management of patients in an intensive care setting.					
Tizanidine (Zanaflex®)	PO	4 mg	q6–8 hours	36 mg/d	2.5	None
	Major side effects: Anxiety, depression, dizziness, sedation, weakness, abdominal pain, diarrhea, dry mouth, dyspepsia, rash, skin ulcers, sweating, hypotension **Monitoring:** Liver function at 1, 3, and 6 months; pain; muscle stiffness; ROM **Dose adjustment:** Increase by 2–4 mg per dose up to 36 mg/d.					

bid, twice daily; IV, intravenously; PO, orally; ROM, range of motion; TD, transdermally.

appendix

14-2

Anticonvulsants (Adult Drug Doses)

Name	Route	Average Dose Range (mg)	Average Dose Interval	Maximal Daily Dose (mg)	Half-Life (hours)	Clinically Important Metabolites (Active)
Note: Drug doses for pain management are less than those for seizure management.						
Carbamazepine	PO	200–400	bid	600	15 ± 5	10,11-epoxide
(Tegretol®, Tegretol-XR®, Epitol®, Carbatrol®)	**Major side effects:** Stevens-Johnson syndrome (patients of Asian ancestry with HLA-B 1502 gene allele are at high risk), neutropenia, aplastic anemia, hepatitis, rash, edema, sedation, ataxia, confusion, hyponatremia **Monitoring:** Plasma drug levels greater than 12 microgram/ml are associated with CNS side effects. Check CBC with platelet count and liver function tests periodically. Use serum creatinine for patients with renal impairment. **Dose adjustment:** Decrease the dose by 75% for creatinine clearance of less than 10 ml/min.					
Gabapentin	PO	300–900	tid	3,600	6.5 ± 1	None
(Neurontin®)	**Major side effects:** Somnolence, ataxia, fatigue, nausea, vomiting, peripheral edema **Monitoring:** Routine monitoring of drug level is not required. Use serum creatinine for patients with renal impairment. **Dose adjustment:** Give an initial dose of 300 mg at bedtime; increase by 300 mg every 3 days. Elderly patients should start at 100 mg at bedtime with dose increases not exceeding 100 mg every 3 days. *Decrease dose based on creatinine clearance.*					
	Creatinine Clearance		Dose Adjusted			
	30–60 ml/min		300 mg bid			
	15–30 ml/min		300 mg/d			
	<15 ml/min		150 mg/d or 300 mg every other day			
	Hemodialysis:		Give 200–300 mg after each 4-hour dialysis			
Lamotrigine	PO	100–150	bid	400	25 ± 10	None
(Lamictal®)	**Major side effects:** Stevens-Johnson syndrome (rare life-threatening rash unlikely with gradual dose titration), nausea, vomiting, sedation, dizziness, ataxia, fever, headache, blurred vision **Monitoring:** Clinical serum concentrations are not well established. Monitor liver function tests periodically. **Dose adjustment:** Initial dose is 25 mg/d; increase by 25–50 mg every 1–2 weeks. Decrease dose based on hepatic impairment.					
		Moderate hepatic impairment: Reduce dose by 50%				
		Severe hepatic impairment: Reduce dose by 75%				
Oxcarbazepine	PO	150–300	bid	1,200	2 ± 1	10-hydroxycarbazepine (half-life 8–13 hours)

(continued)

Name	Route	Average Dose Range (mg)	Average Dose Interval	Maximal Daily Dose (mg)	Half-Life (hours)	Clinically Important Metabolites (Active)
(Trileptal®)	**Major side effects:** Severe sedation, headache, dizziness, abnormal gait, tremor, fatigue, memory impairment, weight gain, nausea, vomiting, diarrhea, constipation					
	Monitoring: Therapeutic drug concentrations have not been established. Use serum creatinine for patients with renal impairment.					
	Dose adjustment: Initial dose is 150–300 bid; increase by 600 mg/wk. Above dose based on recommendations for treatment of trigeminal neuralgia. Dose must be decreased in patients with impaired renal function (creatinine clearance < 30 ml/min), with initiation of therapy starting at 300 mg/d. Adjust the dose based on patient response and side effects.					
Pregabalin (Lyrica®)	PO	50–75	bid-tid	600	6 ± 1	None
	Major side effects: Drowsiness, dizziness, fatigue, nausea, sedation, peripheral edema,					
	Monitoring: Therapeutic drug concentrations have not been established. Use serum creatinine for patients with renal impairment.					
	Dose adjustment: Decrease dose in patients with renal impairment based on creatinine clearance.					
	Creatinine Clearance		Dose Adjusted			
	30–60 ml/min		75 mg PO bid-tid			
	15–30 ml/min		25–50 mg every day to bid			
	<15 ml/min		Dose 25–50 mg every day			
	Hemodialysis:		Supplemental 25-mg dose			
Phenytoin (Dilantin®)	PO	100–200	bid-tid	500	15 ± 10	None
	Major side effects: Drowsiness, slurred speech, lethargy, hirsutism, fever, rash, Stevens-Johnson syndrome, nausea, vomiting, gingival hyperplasia, hepatitis, hematological abnormalities					
	Monitoring: Toxic plasma drug levels are more than 20 μg (micrograms)/ml (signs or symptoms are lethargy, slurred speech, ataxia, and coma). Plasma drug levels of more than 100 μg (micrograms)/ml are lethal. Check CBC with differential, liver function tests, and serum creatinine for patients with impaired renal function.					
	Dose adjustment: Adjust based on drug level and occurrence of side effects. Dose and frequency for status epilepticus is based on intravenous dosing.					
Topiramate (Topamax®)	PO	50–200	bid	400	21 ± 2	None
	Major side effects: Somnolence, fatigue, ataxia, difficulty in concentrating, memory difficulties, psychomotor slowing, speech or language problems, confusion, weight loss, anorexia, nausea, tremor, nephrolithiasis					
	Monitoring: Plasma topiramate concentrations have not been shown to correlate with clinical efficacy. Use serum creatinine for patients with impaired renal function.					
	Dose adjustment: Initial dose is 25 mg PO bid; increase by 25–50 mg/wk. For patients with renal impairment (creatinine clearance < 70 ml/min), reduce usual dose by 50% and titrate slowly.					
Valproic acid (Depakote ER® for migraine prophylaxis)	PO	500	Once daily	1,000	14 ± 3	None
	Major side effects: Drowsiness, confusion, alopecia, carnitine deficiency, nausea, vomiting, diarrhea, pancreatitis (potentially fatal), weight gain, liver failure (potentially fatal), thrombocytopenia, prolonged bleeding time					
	Monitoring: Toxic plasma levels are greater than 100 μg (microgram)/ml (signs or symptoms are nausea, vomiting, loss of appetite, abdominal pain, and weakness). Liver function tests, bilirubin, serum ammonia, and CBC with platelets must be monitored.					
	Dose adjustment: No dose adjustment is needed for patients on hemodialysis. Adjust the dose or discontinue therapy based on liver function and occurrence of side effects.					

bid, twice daily; CBC, complete blood count; CNS, central nervous system; HLA-B, major histocompatibility complex, class I, B; PO, orally; tid, three times per day.

Antidepressants (Adult Drug Doses)

Name	Route	Average Dose Range (mg)	Average Dose Interval	Maximal Daily Dose (mg)	Half-Life (hours)	Clinically Important Metabolites (Active)
Black Box Warning (all antidepressant classes): Antidepressants increase the risk of suicidal thinking and behavior in children, adolescents, and young adults (18–24 years) with major depressive disorder and other psychiatric disorders.						
Amitriptyline (Elavil®)	PO	75–100	At bedtime	300	21 ± 5	Nortriptyline, 10-hydroxy-nortriptyline
	Major side effects: Anticholinergic effects in more than 10% of patients (dizziness, blurred vision, drowsiness, xerostomia, constipation, urinary retention, tachycardia, orthostatic hypotension), arrhythmias, increased risk of seizures, increased appetite, weight gain, sexual dysfunction, cholinergic rebound with abrupt withdrawal (signs or symptoms include dizziness, nausea, diarrhea, insomnia, restlessness)					
	Monitoring: Take EKG, blood pressure, and pulse rate before start of therapy and then blood pressure with pulse during therapy. Evaluate mental status. Monitor weight changes, frequency of bowel movements, and acute toxicity (signs or symptoms include agitation, confusion, urinary retention, hypothermia, hypotension, ventricular tachycardia, and seizures). Monitor amitriptyline and nortriptyline plasma levels in patients with hepatic impairment. Normal plasma level ranges are as follows:					
		Amitriptyline		100–250 ng/ml		
		Nortriptyline		50–150 ng/ml		
	Dose adjustment: Initial dose is 10–25 mg at bedtime. Increase by 10–25 mg/wk. Adjust the dose based on occurrence of side effects and clinical efficacy.					
Amoxapine (Asendin®)	PO	100–150	Every day to tid	400	8	8-hydroxy-amoxapine
	Major side effects: Same as amitriptyline					
	Monitoring: Same as amitriptyline					
	Dose adjustment: Adjust the dose based on occurrence of side effects and clinical efficacy. Plasma concentrations have not been shown to correlate with clinical efficacy.					
Bupropion (Wellbutrin®)	PO	100–150	bid-tid	450	15 ± 5	Bupropion threoaminoalcohol, bupropion morpholinol
	Major side effects: Agitation, insomnia, fever, headache, psychosis, confusion, anxiety, increased risk of seizures, nausea, vomiting, xerostomia, constipation, weight loss, impotence					
	Monitoring: Body weight, acute toxicity (respiratory depression, coma, sedation, convulsions, ataxia)					
	Dose adjustment: Initiate therapy at a lower dose for patients with hepatic or renal impairment. Adjust the dose based on occurrence of side effects and clinical efficacy. Plasma concentrations have not been shown to correlate with clinical efficacy.					

(continued)

Name	Route	Average Dose Range (mg)	Average Dose Interval	Maximal Daily Dose (mg)	Half-Life (hours)	Clinically Important Metabolites (Active)
Black Box Warning (all antidepressant classes): Antidepressants increase the risk of suicidal thinking and behavior in children, adolescents, and young adults (18–24 years) with major depressive disorder and other psychiatric disorders.						
Clomipramine (Anafranil®)	PO	50–100	Every day	250	25 ± 5	None
	Major side effects: Same as amitriptyline **Monitoring:** Same as amitriptyline **Dose adjustment:** Adjust the dose based on occurrence of side effects and clinical efficacy. Plasma concentrations have not been shown to correlate with clinical efficacy.					
Desipramine (Norpramin®)	PO	50–150	At bedtime to tid	300	22 ± 5	2-hydroxydesipramine
	Major side effects: Same as amitriptyline **Monitoring:** Same as amitriptyline, but toxicity is possible at plasma levels greater than 300 ng/ml **Dose adjustment:** Adjust the dose based on occurrence of side effects and clinical efficacy.					
Doxepin (Sinequan®, Adapin®)	PO	50–150	Every day to tid	300	17 ± 6	Desmethyldoxepin
	Major side effects: Same as amitriptyline **Monitoring:** Same as amitriptyline. Plasma concentrations have not been shown to correlate with clinical efficacy. **Dose adjustment:** Adjust the dose based on occurrence of side effects and clinical efficacy.					
Duloxetine (Cymbalta®)	PO	30–60	Every day	120	12 ± 4	None
	Major side effects: Palpitations, fatigue, anxiety, hyperhydrosis, decreased libido, decreased appetite, vomiting, loose stools, erectile dysfunction, muscle cramps, weakness, nasopharyngitis, cough, diaphoresis **Monitoring:** Blood pressure **Dose adjustment:** Use is not recommended in patients with creatinine clearance of less than 30 ml/min or in patients with hepatic impairment.					
Citalopram (Celexa®)	PO	20–40	Every day	60	35 ± 2	Desmethylcitalopram, didesmethylcitalopram
Escitalopram (Lexapro®)	PO	10–20	Every day	20	30 ± 2	Same as citalopram
	Major side effects: Fatigue, insomnia, tremor, anxiety, agitation, headache, tachycardia, hypotension, xerostomia, nausea, vomiting, anorexia, dyspepsia, diarrhea, amenorrhea, sexual dysfunction (ejaculation disorder, decreased libido, impotence) **Monitoring:** Heart rate, blood pressure, liver function tests, CBC periodically, acute toxicity (signs or symptoms of toxicity include SIADH, electrolyte abnormalities, sexual dysfunction) **Dose adjustment:** Adjust the dose based on occurrence of side effects and clinical efficacy. Plasma concentrations have not been shown to correlate with clinical efficacy.					
Fluoxetine (Prozac®)	PO	20–60	Every day to bid	80	53 ± 41	Norfluoxetine (half-life 4–16 days)
	Major side effects: Same as citalopram **Monitoring:** Same as citalopram **Dose adjustment:** Lower or less frequent dosing should be used in patients with hepatic impairment because of a prolonged elimination half-life. Adjust the dose based on occurrence of side effects and clinical efficacy. When switching from fluoxetine to another antidepressant, the dose of the new antidepressant drug must be adjusted over 5 weeks because of the prolonged half-life of fluoxetine.					

(continued)

Name	Route	Average Dose Range (mg)	Average Dose Interval	Maximal Daily Dose (mg)	Half-Life (hours)	Clinically Important Metabolites (Active)
Fluvoxamine (Luvox®)	PO	50–300	Every day to bid	300	20 ± 5	None
	Major side effects: Same as citalopram **Monitoring:** Same as citalopram **Dose adjustment:** Adjust the dose based on occurrence of side effects and clinical efficacy.					
Black Box Warning (all antidepressant classes): Antidepressants increase the risk of suicidal thinking and behavior in children, adolescents, and young adults (18–24 years) with major depressive disorder and other psychiatric disorders.						
Imipramine (Tofranil®)	PO	50–150	tid-qid	300	12 ± 5	2-hydroxydesipramine, desipramine, 2-hydroxyimipramine
	Major side effects: Same as amitriptyline **Monitoring:** Same as amitriptyline. Toxicity is possible at plasma levels greater than 300 ng/ml for desipramine and greater than 500 ng/ml for imipramine. **Dose adjustment:** Adjust the dose based on occurrence of side effects and clinical efficacy.					
Maprotiline (Ludiomil®)	PO	50–150	Every day to tid	225	43 ± 15	Desmethylmaprotiline
	Major side effects: Same as amitriptyline **Monitoring:** Same as amitriptyline. Plasma concentrations have not been shown to correlate with clinical efficacy **Dose adjustment:** Adjust the dose based on occurrence of side effects and clinical efficacy.					
Mirtazapine (Remeron®)	PO	15–30	Every day	45	30 ± 10	Unknown
	Major side effects: Low incidence of anticholinergic side effects, with most common side effects being asthenia, xerostomia, increased appetite, weight gain, constipation, somnolence, dizziness **Monitoring:** Serum creatinine, liver function tests **Dose adjustment:** Make a 30% reduction in clearance in patients with moderate hepatic or renal impairment. Adjust the dose based on occurrence of side effects and clinical efficacy.					
Nefazodone (Serzone®)	PO	100–300	bid	600	2–4	Hydroxynefazodone, desethylhydroxy nefazodone
	Major side effects: Headache, drowsiness, insomnia, agitation, dizziness, confusion, xerostomia, nausea, vomiting, weakness, tremor, postural hypotension **Monitoring:** Monitor heart rate, blood pressure, liver function tests, CBC periodically, acute toxicity (signs or symptoms of toxicity include SIADH, electrolyte abnormalities, and sexual dysfunction). Plasma concentrations have not been shown to correlate with clinical efficacy. **Dose adjustment:** Adjust the dose based on occurrence of side effects and clinical efficacy.					
Nortriptyline (Pamelor®, Aventyl®)	PO	50–150	Every day to qid	300	31 ± 13	10-hydroxynortriptyline
	Major side effects: Same as amitriptyline **Monitoring:** Same as amitriptyline. Daily doses greater than 100 mg should have plasma concentrations periodically monitored (normal plasma level for nortriptyline is 50–150 ng/ml). Toxicity is possible at plasma levels greater than 500 ng/ml. **Dose adjustment:** Adjust the dose based on occurrence of side effects and clinical efficacy.					

(continued)

Name	Route	Average Dose Range (mg)	Average Dose Interval	Maximal Daily Dose (mg)	Half-Life (hours)	Clinically Important Metabolites (Active)
Paroxetine						
(Paxil®)	PO	20–40	Every day	60	26 ± 5	None
(Paxil CR®)	PO	12.5–25	Every day	75	26 ± 5	None
	Major side effects: Same as citalopram					
	Monitoring: Same as citalopram					
	Dose adjustment: Adjust the dose based on occurrence of side effects and clinical efficacy.					
Black Box Warning (all antidepressant classes): Antidepressants increase the risk of suicidal thinking and behavior in children, adolescents, and young adults (18–24 years) with major depressive disorder and other psychiatric disorders.						
Protriptyline (Vivactil®)	PO	5–15	tid-qid	60	54–198	Protriptyline 10,11-epoxide, 10-hydroxy-protriptyline, 10,11-dihydroxyprotriptyline
	Major side effects: Same as amitriptyline					
	Monitoring: Same as amitriptyline. Toxicity is possible at plasma levels greater than 1,000 ng/ml.					
	Dose adjustment: Adjust the dose based on occurrence of side effects and clinical efficacy.					
Sertraline (Zoloft®)	PO	100–200	Every day	200	23	N-desmethylsertraline
	Major side effects: Same as citalopram					
	Monitoring: Same as citalopram					
	Dose adjustment: Adjust the dose based on occurrence of side effects and clinical efficacy. Use with caution in patients with hepatic impairment because of extensive drug metabolism.					
Trazodone (Desyrel®)	PO	100–200	At bedtime to tid	600	6.5 ± 1.8	Meta-chlorophenylpiperazine
	Major side effects: Extremely sedating, dizziness, headache, confusion, bad taste in mouth, constipation, diarrhea, xerostomia, muscle tremors, weakness, blurred vision					
	Monitoring: Heart rate, blood pressure, acute toxicity (signs or symptoms of toxicity include drowsiness, vomiting, tachycardia, incontinence, coma, priapism), although plasma concentrations have not been shown to correlate with clinical efficacy					
	Dose adjustment: Adjust the dose based on occurrence of side effects and clinical efficacy.					
Venlafaxine						
(Effexor®)	PO	75–225	bid-tid	375	4.9 ± 2.4	O-desmethylvenlafaxine
(Effexor XR®)	PO	37.5–75	Every day	225	11 ± 2	Same as venlafaxine
	Major side effects: Headache, asthenia, somnolence, dizziness, blurred vision, hypertension, sinus tachycardia, insomnia, nervousness, nausea, anorexia, vomiting, constipation, weight loss, xerostomia, weakness, tremor, neck pain, diaphoresis, abnormal ejaculation, impotence					
	Monitoring: Blood pressure should be monitored regularly, especially in patients with a high baseline. Liver function tests and serum creatinine are based on occurrence of side effects.					
	Dose adjustments: Reduce the dose for patients with renal or hepatic impairment based on creatinine clearance					
		Renal impairment dose reduction:				
		10–70 ml/min	Decrease total daily dose by 25%			
		<10 ml/min	Decrease total daily dose by 50%			

(continued)

Hepatic impairment dose reduction:

Moderate impairment	Decrease total daily dose by 50%
Severe impairment	Avoid use

bid, twice daily; CBC, complete blood count; EKG, electrocardiogram; PO, orally; qid, four times per day; SIADH, syndrome of inappropriate antidiuretic hormone; tid, three times per day.

appendix

14-4 Antihistamines (Adult Drug Doses)

Name	Route	Average Dose Range (mg)	Average Dose Interval	Maximal Daily Dose (mg)	Half-Life (hours)	Clinically Important Metabolites (Active)
FDA Warning: Antihistamine-containing products are not recommended for administration to children under the age of 4 years due to risk of excessive sedation and respiratory depression.						
Diphenhydramine (Benadryl®)	PO, IV	25–50	q4–6 hours	150	6 ± 4	None
Hydroxyzine (Vistaril®, Atarax®)	PO	25–50	tid-qid	600	5 ± 2	Cetirizine
	Contraindication: Do not give by subcutaneous, intraarterial, or rapid intravenous push administration (risk of infiltration) due to severe tissue damage and necrosis.					
Promethazine (Phenergan®)	PO	12.5–25	q4–6 hours	NA	12 ± 3	None
	Contraindication: Do not give by subcutaneous, intraarterial, or rapid IV push administration (risk of infiltration) due to severe tissue damage and necrosis. **Major side effects:** Dizziness, drowsiness, confusion, hallucinations, paradoxical excitement, blurred vision, xerostomia, thickening of bronchial secretions, difficult urination **Monitoring:** Relief of symptoms and mental status **Dose adjustment:** Reduce dose by 50–75% in elderly patients.					

IV, intravenously; NA, not available; PO, orally; qid, four times per day; tid, three times per day.

appendix

14-5

Anxiolytics (Adult Drug Doses)

Name	Route	Average Dose Range (mg)	Average Dose Interval	Maximal Daily Dose (mg)	Half-Life (hours)	Clinically Important Metabolites (Active)
Alprazolam (Xanax®)	PO	0.25–0.5	tid	10	12 ± 2	4- hydroxyalprazolam, α-hydroxyalprazolam
	Major side effects: Drowsiness, fatigue, memory impairment, rebound anxiety, depression, tachycardia, chest pain, xerostomia, constipation, nausea, vomiting, diaphoresis, decreased libido, physical and psychological drug dependence, increased risk of respiratory depression when combined with opioids, alcohol, or other CNS depressants **Monitoring:** Respiratory function and cardiovascular status, acute toxicity (signs or symptoms include somnolence, confusion, coma, diminished reflexes, hypotension, respiratory depression, cardiac arrhythmias), withdrawal (signs or symptoms include seizures) **Dose adjustment:** Withdrawal symptoms have occurred 18–72 hours after abrupt discontinuation. When discontinuing therapy, decrease the daily dose by no more than 0.5 mg every 3 days. Reduce the daily dose by 50–60% in patients with hepatic impairment. Avoid administration in patients with cirrhosis. The dose for patients with panic disorder should not to exceed 10 mg/d.					
Buspirone (BuSpar®)	PO	10–15	bid	60	2.5 ± 0.5	None
	Major side effects: Dizziness, nausea, headache, nervousness, lightheadedness, low risk of physical drug dependence **Monitoring:** Symptoms of anxiety, mental status **Dose adjustment:** The daily dose should be decreased by 50% for patients with severe hepatic or renal impairment.					
Chlordiazepoxide (Librium®)	PO	15–25	tid–qid	300	10 ± 3.4	Demoxepam, desmethylchlordiazepoxide, desmethyldiazepam, oxazepam
	IV	50–100	q2–4 hours	300	10 ± 3.4	
	Major side effects: Same as alprazolam **Monitoring:** Same as alprazolam **Dose adjustment:** Patients with severe anxiety or acute alcohol withdrawal need to be dosed more frequently and at higher doses (use intravenous chlordiazepoxide). Chlordiazepoxide undergoes extensive liver metabolism to its active form. The half-life is prolonged significantly in patients with cirrhosis or impaired renal function (reduce the daily dose by 50% for these patients).					
Clonazepam (Klonopin®)	PO	0.5–1.0	tid	4	23 ± 5	None

(continued)

Name	Route	Average Dose Range (mg)	Average Dose Interval	Maximal Daily Dose (mg)	Half-Life (hours)	Clinically Important Metabolites (Active)
	Major side effects: Same as alprazolam **Monitoring:** Same as alprazolam, plus CBC, liver function testing. The relationship between serum concentration and seizure control is not well established. Toxicity may occur with plasma concentrations greater than 80 ng/ml. **Dose adjustment:** Withdrawal symptoms have occurred 18–72 hours after abrupt discontinuation. When discontinuing therapy, decrease the daily dose by no more than 0.5 mg every 3 days. Reduce the daily dose by 50–60% in patients with hepatic impairment. Avoid administration in patients with cirrhosis.					
Clorazepate (Tranxene®)	PO	7.5–15	bid–qid	90	72 ± 24	Desmethyldiazepam
(Tranxene® SD)	PO	11.25–22.5	Every day	90	72 ± 24	Oxazepam
	Major side effects: Same as alprazolam **Monitoring:** Same as alprazolam **Dose adjustment:** Patients with severe anxiety or acute alcohol withdrawal need to be dosed more frequently and at higher doses, with a maximal daily dose of 90 mg. Use is not recommended in elderly patients.					
Diazepam (Valium®)	PO	2–10	q4–6 hours	60	43 ± 13	Desmethyldiazepam, hydroxydiazepam, oxazepam
	IV	2–10	q4–6 hours	60	43 ± 13	
	Major side effects: Same as alprazolam **Monitoring:** Same as alprazolam **Dose adjustment:** Patients with severe anxiety, status epilepticus, or acute alcohol withdrawal need to be dosed more frequently and at higher doses (use intravenous diazepam). Muscle relaxant doses are lower (2–5 mg bid-qid) than doses for severe anxiety. Diazepam undergoes extensive liver metabolism to long-acting metabolites. The half-life is prolonged significantly in patients with impaired liver function, cirrhosis, or impaired renal function (reduce the daily dose by 50% for these patients). Withdrawal symptoms have occurred 18–72 hours after abrupt discontinuation. When discontinuing therapy, decrease the daily dose by no more than 0.5 mg every 3 days.					
Flumazenil (Romazicon®) *Antagonist*	IV	0.2–1	q2–10 minutes	5	1 ± 0.5	None
	Major side effects: The risk of seizures is high in patients poisoned with tricyclic antidepressants (amitriptyline, clomipramine, doxepin, imipramine, desipramine, and nortriptyline). Withdrawal symptoms may be precipitated in patients using benzodiazepines for a prolonged period and in whom tolerance, dependence, or both may have developed. This is not effective for reversal of drug overdoses because of tricyclic antidepressants, barbiturates, or opioids. **Monitoring:** Respiratory function and cardiovascular status, benzodiazepine withdrawal (signs or symptoms include seizures) **Dose adjustment:** May repeat within 20–30 minutes if sedation reappears.					
Lorazepam	PO	1–2	q4–6 hours	10	14 ± 5	None
(Ativan®)	IV	0.5–2	q4–6 hours	10	14 ± 5	

(continued)

Name	Route	Average Dose Range (mg)	Average Dose Interval	Maximal Daily Dose (mg)	Half-Life (hours)	Clinically Important Metabolites (Active)
	Major side effects: Same as alprazolam **Monitoring:** Same as alprazolam **Dose adjustment:** Patients with severe anxiety, emesis, or status epilepticus need to be dosed more frequently and at higher doses (use IV lorazepam). Withdrawal symptoms have occurred 18–72 hours after abrupt discontinuation. When discontinuing therapy, decrease the daily dose by no more than 0.5 mg every 3 days.					
Midazolam (Versed®)	IV	0.5–2	q2–3 minutes	5	19 ± 0.6	1-Hydroxymethylmidazolam
	Major side effects: Cardiac arrest, hypotension, bradycardia, respiratory depression, apnea, laryngospasm, bronchospasm, sedation, nausea, vomiting, blurred vision, diplopia, physical and psychological dependence with prolonged use **Monitoring:** Respiratory function and cardiovascular status, acute toxicity (signs or symptoms include somnolence, confusion, coma, diminished reflexes, hypotension, respiratory depression, cardiac arrhythmias), withdrawal (signs or symptoms include seizures) **Dose adjustment:** Reduce the dose by 30% if given concomitantly with opioids or other CNS depressants. This is not for long-term administration; dose as above for short-term use with procedural sedation.					
Oxazepam (Serax®)	PO	10–30	tid-qid	120	8 ± 2.4	None
	Major side effects: Same as alprazolam **Monitoring:** Same as alprazolam **Dose adjustment:** Withdrawal symptoms have occurred 18–72 hours after abrupt discontinuation. When discontinuing therapy, taper the daily dose every 3 days.					

bid, twice daily; CNS, central nervous system; IV, intravenously; PO, orally; qid, four times per day; SD, single dose; tid, three times per day.

appendix

14-6

Hypnotics (Adult Drug Doses)

Name	Route	Average Dose Range (mg)	Average Dose Interval	Maximal Daily Dose (mg)	Half-Life (hours)	Clinically Important Metabolites (Active)
Eszopiclone (Lunesta®)	PO	1–2	At bedtime	2	7 ± 1	Active metabolites
	Major side effects: Chest pain, peripheral edema, somnolence, dizziness, nervousness, confusion, hallucinations, hazardous sleep activities (driving, cooking, etc.), abnormal dreams, migraine, pain, xerostomia, nausea, infection **Monitoring:** Liver function tests, sleep-wake pattern **Dose adjustment:** Eszopiclone is extensively metabolized by the liver. Avoid in patients with severe liver disease.					
Flurazepam (Dalmane®)	PO	15–30	At bedtime	30	74 ± 24	*N*-hydroxyethylflurazepam, *N*-desalkylflurazepam
	Major side effects: Same as alprazolam **Monitoring:** Respiratory function and cardiovascular status, acute toxicity (signs or symptoms include somnolence, confusion, coma, diminished reflexes, hypotension, respiratory depression, cardiac arrhythmias), sleep-wake pattern **Dose adjustment:** Use is not recommended in the elderly. Flurazepam undergoes extensive liver metabolism to long-acting metabolites. The half-life is prolonged significantly in patients with impaired liver function, cirrhosis, or impaired renal function leading to excessive sedation (avoid use of flurazepam in these patients). Withdrawal symptoms have occurred 18–72 hours after abrupt discontinuation. When discontinuing therapy, taper the daily dose every 3 days.					
Ramelteon (Rozerem®)	PO	8	At bedtime	NA	4 ± 2	NA
	Major side effects: Headache, somnolence, fatigue, nausea **Monitoring:** Sleep-wake pattern **Dose adjustment:** Ramelteon is extensively metabolized by the liver. Avoid in patients with severe liver disease.					
Temazepam (Restoril®)	PO	7.5–15	At bedtime	30	11 ± 6	None
	Major side effects: Same as alprazolam **Monitoring:** Same as alprazolam, plus sleep-wake pattern **Dose adjustment:** Withdrawal symptoms have occurred 18–72 hours after abrupt discontinuation. When discontinuing therapy, taper the daily dose every 3 days.					
Triazolam (Halcion®)	PO	0.125–0.25	At bedtime	0.25	2.9 ± 1	None

(continued)

Name	Route	Average Dose Range (mg)	Average Dose Interval	Maximal Daily Dose (mg)	Half-Life (hours)	Clinically Important Metabolites (Active)
	Major side effects: Same as alprazolam **Monitoring:** Same as alprazolam, plus sleep-wake pattern **Dose adjustment:** Do not exceed 0.5 mg/d because of the emergence of increased mental confusion and psychosis. Administer for short-term use of 7–10 days. Avoid use in patients with cirrhosis. Withdrawal symptoms have occurred 18–72 hours after abrupt discontinuation. When discontinuing therapy, taper the daily dose every 3 days.					
Zaleplon (Sonata®)	PO	10	At bedtime	20	1	None
	Major side effects: Same as eszopiclone, with potential for physical and psychological drug dependence **Monitoring:** Sleep-wake pattern **Dose adjustment:** Zaleplon is extensively metabolized by the liver. Avoid use in patients with severe liver impairment or cirrhosis.					
Zolpidem (Ambien®)	PO	5–10	At bedtime	20	2–2.6	None
	Major side effects: Same as eszopiclone, with potential for physical and psychological drug dependence **Monitoring:** Sleep-wake pattern **Dose adjustment:** Zolpidem is extensively metabolized by the liver. Reduce the dose to 5 mg in patients with severe liver impairment or cirrhosis.					

NA, not available; PO, orally.

appendix

14-7

Muscle Relaxants (Adult Drug Doses)

Name	Route	Average Dose Range	Average Dose Interval	Maximal Daily Dose (mg)	Half-Life	Clinically Important Metabolites (Active)
Baclofen (Lioresal®)	PO	5–10 mg	tid	80	2.5–4 hours	None
	IT	100–800 μg/d	Infusion	Dose by response	—	
	Major side effects: Dizziness, drowsiness, fatigue, weakness, nausea, cardiac arrhythmias, urinary frequency. Avoid abrupt withdrawal; potential life-threatening adverse effects include rhabdomyolysis and seizures. **Monitoring:** Pain, hypotension, muscle stiffness, ROM, liver function tests (AST, ALT, Alk phos), renal function **Dose adjustment:** Additive CNS depression occurs with other CNS depressants, including alcohol, antihistamines, opioids, sedatives or hypnotics, and MAOIs (also hypotension). Use with caution in patients with renal impairment.					
Carisoprodol (Soma®), (Soma Compound®)	PO	350 mg	qid	1,400	8 hours	Meprobamate
	Major side effects: Contraindicated in patients with acute intermittent porphyria, allergic, or idiosyncratic reactions to carisoprodol or related compounds of less than four doses (extreme weakness, ataxia, vision loss, euphoria, diplopia, dysarthria, disorientation); dizziness; drowsiness; postural hypotension; risk of physical dependence or psychological dependency **Monitoring:** Pain, muscle stiffness, ROM **Dose adjustment:** Additive CNS depression occurs with other CNS depressants, including alcohol, antihistamines, opioids, and sedatives or hypnotics. Use is not recommended in patients with renal or hepatic insufficiency.					
Chlorzoxazone (Parafon Forte®)	PO	250 mg	tid-qid	750 qid	1.1 hours	None
	Major side effects: GI bleed, agranulocytosis, anemia, dizziness, drowsiness, angioedema, hepatocellular toxicity **Monitoring:** Pain, muscle stiffness, ROM, administration with meals, liver function tests (AST, ALT, Alk phos) **Dose adjustment:** Use is contraindicated in patients with hepatic dysfunction. Additive CNS depression occurs with other CNS depressants, including alcohol, antihistamines, opioids, and sedatives or hypnotics.					
Cyclobenzaprine (Flexeril®)	PO	10 mg	tid	60	1–3 days	None
	Major side effects: Same precautions as with tricyclic antidepressants, plus torsades de pointes with fluoxetine or droperidol, dizziness, drowsiness, confusion, psychosis, dry mouth, urinary retention, myoclonus, weakness **Monitoring:** Pain, muscle stiffness, ROM					

(continued)

Name	Route	Average Dose Range	Average Dose Interval	Maximal Daily Dose (mg)	Half-Life	Clinically Important Metabolites (Active)
	Dose adjustment: Additive CNS depression occurs with other CNS depressants, including alcohol, antihistamines, opioids, and sedatives or hypnotics. Cyclobenzaprine should not be used within 14 days of MAOI (it may cause hyperpyretic crisis, convulsions, and death).					
Metaxalone (Skelaxin®)	PO	800 mg	tid-qid	3,200	2–3 hours	None
	Major side effects: Use is contraindicated in patients with severe hepatic or renal impairment. Metaxalone should not be administered to patients with a known tendency to drug-induced anemias. Side effects include dyspepsia, drowsiness, dizziness, and xerostomia. **Monitoring:** Sedation, mental status, liver function tests (AST, ALT, Alk Phos), renal function **Dose adjustment:** Avoid use in patients at high risk for hemolytic anemias.					
Methocarbamol (Robaxin®)	PO	750 mg	q4 hour	1,500 mg tid	1–2 hours	None
	IM, IV	500–1,000 mg	q8 hours	No more than 3 days of therapy	1–2 hours	
	Major side effects: Seizures, syncope, hypotension, bradycardia, lightheadedness, dizziness, drowsiness, anorexia, GI upset, nausea, xerostomia, urine discoloration **Monitoring:** Pain; muscle stiffness; ROM; allergic reactions such as rash, asthma, hives, wheezing; hypotension after parenteral administration. Monitor renal function if treatment lasts longer than 3 months. **Dose adjustment:** May repeat IV or IM dose after 48-hour rest. The injectable formulation is contraindicated in patients with renal dysfunction due to the presence of polyethylene glycol 300. Additive CNS depression occurs with other CNS depressants, including alcohol, antihistamines, opioids, and sedatives or hypnotics.					
Orphenadrine (Norflex®) (Norgesic®)	PO	100 mg	bid	200	14–16 hours	None
	IV	60 mg	bid	120		
	Major side effects: Drowsiness, dizziness, blurred vision, mental confusion, tachycardia, palpitations, hallucinations, agitation, tremor, nausea, xerostomia, constipation, abdominal distention, vomiting, urinary retention **Monitoring:** Vital signs, frequency of bowel movements, mental status **Dose adjustment:** Use is contraindicated for use in patients with glaucoma, GI obstruction, cardiospasm, or myasthenia gravis. Use with caution in patients with congestive heart failure or cardiac arrhythmias.					
Tizanidine (Zanaflex®)	PO	4 mg	q6–8 hours	36	2.5 hours	None
	Major side effects: Anxiety, depression, dizziness, sedation, weakness, abdominal pain, diarrhea, dry mouth, dyspepsia, rash, skin ulcers, sweating, hypotension **Monitoring:** Liver function at 1, 3, and 6 months; pain; muscle stiffness; ROM **Dose adjustment:** Increase by 2–4 mg per dose up to 36 mg/d.					

bid, twice daily; CNS, central nervous system; GI, gastrointestinal; IM, intramuscular; IT, intrathecal; IV, intravenous; MAOI, monoamine oxidase inhibitor; PO, orally; qid, four times per day; ROM, range of motion; tid, three times per day.

appendix

14-8

Nonsteroidal Anti-inflammatory Drugs (NSAIDs) (Adult Drug Doses)

Name	Route	Average Dose Range (mg)	Average Dose Interval	Maximal Daily Dose (mg)	Half-Life (hours)	Analgesic Efficacy
Aspirin (various OTC)	PO	650–975	q 4–6 hours	4,000	0.25–0.33	Aspirin is hydrolyzed to salicylate by esterases in the GI mucosa during absorption. Plasma and erythrocyte esterases further hydrolyze aspirin. Aspirin does not undergo extensive liver metabolism or accumulate after multiple doses. Aspirin is the analgesic standard for comparison of all NSAIDs.

Major side effects: Dyspepsia, heartburn, epigastric distress, nausea, occult GI bleeding (≥70% of patients using doses greater than 1,000 mg/d of nonenteric-coated aspirin), GI ulcers, tinnitus and hearing loss with high doses, reversible hepatotoxicity, irreversible renal papillary necrosis and interstitial nephritis with long-term therapy, noncardiogenic edema with high doses, irreversible platelet inhibition, prolonged bleeding time, bronchospasm and hypersensitivity reactions (i.e., urticaria, angioedema)

Monitoring: Acute toxicity (signs or symptoms include acid-base electrolyte disturbances, dehydration, hyperpyrexia, hyperglycemia or hypoglycemia, coma, seizures, mental status changes); chronic toxicity (signs or symptoms include tinnitus, hearing loss, dimness of vision, headache, dizziness, mental confusion, lassitude, drowsiness, sweating, thirst, hyperventilation, tachycardia, nausea, vomiting); laboratory monitoring, including serum creatinine for patients at risk for renal complications and serum salicylate level for patients with toxic symptoms; black-tarry stools for GI bleeding

Dose adjustment: Use is not recommended in children and teenagers with chickenpox, influenza, or flulike symptoms. It lacks the peripheral antiinflammatory activity of other NSAIDs. Total daily doses of 3,600–5,400 mg may be needed for treatment of inflammatory diseases (i.e., spondyloarthropathies, arthritis, and pleurisy of systemic lupus erythematosus). Cross-sensitivity of hypersensitivity reactions with other NSAIDs occurs most often with indomethacin, ibuprofen, mefenamic acid, and phenylbutazone. Use is not recommended in patients with renal or hepatic impairment.

(continued)

Name	Route	Average Dose Range (mg)	Average Dose Interval	Maximal Daily Dose (mg)	Half-Life (hours)	Analgesic Efficacy
Black Box Warning (all NSAID classes): NSAIDs may cause an increased risk of serious CV thrombotic events, myocardial infarction, and stroke, which can be fatal. This risk may increase with duration of use. Patients with CV disease or risk factors for CV disease may be at greater risk.						
Celecoxib (Celebrex®)	PO	100–200	bid	400	11	This COX-2 enzyme inhibitor has a lower incidence of gastrointestinal side effects. Celecoxib, at 200 mg every 12 hours, is similar in efficacy to naproxen, at 500 mg every 12 hours, or sustained-release diclofenac, at 75 mg every 12 hours, for arthritis treatment.
	Major side effects: Headache, dyspepsia, diarrhea, abdominal pain, nausea, flatulence, renal ischemia and Na^+ retention, fluid retention, peripheral edema, hypertension, elevation of liver function tests (6% of patients), jaundice, hepatitis (severe and potentially fatal)					
	Monitoring: Acute toxicity (signs or symptoms include lethargy, drowsiness, nausea, vomiting, epigastric pain, hypertension, renal failure), serum creatinine in patients at risk for renal complications, liver function tests for patients with hepatic impairment					
	Dose adjustment: Use is contraindicated in patients with a history of sulfonamide sensitivity or in patients with renal or hepatic impairment. Reduce the dose by 50% for patients with moderate hepatic impairment.					
Choline magnesium trisalicylate (Trilisate®)	PO	1,000–1,500	q 12 hours	3,000	9–17	Longer duration of action than aspirin
	Major side effects: Nausea, vomiting, dyspepsia, diarrhea, abdominal pain, tinnitus at high doses, headache, dizziness, lethargy, rash, but does not increase bleeding time					
	Monitoring: Same as aspirin					
	Dose adjustment: Use is not recommended in children and teenagers with chickenpox, influenza, or flulike symptoms or in patients with renal or hepatic impairment.					
Diclofenac (Voltaren®)	PO	50	q 8 hours	150	2	Superior in efficacy and analgesic duration compared with aspirin at 650 mg
(Voltaren® SR)	PO	75	q 12 hours	150	2	
(Flector® Patch)	TD	1 patch	bid			
		Note: Use the lowest effective dose for the shortest duration is consistent with individual patient treatment goals.				
(Voltaren® Gel)	Topical	Lower extremities: Apply 4 g of 1% gel to affected area four times daily (maximum of 16 g per joint per day). Upper extremities: Apply 2 g of 1% gel to affected area four times daily (maximum of 8 g per joint per day) Note: Maximum total body dose of 1% gel should not exceed 32 g/day.				

(continued)

Name	Route	Average Dose Range (mg)	Average Dose Interval	Maximal Daily Dose (mg)	Half-Life (hours)	Analgesic Efficacy
	Major side effects: Same as other COX-1 enzyme inhibitors (refer to ibuprofen)					
	Monitoring: Same as other COX-1 enzyme inhibitors (refer to ibuprofen)					
	Dose adjustment: Use is not recommended in patients with renal impairment, hepatic dysfunction, or congestive heart failure with marginal cardiac function.					
Black Box Warning (all NSAID classes): NSAIDs may cause an increased risk of serious CV thrombotic events, myocardial infarction, and stroke, which can be fatal. This risk may increase with duration of use. Patients with CV disease or risk factors for CV disease may be at greater risk.						
Etodolac (Lodine®)	PO	200–400	q 6–8 hours	1,200	6–7	Etodolac, at 200 mg, is comparable in efficacy to aspirin, at 650 mg.
	Major side effects: Same as other COX-1 enzyme inhibitors (refer to ibuprofen)					
	Monitoring: Same as other COX-1 enzyme inhibitors (refer to ibuprofen)					
	Dose adjustment: Use is not recommended in patients with renal impairment, hepatic dysfunction, or congestive heart failure with marginal cardiac function.					
Fenoprofen (Nalfon®)	PO	200–600	q 6 hours	3,200	2–3	Comparable to aspirin
	Major side effects: Same as other COX-1 enzyme inhibitors (refer to ibuprofen)					
	Monitoring: Same as other COX-1 enzyme inhibitors (refer to ibuprofen)					
	Dose adjustment: Use is not recommended in patients with renal impairment, hepatic dysfunction, or congestive heart failure with marginal cardiac function.					
Ibuprofen (Motrin®, Advil®)	PO	400–800	q 6–8 hours	2,400	1.8–2.5	Ibuprofen, at 200 mg, has superior analgesia compared with aspirin, at 650 mg.
	Major side effects: Dyspepsia, heartburn, epigastric distress, nausea, occult GI bleeding, GI ulcers (especially with long-term therapy), dizziness, drowsiness, fatigue, malaise, lightheadedness, confusion, jaundice, hepatitis (severe and potentially fatal), elevated liver function tests (15% of patients), bronchospasm and hypersensitivity (i.e., urticaria, angioedema) reactions because of prostaglandin inhibition, decreased hemoglobin (in 17% of patients receiving ≥ 1,600 mg/d and 23% of patients receiving ≥ 2,400 mg/d), reversible inhibitor of platelet aggregation, prolong bleeding time, acute renal tubular necrosis, interstitial nephritis, nephrotic syndrome, renal failure (especially with long-term therapy), peripheral edema, fluid retention, congestive heart failure with marginal cardiac function, blurred or diminished vision, scotoma, changes in color vision					
	Monitoring: Acute toxicity (abdominal pain, GI bleeding, nausea, vomiting, lethargy, drowsiness, tinnitus, acute renal failure, tachycardia or bradycardia); laboratory monitoring, including serum creatinine for patients at risk for renal complications; periodic liver function tests with long-term therapy or patients concurrently consuming alcohol; black-tarry stools for GI bleeding; ophthalmological examination for vision changes					
	Dose adjustment: Use is contraindicated in patients in whom bronchospasm, angioedema, or nasal polyps are precipitated by aspirin or NSAIDs and is contraindicated in patients with peptic ulcer disease, history of peptic ulcer disease, or chronic glucocorticoid steroid use. Use is not recommended in patients with renal impairment, hepatic dysfunction, or congestive heart failure with marginal cardiac function. There is cross-sensitivity of hypersensitivity reactions with aspirin.					

(continued)

Name	Route	Average Dose Range (mg)	Average Dose Interval	Maximal Daily Dose (mg)	Half-Life (hours)	Analgesic Efficacy
Indomethacin						
(Indocin®)	PO	25–50	q 8–12 hours	200	4.5–6	Indomethacin, at 25 mg, is comparable to aspirin, at 650 mg, but not routinely used because of the high incidence of side effects.
(Indocin SR®)	PO	75	q 24 hours	150	4.5–6	
	Major side effects: Same as other COX-1 enzyme inhibitors (refer to ibuprofen)					
	Monitoring: Same as other COX-1 enzyme inhibitors (refer to ibuprofen)					
	Dose adjustment: Use is not recommended in patients with renal impairment, hepatic dysfunction, or congestive heart failure with marginal cardiac function. There is cross-sensitivity of hypersensitivity reactions with aspirin.					
Black Box Warning (all NSAID classes): NSAIDs may cause an increased risk of serious CV thrombotic events, myocardial infarction, and stroke, which can be fatal. This risk may increase with duration of use. Patients with CV disease or risk factors for CV disease may be at greater risk.						
Ketoprofen						
(Orudis®)	PO	25–50	q 6–8 hours	300	1.5–4	Comparable to aspirin
(Oruvail SR®, Actron SR®)	PO	200	q 24 hours	300	—	
	Major side effects: Same as other COX-1 enzyme inhibitors (refer to ibuprofen)					
	Monitoring: Same as other COX-1 enzyme inhibitors (refer to ibuprofen)					
	Dose adjustment: Use is not recommended in patients with renal impairment, hepatic dysfunction, or congestive heart failure with marginal cardiac function.					
Ketorolac (Toradol®)	PO	10	q 4–6 hours	40	4–8	Combined use of intravenous or intramuscular doses with oral doses should not exceed 120 mg/d and should be administered for no more than 5 days because of increased risk of GI bleeding.
	IM, IV	Patients < 65 years of age:	30 mg q 6 hr			Administer no more than 5 days. Use an intramuscular route only if an intravenous one is not available.
		Patients ≥ 65 years of age:	15 mg q 6 hr			Ketorolac is comparable to 6–12 mg of morphine or 100 mg of meperidine.
	Major side effects: Same as other COX-1 enzyme inhibitors (refer to ibuprofen)					
	Monitoring: Same as other COX-1 enzyme inhibitors (refer to ibuprofen)					
	Dose adjustment: Use is not recommended in patients with renal impairment, hepatic dysfunction, or congestive heart failure with marginal cardiac function.					

(continued)

Name	Route	Average Dose Range (mg)	Average Dose Interval	Maximal Daily Dose (mg)	Half-Life (hours)	Analgesic Efficacy
Meloxicam (Mobic®)	PO	7.5	q 24 hours	15	20	Meloxicam, at 7.5 mg, is comparable to diclofenac, at 100 mg, in osteoarthritis. There is less GI irritation with meloxicam.
	Major side effects: Same as other COX-1 enzyme inhibitors (refer to ibuprofen) **Monitoring:** Same as other COX-1 enzyme inhibitors (refer to ibuprofen) **Dose adjustment:** Use is not recommended in patients with renal impairment, hepatic dysfunction, or congestive heart failure with marginal cardiac function.					
Black Box Warning (all NSAID classes): NSAIDs may cause an increased risk of serious CV thrombotic events, myocardial infarction, and stroke, which can be fatal. This risk may increase with duration of use. Patients with CV disease or risk factors for CV disease may be at greater risk.						
Nabumetone (Relafen®)	PO	1,000	q 24 hours	2,000	24	Nabumetone is a prodrug metabolized to active metabolite 6-methoxy-2-naphthylacetic acid. nabumetone, at 1,000 mg, is comparable to aspirin, at 900 mg.
	Major side effects: Same as other COX-1 enzyme inhibitors (refer to ibuprofen) **Monitoring:** Same as other COX-1 enzyme inhibitors (refer to ibuprofen) **Dose adjustment:** Use is not recommended in patients with renal impairment, hepatic dysfunction, or congestive heart failure with marginal cardiac function.					
Naproxen (Naprosyn®)	PO	250	q 6–8 hours	1,000	12–15	Naproxen, at 250 mg, is comparable to aspirin, at 650 mg.
	Major side effects: Same as other COX-1 enzyme inhibitors (refer to ibuprofen) **Monitoring:** Same as other COX-1 enzyme inhibitors (refer to ibuprofen) **Dose adjustment:** Use is not recommended in patients with renal impairment, hepatic dysfunction, or congestive heart failure with marginal cardiac function.					
Piroxicam (Feldene®)	PO	10–20	q 24 hours	20	45–50	Protein binding is 99%. There is a high incidence of GI bleeding with long-term therapy.
	Major side effects: Same as other COX-1 enzyme inhibitors (refer to ibuprofen) **Monitoring:** Same as other COX-1 enzyme inhibitors (refer to ibuprofen) **Dose adjustment:** Use is not recommended in patients with renal impairment, hepatic dysfunction, or congestive heart failure with marginal cardiac function.					

(continued)

Name	Route	Average Dose Range (mg)	Average Dose Interval	Maximal Daily Dose (mg)	Half-Life (hours)	Analgesic Efficacy
Salsalate (Disalcid®)	PO	500	q 4 hours	3,000	7–8	Salsalate is comparable to aspirin for osteoarthritis.
	Major side effects: Nausea, heartburn, epigastric discomfort, dyspepsia, gastrointestinal ulceration, hemolytic anemia, weakness, fatigue, rash **Monitoring:** Acute toxicity (signs or symptoms include dehydration, metabolic acidosis, hyperthermia, coagulopathy, hemorrhage, hypoglycemia, coma, seizures, mental status changes); laboratory monitoring, including serum creatinine for patients at risk for renal complications and serum salicylate level for patients with toxic symptoms; black-tarry stools for GI bleeding **Dose adjustment:** For patients with end-stage renal disease undergoing hemodialysis, adjust to 750 bid with an additional 500 mg after hemodialysis.					
Black Box Warning (all NSAID classes): NSAIDs may cause an increased risk of serious CV thrombotic events, myocardial infarction, and stroke, which can be fatal. This risk may increase with duration of use. Patients with CV disease or risk factors for CV disease may be at greater risk.						
Sulindac (Clinoril®)	PO	150	q 12 hours	400	7.8	Sulindac is a prodrug metabolized to active metabolite, sulfide. Sulindac, at 200–400 mg/d, is comparable to aspirin, at 2,000–4,000 mg/d.
	Major side effects: Same as other COX-1 enzyme inhibitors (refer to ibuprofen) **Monitoring:** Same as other COX-1 enzyme inhibitors (refer to ibuprofen) **Dose adjustment:** Use is not recommended in patients with renal impairment, hepatic dysfunction, or congestive heart failure with marginal cardiac function.					
Tolmetin (Tolectin®)	PO	400	q 8 hours	1,800	1–1.5	Protein binding is 99%. Tolmetin is comparable to aspirin.
	Major side effects: Same as other COX-1 enzyme inhibitors (refer to ibuprofen) **Monitoring:** Same as other COX-1 enzyme inhibitors (refer to ibuprofen) **Dose adjustment:** Use is not recommended in patients with renal impairment, hepatic dysfunction, or congestive heart failure with marginal cardiac function.					

COX, cyclooxygenase; CV, cardiovascular; GI, gastrointestinal; IM, intramuscularly; IV, intravenously; OTC, over-the-counter; PO, orally; TD, transdermally.

appendix

14-9A

Opioid Agonists (Opioid Analgesics) (Adult Drug Doses)

Name	Route	Average Dose Range	Average Dose Interval (hours)	Duration of Action (hours)	Half-Life (hours)	Clinically Important Metabolites (Active)
Disclaimer: **Equianalgesic doses may vary depending on institutional guidelines and practice setting (e.g., acute pain, chronic pain, palliative care, or hospice).**						
Codeine	PO	30–60 mg	q4	4–6	2.5–4	Morphine
(various names)	IV	15–30 mg	q4	4–6		
	Equianalgesic dose: 120 mg of codeine IV = 200 mg of codeine PO = 10 mg of morphine IV (Carroll et al., 2004) **Major side effects:** Same toxic potentials as other opioid agonists (refer to morphine) **Monitoring:** Same as other opioid agonists (refer to morphine) **Dose adjustment:** Use is not recommended in patients with severe renal or hepatic impairment. *FDA Warning:* The FDA has notified health care providers of life-threatening adverse events reported in a nursing infant following maternal use of codeine. Codeine and its metabolite (morphine) are found in breast milk and can be detected in the serum of nursing infants. Exposure to the nursing infant is generally considered to be low. However, excessively high serum concentrations of morphine were reported in a breastfed infant following maternal use of acetaminophen with codeine. The mother was later found to be an "ultrarapid metabolizer" of codeine; symptoms in the infant included feeding difficulty and lethargy, followed by death. The FDA recommends that caution be used when prescribing codeine to nursing women, since most people are not aware if they have the genotype resulting in ultrarapid metabolizer status. When codeine is prescribed, it is recommended to use the lowest dose for the shortest duration and to observe the infant for increased sleepiness, difficulty in feeding or breathing, or limpness.					
Fentanyl	IV	50–100 micrograms	q1	0.5–1	7.5	None
(Sublimaze®)	**Equianalgesic dose:** 0.1 mg of fentanyl IV = 10 mg of morphine IV (Carroll et al., 2004) **Major side effects:** Same toxic potentials as other opioid agonists (refer to morphine) **Monitoring:** Same as other opioid agonists (refer to morphine)					
Fentanyl	Lozenge, oral, as citrate (transmucosal): 200, 400, 600, 800, 1,200, 1,600 micrograms					
Buccal (Actiq®)	The initial dose is 200 micrograms. The second dose may be started 15 minutes after completion of the first dose. Consumption should be limited to no more than 4 units per day.					

(continued)

Name	Route	Average Dose Range	Average Dose Interval (hours)	Duration of Action (hours)	Half-Life (hours)	Clinically Important Metabolites (Active)

Disclaimer: Equianalgesic doses may vary depending on institutional guidelines and practice setting (e.g., acute pain, chronic pain, palliative care, or hospice).

Fentanyl Buccal (Fentora®)

Tablet, for buccal application, as citrate: 100, 200, 300, 400, 600, 800 micrograms

The initial dose is 100 micrograms. A second 100 micrograms dose, if needed, may be started 30 minutes after the start of the first dose.

Equianalgesic dose: Actiq and Fentora are not equivalent in bioavailability and dose unit. Equianalgesic dose guidelines are not available for buccal formulations.

Major side effects: Same toxic potentials as other opioid agonists (refer to morphine)

Monitoring: Same as other opioid agonists (refer to morphine)

FDA Warning: Cephalon, in conjunction with the FDA, has notified health care providers of fatal adverse events that have occurred in patients treated with Fentora, a transmucosal buccal tablet formulation of fentanyl. The fatalities have been attributed to several factors, including improper patient selection, improper dosing, improper product substitution, or a combination of these. The FDA emphasized that Fentora only be used for labeled indications and only in patients who are opioid tolerant. When using Fentora for breakthrough pain, it is recommended that patients not exceed two tablets per breakthrough pain episode and that patients allow at least 4 hours to elapse between doses. In addition, Fentora should not be used in patients with acute pain, postoperative pain, a headache or migraine, or a sports injury. The FDA also stressed that Fentora and Actiq (transmucosal lozenge) are not equivalent and that these products should not be used interchangeably on a microgram-per-microgram basis.

Fentanyl Transdermal (Duragesic®)

Transdermal patch systems: 12.5, 25, 50, 75, 100 micrograms/hr

With the standard dose interval, a new patch should be applied every 72 hours.

Equianalgesic dose: 25 micrograms/hr for each 45 mg of morphine PO (Carroll et al., 2004)

Major side effects: Same toxic potentials as other opioid agonists (refer to morphine)

Monitoring: Same as other opioid agonists (refer to morphine)

FDA Warning: Transdermal fentanyl systems are indicated for use only by opioid-tolerant patients (individuals taking routine, around-the-clock opioid pain medication) with persistent, moderate-to-severe pain. In non-opioid-tolerant patients, use of even low-dose transdermal fentanyl may result in respiratory depression and death. Patients should be instructed on the appropriate use and removal of patches and to avoid heat sources (e.g., heating pads, electric blankets, and saunas) while wearing patches, as heat may increase the absorption of fentanyl, leading to dangerously elevated serum concentrations. In addition, patients should report to their health care provider any fever higher than 102°F while the patch is being worn.

Disclaimer: Equianalgesic doses may vary depending on institutional guidelines and practice setting (e.g., acute pain, chronic pain, palliative care, or hospice).

(continued)

Name	Route	Average Dose Range	Average Dose Interval (hours)	Duration of Action (hours)	Half-Life (hours)	Clinically Important Metabolites (Active)
Hydrocodone with acetaminophen	PO	5–10 mg	q4	4–6	3.3–4.4	Hydromorphone, norcodeine, hydrocodol derivatives, hydromorphol derivatives
(various products)	**Equianalgesic dose:** 30 mg of hydrocodone PO = 30 mg of morphine PO (Carroll et al., 2004) **Major side effects:** Same toxic potentials as other opioid agonists (refer to morphine) **Monitoring:** Same as other opioid agonists (refer to morphine) **Dose adjustment:** Use is not recommended for patients with severe hepatic impairment.					
Hydromorphone (Dilaudid®)	PO	4–8 mg	q3–4	4–6	2–4	None
	PR	3 mg	q6–8	6		
	IV, SC	0.2–0.4 mg	q3–4	4–6		
	Equianalgesic dose: 1.5 mg of hydromorphone IV = 7.5 mg of hydromorphone PO = 10 mg of morphine IV (Carroll, et al., 2004) **Major side effects:** Same toxic potentials as other opioid agonists (refer to morphine) **Monitoring:** Same as other with opioid agonists (refer to morphine) **Dose adjustment:** Use is not recommended in patients with renal impairment.					
Levorphanol (Levo-Dromoran®)	PO	2–4 mg	q6	6–8	12–16	None
	IV	2–4 mg	q6	6–8		
	Equianalgesic dose: Acute pain: 2 mg of levorphanol IV = 4 mg of levorphanol PO (APS, 2008) For chronic pain dosing (McNulty, 2007):					

Oral Morphine Equivalent (mg)	*Oral Morphine-to-Oral Levorphanol Ratio*
<100	12:1
100–299	15:1
300–599	20:1
600–799	25:1
≥800	No data

Name	Route	Average Dose Range	Average Dose Interval (hours)	Duration of Action (hours)	Half-Life (hours)	Clinically Important Metabolites (Active)
	Major side effects: Same toxic potentials as other opioid agonists (refer to morphine), but less nausea or vomiting and more sedation compared with morphine **Monitoring:** Same as other opioid agonists (refer to morphine) **Dose adjustment:** Accumulates in 2–3 days because of long half-life.					
Meperidine (Demerol®, Pethidine®)	PO	Not recommended				
	IV	50–100 mg	q2–3	4	3–4	Normeperidine (half-life 8–20 hours)
	Equianalgesic dose: 100 mg of meperidine IV = 300 mg of meperidine PO = 10 mg of morphine IV (Carroll, et al., 2004) **Major side effects:** There is a risk of seizures because of accumulation of normeperidine metabolite with prolonged administration of more than 48 hours for acute pain or doses greater than 600 mg in 24 hours; otherwise, there are the same toxic potentials as with other opioid agonists (refer to morphine). Has atropine-like characteristics and therefore causes pupil dilation. Normeperidine is the metabolite and while naloxone reverses the CNS-depressing effect of meperidine, it does not reverse the CNS-activating properties of normeperidine and can cause seizures. (APS, 2003, p. 36).					

(continued)

Name	Route	Average Dose Range	Average Dose Interval (hours)	Duration of Action (hours)	Half-Life (hours)	Clinically Important Metabolites (Active)

Monitoring: Same as other opioid agonists (refer to morphine)

Dose adjustment: Avoid administration in patients with hepatic or renal impairment. Administration is contraindicated in patients receiving monoamine oxidase inhibitors during the previous 14 days.

Disclaimer: Equianalgesic doses may vary depending on institutional guidelines and practice setting (e.g., acute pain, chronic pain, palliative care, or hospice).

Name	Route	Average Dose Range	Average Dose Interval (hours)	Duration of Action (hours)	Half-Life (hours)	Clinically Important Metabolites (Active)
Methadone®	PO	5–10 mg	q6–8	6–12	24–36	None
(Dolophine®)	IV	2–5 mg	q6–8	6–12		

Equianalgesic dose: Acute pain: 5 mg of methadone IV = 10 mg of methadone PO (APS, 2003)

For chronic pain dosing (Gazelle & Fine, 2004):

Oral Morphine Equivalent (mg)	*Oral Morphine-to-Oral Methadone Ratio*
<100	3:1
101–300	5:1
301–600	10:1
601–800	12:1
801–1,000	15:1
>1,001	20:1

Major side effects: Sedation increases with repeated administration; same toxic potentials as other opioid agonists (refer to morphine)

Monitoring: Same as other opioid agonists (refer to morphine)

Dose adjustment: Steady state level is achieved in 3–5 days. Use is not recommended for patients with severe renal impairment.

FDA Warning (deaths):

- Deaths, cardiac and respiratory events, have been reported during initiation and conversion of pain patients to methadone treatment from treatment with other opioids
- Cause of death is thought to be related to prolongation of the QT_c interval, which creates ventricular arrhythmias and torsades de pointes. The recommendations for timing of EKG monitoring differ per institution.
- Consensus guidelines state that the clinician (1) inform patients of arrhythmia risk when prescribing methadone; (2) ask patients about any history of structural heart disease, arrhythmia, and syncope; (3) obtain a pretreatment EKG for all patients to measure the QT_c interval, a follow-up EKG within 30 days and annually, and an additional EKG if doses exceed 100 mg/d or patients have unexplained syncope or seizures; (4) if the QT_c interval is greater than 450 milliseconds but less than 500 milliseconds, discuss the potential risk with patients and monitor more frequently or, if the QT_c interval exceeds 500 milliseconds, eliminate drugs that promote hypokalemia or choose an alternative therapy; (5) be aware of interactions of other drugs with methadone and of other drugs that will possess QT interval-prolonging properties or slow the elimination of methadone (Krantz, Martin, Stimmel, Mehta, & Halgney, 2009).
- In some cases, drug interactions with other drugs, both licit and illicit, have been suspected. In other cases, deaths appear to have occurred due to the respiratory or cardiac effects of methadone and overly rapid titration without appreciation for the accumulation of methadone over time.

(continued)

Name	Route	Average Dose Range	Average Dose Interval (hours)	Duration of Action (hours)	Half-Life (hours)	Clinically Important Metabolites (Active)
	• Particular vigilance is necessary during treatment initiation, during conversion from one opioid to another, and during dose titration. • Patients must also be strongly cautioned against self-medicating with CNS depressants during initiation of methadone treatment.					
Disclaimer: Equianalgesic doses may vary depending on institutional guidelines and practice setting (e.g., acute pain, chronic pain, palliative care, or hospice).						
Morphine®	PO	10–20 mg	q4	3–6	2–4	M3G, M6G, normorphine
Short acting	IV, SC	2–8 mg	q4	3–6	6	
(various products)	PR	10–20 mg	q4	8	6	No data
	Equianalgesic dose: 10 mg of morphine IV = 30 mg of morphine PO (APS, 2003) **Major side effects:** Respiratory depression and apnea in opioid-naïve patients or patients receiving concurrent CNS depressants, such as benzodiazepines or alcohol; hypotension; sedation; dizziness; weakness; agitation; restlessness; delirium; mental clouding; seizures; nausea; vomiting; constipation; biliary spasm; urinary retention; impotence, sweating, pruritus, and itching because of histamine release; urticaria; long-term use potentially leading to psychological and physical dependence **Monitoring:** Respiratory function, including oxygen saturation and respiration rate; sedation level (i.e., increased sedation precedes respiratory depression); withdrawal (signs or symptoms occur within 24 hours of abrupt discontinuation, including restlessness, anxiety, lacrimation, rhinorrhea, yawning, sweating, piloerection, mydriasis, with peak intensity of withdrawal in 36–72 hours characterized by muscle spasms, backaches, hot and cold flashes, insomnia, nausea, vomiting, diarrhea, fever, elevated vital signs); frequency of bowel movements **Dose adjustment:** Avoid in patients with renal impairment because of accumulation of M6G metabolite, which can result in enhanced and prolonged opioid activity. Avoid abrupt discontinuation to prevent severe withdrawal symptoms.					

Long-Acting Oral Morphine

Brand Name	Dose Interval (hr)	Black Box Warning:
MS Contin®	8 or 12	Extended/sustained Release Products: [U.S. Boxed Warning]: Extended- or sustained-release dosage forms should not be crushed or chewed. Controlled-, extended-, or sustained-release products are not intended for "as needed" use. MS Contin® in 100- or 200-mg tablets is for use only in opioid-tolerant patients requiring more than 400 mg/d. Kadian® in 100- or 200-mg capsules is for use only in opioid-tolerant patients. Avinza®, Kadian®, and MS Contin® [U.S. Boxed Warning]: are indicated for the management of moderate-to-severe pain when around-the-clock pain control is needed for an extended period.
Oramorph®	8 or 12	
Kadian®	12 or 24	
Avinza®	24	Avinza® [U.S. Boxed Warning]: Do not administer Avinza® with alcoholic beverages or ethanol-containing products, which may disrupt the extended-release characteristic of product.

(continued)

Name	Route	Average Dose Range	Average Dose Interval (hours)	Duration of Action (hours)	Half-Life (hours)	Clinically Important Metabolites (Active)
Disclaimer: Equianalgesic doses may vary depending on institutional guidelines and practice setting (e.g., acute pain, chronic pain, palliative care, or hospice).						
Oxycodone	PO	5–10 mg	q4	4–6	3–4	Noroxycodone, oxymorphone
Short acting (various products)	**Equianalgesic dose:** 20 mg of oxycodone PO = 30 mg of morphine PO (Carroll et al., 2004) **Major side effects:** Same as other opioid agonists (refer to morphine) **Monitoring:** Same toxic potentials as other opioid agonists (refer to morphine) **Dose adjustment:** Oxycontin 80-mg tablets should be used in opioid-tolerant patients who require total daily doses of at least 160 mg of oxycodone product.					
Oxycodone	PO	10–20 mg	q12	4–6	3–4	Noroxycodone, oxymorphone
Long acting (Oxycontin®)	*Black Box Warning:* Controlled-release tablets [U.S. Boxed Warning]: OxyContin® is not intended for use as an "as needed" analgesic or for immediately postoperative pain management (it should be used postoperatively only if the patient has received it before surgery or if severe, persistent pain is anticipated). Do not crush, break, or chew controlled-release tablets. The 60-, 80-, and 160-mg strengths are for use only in opioid-tolerant patients.					
Disclaimer: Equianalgesic doses may vary depending on institutional guidelines and practice setting (e.g., acute pain, chronic pain, palliative care, or hospice).						
Oxymorphone	PO	10–20 mg	q4–6	3–4	7–9	None
Short acting (Opana®)	IV	1–1.5 mg	q4–6	3–4	7–9	None
Oxymorphone						
Long acting (Opana® ER)	PO	5 mg	q12		9–11	None
	Equianalgesic dose: 1 mg of oxymorphone IV = 10 mg of morphine IV (APS, 2008) **Major side effects:** Same as other opioid agonists (refer to morphine) **Monitoring:** Same toxic potentials as other opioid agonists (refer to morphine) **Dose adjustment:** Adjust the dose cautiously in patients with impaired renal function. With creatinine clearance of less than 50 ml/min, reduce the initial dosage of oral formulations (bioavailability increased 57–65%). *Black Box Warning:* Opana ER®: [U.S. Boxed Warnings]: Opana ER® is an extended-release oral formulation of oxymorphone and is not suitable for use as an "as needed" analgesic. Tablets should not be broken, chewed, dissolved, or crushed; tablets should be swallowed whole. Opana ER® is intended for use in long-term, continuous management of moderate-to-severe chronic pain. It is not indicated for use in the immediate postoperative period (12–24 hours). The coingestion of ethanol or ethanol-containing medications with Opana ER® may result in accelerated release of drug from the dosage form, abruptly increasing plasma levels, which may have fatal consequences.					

(continued)

Name	Route	Average Dose Range	Average Dose Interval (hours)	Duration of Action (hours)	Half-Life (hours)	Clinically Important Metabolites (Active)
Propoxyphene (Darvocet®, Darvon®, various names)	PO	65–130 mg	q4	4–6	8–24	Norpropoxyphene 130 (HCl salt), norpropoxyphene 200 (napsylate salt)
	Major side effects: Same as other opioid agonists (refer to morphine) **Monitoring:** Same toxic potentials as other opioid agonists (refer to morphine) **Dose adjustment:** Avoid use in patients with renal impairment; propoxyphene is not dialyzable and norpropoxyphene half-life is at least 34 hours, which can accumulate and cause seizures. Use is not recommended in patients with hepatic impairment. The maximum daily dose should not exceed 390 mg with HCl salt and 600 mg with napsylate salt. With products that combine propoxyphene with acetaminophen, know how much acetaminophen use the patient has with other medications that combine with acetaminophen and adjust the dose accordingly. Both propoxyphene and norpropoxyphene have direct cardiac effects, including decreases in heart rate, contractility, and electrical conductivity. Norpropoxyphene is more potent in this regard, and these symptoms are not reversed with naloxone. Both propoxyphene and norpropoxyphene have local anesthetic effects (Bredgaard Sorensen, Strom, Sloth Madsen, Angelo, & Reiz, 1984; Sloth Madsen, Strom, Reiz, & Bredgaard Sorensen, 1984; Nickander, Smits, & Steinberg, 1977; Nickander, Emmerson, Hynes, Steinberg, & Sullivan, 1984).					

CNS, central nervous system; EKG, electrocardiogram; FDA, U.S. Food and Drug Administration; HCl, hydrochloride; IV, intravenously; M3G, morphine-3-glucuronide; M6G, morphine-6-glucuronide; PO, orally; PR, per rectum; SC, subcutaneously.

appendix

14-9B

Partial Opioid Agonists or Antagonists (Adult Drug Doses)

Name	Route	Average Dose Range (mg)	Average Dose Interval	Duration of Action (hours)	Half-Life (hours)	Clinically Important Metabolites (Active)
Buprenorphine						
(Buprenex®)	IV	0.3	q6 hours	4–8	2–3	None
(Subutex®)	SL	6–8	tid-qid	6–8		
	Equianalgesic dose: 0.4 mg of buprenorphine IV = 10 mg of morphine IV (APS, 2008) **Major side effects:** Similar to other opioid agonists (refer to morphine) **Monitoring:** Similar toxic potentials (including withdrawal syndrome) as other opioid agonists (refer to morphine) **Dose adjustment:** The subcutaneous route is not recommended. Use cautiously in patients with hepatic impairment. Buprenorphine is not for long-term use. The maximum daily dose for chronic pain management should not exceed 32 mg (Heit & Gourlay, 2008).					
Butorphanol	IV	0.5–2	q3–4 hours	3–4	2.5–4	None
(Stadol®)	Nasal spray	1 mg (1 spray) per nostril	May repeat in 1–1.5 hours	4–5		
	Equianalgesic dose: 2 mg of butorphanol IV = 10 mg of morphine IV (APS, 2008) **Major side effects:** Drowsiness (avoid use with alcohol because of additive sedative effects), facial flushing, hypotension, dizziness, lightheadedness, nausea, vomiting, decreased urination, increased diaphoresis **Monitoring:** Similar toxic potentials (including withdrawal syndrome) as other opioid agonists (refer to morphine) **Dose adjustment:** Reduce dose for patients with renal impairment. For creatinine clearance of 10–50 ml/min, administer 75% of the usual dose. If creatinine clearance is less than 10 ml/min, administer 50% of the usual dose.					
Nalbuphine	IV, SC	10 mg per 70 kg	q3–6 hours	3–6	3.5–5	None
(Nubain®)	**Equianalgesic dose:** 10 mg of nalbuphine IV = 10 mg of morphine IV (APS, 2008) **Major side effects:** Drowsiness (avoid use with alcohol because of additive sedative effects), paradoxical CNS stimulation, facial flushing, hypotension, dizziness, lightheadedness, nausea, vomiting, xerostomia, decreased urination, increased diaphoresis, pulmonary edema **Monitoring:** Similar toxic potentials (including withdrawal syndrome) as other opioid agonists (refer to morphine)					

(continued)

Name	Route	Average Dose Range (mg)	Average Dose Interval	Duration of Action (hours)	Half-Life (hours)	Clinically Important Metabolites (Active)
	Dose adjustment: The total daily dose should not to exceed 160 mg. Single doses should not exceed 20 mg. Use is not recommended for patients with hepatic impairment.					
Pentazocine (Talwin®)	PO	50–100	q3–4 hours	4–5	2–3	None
	Equianalgesic dose: 30 mg of pentazocine IV = 50 mg of pentazocine PO = 10 mg of morphine IV (APS, 2008) **Major side effects:** Euphoria, drowsiness, nausea, vomiting, weakness, hypotension, malaise, xerostomia, ureteral spasm, blurred vision, dyspnea **Monitoring:** Similar toxic potentials (including withdrawal syndrome) as other opioid agonists (refer to morphine) **Dose adjustment:** The total daily dose should not to exceed 600 mg. Use is not recommended for patients with hepatic impairment. Reduce the dose for patients with renal impairment. For creatinine clearance of 10–50 ml/min, administer 75% of the usual dose. If creatinine clearance is less than 10 ml/min, administer 50% of the usual dose.					

CNS, central nervous system; IV, intravenously; PO, orally; qid, four times per day; SC, subcutaneously; SL, sublingually; tid, three per day.

14-9C

Opioid Antagonists (Adult Drug Doses)

Name	Route	Average Dose Range	Average Dose Interval	Duration of Action (hours)	Plasma Half-Life (hours)
Nalmefene (Revex®)	IV	0.25 micrograms/kg for postoperative respiratory depression; 1 microgram/kg for overdose	Titrate dose every 2–5 minutes	4–8 (longer duration than naloxone more suitable for reversal of long-acting opioids)	10
	Major side effects: Symptoms of acute withdrawal (nausea, vomiting, agitation, tachycardia, hypertension, fever, dizziness, acute pain), increased risk of seizures with coadministration of nalmefene and flumazenil **Monitoring:** Vital signs for recurrence of respiratory depression, withdrawal symptoms, level of pain, cardiac function in patients with cardiovascular disorders (i.e., preexisting hypertension, arrhythmias) **Dose adjustment:** Administration is not approved in children. Do not administer IM or SC in apneic patients because of prolonged time to maximal affect. The blue-label product (100 micrograms/ml) is for postoperative respiratory depression; the green label product (1,000 micrograms/ml) is for opioid overdose.				
Naloxone (Narcan®)	IV	0.4–2 mg for adults; 0.2 mg per dose for children older than 5 years or at least 20 kg	Titrate dose every 2–3 minutes; bolus dose if patient is apneic	0.3–1	1–1.5, adults; 1.2–3, neonates
	Major side effects: Symptoms of acute withdrawal (nausea, vomiting, agitation, tachycardia, hypertension, fever, dizziness, acute pain), increased risk of seizures with coadministration of nalmefene and flumazenil **Monitoring:** Vital signs for recurrence of respiratory depression, withdrawal symptoms, level of pain, cardiac function in patients with cardiovascular disorders (i.e., preexisting hypertension, arrhythmias) **Dose adjustment:** Titrate to effect.				

(continued)

Name	Route	Average Dose Range	Average Dose Interval	Duration of Action (hours)	Plasma Half-Life (hours)
Alvimopan (Entereg®)	Postoperative ileus, following partial large or small bowel resection surgery with primary anastomosis: 12 mg PO 30 minutes to 5 hours before surgery, followed by 12 mg PO twice daily beginning the day after surgery for up to 7 days or until hospital discharge for a maximum of 15 doses				
	Major side effects: Hypokalemia, flatulence, indigestion, backache, anemia, urinary retention, myocardial infarction **Monitoring:** GI motility, loose stools **Dose adjustment:** Alvimopan is not recommended in renal or hepatic insufficiency.				
Methylnaltrexone (Relistor®)	Use for opioid-induced constipation in patients with advanced illness receiving palliative care after failing laxative therapy. Give one dose (weight-based) subcutaneous every other day as needed. Do not exceed a maximum of one dose in a 24-hour period.				
		Weight < 38 kg	0.15 mg/kg per dose		
	Calculate injection volume by multiplying above weight (in kilograms) by 0.0075 and rounding up to the nearest 0.1 ml.				
		Weight 38 kg to < 62 kg:	8 mg per dose (0.4 ml)		
		Weight 62–114 kg:	12 mg per dose (0.6 ml)		
	Major side effects: Contraindicated in patients with mechanical gastrointestinal obstruction, abdominal pain, flatulence, nausea, dizziness **Monitoring:** GI motility, loose stools, renal function **Dose adjustment:** For subcutaneous use only: inject in the upper arm, abdomen, or thigh. For creatinine clearance of less than 30 ml/min, reduce the dose by 50%.				

GI, gastrointestinal; IM, intramuscularly; IV, intravenously; PO, orally; SC, subcutaneously.

14-10A

Glucocorticoid Steroids (Adult Drug Doses)

Name	Route	Average Dose Range (mg)	Average Dose Interval (hours)	Plasma Half-Life (hours) Plasma	Biological
Betamethasone (Celestone®)	PO	0.6–2.4	q 6–12	>5	36–54
	Major side effects: Adrenal insufficiency with use more than 10 consecutive days (do not abruptly discontinue if used ≥ 10 days), immunosuppression (contraindicated for use in patients with systemic fungal infections), insomnia, increased appetite, weight gain, blurred vision, confusion, dyspepsia, peptic ulcer, hyperglycemia, hypertension, Na^+ retention, hypertrichosis, impaired wound healing, skin atrophy, acneiform eruptions, myalgia and muscle weakness, bone growth suppression, sterile abscess (with intramuscular or local injections), osteoporosis and compression fractures with long-term use **Monitoring:** Blood glucose, blood pressure, weight, mental status, black-tarry stools for gastrointestinal bleeding **Dose adjustment:** Dose must be tapered off if administered at least 10 days (fatal adrenal insufficiency can result from abrupt discontinuation). Use with caution in patients with hypothyroidism, cirrhosis, or ulcerative colitis. Dose can be administered via other routes, including intramuscular, inhalation, joint injections, and topical.				
Dexamethasone (Decadron®)	PO, IV	2–6	q 6–12	1.8–3.5	36–54
	Major side effects: Same as other glucocorticoids (refer to betamethasone) **Monitoring:** Same as other glucocorticoids (refer to betamethasone) **Dose adjustment:** Dose can be administered via other routes, including intramuscular, joint injections, and topical.				
Methylprednisolone (Medrol®)	PO	2–16	q 6–24	1.3–3	18–36
	IV	10–40	q 4–6 for 48 hours		
	Major side effects: Same as other glucocorticoids (refer to betamethasone) **Monitoring:** Same as other glucocorticoids (refer to betamethasone) **Dose adjustment:** Dose can be administered via other routes, including intramuscular, joint injections, and topical. Dose varies depending on inflammatory condition.				
Prednisone (Deltasone®)	PO	5–15	q 6–24	1	18–36
	Major side effects: Same as other glucocorticoids (refer to betamethasone) **Monitoring:** Same as other glucocorticoids (refer to betamethasone) **Dose adjustment:** Dose varies depending on inflammatory condition.				
Triamcinolone (Aristocort,® Kenalog®)	Joint injection	10–40	—	>3	18–36
	Major side effects: Same as other glucocorticoids (refer to betamethasone) **Monitoring:** Same as other glucocorticoids (refer to betamethasone) **Dose adjustment:** Dose can be administered via other routes, including intramuscular, inhalation, and topical. Dose varies depending on inflammatory condition.				

IV, intravenously; Na^+, sodium; PO, orally.

appendix

14-10B

Mineralocorticoid Steroids (Adult Drug Doses)

Name	Route	Average Dose Range (mg)	Average Dose Interval (hours)	Plasma Half-Life (hours) Plasma	Biological	Anti-Inflammatory Potency	Mineralocorticoid Potency
Cortisone (Cortizone®, Cortone®)	PO	25–150	q 12–24	0.5	8–12	0.8	Yes
	Major side effects: Same as other mineralocorticoids (refer to fludrocortisone) **Monitoring:** Same as other mineralocorticoids (refer to fludrocortisone) **Dose adjustment:** Dose varies depending on inflammatory condition.						
Fludrocortisone (Florinef®)	PO	0.1–0.2	q 24	0.5	18–36	No data	Most potent
	Major side effects: Adrenal insufficiency with use more than 10 consecutive days (do not abruptly discontinue if used ≥ 5 days), immunosuppression (contraindicated for use in patients with systemic fungal infections), hypertension, edema, congestive heart failure, acne, rash, bruising, hypokalemic alkalosis, suppression of growth, hyperglycemia, peptic ulcer, muscle weakness, cataracts, diaphoresis, increased appetite, weight gain, osteoporosis and compression fractures with long-term use **Monitoring:** Blood glucose, blood pressure, weight, mental status, black-tarry stools for gastrointestinal bleeding **Dose adjustment:** Dose must be tapered off if administered at least 5 days (fatal adrenal insufficiency can result from abrupt discontinuation).						
Hydrocortisone (Cortef®)	PO	25–240	q 12–24	1.3–2	8–12	1	2
	Major side effects: Same as other mineralocorticoids (refer to fludrocortisone) **Monitoring:** Same as other mineralocorticoids (refer to fludrocortisone) **Dose adjustment:** Dose varies depending on inflammatory condition. Dose can be administered via other routes including intramuscular, joint injections, and topical.						

PO, orally.

Steroid Potencies

Steroid	Equivalent Dose (mg)	Antiinflammatory	Sodium Retaining
Betamethasone	0.65	25	0
Cortisone	25	0.8	2
Dexamethasone	0.75	25	0
Hydrocortisone	20	1	2
Methylprednisolone	4	5	0
Prednisone	5	4	1
Triamcinolone	4	5	0

appendix

14-11

Serotonin Agonists and Antagonists (Adult Drug Doses)

Name	Route	Average Dose Range (mg)	Average Dose Interval	Maximal Daily Dose	Plasma Half-Life
Dihydroergotamine (Migranal®, DHE)	Intranasal	2	1 spray each nostril; repeat once in 15 minutes as needed; may repeat cycle every 8 hours	4 sprays every 24 hours	10 hours
	IV	0.5	May repeat once in 1 hour (administer IV over 1 minute)	Not to exceed 2 mg/d or 6 mg/wk	Two phases: first phase is 2.3 minutes to 1.45 hours, second phase is 10–32 hours
	IM, SC	1	May repeat every hour	3 mg/d or 6 mg/wk	Two phases: first phase is 2.3 minutes to 1.45 hours, second phase is 10–32 hours
	Major side effects: Do not use in patients with CAD or who are at risk for CAD, as doing so may precipitate a myocardial infarction; cold, numb fingers and toes; nausea; vomiting; xerostomia; diarrhea headache; muscle pain; or weakness. **Monitoring:** Effect is seen in 15 minutes, with a recurrence rate in 14% of patients. Monitor blood pressure and peripheral pulses during treatment, and report hypertension. Monitor acute toxicity (signs or symptoms include peripheral ischemia, paresthesia, headache, nausea, and vomiting). **Dose adjustment:** Give the initial dose in the physician's office. Do not use triptans within 8 hr of ergotamine and do not use triptans when ergotamine has been used within 8 hours.				
Ergoloid mesylate (Hydergine®)	PO	1	Up to tid	12 mg/d for ≤ 6 month	3.5
	Major side effects: Nausea, sublingual irritation **Monitoring:** Blood pressure, heart rate, acute toxicity (signs or symptoms include sinus bradycardia, blurred vision, headache, stomach cramps), chronic toxicity (signs or symptoms include extremity or organ ischemia) **Dose adjustment:** Do not use triptans within 8 hr of ergotamine and do not use triptans when ergotamine has been used within 8 hours.				

(continued)

Name	Route	Average Dose Range (mg)	Average Dose Interval	Maximal Daily Dose	Plasma Half-Life
Ergotamine tartrate (Ergomar®, Bellergal-S®, Cafergot®)	PO, SL	1–2 initially	1–2 mg every 30 minutes until headache subsides	6 mg; should not be used more than twice a week, with at least 5 days between courses	Two phases: first phase is 2.7 hours, second phase is 21 hours
	Major side effects: Do not use in patients with CAD or who are at risk for CAD, as doing so may precipitate a myocardial infarction, tachycardia, bradycardia, arterial spasm, claudication and vasoconstriction, rebound headache, local edema, and numbness and tingling of fingers and toes. Other side effects include drowsiness, dizziness, nausea, vomiting, xerostomia, and diarrhea. **Monitoring:** Effect is seen in 15 minutes, with a recurrence rate in 14% of patients. Monitor blood pressure and peripheral pulses during treatment, and report hypertension. Monitor acute toxicity (signs or symptoms include nausea, vomiting, vasospastic effects, lassitude, impaired mental function, hypotension or hypertension, unconsciousness, seizures, and shock). **Dose adjustment:** Do not use triptans within 8 hr of ergotamine and do not use triptans when ergotamine has been used within 8 hours.				
Almotriptan (Axert®)	PO	6.25–12.5	Repeat in 2 hours; no more than four headache treatments in 1 month	Not to exceed 2 doses every 24 hours	3–4 hours
	Major side effects: Tingling; nausea; dry mouth; drowsiness. Contraindicated in patients with hemiplegic or basilar migraine; cluster headache; known or suspected ischemic heart disease (angina pectoris, myocardial infarction, documented silent ischemia, coronary artery vasospasm, Prinzmetal's variant angina); peripheral vascular syndromes (including ischemic bowel disease); uncontrolled hypertension. Do not use within 24 hours of another 5-HT_1 agonist. Do not use within 24 hours of an ergotamine derivative. Do not administer concurrently or within 2 weeks of discontinuing an MAOI, specifically MAOI type A inhibitors. **Monitoring:** Liver and renal function before initiation, blood pressure **Dose adjustment:** For patients with renal or hepatic impairment, the initial dose is 6.25 mg in a single dose and the maximum daily dose is no more than 12.5 mg.				
Eletriptan (Relpax®)	PO	20–40	Repeat in 2 hours	Not to exceed 80 mg in 24 hours	4 hours
	Major side effects: Dizziness; drowsiness; nausea; dry mouth; paresthesia; chest or abdominal tightness; vomiting; dysphagia. Contraindicated in patients with ischemic heart disease or signs or symptoms of ischemic heart disease (including Prinzmetal's angina, angina pectoris, myocardial infarction, silent myocardial ischemia); cerebrovascular syndromes (including strokes, transient ischemic attacks); peripheral vascular syndromes (including ischemic bowel disease); uncontrolled hypertension; severe hepatic impairment. Do not use within 24 hours of ergotamine derivatives. Do not use within 24 hours of another 5-HT_1 agonist. Do not use within 72 hours of potent CYP3A4 inhibitors. Do not use to manage a hemiplegic or basilar migraine. **Monitoring:** Liver and renal function before initiation, blood pressure **Dose adjustment:** None recommended.				

(continued)

Name	Route	Average Dose Range (mg)	Average Dose Interval	Maximal Daily Dose	Plasma Half-Life
Frovatriptan (Frova®)	PO	2.5	Repeat in 2 hours; no more than four headache treatments in 1 month	Not to exceed 7.5 mg in 24 hours; no more than 4 HA treatment in 1 month	26 hours
	Major side effects: Chest tightness; flushing; dizziness; tingling; fatigue. Contraindicated in patients with ischemic heart disease or signs or symptoms of ischemic heart disease (including Prinzmetal's angina, angina pectoris, myocardial infarction, silent myocardial ischemia); cerebrovascular syndromes (including strokes, transient ischemic attacks); peripheral vascular syndromes (including ischemic bowel disease); uncontrolled hypertension; severe hepatic impairment. Do not use within 24 hours of ergotamine derivatives. Do not use within 24 hours of another 5-HT_1 agonist. Do not use to manage a hemiplegic or basilar migraine. **Monitoring:** Liver and renal function before initiation, blood pressure **Dose adjustment:** None recommended				
Naratriptan (Amerge®)	PO	2.5	No more than four headache treatments in 1 month	5 mg every 24 hours, no more than 4 HA treatments in 1 month	6 hours; however, increased in renal dysfunction
	Major side effects: Chest or throat tightness; tingling; flushing; dizziness; nausea. Contraindicated in patients with hemiplegic or basilar migraine; cluster headache; known or suspected ischemic heart disease (angina pectoris, myocardial infarction, documented silent ischemia, coronary artery vasospasm, Prinzmetal's variant angina); peripheral vascular syndromes (including ischemic bowel disease); uncontrolled hypertension. Do not use within 24 hours of another 5-HT_1 agonist. Do not use within 24 hours of an ergotamine derivative. **Monitoring:** Liver and renal function before initiation, blood pressure **Dose adjustment:** For creatinine clearance of 18–39 ml/min, use an initial dose of 1 mg and do not exceed 2.5 mg in 24 hours. If the creatinine clearance is less than 15 ml/min, do not use. The maximum dose is 2.5 mg in 24 hours for patients with mild or moderate liver failure.				
Rizatriptan (Maxalt®)	PO	5–10	Repeat in 2 hours	Not to exceed 15 mg in 24 hours	
	Major side effects: Somnolence; myocardial infarction; ventricular fibrillation; ventricular tachycardia; coronary artery vasospasm. Contraindicated in patients with documented ischemic heart disease or Prinzmetal's angina; uncontrolled hypertension; basilar or hemiplegic migraine. Do not use during or within 2 weeks of MAOIs. Do not use during or within 24 hours of treatment with another 5-HT_1 agonist or an ergot-containing or ergot-type medication (e.g., methysergide or dihydroergotamine). **Monitoring:** Liver and renal function before initiation, blood pressure **Dose adjustment:** Use lower dose in patients receiving propranolol.				
Sumatriptan (Imitrex®)	PO	25–50	q 2 hr	300 mg/d	2 hours
	SC	6	q 1 hr	12 mg/d	2 hours

(continued)

Name	Route	Average Dose Range (mg)	Average Dose Interval	Maximal Daily Dose	Plasma Half-Life
	Nasal	5, 10, 20 in one nostril	Do not administer second dose if there was no relief with the first dose	40 mg/d or no > 5 episodes per month	2 hours
	Major side effects: Myocardial infarction; dizziness; vertigo; tingling; warm sensation. Contraindicated in patients with patients with ischemic heart disease or signs or symptoms of ischemic heart disease (including Prinzmetal's angina, angina pectoris, myocardial infarction, silent myocardial ischemia); cerebrovascular syndromes (including strokes, transient ischemic attacks); peripheral vascular syndromes (including ischemic bowel disease); uncontrolled hypertension; severe hepatic impairment. Do not use within 24 hours of ergotamine derivatives. Do not use within 24 hours of another 5-HT_1 agonist. Do not administer concurrently or within 2 weeks of discontinuing an MAOI, specifically MAOI type A inhibitor. Do not use to manage a hemiplegic or basilar migraine. Do not administer IV. **Monitoring:** Liver and renal function before initiation, blood pressure **Dose adjustment:** Administer with caution in patients with renal or liver impairment.				
Zolmitriptan (Zomig®)	PO	2.5–5	Repeat in 2 hours	Not to exceed 10 mg in 24 hours	3
	Nasal	5 mg in one nostril	Repeat in 2 hours	Not to exceed 10 mg in 24 hours	3
	Major side effects: Chest pain, pressure, tightness, heaviness, hypertension, palpitations. Contraindicated in patients with ischemic heart disease or Prinzmetal's angina; signs or symptoms of ischemic heart disease; uncontrolled hypertension; symptomatic Wolff-Parkinson-White syndrome or arrhythmias associated with other cardiac accessory conduction pathway disorders. Do not use with or within 24 hours of ergotamine derivatives. Do not use within 24 hours of another 5-HT_1 agonist. Do not administer concurrently or within 2 weeks of discontinuing an MAOI. Do not use to manage a hemiplegic or basilar migraine. **Monitoring:** Liver and renal function before initiation, blood pressure **Dose adjustment:** No dose recommendation is given for renal impairment. Administer with caution in patients with liver disease, generally using doses less than 2.5 mg. Patients with moderate-to-severe hepatic impairment may have decreased clearance of zolmitriptan, and significant elevation in blood pressure was observed in some patients.				

5-HT, 5-hydroxytryptamine; CAD, coronary artery disease; CYP3A4, cytochrome P3A4; IM, intramuscularly; IV, intravenously; MAOI, monoamine oxidase inhibitor; SC, subcutaneously; SL, sublingually; PO, orally; tid, three times per day; HA, headache.

appendix

14-12A

Acetaminophen (Adult Drug Doses)

Name	Route	Average Dose Range (mg)	Average Dose Interval (hours)	Maximal Daily Dose (mg)	Half-Life (hours)	Analgesic Efficacy
Acetaminophen (Tylenol®)	PO, PR	325–650	q 4–6	4,000	1–3	Analgesia comparable to aspirin but weak antiinflammatory activity

Major side effects: The incidence of adverse effects is low (<1%) at the normal daily dose.

Monitoring: Monitor acute toxicity from large doses of 7,500–10,000 mg daily for 1–2 days (signs or symptoms include dose-dependent hepatic necrosis that is potentially fatal and associated with acetaminophen blood levels > 200 micrograms/ml at 4 hours and 50 micrograms/ml at 12 hours postingestion; nausea, vomiting, and abdominal pain within 2–3 hours of ingestion of toxic dose; methemoglobinemia resulting in cyanosis of the skin, mucosa, and fingernails; hypoxia, shock, and coma). Laboratory monitoring includes serum creatinine for patients at risk for renal complications and periodic liver function tests with long-term therapy or patients concurrently consuming alcohol.

Dose adjustment: The maximal daily dose is 2,400 mg for patients who consume at least 2 drinks per day containing alcohol. The dosing interval is reduced for patients with renal impairment, based on creatinine clearance, as follows:

Creatinine clearance 10–50 ml/min	Administer every 6 hours
Creatinine clearance <10 ml/min	Administer every 8 hours
Hemodialysis:	Moderately dialyzable (20–50%)

PO, orally; PR, per rectum.

14-12B

Tramadol (Adult Drug Doses)

Name	Route	Average Dose Range (mg)	Average Dose Interval (hours)	Maximal Daily Dose	Half-Life (hours)	Analgesic Efficacy
Tramadol						
(Ultram®)	PO	50–100	q 4–6	400 mg	6–8	Tramadol, at 100 mg, is comparable to morphine, at 10 mg IV, but with a higher incidence of nausea or vomiting.
(Ultracet®)	PO	1–2 tabs	q 4–6	8 tabs	6–8	
	1 tab contains 37.5 mg of tramadol and 325 mg acetaminophen					

Major side effects: Dizziness, somnolence, restlessness, nausea, diarrhea, constipation, vomiting, dyspepsia, weakness, diaphoresis, seizures, respiratory depression (not completely reversible with naloxone)

Monitoring: Acute toxicity (signs or symptoms include respiratory depression, seizure, miosis, vomiting), serum creatinine for patients with renal impairment, liver function tests periodically for patients with hepatic impairment of cirrhosis

Dose adjustment: The dose must be adjusted in patients with renal or hepatic impairment. For patients with creatinine clearance of less than 30 ml/min or hepatic cirrhosis, tramadol should be dosed at 50–100 mg every 12 hours, not to exceed 200 mg/d. When used as a combination product with acetaminophen, consider the 24-hour use of acetaminophen with other combination products. Ultracet® (contains acetaminophen) is not recommended for patients with liver failure.

IV, intravenous; PO, oral.

chapter

15

Integrative Therapies Used in Pain Management Nursing

Susan O'Conner-Von, PhD, RN
Hob Osterlund, APRN, BC
Linda Shin, MN, ACNS-BC
Melanie H. Simpson, PhD, RN-BC, OCN, CHPN

Objectives

After studying this chapter, the reader should be able to:

1. Define the terms integrative therapy, complementary therapy, and alternative therapy.
2. Describe the four domains of complementary and alternative medicine (CAM) according to the National Institutes of Health National Center for Complementary and Alternative Medicine.
3. Identify the potential benefits of integrative therapies.
4. Describe the use of acupuncture, chiropractic, humor, and massage for patients in pain.
5. Describe the use of integrative therapies for pediatric pain management.

For centuries, nurses have embraced the use of complementary therapies. Although not identified as such, nurses have used therapies such as music, humor, and massage to provide comfort for their patients. More recently, other health care professions have recognized the value of complementary therapies, yet many conclude that there is insufficient evidence for the efficacy of these therapies due to the lack of the scientific rigor of randomized, controlled clinical trials. Pain management nurses can play a critical role in promoting the use of complementary therapies, and engaging in the much-needed research that will establish a scientific base to support the use of these therapies for our patients in pain.

I. Definition of Terms

A. Although these terms *are often used interchangeably,* the following are definitions from the National Institutes of Health (NIH) National Center for Complementary and Alternative Medicine (NCCAM) (NIH, 2009):
   1. *Complementary:* a therapy *used with* conventional medicine
   2. *Alternative:* a therapy *used in place of* conventional medicine
   3. *Integrative:* a *combination* of conventional medicine and complementary or alternative therapy for which there is solid evidence of safety and effectiveness

B. *Complementary and alternative medicine (CAM)* is a group of diverse medical and health care systems, practices, and products that are not presently considered to be part of conventional medicine. The list of what is considered to be CAM is in constant flux as those therapies that are found to be safe and effective become adopted into conventional health care.

C. *Integrative medicine* is a comprehensive, primary care system in which wellness and healing of the whole person are the major goals, as opposed to the basic suppression of symptoms or disease (Bell et al., 2002).

II. National Center for Complementary and Alternative Medicine (NCCAM)

A. NCCAM is the U.S. government's leading agency for scientific research on CAM.

B. NCCAM is 1 of 27 institutes and centers that make up the NIH.

C. The mission of NCCAM is to
   1. Explore complementary and alternative healing practices in the context of rigorous science.
   2. Educate complementary and alternative therapies researchers.
   3. Disseminate authoritative information to professionals and the public.

D. Four domains of CAM have been established by NCCAM (NIH, 2009).
   1. *Mind-body therapy* involves the use of various techniques to enhance bodily function or relieve symptoms. Examples include humor, imagery, meditation, prayer, and yoga.
   2. *Biologically based practices* involve the use the substances found in nature. Examples include herbs, vitamins, and nutritional supplements.
   3. *Manipulative and body-based practices* involve the movement of one or more body parts. Examples include acupuncture, chiropractic, hydrotherapy, Rolfing, and massage.
   4. *Energy therapy* involves the use of energy fields. Examples include healing touch, therapeutic touch, Reiki, and magnets.

E. Use of CAM in the United States
   1. More than 1,800 complementary and alternative therapies have been identified (Kreitzer & Jensen, 2000).
   2. Based on a survey of 31,044 adults 18 years and older in the United States, 36% use some form of CAM (NIH, 2009).
   3. When prayer for health reasons was added to the definition of CAM in this survey, the percentage of U.S. adults using CAM rose to 62%.
   4. The most commonly reported conditions of those seeking complementary and alternative therapies were the following: back problems, neck problems, cancer, chronic pain, HIV, anxiety, depression, headaches, arthritis, and fatigue (NIH, 2002).
   5. According to the survey, CAM was used more often by
      a. Women than men.

b. People with higher educational levels.
c. People who had been hospitalized within the year.

III. Potential Benefits of CAM

A. Researchers have identified the neuroanatomic pathways and neurochemical mechanisms involved in the pain experience (see the chapter on Neurophysiology of Pain); however, the subjective nature of pain presents a challenge for those treating pain.
B. Although pharmacological interventions are primary in caring for most patients in pain, complementary therapies can be used in addition and may reduce the need for excessive analgesics, thus reducing potential side effects (Acute Pain Management Guideline Panel, 1992).
C. CAM may have a physiological effect: decrease stimulation of the sympathetic nervous system, produce muscle relaxation, lower heart rate, improve oxygenation, lower blood pressure, and release endogenous pain-relieving substances (McCaffery & Pasero, 1999).
D. CAM require the health care professional to interact with the patient in a manner that offers hope of pain relief, establishes an empathetic relationship, and requires time to be spent working directly with the patient.

IV. Nurses' Role in the Use of Integrative Therapies in Pain Management

A. Nurses must be aware of the reasons patients turn to complementary and alternative therapies. The following are some of the reported reasons:
   1. Financial, cultural, and geographic barriers to conventional care
   2. Seeking a sense of hope, control, personal attention, regard for the whole person, and decreased use of medications (Fontaine, 2005)
B. Nurses must assess and document which complementary and alternative therapies patients are using, how often, and when they are being used.
   1. It is important for nurses to screen for CAM use, assess for safety and efficacy, identify any potential interactions, and be alert for any adverse effects.
C. Nurses must educate their patients regarding the importance of seeking out qualified and licensed CAM practitioners.
   1. Most state nurse practice acts are silent on complementary and alternative therapies; they do not preclude nurses from practicing these approaches.
   2. Nurses can seek additional education and certification in several of these therapies, such as massage, Reiki, and therapeutic touch.
D. Although patients can use various therapies to manage their pain, visits to chiropractors and massage therapists combined represent 50% of all visits to CAM practitioners in the United States (Eisenberg et al., 1998). These two therapies will be addressed as they pertain to pain management, along with the use of acupuncture and humor.

V. Acupuncture

A. Included in the NCCAM domain of manipulative-body based practices, acupuncture is an ancient therapeutic technique that involves the insertion of needles into the body to promote health and for various illnesses.
B. Theory
   1. There are patterns of energy flow (Qi) (pronounced "Chee") through the body that are essential for health.
   2. Disruptions of Qi are thought to be responsible for disease.
   3. Acupuncture corrects these imbalances of Qi using the meridian system, which is difficult to explain in Western medicine.
C. Indications (NIH, 1997)
   1. Fibromyalgia
   2. Headache
   3. Menstrual cramps
   4. Myofascial pain

5. Osteoarthritis
6. Low back pain
7. Carpal tunnel syndrome

D. Efficacy (Barlas & Lundeberg, 2006)
1. The data in support of acupuncture are as strong as those for many accepted Western medical therapies.
2. The incidence of adverse effects is lower than that of many drugs and accepted medical procedures used for the same conditions.

E. Biological effects of acupuncture (Leung, 2005)
1. Considerable evidence supports the claim that opioid peptides are released during acupuncture and that opioid antagonists such as naloxone reverse the analgesic effects of acupuncture.
2. Stimulation of acupuncture needles activates the hypothalamus and pituitary gland, resulting in systemic effects, including regulation of blood flow centrally and peripherally.

F. Who can perform acupuncture in the United States
1. Training and credentialing of acupuncture practitioners are by the appropriate state agencies.
2. Education standards are established for training physicians and nonphysician acupuncturists.

VI. Chiropractic

A. Chiropractic is included in the NCCAM domain of manipulative and body-based practices that involve the movement of one or more body parts. Chiropractic is defined as a health care discipline that emphasizes the inherent recuperative power of the body to heal itself without the use of drugs or surgery (Redwood, 2008). Chiropractic was promoted in early 20th-century medicine by Andrew Still and David Palmer and was an important influence on the use of complementary therapies for health care (Spencer & Jacobs, 2003). Chiropractic is the third largest independent health profession in the United States, after conventional medicine and dentistry (Fontaine, 2005). Approximately 3% to 16% of adults receive chiropractic care in the United States every year (NIH, 2009).

B. Theory
1. Theoretical underpinnings of chiropractic care include the following:
   a. Structure and function exist in intimate relation to each other.
   b. Structural distortions can cause functional abnormalities.
   c. The nervous system occupies a preeminent role in the restoration and maintenance of proper bodily function.
   d. A vertebral subluxation influences bodily function primarily through neurological means (Redwood, 2008).
2. The major focus is adjustment of the spinal column, which is proposed to improve health, arrest disease, or both (Spencer & Jacobs, 2003).

C. Indications
1. Of patients who seek the care of chiropractors, 90% do so for musculoskeletal pain such as backache, neck ache, and headache (Redwood, 2008).
2. Chiropractic was included as oft-used therapy to treat pain according to a national study examining the use of complementary therapies (Eisenberg et al., 1998).

D. Efficacy
1. Research supports the use of chiropractic for low back pain (Assendelft, Koes, Knipschild, & Bouter, 1995) and neck pain (Hurwitz et al., 2002).

E. Who can perform chiropractic care in the United States
1. Chiropractors are licensed in every state, and most major health insurance companies reimburse for chiropractic care.

VII. Humor

A. Included in the NCCAM mind—body therapy domain, humor is defined by the Association for Applied and Therapeutic Humor (2008) as any intervention that promotes health and wellness by stimulating a playful discovery, expression, or appreciation of the absurdity or incongruity of life's situations.

B. Indications
   1. Humor may enhance health or be used as a complementary treatment of illness to facilitate healing or coping, whether physical, emotional, cognitive, social or spiritual (http://www.aath.org).
   2. Humor is present in 85% of home hospice visits (Adamle & Ludwick, 2005).
   3. Humor is a CAM option, used in 34% of patients with primary brain tumors (Armstrong et al., 2006).
   4. Up to 75% of breast cancer patients report using various CAMs, of which humor is included (Astin, Reilly, Perkins, & Child, 2006).
   5. Up to 54% of cancer patients use for cancer symptom management in palliative care (Mansky & Wallerstedt, 2006).
   6. Humor is used in a large proportion of patient encounters with physicians, independent of patient characteristics (Granek-Catarivas, Goldstein-Ferber, Azuri, Vinker, & Kahan, 2005).
   7. It is an important coping factor and plays a significant role in spirituality, purpose, and meaning of life (Johnson, 2002).
C. Efficacy
   1. Relationships between sense of humor and self-reported measures of physical well-being are supported (Bennett & Lengacher, 2006a, 2006b).
   2. Sense of humor predicts quality of life and depression levels in head and neck cancer patients (Aarstad, Aarstad, Heimdal, & Olofsson, 2005).
   3. An individual's humorous personality trait or receptivity to humor may play an important role in the effects of humor on diminishing pain and other symptoms (Hudak, Dale, Hudak, & DeGood, 1991).
   4. Although humor is a popular topic in the lay literature, there are limited data from randomized trials addressing the effect of humor on pain.
D. Biological effects of humor
   1. Both mirthful laughter and the expectation of mirthful laughter boost endorphins (Berk, Tan, & Westengard, 2006).
   2. There are significant increases in discomfort thresholds in humorous treatment versus non-humorous condition (Hudak et al., 1991).
   3. Humor and relaxation raises discomfort thresholds (Mahony, Burroughs, & Hieatt, 2001).
   4. Laughter significantly increases pain thresholds (Cogan, Cogan, Waltz, & McCue, 1987).
   5. All categories of CAM are used to reduce physical symptoms and side effects from breast cancer and its treatment (Lengacher et al., 2006).
   6. Individuals with low humor traits have lower pain thresholds, whereas those with high humor traits have higher pain thresholds (Hudak et al., 1991).
   7. Humorous film increases pain tolerance (Weisenberg, Raz, & Hener, 1998).
   8. Sense of humor may not affect discomfort thresholds; successful clinical use may be due to patients' existing beliefs (Mahony et al., 2001).
E. Who can use humor when caring for patients dealing with pain
   1. All nurses can use humor.
   2. Humor was promoted by Florence Nightingale in *Notes on Nursing:* "painful impressions are far better dismissed by a real laugh" (Christie & Moore, 2004).

VIII. Massage Therapy

A. Included in the NCCAM domain of manipulative and body-based practices, massage therapy is defined as manual soft tissue manipulation that includes holding, causing movement, and applying pressure to the body for the purpose of easing pain or increasing relaxation. In one survey, 36% of Americans said they received a massage for stress management, relaxation, or both within the last 5 years, compared to 22% in the prior year (American Massage Therapy Association, 2008). A national survey by the American Hospital Association in 2003 showed that 82% of hospitals offering CAM included massage therapy for pain management and pain relief (Barnes, Powell-Griner, McFann, & Nahini, 2004).
B. Indications (Calenda & Weinstein, 2008)
   1. Stress management

2. Pain management
3. Improved mobility

C. Efficacy
1. Massage therapy is considered to be safe with few negative effects; however, there have been few clinical trials evaluating the effectiveness of massage in the treatment of pain (NIH, 2009).
2. One randomized, controlled trial examined the impact of massage, with 605 adult patients undergoing abdominal or thoracic surgery. Patients receiving massage therapy every day during the postoperative hospital stay had overall improvements in pain relief and anxiety (Mitchinson et al., 2007).

D. Biological effects
1. Effects include increased blood circulation to the muscles, decreased stress, decreased muscle tension, and improved range of motion (Ernst, 2004).
2. Massage effectively reduces lymphedema in cancer patients.
3. Contraindications for massage therapy include bone fractures, open wounds, burns, and deep vein thrombosis.

E. Who can perform massage therapy in the United States
1. A surge in the regulation of profession began in the 1990s.
2. Currently, massage therapists are licensed in 38 states.
3. Basic Swedish massage techniques used to provide a back rub are included in most nursing curricula.

IX. Use of CAM for Pediatric Pain

A. Developmental considerations
1. A child's cognitive and psychosocial development influences the child's ability to communicate and cope with pain.
2. As children age, they shift from using passive coping strategies to active coping strategies (Sharrer & Ryan-Wenger, 1995).

B. Indications
1. The use of CAM techniques is a cornerstone of providing care for acute (procedural, postoperative) and chronic pain.
2. CAM interventions such as cognitive-behavioral therapies can increase the child's feelings of control, restructure negative feelings that can amplify pain perception and behaviors, and teach the child how to cope during painful procedures.
3. Mind-body interventions such as cognitive-behavioral therapies (i.e., distraction, music, guided imagery, and hypnosis) have been used for decades with the pediatric cancer population to reduce procedural pain, anxiety, and distress (Post-White, Sencer, Fitzgerald, & Miranda, 2000).

C. Efficacy
1. In general, active coping strategies such as distraction, relaxation, and imagery are effective in reducing a child's pain response when measured by self-report, parent report, and child behavior (Vessey & Carlson, 1996). These strategies are most effective when the child and parent work together (Blount, Landolf-Fritsche, Powers, & Sturgis, 1991).

D. Biological effects
1. Biologically based therapies have the greatest potential for harm due to interactions with medications, cancer treatment (chemotherapy), or liver and renal toxicities. Children are especially vulnerable to products with heavy-metal impurities because of their developing organs and smaller body mass.

E. Nursing considerations when working with children
1. In a study of 120 pediatric patients with cancer who were using complementary and alternative therapies, 28% of the families never reported their use of CAM to their health care team. This was because they were never asked (Post-White et al., 2000).
    a. Assess and document the following:
        (1) Use of CAM at initial visit and throughout course of care
        (2) The child's response to CAM and the effectiveness in pain management
        (3) Any negative effects of CAM and needed follow-up

b. Educate the child and family about the availability of CAM.
   (1) Teach the child and family proper use of CAM before pain is present, if possible.
c. Provide the child and family with reliable resources for CAM professionals with pediatric expertise.
   (1) Assist the family to find resources providing financial assistance or insurance reimbursement for CAM.

Summary

It is evident that patients are interested in and use complementary and alternative therapies to manage pain. According to the Institute of Medicine (2002), the number of annual visits to CAM providers in the United States outnumbers the number of annual visits to primary care providers. In addition, it is estimated that annual out-of-pocket costs for CAM exceed $27 billion. There are many complementary and alternative therapies available to assist patients in the management of acute and chronic pain; however, additional research is needed to examine the safety and effectiveness of these therapies and to protect patients from potential harm. As patient demand for complementary and alternative therapies increases, it is imperative that pain management nurses remain committed to providing high-quality, evidence-based care. Pain management nurses are in a key position to promote a truly integrative healing environment with the use of safe and effective complementary and alternative therapies, along with conventional care.

References

Aarstad, H. J., Aarstad, A. K., Heimdal, J. H., & Olofsson, J. (2005). Mood, anxiety and sense of humor in head and neck cancer patients in relation to disease stage, prognosis and quality of life. *Acta Otolaryngology, 125*(5), 557–565.

Acute Pain Management Guideline Panel. (1992). *Acute pain management: Operative or medical procedures and trauma.* Clinical Practice Guideline No. 1. (AHCPR Publication No. 92-0032.) Rockville, MD: Agency for Health Care Policy and Research.

Adamle, K. N., & Ludwick, R. (2005). Humor in hospice care: Who, where, and how much? *American Journal Hospice & Palliative Care, 22*(4), 287–290.

American Massage Therapy Association. (2008). *2008 massage therapy consumer survey fact sheet.* Retrieved December 19, 2008, from http://www.amtamassage.org/media/consumersurvey_factsheet-2008.html.Armstrong, T., Cohen, M. Z., Hess, K. R., Manning, R., Lee, E. L., Tamayo, G., Baumgartner, K., Min, S., Yung, A., & Gilbert, M. et al. (2006). Complementary and alternative medicine use and quality of life in patients with primary brain tumors. *Journal of Pain and Symptom Management, 32*(2), 148–154.

Assendelft, W., Koes, B., Knipschild, P., & Bouter, L. (1995). The relationship between methodological quality and conclusions in reviews of spinal manipulation. *Journal of the American Medical Association, 274*(24), 1942–1948.

Association for Applied and Therapeutic Humor. (2008). *Definition of therapeutic humor.* Retrieved June 10, 2008, from http://www.aath.org.

Astin, J. A., Reilly, C., Perkins, C., & Child, W. L. (2006). Breast cancer patients' perspectives on and use of complementary and alternative medicine: A study by the Susan G. Komen Breast Cancer Foundation. *Journal of the Society for Integrative Oncology, 4*(4), 157–169.

Barlas, P., & Lundeberg, T. (2006). Transcutaneous electrical nerve stimulation and acupuncture. In S. B. McMahon & M. Koltzenburg (Eds.), *Textbook of pain* (5th ed., pp. 19–835). Philadelphia: Elsevier.

Barnes, P., Powell-Griner, E., McFann, K., & Nahini, R. (2004). Complementary and alternative medicine use among adults: United States, 2002. *Seminars in Integrative Medicine, 2,* 54–71.

Bell, I., Caspi, C., Schwartz, G., Grant, K., Gaudet, T., Rychener, D., Maizes, V., & Weil, A. (2002). Integrative medicine and systemic outcomes research: Issues in the emergence of a new model for primary health care. *Archives of Internal Medicine, 162,* 133–140.

Bennett, M. P., & Lengacher, C. A. (2006a). Humor and laughter may influence health. I. History and background. *Evidence-Based Complementary and Alternative Medicine, 3*(1), 61–63.

Bennett, M. P., & Lengacher, C. (2006b). Humor and laughter may influence health. II. Complementary therapies and humor in a clinical population. *Evidence-Based Complementary and Alternative Medicine, 3*(2), 187–190.

Berk, L., Tan, S., & Westengard, J. (2006). *Beta-endorphin and HGH increase are associated with both the anticipation and experience of mirthful laughter.* Paper presented at the meeting of the American Physiological Society. Abstract 233.18.

Blount, R., Landolf-Fritsche, B., Powers, S., & Sturgis, J. (1991). Differences between high and low coping children and between parent and staff behaviors during painful medical procedures. *Journal of Pediatric Psychology, 16*(6), 795–809.

Calenda, E., & Weinstein, S. (2008). Therapeutic massage. In M. Weintraub, R. Mamtani, & M. Micozzi (Eds.), *Complementary and integrative medicine in pain management* (pp. 139–161). New York: Springer.

Christie, W., & Moore, C. (2004). The impact of humor on patients with cancer. *Clinical Journal of Oncology Nursing, 9*(2), 211–218.

Cogan, R., Cogan, D., Waltz, W., & McCue, M. (1987). Effects of laughter and relaxation on discomfort thresholds. *Journal of Behavioral Medicine, 10,* 139–144.

Eisenberg, D., Davis, R., Ettner, S., Appel, S. Wilkey, S., Van Rompay, M., & Kessler, R. (1998). Trends in alternative medicine use in the United States: Results of a follow-up national survey. *Journal of the American Medical Association, 280*(18), 1569–1575.

Ernst, E. (2004). Manual therapies for pain control: Chiropractic and massage. *Clinical Journal of Pain, 20*(1), 8–12.

Fontaine, K. (2005). *Complementary & alternative therapies for nursing practice.* Upper Saddle River, NJ: Prentice Hall Health.

Granek-Catarivas, M., Goldstein-Ferber, S., Azuri, Y., Vinker, S., & Kahan, E. (2005). Use of humour in primary care: Different perceptions among patients and physicians. *Postgraduate Medicine Journal, 81*(952), 126–130.

Hudak, D. A., Dale, J. A., Hudak, M. A., & DeGood, D. E. (1991). Effects of humorous stimuli and sense of humor on discomfort. *Psychological Reports, 69*(3, Pt. 1), 779–786.

Hurwitz, E., Morgenstern, H., Harber, P., Kominski, G., Yu, P., & Adams, A. (2002). A randomized trial of chiropractic manipulation and mobilization for patients with neck pain. *American Journal of Public Health, 92*(10), 1634–1641.

Institute of Medicine. (2002). *Executive summary: Complementary and alternative medicine in the United States.* Committee on the Use of Complementary and Alternative Medicine by the American Public. Washington, DC: National Academies Press.

Johnson, P. (2002). The use of humor and its influences on spirituality and coping in breast cancer survivors. *Oncology Nursing Forum, 29*(4), 691–695.

Kreitzer, M. J., & Jensen, D. (2000). Healing practices: Trends, challenges, and opportunities for nurses in acute and critical care. *AACN Clinical Issues, 11,* 7–16.

Lengacher, C. A., Bennett, M. P., Kip, K. E., Gonzalez, L., Jacobsen, P., & Cox, C. E. (2006). Relief of symptoms, side effects, and psychological distress through use of complementary and alternative medicine in women with breast cancer. *Oncology Nursing Forum, 33*(1), 97–104.

Leung, A. Y. (2005). Acupuncture. In M. S. Wallace & P. S. Staats (Eds.), *Pain medicine & management: Just the facts* (pp. 260–266). New York: McGraw-Hill.

Mahony, D. L., Burroughs, W. J., & Hieatt, A. C. (2001). The effects of laughter on discomfort thresholds: Does expectation become reality? *Journal of General Psychology, 128*(2), 217–226.

Mansky, P. J., & Wallerstedt, D. B. (2006). Complementary medicine in palliative care and cancer symptom management. *Cancer Journal, 12*(5), 425–431.

McCaffery, M., & Pasero, C. (1999). *Pain: Clinical manual.* St. Louis: Mosby.

Mitchinson, A. R., Kim, H. M., Rosenberg, J. M., Geisser, M., Kirsh, M., Cikrit, D., & Hinshaw, D.B. (2007). Acute postoperative pain management using massage as an adjuvant therapy. *Archives of Surgery, 142*(12), 1158–1167.

National Institutes of Health. (1997). Acupuncture: Consensus statement. *National Institutes of Health, 15,* 1–34.

National Institutes of Health. (2002). *White House Commission on Complementary and Alternative Medicine Policy.* Washington, DC: U.S. Government Printing Office.

National Institutes of Health. (2009). *National Center for Complementary and Alternative Medicine.* Retrieved May 24, 2009, from http://www.nccam.nih.gov.

Post-White, J., Sencer, S., Fitzgerald, M., & Miranda, M. (2000). Complementary therapy use in pediatric cancer. *Oncology Nursing Forum, 27,* 342–343.

Redwood, D. (2008). Chiropractic. In M. Weintraub, R. Mamtani, & M. Micozzi (Eds.), Complementary *and integrative medicine in pain management* (pp. 175–199). New York: Spring Publishing.

Sharrer, V., & Ryan-Wenger, N. (1995). A longitudinal study of age and gender differences of stressors and coping strategies in school-aged children. *Journal of Pediatric Health Care, 9,* 123–130.

Spencer, J., & Jacobs, J. (2003). *Complementary and alternative medicine: An evidence-based approach.* St. Louis: Mosby.

Vessey, J., & Carlson, K. (1996). Nonpharmacological interventions to use with children in pain. *Issues in Comprehensive Pediatric Nursing, 19*(3), 169–182.

Weisenberg, M., Raz, T., & Hener, T. (1998). The influence of film-induced mood on pain perception. *Pain, 76*(3), 365–375.

Websites

The American Chiropractic Association is the largest professional association in the world representing doctors of chiropractic. The association provides professional and educational opportunities for doctors of chiropractic, funds research, and offers leadership for the profession.

http://www.acatoday.org

The American Holistic Nurses Association is a nonprofit membership association for nurses and other holistic health care professionals, serving more than 4,000 members across the United States. This organization promotes the education of nurses and the public in all aspects of holistic caring and healing.

http://www.ahna.org

Healing Touch International is the professional nonprofit organization for healing touch. This organization sets healing touch standards for practice, administers certification, coordinates research and health integration, and provides education.

http://www.healingtouchinternational.org/index.php

The National Institutes of Health National Center for Complementary and Alternative Medicine provides information on complementary and alternative medicine, including publications and searches of federal databases of scientific literature.

http://www.nccam.nih.gov

The National Institutes of Health Office of Dietary Supplements provides information on dietary supplements, evaluates scientific information, and educates professionals and the public.

http://www.ods.od.nih.gov

University of Minnesota, Center for Spirituality & Healing website provides interdisciplinary education, research, and provides innovative programs that advance integrative health and healing.

http://www.csh.umn.edu

Suggested Readings

Antall, G., & Kresevic, D. (2004). The use of guided imagery to manage pain in an elderly orthopaedic population. *Orthopedic Nursing, 23*(5), 335–340.

Astin, J., Berman, B., Bausell, B., Lee, W., Hochberg, M., & Forys, K. (2003). The efficacy of mindfulness meditation plus Qigong movement therapy in the treatment of fibromyalgia: A randomized controlled trial. *Journal of Rheumatology, 30,* 2257–2262.

Buckle, J. (1999). Use of aromatherapy as a complementary treatment for chronic pain. *Alternative Therapies, 5*(5), 42–51.

Burns, E., Blamey, C., Ersser, S., Barnetson, L., & Lloyd, A. (2000). An investigation into the use of aromatherapy in intrapartum midwifery practice. *Journal of Alternative and Complementary Therapies, 6*(2), 141–147.

Cross, J. (2000). *Acupressure: Clinical applications in musculo-skeletal conditions.* Boston: Butterworth-Heinemann.

Cuellar, N. (2006). *Conversations in complementary and alternative medicine.* Boston: Jones and Bartlett.

Dennison, B. (2004). Touch the pain away: New research on therapeutic touch and persons with fibromyalgia syndrome. *Holistic Nursing Practice, 18*(3), 142–151.

Dillard, J., & Knapp, S. (2005). Complementary and alternative pain therapy in the emergency department. *Emergency Medicine Clinics of North America, 23,* 529–549.

Dossey, B., & Keegan, L. (Eds.). (2009). *Holistic nursing: A handbook for practice.* Sudbury, MA: Jones and Bartlett.

Field, T. (2008). Pregnancy and labor alternative therapy research. *Alternative Therapies in Health & Medicine, 14*(5), 28–34.

Freeman, L. (2004). *Mosby's complementary and alternative medicine: A research-based approach.* St. Louis: Mosby.

Good, M., Anderson, G., Stanton-Hicks, M., Grass, J., & Makii, M. (2002). Relaxation and music reduces pain after gynecologic surgery. *Pain Management Nursing, 3,* 61–70.

Good, M., Picot, B., Salem, S., Chin, C., & Lane, D. (2000). Cultural differences in music chosen for pain relief. *Journal of Holistic Music, 18*(3), 245–260.

Hinman, M., Ford, J., & Heyl, H. (2002). Effects of static magnets on chronic knee pain and physical function: A double-blind study. *Alternative Therapies in Health & Medicine, 8*(4), 50–55.

Institute of Medicine. (2005). *Complementary and alternative medicine in the United States.* Washington, DC: National Academies Press.

Keefer, L., & Blanchard, E. (2002). A one year follow-up of relaxation response meditation as a treatment for irritable bowel syndrome. *Behavior Research & Therapy, 40,* 541–546.

Knutson, L., & Weiss, P. (2009). Exploring integrative medicine: The story of a large, urban, tertiary care hospital. In B. Dossey & L. Keegan (Eds.), *Holistic nursing: A handbook for practice.* Boston: Jones and Bartlett.

Kwekkeboom, K., Kneip, J., & Pearson, L. (2003). A pilot study to predict success with guided imagery for cancer pain. *Pain Management Nursing, 4*(3), 112–123.

Lee, M. (2008). Is Reiki beneficial for pain management? *Focus on Alternative and Complementary Therapies, 13*(2), 78–81.

Micozzi, M. (2006). *Fundamentals of complementary and integrative medicine.* St. Louis: Saunders Elsevier.

Micozzi, M. (2007). *Complementary and integrative medicine in cancer care and prevention.* New York: Springer.

Olson, K., & Hanson, J. (2003). A phase II trial of Reiki for the management of pain in advanced cancer patients. *Journal of Pain and Symptom Management, 26*(5), 990–997.

Post-White, J., Fitzgerald, M., Hageness, S., & Sencer, S. (2009). Complementary and alternative medicine use in children with cancer and general and specialty pediatrics. *Journal of Pediatric Oncology Nursing, 26*(1), 7–15.

Post-White, J., Fitzgerald, M., Savik, K., Hooke, M., Hannahan, A., & Sencer, S. (2009). Massage therapy for children with cancer. *Journal of Pediatric Oncology Nursing, 26*(1), 16–28.

Rossi, P., Torelli, P., Lorenzo, C., Sances, G., Manzoni, G., Tassorelli, C., & Nappi, G. (2008). Use of complementary and alternative medicine by patients with cluster headache: Results of a multi-centre headache clinic survey. *Complementary Therapies in Medicine, 16*(4), 220–227.

Snyder, M., & Lindquist, R. (2006). *Complementary/alternative therapies in nursing.* New York: Springer.

Stephenson, L., Dalton, J., & Carlson, J. (2003). The effect of foot reflexology on pain in patients with metastatic cancer. *Applied Nursing Research, 16,* 284–286.

Tekur, P., Singphow, C., Nagendra, H., & Raghuram, N. (2008). Effect of short-term intensive yoga program on pain, functional disability and spinal flexibility in chronic low back pain: A randomized control study. *Journal of Alternative & Complementary Medicine, 14*(6), 637–644.

Wahbeh, H., Elsas, S., & Oken, B. (2008). Mind-body interventions: Applications in neurology. *Neurology, 70,* 2321–2328.

Wardell, D., & Weymouth, K. (2004). Review of studies of healing touch. *Journal of Nursing Scholarship, 36*(2), 147–154.

Weintraub, M., Mamtani, R., & Micozzi, M. (2008). *Complementary and integrative medicine in pain management.* New York: Springer.

Winstead-Fry, P., & Kijek, J. (1999). An integrative review and meta-analysis of therapeutic touch research. *Alternative Therapies, 5,* 58–67.

Acupuncture

Ernst, E., & White, A. R. (1998). Acupuncture for back pain: A meta-analysis of randomized controlled trials. *Archives of Internal Medicine, 158,* 2235–2241.

Eshkevari, L., & Heath, J. (2005). Use of acupuncture for chronic pain: Optimizing clinical practice. *Holistic Nursing Practice, 19*(5), 217–221.

Goldman, R. Stason, W., Park, S., Kim, R., Schnyer, R., Davis, R., Legedza, A., & Kaptchuk, T. (2008). Acupuncture for treatment of persistent arm pain due to repetitive use: A randomized controlled clinical trial. *Clinical Journal of Pain, 24*(3), 211–218.

Kwon, Y., Pittler, M., & Ernst, E. (2006). Acupuncture for peripheral joint osteoarthritis: A systematic review and meta-analysis. *Rheumatology, 45*(11), 1331–1337.

Marklow, M. J., & Secor, E. R. (2003). Acupuncture for the pain management of osteoarthritis of the knee. *Techniques in Orthopaedics, 18*(1), 33–36.

Selfe, T., & Taylor, A. (2008). Acupuncture and osteoarthritis of the knee: A review of randomized, controlled trials. *Family Community Health, 31*(3), 247–254.

Sierpina, V. S., & Frenkel, M. A. (2005). Acupuncture: A clinical review. *Southern Medical Journal, 98*(3), 330–337.

Wang, S. M., Kain, Z. N., & White, P. (2008). Acupuncture analgesia: The scientific basis. *Pain Medicine, 106*(2), 602–610.

Chiropractic

Vinjamury, S., Singh, B., Khorsan, R., Comberiati, R., Meier, M., & Holm, S. (2008). Chiropractic treatment of temporo-mandibular disorders. *Alternative Therapies in Health & Medicine, 14*(4), 60–63.

Wilkey, A., Gregory, M., Byfield, D., & McCarthy, P. (2008). A comparison between chiropractic management and pain clinic management for chronic low-back pain in a National Health Service outpatient clinic. *Journal of Alternative & Complementary Medicine, 14*(5), 465–473.

Humor

Matz, A., & Brown, S. T. (1998). Humor and pain management: A review of current literature. *Journal of Holistic Nursing, 16*(1), 68–75.

Swarup, A. B., Barrett, W., & Jazieh, A. R. (2006). The use of complementary and alternative medicine by cancer patients undergoing radiation therapy. *American Journal of Clinical Oncology, 29*(5), 468–473.

Zillman, D., Rockwell, S., Schweitzer, K., & Sundar, S. (1993). Does humor facilitate coping with physical discomfort? *Motivation and Emotion, 17,* 1–21.

Massage Therapy

Anderson, P. G., & Cutshall, S. M. (2007). Massage therapy: A comfort intervention for cardiac surgery patients. *Clinical Nurse Specialist, 21*(3), 161–165.

Chang, M., Wang, S., & Chen, C. (2002). Effects of massage on pain and anxiety during labour: A randomized controlled trial in Taiwan. *Journal of Advanced Nursing, 38,* 68–73.

Currin, J., & Meister, E. (2008). A hospital-based intervention using massage to reduce distress among oncology patients. *Cancer Nursing, 31*(3), 214–221.

Dryden, T., Baskwill, A., & Preyde, M. (2004). Massage therapy for the orthopaedic patient. *Orthopaedic Nursing, 23*(5), 327–332.

Kolcaba, K., Dowd, T., Steiner, R., & Mitzel, A. (2004). Efficacy of hand massage for enhancing the comfort of hospice patients. *Journal of Hospice and Palliative Nursing, 6*(2), 91–102.

Liu, Y., & Fawcett, T. (2008). The role of massage therapy in the relief of cancer pain. *Nursing Standard, 22*(21), 35–40.

McCaffery, R., Frock, T. L., & Garguilo, H. (2003). Understanding chronic pain and the mind–body connection. *Holistic Nursing Practice, 17*(6), 281–289.

MacDonald, G. (1999). *Medicine hands: Massage therapy for people with cancer.* Tallahassee, FL: Findhorn Press.

Salvo, S. (1999). *Massage therapy: Principles and practice.* Philadelphia: W. B. Saunders.

Wang, H., & Keck, J. (2004). Foot and hand massage as an intervention for postoperative pain. *Pain Management Nursing, 5,* 59–65.

Weiner, D. K., & Ernst, E. (2004). Complementary and alternative approaches to the treatment of persistent musculoskeletal pain. *Clinical Journal of Pain, 20*(4), 244–255.

Pediatric

American Pain Society. (2005). *Guideline for the management of cancer pain in adults and children.* Glenview, IL: Author.

Anbar, R. (2001). Self-hypnosis for the treatment of functional abdominal pain in childhood. *Clinical Pediatrics, 40*(8), 447–451.

Ball, T., Shapiro, D., Monheim, C., & Wydert, J. (2003). A pilot study of the use of guided imagery for the treatment of recurrent abdominal pain in children. *Clinical Pediatrics, 42*(6), 527–532.

Baumann, R. (2002). Behavioral treatment of migraine in children and adolescents. *Pediatric Drugs, 4*(9), 555–561.

Bligen, H., & Ozek, E. (2002). Comparison of sucrose, expressed breast milk, and breast-feeding on the neonatal response to heel prick. *Journal of Pain, 2*(5), 301–305.

Boyle, E., Freer, Y., Khan-Orakzai, Z., Watkinson, M., Ainsworth, J., & McIntosh, N. (2006). Sucrose and non-nutritive sucking for the relief of pain in screening for retinopathy of prematurity: A randomized controlled trial. *Archives of Disease in Childhood: Fetal and Neonatal Edition, 91,* 166–168.

Butler, L., Symons, B., Henderson, S., Shortliffe, L., & Spiegel, D. (2005). Hypnosis reduces distress and duration of an invasive medical procedural for children. *Pediatrics, 115*(1), 77–85.

D'Apolito, K. (2006). State of the science: Procedural pain management in the neonate. *Journal of Perinatology & Neonatal Nursing, 20*(1), 56–61.

Evans, S., Tsao, J., & Zeltzer, L. (2008). Complementary and alternative medicine for acute procedural pain in children. *Alternative Therapies in Health & Medicine, 14*(5), 52–56.

Field, T., Henteleff, T., Hernandez-Reif, M., Martinez, E., Mavunda, K., Kuhn, C., Schanberg, S. (1998). Children with asthma have improved pulmonary function after massage. *Journal of Pediatrics, 132,* 854–858.

Golianu, B. (2007). Non-pharmacological techniques for pain management in neonates. *Seminars in Perinatology, 31*(5), 318–322.

Harvey, S., Bauer-Wu, S., Hawks, R., Kelly, K., Laizner, A., & Post-White, J. (2005). Consensus statement: Complementary and alternative medicine in pediatric oncology. *Seminars in Oncology Nursing, 21*(2), 122–124.

Jindal, V., Ge, A., & Mansky, P. (2008). Safety and efficacy of acupuncture in children: A review of the evidence. *Journal of Pediatric Hematology/Oncology, 30*(6), 431–442.

Kemper, K., Sarah, R., Silver-Highfield, E., Barnes, L., & Berde, C. (2000). On pins and needles? Pediatric pain patients' experience with acupuncture. *Pediatrics, 105*(4), 941–947.

King, P. (2003). Listen to the children and honor their pain. *Oncology Nursing Forum, 30*(5), 797–800.

Kundu, A., & Berman, B. (2007). Acupuncture for pediatric pain and symptom management. *Pediatric Clinics of North America, 54,* 885–899.

Lassetter, J. (2006). The effectiveness of complementary therapies on the pain experience of hospitalized children. *Journal of Holistic Nursing, 24,* 196–208.

Liossi, C. (2000). Clinical hypnosis in pediatric oncology: A critical review of the literature. *Sleep and Hypnosis, 2*(3), 125–131.

Liossi, C., & Hatira, P. (1999). Clinical hypnosis versus cognitive behavioral training for pain management with pediatric cancer patients undergoing bone marrow aspirations. *International Journal of Clinical Hypnosis, 47*(2), 104–116.

Liossi, C., White, P., & Hatira, P. (2006). Randomized clinical trial of local anesthetic versus a combination of local anesthetic with self-hypnosis in the management of pediatric procedural pain. *Health Psychology, 25*(3), 307–315.

McCarthy, A., Cool, V., & Hanrahan, K. (1998). Cognitive behavioral interventions for children during painful procedures: Research challenges and program development. *Journal of Pediatric Nursing, 13*(1), 55–63.

Post-White, J. (2006). Complementary and alternative medicine in pediatric oncology. *Journal of Pediatric Oncology Nursing, 23*(5), 244–253.

Rheingans, J. (2007). A systematic review of nonpharmacologic adjunctive therapies for symptom management in children with cancer. *Journal of Pediatric Oncology Nursing, 24,* 81–94.

Richardson, J., Smith, J.E., McCall,G., & Pilkington, K. (2006). Hypnosis for procedure-related pain and distress in pediatric cancer patients: A systematic review of effectiveness and methodology related to hypnosis interventions. *Journal of Pain and Symptom Management, 31*(1), 70–84.

Steggles, S., Damore, S., Maxwell, J., & Lightfoot, N. (1997). Hypnosis for children and adolescents with cancer. *Journal of Pediatric Oncology Nursing, 14*(1), 27–32.

Styles, J. (1997). The use of aromatherapy in hospitalized children with HIV disease. *Complementary Therapies in Nursing, 3,* 16–20.

Van Epps, S., Zempsky, W., Schechter, N., & Laner, T. (2007). The effects of a two-week trial of transcutaneous electrical nerve stimulation for pediatric chronic back pain. *Journal of Pain and Symptom Management, 34*(2), 115–117.

Waterhouse, M., Stelling, C., Powers, M., Levy, S., & Zeltzer, L. (1999–2000). Acupuncture and hypnotherapy in the treatment of chronic pain in children. *Clinical Acupuncture and Oriental Medicine, 1*(3), 139–150.

chapter 16

Moderate Sedation/Analgesia

Melanie H. Simpson, PhD, RN-BC, OCN, CHPN

Objectives

After studying this chapter, the reader should be able to:

1. Define moderate sedation/analgesia.
2. List two goals for moderate sedation/analgesia.
3. Identify medications used to achieve moderate sedation/analgesia.

Moderate sedation/analgesia is the administration of pharmacological agents for the relief of discomfort, pain or anxiety that may be experienced during invasive, manipulative, or constraining procedures. The goal is for the patient to have a depressed level of consciousness yet independently maintain a patent airway and be able to respond appropriately to verbal commands or physical stimulation (Youmans, 2001). The difference in moderate sedation/analgesia and analgesia is the *intent.* With moderate sedation/analgesia, the intent is to produce an altered mental state. With analgesia, the intent is to provide pain relief with minimal side effects.

I. Four Levels of Sedation, as Defined by the American Society of Anesthesiologists (ASA) Task Force (2002)

A. Minimal sedation (anxiolysis)
  1. The patient is awake or arouses easily yet is under the influence of the drug administered.
  2. The patient maintains normal respiration, eye movements, and intact protective reflexes.
  3. Amnesia may or may not be present.

B. Moderate sedation/analgesia (conscious sedation)
  1. The patient is in a pharmacologically controlled state of limited or minimally depressed consciousness.
  2. The patient independently and continuously maintains protective reflexes and a patent airway.
  3. The patient responds appropriately to physical stimulation and verbal commands.
  4. *This level is the topic of this chapter.*

C. Deep sedation/analgesia
  1. Deep sedation/analgesia is a controlled state of depressed consciousness.
  2. Patients are not easily aroused.
  3. Partial or complete loss of protective reflexes occurs, including ability to independently maintain airway.

D. General anesthesia
  1. General anesthesia is a controlled state of unconsciousness.
  2. There is loss of protective reflexes.
  3. The patient is unable to respond to physical stimuli or verbal commands.

II. Moderate Sedation/Analgesia, Previously Known as Conscious Sedation

A. Goals of moderate sedation/analgesia (Odom-Forren & Watson, 2005)
  1. Reduce the patient's anxiety and discomfort.
  2. Facilitate cooperation of the patient.

B. Objectives (Kost & Odom-Forren, 2007)
  1. Alteration in mood
  2. Maintenance of consciousness
  3. Elevation of pain threshold
  4. Minimal variation of vital signs
  5. Some degree of amnesia
  6. Rapid and safe return to activities of daily living

C. Patient selection
  1. Complete and thorough assessment (Kost & Odom-Forren, 2007; Waring et al., 2003)
     a. Medical and anesthetic history
     b. Nothing-by-mouth (NPO) status (Table 16-1)
     c. Baseline vital signs
     d. Weight
     e. Current medications
     f. Allergies
     g. Mental status
     h. History of substance abuse: alcohol, tobacco, and illicit substances

i. Airway assessment because positive pressure ventilation may be necessary if respiration is compromised
   (1) History of stridor, snoring, sleep apnea, and problems with anesthesia
   (2) Significant obesity
   (3) Facial abnormalities
   (4) Head, neck, and jaw deformities
      (a) Short neck
      (b) Limited neck extension
      (c) Neck mass
      (d) Cervical spine disease
      (e) Tracheal deviation
   (5) Mouth deformities
      (a) Nonvisible uvula
      (b) Tonsillar hypertrophy
      (c) Small mouth opening
      (d) Protruding incisors
      (e) Loose or capped teeth
      (f) High, arched palate

2. Cooperative patient
3. Patient able to follow commands
4. Unsuitable candidates
   a. Severe cardiovascular disease
   b. Severe respiratory problems

D. The nurse monitoring the patient should (Youmans, 2001)
   1. Have no other responsibilities.
   2. Be clinically competent to identify any complications.
   3. Understand the pharmacology of the administered agents.
   4. Understand the role of pharmacological reversal agents for opioids and benzodiazepines.
   5. Maintain certification in cardiopulmonary resuscitation.
   6. Have a clinician with certification in advanced cardiac life support be immediately available (ASA Task Force, 2002).

Table 16-1 NPO Recommendation for Sedation/Analgesia

Ingested Material	Minimum Fasting Time
Clear liquids	2 hours
Breast milk	4 hours
Infant formula	6 hours
Nonhuman milks	6 hours
Light meal	6 hours

- NPO is nothing by mouth.
- Recommendations apply to healthy patients who are undergoing elective procedures.
- Examples of clear liquids include water, fruit juices without pulp, carbonated beverages, clear tea, and black coffee.
- A light meal is typically toast and clear liquids. Meals that include fried or fatty foods may prolong gastric emptying.

Data from American Society of Anesthesiologists Task Force. (2002). Practice guidelines for sedation and analgesia by non-anesthesiologists. *Anesthesiology, 96*(4), 1004–1017.

Table 16-2 Level of Consciousness Scale for Monitoring Mental Status

Level	Patient Response
I	Alert
II	Sleepy
III	Lethargic
IV	Responds only to maximal stimulation; response to painful stimulus still present
V	Coma

E. Equipment must be in the room before administration of any medication.
   1. Oxygen
   2. Oxygen delivery devices
   3. Suction apparatus
   4. Noninvasive blood pressure device
   5. Electrocardiograph
   6. Pulse oximeter
   7. An emergency cart must be immediately available.
      a. Resuscitative medications
      b. Opioid and sedative reversal agents
      c. Defibrillator

F. Monitoring during the procedure (Kost & Odom-Forren, 2007)
   1. Respiratory rate
   2. Oxygen saturation
   3. Blood pressure
   4. Cardiac rate and rhythm
   5. Level of consciousness (Table 16-2)
   6. Skin condition
   7. Continuous IV access
   8. Continuous electrocardiograph for high-risk patients only
   9. Changes in condition immediately reported to the physician

G. Pharmacology agents used for sedation/analgesia depend on the type, duration, and intensity of the procedure (University of Kansas Hospital, 2005; Youmans, 2001).
   1. Nurse responsibility
      a. Consider the patient's health status.
      b. Validate the physician's orders.
      c. Obtain medications.
      d. Ensure proper administration of medications.
   2. Benzodiazepines have anticonvulsant, antianxiety, sedative, muscle relaxant, and amnesic properties and can be administered before, during, and after procedure.
      a. Midazolam (Versed) (see the chapter on Overview of Pharmacology)
         (1) Midazolam is the most commonly used in moderate sedation/analgesia (Waring et al., 2003).
         (2) Midazolam is short acting, for short-term procedures.
         (3) It is a central nervous system (CNS) depressant and sedative hypnotic.
         (4) It should be administered intravenously, orally, rectally, or nasally.
         (5) Midazolam must be given slowly by IV route.
         (6) Elderly, debilitated, or chronically ill patients should receive lower doses.
         (7) Slurred speech is an excellent indicator of an adequate dose.
         (8) Doses should be individualized (Table 16-3). Refer to Appendix 14-5.

Table 16-3 Moderate Sedation/Analgesia: Adult Medications

Drug	Age	Route	Dose or Titration	Onset	Duration	Side Effects or Precautions
Opioids: for pain control only; not appropriate for sedation, amnesia, or relief of anxiety						
Morphine (various brands)	Adults	PO PR IV	10–30 mg 10–20 mg 2 mg given slowly initially, 5–20 mg total dose	PO: 60 minutes IV: 5–10 minutes	PO or IV: 7 hours $T_{1/2}$ = 2–4 hours	Dose dependent: respiratory depression, orthostatic hypotension, nausea, itching, painful injection Decrease doses in hepatic and renal insufficiency and in elderly, debilitated patients
Fentanyl (various brands)	Adults	IV	1–2 µg/kg in 25-µg increments, slowly titrated over 1–2 minutes	IV: 1–3 minutes	IV: <60 minutes $T_{1/2}$ = 2–4 hours	Respiratory depression, apnea, hypotension, bradycardia, dizziness, nausea Decrease doses in hepatic and renal insufficiency and in elderly, debilitated patients
Opioid Reversal Agent						
Naloxone (Narcan®)	Adults	IV	Dilute 1 ampule or 0.4 mg of naloxone in 9 ml of normal saline to create a total of 10 ml and titrate to effect Maximum of 2 mg in adults	1–2 minutes	1–4 hours $T_{1/2}$ = 15 hours	Pulmonary edema, nausea, sweating, tachycardia, pain
Benzodiazepines: for sedation, amnesia, and relief of anxiety only; not for pain control						
Midazolam (Versed®)	Adults	IV	0.5–2 mg, given in no more than 1 mg increments over 2 minutes titrated to effect	IV: 1–5 minutes	IV: 2–6 hours $T_{1/2}$ = 1–4 hours	Respiratory depression, hypotension, bradycardia, hiccups, apnea Decrease doses in hepatic and renal insufficiency; in elderly, debilitated patients; and when given concurrently with other CNS depressants
Benzodiazepine Reversal Agent						
Flumazenil (Romazicon®)	Adults	IV	0.2 mg/min in incremental doses up to 1 mg	IV: 1–3 minutes	45–90 minutes $T_{1/2}$ = 30–90 minutes	Hypoventilation, may precipitate seizure
Other Agents						
Chloral Hydrate (Various Brands)	Adults	PO	500–1,000 mg for 30 minutes before procedure Maximum dose of 2 g in 24 hours	0.5–1 hours	4–8 hours $T_{1/2}$ = 8–11 hours	GI irritation, nausea, vomiting, diarrhea, disorientation, drowsiness Decrease doses in patients with renal insufficiency and avoid in hepatic impairment

CNS, central nervous system; GI, gastrointestinal; IV, intravenous, PO, oral; PR, as needed.

Adapted from Uiversity of Kansas Hospital (2005). *Policy on moderate sedation/analgesia (conscious sedation): Management of patient undergoing procedures* (revised 8-05). Lawrence, Kansas: Author.

(a) IV dose is 0.5 to 2 mg, dose adjusted by 30% when given with opioids and other CNS depressants.
(b) Give the IV dose in 1 mg increments or less every 2 to 3 minutes, titrate to effect a maximum daily dose of 5 mg.
(9) Use is contraindicated in patients with a known hypersensitivity to benzodiazepines or narrow angle glaucoma.
(10) Use with caution in patients with impaired liver or kidney function.
(11) Adverse reactions with the IV route include respiratory depression, hypotension, bradycardia, hiccups, apnea, and pain at injection site.

b. Diazepam (Valium®) (see the chapter on Overview of Pharmacology)
(1) Diazepam is long acting for longer procedures.
(2) It is a CNS depressant and anticonvulsant.
(3) It can be administered intravenously, orally, or rectally.
(4) Diazepam must be given slowly by an IV route.
(5) Elderly, debilitated, or chronically ill patients should receive lower doses.
(6) Slurred speech is an excellent indicator of an adequate dose.
(7) Doses should be individualized (see Appendix 14-5).
(a) The initial IV dose is 2 to 5 mg and may be repeated every 5 to 10 minutes.
(b) The maximum IV dose should not exceed 30 mg in 2 hours.
(8) Use is contraindicated in patients with a known hypersensitivity to benzodiazepines.
(9) Use with caution in patients with impaired liver or kidney function.
(10) Adverse reactions include drowsiness, nausea, bradycardia, venous thrombosis, phlebitis, apnea, hypotension, headache, blurred vision, syncope, vertigo, skin rash, hiccups, and changes in salivation.

c. Lorazepam (Ativan®) (see the chapter on Overview of Pharmacology)
(1) Lorazepam is long acting for longer procedures.
(2) It is a CNS depressant, anxiolytic, and sedative hypnotic.
(3) It can be administered intravenously or orally.
(4) Lorazepam must be given slowly by an IV route.
(5) Doses should be individualized (see Appendix 14-5).
(a) The initial IV dose is 0.5 to 2 mg, 15 to 20 minutes before the procedure.
(b) The initial oral dose is 1 to 2 mg, 2 hours before procedure.
(c) Half of the initial dose may be repeated every 10 to 15 minutes.
(d) The maximum adult dose by all routes is 10 mg.
(6) Use is contraindicated in patients with a known hypersensitivity to benzodiazepines or acute narrow-angle glaucoma.
(7) Use with caution in patients who are elderly, are debilitated, or have limited pulmonary reserve.
(8) Adverse reactions include excessive drowsiness and sleepiness, hallucinations, dizziness, hypertension or hypotension, nausea and vomiting, blurred vision, diplopia, depressed hearing, and skin rash.

d. When used with opioids or other CNS depressants, doses should be decreased by 30%.

3. Flumazenil (Romazicon®) (see the chapter on Overview of Pharmacology)
a. This benzodiazepine reversal agent selectively blocks the binding of benzodiazepines to its receptor site.
b. Indication is for the partial or complete reversal of the sedative effects of benzodiazepines.
c. The IV dose is 0.2 mg every 45 to 60 seconds.
(1) Continue until the desired effect is achieved.
(2) Continue until 1 mg is given.
(3) The dose can be repeated every 20 minutes if sedation reappears.
(4) No more than 3 mg should be given in a 1-hour period.
d. Flumazenil does not reverse hypoventilation or cardiac depression.

e. Use with extreme caution with patients who
   (1) Have a history of seizures.
   (2) Are dependent on benzodiazepines (increased risk of grand mal seizure, also known as tonic–clonic seizure).
   (3) Have impaired hepatic or kidney function.
f. Use is contraindicated in patients with a known hypersensitivity to benzodiazepines.
g. Adverse reactions include nausea and vomiting, dizziness, injection site pain or inflammation, agitation, headache, cutaneous vasodilation, paresthesia, labile emotion, fatigue, abnormal vision, and seizures.

4. Opioids may be administered as a premedication to provide sedation and analgesia by elevating the pain threshold.
   a. Fentanyl citrate (see the chapter on Overview of Pharmacology)
      (1) Fentanyl citrate is a synthetic opioid used for short-term analgesia.
      (2) It has a rapid onset of action.
      (3) It has a short duration of action.
      (4) Fentanyl citrate can be administered intravenously or orally.
      (5) It must be given slowly by an IV route to prevent chest wall rigidity.
      (6) Doses should be individualized (see Appendix 14-9A).
         (a) The initial IV dose of 1 to 2 μg/kg is given in 25-μg increments.
         (b) Slowly titrate over 1 to 2 minutes.
      (7) Use is contraindicated in patients with a known hypersensitivity.
      (8) Fentanyl citrate can be stored in fat and muscle tissue and thus can result in delayed-onset respiratory depression.
      (9) Use with caution in patients who are elderly or debilitated or who have supraventricular arrhythmia or bradycardia, head injury, renal or hepatic dysfunction, and pulmonary disease.
      (10) Adverse reactions include sedation, nausea and vomiting, dizziness, delirium, euphoria, blurred vision, apnea, hypotension, bradycardia, and respiratory depression.
   b. Morphine (see the chapter on Overview of Pharmacology)
      (1) Morphine can be administered intravenously or orally.
      (2) It must be given slowly by an IV route.
      (3) Doses should be individualized (see Appendix 14-9A).
         (a) The initial IV dose is 2.5 mg.
         (b) The total dose is 5 to 20 mg.
      (4) Use is contraindicated in patients with a known hypersensitivity to morphine or phenanthrene opioids.
      (5) Use with caution in patients who are elderly or debilitated or who have supraventricular arrhythmia, head injury, intracranial pressure, renal or hepatic dysfunction, and pulmonary disease.
      (6) Adverse reactions include sedation, nausea and vomiting, dizziness, delirium, euphoria, blurred vision, hypotension, bradycardia, rash, itching, flushing, and respiratory depression.

5. Naloxone (Narcan®) (see Appendix 14-9C)
   a. This opioid reversal agent reverses the effect of opioids, including sedation, respiratory depression, and analgesia by competing for the same receptor sites.
   b. Indication is for the partial or complete reversal of respiratory depression induced by opioids.
   c. A mixture of 0.4 mg is diluted in 9 ml of normal saline for a total of 10 ml.
   d. Give in 1-ml (or 0.04-mg) increments slowly and titrate to effect.
   e. Give a maximum of 2 mg in adults.
   f. If given too quickly, the immediate return of pain can cause significant sympathetic and cardiovascular stimulation, which can cause
      (1) Respiratory depression.
      (2) Hypertension or hypotension.

(3) Pulmonary edema.
(4) Nausea.
(5) Sweating.
(6) Tachycardia.
(7) Stroke.
(8) Congestive heart failure.
(9) Cardiac arrest.

H. Managing complications
1. The most common complication is respiratory depression or arrest.
a. Prevention
(1) Observe constantly.
(2) Monitor the patient's respiratory rate and pulse oximetry.
b. Treatment
(1) Administer oxygen.
(2) Stimulate the patient: verbal or painful stimulus.
(3) Instruct the patient to take a deep breath.
(4) If no spontaneous respiration occurs,
(a) use a head tilt-jaw lift maneuver.
(b) use positive-pressure ventilation.
(c) the patient may require artificial airway.
2. Notify the physician immediately of the following:
a. Rise or fall in systolic blood pressure of 20 to 30 mm Hg from baseline
b. Tachycardia (more than 150 bpm) or bradycardia (less than 50 bpm)
c. Excessive rise or fall in respiratory rate
d. Oxygen saturation of less than 90% or significantly below presedation level
e. Marked decrease in patient responsiveness to verbal or painful stimulation
f. Signs or symptoms of medication intolerance or allergy
g. Unmet discharge parameters

I. Postprocedural care and discharge
1. Monitor and document vital signs, pulse oximetry, and mental status until stable at presedation levels or at least 30 minutes after the last sedating medications are given.
2. The patient must meet specific discharge criteria.
a. Stable vital signs
b. Intact mental status
c. Relative freedom from pain
d. Denial of nausea or vomiting
e. Ability to void and take fluids
3. Provide verbal and written discharge instructions to patient and escort.
a. Home medication administration
b. Dietary requirements
c. Activity limitations
d. Signs and symptoms of complications
e. Emergency numbers
f. Follow-up appointment if applicable
4. Patient should not drive home.

References

American Society of Anesthesiologists Task Force. (2002). Practice guidelines for sedation and analgesia by non-anesthesiologists. *Anesthesiology, 96*(4), 1004–1017.

Kost, M., & Odom-Forren, J. S. (2007). *Administration of moderate sedation/analgesia.* Retrieved May 24, 2009 from http://www.nurse.com/ce/CE159-60/CoursePage/.

Odom-Forren, J., & Watson, D. (2005). *Practical guide to moderate sedation/analgesia* (2nd ed.). St. Louis: Elsevier Mosby.

University of Kansas Hospital. (2005). *Policy on moderate sedation/analgesia (conscious sedation): Management of patient undergoing procedures.* Lawrence, Kansas: Author.

Waring, J. P., Baron, T. H., Hirota, W. K., Goldstein, J. L., Jacobson, B. C., Leighton, J. A., Mallery, J. S., & Faigel, D. O. (2003). Guidelines for conscious sedation and monitoring during gastrointestinal endoscopy. *Gastrointestinal Endoscopy, 58*(3), 317–322.

Youmans, L. (2001). Conscious sedation. In J. Hankins, R. A. Waldman Lonsway, C. Hedrick, & M. B. Perdue (Eds.), *Infusion therapy in clinical practice* (2nd ed., pp. 604–615). Philadelphia: Saunders.

chapter

17

Acute Pain Management

Nancy Eksterowicz, RN-BC, MSN, CNS
Ann Quinlan-Colwell, RN-BC, FAAPM, PhD Candidate
Barbara L. Vanderveer, MSN, RN-BC, ARNP
John A. Menez, MS, RN-BC, CMSRN

Objectives

After studying this chapter, the reader should be able to:

1. Classify acute pain based on pathophysiology and assessment of characteristics.
2. Identify the principles and rationale for multimodal therapy.
3. Identify the principles of interventions based on mechanism of action as it relates to acute pain.
4. Identify the safety and monitoring issues associated with interventions.
5. Review treatment of acute pain in the presence of opioid tolerance or persistent chronic pain.
6. Review the important features of an acute pain service and the process for establishing one.

"Excuses for inadequate pain control appear to have run their course and will no longer be accepted because poor pain control is unethical, clinically unsound, and economically wasteful." (Phillips, 2000)

> *"Cultural, attitudinal, educational, political, religious, and logistical reasons have a major impact on the undertreatment of pain. This is despite major physiological, psychological, economic, and social ramifications for patients, their families, and society."*
>
> (Brennan, Carr, & Cousins, 2007)

Pain is the most common reason Americans access the health care system and is a leading contributor to health care costs. It is a principal cause of lost productivity, and temporary and permanent disability of the American workforce (National Pain Care Policy Act, 2008). As well, unrelieved pain can result in longer hospital stay, increased rates of recurrent hospitalization, and increased numbers of outpatient visits. Decreased productive function also results in lost wages and costing employers 60 to 100 billion dollars annually in insurance coverage (American Academy of Pain Medicine, 2007).

I. Overview of Acute Pain: The Nurse's Role

A. Despite an increased focus on pain management programs and the development of new standards for pain management, current studies show that physicians continue to underprescribe analgesic agents, nurses continue to administer fewer analgesics than prescribed, patients continue to request fewer analgesic medications than they need, and as-needed (PRN) regimens continue to dominate treatment for acute pain in the inpatient settings (Apfelbaum, Chen, Mehta, & Gan, 2003).

B. Nurses as frontline patient caregivers play a vital role in acute pain management. This role includes
   1. Obtaining a comprehensive pain history that consists of previous pain levels and effective pain management techniques.
   2. Educating the patient about using acceptable pain intensity scales and setting safe goals.
   3. Balancing analgesia and side effects for optimal pain control.
   4. Initiating nonpharmacological measures to complement pharmacological measures.
   5. Working collaboratively with the members of the health care team for optimum acute pain management.
   6. Continuously evaluating the effectiveness of the acute pain management regimen.

C. *Goals:* As nurses oversee and advocate for patients who suffer pain, they should be cognizant of
   1. Adequacy of prescribed analgesics (see the chapter on Overview of Pharmacology).
   2. Optimal use of appropriate multimodal analgesia.
   3. Frequent use of appropriate pain assessment scales (see the chapter on Pain Assessment).
   4. Use of regularly scheduled analgesics as opposed to PRN.

D. As pain management nurses grow in numbers, their collaboration with other members of the health care team will help provide adequate pain management.
   1. Acute pain is a symptom that serves the purpose of warning the body that something is wrong. Once it serves that purpose, it should be relieved (St. Marie, 1995). Treating acute pain while pain is being assessed will not impede assessment.
   2. Unrelieved acute pain may result in clinical and psychological changes that increase morbidity, mortality, and costs. Unrelieved acute pain may result in persistent pain. This is a result of neuronal remodeling (Dunwoody, Krenzischek, Pasero, Rathmell, & Polomano, 2008).
   3. The health care team can be held accountable for inadequate pain control (see the chapter on Social, Political, and Ethical Forces Influencing Nursing Practice).

II. Physical Impact of Acute Pain

A. Acute pain initially triggers physiological stress responses that activate the sympathetic nervous system. These responses provide immediate protection preventing further damage, such as
   1. Minimizing organ damage.
   2. Limiting blood loss.
   3. Optimizing perfusion to life-sustaining organs.
   4. Preventing infection (Pasero, Paice, & McCaffery, 1999).

B. When acute pain is prolonged or unrelieved, the physiological stress response has harmful physical consequences to the various systems of the body.
   1. Pulmonary system
      a. Potential problems include increased atelectasis progressing to pneumonia, hypoxemia, and decreased oxygen saturation.
      b. There may also be decreased tidal volumes, higher pressures, decreased vital lung capacity and alveolar ventilation, shunting, and decreased cough.
      c. Nursing implications
         (1) Observe for splinting, poor cough, decreased breath sounds, infection from pneumonia, and poor wound oxygenation.
         (2) Treat pain while monitoring respiratory rate and quality, oxygen saturation through pulse oximetry, capnography, and ease of productive cough and mobility. Observe for sustained temperature elevation.
            (a) Encourage the use of incentive spirometry, frequent turning, coughing, sitting in a chair, and walking in a room or hallway, if able.
         (3) Monitor for sudden onset of chest pain or shortness of breath.
   2. Cardiovascular system
      a. Potential problems include
         (1) Increased heart rate, increased blood pressure, increased workload, and oxygen demands (reports of chest pain or angina) caused by activation of the sympathetic nervous system.
         (2) Hypercoagulation due to decreased fibrinolysis. This increases the risk for deep vein thrombosis, thereby increasing postoperative morbidity and mortality due to thrombosis and myocardial ischemia.
         (3) Increased peripheral, systemic, and coronary vascular resistance (Pasero et al., 1999).
      b. Nursing implications
         (1) Monitor vital signs, including pain status, at regular intervals, especially with patients who have a significant cardiac history.
            (a) Preintervention assessments and documentation
            (b) Intervention with multimodal analgesics
            (c) Postintervention assessments and documentation
         (2) To reduce thromboembolic and cardiac complications, provide aggressive pain control directed toward
            (a) Decreasing cardiac workload.
            (b) Decreasing hypercoagulation.
            (c) Increasing myocardial oxygen supply.
            (d) Increasing perfusion to the lungs.
            (e) Increasing perfusion to the extremities (Pasero et al., 1999).
         (3) Intermittent pneumatic compression is a commonly applied tool used to reduce stasis and improve venous return from the lower extremities.
         (4) Develop a plan to prevent pain using around-the-clock dosing of analgesic agents and supplemental doses for breakthrough pain using a parenteral or oral opioid. Incorporate the principles of multimodal analgesia (see X. Principles of Preemptive and Multimodal Analgesia and the chapter on Overview of Pharmacology).
            (a) When opioids are given on a schedule, the care plan should include the statement "hold if sedated" to prevent accidental overmedication.

(5) Assess for other means of comfort.
(a) Providing soft music, a humor television channel, and soft lighting
(b) Being a visible presence for the patient
(c) Limiting visitors, or having appropriate visitors (as defined by the patient)

3. Musculoskeletal system
a. Potential problems include
(1) Refractory muscle spasms.
(2) Impaired muscle function, fatigue, and immobility.
(3) Muscle disuse syndrome.
(4) Inability to perform rehabilitation therapy.
b. Nursing implications
(1) Treat pain while monitoring ease of mobility; treat spasms with muscles relaxants or antispasmodics.
(a) Massage therapy (see the chapter on Integrative Therapies Used in Pain Management Nursing)
(b) Topical analgesic agents over tight muscles (see the chapter on Overview of Pharmacology)
(2) Use around-the-clock dosing of analgesic agents and supplemental doses for breakthrough pain and before and during times of expected discomfort, which can improve the patient's performance of the activities needed for a faster and smoother recovery (Pasero et al., 1999).
(3) Use hot–cold application and ultrasound, which can provide effective analgesia, along with rehabilitative therapies, to improve function (Ross, 2004).

4. Gastrointestinal system
a. Potential problems include
(1) An increase in intestinal secretions and smooth muscle tone and a decrease in gastric emptying and intestinal motility as a result of increased sympathetic nervous system activity.
(2) Possible ileus as a result of unrelieved pain and stress from the acute injury or surgery.
b. Nursing implication
(1) Monitor bowel activity, and start physical activity as soon as possible.
(2) Evidence shows postoperative epidural analgesia with the use of a combination of local anesthetics and opioids can shorten duration of ileus (Kehlet, 2005).

5. Endocrine and metabolic systems
a. Potential problems include
(1) Stress from pain causing release of hormones, including cortisol, adrenocorticotropic hormone, growth hormone, catecholamines, and glucagon, and decreases in insulin and testosterone.
(2) Altered metabolism due to destruction of carbohydrates, protein, and fat, resulting in hyperglycemia, weight loss, tachycardia, fever, shock, and even death (Kehlet, 1998).
(3) Possible gluconeogenesis, glucose intolerance, insulin resistance, and increased lipolysis (Pasero et al., 1999).
b. Nursing implications
(1) Reduce pain.
(2) Limit external stressors.
(3) Monitor for heart rate, temperature, glucose, and blood pressure.

6. Immune system (see the chapter on Immunity and Pain)
a. Stress that results from pain can suppress the immune system through the suppression of natural killer cells (NK cells) (Page, 2005).
(1) Immunosuppression can predispose patients to postoperative infections, including pneumonia, wound infections, and sepsis (Pasero, et al., 1999).

b. Nursing implications
   (1) Monitor postoperative patients for signs of infection.
   (2) Treat pain while monitoring for changes in sedation and cognition.
   (3) Use regional anesthetics and epidurals with local anesthetics to reduce suppression of the immune consequences of surgery (Page, 2005).

7. Cognitive function
   a. Pain may increase the risk of postoperative delirium, especially in the elderly (Lynch et al., 1998).
   b. Nursing implications
      (1) Monitor for pain by observing behavioral signs of pain.
      (2) Treat pain preventatively. Improving pain management practices is one way to reduce confusion among elders after surgery (Pasero et al., 1999).
      (3) Reorient confused patients often (see the chapter on Gerontology Pain Management).
      (4) Note a patient's history of alcohol and drug use before surgery. Alcohol withdrawal can change a normal postoperative course into a life-threatening situation in which the patient requires intensive care unit (ICU) treatment (Spies & Rommelspacher, 1999).
8. Developmental
   a. The long-term effects of untreated pain may result in the decrease of pain threshold, problematic behaviors in children, vulnerability to stress disorders, addictive behaviors, and anxiety states despite the resolution of pain (Pasero, et al., 1999).
   b. Nursing implications
      (1) Monitor and prevent pain through the use of analgesia and anesthesia techniques.
      (2) Establish institutional procedural pain treatment and assessment guidelines (see the chapter on Moderate Sedation/Analgesia).
9. Psychological and behavioral
   a. Pain is associated with physical, psychological, and emotional distress.
   b. The consequences of unmanaged pain, even in healthy individuals, can prolong rehabilitation, delay the patient's return to work, prolong dependency, and decrease independence (Ross, 2004).
   c. Nursing implications
      (1) Establish a trusting working relationship with the patient.
      (2) Identify the patient's coping skills, and encourage the use of positive coping skills.
      (3) Identify and validate pain, depression, and anxiety.
      (4) Involve other members of the interdisciplinary team in formulating a collaborative plan of care.
      (5) Monitor the patient for behaviors that pose a risk to self or others.
      (6) Apply therapeutic communication techniques in talking with the patient.
      (7) Modify the environment to ensure healing and comfort.

III. Goal of Pain Management

A. Goals of the patient
   1. Goals are written in the plan of care.
   2. They should be specific, measurable, and patient centered.
   3. Goals of the patient have been met if the patient
      a. Expresses adequate pain relief.
      b. Experiences minimal side effects from the analgesic regimen.
      c. Maintains or improves functional status.
      d. Expresses satisfaction with pain management (Farrar, Berline, & Strom, 2003).

B. Goals of the health care team
   1. Set comfort goals that include
      a. A focus on prevention of pain, quick relief when pain occurs, and relief to allow improvement of function.

b. The restoration of health and quality of life.
c. An individualized approach.
2. The end results of an effective pain management plan are
a. Minimal to no psychological and physiological stress response generated by nociception.
b. Optimal patient recovery and reduced hospital length of stay.
c. Minimal development of chronic pain syndromes caused by untreated acute injury or trauma.
d. Improved quality of life.

IV. Surgical and Trauma Pain Etiology

A. Initiating nociception
1. Pain is a predictable consequence of surgery or trauma. There are more than 23 million surgical procedures each year in the United States. Pain is inadequately treated in half of all surgical procedures (Dunwoody et al., 2008).
a. Surgery and trauma produce tissue damage and subsequent release of neurotransmitters that stimulate the A δ and C nerve fibers generating noxious stimuli to the high centers of the cortical center by way of the spinal cord (Grass, 2000). Pain from surgery or trauma can be somatic or visceral. Musculoskeletal or myofascial pain can be manifested following trauma.
b. Pain from trauma or surgery stimulates inflammatory mediators. Intense or repeated noxious stimulation can decrease the threshold for nerve activation, leading to hyperalgesia (Byers & Bonica, 2001).

B. Postsurgical pain diagnoses
1. Phantom pain (see the chapter on Persistent Pain)
a. Phantom pain is perceived pain in the missing body part after amputation (Jensen & Nikolajsen, 1999).
b. Persistent pain has been reported in up to 80% of patients after limb amputation.
c. The mechanisms are not fully understood but involve nerve injury during amputation (Wilson, Nimmo, Fleetwood-Walker, & Colvin, 2008) and changes in the ascending nociceptive pathways.
d. Amputees experience phantom sensations and phantom pain within 1 month after amputation; a second peak occurs 12 months after amputation (Schley et al., 2008).
2. Postthoracotomy pain (see the chapter on Persistent Pain Management)
a. Pain from intercostal nerve damage appeared no different than pain from a peripheral nerve injury, leading to a neuropathic syndrome (Wallace & Wallace, 1997).
b. The exact cause of chronic pain after thoracic surgery has not been established (Maguire, Latter, Mahajan, Beggs, & Duffy, 2006); however, the cause of postthoracotomy neuralgia is believed to be from intercostal nerve injury due to rib retraction during surgery.
c. A multimodal perioperative pain management regimen should begin before surgical incision and continued through the postoperative period to prevent postthoracotomy pain syndrome (Karmakar & Ho, 2004).
3. Compartment syndrome
a. Description
(1) Compartment syndrome is a condition in which swelling occurs and an increase in pressure within a limited space (a compartment) presses on and compromises blood vessels, nerves, tendons, or a combination of these that run through that compartment. Hence, the function of tissue within that compartment is compromised.
(2) This can commonly occur after long bone fractures or following vascular injury when perfusion pressure falls below tissue pressure in a closed anatomical space; as intracompartmental pressure rises, autoregulatory mechanisms are overwhelmed, and a cascade of injury develops (Paula, 2006).
(3) Untreated compartment syndrome leads to tissue necrosis, loss of limb, and permanent functional impairment. If severe, renal failure and death can result.

(4) Surgical treatment (fasciotomy) is considered an emergency (Paula, 2006).

b. Nursing implications
   (1) Monitor for severe pain at rest or with any movement. This occurrence should raise suspicion.
   (2) After initial symptoms of pain or burning, observe for decreased strength. Paralysis of the affected extremity may result if this problem is left unattended.
   (3) Monitor for progression of symptoms. The affected limb may begin to feel tense or hard, as if filling with fluid. Compare the affected limb to the unaffected limb.
   (4) Do not elevate the affected extremity.
   (5) Administer additional oxygen.

V. Pain in the Emergency Department Setting

A. Pain continues to be the most common reason for seeking health care in the emergency room (Todd et al., 2007).

B. Appropriate assessment of pain leads to correct diagnosis and treatment. Therefore, assessment and treatment can occur immediately since it is generally accepted that the reduction or suppression of acute pain does nothing to change ability to determine cause (Tamchèsa et al., 2007).
   1. The use of visual analogue scales is helpful in assessing pain in the emergency department; however, if the patient cannot communicate, nonverbal assessment tools are needed (Todd et al., 2007).
   2. If intravenous opioids are chosen as treatment, titration should be considered the standard of care (Ducharme et al., 2007).
      a. This provides analgesia to allow the patient to lie still for tests to ensure the accuracy of tests.
      b. Evidence suggests that pain is reduced and safety is enhanced when appropriately trained health professionals follow protocol-driven pain treatment algorithms in the emergency department (Tamchèsa et al., 2007).

C. Nursing implications
   1. Regular assessment of heart rate, respiratory rate and effort, blood pressure, level of consciousness, and oxygen saturation needs to occur when parenteral opioids are used for managing acute traumatic pain by skilled health care professionals (Thierbach, Lipp, & Daublander, 1999).
   2. Titrate opioids to effect.
   3. Use multimodal analgesia to optimize pain management.

D. Common pain-related admissions in the emergency room
   1. Ischemic pain and myocardial infarction
      a. Ischemia may be manifested in any blood vessel, causing acute ischemic pain when there is obstruction of blood flow through vessels.
      b. During cardiac ischemia, an imbalance occurs between myocardial oxygen supply and demand. Ischemia may manifest as anginal pain.
      c. The increase in sympathetic impulses heightens the workload on the heart and increases oxygen consumption.
      d. Nursing implications
         (1) Pharmacological treatment of coronary artery disease can be divided into agents that prolong survival (e.g., aspirin, statin drugs, angiotensin-converting enzyme (ACE) inhibitors, and β-blockers) and those that treat symptoms (e.g., calcium channel blockers, nitrates, and opioids).
         (2) Administer oxygen and morphine sulfate (see the chapter on Overview of Pharmacology) to decrease pain and improve left ventricular function. Morphine sulfate at 8 to 15 mg intravenously produces a decrease in the oxygen consumption, left ventricular and diastolic pressure, and cardiac work (Gutstein & Akil, 2006, p. 561). Morphine produces cardioprotective effects by decreasing preload, inotropy, and chronotropy, thus favorably altering myocardial oxygen consumption and helping relieve ischemia and pain (Gutstein & Akil, 2006, p. 561).

(3) Caution should be taken in the use of morphine in the presence of hypotension, bradycardia, and respiratory depression, which may result in cerebrovascular hypoperfusion (Barclay, 2005).

2. Acute abdominal pain
   a. Incidence
      (1) Abdominal pain is the primary complaint in 25% of all general surgery admissions (Tait, Ionescu, & Cuschieri, 1999).
      (2) Yearly, a total of 5 million patients present to an emergency department due to abdominal pain in the United States. This accounts for 5% to 10% of all emergency department visits in the U.S. (Thierbach et al., 1999).
      (3) The incidence of newly diagnosed and unspecified abdominal pain in the U.S. was 22.3 per 1,000 person-years (Wallander, Johansson, Ruigómez, & García Rodríguez, 2007).
   b. Causes include
      (1) Visceral disorders within the abdominal cavity cause abdominal pain.
      (2) Cardiovascular causes such as myocardial infarction, pericarditis, aortic dissection, and mesenteric ischemia.
      (3) Gastrointestinal causes such as esophagitis, gastritis, peptic ulcer, and appendicitis.
      (4) Biliary causes such as cholecystitis, cholelithiasis, and cholangitis.
      (5) Pancreatic causes such as mass and pancreatitis (acute and chronic).
      (6) Abdominal wall causes such as herpes zoster, muscle strain, and hernia.
      (7) Localized abdominal pain such as bowel obstruction, mesenteric ischemia, peritonitis, opioid withdrawal, sickle cell crisis, porphyria, irritable bowel disorder, or heavy metal poisoning (Barclay, 2008).
   c. Nursing implications
      (1) Treating the cause of pain is the primary goal.
      (2) Opioid administration has not been shown to obscure clinical assessment; rather, it aids in the physical examination.
      (3) Opioids help reduce pain and anxiety, relaxing the abdominal muscles and improving palpation methods used in assessment. Opioids relieve pain but not palpation tenderness (Thierbach et al., 1999).
      (4) Caution should be used when administering continuous opioids in the presence of opioid-induced constipation. Encourage physical activity, liquids if possible, and stool softeners. Laxatives may also be needed to stimulate evacuation.

VI. Burns and Wounds

A. Description
   1. Pain caused by severe burns or deep wounds is not limited to one category of pain, such as somatosensory or neuropathic, but can be caused by multiple mechanisms. Treatments of burns or wounds and the subsequent healing may precipitate a painful response.
   2. The management of pain from a burn or wound depends on the underlying cause. Determine whether the pain is continuous pain, breakthrough pain, procedural pain such as debridement and dressing changes, postoperative pain, pain from infection, or pain associated with healing.
   3. Recovery and restoration from burns or other types of wounds is a long process. The cause of pain may vary (i.e. somatosensory, visceral, neuropathic) and should be assessed often (Summer, Puntillo, Miaskowski, & Green, 2007).

B. Burns
   1. Incidence (Summer et al., 2007)
      a. In the United States, unrelieved pain from burns is a significant public health problem.
      b. More than 1 million people sustain burn injuries per year.
      c. Of these, two-thirds obtain care in the emergency department. Of people with burn injuries, 25% to 30% require hospitalization. Between 25% and 30% of those patients require prolonged hospitalization.

d. Pain is the most common complaint of burn-injured patients (Summer et al., 2007).
   (1) Full-thickness burns involve the destruction of nerve fibers and do not result in pain.
   (2) Extensive full-thickness burns produce pain only from tissues at the margins of the burned areas (Summer et al., 2007).
   (3) Partial thickness burns have damaged but functioning nerve fibers that are exposed at the surface of the skin (Supple, 2004).

2. Burns induce mechanical and thermal hyperalgesia in human skin. However, primary mechanical hyperalgesia, induced by mechanical stimulation of the injured site, is also a major source of severe pain (Summer et al., 2007).
   a. Activation of nociceptive and inflammatory mediators alters the response to further stimulation, resulting in hyperalgesia and temporal summation.
   b. Temporal summation is the summing of impulses to reach action potential (Chu, Angst, & Clark, 2008).
3. The classes of medications normally used in the treatment of burns are
   a. Opioids.
   b. Nonsteroidal antiinflammatory drugs (NSAIDs).
   c. Ketamine.
   d. Clonidine.
   e. Local anesthetics.
   f. Regional analgesia.

C. Wounds and pressure ulcers
   1. Incidence
      a. The incidence of painful wounds is not well documented.
   2. Special considerations
      a. Wound infection can cause pain and distress to patients and may lead to prolonged hospital stays with accompanying increases in health care and personal costs (Santy, 2008).
      b. While a wound is healing, clinical observations suggest that hyperalgesia is likely to be severe and variable (Summer et al., 2007).
         (1) The clinical practice guidelines on pressure ulcers establish pain assessment and intentional analgesia as standard (Vanderwee et al., 2008).
            (a) Treatment of persistent pressure ulcer pain (nociceptive) includes
               (i) Local anesthetics.
               (ii) Antidepressants (tricyclic antidepressants or serotonin-norepinephrine reuptake inhibitors).
               (iii) Anticonvulsants (pregabalin or gabapentin).
               (iv) Transcutaneous nerve stimulation around the wound edge, avoiding open skin.
               (v) Warm applications.
            (b) As peripheral nerves regenerate, immature nerve buds are hypersensitive to stimuli. This contributes to pain during wound care procedures and while using cleansing products.

D. Nursing implications for burns and wound (see the chapter on Overview of Pharmacology)
   1. "To ignore the pain and suffering that accompany burn injuries is not only inhumane but also dismisses decades of research documenting the deleterious effects of pain" (Henry & Foster, 2000).
   2. An intravenous route is preferred because of the possibility of delayed absorption with decreased peak concentrations and decreased bioavailability of opioids by other routes.
      a. Opioid therapy remains the mainstay during the acute phase.
      b. Ketamine in analgesic doses for wound care consists of a 5- to 10-mg intravenous push over 3 minutes, 15 minutes before the dressing change (Schmid, Sandler, & Katz, 1999; Thierbach et al., 1999).
      c. Anticonvulsants, such as gabapentin, reduce opioid consumption, decrease hyperalgesia, and lower pain scores in sustained painful conditions such as burns and wound pain (Cuignet, Pierson, Soudon, & Zizi, 2007).

3. Topical application of local anesthetics inhibits transduction of the primary afferent nerve (Van Rijswijk, 1999).
   a. Topical morphine preparations may provide analgesia. The pain management care plan is to be developed in collaboration with the health care team, that is, wound specialists and physicians.
4. Nonpharmacological methods of managing pain include hydrotherapy, cognitive interventions, and behavioral techniques.
   a. Psychological support can reduce pain and increase patient satisfaction. There are potential benefits of psychological assistance during dressing changes, particularly in burned patients (Frenay, Faymonville, Devlieger, Albert, & Vanderkelen, 2001). Integrative therapies may provide help in alleviating pain (see the Integrative Therapies Used in Pain Management Nursing).
5. Pain assessment should be performed regularly with a consistent rating scale assessing location and quality of pain.
   a. In determining the quality of pain, ask patients to describe their pain. The words patients use to describe their pain can help guide the treatment.
   b. Document pain intensity before intervention, then intervene and document pain intensity after the intervention.

VII. Procedural Pain

A. Description
   1. If procedural pain is not treated adequately, pain levels may be perceived by the patient as being higher when subsequent procedures are performed (Ducharme, 2000) (see the chapter on Moderate Sedation/Analgesia).

B. Common examples
   1. Intravenous cannula placement
      a. Special considerations
         (1) Local anesthetic intradermal injection before cannula insertion decreases insertion pain.
         (2) Injection with intradermal 0.9% sodium chloride adjacent to the vein before cannulation produces an anesthetic effect (Windle et al., 2006).
         (3) Topical local anesthetics are an option (see the chapter on Overview on Pharmacology).
            (a) Nursing implications
               (i) Monitor for allergic reaction from local anesthetic and possible inadvertent injection of the local anesthetic into the vascular system.
   2. Chest tube placement and removal
      a. Special considerations
         (1) Premedicate with fast-acting opioid before chest tube placement or removal.
         (2) Consider ketorolac injections 3.5 hours before removal of the chest tube (Puntillo et al., 2002).
      b. The acute pain guidelines (U.S. Agency for Health Care Policy and Research, 1992) advocate the use of techniques such as intercostal nerve blocks to provide analgesia. These can be used by skilled clinicians to prevent pain upon insertion of chest tubes.
      c. Nursing implications
         (1) Monitor for undermedication, sedation, respiratory depression related to opioids, and allergic reaction to local anesthetics.
         (2) Avoid ketorolac in the presence of elevated creatinine (renal insufficiency or renal failure), peptic ulcer disease and poor platelet function.
         (3) Monitor the patient for a minimum of 10 minutes after short-acting opioid injection.
   3. Intubation
      a. Special considerations and nursing implications
         (1) Patient should be sedated before intubation and given analgesia to provide comfort. Liu,

Block, and Wu (2004) noted improved pain scores, along with associated improvements including faster time to extubation.

(2) The method of communication of pain needs to be determined. If the patient is alert but unable to communicate, a nonverbal tool such as pen and paper can be used to report pain or discomfort.

(3) If the patient is unresponsive, watch for behavioral cues or assume pain is present (Herr et al., 2006) (see the chapter on Pain Assessment).

VIII. Pain in Pregnancy, Labor, and Delivery

A. Pain in the pregnant patient with sickle cell disease

1. Vasoocclusive crisis is the most common maternal complication. Recurrent sudden attacks of pain, usually involving the abdomen, chest, vertebrae, and extremities, may occur. In patients with sickle cell disease, painful episodes occurred at some time during 50% of pregnancies (Smith et al., 1996).
2. For treatment of pain related to sickle cell disease, see the Chapter on Persistent Pain Management.

B. Acute back pain in pregnancy

1. Backache is a common symptom in women of childbearing age.
2. With as many as half of women reporting back pain at some stage during pregnancy, sacroiliac subluxation or a herniated disc may result from weight gain and postural changes (Russell & Reynolds, 1997).
   a. Treatment includes
      (1) Physical therapy.
      (2) Instruction in body mechanics.
      (3) Instruction in low back exercises.
      (4) Aquatic exercise programs.
      (5) Massage.
      (6) Surface application of heat or ice.
      (7) Transcutaneous electrical nerve stimulation.
      (8) Epidural steroid injection.
         (a) Use in pregnancy is controversial because of the potential risk to the fetus.
         (b) Current thinking is that a single dose of corticosteroid seems low risk; however, epidural steroid injection should be reserved for pregnant women with new onset of neurological signs that are consistent with lumbar nerve root compression such as unilateral loss of deep tendon reflex or sensory or motor change in a dermatomal distribution (Rathmell, Viscomi, & Ashburn, 1997).

C. Migraines in pregnancy (see the chapter on Persistent Pain Management for other causes of migraine and their treatments)

1. Description
   a. A higher percentage of women with menstrual migraines improve during pregnancy.
   b. The positive effects and possible worsening postpartum are probably related to the uniformly high and stable estrogen levels during pregnancy and the rapid decline thereafter.
   c. Migraine may appear for the first time during pregnancy.
   d. The greatest frequency of migraine attacks occurs during the first trimester.
   e. Migraine during pregnancy is associated with a 19-fold increased risk for stroke and a significant increased risk for other types of vascular disease (Bushnell, 2007).
2. Treatment (see the chapter on Persistent Pain Management)
   a. Treat first with nonpharmacological techniques such as massage, relaxation, biofeedback, and the elimination of certain foods or environmental triggers.
   b. If pharmacological therapy is warranted, ergotamine preparations should be avoided during pregnancy and lactation.
   c. An intravenous or oral opioid may be needed as a last resort, understanding that analgesic rebound headache may occur.

D. Pain in labor and delivery
   1. Description
      a. Labor is one of the most painful experiences a woman can undergo (Melzack, 1984).
      b. Few pain specialists would dispute that labor and delivery have nociceptive sensations resulting in pain (Melzack, 1984).
   2. Causes of pain
      a. Pressure may be placed on nerve endings between the muscle fibers of the body and the fundus of the uterus.
      b. Pain in the first stage of labor is mainly a result of dilation of the cervix and lower uterine segment. This is followed by distention, stretching, and tearing of these structures during contractions.
      c. Pain originates from the T11 and T12 nerve root exits and distributes pain sensation along the T11 and T12 dermatomes.
      d. Pain in the second and third stages of labor no longer results from the cervix but instead results from the body of the uterus and distention of the lower uterine segment. With the distention of the outlet and perineum, new sources of pain occur. This involves the pudendal nerve and other nerves derived from S2 through S4.
      e. Afferent nerves that innervate the uterine cervix sprout into this tissue during late pregnancy, and estrogen increases excitability of these mechanosensitive afferents (Liu, Tong, & Eisenach, 2008).
   3. Treatment
      a. Intravenous or oral opioids
         (1) Opioids are used to promote rest without causing muscle weakness and may promote sedation.
         (2) Opioids may cause sleepiness and temporarily depress neonatal respirations.
         (3) Most analgesic agents commonly used to alleviate labor pain readily transfer to the fetus via the placenta. The current evidence on the safety of maternal analgesia (parenteral opioids or epidural or combined epidural–spinal) and the effects on the neonate are limited (Mercer, Erickson-Owens, Graves, & Haley, 2007).
      b. Epidural analgesia
         (1) The epidural is the most efficient way of reducing labor pain (Tournaire & Theau-Yonneau, 2007).
         (2) Continuous epidural infusions do not significantly slow labor and can be used for vaginal delivery, as well as cesarean sections (Wong et al., 2005).
         (3) Compared with continuous epidural infusion, patient-controlled epidural analgesia resulted in identical safety and side-effect profiles to both mother and fetus but failed to demonstrate significant differences in pain scores or patient satisfaction (Vallejo, Ramesh, Phelps, & Sah, 2007).
         (4) Potential complications associated with epidural analgesia are dural puncture creating spinal headache, hemodynamic alterations, nausea, pruritus, and high sensory and motor blockade (Cappiello, O'Rourke, Segal, & Tsen, 2008). Epidural hematoma is the most serious potential complication.
      c. Spinal (intrathecal) blocks
         (1) Spinal blocks are effective for complete pain control but may decrease blood pressure and potentially slow the fetal heart rate when using a single bolus (Mardirosoff, Dumont, Boulvain, & Tramer, 2002).
         (2) Spinal headache from the dural puncture required for intrathecal access is possible.
         (3) There may also be a temporary loss of bladder control. It may cause lightheadedness and nausea.
      d. Pudendal blocks
         (1) Local anesthetics are injected in perineal tissue.
         (2) A pudendal block may be used to numb the vaginal area for episiotomy or to repair a vaginal tear.

(3) A pudendal block relieves pain at the perineum, vulva, and vagina.
(4) It is used less often with the increased preference for epidurals.
(5) This block is usually given in the second stage of labor and offers quick relief (DeCherney, Pernoll, & Nathan, 2002).

e. Complementary alternative therapies (see the chapter on Integrative Therapies Used in Pain Management Nursing)
(1) While commonly recommended, few scientific studies conclude that labor pain is significantly reduced using complementary alternative therapies. Evidence regarding patient satisfaction varies (Tournaire & Theau-Yonneau, 2007).
(2) Several methods are preferred by women based on cultural and personal preferences.
(3) Complementary alternative therapies include hypnosis, massage, therapeutic touch, biofeedback, distraction, music therapy, relaxation therapy (e.g., Lamaze), acupressure and acupuncture, transcutaneous electrical nerve stimulation, sterile water blocks, and hydrotherapy.
(4) Tournaire and Theau-Yonneau (2007) performed a meta-analysis to evaluate the effect of complementary and alternative medicine on pain during labor with conventional scientific methods using electronic databases through 2006 and found efficacy in acupressure and hydrotherapy.

IX. Shingles

A. Description
1. Herpes zoster (shingles) is a neurocutaneous disease caused by the varicella-zoster virus and is associated with significant morbidity and long-term sequelae in older adults.
2. Surfacing of the varicella-zoster virus causes inflammation, a painful, unilateral, localized rash at the corresponding dermatome. It is often a serious, debilitating neuralgia (postherpetic neuralgia).
3. The rash is initially erythematous, with numerous maculopapular lesions that eventually become vesicular.
4. Vesicles may continue to appear for as long as 7 days. Pustulation and crustation of the lesions usually occur 2 to 3 days and 2 to 3 weeks, respectively, after eruption. Occasionally, a skin eruption never occurs (Kockler & McCarthy, 2007).
5. Pain is characterized as burning, continuous, or lancinating sensations.

B. Treatment
1. Treatment of the acute viral infection (Stankus, Dlugopolski, & Packer, 2000)
a. With antiviral agents, it is best if treatment begins within 72 hours of the onset of the rash.
b. An ophthalmology consultation is advised if there is eye involvement.
2. Treatment of the acute pain associated with herpes zoster
a. Pain may be mild to severe.
(1) For mild to moderate pain, use over-the-counter analgesics.
(2) For severe pain, use opioids with regular dosing schedule.
(a) Tricyclic antidepressant medicine can be used to facilitate pain control and sleep.
(b) NSAIDs may reduce inflammation around the nerve and surrounding tissue.
(c) Anticonvulsants (e.g., gabapentin and pregabalin) may also decrease pain.
(d) Opioids may be required initially and short term.
(e) Topical agents provide benefit after lesions heal. A lidocaine (Lidoderm® 5%) patch applied for twelve hours a day could serve as a well-tolerated and effective modality to relieve moderate to severe pain associated with acute herpes zoster, presumably through its pharmacological action and physical barrier effect on sensitized skin (Lin et al., 2008).

C. Prevention
1. Vaccination for the prevention of herpes zoster (shingles) reduces the incidence of postherpetic neuralgia.

2. Zoster vaccine is the first vaccine approved for the prevention of herpes zoster.
3. It was approved by the U.S. Food and Drug Administration (FDA) for adults 60 years or older.
4. Results of the Shingles Prevention Study demonstrated that, in older individuals, administration of zoster vaccine reduces the burden of illness associated with herpes zoster by 61.1%, the frequency of herpes zoster pain and discomfort by 51.3%, and the frequency of postherpetic neuralgia by 66.5% (Kockler & McCarthy, 2007).

X. Principles of Preemptive and Multimodal Analgesia

A. Preemptive analgesia
   1. Preemptive analgesia involves initiating the analgesic process before the nociceptive event, that is, procedures and surgery.
   2. Preemptive analgesia is an antinociceptive treatment that prevents the establishment of altered central processing of afferent input, which amplifies postoperative pain. It decreases the incidence of hyperalgesia and allodynia by decreasing the altered central sensory processing (Ong, Lirk, Seymour, & Jenkins, 2005).
   3. Using a multimodal approach with three drug groups (NSAIDs, opioids, and local anesthetics) may be one method to apply preemptive analgesia (Woolf & Chong, 1993).
      a. Animal studies show consistent positive results; however, in a meta-analysis of current research in humans there are varying results, so efficacy remains controversial (Ong et al., 2005).
      b. Further studies are needed to evaluate whether preemptive analgesia improves pain intensity scores for the first 24 to 48 hours, reduces total supplemental postoperative analgesic requirement, and increases the time to first-rescue analgesic (Pogatzki-Zahn & Zahn, 2006).
   4. Studies on preemptive analgesia show that a redirection from timing of the analgesia to duration and efficacy of an analgesic and antihyperalgesic intervention may offer protective analgesia aimed at the prevention of pain hypersensitivity (Moiniche, Kehlet, & Dahl, 2002; Pogatzki-Zahn & Zahn, 2006).
      a. Extending multimodal analgesia into the postoperative period may be superior to preemptive analgesia in providing protective analgesia (Pogatzki-Zahn & Zahn, 2006).
   5. D'Arcy (2009) suggested that when trying to determine whether preemptive analgesia works for a particular condition practitioners should read the literature and use the best evidence available. The following are examples of where the guidelines are evolving:
      a. Practice guidelines are key (Ashburn et al., 2004). The American Society of Anesthesiologists (ASA) appointed a task force of nine anesthesiologists to review the published evidence and build consensus for perioperative management of pain. Some recommendations are highlighted here that would enhance the practice of preemptive analgesia or preventive analgesia for pain management nurses.
         (1) Obtain a pain management history, including description of persistent pain location, frequency, intensity, and duration.
         (2) Adjust or continue "analgesic medications whose sudden cessation may provoke a withdrawal syndrome" (Ashburn et al., 2004, p. 1575).
         (3) "Treatments [should be used] to reduce preexisting pain and anxiety" (Ashburn et al., 2004, p. 1575).
         (4) Premedicate before surgery as part of a multimodal analgesic pain management program (Ashburn et al., 2004, p. 1575).
         (5) Include the patient and family in education of analgesic methods, including behavioral pain control and integrative therapies.
            (a) Literature supports patient education in reducing anxiety and decreasing time to discharge.
            (b) Literature is vague on whether patient education in pain management reduces the patient's pain intensity, but it does support a reduction in total dosages of analgesics used by a patient receiving preoperative education (Ashburn et al., 2004, p. 1575).

b. In a meta-analysis of the literature, Ong and colleagues (2005) conclude that preemptive analgesia supports the use of epidural analgesia, local wound infiltrations, and systemic NSAID administration (Ong et al., 2005).
   (1) To optimize preemptive analgesia with an NSAID, it should be given 1 to 2 hours before surgical incision.
   (2) When NSAIDs are used in preemptive analgesia, it should be noted that NSAIDs inhibit platelet aggregation for the duration of serum level of the drug. However, a meta-analysis by Moiniche, Romsing, Dahl, and Tramer (2003) concluded that it is ambiguous as to whether NSAIDs increase the incidence of bleeding after surgery.

B. Multimodal analgesia
1. A definition of multimodal analgesia is found in the chapter on Taxonomy for Pain Management Nursing.
   a. The literature supports the administration of two analgesic agents by a single route that act by different mechanisms to provide superior analgesia with reduced adverse effects.
      (1) The ASA Task Force recommends using NSAIDs, cyclooxygenase (COX)–2, or acetaminophen. In doing this, the doses for systemically administered opioids can be reduced (Ashburn et al., 2004).
   b. The literature also indicates that two routes of administration of analgesic agents may be more effective in providing perioperative analgesia.
2. Recommendations of the ASA Task Force
   a. "Whenever possible, anesthesiologists should employ multimodal pain management therapy. Unless contraindicated, all patients should receive an around-the-clock regimen of NSAIDs, COX-2, or acetaminophen. In addition, regional blockade with local anesthetics should be considered. Dosing regimens should be administered to optimize efficacy while minimizing the risk of adverse events. The choice of medication, dose, route, and duration of therapy should be individualized" (Ashburn et al., 2004, p. 1577).
   b. Examples of multimodal analgesia (Ashburn et al., 2004) include the following:
      (1) Epidural opioids administered in combination with epidural local anesthetics or clonidine.
      (2) Intravenous opioids in combination with ketorolac or ketamine.
      (3) Intravenous opioids combined with oral NSAIDs, COX-2 inhibitors, or acetaminophen.
      (4) Epidural or intrathecal opioid analgesia combined with intravenous, oral, transdermal, or subcutaneous analgesics.
3. Components of multimodal analgesia
   a. Acetaminophen (see the chapter on Overview of Pharmacology)
      (1) Nursing implications
         (a) "The American Liver Foundation recommends that people not exceed three grams of acetaminophen a day for any prolonged period of time" (American Liver Foundation, 2008; Watkins et al., 2008).
         (b) Caution should be used with patients with liver disease, alcoholism, and malnutrition (Strassels, McNichol, & Suleman, 2005).
   b. NSAIDs (see the chapter on Overview of Pharmacology)
      (1) NSAIDs decrease the inflammatory response (see the chapter on Neurophysiology of Pain).
      (2) Nursing implications
         (a) Different NSAIDs have particular onsets, durations of action, ceiling effects, and potencies.
         (b) Responses to NSAIDs are variable; if one NSAID is not effective, another may be effective.
         (c) NSAIDs can cause gastrointestinal disturbances; therefore, use with caution in people with a history of gastrointestinal bleeding or distress.
         (d) Avoid NSAIDs in the presence of acute renal compromise (Strassels et al., 2005). Check for elevated serum creatinine before administration.

c. Intravenous opioid administration
   (1) Because of the frequency of intravenous administration (via central or peripheral venous access) of opioids in the acute care setting, intravenous administration is the route discussed here. Other routes of analgesia, such as oral, rectal, buccal, transdermal, and sublingual, are discussed in the chapter on Overview of Pharmacology.
   (2) Indications
      (a) The patient is intolerant of oral pain medications or cannot have medications orally.
      (b) Rapid analgesia is necessary.
   (3) The physician, advanced practice nurse, or physician's assistant (depending on state regulations) may order intermittent injections to be administered by the nurse, constant infusions, or patient-controlled analgesia (PCA).
   (4) Nursing implications
      (a) The affinity of opioid agonists corresponds well with analgesic potency. No ceiling effect exists on analgesia.
         (i) Side effects are related to receptor affinity, dose, and lack of tolerance.
         (ii) Monitor for central nervous system effects, such as sedation or respiratory depression. These may occur easily with a patient who is opioid naïve.
         (iii) Opioids can be titrated until effective analgesia or unacceptable side effects occur (Strassels et al., 2005).
d. Local anesthetics via neuraxial, peripheral, or both types of nerve blocks
   (1) Local anesthetics interrupt sensory input, resulting in altered sensory perception.
   (2) They block the transmission of nociception by preventing the rapid influx of sodium ions into nerve axons, thus preventing the production of an action potential.
e. Ketamine
   (1) Ketamine is an *N*-methyl-D-aspartate receptor antagonist.
   (2) In the first 24 hours after surgery, low-dose ketamine reduces pain scores and analgesia requirements.
   (3) In low doses, undesirable side effects are not as common as they are at higher doses (Pyati & Gan, 2007).
   (4) Nursing implications
      (a) Be aware of side effects.
      (b) Monitor for side effects.
f. Gabapentin, pregabalin, and other antiepileptics
   (1) Anticonvulsants reduce the need for opioids and improve analgesia.
   (2) Reduced postoperative vomiting has been reported (Pyati & Gan, 2007).
   (3) Nursing implications
      (a) Some increased risk of sedation has been reported.
g. Nonpharmacological interventions
   (1) Environmental controls used to promote comfort include noise, temperature, and lighting.
   (2) Identify methods the patient generally uses to manage pain.
   (3) Coach the patient in the use of breathing, distraction, relaxation, and guided imagery.
   (4) Offer therapeutic touch, massage, music therapy, humor therapy, acupressure, reflexology, and hypnosis as available.
   (5) Caution the patient about unapproved use of herbal medications because they may interact with prescribed analgesic agents.

4. Nursing implications of multimodal analgesia
   a. Know the pharmacokinetics and pharmacodynamics of all medications used.
   b. Know and assess the patient for side effects, drug-drug interactions, and food-drug interactions of all medications used.
   c. Know and assess for any untoward effects of nonpharmacological interventions.

d. Educate the patient and family about multimodal analgesia and the individual interventions used.
e. Reassess the patient within 1 hour following any intervention.

XI. Regional and Localized Acute Pain Management Modalities

A. Terms used for intraspinal opioid analgesia (epidural and intrathecal)
1. Basic concepts: epidural
   a. The epidural space is a potential space that lies between a tough ligament and the dura mater.
   b. It contains a venous network of veins that are large bore and thin walled.
   c. It contains fat that is proportional to the individual's body fat.
   d. It contains nerve extensions from the spinal cord.
   e. Other terms used to describe the epidural space include
      (1) Peridural.
      (2) Extradural.
2. Basic concepts: intrathecal
   a. The intrathecal space surrounds the spinal cord.
   b. It contains cerebrospinal fluid.
   c. Other terms used to describe the intrathecal space include
      (1) Spinal space.
      (2) Subarachnoid space.
3. Dermatome is segmental distribution of the spinal nerves.
   a. Dermatome levels are labeled according to the exit point on the spinal cord.
   b. Dermatome levels are sensory levels (see the chapter on Taxonomy for Pain Management Nursing for a dermatome chart).
   c. Understanding dermatome levels is important for the evaluation of numbness or weakness while patients have local anesthetic in their epidural infusions.
4. The term ***intraspinal*** is used to describe both the intrathecal and the epidural spaces.

B. Intraspinal pharmacokinetics (St. Marie, 1995)
1. Epidural and intrathecal opioids bind at their respective opioid receptor sites at the substantia gelatinosa in the dorsal horn.
   a. Epidural opioid is instilled or infused into the epidural space.
   b. Some of the opioid is absorbed through the epidural veins in the epidural space. This is called ***vascular uptake.***
   c. The epidural opioid diffuses through the dura and accesses the opioid receptors of the spinal cord.
   d. The opioid spreads up the neuraxis in the cerebrospinal fluid. This is called ***rostral spread.***
   e. Lipophilic medications
      (1) Lipophilic opioids diffuse rapidly through the dura and bind at the opioid receptors at the dorsal horn of the spinal cord.
      (2) Such drugs include fentanyl citrate and sufentanil citrate.
      (3) They create a narrow segment of analgesia as a result of less rostral spread.
   f. Hydrophilic medications
      (1) Hydrophilic opioids diffuse more slowly through the dura and bind at the opioid receptors at the dorsal horn of the spinal cord.
      (2) Such drugs include morphine.
      (3) Morphine creates a wider segment of analgesia as a result of more rostral spread.
   g. Intraspinal opioids provide pain relief with fewer sedative effects and respiratory depression than are associated with intravenous and intramuscular opioids (Slack & Faut-Callahan, 1991; Wild & Coyne, 1992).
   h. Meta-analysis of epidural analgesia
      (1) Epidural with local anesthetics with or without opioids gives better analgesia than epidural with opioid alone.

(2) The benefit may be felt for only 4 to 6 hours with single injection after surgery.
(3) Epidural analgesia with the epidural catheter in place may delay the administration of anticoagulant therapy (Choi, Bhandari, Scott, & Douketis, 2003).

2. Side effects and treatments
  a. Respiratory depression
    (1) Because of the vascular uptake, respiratory depression is a possibility, although it is less likely because of the lower doses.
    (2) Hydrophilic opioids cause delayed respiratory depression when the opioid has spread up the neuraxis, affecting the respiratory drive at the medulla.
    (3) By observing mental status, the nurse can predict respiratory complications more effectively. Sedation is the earliest sign of impending respiratory depression or arrest.
  b. Nausea can be treated with antiemetics or serotonin (5-hydroxytryptamine [5-HT_3]) antagonists.
  c. If sedation occurs at higher opioid dosages, reduce opioid dosage and add multimodal analgesia (see the chapter on Overview of Pharmacology).
  d. Urinary retention is most likely caused by the ability of the opioid to relax the detrusor muscle at the floor of the bladder. It can be treated with catheterization, naloxone hydrochloride (Narcan®), or bethanechol chloride (Rosow et al., 2007).
  e. Pruritus
    (1) Pruritus is not related to histamine release but rather to the action of the opioid at the opioid receptor at the substantia gelatinosa.
    (2) Treatment with diphenhydramine (Benadryl®) causes sedation.
    (3) Treatment with a low-dose antagonist (nalbuphine hydrochloride [Nubain®] or naloxone hydrochloride [Narcan®]) or with nalmefene hydrochloride (Revex®) reverses the side effect without reversing the analgesia.
  f. There is a 20% incidence of back, pelvic, or leg pain during an epidural injection or infusion. This pain is believed to be due to the compression of an adjacent nerve root by the injected fluid (Cherny, 1998).

3. Local anesthetics
  a. Local anesthetics affect the pain pathway at the sympathetic chain ganglion outside of the spinal cord (St. Marie, 1995).
    (1) By administering local anesthetics, the opioid doses are reduced.
      (a) The most commonly administered local anesthetic is bupivacaine.
    (2) Benefits of local anesthetic agents via the epidural or intrathecal route include
      (a) Fewer opioid side effects.
      (b) Improved vascular graft blood flow.
      (c) Reduced incidence of thrombophlebitis.
      (d) Reduced incidence of paralytic ileus.
      (e) Improved resistance to infection.
    (3) Outcome studies show superior results (Choi et al., 2003).
  b. Intraspinal local anesthetic side effects and their treatments
    (1) Postural hypotension
      (a) Postural hypotension can be treated with intravenous fluids and medications such as ephedrine or phenylephrine (Neo-Synephrine®).
      (b) Patients should be watched and supported carefully when first sitting up in bed, standing by the bedside, and ambulating.
      (c) If patients report feeling lightheaded, they should wait before proceeding with standing by the bedside.
      (d) The hypotension may create a feeling of nausea. Most postural hypotension is self-limited.
    (2) Numbness
      (a) Numbness at the dermatome level covered by the local anesthetics is treated by using a more dilute infusion of local anesthetic.

(b) The local anesthetic may accumulate over an infusion of several hours, and numbness may appear later in the course of an infusion.

(3) Weakness

(a) Nurses should be aware of the patient's lower extremity strength while receiving local anesthetic.

(b) The most problematic complication of epidural local anesthetic is the patient falling. This occurs more readily if the dermatomes of L2 to L3 or lower are affected.

(c) The nerves that exit from the second and third lumbar vertebral foramina innervate the anterior thigh. If these nerves predominately are anesthetized, the knees buckle when the patient attempts ambulation.

(d) The strength of the upper and lower legs should be tested before ambulation. If weakness is present, the anesthesiologist should be notified.

(e) Removing the local anesthetics from the infusion may be necessary; the numbness should then resolve in 4 hours. If numbness increases or does not resolve, this could be a hematoma and the physician should be notified immediately. If it is determined that a hematoma is causing the numbness, surgical intervention should occur in less than 8 hours to avoid injury to the spinal cord (Christie & McCabe, 2007). Administering less concentrated local anesthetic may also resolve this problem.

C. Anticoagulation considerations

1. Low-molecular-weight heparin (LMWH) creates a risk of epidural or intrathecal hematoma (U.S. FDA, 1997).

a. The LMWH dose should be held for at least 2 hours after the catheter has been discontinued.

2. The second American Society of Regional Anesthesia and Pain (ASRA) consensus conference on neuraxial anesthesia and anticoagulation (Horlocker et al., 2003) stated the following.

a. Recommendations are based on current best evidence, but in some cases data are sparse.

b. Although patient safety and quality of care are of utmost concern, no specific outcome is guaranteed.

c. Unfractionated heparin may be associated with an increased risk of epidural hematoma.

d. Heparin should be discontinued for 2 to 4 hours before neuraxial catheter removal.

e. Coagulation status should be assessed before manipulation of the catheter.

f. Neurological assessment of sensory and motor function in the lower extremities should be continued for at least 12 hours following the catheter removal.

g. In patients receiving LMWH (e.g., enoxaparin) "the catheter should be removed a minimum of 10 to 12 hours after the last dose of LMWH. Subsequent LMWH dosing should occur a minimum of 2 hours after catheter removal" (Horlocker et al., 2003, p. 181).

h. Patients on warfarin therapy

(1) The warfarin should be stopped 4 to 5 days before any planned neuraxial procedure.

(2) The international normalized ratio (INR) and bleeding time should be

(a) Checked before neuraxial block.

(b) Monitored daily if a neuraxial catheter is in place.

(c) Checked before catheter removal.

(d) Checked if warfarin is administered within 36 hours of surgery (Horlocker et al., 2003).

(3) Other medication may increase the risk of bleeding without affecting the INR because they work through other clotting mechanisms. Aspirin, NSAIDs, ticlopidine, clopidogrel, unfractionated heparin, and LMWH are among these medications.

i. Patients with neuraxial catheters on warfarin therapy

(1) Catheters can be removed when the INR is less than 1.5 under the direction of an anesthesiologist.

(2) Neurological checks should be performed a minimum of 24 hours after catheter removal, longer if the INR was higher than 1.5 when the catheter was removed.

(3) Stopping or reducing the dose of warfarin should be considered if the INR is greater than 3 or per physician's orders.

j. Indwelling catheters should not be removed in the presence of therapeutic anticoagulation.
   (1) Vigilance in monitoring anticoagulation is critical to allow early evaluation of neurological dysfunction and prompt intervention.
   (2) In the presence of pathologies that alter coagulation (e.g., liver resections or liver disease), greater vigilance is needed in monitoring for epidural hematoma.
k. Recommendations for plexus blocks and peripheral techniques are not yet defined.
l. The ASRA had its third consensus conference in 2007. At the time of writing this chapter, the statement was not yet in print.

D. Indications for epidural and intrathecal analgesia
   1. Epidural and intrathecal analgesia are indicated in a wide variety of surgical procedures, including
      a. Any surgical situation in which uncontrolled pain would lead to pulmonary complications (e.g., gastrectomy, hip surgery, and thoracotomy).
      b. Abdominal and chest wall trauma.
      c. Painful medical conditions.
      d. When oral or parenteral analgesics are ineffective or when the side effects cannot be adequately controlled.

E. Types of epidural or intrathecal administration
   1. Bolus dose only
      a. The medication is intermittently injected into the epidural space.
      b. If an epidural or intrathecal catheter is left in place, intermittent boluses of preservative-free opioids can be administered.
   2. Patient-controlled epidural analgesia
      a. Studies compared the effectiveness of several epidural opioids administered on demand.
      b. Significantly less self-administered epidural morphine was required to provide analgesia than the amount of either continuous epidural infusion or intravenous PCA (Ready, 2001; Standl et al., 2003).
   3. Continuous infusion only
      a. The medication is infused via a pump.
      b. Infusions include opioid alone or with local anesthetic agent.

F. Protocol considerations (Pasero, Eksterowicz, Primeau, & Cowley, 2007)
   1. What are the criteria for patient selection?
   2. When is the catheter placed?
   3. What area in the hospital is used for catheter placement?
   4. Who tests placement of the epidural catheter?
   5. What is the appropriate infusion device?
   6. Who attaches the infusion or injects the epidural catheter?
   7. Who adjusts the infusion rate? Where do the orders come from: surgery or anesthesiology?
      a. Establish consistency of use and dosage.
   8. How is the patient monitored?
   9. Who manages side effects?
      a. Take ambulation precautions.
      b. Decide what to do for breakthrough pain.
   10. What will be the avenue of communication between the patient and the nurse to determine the quality of pain relief experienced by the patient?
   11. Who discontinues the epidural catheter?
      a. Consider anticoagulants and epidural catheter placement, maintenance, and discontinuation.
   12. What are the state board of nursing regulations for epidural care?

G. Patient selection criteria
   1. No infection
   2. No coagulopathies
   3. Informed consent

H. Contraindications
   1. Do not use this technique for patients with head injuries (e.g., increased intracranial pressure) in whom mental status is difficult to monitor.
   2. Do not use for patients with coagulopathies, infections, spinal fractures, or tumor infiltration.

I. Proper equipment for epidural analgesia
   1. Infusion pumps must allow epidural use and be well marked for epidural use.

J. Concepts of patient teaching
   1. To help the patient understand where the catheter is placed, say, "in the tissue surrounding the spinal cord".
   2. Tell the patient what medication is going to be infused.
   3. Explain what the patient should do if there is pain while receiving epidural analgesia.
   4. If local anesthetic agents are used, tell the patient to take ambulation precautions, such as testing the strength of the legs before getting out of bed to ambulate.
   5. The patient should move slowly from lying to sitting to standing to prevent orthostatic hypotension.

K. Expected outcomes
   1. Provide better analgesia with fewer side effects.
   2. Allow early ambulation with less pain.
   3. Have fewer cardiac, pulmonary and vascular complications posttrauma and postoperatively.
   4. Decrease the stress response evident in patients with pain.
   5. Shorten the ICU stay.
   6. Facilitate earlier hospital discharge.

L. Potential complications (Pasero, 2005)
   1. Dural puncture
      a. Inadvertent puncture may occur through the dura at the time of catheter insertion.
      b. Symptoms
         (1) Symptoms include a dull aching or throbbing headache. It may be frontal, occipital or diffuse in location.
            (a) The headache is usually of moderate to severe intensity.
            (b) It may be accompanied by a stiff neck, photophobia, visual disturbances, and nausea and vomiting.
            (c) The headache may worsen with movement, sitting, or standing; the patient may feel better when lying down. This is called a positional headache.
      c. Treatment
         (1) The main treatment is a blood patch, when the anesthesiologist injects the patient's blood into the epidural space.
   2. Epidural catheter displacement
      a. The catheter may be inadvertently pulled out.
      b. Treatment
         (1) Notify anesthesiology to discuss whether to replace the catheter or leave it out.
         (2) Document if the tip is intact.
   3. Epidural catheter migration
      a. The catheter may move from the epidural space to the subarachnoid space or into a vascular space. This movement may result in too much or too little analgesia.
   4. Tissue trauma related to epidural needle or catheter
      a. Such trauma is rare, and its exact cause is unknown.
      b. Symptoms
         (1) Severe, sharp pain can radiate along the nerve at which the catheter was placed.
         (2) Tissue trauma is more common with long-term placement of the catheter.
      c. Treatment
         (1) Report new pain symptoms to the anesthesiologist.
         (2) Provide symptomatic treatment.

Box 17-1 Suggestions for Prevention of Epidural Neurotoxicity

The following measures may be helpful in preventing inadvertent injection or infusion of neurotoxic agents into the epidural space.

- Do not use agents from a multiple-dose vial; it is wise to assume that all multiple-dose vials contain preservatives.
- Use only nonneurotoxic agents to disinfect epidural catheter connections or ports. For example, alcohol often is used to cleanse skin of drainage but should not be used to disinfect catheter connections or ports.
- Boldly label indwelling epidural catheters used for intermittent analgesic bolusing.
- Do not use infusion lines with injection ports for epidural analgesia; if such tubing must be used, tape over every injection port.
- Use color-coded infusion lines made specifically for epidural analgesia.
- Label infusion lines when patients have several.
- Double-check the labels of epidural analgesia drug reservoirs for wording that indicates the solution is free of preservatives and has been prepared for intraspinal use.
- Return to the pharmacy any drug reservoirs or agents that are unclearly labeled, cloudy, or contain particulate matter.

Pasero, C. (2005). *Self-directed learning program: Epidural analgesia for acute pain management in adults.* Pensacola, FL: American Society for Pain Management Nursing, p. 55.

5. Injection or infusion of neurotoxic agents (Box 17–1)
    a. Prevention is the most important.
6. Infection
    a. Prevention is the best therapy.
    b. Symptoms
        (1) Early signs may be difficult to detect.
        (2) Diffuse back pain may increase.
        (3) Pain or paresthesia may occur on injection.
        (4) Bowel or bladder dysfunction is possible.
        (5) Inadequate analgesia may occur.
        (6) The patient may have gradually increasing motor or sensory deficits.
        (7) Inflammation, edema, drainage, pain, or a combination of these may be found at the entry site.
    c. Treatment
        (1) Early detection and treatment of the infection is advised.
7. Epidural hematoma
    a. Pressure on the spinal cord by accumulating blood may develop.
    b. Symptoms
        (1) Early signs may be difficult to detect.
        (2) Diffuse increasing back pain or tenderness may occur.
        (3) The patient can have pain or paresthesia on epidural injection.
        (4) Bowel or bladder dysfunction is possible.
        (5) Increasing sensory deficits, motor deficits, or both may occur.
    c. Treatment
        (1) Prevent by paying attention to the timing of removal as related to anticoagulant medications.
        (2) Immediate surgical removal of the hematoma is indicated.

M. Advantages
1. A study showed the combination of opioid with local anesthetic produced analgesia superior to either medication alone in the epidural space (McQuay & Moore, 1999).

N. Disadvantages
   1. Knowledge of catheter placement is a learned and mentored process.
   2. Knowledge of lipid- and water-soluble medication used in the epidural space is not taught in nursing schools.
   3. Dosing of epidural analgesia is not well defined.

XII. Interpleural Administration of Local Anesthetic (Ditonto & deLeon-Casasola, 1998; Dravid & Paul, 2007a, 2007b)

1. Indications
   a. Local anesthetic is used to treat visceral pain anywhere from the head and upper extremity to the abdomen. Examples of situations in which interpleural administration of local anesthetics is used include breast surgery, chest wall trauma, herpes zoster, cholecystectomy, and pancreatitis.
2. Technique
   a. Insert a needle or catheter into the seventh intercostal space approximately 10 cm lateral to the midline.
   b. This technique involves using a passive loss of resistance technique (i.e., when the needle tip is in the pleural space, injection will be easy) to inject local anesthetic solution between the parietal and the visceral pleura, which blocks multiple thoracic dermatomes.
3. Medications
   a. Local anesthetic is used.
   b. Morphine has been shown to be of no additional benefit.
   c. Clonidine has been used in a few trials but needs further investigation.
4. Nursing implications
   a. Observe for pneumothorax (chest pain or shortness of breath).
   b. The catheter should be pliable; a stiff catheter increases the chance of pneumothorax.
      (1) Check catheter placement before use.
      (2) Maintain catheter security and placement.
   c. Evaluate for systemic local anesthetic toxicity.
      (1) Monitor for signs and symptoms of toxicity.
      (2) Local anesthetics readily cross the blood-brain barrier.
      (3) Central nervous system toxicity may occur from systemic absorption or direct vascular injection.
      (4) For plasma concentration,
         (a) 1 to 5 mg/ml produces analgesia.
         (b) 5 to 10 mg/ml produces lightheadedness, tinnitus, and numbness of the tongue.
         (c) 10 to 15 mg/ml produces seizures and unconsciousness.
         (d) 15 to 25 mg/ml produces coma and respiratory arrest.
         (e) Greater than 25 mg/ml produces cardiovascular depression (Liu, 1998).
   d. Evaluate for signs and symptoms of pleural effusion.
      (1) These may be absent or may include
         (a) Cough, usually dry and nonproductive.
         (b) Dyspnea, gradually increasing over time.
         (c) Pleuritic chest pain.
   e. Evaluate for catheter dislodgement, disconnection, or kinking.
   f. Evaluate for phrenic nerve paralysis (rare) as evidenced by respiratory depression or paralysis. This is usually screened by chest imaging and diaphragm screening. Diaphragm paralysis following cardiac surgery may be the result of phrenic nerve injury (Efthimiou, Butler, Woodham, Benson, & Westaby, 1991).
   g. Notify the physician of signs or symptoms of potential complications.

XIII. Peripheral Nerve Blocks (Greengrass & Nielsen, 2005; Grossi & Allegri, 2005; Grossi & Urmey, 2003; Murauski & Gonzalez, 2002; New York School of Regional Anesthesia [NYSORA], 2008a–2008e; Waldman, 2004a–2004k)

A. Peripheral nerve blocks are used for moderate to severe acute pain.

B. Types

1. Continuous peripheral local anesthetic nerve blocks
2. Single injection peripheral local anesthetic nerve blocks

C. Location

1. Upper extremity blocks or brachial plexus blocks (NYSORA, 2008a–2008c, 2008e; Waldman, 2004a–2004c, 2004k)
   a. Basic concepts
      (1) The anterior rami of the spinal nerves of C5 through C8 and T1 form the roots of the brachial plexus.
      (2) The brachial plexus supplies the shoulder and upper arm, branching into a network of nerves derived from the anterior rami of the lower four cervical and the first thoracic spinal nerves.
      (3) The anterior rami give rise to three trunks (superior, middle, and inferior) that emerge between the scalenus medius and scalenus anterior on the posterior triangle of the neck.
      (4) The trunks are covered by its lateral extension, the axillary sheath; each trunk divides onto an anterior and a posterior division behind the clavicle, at the apex of the axilla.
      (5) The brachial plexus can be blocked by various methods depending on the area affected and length of time the block is needed.
   b. Techniques
      (1) Interscalene (NYSORA, 2008c; Waldman, 2004b)
         (a) The block is infused into the interscalene groove.
         (b) Indications include shoulder, arm, or elbow trauma, disease, or surgery.
      (2) Infraclavicular (NYSORA, 2008b)
         (a) The block is infused into a deeper location.
         (b) The infraclavicular technique decreases the risk of accidental catheter dislodgement.
         (c) It should be avoided in patients with coagulation risks secondary to close subclavian and axillary artery and vein.
         (d) Indications include hand, wrist, elbow, or distal wrist trauma, disease, or surgery.
         (e) The nurse must be sure to check for proper placement before beginning infusion to prevent complications.
      (2) Supraclavicular (NYSORA, 2008e; Waldman, 2004k)
         (a) The block is infused above the clavicle, where the three main nerve structures (sensory, motor, and sympathetic) are confined to a small area.
         (b) The indication is typically a rapid onset, predictable dense block that covers almost the entire upper extremity except the shoulder. The supraclavicular technique is especially good for elbow or hand surgery.
         (c) This technique typically is not used for continuous infusions unless the block is tunneled. This is because of proximity to the neck and risk of dislodgement.
         (d) Few articles are currently in the literature regarding the continuous use of this block.
      (3) Axillary (NYSORA, 2008a; Waldman, 2004a)
         (a) This block is infused along the axillary brachial plexus sheath.
         (b) Indications include forearm and hand trauma or surgery.
         (c) This is a highly vascular area with potential for inadvertent intravascular administration of local anesthetic.
         (d) The nurse must be sure to check for proper placement before beginning infusion.

2. Lower extremity (NYSORA, 2008d; Waldman, 2004d–2004j)
   a. Basic concepts
      (1) Lumbar plexus consists of five nerves on each side; the first emerges between the first and the second lumbar vertebra and the last between the last lumbar vertebra and the base of the sacrum.
      (2) As the L2 through L4 roots split off their spinal nerves, they immediately become embedded in the psoas major muscle.
      (3) Within the muscle, they split into anterior and posterior divisions, which then reunite to form the individual nerves or branches of the plexus.
      (4) The major branches of the plexus are genitofemoral, lateral femoral cutaneous, femoral, and obturator.
   b. Techniques
      (1) Lumbar plexus (NYSORA, 2008d; Waldman, 2004f, 2004g).
         (a) This block is infused into the deep muscle bed to provide analgesia along the entire plexus, including the thigh, knee, and below the knee.
         (b) Indications include hip, anterior thigh, and knee trauma, disease, or surgery.
         (c) This technique may need to be combined with a sciatic nerve block to obtain anesthesia for the entire leg.
         (d) When this wears off, the patient may have pain along this area and may need supplementation with oral or intravenous opioids.
      (2) Femoral nerve (NYSORA, 2008d; Waldman, 2004d)
         (a) This block is infused into the femoral nerve sheath.
         (b) Indications include anterior thigh and knee trauma or surgery.
         (c) Nursing implications
            (i) Due to risk of femoral artery or vein puncture, INR should be monitored.
            (ii) The patient should be instructed on their ability to bear weight on blocked extremity if a dense block is maintained postoperatively.
      (3) Fascia iliac (femoral and lateral femoral cutaneous) (Cuignet, Pierson, Boughrouph, & Duville, 2004; NYSORA, 2008d; Waldman, 2004e)
         (a) The block is infused along the fascia iliaca.
         (b) Indications include knee trauma or surgery as well as anterior or lateral thigh trauma or surgery.
            (i) This was first used in pediatric patients.
            (ii) Early reports were of 100% blockage along the femoral and femorocutaneous nerves and 88% blockage along the obturator nerve in children.
            (iii) This is a more lateral approach than the three-in-one block described below.
         (c) This block is not as successful in adults but does block the lateral femorocutaneous and femoral nerves while sparing the obturator nerve.
      (4) Three-in-one (Capdevila et al., 2005; Marhofer, Greher, & Kapral, 2005; NYSORA, 2008d; Waldman, 2004g)
         (a) Blockage is of the femoral, obturator, and lateral cutaneous femoral nerves with a single inguinal perivascular injection.
            (i) This block was first used 30 years ago.
            (ii) It has an 80% success rate.
            (iii) It is not generally used as a continuous infusion since the obturator nerve is not consistently blocked; therefore, pain management to the hip and knee may be spotty.
      (5) Sciatic nerve (NYSORA, 2008d; Waldman, 2004h–2004j)
         (a) The block is infused along the sciatic nerve.
            (i) This can result in analgesia of the entire leg below the knee, with the exception of the medial aspect of the lower leg.

(ii) A femoral nerve catheter may be needed depending on the level of injury or surgery.

(b) Indications include surgery or trauma of the knee, tibia, ankle, or foot.

3. Other peripheral nerves
   a. Thoracic paravertebral (Boezaart & Raw, 2006)
      (1) The block is infused into the paravertebral space.
      (2) Mechanism of action
         (a) Local anesthetic is directly infiltrated into the spinal nerves.
         (b) Lateral extension occurs along the intercostal nerve.
         (c) Medial extension is through the intervertebral foramina.
      (3) Indications include breast or thoracic surgery or rib fractures.
         (a) Note that the risk of pneumothorax is nonexistent when patients already have a chest tube inserted.

D. Settings of a peripheral nerve block (Buckenmaier & Bleckner, 2005; Cheng, Choy, & Ilfeld, 2008; Le-Wendling & Enneking, 2008)
   1. Inpatient
   2. Outpatient
   3. Setting is generally dependent on the patient's overall health condition, the type of surgery performed, and the patient's ability to manage at home.

E. Benefits include (Buckenmaier & Bleckner, 2005; Cheng et al., 2008; Le-Wendling & Enneking, 2008)
   1. Superior pain control.
   2. Improved patient satisfaction.
   3. Decreased stress response to surgery.
   4. Reduced operative and postoperative nausea and vomiting.
   5. Potentially shorter hospital stays and, possibly, reduced costs.
   6. Less pruritus.
   7. Less hypotension.
   8. Less urinary retention.
   9. Less lateralization of the blockade to the contralateral side.

F. Possible complications and side effects include (Buckenmaier & Bleckner, 2005; Capdevila et al., 2005; Le-Wendling & Enneking, 2008)
   1. Intravascular injection (see the chapter on Overview of Pharmacology for signs and symptoms of local anesthetic toxicity).
   2. Block failure (inadequate or spotty analgesia).
   3. Technical complications such as
      a. Displaced catheters.
      b. Knotted or kinked catheters.
      c. Catheter shearing or breakage.
      d. Dislodged catheters.
      e. Disconnections.
   4. Pneumothorax (thoracic paravertebral).
   5. Possible nerve injury.
   6. Hematoma (see the ASRA anticoagulation guidelines in XI. Regional and Localized Acute Pain Management Modalities).
   7. Infection.
   8. Horner's syndrome, a possible short-term side effect of brachial plexus blocks manifested by drooping eyelid, constricted pupil, and absence of facial sweating.

G. Assessment during infusion
   1. Check vital signs.
      a. Numerous studies involving continuous peripheral local anesthetic nerve blocks in children, have been completed without major morbidity and with few comorbidities (Le-Wendling &

Enneking, 2008; Ludot et al., 2008; Raimer et al., 2007; Richman et al., 2006; Zaric et al., 2006).

b. These studies support the safety of these patients on the normal medical or surgical ward.

c. Note respiratory status, especially if a thoracic paravertebral block is used, as pneumothorax is possible.

2. Assess the catheter and access site for
   a. Catheter placement.
   b. Intact dressing.
   c. Signs or symptoms of hematoma.
   d. Signs or symptoms of infection.
   e. Previously described technical complications.
3. Assess the patient for pain relief.
4. Check for muscle weakness.
   a. Ambulation precautions may be necessary, especially the first time the patient is out of bed.

H. Protocol considerations
1. What are the criteria for patient selection?
2. What are the anticoagulant considerations regarding placement, maintenance, and discontinuation?
3. Where and when should the block or catheter placement be performed?
4. Which infusion device should be selected?
5. Who attaches the device or injects the block?
   a. Who adjusts the rate or changes the orders?
   b. Who changes dressings or discontinues the catheter?
6. What are the state nursing board regulations regarding care of patients with blocks?

XIV. Preventing Persistent (Chronic) Pain after Surgery

A. Much attention has been given to the development of postsurgical persistent (chronic) pain.

B. Review articles on the subject have been vague, with some demonstrating no beneficial effect (Moiniche et al., 2002).

C. Another study concluded there is possible efficacy in selected analgesic regimes (Ong et al., 2005).

XV. Delivery Systems of Systemic Opioid Analgesia

A. Continuous delivery systems
1. Delivery options are
   a. Sustained release or long-acting oral medications.
   b. Intravenous infusions.
   c. Subcutaneous infusions.
   d. Transdermal.
2. Indications are as follows:
   a. If the patient was receiving this opioid medication before the acute situation.
   b. Continuous systemic opioid analgesia should not be initiated in acute situations with opioid-naïve patients (U.S. FDA, 2007).
   c. Continuous systemic analgesia is given for patients when pain management is desired at a steady state, including
      (1) Traumatic injury.
      (2) Postsurgical.
      (3) Acute medical disorders.
      (4) Coverage for baseline requirements of opioid tolerant/dependent patients.
3. Titrate to effect.
   a. Begin continuous infusion by titrating to effect. To do this, administer small doses of opioid frequently until the proper blood level is achieved to control pain.
   b. Titration is the rapid escalation of opioid.
   c. Once a safe and effective dose is achieved, the continuous infusion begins.

d. Concentration of the opioid during the continuous infusion must be determined based on the volume the dosage is to be delivered.
4. Nursing implications
a. Continuous systemic analgesia provides steady-state analgesia, thus minimizing the end-of-dose pain escalation of the intermittent dosing.
b. Assessment includes the following:
(1) Assess respiratory status, including rate, rhythm, quality, and characteristics of respirations.
(2) The sedation level may increase due to accumulation of opioid, resulting in oversedation and respiratory depression.
(3) Evaluate analgesia adequacy (patient satisfaction balanced with patient safety).
(4) Evaluate other side effects.

B. Intermittent dosing
1. Indications
a. Pain is episodic.
b. This dosage method is used when pain is intermittent (e.g., renal calculi produce intermittent yet severe pain).
c. Rescue doses may be needed intermittently during continuous infusions.
d. Intermittent dosing may be needed preemptively before painful procedures or activities.
2. Techniques
a. Fast-acting opioids are effective for short periods.
b. Frequent, intermittent doses of opioid can be administered by the nurse or patient.
3. Nursing implications
a. Intermittent dosing is feasible for critical care settings and postanesthesia care units (PACU).
b. It is often not feasible for nurses who work on postsurgical, oncology, or medical-surgical units, where the patient-to-nurse ratio is larger and patients require frequent dosing.
c. Administering opioids in larger doses less often can create periods of oversedation interrupted by periods of inadequate pain relief (Owens, Szekely, & Plummer, 1989).

C. Around-the-clock analgesic dosing
1. Indications
a. Pain anticipated to last more than 12 to 24 hours requires scheduled dosing of analgesic agents.
b. The patient is not a candidate for PCA.
2. Goals
a. Prevent recurrence of pain.
b. Reduce anxiety of anticipating the return of pain.
c. Reduce the total dose required to manage pain (Bonica, 1990; Twycross & McQuay, 1989).
d. Possibly replace around-the-clock dosing with PRN dosing as acute pain begins to resolve (McCaffery & Portenoy, 1999).
3. Nursing implications
a. Intent is to provide steady-state analgesia, thus minimizing end-of-dose pain escalation.
b. Important assessment includes
(1) Respiratory status, including rate, rhythm, quality, and characteristics of respirations.
(2) Possible increased level of sedation due to opioid accumulation, resulting in the patient feeling oversedated and at risk for developing respiratory depression. An example of creating safety in this type of medication administration would be to state "hold if sedated" in the protocol.
(3) Adequacy of analgesia (patient satisfaction balanced with patient safety).
(4) Monitoring for side effects.

D. Patient-controlled analgesia
1. PCA is a method of analgesia in which the patient self-administers a predetermined amount of analgesia through a specialized delivery administration system (Momeni, Crucitti, & De Kock, 2006).

2. The routes of administration are (Momeni et al., 2006)
   a. Intravenous.
   b. Epidural.
   c. Regional.
   d. Subcutaneous.
3. Indications are
   a. For intermittent and steady-state analgesia.
   b. Postsurgical, traumatic injuries, acute medical disorders, and procedural pain.
4. The method of analgesia administered is a patient-activated bolus dose only.
   a. Description
      (1) The opioid is delivered when the patient pushes a bolus button.
      (2) This is a demand dose at a single interval (Stanik, 1991).
      (3) The lockout is the time set between consecutive PCA doses.
      (4) PCA allows the patient control over opioid administration.
   b. Advantages
      (1) PCA avoids the peaks and valleys of analgesia, sedation, and pain (Mather & Owen, 1988).
      (2) It minimizes accumulation of the opioid.
   c. Disadvantages
      (1) The patient needs to be awake to push the bolus button to receive the opioid dose.

E. Continuous infusion with a bolus capability
   1. Description
      a. This is a constant low-dose infusion of an opioid.
      b. It is also called a background or basal rate.
      c. Continuous infusion is designed to prevent a subtherapeutic plasma concentration (Stanik, 1991).
      d. It allows patient control over opioid administration beyond the continuous infusion.
   2. Advantages
      a. Continuous infusion avoids the peaks and valleys of analgesia, sedation, and pain.
      b. It maintains an effective analgesia concentration.
      c. A bolus dose alone may allow peaks and valleys in a therapeutic concentration; a continuous infusion along with a bolus dose may be more effective (Glass, 1997). The above may be especially true for the first 24 to 48 hours postoperatively.
      d. The patient does not need to be awake to receive the opioid.
   3. Disadvantages
      a. Continuous infusion is more likely to accumulate opioid.
      b. The patient must be assessed at regular intervals for mental status changes and respiratory effects. Continuous monitoring may be needed.
      c. There may be more serious side effects associated with continuous infusions, such as nausea and vomiting, itching, urinary retention, sedation, and respiratory depression (White, 1988).

F. Protocol considerations
   1. General considerations
      a. The goal of safety is mandatory while providing adequate pain relief (Parker, Holtmann, & White, 1991; White, 1988).
      b. Define the type of patient who can use PCA devices, and prepare a list of teaching tools.
      c. Select the appropriate equipment.
      d. Select the medications and concentrations used.
      e. Establish consistency of use and dose.
      f. Define who manages the side effects.
      g. Provide an avenue of communication between the patient and the nurse to determine the quality of pain relief experienced by the patient.

h. Provide the required educational competency for nursing staff.
i. Provide patient and family education.
j. Establish monitoring, assessment, and documentation protocols.
k. Use a single concentration of opioid (this is strongly recommended) (Hutchinson, 2007; Viscusi & Schechter, 2006).
l. Educate patients with sleep apnea regarding the importance of using continuous positive airway pressure equipment postoperatively (Adams & Murphy, 2000).

2. Patient selection criteria
   a. It is anticipated that the pain may be severe yet intermittent and acute (i.e., renal calculi) or intermittent pain related to chronic illnesses (i.e., cancer).
   b. Constant pain increases in intensity with activity.
   c. The patient can comprehend the concepts and technique of PCA (Viscusi & Schechter, 2006).
   d. The patient has the physical capability to manipulate the dose button.
   e. The patient and family members are capable of understanding instructions and safety issues concerning PCA and they have met the standards of instructions applied at the institution.
   f. The patient is motivated to use the system (Viscusi & Schechter, 2006).
   g. The patient is not sedated from other medications.
   h. The patient cannot be well managed on oral medications.
   i. The patient is in moderate to severe pain.
   j. Care and additional monitoring are needed for a patient at risk for oversedation related to a comorbid diagnosis (i.e., sleep apnea or morbid obesity) or concurrently administered medications (e.g., benzodiazepines).
3. Nursing implications
   a. It is extremely important to teach the patient and family that with PCA only the patient can press the bolus button to administer the analgesia.
   b. Choose proper equipment for PCA administration.
      (1) The rate of use and doses can be programmed and locked into the delivery system.
      (2) Opioid can be locked to the infusion pump delivery system to minimize tampering.
      (3) Continuous infusion with a bolus capability is available.
      (4) The delivery system measures and records the amount used by the patient.
      (5) The delivery system can be either mounted to a pole or used in an ambulatory manner.
      (6) The delivery system is reliable, durable, affordable, and simple to program.
      (7) A nurse-activated bolus is available when a loading dose or rescue dose is prescribed.
   c. Assess the patient for effectiveness of analgesia and medication specific side effects.
      (1) Monitor the following when taking care of a patient on PCA:
         (a) Sedation level
         (b) Mental status
         (c) Respirations
            (i) Assess rate, rhythm, and depth (shallow versus deep).
            (ii) Note trends and changes in respirations.
         (d) Oxygen saturation
            (i) Pulse oximetry is one method to measure oxygen saturation; however, patients may not become hypoxic until after significant hypercarbia (also called hypercapnia) develops.
            (ii) Two systematic reviews noted that while pulse oximetry did reduce the amount of hypoxemia events postoperatively it did not significantly reduce the number of postoperative complications (Pedersen, Moller, & Pedersen, 2003; Young & Griffiths, 2006).
            (iii) Frequent monitoring of the patient is preferred and should not be substituted with pulse oximetry monitoring (Viscusi & Schechter, 2006).

(e) Capnography
(i) Potential exists for improving patient safety through early detection of respiratory events (Kodali, 2005).
(ii) Capnography may be an effective addition for monitoring patients who are at high risk for respiratory depression secondary to analgesics.
(iii) Additional studies are needed to ascertain general effectiveness of capnography (Hutchinson, 2007; Viscusi & Schechter, 2006).

d. Monitor the PCA delivery system.
(1) Have two nurses make independent double-checks.
(2) Reassess the delivery system (pump) settings.
(3) Reassess the medication and concentration.
(4) Reassess the delivery route lines and connections (Hutchinson, 2007).

e. Teach the patient
(1) To become familiar with the PCA infusion device before surgery.
(2) How to use PCA.
(3) When to push the bolus button.
(4) That only the patient may push the bolus button.
(5) When to communicate with the nurse (e.g., the patient is not controlled with PCA or is feeling sedated).
(6) Addressing fear of administering too much medication.
(7) Addressing fear of addiction to opioid with PCA therapy.
(8) The expected outcomes in terms of pain intensity or function.

f. Initiate PCA.
(1) In the surgical patient, the quality of intraoperative analgesia determines the amount of opioid required for pain control subsequently.
(a) The anesthesiology team may have injected the surgical site with local anesthetic agent or placed a disposable infusion system at the surgical site for continuous infusion of local anesthetic agent.
(2) Opioid administration continues in the PACU.
(a) Titration to effect is the common method of administering fast-acting opioid using a rapid acceleration.
(b) The purpose of titration to effect is to elevate the serum opioid level to provide the patient with proper analgesia.
(c) Dosage and frequency of opioid analgesia depend on opioid pharmacokinetics and pharmacodynamics (see the chapter on Overview of Pharmacology).
(d) Individual features of the patient, such as pain intensity, age, mental status, type of surgery, pain history, analgesia history, and comorbidities including pulmonary, renal, and hepatic function need to be considered while opioid administration is given. Dosage adjustments may be necessary.
(e) Hospital policies and procedures that take into account the clinical setting of titration to effect are occurring (e.g., in a PACU, ICU, and general medicine unit) (Pico, Hernot, Negre, Samil, & Fletcher, 2000; Stamer, Grond, & Maier, 1999).
(3) The nurse-to-patient ratio needs to be considered when initiating PCA.
(a) Nursing observation of the patient includes pain rating; mental status; respiratory rate, depth, and quality; and sedation. Sedation precedes respiratory depression.
(b) The pain rating must be documented (e.g., the fifth vital sign) (see the chapter on Social, Political, and Ethical Forces Influencing Nursing Practice).

g. Expect the following outcomes.
(1) The patient has improved pain relief.
(2) The patient has control in pain relief.

(3) The patient is able to keep the opioid serum level within a therapeutic range to prevent the peaks and valleys of analgesia that are common in intramuscular or short-acting oral opioid therapy (Lefkowitz & Lebovits, 1996).
(4) The patient can breathe deeply and ambulate early.
(5) PCA use has been shown to significantly shorten the length of hospital stay after major surgery (Stanik, 1991).

h. Advantages
(1) PCA enables patients to actively participate in managing pain.
(2) The intravenous route is familiar to nurses.
(3) There is rapid onset of action.
(4) It is easy to titrate for effective pain relief, especially as pain is escalating.
(5) PCA is safe to use when safe dosing guidelines are followed and only the patient administers the analgesia.
(6) It is used commonly in children older than 5 years of age (Berde & Kain, 1996).
(7) PCA has become the standard of care for pain management (Glass, 1997).

i. Disadvantages
(1) Intravenous access is difficult to maintain.
(2) The accumulation of intravenous opioid may not be predictable.
(3) Side effects such as somnolence may interfere with deep breathing and ambulation.
(4) The nurse may decide PCA liberates him or her from the role as the patient's primary pain manager (McCaffery & Pasero, 1999).
(5) Increased nursing vigilance is necessary.

G. Authorized agent-controlled analgesia (AACA)

1. Description
a. AACA is a method of pain control in which a consistently available and competent individual is authorized and properly educated by a prescriber to activate the dosing button of an analgesic infusion pump, when a patient is unable to do so, in response to that patient's pain (Wuhrman et al., 2007).
b. Individuals authorized to activate the analgesic infusion pump by the prescriber include the nurse taking care of the patient (nurse-controlled analgesia [NCA]) or a caregiver who is properly educated in the pain control method; this could be a parent or a significant other (caregiver-controlled analgesia [CCA]).
c. Its use is limited to individuals who cannot safely administer analgesic medications via analgesic infusion pump because of cognitive or physical impairment (Wuhrman et al., 2007).
(1) PCA by proxy, by standards of the American Society of Pain Management Nurses (Wuhrman, et al., 2007), is the use of an analgesic infusion pump by an ***unauthorized*** individual to administer medication to the patient.
(2) It is important to note that the American Society of Pain Management Nurses "does not support the use of unauthorized agent-controlled analgesia (UACA) or 'PCA by proxy' in which an unauthorized person activates the dosing mechanism of an analgesic infusion pump and delivers analgesic medication to the patient, thereby increasing the risk for potential patient harm" (Wuhrman et al., 2007).

2. Advantages (Wuhrman et al., 2007)
a. The greatest advantage is that it enables the patient to receive timely, effective, opioid analgesia without loss of dignity, periods of uncontrolled pain, or the high side effect burden.
b. AACA reduces the potential for medication errors.
c. Delay in administering analgesia is reduced.
d. Entry of infection through intravenous sites is decreased.
e. AACA reduces waste of unused opioids.

3. Protocol considerations
a. The agency must have clear guidelines that outline
(1) Conditions under which AACA may be implemented.

(2) Monitoring procedures that ensure safe use.
(3) Specific education requirements and materials.
(4) The requirement of a competent and consistently available person (agent).
(5) That the person (agent) must be authorized by a prescriber.
(6) That the agent must demonstrate proper education in delivering the proper medication in response to the patient's pain.

4. Key points regarding AACA are given in Box 17-2 (Wuhrman et al., 2007).
   a. All professionals and caregivers involved with AACA must know the requirements, guidelines, and rules as stipulated by the institution.
   b. PCA is a type of therapy. PCA is not the description of or name of the pump or delivery system.
   c. AACA is not an appropriate mode of therapy if the patient is appropriate to use PCA.
   d. Either AACA or PCA may be the mode of therapy. They cannot be use simultaneously.
   e. The medical record should prescribe PCA or AACA, indicating the NCA, CCA, or CCA with NCA coverage.
   f. Identify and educate all authorized agents.
   g. Identify all authorized agents and the method of analgesia in the care of the patient.

Box 17-2 Authorized Agent Controlled Analgesia (AACA)

Currently, the use of AACA in the adult population is based on expert panel recommendations. The safety and efficacy of this practice is based on the best-available literature and clinical anecdotes rather than scientific evidence. The Joint Commission and Institute for Safe Medication Practices have made clear statements prohibiting PCA by proxy because that practice lacked the necessary limitations to ensure patient safety (Joint Commission, 2004). Before the position paper was published, Paul Schieve, then vice president for patient safety at the Joint Commission, indicated it met the requirements for patient safety so long as the following points were highlighted (Wuhrman et al., 2007, p. 8):

- Everyone (patient, professionals, and visitors) should know the ground rules.
- PCA is a method of analgesia therapy, ***not*** the analgesic delivery pump.
- AACA is not appropriate if the patient is determined to be able to use PCA.
- Therapy is either PCA or AACA but not both.
- If method of therapy is to be changed, the medication order should be changed and documented in the patient record.
- The medical order should designate the following:
  - PCA
  - AACA (specifying Nurse Controlled Analgesia (NCA), Caregiver Controlled Analgesia (CCA), or CCA with NCA coverage)
- Avoid UACA (unauthorized agent controlled analgesia, also known as PCA by proxy).
- Identify the authorized agent or agents to the patient, family, visitors, and other caregivers.
- Identify the therapy to all agency personnel involved with the patient by a visual method (e.g., sign or label).
- Inform all unauthorized people that they must not activate the dosing button even in the absence of the authorized agent.
- It remains the responsibility of the health care team to continue to assess pain and treatment effectiveness.

Key points derived from Joint Commission. (2004). *Patient controlled analgesia by proxy.* Sentinel Event Alert No. 33. Retrieved December 29, 2008, from http://www.jointcommission.org/SentinelEvents/SentinelEventAlert/sea_33.htm. Emphasis recommended by the executive director for patient safety initiatives at the Joint Commission (Richard Croteau, personal communication, August 7, 2006).

h. Educate all family and visitors that they must not activate the analgesia when the authorized agent is not present.
   (1) Provisions should be made for nurses and health care staff to document the identity of the authorized caregiver, authorized caregiver education and feedback, amount of medication given over a specified period, and assessment and reassessment of therapy (Wuhrman et al., 2007).
i. The health care team continues to be responsible for the assessment and management of the patient's pain.
   (1) Use of AACA does not preclude nursing observation, assessment, and interventions that are standard in caring for a patient receiving analgesic infusion therapies (Wuhrman et al., 2007).

H. Subcutaneous analgesia: continuous infusion, PCA, or both
1. Indications
   a. The patient is intolerant to oral pain medications.
   b. Vascular access is not desirable or reliable.
2. Administration
   a. Subcutaneous and intravenous opioid infusions produce similar serum levels and provide comparable analgesia and side effects (Moulin, Kreeft, Murray-Parson, & Bouquillon, 1991; Storey & Hill, 1990).
   b. Plasma concentrations of subcutaneous and intravenous opioid infusions are similar at 24 hours, but at 48 hours the plasma concentration of the subcutaneous infusion decreases to 78% of the intravenous infusion (Moulin et al., 1991; Storey & Hill, 1990).
   c. Reevaluation may be necessary during the second day for dosage increase.
   d. The subcutaneous tissue can tolerate opioid infusions with less trauma and irritation if the infusion rate is less than 2 to 3 ml/hr (Coyle, Mauskop, Moggard, & Foley, 1986).
3. Patient selection criteria
   a. Intravenous access is poor.
   b. The patient and caregivers are willing to work with this means of administering opioid.
   c. Insurance covers maintenance of this technique.
4. Protocol considerations
   a. Opioids used (see the chapter on Overview of Pharmacology)
      (1) Morphine sulfate is commonly used.
      (2) Hydromorphone hydrochloride is commonly used.
         (a) Hydromorphone hydrochloride has high analgesic potency per milliliter that is five to six times higher than that of morphine.
         (b) This property minimizes the volume of infusion and is useful in opioid-tolerant patients who require higher hourly dosages for adequate pain relief.
      (3) Levorphanol tartrate is an option.
      (4) Methadone hydrochloride can be used.
   b. Technique for subcutaneous access
      (1) Prepare the skin with a povidone-iodine swab over the access site.
      (2) Common sites are the subclavicular area, anterior chest wall, and abdomen (Storey & Hill, 1990).
      (3) The insertion technique varies depending on equipment used.
         (a) With a small-gauge scalp vein needle, insert the needle at an angle under the skin. (In addition, there are 90-degree needles with a circular adhesive patch surrounding the needle specially designed for subcutaneous use.)
         (b) Stabilize by covering with a transparent dressing.
         (c) With a polytef (Teflon) catheter, the insertion is at a 90-degree angle to the skin and then the needle is removed, leaving the Teflon catheter in place.
         (d) It is recommended that the site be changed twice per week.

(e) Monitor the site for infection, infiltration, and local reactions (Walsh, Smyth, Currie, Glare, & Schneider, 1992).

c. Proper equipment for subcutaneous administration
   (1) Choose the appropriate needle.
   (2) Use an extension catheter if one is not attached to needle.
   (3) Use a povidone–iodine swab.
   (4) An adhesive bandage or transparent dressing should be applied.
d. The rate of infusion, frequency of site monitoring, and dressing changes must be consistent with physician orders and agency policy (Millam & DuFour, 2002).
e. Expected outcomes
   (1) Steady-state analgesia should be achieved with continuous infusion and bolus capability.
   (2) The delivery system should be easy to use.
f. Advantages
   (1) Subcutaneous analgesia is less invasive.
   (2) It is less expensive.
   (3) Nursing management is less complicated than the intravenous route due to easier access.
   (4) Opioids and antiemetics can be delivered simultaneously by subcutaneous infusion (Storey & Hill, 1990).
   (5) The metabolites of morphine-6-glucuronide and morphine-3-glucuronide levels were lower in subcutaneous than in intravenous administration of morphine (Stuart-Harris, 2000).
g. Disadvantages
   (1) The effects of subcutaneous infusions or boluses of opioid are limited to the absorption of the opioid at the subcutaneous site; thus, reduced infusate volume or more frequent site rotation may be needed.
   (2) Absorption from injections of subcutaneous or intramuscular opioid follows comparable time frames (Coyle et al., 1986; Stuart-Harris, 2000).
   (3) Local toxicity from mechanical or chemical irritation of the opioid is uncommon but is more likely to occur with the extremes of higher volume infusions and higher concentrations of opioid.
   (4) Problems associated with skin irritation at the needle insertion site include
      (a) Subcutaneous scarring.
      (b) Variable absorption.
      (c) Unpredictable analgesia.

XVI. Systemic Opioid Considerations: Monitoring

A. Monitoring requires nursing documentation, on a flow sheet, of
   1. Pain intensity (the fifth vital sign) pre intervention and post intervention.
   2. Blood pressure, pulse, respiration rate and depth, and oxygen saturation.
   3. Side effects.
B. Nurses should evaluate response to intervention.
C. Nurses must have knowledge of pharmacological implications of the medications, along with baseline information about the patient related to
   1. Known drug allergies.
   2. Renal function.
   3. Liver function.
   4. Past opioid use.
   5. Health habits, including alcohol intake and recreational drug use.
   6. Baseline mental status.
   7. Other medications taken.
   8. Bowel and bladder function.

D. Avoid inadequate pain relief.
   1. Believe the patient's report of pain.
   2. Be mindful of not making the patient feel stigmatized for expressing inadequate pain relief after intervention.
   3. The patient may fall asleep from the opioid but then awaken in pain.
   4. Treating pain with small, repetitive doses of intravenous opioid is safe, effective practice that should be used routinely until the medication can be adjusted or the technique of pain management altered.
   5. While providing this type of intervention, the nurse should monitor the patient continually and keep track of the pain medication used (i.e., document amount, type, time, and patient response).
   6. Assess to ensure that the pain being treated is opioid responsive. Neuropathic pain (described as burning, prickling, or tingling) is less responsive to opioid therapy and may need analgesic agents other than opioid.

E. Respiratory depression
   1. Respiratory depression is a serious complication resulting from too high an opioid dose.
   2. It can occur with any route of opioid.
   3. Respiratory depression is uniformly preceded by changes in mental status (e.g., confusion or sedation).
   4. If mental status is monitored regularly (e.g., every hour), the potential problem of respiratory depression can be identified earlier, allowing for opioid dosage to be reduced or stopped.
   5. Even if breathing is not slowed, confusion and somnolence are reasons to identify alternatives of analgesia (e.g., reducing dosage, identifying drug-drug interaction, changing the opioid, or identifying other causes for confusion or somnolence, such as hyponatremia).
      a. Count the respiratory rate for 1 full minute for accuracy.
      b. Determine the quality of respirations.
      c. If the respiratory rate drops below the predefined rate (e.g., eight respirations per minute) or becomes shallow with poor quality and patient becomes difficult to arouse, the opioid should be stopped; reversal with naloxone is indicated.

F. Reversal of opioid with naloxone
   1. Reversal is indicated if the mental status is markedly abnormal or there is poor-quality respiratory status.
   2. Reversal of opioid overdose can occur with pure antagonist or agonist-antagonist opioid (if the primary opioid combines with the μ-receptor).
   3. Intravenous naloxone can be administered in small increments frequently.
   4. An abrupt reversal of all analgesia may produce an increase in sympathetic drive, creating hypertension, tachycardia, rapid respirations, decreased gastrointestinal motility, and hypercoagulability (Zuckerman & Ferrante, 1998) (Box 17-3).
   5. By titrating naloxone hydrochloride slowly, the nurse can reverse the side effects without reversing the analgesia (Box 17-4).

Box 17-3 Administering Naloxone: Emergent

- IV push dosage: Dilution of naloxone with normal saline is optional. An ampule or prefilled syringe of naloxone contains 0.4 mg/ml.
- Administration: Administer 0.2 to 0.4 mg of undiluted naloxone. This may be repeated every 1 to 5 minutes as necessary. Maximum dosage is 10 mg, however opioid cause for respiratory depression may be questioned before this dose is reached.

From Rothley, B. B., & Therrien, S. R. (2002). Acute pain management. In B. St. Marie (Ed.), *Core curriculum for pain management nursing*. Philadelphia: Elsevier, p. 261.

Box 17-4 Administering Naloxone: Nonemergent

- One ampule of naloxone contains 0.4 mg/ml. Dilute the naloxone with normal saline to a total volume of 10 ml.
- Give 1 ml (or 0.04 mg) every minute until the patient is responsive.
- Assess responsiveness.
- If patient is not responsive after administering 0.8 mg of naloxone (two ampules), consider other causes for unresponsiveness.

From Dunwoody, C. J., & Arnold, R. (2005). *Fast fact and concept No. 039: Using naloxone.* Retrieved December 13, 2008, from http://www.eperc.mcw.edu/fastFact/ff_39.htm.

6. When reversal takes place, the patient should continue to be monitored for a return of a decrease in mental status and respiration because the duration of some opioids can be longer than the duration of naloxone. Naloxone may need to be repeated; consider low-dose naloxone infusion (Box 17-5).

G. Apnea monitor
   1. The apnea monitor is a plethysmographic device that detects movement of the thorax, which is recorded as ventilation rate.
   2. Reliability varies from one patient to another.
   3. The monitor emits false alarms that disrupt normal sleep.
   4. Patients may develop progressive respiratory depression characterized by rapid, shallow breathing that is not detected by plethysmographic apnea monitors (St. Marie, 1995).

H. Other side effects
   1. Nausea
      a. Causes
         (1) Nausea may occur from causes not related to opioid or other analgesic agents.
         (2) An opioid of any route may be one cause of nausea.
         (3) Opioid-related nausea tends to occur as the result of medullary chemoreceptor trigger zone stimulation, gastric stasis, or enhanced labyrinthine sensitivity (McNicol et al., 2003).
         (4) Nausea may result in patients with small doses of morphine sulfate and very mild renal insufficiency. This has been cited as related to morphine-6-glucuronide metabolite (Hagen, Foley, Cerbone, Portenoy, & Intrussi, 1991).
      b. Options for intervention
         (1) Change to another opioid agent.
         (2) Antiemetics may be administered.
            (a) These should be used in low doses.
            (b) Antihistamine agents may potentiate sedation.
            (c) Ondansetron may be administered (Heui-Ming et al., 2000).

Box 17-5 Prolonged and Continued Respiratory Depression

After initial parenteral administration, the central nervous system depressant effects of the opioid may have longer duration than the effects of reversal with naloxone. Intravenous infusion of naloxone may be necessary. The recommended concentration for intravenous infusion is 4 micrograms/ml, with an infusion rate of 2.5 to 3.5 micrograms/kg/hr.

From Rothley, B. B., & Therrien, S. R. (2002). Acute pain management. In B. St. Marie (Ed.), *Core curriculum for pain management nursing.* Philadelphia: Elsevier, p. 262

(3) Decrease the individual bolus dose per PCA or the infusion rate of the opioid.
(4) Modify the nausea with an antagonist, such as nalbuphine or naloxone, in low doses that will not reverse analgesia (Gan et al., 1997).

2. Urinary retention
   a. Causes
      (1) Urinary retention is common with a systemically administered opioid.
      (2) It is caused by a relaxation of the detrusor muscle at the floor of the bladder.
      (3) A physician or advanced practice nurse needs to evaluate a cause other than medication, such as mechanical urinary obstruction.
   b. Options for intervention
      (1) Reduce or change the opioid.
      (2) Treat with medications that contract the bladder, such as bethanechol chloride.
      (3) Single bladder catheterization relieves the problem but may expose the patient to the risk of urinary tract infection.
3. Pruritus
   a. Causes
      (1) Systemic opioid-induced pruritus is usually related to sensitivity or allergy to the drug or its vehicle.
      (2) True sensitivity or allergy to an opioid is rare.
   b. Options for intervention
      (1) Stop the opioid.
      (2) Antihistamine may be administered.
         (a) This should be done in low doses.
         (b) Antihistamine agents may potentiate sedation.
4. Constipation
   a. Causes
      (1) Pain slows bowel peristalsis.
      (2) The opioid slows bowel peristalsis.
      (3) Immobility, poor diet, and dehydration also slow bowel peristalsis.
   b. Monitor for
      (1) Bowel sounds.
      (2) Elimination patterns.
   c. Educate the patient and family that
      (1) Constipation is a side effect of opioid analgesia.
      (2) Dietary methods, including adequate hydration, can promote evacuation.
      (3) Activity promotes evacuation.
      (4) If patient has difficulty with bowel movements, discuss this with a nurse.
   d. Options for intervention are
      (1) Hydration.
      (2) Ambulation.
      (3) A high-fiber diet.
      (4) A stool softener given routinely.
      (5) A peristaltic agent.
      (6) A hyperosmotic laxative.
      (7) Oral naloxone for reversal of constipation secondary to the opioid.
         (a) Oral naloxone has systemic bioavailability of less than 3% due to extensive first-pass hepatic metabolism.
         (b) A study showed that oral naloxone did not change pain intensity, improved constipation symptoms associated with opioid, and reduced laxative use (Meissner, Schmidt, Hartmann, Kath, & Reinhart, 2000).
         (c) Methylnaltrexone given subcutaneously at 0.3 mg/kg is reported to be effective in advanced illness situations such as in palliative care (Thomas et al., 2008).

5. Urinary retention
   a. Causes
      (1) Urinary retention may be caused by various factors.
      (2) It has been associated with opioid administration.
      (3) It has been associated with increasing age, male gender, and opioids.
   b. Monitor for urine output.
      (1) A Foley catheter may be necessary to ensure adequate bladder emptying (Momeni et al., 2006).
6. Confusion
   a. Causes
      (1) Confusion may be caused by various factors.
      (2) It has been associated with opioid administration, especially when there is impaired renal function.
      (3) Confusion has also been associated with inadequately treated pain (Momeni et al., 2006).
   b. Monitor to
      (1) Determine baseline.
      (2) Assess for changes from baseline.
      (3) Assess for etiology.
   c. Options for intervention
      (1) If inadequate analgesia is the cause, adjust analgesia appropriately.
      (2) If the opioid is the cause, decrease the opioid dose and use multimodal analgesia, such as adding acetaminophen orally or rectally.
      (3) Consider other analgesia options.

I. Disposal of unused opioids
   1. State and federal regulations require that controlled substances be discarded and documented appropriately.
   2. Nurses' actions must support the institution and home health care policy and procedure.

XVII. Special Considerations in the Management of Acute Pain of Patients with Chronic Pain on Chronic Opioid Therapy or Have Opioid Addiction

A. Basic concepts
   1. An increasing number of individuals are living with chronic pain. In addition, they may experience acute pain related to surgical or nonsurgical trauma (Gordon et al., 2008).
   2. While not all patients who use opioids for long periods develop tolerance or experience dose escalation, the need can arise to increase doses over time.
   3. Dose escalation may be the result of progressive severity of pain or tolerance.
   4. Opioid tolerance occurs when patients need increasing doses of analgesia to attain and maintain the same analgesic effect.
   5. Tolerance develops in response to both prescribed and illicitly obtained opioids.
   6. Types of tolerance to opioids
      a. Innate tolerance is a genetically determined insensitivity that is present before the initial administration of the medication (Mitra & Sinatra, 2004).
      b. Pharmacokinetic tolerance occurs when the distribution or metabolism of the opioid is altered, resulting in an acceleration of the metabolism of the medication (Mitra & Sinatra, 2004).
      c. Pharmacodynamic tolerance occurs when neuroadaptive changes occur on two physiological levels (Mitra & Sinatra, 2004).
      d. Long-term tolerance occurs in individuals who develop an unrelenting neural adaptation that lasts for extended periods following cessation of prolonged opioid use (Mitra & Sinatra, 2004).

B. Opioid-induced hyperalgesia occurs when changes in the Central Nervous System result in increased sensitivity to pain (Chu, Clark, & Angst, 2005; Gordon et al., 2008).

C. Cross-addiction or polysubstance abuse occurs in individuals who routinely use nicotine, alcohol, or marijuana who may have greater dependence on opioids or other medications (Mitra & Sinatra, 2004).

D. Patient assessment
   1. Assess current use of opioids (prescribed or obtained from other sources).
   2. Establish a safe and nonthreatening relationship.
   3. Ask for names of all substances taken.
   4. Determine the actual doses (not prescribed dose) taken by the patient.
   5. Ask the patient or family about the usual 24-hour dose total. (If there is a range of dosing, establish the range.)
   6. Assess for use of other medications and substances that have a potential for dependency, including nicotine, marijuana, alcohol, benzodiazepines, anxiolytics, and cocaine (Mitra & Sinatra, 2004).
   7. Assess concerns and anxieties that the patient has regarding postoperative analgesia.
   8. Accurate assessment is imperative to adequately manage pain.

E. Patient treatment (Alford, Compton, & Samet, 2006)
   1. Preoperative intervention
      a. Reassure the patient.
      b. Instruct the patient to take baseline medications (both chronic pain medications and detoxification [methadone] maintenance program medications) the morning of surgery. For example, continue transdermal fentanyl patches during surgery.
      c. Maintain baseline opioid therapy if the patient is receiving opioids via epidural or intrathecal infusions. The patient should continue baseline medications to prevent withdrawal.
      d. A patient who did not take their baseline medications should receive an equivalent medication before surgery.
      e. A patient being treated with naltrexone should discontinue this use 24 hours or more before surgery.
      f. A patient being treated with methadone or buprenorphine maintenance therapy and needs treatment for acute pain must have higher levels of opioid to maintain baseline requirements of opioids plus the analgesia for the acute pain (see dosage adjustment estimates given later).
         (1) It is essential to adequately address, in a nonjudgmental manner, acute pain situations being experienced.
         (2) A patient receiving methadone maintenance needs to continue the maintenance dose and augment it with a short-acting opioid.
      g. A patient receiving buprenorphine therapy may be treated in one of four ways:
         (1) Continue maintenance therapy and augment with short-acting opioids.
         (2) Divide the maintenance dose of buprenorphine into three or four doses given every 6 to 8 hours.
         (3) Stop the buprenorphine maintenance therapy and treat with opioids (when able stop the opioids and resume the buprenorphine maintenance therapy).
         (4) A patient who is hospitalized may stop the buprenorphine maintenance therapy and treat with methadone augmented with short-acting opioids. When the patient is able stop the opioids, resume the buprenorphine maintenance therapy before hospital discharge (Alford et al., 2006, p. 130).
   2. Intraoperative
      a. Maintain baseline opioids.
      b. Upwardly adjust intraoperative usual opioids to compensate for tolerance.
      c. Consider using local anesthesia through spinal, epidural, or peripheral nerve blocks.
   3. Postoperative pain management
      a. Maintain baseline opioids.
      b. Consider using local anesthetic agents via intrathecal, epidural, or peripheral nerve continuous or PCA infusions.
      c. Consider administering opioids via the epidural route.

4. Dosing must be individualized.
   a. Opioid doses to manage postoperative pain and "analgesic requirements are affected by receptor down-regulation" (Mitra & Sinatra, 2004, p. 220).
   b. Postoperative doses may need to be 30% to 100% greater than those for comparable patients who are opioid naïve (Mitra and Sinatra, 2004, p. 220).
5. Employ multimodal analgesia that includes nonopioid medications and nonpharmacological comfort techniques.
6. Opioid delivery
   (1) Opioids can be delivered via PCA doses. PCA can be used effectively by patients who are recovering from opioid addiction when pain and opioid use are appropriately assessed.
   (2) Delivery can be the continuous infusion equivalent to the hourly dose of baseline medications. Multimodal analgesia is employed, including intravenous opioids, local anesthetics through various routes, and NSAIDs.
7. Rehabilitation maintenance
   a. Patients maintaining their rehabilitation from opioid use with buprenorphine should continue on that medication if it is adequate. The equianalgesic conversion of 0.8 mg of buprenorphine is approximately 20 mg of oral methadone (Mitra & Sinatra, 2004; Alford et al., 2006). Another reference states the equianalgesic conversion of 8 to 24 mg of sublingual buprenorphine is approximately 20 to 100 mg of oral methadone (Heit & Gourlay, 2008, p. 96).
   b. Patients maintaining with buprenorphine can be managed with additional methadone or morphine to achieve effective analgesia (Mitra & Sinatra, 2004).
8. Withdrawal concerns
   a. Opioid antagonists (i.e., naltrexone and naloxone) can cause withdrawal and should be avoided in opioid tolerant patients.
   b. The acute postoperative or posttrauma period is not the appropriate time to initiate detoxification or rehabilitation.
   c. Withdrawal from opioids is painful and increases the postoperative pain experience.
   d. "It is important to note that although the addition of a partial μ-agonist to a fully μ-dependent patient may precipitate severe withdrawal, the reverse is not true. Although analgesic response may be blunted, full μ-agonists can always be added to buprenorphine-maintained patients without fear of precipitating withdrawal. Care, however, should be exercised during titration due to potentially unpredictable μ-sensitivity" (Heit & Gourlay, 2008, p. 95).
9. Preparation for discharge
   a. During recovery, taper opioids.
   b. Do not abruptly decrease or discontinue opioids.
   c. Develop a plan of pain management.
   d. Arrange an appropriate and well-timed outpatient pain management consultation appointment.
      (1) Consider this appointment when prescribing adequate opioid and nonopioid medication (Ashraf, Wong, Ronayne, & Williams, 2004; Gordon et al., 2008; Mitra & Sinatra, 2004).
      (2) Have the discharge opioids given on a schedule and avoid PRN.
      (3) Talk with the patient about the schedule of the opioid, and talk with a trusted individual who will help in the opioid administration.
         (a) It is possible to set up taper schedule under the advice of a pain specialist.
         (b) For example, have the patient reduce the total opioid 24-hour dose by 10% to 20% every 3 days.
      (4) Instruct the patient to lock up the opioid in a lockbox or a tackle box with a padlock.
         (a) This allows the opioid to be safe from children or visitors.
         (b) This prevents theft of a prescription opioid.

XVIII. Acute Pain Services: Benefits and Processes

A. Benefits of acute pain services
   1. Benefits include relief of postoperative pain (see the chapter on Benefits of State-of-the-Art Pain Management).
   2. Surgical stress response decrease.
   3. Optimal analgesia can be provided using preemptive analgesia and a multimodal approach that uses rational pharmacology and multidisciplinary interventions.
   4. The complexities of pain are manageable for
      a. People with a history or current substance dependence.
      b. People with coexisting medical conditions and multiple drug administration.
      c. Postoperative pain that is refractory to conventional approach to pain.
      d. Postoperative pain in the context of persistent (chronic) pain.
      e. People in the age extremes (i.e., the very old and the very young).
      f. Pain from numerous etiologies.

B. Assessment of need
   1. Has a group of practitioners identified the undertreatment of inpatient pain?
   2. Is there a model that meets the needs of the institution (i.e., anesthesiology-based practice, advanced practice nurse consult service, pain resource nurse model, multidisciplinary model, or interdisciplinary model)?
      a. Anesthesiology-based practice
         (1) This service provides regional analgesia techniques for postoperative pain. It may also incorporate intravenous PCA (St. Marie & Schultz, 1991).
         (2) It is initiated in the perioperative setting and may continue throughout the postoperative period.
         (3) This model can be nurse based with anesthesiology supervision.
         (4) It offers cost-effective methods. The usual approach is regional analgesia, neuroaxial analgesia, and PCA. It may be supervised by anesthesiologists who are also managing operating rooms or pain services within anesthesiology.
      b. Advanced practice nurse consult service
         (1) This service requires an advanced practice nurse (clinical nurse specialist, nurse practitioner, or doctor of nursing practice) with a strong clinical background and interest and training in pain management.
         (2) Consult includes review of medical records; discussion with physicians involved in care; assessment of the patient (see the chapter on Pain Assessment), including previous opioid use; review of systems; physical examination; differential diagnosis, including pain diagnosis; and treatment plan.
         (3) There should be documentation, dictation, or both in the medical records. Prescribing may be necessary.
         (4) This is a billable consult, and follow-up is necessary to evaluate the efficacy of treatment plan.
      c. Pain resource nurse model
         (1) A registered nurse with advanced training in pain management is needed.
         (2) The concept of the pain resource nurse was first introduced at the City of Hope National Medical Center in Duarte, California (Jerin, 2002).
         (3) The goals are
            (a) To have one or two nurses assume an active role in guiding pain management in the clinical setting.
            (b) To increase general awareness of pain and barriers to pain management.
         (4) The model may have registered nurses trained for 24-hour coverage.
         (5) This is not a billable service; however, it is advantageous in its mentoring capability.
      d. Multidisciplinary model
         (1) A multidisciplinary model uses individuals from various disciplines.

(2) Each discipline provides recommendations to the physician who is the primary treating physician.
(3) Disciplines include pharmacy, nursing, rehabilitation specialists (e.g., physical therapy, occupational therapy, or music therapy), and mental health specialists (e.g., psychiatry, psychology, social work, chaplaincy, or chemical dependency).

e. Interdisciplinary model
(1) Individuals from various disciplines meet as a unit to provide their recommendations and collaborate to achieve a common goal (Jerin, 2002, p. 492).
(2) The Joint Commission requires an interdisciplinary model.
(3) Members of the interdisciplinary model depend on the needs of the patient.
(4) Limitations are extensive time for discussions to develop treatment plan. This time takes away from billable hours and limits access for each discipline involved (Jerin, 2002, p. 492).

C. Further needs assessment
1. Determine the size of the population.
2. Discover the willingness of physicians to refer their patients to the acute pain service.
3. Ensure the availability of disciplines to collaborate in caring for the patient.

D. Domains of the acute pain service
1. After the model has been determined, resources have been defined, the mission statement coincides with the model and resources, and people have been hired and trained, the domains of the acute pain service are then defined.
2. These domains may be prioritized according to the mission statement of the acute pain service.
3. Domains include clinical practice, research, education, and administrative.

a. Clinical practice
(1) Treat patients within the institution who need help with pain.
(a) According to Jerin (2002, p. 494), "70% of patients experience pain while hospitalized."
(b) Clinical systems of care that focus on pain prevention and intervention start in the perioperative and emergency department sites and continue through to discharge from the facility with a plan for continued outpatient pain care.
(2) Communication among the collaborative team ensures both patient satisfaction and physician referral satisfaction (Minzter & Cahana, 2008).

b. Research (see the chapter on Research Utilization in Pain Management Nursing)
(1) Research can include outcome measures of interventions used, patient satisfaction with care, and knowledge and attitudes of the health care team.
(2) Funding for research can be obtained both through the institution (i.e., auxiliary department funds), and outside the institution (i.e., Robert Woods Johnson Foundation, http://www.rwjf.org).

c. Education (see the chapter on The Pain Management Nurse as an Educator)
(1) With the advent of preemptive analgesia and multimodal analgesia, the development of a plan by the acute pain service in implementing these modalities must be orchestrated.
(2) Education must occur at all levels of care, including all disciplines of physicians, nurses, and pharmacists.
(3) Safety features must be redesigned (i.e., capnography monitoring versus apnea monitoring or oxygen saturation monitoring).

d. Administrative
(1) Business plan development
(a) Create a narrative mission statement, structure and responsibilities of the service, including
(i) Job descriptions.
(ii) Facility requirements.
(iii) Marketing plan.

(b) Prepare a spreadsheet (this may require assistance of business or administrative adviser), including
    (i) Estimates for fixed and variable incomes.
    (ii) Start-up capital.
    (iii) Month-to-month expenditure estimates for at least 1 year, including an analysis of reimbursement issues within the community.

(2) Centers of Medicare and Medicaid Services (CMS) guidelines
  (a) Guidelines for documentation
  (b) Guidelines for billing and collection
    (i) Efficient billing and collection services must be instituted at the time the service is formed. This is imperative for the service to succeed.
    (ii) This can be done in-house or through an outside billing and collection service with a percentage-based contract (Minzter & Cahana, 2008).
    (iii) Predesignated current procedural terminology (CPT) codes can be used to document billing.
  (c) Payment for service versus managed care model
    (i) If payment for services is changing to a managed care model, data are necessary to ensure funding is maintained.
    (ii) By tracking CPT codes and defining case mix, the managed care transition may have less financial impact.
    (iii) Analysis of "actual CPT reimbursement must be calculated to define a negotiating basis with insurers" (Minzter & Cahana, 2008, p. 26).

Summary

Establishment of an acute pain service must be well thought out, well planned, and supported by the administration of the facility to close the gap between the clinical need and the ability to meet that need (Pasero, Eksterowicz, & McCaffery, 2009; St. Marie & Schultz, 1991).

References

Adams, J. P., & Murphy, P. G. (2000). Obesity in anaesthesia and intensive care. *British Journal of Anaesthesia, 85,* 91–108.

Alford, D. P., Compton, P., & Samet, J. H. (2006). Acute pain management for patients receiving maintenance methadone or buprenorphine therapy. *Annals of Internal Medicine, 144,* 127–134.

American Academy of Pain Medicine. (2007). *AAPM facts and figures on pain.* Retrieved January 4, 2009, from http://www.painmed.org/patient/facts.html.

American Liver Foundation. (2008). *The American Liver Foundation issues a warning on dangers of excess acetaminophen.* Retrieved November 22, 2008, from http://www.liverfoundation.org/about/news/33/.

Apfelbaum, J. L., Chen, C., Mehta, S. S., & Gan, T. J. (2003). Postoperative pain experience: Results from a national survey suggest postoperative pain continues to be undermanaged. *Anesthesia & Analgesia, 97,* 534–540.

Ashburn, M. A., Caplan, R. A., Carr, D. B., Connis, R. T., Ginsberg, B., Green, C. R., Lema, M. J., Nickinovich, D. G., & Rice, L. J. (2004). Practice guidelines for acute pain management in the perioperative setting: An updated report by the American Society of Anesthesiologists Task Force on Acute Pain Management. *Anesthesiology, 100*(6), 1573–1581.

Ashraf, W., Wong, D. T., Ronayne, M., & Williams, D. (2004). Guidelines for perioperative administration of patient's home medications. *Journal of PeriAnesthesia Nursing, 19,* 228–233.

Barclay, L. (2005). *Intravenous morphine may increase mortality in non-ST segment elevation acute coronary syndromes CME: Medscape medical news.* Retrieved January 18, 2009, from http://www.medscape.com/viewarticle/504519.

Barclay, L. (2008). *Evaluation of acute abdominal pain reviewed: Medscape medical news.* Retrieved January 19, 2008, from http://www.medscape.com/viewarticle/57320.

Berde, C. B., & Kain, Z. N. (1996). Pain management in infants and children. In E. K. Motoyama & P. J. Davis (Eds.), *Smith's anesthesia for infants and children* (pp. 385–402). St. Louis: Mosby.

Boezaart, A. P., & Raw, R. M. (2006). Continuous thoracic paravertebral block for major breast surgery. *Regional Anesthesia and Pain Medicine, 31*(5), 470–476.

Bonica, J. J. (1990). *The management of pain* (2nd ed.). Philadelphia: Lea & Febiger.

Brennan, F., Carr, D., & Cousins, M. (2007). Pain management: A fundamental human right. *Anesthesia & Analgesia, 105*(1), 205–221.

Buckenmaier, C. C., & Bleckner, L. L. (2005). Anaesthetic agents for advances regional anaesthesia: A North American perspective. *Drugs, 65*(6), 745–759.

Bushnell, C. (2007). American Academy of Neurology 59th Annual Meeting. Abstract P03.083.

Byers, M., & Bonica, J. J. (2001). Peripheral pain mechanisms and nociceptor plasticity. In J. D. Loeser, S. H. Butler, & C. R. Chapman (Eds.). *Bonica's management of pain* (3rd ed., pp. 26–72.). Baltimore: Lippincott Williams & Wilkins.

Capdevila, X., Pirat, P., Bringuler, S., Gaertner, E., Singelyn, F., Bernard, N., Choquet, O., Bouaziz, H., & Bonnet, F. (2005). Continuous peripheral nerve blocks in hospital wards after orthopedic surgery: A multicenter prospective analysis of the quality of postoperative analgesia and complications in 1,416 patients. *Anesthesiology, 103*(5), 1035–1045.

Cappiello, E., O'Rourke, N., Segal, S., & Tsen, L. C. (2008). A randomized trial of dural puncture epidural technique compared with the standard epidural technique for labor analgesia. *Anesthesia & Analgesia, 107*(5), 1646–1651.

Cheng, G. S., Choy, L. P., & Ilfeld, B. M. (2008). Regional anesthesia at home. *Current Opinion in Anaesthesiology, 21*(4), 488–493.

Cherny, N. I. (1998). Cancer pain: Principles of assessment and syndromes. In A. Berger, R. K. Portenoy, & D. Weissman (Eds.), *Principles and practice of supportive oncology.* Philadelphia: Lippincott-Raven.

Choi, P., Bhandari, M., Scott, J., & Douketis, J. D. (2003). Epidural analgesia for pain relief following hip or knee replacement. *Cochrane Database of Systematic Reviews,* Issue 3. Retrieved January 11, 2008, from http://www.cochrane.org/reviews/en/ab003071.html.

Christie, I. W., & McCabe, S. (2007). Major complications of epidural analgesia after surgery: Results of a six-year survey. *Anaesthesia, 62*(4), 335–341.

Chu, L. F., Angst, M. S., & Clark, D. J. (2008). Opioid-induced hyperalgesia in humans: Molecular mechanisms and clinical considerations. *Clinical Journal of Pain, 24*(6), 479–496.

Chu, L. F., Clark, D. J., & Angst, M. S. (2005). Opioid tolerance and hyperalgesia in chronic pain patients after one month of oral morphine therapy: A preliminary prospective study. *Journal of Pain, 7*(1), 43–48.

Coyle, N., Mauskop, A., Moggard, J., & Foley, K. M. (1986). Continuous subcutaneous infusions of opiates in cancer patients with pain. *Oncology Nursing Forum, 13,* 53.

Cuignet, O., Pierson, J., Boughrouph, J., & Duville, D. (2004). The efficacy of continuous fascia iliaca compartment block for pain management in burn patients undergoing skin grafting procedures. *Anesthesia & Analgesia, 98*(4), 1077–1081.

Cuignet, O., Pierson, J., Soudon, O., & Zizi, M. (2007). Effects of gabapentin on morphine consumption and pain in severely burned patients. *Burns, 33*(1), 81–86.

D'Arcy, Y. (2009). First strike: Does preemptive analgesia work? *OR Nurse, 3*(1), 46–50.

DeCherney, A. D., Pernoll, M. L., & Nathan, L. (2002). *Current obstetric & gynecologic diagnosis & treatment* (9th ed., p. 491). New York City, N.Y.: McGraw-Hill Professional.

Ditonto, E. D., & deLeon-Casasola, O. A. (1998). Neurolytic blockade for the management of pain associated with cancer. In M. A. Ashburn & L. J. Rice (Eds.), *The management of pain.* New York: Churchill Livingstone.

Dravid, R. M., & Paul, R. E. (2007a). Interpleural block: Part 1. *Anaesthesia, 62*(10), 1039–1049.

Dravid, R. M., & Paul, R. E. (2007b). Interpleural block: Part 2. *Anaesthesia, 62*(11), 1143–1153.

Ducharme, J. (2000). Acute pain and pain control: State of the art. *Annals of Emergency Medicine, 35*(6), 592–603.

Ducharme, J., Choiniere, M., Crandall, C., Fosnocht, D., Homel, P., & Tanabe, P. (2007). Pain in the emergency department: Results of the pain and emergency medicine initiative (PEMI) multicenter study. *Journal of Pain, 8,* 460–466.

Dunwoody, C. J., & Arnold, R. (2005). *Fast fact and concept No. 039: Using naloxone.* Retrieved December 13, 2008, from http://www.eperc.mcw.edu/fastFact/ff_39.htm.

Dunwoody, C. J., Krenzischek, D. A., Pasero, C., Rathmell, J. P., & Polomano, R. C. (2008). Assessment, physiological monitoring, and consequences of inadequately treated acute pain. *Pain Management Nursing, 9*(1 Suppl. 1), 11–21.

Efthimiou, J., Butler, J., Woodham, C., Benson, M. K., & Westaby, S. (1991). Diaphragm paralysis following cardiac surgery: Role of phrenic nerve cold injury. *Annals of Thoracic Surgery, 52*(4), 1005–1008. Retrieved January 8, 2009, from http://www.medscape.com/medline/abstract/1929616.

Farrar, J. T., Berline, J. A., & Strom, B. L. (2003). Clinically important changes in acute pain outcome measures: A validation study. *Journal of Pain and Symptom Management, 25*(5), 406–411.

Frenay, M. C., Faymonville, M. E., Devlieger, S., Albert, A., & Vanderkelen, A. (2001). Psychological approaches during dressing changes of burned patients: A prospective randomised study comparing hypnosis against stress reducing strategy. *Burns, 27*(8), 793–799.

Gan, T. J., Ginsberg, B., Glass, P., Fortney, J., Jhaveri, R., & Perno, R. (1997). Opioid-sparing effects of a low-dose infusion of naloxone in patient administered morphine sulfate. *Anesthesiology, 87,* 1075–1081.

Glass, P. S. (1997). *Managing postoperative events.* Huntsville, TX.: Teleconference Educational Network.

Gordon, D., Inturrisi, C. E., Greensmith, J. E., Brennan, T. J., Goble, L., & Kerns, R. D. (2008). Perioperative pain management in the opioid-tolerant individual. *Journal of Pain, 9,* 383–387.

Grass, J. A. (2000). The role of epidural anesthesia and analgesia in postoperative outcome. *Anesthesiology Clinics of North America, 18,* 407–428.

Greengrass, R. A., & Nielsen, K. C. (2005). Management of peripheral nerve block catheters at home. *International Anesthesiology Clinics, 43*(3), 79–87.

Grossi, P., & Allegri, M. (2005). Continuous peripheral nerve blocks: State of the art. *Current Opinion in Anaesthesiology, 18*(5), 522–526.

Grossi, P., & Urmey, W. F. (2003). Peripheral nerve blocks for anaesthesia and postoperative analgesia. *Current Opinion in Anaesthesiology, 16*(5), 493–501.

Gutstein, H. B., & Akil, H. (2006). Opioid analgesics. In Brunton, L. (Ed.), *Goodman and Gilman's the pharmacological basis of therapeutics* (11th ed., pp. 521-552). New York: McGraw-Hill.

Hagen, N. A., Foley, K. M., Cerbone, D. F., Portenoy, R. K., & Intrussi, C. E. (1991). Chronic nausea and morphine-6-glucuronide. *Journal of Pain and Symptom Management, 6,* 125–128.

Heit, H. A., & Gourlay, D. L. (2008). Buprenorphine: New tricks for an old molecule for pain management. *Clinical Journal of Pain, 24,* 93–97.

Henry, D., & Foster, R. (2000). Burn pain management in children. *Pediatric Clinics of North America, 47*(3), 681–698.

Herr, K., Coyne, P. J., Key, T., Manworren, R., McCaffery, M., Merkel, S., Pelosi-Kelly, J., & Wild, L. (2006). Pain assessment in the nonverbal patient: Position statement with clinical practice recommendations. *Pain Management Nursing, 7*(2), 44–52.

Heui-Ming, Y., Li-Kuei, C., Chen-Jung, L., Wei-Hung, C., Yen-Po, Chou-Shun, L., Wei-Zen, S., Ming-Jiuh, W., & Shen-Kou, T. (2000). Prophylactic intravenous ondansetron reduces the incidence of intrathecal morphine-induced pruritus in patients undergoing cesarean delivery. *Anesthesia & Analgesia, 91,* 172–175.

Horlocker, T. T., Wedel, D. J., Benzon, H., Brown, D. L., Enneking, F. K., Heit, J. A., Mulroy, M. F., Rosenquist, R. W., Rowlingson, J., Tryba, M., & Yuan, C. S. (2003). Regional anesthesia in the anticoagulated patient: Defining the risks. The 2nd ASRA Consensus Conference on Neuraxial Anesthesia and Anticoagulation. *Regional Anesthesia and Pain Medicine, 28,* 172–197.

Hutchinson, R. W. (2007). Challenges in acute post-operative pain management. *American Journal of Health-System Pharmacy, 64,* S2–S5.

Jensen, T. S., & Nikolajsen, L. (1999). Phantom pain and other phenomena after amputation. In P. D. Wall & R. Melzack (Eds.), *Textbook of pain* (4th ed.). New York: Churchill Livingstone.

Jerin, L. (2002). Care delivery models for pain management. In B. J. St. Marie (Ed.), *Core curriculum for pain management nursing* (pp. 491–497). Philadelphia: W. B. Saunders/Elsevier.

Joint Commission. (2004). *Patient controlled analgesia by proxy.* Sentinel Event Alert No. 33. Retrieved December 29, 2008, from http://www.jointcommission.org/SentinelEvents/SentinelEventAlert/sea_33.htm.

Karmakar, M. K., & Ho, A. M. (2004). Postthoracotomy pain syndrome. *Thoracic Surgery Clinics, 14*(3), 345–352.

Kehlet, H. (1998). Modification of responses to surgery by neural blockade. In M. J. Cousins & P. O. Bridenbaugh (Eds.), *Neural blockade.* Philadelphia: Lippincott-Raven.

Kehlet, H. (2005). Preventive measures to minimize or avoid postoperative ileus. *Seminars in Colon and Rectal Surgery, 6,* 203–206.

Kockler, D. R., & McCarthy, M. W. (2007). Zoster vaccine live. *Pharmacotherapy, 27*(7), 1013–1019.

Kodali, B. S. (2005). Capnogram shape in obstructive lung disease. *Anesthesia & Analgesia, 100,* 884–888.

Lefkowitz, M., & Lebovits, A. H. (1996). *A practical approach to pain management.* Boston: Little, Brown.

Le-Wendling, L., & Enneking, F. K. (2008). Continuous peripheral nerve blockade for postoperative analgesia. *Current Opinion in Anaesthesiology, 21*(5), 602–609.

Lin, P. L., Fan, S. Z., Huang, C. H., Huang, H. H., Tsai, M. C., Lin, C. J., & Sun, W. Z. (2008). Analgesic effect of lidocaine patch 5% in the treatment of acute herpes zoster: A double-blind and vehicle-controlled study. *Regional Anesthesia and Pain Medicine, 33*(4), 320–325.

Liu, S. S. (1998) Local anesthetics and analgesia. In M. A. Ashburn & L. J. Rice (Eds.), *The management of pain*. New York: Churchill Livingstone.

Liu, S. S., Block, B. M., & Wu, C. L. (2004). Effects of perioperative central neuraxial analgesia on outcome after coronary artery bypass surgery: A meta-analysis. *Pain and Regional Anesthesia Anesthesiology, 101*(1), 153–161.

Liu, B., Tong, C., & Eisenach, J. (2008). Pregnancy increases excitability of mechanosensitive afferents innervating the uterine cervix. *Pain and Regional Anesthesia, 108*(6), 1087–1092.

Ludot, H., Berger, J., Pichenot, V., Belouadah, M., Madi, K., & Malinovsky, J. M. (2008). Continuous peripheral nerve block for postoperative pain control at home: A prospective feasibility study in children. *Regional Anesthesia and Pain Medicine, 33*, 52–56.

Lynch, E. P., Lazor, M. A., Gellis, J. E., Orav, J., Goldman, L., & Marcantonio, E. R. (1998). The impact of postoperative pain on the development of postoperative delirium. *Anesthesia & Analgesia, 86*(4), 781–785.

Maguire, M. F., Latter, J., Mahajan, R., Beggs, F., & Duffy, J. (2006). A study exploring the role of intercostal nerve damage in chronic pain after thoracic surgery. *European Journal of Cardiothoracic Surgery, 29*, 873–879.

Mardirosoff, C., Dumont, L., Boulvain, M., & Tramer, M. R. (2002). Fetal bradycardia due to intrathecal opioids for labor analgesia: A systematic review. *BJOG, 109*, 274–281.

Marhofer, P. Greher, M., & Kapral, S. (2005). Ultrasound guidance in regional anaesthesia. *British Journal of Anaesthesia, 94*(1), 7–17.

Mather, L. E., & Owen, H. (1988). The scientific basis of patient-controlled analgesia. *Anaesthesia and Intensive Care, 16*, 427–436.

McCaffery, M., & Pasero, C. (1999). *Pain: Clinical manual* (2nd ed.). St. Louis: Mosby.

McCaffery, M., & Portenoy, R. (1999). Overview of three groups of analgesics. In M. McCaffery & C. Pasero (Ed.), *Pain: Clinical manual* (2nd ed., p. 63). St. Louis: Mosby.

McNicol, E., Horowicz-Mehler, N., Fisk, R. A., Bennett, K., Gialeli-Goudas, M., Chew, P. W., Lau, J., & Carr, D. (2003). Management of opioid side effects in cancer-related and chronic noncancer pain: A systematic review. *Journal of Pain, 4*, 231–256.

McQuay, H. J., & Moore, R. A. (1999). Local anaesthetics and epidurals. In P. D. Wall & R. Melzack (Eds.), *Textbook of pain* (4th ed.). New York: Churchill Livingstone.

Meissner, W., Schmidt, U., Hartmann, M., Kath, R., & Reinhart, H. (2000). Oral naloxone reverses opioid-associated constipation. *Pain, 84*(1), 105–109.

Melzack, R. (1984). The myth of painless childbirth (the John J. Bonica lecture). *Pain, 19*, 321–337.

Mercer, J. S., Erickson-Owens, D. A., Graves, B., & Haley, M. M. (2007). Evidence-based practices for the fetal to newborn transition. *Midwifery Women's Health, 52*(3), 262–272.

Millam, D. A., & DuFour, J. L. (2002). IV therapy. In H. N. Holmes (Ed.), *Illustrated manual nursing practice* (3rd ed., p. 115). Springhouse, PA: Lippincott Williams & Wilkins.

Minzter, B. H., & Cahana, A. (2008). Organizing an inpatient acute pain management service. In H. T. Benzon, J. P. Rathmell, C. L. Wu, D. C., Turk, & C. D. Argoff (Eds.), *Raj's practical management of pain* (pp. 19–27). Philadelphia: Mosby/Elsevier.

Mitra, S., & Sinatra, R. S. (2004). Perioperative management of acute pain in the opioid-dependent patient. *Anesthesiology, 101*, 212–227.

Moiniche, S., Kehlet, H., & Dahl, J. B. (2002). A qualitative and quantitative systematic review of preemptive analgesia for postoperative pain relief: The role of timing of analgesia. *Anesthesiology, 96*(3), 725–741.

Moiniche, S., Romsing, J., Dahl, J. B., & Tramer, M. R. (2003). NSAIDs and the risk of operative site bleeding after tonsillectomy: A quantitative systematic review. *Anesthesia & Analgesia, 96*, 68–77.

Momeni, M., Crucitti, M., & De Kock, M. (2006). Patient-controlled analgesia in the management of postoperative pain. *Drugs, 66*, 2321–2337.

Moulin, E., Kreeft, J., Murray-Parson, N., & Bouquillon, A. I. (1991). Comparison of continuous subcutaneous and intravenous hydromorphone infusions for management of cancer pain. *Lancet, 337*, 465–468.

Murauski, J. D., & Gonzalez, K. R. (2002). Peripheral nerve blocks for postoperative analgesia. *AORN Journal, 75*(1), 134, 136–140, 142–151, 153–154.

National Pain Care Policy Act of 2008, S. 3387, 110th Cong. (2008).

New York School of Regional Anesthesia. (2008a). *Axillary brachial plexus block.* Retrieved January 23, 2008, from http://www.nysora.com/posts/view/177/axillary.

New York School of Regional Anesthesia. (2008b). *Continuous infraclavicular brachial plexus block.* Retrieved January 23, 2008, from http://www.nysora.com/posts/view/113.

New York School of Regional Anesthesia. (2008c). *Interscalene brachial plexus block.* Retrieved January 23, 2008, from http://www.nysora.com/posts/view/99.

New York School of Regional Anesthesia. (2008d). *Lower extremity nerve blocks: an update.* Retrieved January 23, 2008, from http://www.nysora.com/posts/view/148/lumbar%20plexus.

New York School of Regional Anesthesia. (2008e). *Supraclavicular brachial plexus block.* Retrieved January 23, 2008, from http://www.nysora.com/posts/view/105/supraclavicular.

Ong, C. K., Lirk, P., Seymour, R. A., & Jenkins, B. J. (2005). The efficacy of preemptive analgesia for acute postoperative pain management: A meta-analysis. *Anesthesia & Analgesia,* 100 (3), 757–773.

Owens, H., Szekely, S. M., & Plummer, J. L. (1989). Variables of patient-controlled analgesia: Bolus size. *Anesthesia, 44,* 7–10.

Page, G. G. (2005). Surgery-induced immunosuppression and postoperative pain management. *AACN Clinical Issues, 16*(3), 302–309.

Parker, R. K., Holtmann, B., & White, P. F. (1991). Patient-controlled analgesia: Does a concurrent opioid infusion improve pain management after surgery? *Journal of the American Medical Association, 266,* 1947–1952.

Pasero, C. (2005). *Self-directed learning program: Epidural analgesia for acute pain management in adults.* Pensacola, FL: American Society for Pain Management Nursing.

Pasero, C., Eksterowicz, N., & McCaffery, M. (2009). The nurse's perspective on acute pain management. In R. Sinatra, O. de Leon Casasola, E. Viscusi, & B. Ginsberg (Eds.), *Acute pain management.* New York: Cambridge University Press.

Pasero, C., Eksterowicz, N., Primeau, M., & Cowley, C. (2007). Registered nurse management and monitoring of analgesia by catheter techniques: Position statement. *Pain Management Nursing, 8*(2), 48–54.

Pasero, C., Paice, J. A., & McCaffery, M. (1999). Basic mechanisms underlying the causes and effects of pain. In M. McCaffery & C. Pasero (Eds.), *Pain clinical manual* (2nd ed., pp. 15–34). St. Louis: Mosby.

Paula, R. (2006). Compartment syndrome, extremity. Retrieved November 11, 2008, from http://www.emedicine.com/EMERG/topic739.htm.

Pedersen, T., Moller, A. M., & Pedersen, B. D. (2003). Pulse oximetry for perioperative monitoring: Systematic review of randomized, controlled trials. *Anesthesia & Analgesia, 96,* 426–431.

Phillips, D. M. (2000). JCAHO pain management standards are unveiled. *Journal of the American Medical Association, 284*(4), 428–429.

Pico, L., Hernot, S., Negre, I., Samil, K., & Fletcher, D. (2000). Perioperative titration of morphine improves immediate postoperative analgesia after total hip arthroplasty. *Canadian Journal of Anaesthesia, 47,* 309–314.

Pogatzki-Zahn, E., & Zahn, P. (2006). From preemptive to preventive analgesia. *Current Opinion in Anaesthesiology, 19*(5), 551–555.

Puntillo, K. A., Wild, L. R., Morris, A. B., Stanik-Hutt, J., Thompson, C. L., & White, C. (2002). Practices and predictors of analgesic interventions for adults undergoing painful procedures. *American Journal of Critical Care, 11,* 415–429.

Pyati, S., & Gan, T. J. (2007). Perioperative pain management. *CNS Drugs, 21,* 185–211.

Raimer, C., Priem, K., Wiese, A. A., Birnbaum, J., Dirkmorfeld, L. M., Mossner, A., Matziolis, G., Perka, C., & Volk, T. (2007). Continuous psoas and sciatic block after knee arthroplasty: Good effects compared to epidural analgesia or IV opioid analgesia—a prospective study of 63 patients. *Acta Orthopaedica, 78,* 193–200.

Rathmell, J. P., Viscomi, C. M., & Ashburn, M. A. (1997). Acute and chronic pain management in the pregnant patient. *Anesthesia & Analgesia, 85,* 1074–1087.

Ready, L. B. (2001). Regional analgesia with intraspinal opioids. In J. D. Loeser (Ed.), *Bonica's management of pain* (3rd ed., pp. 1953–1966). Philadelphia: Lippincott Williams & Wilkins.

Richman, J. M., Liu, S. S., Courpas, B. A., Wong, R., Rowlingson, A. B., McGready, J., Cohen, S. R., & Wu, C. L. (2006). Does continuous peripheral nerve block provide superior pain control to opioids? A meta-analysis. *Anesthesia & Analgesia, 102,* 248–257.

Rosow, C. E., Gomery, P., Chen, T. Y., Stefanovich, P., Stambler, N., & Israel, R. (2007). Reversal of opioid-induced bladder dysfunction by intravenous naloxone and methylnaltrexone. *Clinical Pharmacology & Therapeutics, 82*(1), 48–53.

Ross, E. L. (2004). *Hot topics: Pain management.* Philadelphia: Hanley and Belfus.

Rothley, B. B., & Therrien, S. R. (2002). Acute pain management. In B. St. Marie (Ed.), *Core curriculum for pain management nursing.* Philadelphia: Elsevier.

Russell, R., & Reynolds, F. (1997). Editorial: Back pain, pregnancy, and childbirth. *British Medical Journal, 12*(314;7087), 1062–1063.

Santy, J. (2008). Recognizing infection in wounds. *Nursing Standard, 23*(7), 53–60.

Schley, M. T., Wilms, P., Toepfner, S., Schaller, H. P., Schmelz, M., Konrad, C. J., & Birbaumer, N. (2008). Painful and non-painful phantom and stump sensations in acute traumatic amputees. *Journal of Trauma, 65*(4), 858–864.

Schmid, R. L., Sandler, A. N., & Katz, J. (1999). Use and efficacy of low-dose ketamine in the management of acute postoperative pain: A review of current techniques and outcomes. *Pain, 82*(2), 111–125.

Slack, J. F., & Faut-Callahan, M. (1991). Efficacy of epidural analgesia for pain management of critically ill patients and the implications for nursing care. *AACN Clinical Issues, 2*(4), 729–739.

Smith, J. A., Espeland, M., Bellevue, R., Bonds, D., Brown, A.K., & Koshy, M. (1996). Pregnancy in sickle cell disease: Experience of the cooperative study of sickle cell disease. *Obstetrics and Gynecology, 87,* 199–204.

Spies, C. D., & Rommelspacher, H. (1999). Alcohol withdrawal and the surgical patient: Prevention and treatment. *Anesthesia & Analgesia, 88*(4), 946–954.

Stamer, U. M., Grond, S., & Maier, C. (1999). Responders and non-responders to post-operative pain treatment: The loading dose predicts analgesic needs. *European Journal of Anaesthesiology, 16,* 103–110.

Standl, T., Burmeister, M., Ohnesorge, H., Wilhelm, S., Striepke, M., Gottschalk, A., Horn, E.P., & Schulte, J. (2003). Patient-controlled epidural analgesia reduces analgesic requirements compared to continuous epidural infusion after major abdominal surgery. *Regional Anesthesia & Pain Medicine, 50*(3), 258–264.

Stanik, J. A. (1991). Patient-controlled analgesia and critically ill patients. *AACN Clinical Issues, 2*(4), 741–744.

Stankus, S. J., Dlugopolski, M., & Packer, D. (2000) Management of herpes zoster (shingles) and postherpetic neuralgia. *American Family Physician, 61*(8), 2437–2444, 2447–2448.

St. Marie, B. (1995). Pain management. In J. Terry, L. Baranowski, R. A. Lonsway, & C. Hedrick (Eds.), *Intravenous therapy: Clinical principles and practice.* Philadelphia: W. B. Saunders.

St. Marie, B., & Schultz, D. (1991). *Acute pain service manual.* Developed for Anesthesiology, P. A., at North Memorial Medical Center, Minneapolis, Minnesota.

Storey, P., & Hill, H. (1990). Subcutaneous infusions for control of cancer symptoms. *Journal of Pain and Symptom Management, 5,* 33–41.

Strassels, S. A., McNichol, E., & Suleman, R. (2005). Postoperative pain management: A practical review, part 1. *American Journal of Health-System Pharmacy, 62,* 1904–1916.

Stuart-Harris, R. (2000). The pharmacokinetics of morphine and morphine glucuronide metabolites after subcutaneous bolus injection and subcutaneous infusion of morphine. *British Journal of Clinical Pharmacology, 49*(3), 207–214.

Summer, G. J., Puntillo, K. A., Miaskowski, C., & Green, P. G. (2007). Burn injury pain: The continuing challenge. *Journal of Pain, 8*(7), 533–548.

Supple, K. G. (2004). Physiologic response to burn injury. *Critical Care Nursing Clinics of North America, 16*(1), 119–126.

Tait, I. S., Ionescu, M. V., & Cuschieri, A. (1999). A. Do patients with acute abdominal pain wait unduly long for analgesia? *Journal of the Royal College of Surgeons of Edinburgh, 44,* 181.

Tamchèsa, E., Buclinb, T., Huglia, O., Decosterdc, I., Blancc, C., Mouhsinee, E., Givelf, J. C., & Yersina, B. (2007). Acute pain in adults admitted to the emergency room: Development and implementation of abbreviated guidelines *Swiss Medical Weekly, 137,* 223–227.

Thierbach, A. R., Lipp, M. D., & Daublander, M. (1999). Pain management in the emergency room: Initial evaluation and interventions. In A. D. Rosenberg, C. M. Grande, & R. L. Bernstein (Eds.), *Pain management and regional anesthesia in trauma* (pp. 119–129). St. Louis: W. B. Saunders.

Todd, K. H., Ducharme, J., Choiniere, M., Crandall, C. S., Fosnocht, D. E., Homel, P., & Tanabe, P. (2007). PEMI Study Group. Pain in the emergency department: Results of the pain and emergency medicine initiative (PEMI) multicenter study. *Journal of Pain, 8,* 460–466.

Tournaire, M., & Theau-Yonneau, A. (2007). Complementary and alternative approaches to pain relief during labor. *Evidence-based Complementary and Alternative Medicine, 4,* 409–417.

Twycross, R. G., & McQuay, H. J. (1989). Opioids. In P. D. Wall & R. Melzack (Eds.), *Textbook of pain* (2nd ed., pp. 686–701). New York: Churchill Livingstone.

U.S. Agency for Health Care Policy and Research. (1992). *Acute pain management: Operative or medical procedures and trauma.* Clinical Practice Guideline. (AHCPR Guidelines.) Rockville, MD.: Author.

U.S. Food and Drug Administration. (1997). FDA public health advisory: Reports of epidural and spinal hematomas with the concurrent use of low molecular with heparin and spinal/epidural anesthesia or spinal puncture [Brochure]. Rockville, MD: U.S. Department of Health and Human Services.

U.S. Food and Drug Administration. (2007). Information for healthcare professionals fentanyl transdermal system (marketed as Duragesic and genetics). *FDA Alert, 7/15/2005, updated 12/21/2007,* 1–3.

Vallejo, M. C., Ramesh, V., Phelps, A. L., & Sah, N. (2007). Epidural labor analgesia: Continuous infusion versus patient-controlled epidural analgesia with background infusion versus without a background infusion. *Journal of Pain, 8,* 970–975.

Vanderwee, K., Clark, M., Dealey, C., Defloor, T., Schoonhoven, L., Witherow, A., Baharestani, M., Black, J., Cuddigan, J., Edsberg, L., Garber, S., Langemo, D., Posthauer, M. E., Ratliff, C., & Taler, G. (2008). Development of clinical practice guideline on pressure ulcers. *EWMA Journal, 7*(3), 44–46. Retrieved January 10, 2009, from http://pressureulcerguidelines.org/therapy/docs/pain_assessment_and_management.pdf.

Van Rijswijk, L. (1999). Wound pain. In M. McCaffery & C. Pasero (Eds.), *Pain: Clinical manual* (2nd ed.). St. Louis: Mosby.

Viscusi, E. R., & Schechter, L. N. (2006). Patient-controlled analgesia: Finding a balance between cost and comfort. *American Journal of Health System Pharmacy, 63,* S3–S13.

Waldman, S. D. (2004a). Brachial plexus block: Axillary approach. In *Atlas of interventional pain management* (2nd ed., pp. 159–162). Philadelphia: Saunders.

Waldman, S. D. (2004b). Brachial plexus block: Interscalene approach, In *Atlas of interventional pain management* (2nd ed., pp. 150–154). Philadelphia: Saunders.

Waldman, S. D. (2004c). Brachial plexus block: Supraclavicular approach. In *Atlas of interventional pain management* (2nd ed., pp. 155–158). Philadelphia: Saunders.

Waldman, S. D. (2004d). Femoral nerve block. In *Atlas of interventional pain management* (2nd ed., pp. 449–453). Philadelphia: Saunders.

Waldman, S. D. (2004e). Lateral femoral cutaneous nerve block. In *Atlas of interventional pain management* (2nd ed., pp. 454–457). Philadelphia: Saunders.

Waldman, S. D. (2004f). Lumbar plexus nerve block: Psoas compartment technique. In *Atlas of interventional pain management* (2nd ed., pp. 443–448). Philadelphia: Saunders.

Waldman, S. D. (2004g). Lumbar plexus nerve block: Winnie 3-in-1 technique. In *Atlas of interventional pain management* (2nd ed., pp. 440–442). Philadelphia: Saunders.

Waldman, S. D. (2004h). Sciatic nerve block: Anterior approach. In *Atlas of interventional pain management* (2nd ed., pp. 463–467). Philadelphia: Saunders.

Waldman, S. D. (2004i). Sciatic nerve block: Lithotomy approach. In *Atlas of interventional pain management* (2nd ed., pp. 473–477). Philadelphia: Saunders.

Waldman, S. D. (2004j). Sciatic nerve block: Posterior approach. In *Atlas of interventional pain management* (2nd ed., pp. 468–472). Philadelphia: Saunders.

Waldman, S. D. (2004k). Suprascapular nerve block. In *Atlas of interventional pain management* (2nd ed., pp. 163–165). Philadelphia: Saunders.

Wallace, A. M., & Wallace, M. S. (1997). Pain: Nociceptive and neuropathic mechanisms—postmastectomy and postthoracotomy pain. *Anesthesiology Clinics of North America, 15,* 353–370.

Wallander, M. A., Johansson, S., Ruigómez, A., & García Rodríguez, L. A. (2007). Unspecified abdominal pain in primary care: The role of gastrointestinal morbidity. *International Journal of Clinical Practice, 61*(10), 1663–1670.

Walsh, T. D., Smyth, E. M., Currie, K., Glare, P. A., & Schneider, J. (1992). A pilot study, review of the literature, and dosing guidelines for patient-controlled analgesia using subcutaneous morphine sulphate for chronic cancer pain. *Palliative Medicine, 6,* 217–226.

Watkins, P. B., Kaplowitz, N., Slattery, J. T., Colonese, C. R., Colucci, S. V., Stewart, P. W., & Harris, S. C. (2008) Aminotransferase elevations in healthy adults receiving 4 grams of acetaminophen daily: A randomized controlled trial. *Journal of the American Medical Association, 296*(1), 87–93.

White, P. F. (1988). Use of patient-controlled analgesia for management of acute pain. *Journal of the American Medical Association, 259,* 243–247.

Wild, L., & Coyne, C. (1992). The basics and beyond: Epidural analgesia. *American Journal of Nursing, 92,* 26–36.

Wilson, J. A., Nimmo, A. F., Fleetwood-Walker, S. M., & Colvin, L. A. (2008). A randomised double blind trial of the effect of pre-emptive epidural ketamine on persistent pain after lower limb amputation. *Pain, 135*(1–2), 108–118.

Windle, P. E., Kwan, M. L., Warwick, H., Sibayan, A., Espiritu, C., & Vergara, J. (2006). Comparison of bacteriostatic normal saline and lidocaine used as intradermal anesthesia for the placement of intravenous lines., *Journal of PeriAnesthesia Nursing, 21*(4), 251–258.}

Wong, C. A., Scavone, B. M., Peaceman, A. M., McCarthy, R. J., Sullivan, J. T., Diaz, N. T., Yaghmour, E., Marcus, R. J. L., Sherwani, S. S., Sproviero, M. T., Yilmaz, M., Patel, R., Robles, C., & Grouper, S. (2005). The Risk of cesarean delivery with neuraxial analgesia given early versus late in labor. *New England Journal of Medicine, 352,* 655.

Woolf, C. J., & Chong, M. S. (1993). Preemptive analgesia: Treating postoperative pain by preventing the establishment of central sensitization. *Anesthesia & Analgesia, 77,* 362–379.

Wuhrman, E., Cooney, M. F., Dunwoody, C. J., Eksterowicz, N., Merkel, S., & Oakes, L. L. (2007). Authorized and unauthorized ("PCA by proxy") dosing of analgesic infusion pumps. American Society for Pain Management Nursing position paper. *Pain Management Nursing, 8*(1), 4–11.

Young, D., & Griffiths, J. (2006). Clinical trials of monitoring anaesthesia, critical care and acute ward care: A review. *British Journal of Anaesthesia, 97,* 39–45.

Zaric, D., Boyson, K., Christiansen, C., Christiansen, J., Stephensen, S., & Christensen, B. (2006). A comparison of epidural analgesia with combined continuous femoral-sciatic nerve blocks after total knee replacement. *Anesthesia & Analgesia, 102,* 1240–1246.

Zuckerman, L. A., & Ferrante, F. M. (1998). Nonopioid and opioid analgesics. In M. A. Ashburn & L. J. Rice (Eds.), *The management of pain* (pp. 111–135). New York: Churchill Livingstone.

Suggested Readings

American Pain Foundation. (2007). *Pain facts and figures.* Retrieved January 4, 2009, from http://www.painfoundation.org/page.asp?file=Newsroom/PainFacts.htm.

Department of Health and Human Services. (2008). *Hospital process of care measures.* Retrieved January 4, 2009, from http://www.hospitalcompare.hhs.gov/Hospital/Static/ConsumerInformation_tabset.asp?activeTab=2&Language=English&version=default&subTab=4.

Pasero, C., & McCaffery, M. (2000). Reversing respiratory depression with naloxone. *American Journal of Nursing, 100*(2), 26.

Rozen, D., Ling, C., & Schade, C. (2005). Coadministration of an opioid agonist and antagonist for pain control. *Pain Practice, 5*(1), 11–17.

Todd, K. H., Thomas, J., Karver, S., Cooney, G. A., Chamberlain, B. H., Watt, C. K., Slatkin, N. E., Stambler, N., Kremer, A. B., & Israel, R. J. (2008). Methylnaltrexone for opioid-induced constipation in advanced illness. *New England Journal of Medicine, 358,* 2332–2343.

chapter

18

Persistent Pain Management

Janette E. Elliott, RN-BC, MSN, AOCN
Melanie H. Simpson, PhD, RN-BC, OCN, CHPN

Objectives

After studying this chapter, the reader should be able to:

1. Differentiate persistent pain diagnoses.
2. Identify appropriate interventions for each type of pain.
3. Discuss the goals of treatment in persistent pain.
4. Describe the pharmacological and nonpharmacological modalities appropriate in the treatment of persistent pain.
5. Identify appropriate nonneuroablative interventional techniques used in the management of persistent pain syndromes.
6. Discuss appropriate neuroablative techniques used in the management of persistent pain syndromes.
7. Discuss appropriate use of implantable therapies in the management of persistent pain syndromes.

The pathophysiology of the persistent pain process continues to be the object of intense research. With much still unknown, treatment possibilities and options and resolution of the pain are unpredictable. The impact of persistent pain on people's lives motivates neuroscientists, clinical practitioners, and complementary medicine researchers to move forward to resolve the problems persistent pain patients face. This chapter serves as a guide to recognize certain pain syndromes and provides the clinician with an armamentarium of approaches to persistent pain problems.

A high prevalence of persistent pain occurs in patients with posttraumatic stress disorder (PTSD) (Geisser, Roth, Bachman, & Eckert, 1996). It has even been postulated that uncontrolled pain following physical injury is the core trauma in PTSD (Schreiber & Galai-Gat, 1993). It has also been postulated that persistent pain and PTSD might be mutually maintaining syndromes (Sharp & Harvey, 2001). Therefore, an evaluation for PTSD is warranted in all patients with persistent pain.

PART ONE: PERSISTENT PAIN DIAGNOSES

Persistent pain is pain that lasts longer than typical healing time (thought to be between 3 and 6 months) or recurs intermittently (see the chapter on Taxonomy for Pain Management Nursing). Acute pain decreases with time. In some cases, acute exacerbations of persistent pain problems occur. These situations and persistent pain diagnoses are discussed in this section.

I. Low Back Pain

A. Diagnosing the cause of low back pain may be difficult. Back pain can originate from musculoskeletal problems, may be referred from viscera (kidney or uterus), or may be enigmatic.

B. *Ankylosing spondylitis* is inflammation causing stiffening of the joint structure in the low back and pelvis.

1. Signs and symptoms
   a. Chronic inflammatory changes result in gradual onset of low back aching and stiffness. Ankylosing spondylitis is nine times more common in men than women, with onset in their 20s to 30s.
   b. Aching in lower back and stiffness with gradual onset results from chronic inflammatory change.
   c. Stiffness and pain occur in the morning and after episodes of inactivity.
   d. Associated symptoms may include peripheral joint disease, conjunctivitis, and iritis (inflammation of the iris).
   e. The New York diagnostic criteria for ankylosing spondylitis (Arnett, 1998; MD Consult, 2007) are as follows:
      (1) Limitation of motion of the lumbar spine in all three planes (i.e., anterior flexion, lateral flexion, and extension)
      (2) History of presence of pain at the dorsolumbar junction or in the lumbar spine
      (3) Limitation of chest expansion to 2.5 cm (1 inch) or less, measured at the level of the fourth intercostal space
2. Diagnostic workup
   a. It has been found that 90% of patients have positive HLA-B27 (a genetic marker) (Arnett, 1998).
   b. A radiograph shows bilateral symmetrical sacroiliitis (inflammation of the sacroiliac joint).
      (1) Grade 3 (sclerosis and erosions of the joint margins)
      (2) Grade 4 (fusion across the joint) (Arnett, 1998)
3. Treatment
   a. Educate the patient about the disease.
   b. Encourage physical measures of stretching and strengthening of the pelvic girdle and of pacing activities to prevent injury, reduce pain, and maintain range of motion in affected areas.
   c. Nonsteroidal antiinflammatory drugs (NSAIDs) can be used to reduce pain and stiffness.

C. *Arachnoiditis* is irritation of the arachnoid meningeal layer of the spinal cord. Irritation could have many causative factors: bacterial or viral infections, direct spinal injury, surgery or other invasive spinal procedures, and chemical irritation caused by accidental intrathecal administration of certain medications or solutions, such as povidone–iodine, hyperalimentation, potassium chloride, or myelographic contrast agents (Dawson, 2008; Dworkin et al., 2007; Kafiluddi & Hahn, 2000; National Institute of Neurological Disorders and Stroke [NINDS], 2007). Adhesions and scar tissue may form due to the inflammation, causing the spinal nerves to "stick" together.
  1. Signs and symptoms
     a. Pain starts as local, continuous, dull, or aching and then progresses to an intense, painful, burning sensation.
     b. Neck stiffness and sensory and motor impairments may occur.
     c. Severe pain may occur in the upper limb or be diffused with widespread bilateral symptoms.
     d. When the low back is the focal point, the pain is distributed to both legs.
     e. Pain is aggravated by movement, coughing, and sneezing and is more intense with bed rest and in the morning.
     f. Pain is described as a bandlike, constricting sensation with increasing pain or as stinging, burning, aching, or gnawing.
     g. This often leads to severe chronic pain.
     h. Muscle cramps, twitches, or spasms may occur and may become debilitating.
     i. It may affect bladder, bowel, and sexual function.
  2. Diagnostic workup
     a. Blood and cerebrospinal fluid (CSF) studies are consistent with infection.
     b. Magnetic resonance imaging (MRI) or high-resolution computed tomography (CT) can depict changes characteristic of arachnoiditis (Dubuisson, 1994).
  3. Treatment
     a. For acute episodes,
        (1) Hospitalize.
        (2) Use an orthopedic brace to immobilize.
     b. For persistent pain management,
        (1) Recommend rest.
        (2) Have the patient avoid activities that may increase symptoms.
        (3) Apply heat.
        (4) Use transcutaneous electrical nerve stimulation (TENS).
     c. Pharmacological interventions include
        (1) Opioids.
        (2) NSAIDs.
        (3) Muscle relaxants.
        (4) Tricyclic antidepressants.
        (5) Anticonvulsants.
        (6) Oral local anesthetic agents (e.g., mexiletine) (Challapalli, Tremont-Lukats, McNicol, Lau, & Carr, 2008).
     d. Spinal cord stimulation can be used in chronic cases.
     e. A cognitive-behavioral program may be beneficial.

D. *Facet syndrome* consists of degenerative changes and associated muscle spasms caused by a forced or traumatic twisting sprain of the facet joint. This trauma can occur at all intraarticular facet joint levels. The facet joint is an articulation formed by the superior articular facet (smooth area of the bone) of one vertebra and the inferior articular facet of the adjacent vertebra. This joint is heavily innervated (Neumann & Raj, 2000). When this sprain occurs, it causes the cascade of chemical releases of bradykinin, serotonin, histamine, and prostaglandin (Cavanaugh & Weinstein, 1994).
  1. Signs and symptoms (Clemans & Benzon, 2005)
     a. Lumbar

(1) Pain is described as a dull ache that radiates into the low back or hip, buttock, and posterior or lateral thigh down to the knee; it does not occur below the knee.
(2) Low back pain or stiffness occurs with or without radiation.
(3) The examination should focus on
(a) Local paralumbar tenderness.
(b) Absence of paresthesia.
(c) Pain on hyperextension of the spine.
(d) Hamstring pain and muscle spasm in the hip, buttock, or low back with a straight-leg raise (Benzon, 1996; Lippit, 1984).
(e) Depressed deep tendon reflexes; however, there is usually an absence of nerve root tension signs.

b. Cervical
(1) Neck pain
(2) Headaches
(3) Shoulder pain
(4) Difficulty rotating the head

2. Diagnostic workup
a. Radiological evaluation
(1) Plain films show poor correlation with symptoms.
(2) A CT scan is correlated better with symptoms of diagnostic value.
(3) MRI can be used to rule out fractures or disc herniations.
b. Facet arthropathy with injection of local anesthetic agent and antiinflammatory agent is diagnostic and therapeutic (Brummett & Cohen, 2008).

3. Treatment
a. Correct posture.
b. Modify activity.
c. Recommend exercise or physical therapy.
d. Inject facet with steroids.
e. Prescribe antiinflammatory agents
f. Use local anesthetic agents with steroid injected into the facet joint (facet arthropathy blockade).
g. A good response to facet arthropathy blockade may indicate that the patient may be a candidate for facet denervation using radiofrequency lesioning or ablation.

E. A ***herniated intervertebral disc*** is a disc that places mechanical pressure on the nerve root and causes irritation. The intervertebral disc normally comprises the annulus fibrosus and the nucleus pulposus. A tear in the annulus creates a bulging of the nucleus pulposus and can result in inflammation or compression of the nucleus contents or both. Approximately 90% of herniations occur in the lumbar spine, 8% are in the cervical spine, and 1% to 2% are in thoracic spine (American College of Occupational and Environmental Medicine, 2004; Armon, Argoff, Samuels, & Backonja, 2007; Freedman, 2006).

1. Signs and symptoms
a. Lumbar
(1) Pain is sudden and severe.
(2) It is described as a sharp, lancinating pain in the back.
(3) Pain may radiate in the anatomical distribution of the affected nerve root. Compression of the nucleus contents at L4 to L5 may cause pain radiating to the lower portion of the legs (Boden & Wiesel, 1992).
(4) Pain may be associated with neurological symptoms, such as weakness or loss of motor function, diminished or absent deep tendon reflexes, or loss of sensation to affected extremity.
b. Cervical pain includes
(1) Neck pain.
(2) Deep pain over shoulder blade on the affected side.

(3) Radiation of pain into the shoulder, upper arm, and forearm but rarely into the hand, fingers, or chest.
(4) Worsened pain with coughing, laughing, or straining.
(5) Neck muscle spasms.
(6) Worsened pain with neck bending or turning the head to the side.
(7) Arm muscle weakness.

2. Diagnostic workup
   a. History
   b. Physical examination may indicate a decrease or loss of motor function, deep tendon reflexes, or sensation.
   c. Radiological examination may help narrow the differential diagnosis. Options include
      (1) Plain radiographs.
      (2) MRI.
      (3) CT scan.
3. Treatment
   a. Recommend a short period of rest.
   b. Recommend medications, such as the following:
      (1) NSAIDs
      (2) Muscle relaxants if the patient has back spasms
      (3) Steroids, intravenous or oral (rarely)
      (4) Opioid analgesics for no longer than 2 weeks
      (5) Epidural injection of steroids
   c. Suggest lifestyle changes, such as the following:
      (1) Physical therapy
      (2) Weight loss
   d. Pain that continues after 3 to 4 weeks of physical therapy requires electromyography (EMG) and referral to an orthopedic surgeon or neurosurgeon.
      (1) EMG records electrical activity from muscles.
      (2) Needle EMG is required and differentiates between primary muscle disease and abnormalities of the anterior horn cell or motor axon (Newham, Edwards, & Mills, 1994).
      (3) EMG can be helpful in determining which nerve roots are affected.
   e. Progressive decrease in motor function, deep tendon reflexes, or sensation requires immediate referral to an orthopedic surgeon or neurosurgeon.

F. *Lumbar spondylolysis* is a stress fracture of the pars interarticularis of the vertebrae, not affecting the articular processes. It is often called a *pars defect* (Orthogate, 2006; Pediatric Orthopaedic Society of North America, 2007).
   1. Signs and symptoms
      a. Lumbar spondylolysis occurs most commonly in the L5 vertebra; however, this defect does not always cause pain.
      b. It is common in active individuals (more so in males) in their teens.
      c. Symptoms are commonly bilateral low back pain and sciatica.
      d. Pain is typically a deep ache, poorly localized in the lumbosacral region, that gradually recedes with time.
      e. Symptoms usually diminish with decreased activity.
   2. Diagnostic workup includes a radiograph, MRI, or CT scan of lumbar spine.
   3. Treatment
      a. Facet joint blockade may be indicated to control symptoms.
      b. Rehabilitation can occur through physical therapy, relaxation techniques, and pool therapy.
      c. Occasionally, if there is no response to aforementioned modalities, surgical stabilization may be indicated.
      d. Surgical replacement of facet joints is in the experimental stages (Fallin et al., 2007; Ziger, 2005).

G. *Radiculopathy* is a disorder of the spinal nerve root. Causes may be compression of the nerve root or diabetes mellitus, herpes zoster, carcinoma, or infectious processes (Abrams, 2000).
   1. Signs and symptoms
      a. Pain follows a particular nerve or nerve group distribution.
      b. Paresthesia (an abnormal sensation) and dysesthesia (an unpleasant abnormal sensation) occur, such as burning, prickling, tingling, or weakness.
      c. Hyperalgesia (an increased response to normally painful stimuli) and allodynia (extremely sensitive to nonpainful stimuli) are possible.
      d. The patient may or may not have loss of sensation or motor function (Haddox, 1996).
   2. Diagnostic workup includes an EMG, which indicates impairment of a nerve, localizes the lesion to one or more roots, and measures the severity of the condition.
   3. Treatment
      a. Treat the source of the pain when possible.
      b. Epidural steroid injections may yield some improvement if used between 2 and 6 weeks; however, the amount of evidence is small (Armon et al., 2007).
      c. Surgical interventions may be necessary if nerve root impingement is found or symptoms are unresolving or progressing.
      d. Spinal cord stimulation has weak evidence (Cruccu et al., 2007).

H. *Spinal stenosis* is narrowing of the space available for the neural elements (Spangfort, 1994). The most common cause is osteoarthritis causing spinal degeneration. Other causes may be disc herniations, ligament thickening, tumors, direct spine injury, Paget's disease, and achondroplasia (a genetic disorder that slows bone growth) (Mayo Clinic, 2008b).
   1. Signs and symptoms
      a. Chronic back pain and pain in the legs and buttocks increase gradually.
      b. Pain is described as deep aching with a heavy and numb feeling in the leg from the buttock to the foot.
      c. Pain is worse with activity; in particular, walking causes aching in legs. There is a sense of heaviness and clumsiness, which may be associated with frequent falls.
      d. Associated signs and symptoms are dermatomal paresthesia and bowel and bladder disturbance or impotence.
   2. Diagnostic workup
      a. Examination shows increase pain with extension of the spine, improving with flexion. This may result in a markedly flexed posture of the trunk.
      b. Radiological examination
         (1) A radiograph shows diffuse, severe, degenerative disease with facet hypertrophy and a decreased anteroposterior diameter of the lumbar canal.
         (2) MRI, CT scan, and myelography may indicate narrowing of the spinal canal, the osteophytes on the intervertebral foramina or both.
   3. Treatment options are as follows:
      a. Surgical decompression
      b. NSAIDs
      c. Epidural injection of steroids
      d. Gabapentin (Yaksi, Ozgonenel, & Ozgonenel, 2007)

I. A combined panel of the American College of Physicians and the American Pain Society (APS) completed an extensive review of the literature concerning the diagnosis and treatment of low back pain. This review resulted in seven clinical recommendations (Box 18–1) (Chou & Huffman, 2007).

J. A task force of spine surgeons from several major universities reviewed the literature on neck pain and its associated disorders (e.g., radiculopathy) (Box 18–2).

II. Myofascial Pain

A. *Myofascial pain syndrome* is a chronic muscle pain disorder in one or more muscles and is associated with focal tenderness or trigger points (Naja et al., 2007).

Box 18-1 Recommendations for the Diagnosis and Treatment of Low Back Pain

- "Clinicians should conduct a focused history and physical examination. . . . The history should include assessment of psychosocial risk factors, which predict risk for chronic disabling back pain.
- "Clinicians should not routinely obtain imaging or other diagnostic tests in patients with nonspecific low back pain.
- "Clinicians should perform diagnostic imaging and testing for patients with low back pain when severe or progressive neurologic deficits are present or when serious underlying conditions are suspected on the basis of history and physical examination.
- "Clinicians should evaluate patients with persistent low back pain and signs or symptoms of radiculopathy or spinal stenosis with magnetic resonance imaging (preferred) or computed tomography only if they are potential candidates for surgery or epidural steroid injection.
- "Clinicians should provide patients with evidence-based information on low back pain with regard to their expected course, advise patients to remain active, and provide information about effective self-care options.
- "For patients with low back pain, clinicians should consider the use of medications with proven benefits in conjunction with back care information and self-care. Clinicians should assess severity of baseline pain and functional deficits, potential benefits, risks, and relative lack of long-term efficacy and safety data before initiating therapy.
- "For patients who do not improve with self-care options, clinicians should consider the addition of nonpharmacologic therapy with proven benefits. These include spinal manipulation, massage therapy, yoga, cognitive-behavioral therapy, or progressive relaxation."

From Chou, R., Qaseem, A., Snow, V., Casey, D., Cross, J. T., Shekelle, P., & Owens, D. K. (2007). Diagnosis and treatment of low back pain: A joint clinical practice guideline from the American College of Physicians and the American Pain Society. *Annals of Internal Medicine, 147*(7), 478–479.

Box 18-2 Conclusions Concerning the Treatment of Neck Pain and Associated Disorders

- "Radiofrequency neurotomy, cervical facet injections, cervical fusion and cervical arthroplasty for neck pain without radiculopathy are not supported by current evidence.
- "There is support for short-term symptomatic improvement of radicular symptoms with epidural corticosteroids.
- "It is not clear from the evidence that long-term outcomes are improved with the surgical treatment of cervical radiculopathy compared to nonoperative measures. However, relatively rapid and substantial symptomatic relief after surgical treatment seems to be reliably achieved.
- "Cervical foraminal or epidural injections are associated with relatively frequent minor adverse events (5% to 20%); however, serious adverse events are very uncommon (<1%). After open surgical procedures on the cervical spine, potentially serious acute complications are seen in approximately 4% of patients.
- "Surgical treatment and limited injection procedures for cervical radicular symptoms may be reasonably considered in patients with severe impairments. Percutaneous and open surgical treatment for neck pain alone, without radicular symptoms or clear serious pathology, seems to lack scientific support."

From Carragee, E. J., Hurwitx, E. L., Cheng, I., Carroll, L. J., Nordin, M., Guzman, J., Peloso, P., Holm, L. W., Cote, P., Hogg-Johnson, S., van der Velde, G., Cassidy, J. D., & Haldeman, S. (2008). Treatment of neck pain: Injections and surgical interventions. Results of the Bone and Joint Decade 2000–2010 Task Force on Neck Pain and Its Associated Disorders. *Spine, 33*(45), S153).

1. Signs and symptoms include
   a. Regional body pain and stiffness.
   b. Limited range of motion of the affected muscle.
   c. Twitch response that produces a taut band.
   d. Demonstration of trigger points that may develop within the same area of initial pain.
2. Diagnostic workup
   a. For criteria for diagnosis, see the chapter on Taxonomy for Pain Management Nursing
   b. Examination (Gerwin, 2005)
      (1) A primary trigger zone may reproduce the patient's pain.
      (2) The patient may have a palpable, tender, taut band of muscle.
      (3) Limited range of motion is possible.
      (4) The patient may have referred pain.
   c. No laboratory tests support the clinical diagnosis of myofascial pain syndrome.
3. Treatment (Gerwin, 2005)
   a. Manual inactivation of the trigger points includes
      (1) Stretch and spray techniques using a vapocoolant or ice.
      (2) Trigger point compressions.
      (3) Physical therapy.
      (4) Massage.
      (5) Muscle reeducation.
   b. Trigger point injection of local anesthetic or dry needling can be used.
   c. Recommend ultrasound.
   d. Use electrical stimulation.
   e. Consider a paravertebral block (Naja et al., 2007).
   f. Acupuncture is an option.
   g. Psychological options include
      (1) Education.
      (2) Cognitive-behavioral therapy.
   h. Pharmacological options are
      (1) NSAIDs.
      (2) Antidepressants.
      (3) Muscle relaxants.
      (4) Antispasticity medications.
      (5) Anticonvulsants.
      (6) Opioid analgesics (preferably long acting).
      (7) Botulinum toxin (Jeynes & Gauci, 2008).

B. *Fibromyalgia syndrome* is a common, chronic pain condition characterized by moderate to severe soft-tissue pain and allodynia. The painful symptoms involve central sensitization, which leads to an amplified perception of pain (Russell, 2008).
   1. Signs and symptoms
      a. Pain is continuous, although it may fluctuate in intensity from day to day.
      b. Stiffness appears toward the end of range of motion.
      c. Dysfunctional sleep is common.
      d. Fibromyalgia syndrome is associated with chronic exhaustion.
      e. Comorbidities include cognitive dysfunction, depression, anxiety, recurrent headaches, dizziness, dysesthesia, and irritable bowel syndrome.
   2. Diagnostic workup (Burckhardt et al., 2005)
      a. Diagnostic criteria for fibromyalgia syndrome
         (1) Widespread pain occurs for at least 3 consecutive months.
         (2) Pain is found in all four body quadrants, along with axial pain.
         (3) Disturbed sleep is combined with morning fatigue and stiffness.
         (4) Spinal fluid levels of substance P, nerve growth factor, or both are elevated.

b. Use the American College of Rheumatology (1990) criteria for the classification of fibromyalgia (Wolfe et al., 1990); see the chapter on Taxonomy for Pain Management Nursing for the criteria of the American College of Rheumatology.
c. Examination (Burckhardt et al., 2005; Wolfe et al., 1990)
   (1) Pain occurs on digital palpation in at least 11 of 18 tender points. *Tender* is not considered painful. For a palpated site to be positive, the individual must state that it is painful.
      (a) Bilateral occiput is found at the insertion of the suboccipital muscle.
      (b) Bilateral lower cervical is found at the anterior aspect of the intertransverse spaces at C5 to C7.
      (c) Bilateral trapezius is found at the midpoint of the upper border.
      (d) Bilateral supraspinatus is found above the scapular spine near the medial border.
      (e) Bilateral second rib is found at the second costochondral junction, just lateral to the junction on the upper surface.
      (f) Bilateral lateral epicondyle is 2 cm distal to the epicondyle.
      (g) Bilateral gluteal is found in the upper outer quadrant of the buttock in the anterior fold of muscle.
      (h) Bilateral greater trochanter is posterior to the trochanteric prominence.
      (i) Bilateral knee at the medial fat pad is proximal to the joint line.
   (2) No laboratory evidence points to inflammation or muscle damage.
   (3) Give a complete joint examination.
   (4) Recommend manual muscle-strength testing.
   (5) Give a neurological examination.
   (6) Evaluate for mood and cognitive disturbance.
   (7) Assess functional status (physical, emotional, and overall quality of life).

3. Treatment
   a. Pharmacological therapies include
      (1) Anticonvulsants ($\alpha_2\delta$ ligands) (Arnold, 2006) (see the chapter on Overview of Pharmacology).
      (2) Low-dose tricyclic antidepressant or cyclobenzaprine at bedtime.
      (3) Selective serotonin reuptake inhibitors.
      (4) Serotonin and norepinephrine reuptake inhibitors (Arnold, 2006).
      (5) Sleep and anxiety medications
      (6) Hormone therapy
      (7) NSAIDs and acetaminophen should not be used as the primary pain medication but may be helpful if they are used with other medications.
      (8) Tramadol can be used alone or in combination with acetaminophen.
      (9) Opioids may be used only after all other pharmacological and nonpharmacological therapies have been exhausted.
   b. Nonpharmacological therapies include
      (1) Education about pain management and self-management programs (stress reduction, weight management, and smoking cessation, etc.).
      (2) Cognitive-behavioral therapy.
      (3) Moderately intense aerobic exercise; progression should be slow and gradual.
      (4) Muscle-strengthening exercises.
      (5) Clinician-assisted treatments such as hypnosis, biofeedback, acupuncture, chiropractic manipulation, and therapeutic massage.
   c. Local trigger point injections can be used.

C. *Temporomandibular disorders* refer to various clinical dysfunctions of the temporomandibular joint, muscles of mastication, associated structures, or a combination of these. The causes are thought to be multifactorial with various predisposing, precipitating, and perpetuating factors (Royal College of Dental Surgeons of Ontario, 2006, p. 1). Differential diagnosis should also take into consideration other disease entities, for example, neuralgias, tumors, different types of headaches, dentoalveolar disease, sinus disease, ear disease, salivary gland disease, and psychological or psychiatric disorder (Royal College of Dental Surgeons of Ontario, 2006, p. 2).

1. Signs and symptoms
   a. Persistent orofacial pain
      (1) Pain comes with a neuropathic or atypical component.
      (2) Musculoskeletal pain occurs.
      (3) Pain occurs in the face, jaw joint area, neck, and shoulders and in or around the ear with chewing or speaking.
      (4) The patient has a limited ability to open the mouth widely.
      (5) Clicking, popping, or grating sounds in jaw accompany chewing or speaking.
      (6) Swelling occurs on the side of the face.
   b. Cyclic fluctuations in symptoms
5. Diagnostic workup should include
   a. Patient history and physical examination.
   b. Cranial nerve examination to exclude tumors.
   c. X-rays, MRI, and CT scan.
6. Treatment (Dionne, Kim, & Gordon, 2006)
   a. Pharmacological options are
      (1) NSAIDs or cyclooxygenase (COX–2 inhibitors).
      (2) Corticosteroids.
      (3) Benzodiazepines.
      (4) Muscle relaxants.
      (5) Anticonvulsants.
      (6) Opioids.
      (7) Antidepressants.
      (8) Botulinum toxin.
   b. Nonpharmacological options are
      (1) Moist heat or cold packs.
      (2) Wearing a splint or night guard.
      (3) Corrective dental treatments (crowns or braces).
      (4) TENS.
      (5) Ultrasound.
      (6) Trigger point injections.
      (7) Temporomandibular joint implants.
      (8) Dental consult or orthodontia consult.
      (9) Psychology or psychiatry consult.
      (10) Surgical consult for some.

III. Neuropathic Pain: Peripheral Mononeuropathies

A. Syndromes related to inflammation of peripheral nerves
   1. *Postherpetic neuralgia* is pain persisting past the stage of healing lesions after acute herpes zoster. Pain usually diminishes with time (3 months) (Dubinsky, Kabbani, El-Chami, Boutwell, & Ali, 2004; Scadding, 1994; Schmader & Dworkin, 2008; Wu & Raja, 2008).
      a. Signs and symptoms
         (1) Chronic pain accompanies skin changes in a dermatomal distribution after acute herpes zoster.
         (2) The pain follows the dermatomal distribution of the herpes zoster lesions.
         (3) Pain is mild to severe with burning, sharp, and brief, intense, shooting pains.
         (4) Other words used to describe the pain are *twisting, boring, jabbing,* and *buzzing.*
         (5) Dysesthesia, allodynia, hyperesthesia occur (see the chapter on Taxonomy for Pain Management Nursing).

b. Diagnostic workup
   (1) Thermograms may show heat emission in affected dermatomes.
   (2) Viral cultures during active phase may indicate herpetic infection.
c. Treatment (see the chapter on Overview of Pharmacology)
   (1) Antiviral agents with early detection are most effective if started within 72 hours after the onset of rash (Stankus, Dlugopolski, & Packer, 2000).
   (2) The following treatments can be used:
      (a) Tricyclic antidepressants (e.g., amitriptyline [Elavil®])
      (b) Serotonin norepinephrine reuptake inhibitors (e.g., duloxetine [Cymbalta®])
      (c) Anticonvulsants (e.g., gabapentin [Neurontin®] or pregabalin [Lyrica®])
      (d) Oral local anesthetic agents (e.g., mexiletine [Mexitil®])
      (e) Application of capsaicin cream (Zostrix®) after lesions resolve
      (f) Application of topical local anesthetic (e.g., lidocaine [Lidoderm®]) after the lesions resolve
   (3) Occupational therapy can be used to decrease edema through manual lymphatic drainage and to facilitate fine motor function (Foldi & Strossenreuther, 2008).
   (4) Physical therapy can be used to improve circulation, increase muscle tone and balance, and facilitate large motor function.
d. Prevention
   (1) Zoster vaccine (Zostavax®) is indicated for people 60 years or older without compromised immune function (Mitra, 2006; Oxman et al., 2005).
      (a) The vaccine reduces the incidence of zoster outbreak by 51.3%.
      (b) It reduces illness severity by 61.1%.
      (c) It reduces the incidence of postherpetic neuralgia by 66.5%.

B. Syndromes related to inflammation, ischemia, infarction, or compression injuries of peripheral nerves
   1. *Peripheral neuropathy* consists of damage to the peripheral nervous system. More than 100 types have been identified, each with its own set of symptoms, development, and prognosis. Peripheral neuropathy is related to damage of a specific peripheral nerve. Causes may be inherited (e.g., Charcot-Marie-Tooth disease) or acquired. Acquired causes include physical injury (trauma), tumors, toxins, autoimmune responses, nutritional deficiencies, alcoholism, certain medications and chemotherapy agents, and vascular and metabolic disorders. Damage may occur as a result of disease processes or trauma (Mailes & Bennett, 1999; NINDS, 2008d). In many cases a cause cannot be identified (Cimino, 1999; NINDS, 2008d).
      a. Signs and symptoms
         (1) Signs and symptoms vary depending on what nerve or nerves are involved.
         (2) Constant or transient burning, aching, or lancinating limb pain results from disease of peripheral nerves, usually in the feet (socklike distribution) or hands (glovelike distribution). The patient can have deep aching pain, especially at night.
         (3) Peripheral neuropathy is associated with sensory loss, especially to pinprick or dull stimuli and temperature; diminished vibratory sense, occasionally with weakness and muscle atrophy; and loss of reflex, sympathetic tone, or both with development of smooth, fine skin and hair loss.
         (4) In extreme cases muscle wasting, paralysis, or organ or gland dysfunction may occur. People may be unable to digest food easily, maintain safe levels of blood pressure, sweat normally, or experience normal sexual function. In the most extreme cases, breathing may become difficult or organ failure may occur (NINDS, 2008d).
      b. Diagnostic workup consists of
         (1) History.
         (2) Physical examination with attention to neurological examination.
         (3) EMG and nerve conduction studies.

(4) CT scans.
(5) MRI.
(6) Nerve and skin biopsies.

c. Treatment
(1) Treat or stabilize the underlying disease (i.e., with diabetes, control blood glucose).
(2) Eliminate the underlying cause (i.e., toxins or vitamin deficiencies).
(3) Limit or avoid alcohol consumption.
(4) Quit smoking.
(5) Use anticonvulsant agents.
(6) Use tricyclic antidepressants.
(7) Apply capsaicin cream.
(8) Apply a topical local anesthetic (e.g., lidocaine or EMLA® cream).
(9) Take an oral local anesthetic agent (e.g., mexiletine).
(10) Use occupational therapy.
(11) Start physical therapy.
(12) Use spinal cord stimulation.

2. *Mononeuropathies or plexopathies* include brachial plexus neuropathies, brachial mononeuropathies, lumbosacral plexopathies, crural mononeuropathies, and entrapment neuropathies (Adams, Victor, & Ropper, 1997).

a. Signs and symptoms
(1) The patient has constant or transient burning, aching, stabbing, shooting, electrical, hot, cold, or lancinating pain involving the area supplied by the nerve. The patient can have deep aching pain, especially at night.
(2) Mononeuropathies and plexopathies are associated with sensory loss, especially to pinprick or dull touch and temperature; diminished vibratory sense, sometimes with weakness; and muscle atrophy. Occasionally, there is loss or diminished deep tendon reflex, sympathetic tone, or both with development of smooth, fine skin and hair loss in affected area. Muscle atrophy occurs at later stages.

b. Diagnostic workup
(1) Patient history is needed.
(2) The physical examination should include attention to neurological examination.
(3) EMG and nerve conduction studies indicate muscle denervation.

c. Treatment includes the following (see the chapter on Overview of Pharmacology):
(1) Anticonvulsants
(2) Tricyclic antidepressants
(3) Oral local anesthetic agents
(4) Topical capsaicin cream
(5) Topical local anesthetic (e.g., lidocaine or EMLA® cream)
(6) Occupational therapy
(7) Physical therapy

C. Painful mononeuropathy of the orofacial region

1. *Trigeminal neuralgia (tic douloureux)* consists of pain along the second or third division of the trigeminal nerve (e.g., fifth cranial nerve). It may be caused by pressure from a blood vessel on the trigeminal nerve as it exits the brain stem. It may also be caused by other disorders that damage the nerve sheath (NINDS, 2008c).

a. Signs and symptoms
(1) Sudden-onset, brief, stabbing, recurrent pain occurs in distribution of the fifth cranial nerve.
(2) Pain is more frequent on right side.
(3) It is described as sharp, agonizing, electric shock-like stabs of pain felt superficially in the skin or buccal mucosa
(4) Pain is triggered by light mechanical contact.

(5) It characteristically occurs in brief, repetitive bursts for several seconds to 1 or 2 minutes, followed by a refractory period of 30 seconds to a few minutes. Episodes occur at intervals of several or many times daily and are rarely continuous. Duration is of a few weeks to 2 months, followed by a pain-free period and then recurrence. Intensity is severe; this is the most intense of acute chronic pains (Graham & Bana, 1992).
(6) Pain is associated with mild flush during the episode.

b. Diagnostic workup
(1) The neurological examination is negative.
(2) During the flare, there is hypoesthesia on the face or absence of the corneal reflex.
(3) If sensory deficit is present, a diagnostic workup for causation needs to be done.

c. Treatment (see the chapter on Overview of Pharmacology)
(1) During flare, pressure around the area, but not on top of the area, may be helpful.
(2) Protect the area from cold wind.
(3) Use anticonvulsant agents (e.g., carbamazepine [Tegretol®]).
(4) Use tricyclic antidepressants.
(5) NSAIDs can be used.
(6) Antispasticity drugs (e.g., baclofen [Lioresal®]) can be effective (Sindrup & Jensen, 2002).
(7) Apply topical lidocaine or EMLA® cream.
(8) Give an anesthesiology or surgical referral for local infiltration into the trigeminal ganglion, glycerol injections into the trigeminal cistern, trigeminal thermocoagulation, or radiofrequency rhizotomy (Gellner et al., 2008; Mayo Clinic, 2008c).

D. Syndromes associated with neuroma formation or surgical resection

1. A *neuroma* is an abnormal growth on damaged nerve endings that can cause pain (Cimino, 1999; Mayo Clinic, 2008a).

2. *Residual limb pain* (formerly known as stump pain) is pain located in the remaining part of an amputated limb and is due to neuroma formation (Beth Israel University Hospital and Manhattan Campus for the Albert Einstein College of Medicine, 2008).

a. Signs and symptoms
(1) Pain is described as sharp, shooting, or electrical.
(2) Skin is sensitive.

b. Diagnostic workup includes the following:
(1) History
(2) Examination of the residual limb site

c. Treatment options include the following (see the chapter on Overview of Pharmacology):
(1) Tricyclic antidepressants (e.g., amitriptyline or nortriptyline)
(2) Anticonvulsants (e.g., gabapentin or carbamazepine)
(3) Local anesthetics (e.g., mexiletine)
(4) α_2 adrenergic receptor agonists (e.g., clonidine or tizanidine)
(5) Others, including calcitonin, baclofen, or dextromethorphan
(6) Opioids
(7) Nerve blocks
(8) TENS
(9) Surgical removal is often ineffective. Some patients actually have more pain because the neuroma grows back.
(10) Cognitive therapies can be used.
(11) A prosthesis can be revised.

3. *Postmastectomy pain syndrome (nonmalignant)* is pain caused by operative trauma to the intercostobrachial and other upper thoracic nerves. It also may occur at the brachial plexus during axillary node dissection (Johnson, 2000; Reuben, 2006a; Smith, Bourne, Squair, Phillips, & Chambers, 1999).

a. Incidence (Smith et al., 1999)
(1) Pain occurs in 64.8% women age 30 to 49.

(2) It occurs in 40.3% women age 50 to 69.
(3) It occurs in only 25.5% women age 70 and older.

b. Signs and symptoms
(1) Persistent pain starts after mastectomy on same side as the mastectomy. Pain may involve the ipsilateral arm (same side), axilla, and anterior chest, and it may be in the area of the surgical scar.
(2) Pain is described as burning, constant, tingling, stabbing, numbness, pins and needles, like threads pulling, and unresponsive to analgesics. Pain intensity is moderate to severe.
(3) Pain may begin immediately or start many months after surgery and may last for years.
(4) It is aggravated by prosthesis, clothing, straining, sudden movement, tiredness, cold weather, coughing, or touch.
(5) Pain may be associated with emotional lability and avoidance of sexual encounters.
(6) The patient has hyperesthesia to pinprick, patchy anesthesia, and allodynia.
(7) Trigger point tenderness occurs over the area.

c. Risk factors (Smith et al., 1999)
(1) Age is a key factor (see incidence given earlier).
(2) Risk is higher with a greater body mass index.
(3) Taller height is a factor.
(4) Risk is higher in those with preoperative chemotherapy, radiation therapy, and tamoxifen, although these therapies may have been related to the increased stage of the disease.

d. Diagnostic workup includes
(1) History.
(2) Examination of surgical site.
(3) MRI, CT scan, or bone scan to rule out presence of recurrent tumor or metastases.

e. Treatment options include (see the chapter on Overview of Pharmacology)
(1) Tricyclic antidepressants (e.g., amitriptyline [Elavil®]).
(2) Anticonvulsant (e.g., gabapentin [Neurontin®]).
(3) Capsaicin cream.
(4) Lidocaine patch or EMLA® cream.
(5) Physical therapy to mobilize arms.
(6) Psychotherapy may be helpful for adjustment difficulties.

4. *Postthoracotomy pain syndrome* results from operative trauma to the intercostal nerves. It may involve intrinsic and extrinsic chest wall musculature (de Leon-Casasola, 2007; Johnson, 2000; Reuben, 2006b).

a. Signs and symptoms
(1) Pain recurs or persists along a thoracotomy scar for at least 2 months after surgery.
(2) Pain is described as an aching sensation in the distribution of the incision.
(3) Pain beyond this time may have a burning dysesthetic component.
(4) Pain may have pleuritic component.
(5) Movement of the ipsilateral (same side) shoulder increases pain.
(6) Sensory loss and absence of sweating occur along surgical scar.

b. Diagnostic workup includes the following:
(1) History
(2) Examination of surgical site
(3) CT scan to rule out presence of recurrent tumor or metastases

c. Treatment options include the following:
(1) Tricyclic antidepressants
(2) Anticonvulsants
(3) Topical lidocaine, EMLA® cream, or capsaicin cream
(4) Intercostal nerve block
(5) Epidural steroid injection

(6) Radiation therapy, if malignancy is involved
(7) Physical therapy

5. *Postradical neck dissection pain syndrome (nonmalignant)* is pain caused by operative trauma to superficial cervical plexus. It also may involve regional myofascial pain. Some patients experience both types of pain (Sist, Miner, & Lema, 1999).
   a. Signs and symptoms
      (1) Persistent moderate or severe pain starts after radical neck dissection.
      (2) Pain may be reported within the distribution of the superficial cervical plexus: the trigeminal nerve distribution, the C2 to C4 distributions, the mandibular angle and inferior border of the jaw, and the lateral side of the neck.
      (3) Duration can be years. Sometimes pain decreases with time.
      (4) Pain is aggravated by prosthesis, clothing, or touch.
      (5) Patchy anesthesia may be present.
      (6) Trigger point tenderness in the sternocleidomastoid, trapezius, splenius capitis, splenius cervicis, and semispinalis cervicis muscles may be present.
      (7) Pain is described as burning or shooting; it may be constant or variable.
      (8) Allodynia is present.
      (9) Pain is unremitting to opioid analgesics.
   b. Diagnostic workup includes history and physical examination.
   c. Treatment includes
      (1) Tricyclic antidepressants.
      (2) Anticonvulsant agents.
      (3) Oral local anesthetic agents.
      (4) Muscle relaxants (e.g., baclofen).
      (5) NSAIDs.
      (6) Trigger point injections.
      (7) Capsaicin cream.
      (8) Lidocaine patch.
      (9) Physical therapy to mobilize arms.
      (10) Phenol neurolysis of the superior cervical plexus nerve as a possible last resort (Sist et al., 1999).

E. *Reflex sympathetic dystrophy/complex regional pain syndrome (RSD/CRPS)* is a severe pain, described as burning and persisting longer than would be expected after an initial injury, and accompanied by one or more of the following: sympathetic nervous system activity, swelling, movement disorder, or changes in tissue growth (dystrophy or atrophy) (International Research Foundation for RSD/CRPS, 2003; NINDS, 2001, 2008b) (see the chapter on Taxonomy for Pain Management Nursing for a definition of CRPS-I and CRPS-II).
   1. Signs and symptoms
      a. Pain
         (1) Initial pain is in one or more extremities and is described as a severe, continuous burning, a deep ache, or both without involvement of a major nerve.
         (2) All tactile sensation may be painful (allodynia).
         (3) Repetitive tactile stimulation may cause increasing pain with each tap, and the pain may continue after the stimulation is stopped (hyperpathia).
         (4) The muscles of affected area may have diffuse tenderness or point-tender spots due to small muscle spasms called *muscle trigger points* (myofascial pain syndrome).
         (5) Spontaneous, sharp jabs of pain that seem to come from nowhere may occur in the affected region (paroxysmal dysesthesias and lancinating pains).
         (6) Pain is aggravated by use of the affected part and relieved by immobilization.
      b. Edema
         (1) Diffuse edema is pitting or hard and localized to the painful and tender region.
         (2) If the edema is sharply demarcated on the surface of the skin along a line, it is almost proof that the patient has RSD/CRPS.

c. Skin changes
   (1) Atrophy of skin appendages and cool, red, clammy skin may be variably present.
   (2) Skin may appear shiny, dry, or scaly.
   (3) Nails may grow faster initially and then grow slower.
   (4) Faster-growing nails are almost proof of RSD/CRPS.
   (5) Hair may grow coarse and then thin.
   (6) Skin may be white and mottled to red or blue in appearance.
   (7) RSD/CRPS is associated with skin disorders such as rashes, ulcers, and pustules.
   (8) It is associated with sympathetic hyperactivity (Johnson, 2000).
      (a) Initially, the patient has vasodilation with increasing temperature of affected area or with hyperhidrosis (excessive sweating) and edema.
      (b) Atrophy of skin appendages and cool, red, clammy skin may be variably present.

d. Movement disorder
   (1) Movement causes pain.
   (2) A direct inhibitory effect on muscle contraction is possible.
   (3) Patients have difficulty initiating movement and describe "stiff" joints.
   (4) Tremors and involuntary jerks may be present.
   (5) Debilitating, severe muscle cramps with a sudden onset may occur.
   (6) Increased muscle tone in the extremity, described by some patients as a slow "drawing up of muscles," may result in the hand and fingers or foot and toes drawing into a fixed position (dystonia).
   (7) Psychological distress may exacerbate symptoms.
   (8) Patients can exhibit seemingly bizarre movements and might be inaccurately diagnosed with a psychogenic movement disorder.

e. Symptoms may be progressive and may spread to other limbs.
   (1) Progressive symptoms include persistent coldness, pallor, cyanosis, Raynaud's phenomenon, atrophy of the skin and nails, loss of hair in affected area, atrophy of tissues, and stiffness of joints.
   (2) With progression, disuse atrophy as in Sudeck atrophy (demineralization) of bone may occur.

f. A patient may not exhibit all symptoms together.

2. Diagnostic workup
   a. Advanced cases may show bone atrophy on plain radiograph or bone scan.
   b. Sympathetic block may be diagnostic.
3. Treatment can include
   a. Sympathetic block.
   b. Regional block (Bier block).
   c. Physical therapy.
   d. Anticonvulsants.
   e. Tricyclic antidepressants.
   f. Oral local anesthetic agent.
   g. NSAIDs.
   h. Opioids.
   i. Spinal cord stimulation.
   j. Sympathectomy if long-term results are not achieved with repeated, successful sympathetic blocks.
   k. Early phases may respond to high doses of corticosteroids (i.e., 50 mg of prednisone for 5 days).
   l. Occupational therapy can be used to promote fine motor function.
4. The duration of RSD/CRPS varies from weeks in mild cases to indefinitely in others. Some patients may have remissions from weeks, months, or years followed by exacerbations.

F. *Phantom pain* may be associated with residual limb (stump) pain, but the cause of phantom pain is unclear and seems to originate in the brain (Cimino, 1999; Mayo Clinic, 2008a).

1. Signs and symptoms
   a. Pain occurs in an absent body part.
   b. It follows amputation and may start at time of amputation or occur months to years later.
   c. Severity varies among individuals.
   d. Pain persists indefinitely and often with gradual reduction over years.
   e. Pain may be intermittent or continuous.
   f. It is described as cramping, aching, or burning with transient shocklike pain.
   g. Pain may be associated with a distorted image of the lost part.
   h. It may be triggered by weather changes, pressure on the remaining part of the limb, or emotional stress.
2. Diagnostic workup includes patient history and examination.
3. Treatment options include the following (see the chapter on Overview of Pharmacology):
   a. TENS
   b. Anticonvulsants
   c. Tricyclic antidepressants
   d. Phenothiazines
   e. Oral local anesthetic agents (e.g., mexiletine)
   f. Memantine (Hackworth, Tokarz, Fowler, Wallace, & Stedje-Larsen, 2008)
   g. Sympathetic nerve block
   h. Surgical procedures
   i. Spinal cord stimulation
   j. Physical therapy for myofascial release and range of motion
   k. Comfort measures for prosthetic application
   l. Mirror therapy, which holds some promise (Chan et al., 2007; MacIver, Lloyd, Kelly, Roberts, & Nurmikko, 2008)
   m. Occupational therapy for pacing instructions and management of edema (if present)

G. *Central pain syndrome (thalamic pain)* involves pain associated with lesion or ischemia in the central nervous system: brain, brain stem, or spinal cord. It may be caused by stroke, multiple sclerosis, tumors, epilepsy, brain or spinal cord trauma, or Parkinson's disease (Cimino, 1999; NINDS, 2008a).
   1. Signs and symptoms
      a. Pain differs widely among individuals.
      b. Pain is usually constant, diffuse, unilateral, and severe; usually occurs on half of the body; and is contralateral to a cerebral lesion.
      c. Pain most often occurs within a few weeks to 2 years after an initial injury but may start months or years later, especially after a stroke.
      d. It is localized to the skin, muscle, or bone in most patients.
      e. Pain is described as burning with allodynia, hypoesthesia, hypoalgesia, hyperpathia, dysesthesia, and neurological signs of damage to the affected region. It is also described as stabbing and often aching.
      f. Pain is evoked by light touch, heat, cold, movements, TENS, visceral activity such as micturition, increased anxiety, and emotional arousal.
      g. It may be made worse with auditory or visual stimuli.
      h. It may be associated with typical hemiparesis, most often with motor impairments, and sensory deficits in the affected areas. Sensation associated with light touch is impaired.
      i. Vasomotor and sudomotor atrophic changes are often present.
      j. Anxiety and depression often occur.
      k. This syndrome may be intractable to any therapy available today.
   2. Diagnostic workup with a CT scan shows a relevant lesion in the thalamus.
   3. Treatment includes the following:
      a. Centrally active medications, such as phenothiazines and tricyclic antidepressants
      b. Anticonvulsants (e.g., carbamazepine or diphenylhydantoin)
      c. Mexiletine (Attal et al., 2006)

H. *Spinal cord injury (SCI)* involves pain associated with injury to the spinal cord (Borsook, LeBel, Stojanovic, & Fishman, 1998; Tasker, 1999; Ullrich, Jensen, Loeser, & Cardenas, 2008)
   1. Signs and symptoms
      a. Signs and symptoms are variable; they may be localized, radicular, or diffuse; constant or intermittent; and above the injury or below the injury.
      b. People with injuries at higher spinal areas are more likely to report upper extremity pain consistent with the dermatome distribution of pain at the level of the injury.
      c. Lower body pain tends to be reported as more intense.
      d. People with SCI "tend to experience high pain intensity over multiple body locations" (Ullrich et al., 2008, p. 451).
      e. "Only SCI level was associated with the site(s) of pain" (Ullrich et al., 2008, p. 455).
      f. "Multiple pain with different characteristics may be experienced simultaneously in different regions of the body" (Widerstrom-Noga et al., 2008).
      g. Most SCI is due to trauma (e.g., motor vehicle accidents or diving accidents). This pain is felt most commonly below the level of injury, occurring in the torso, hips, and groin; pain may extend to the legs, feet, and toes. Patients may state that they feel cramping in the feet or "like they are deformed." Uncommonly, patients state that they feel as though they have a mass in the rectum or like they are "sitting on a hot fire."
         (1) Other causes are vascular pathology, inflammatory lesions, skeletal pathology, neoplasms, demyelinating diseases (multiple sclerosis), iatrogenic perisurgical causes, abscesses, and congenital lesions.
         (2) Pain may be aggravated by pressure sores or increases in spasticity.
         (3) It may be described as burning, aching, lancinating, stabbing, prickling, squeezing, cutting, electric shock-like, or pins and needles. Other descriptions include gripping, constant, intense, sharp, shooting, or occurring in waves.
         (4) See Table 18-1 for a description of pain related to SCI.
         (5) See Table 18-2 for a classification of pain related to SCI.
   2. Diagnostic workup
      a. Examination shows allodynia, hypoesthesia, hypoanalgesia, hyperpathia, dysesthesia, and neurological signs of damage to affected region.
      b. Imaging studies should be used.
      c. Use a biopsy as indicated.
      d. Use cultures as indicated.

Table 18-1 Tier Two Groupings of Pain Related to Spinal Cord Injury

Term	Distinguishing Features
Musculoskeletal	Dull, aching, movement related, eased by rest, responsive to opioids and NSAIDs Located in musculoskeletal structures
Visceral	Dull, cramping, responsive to opioids, may or may not be responsive to NSAIDs Located in the abdominal region with preserved innervation Includes dysreflexic headache (vascular)
Neuropathic	Sharp, shooting, burning, electrical abnormal responsiveness (hyperesthesia, hyperalgesia); may be responsive to anticonvulsant agents
Above level	Located in the region of sensory preservation
At level	Located in a segment pattern at the level of injury
Below level	Located diffusely below the level of injury

Siddall PJ, Yezierski RP, Loeser JD from *IASP Newsletter*, 2000 (3). Used with permission from IASP.

Table 18-2 Proposed Classification of Pain Related to Spinal Cord Injury

Broad Type	Broad System	Specific Structures or Pathology
Nociceptive	Musculoskeletal	Bone, joint, muscle trauma or inflammation
		Mechanical instability
		Muscle spasm
		Secondary overuse syndromes
	Visceral	Renal calculus, bowel, sphincter dysfunction
		Dysreflexic headache
Neuropathic	Above level	Compressive mononeuropathies
		Complex regional pain syndromes
	At level	Nerve root compression (including cauda equina)
		Syringomyelia
		Spinal cord trauma or ischemia (transitional zone)
		Dual-level cord and root trauma (double lesion syndrome)
	Below level	Spinal cord trauma or ischemia (central dysesthesia syndrome)

Siddall PJ, Yezierski RP, Loeser JD from *IASP Newsletter*, 2000 (3). Used with permission from IASP.

3. Treatment of this pain can be difficult.
   a. Treat the primary condition as indicated.
   b. Use tricyclic antidepressants.
   c. Use anticonvulsants.
   d. Local anesthetic agents should be given orally.
   e. Use phenothiazines. (Siddall, et al., 2000)
   f. Use opioids.
   g. Neurolytic therapies are controversial in their effectiveness.
   h. Long-term stimulation therapies are controversial (Borsook et al., 1998; Tasker, 1999).
4. Reporting to the international spinal cord injury pain basic data set (ISCIPBDS) (Widerstrom-Noga et al., 2008)
   a. The ISCIPBDS "contains core questions about clinically relevant information concerning SCI-related pain that can be collected by health care professionals with expertise in SCI in various clinical settings" (Widerstrom-Noga et al., 2008, p. 818).
   b. The ISCIPBDS is "an effort to provide a standardized way of evaluating and reporting the diverse pain in persons with SCI" (Widerstrom-Noga et al., 2008, p. 821).
   c. "The basic pain database set is intended to be used to evaluate pain in the daily clinical practice at both inpatient and outpatient SCI clinics around the world" (Widerstrom-Noga et al., 2008, p. 821).
   d. Those pain clinics with significant numbers of SCI patients should consider using this evaluating tool and submitting information to this data set. Pain in the SCI population remains difficult to treat. Future research using this data set may be helpful in determining better therapies.
   e. The syllabus and data set forms are posted on the following websites: http://www.iscos.org.uk and http://www.asia-spinalinjury.org.

I. *Syringomyelia (syrinx)* is a disorder in which a fluid-filled cavitation or cyst is formed within the spinal cord. The cyst expands and elongates over time, resulting in the destruction of the spinal cord from the center outward.

1. "A number of medical conditions can cause an obstruction in the normal flow of CSF, redirecting it into the central canal, and ultimately into the spinal cord itself. For reasons that are only now becoming clear, this redirected CSF fills the expanding central canal and results in syrinx formation. Pressure differences along the spine cause the fluid to move within the cyst. Physicians believe that it is this continual movement of fluid that builds pressure around and inside the spinal cord, and results in cyst growth and further damage to the spinal cord tissue" (NINDS, 2008e, p. 1).
2. Chiari I malformations (anatomical abnormalities that cause the lower part of the cerebellum to protrude from its normal location in the back of the head into the cervical or neck portion of the spinal canal) are the most common cause of syringomyelia (Todor, Mu, & Milhorat, 2000).
3. Signs and symptoms (NINDS, 2008e; Todor et al., 2000)
   a. Syrinx symptoms, especially those related to Chiari I malformations, may begin in young adulthood. Signs of the disorder tend to develop slowly, although sudden onset may occur with coughing or straining.
   b. Symptoms differ depending on the location and size of the syrinx and which spinal nerves are involved.
   c. Pain that accompanies syrinx is a neuropathic, dysesthetic pain similar to CRPS or radicular pain. When syrinx is in the cervical area, the pain may be in "capelike" distribution.
   d. Pain may be experienced as interscapular pain. Pain may spread upward from the site of injury.
   e. It may be described as a sensation of "skin stretching."
   f. Headaches may be experienced.
   g. The person may experience stiffness in the back, shoulder, arms, or legs.
   h. Numbness may also spread upward from the site of the injury.
   i. Weakness may be experienced, similar to other spinal cord injuries.
   j. Disruption in temperature sensation, including the ability to feel extremes or hot or cold, may occur on one or both sides of the body.
   k. Similar to CRPS sweating, skin coldness or pallor may be experienced.
   l. Sexual function and, later, bladder and bowel control may be impaired.
4. Diagnostic workup
   a. MRI usually makes other testing unnecessary.
   b. EMG can be used.
   c. Lumbar puncture tests CSF pressure and analyzes CSF.
   d. CT scan can be helpful.
5. Treatment
   a. Do not treat if the patient is asymptomatic.
   b. If the person is symptomatic, surgery is the therapy. If symptomatic syrinx is not treated surgically, syringomyelia often leads to SCI with incumbent symptoms and persistent, severe pain.
   c. Conventional analgesics and antineuropathic medication provide little or no relief.
   d. Sympathetic nerve blocks (stellate ganglion block or lumbar sympathetic blocks) may be useful for some.

IV. Headache

A. The second edition of the international classification of headache disorders, ICHD-2 (International Headache Society, 2004), separates headache into 12 categories.

B. There are 4 categories of primary headaches and 8 categories of secondary headaches (Bigal & Lipton, 2006).
   1. Primary headaches
      a. *Migraine* is a chronic disorder characterized by episodic attacks of headache with a combination of neurological, gastrointestinal, and autonomic symptoms. The pain is tightly associated with changes in the cranial vasculature. Migraine is divided into six major categories; migraine without aura and migraine with aura are the most important (Goadsby, 2006).

(1) Migraine without aura
  (a) Signs and symptoms are
    (i) Usually unilateral pain, but not always.
    (ii) A pulsating quality.
    (iii) Moderate to severe pain intensity.
    (iv) Nausea, vomiting, or both.
    (v) Photophobia or phonophobia.
  (b) Diagnostic criteria (ICHD-2) are
    (i) At least five attacks (with the criteria of the first four signs and symptoms described previously).
    (ii) Headache attacks lasting 4 to 72 hours and occurring less than 15 days per month.
    (iii) Headache with at least two of the following: unilateral location, pulsating quality, moderate to severe pain intensity, and aggravation by routine physical activity.
    (iv) Headache causing at least one of the following: nausea, vomiting, or both; photophobia; or phonophobia.
    (v) Not attributed to another disorder.

(2) Migraine with aura
  (a) Signs and symptoms include
    (i) Focal neurological phenomena that can proceed or accompany a headache.
    (ii) Aura symptoms developed over 5 to 20 minutes and lasting 20 minutes on the average.
    (iii) Visual aura (the most common), with a crescent-shaped, bright, jagged edge; visual distortions; or double vision.
    (iv) Sensory symptoms (the second most common), with numbness, tingling, and paresthesia; weakness; language problems, such as difficulty finding or using words; or vertigo.
  (b) Diagnostic criteria (ICHD-2) are
    (i) At least two attacks (with the second through fourth symptom criteria given previously).
    (ii) Fully reversible visual, sensory, and speech symptoms but no motor weakness.
    (iii) At least two of the following:
      (a) Visual symptoms: flickering lights, spots and lines, or loss of vision
      (b) Sensory symptoms: feeling of pins and needles or numbness
      (c) At least one symptom developing gradually over more than 5 minutes, different symptoms occurring in succession, or both
      (d) Each symptom lasting more than 5 minutes and less than 60 minutes.
    (iv) Headache that meets criteria for migraine without aura.
    (v) Not attributed to another disorder.
  (c) Diagnostic workup
    (i) Take a history, and make a physical examination.
    (ii) Check vital signs: temperature, blood pressure, and pulse.
    (iii) Examine motor function, sensory testing, and coordination.
    (iv) The patient may need a CT scan, MRI, magnetic resonance angiography, lumbar puncture, electroencephalography, and erythrocyte sedimentation rate if temporal arteritis is part of the differential diagnosis. Where appropriate, diagnostic tests exclude a secondary cause (Silberstein, Lipton, Goadsby, & Smith, 1999).
  (d) Treatment
    (i) Avoid offending agents (i.e., follow a tyramine-free diet).
    (ii) Use abortive measures, such as triptans; ergotamine; dihydroergotamine;

NSAIDs; combination therapy of aspirin, acetaminophen, and caffeine; antiemetics; or intranasal lidocaine.

(iii) Use preventative medications (Goadsby, 2006) (see the chapter on Overview of Pharmacology), such as amine modulators, propranolol, tricyclic antidepressants, anticonvulsant (valproic acid, flunarizine, gabapentin, or topiramate).

(iv) Avoid opioids and barbiturates (Bigal et al., 2008).

(v) Regulate lifestyle factors, ensuring regular sleep, regular exercise, regular meals, and limited alcohol and caffeine.

(vi) Use biofeedback and relaxation techniques.

(vii) Apply a cold pack.

(viii) Give botulinum toxin (Botox®) injections (Freund & Schwartz, 2000; Jankovic et al., 2006; Rollnik et al., 2000; Silberstein, Mathew, Saper, & Jenkins, 2000).

b. *Tension-type headache* is the most common form of headache. It is ill defined because the diagnosis is mainly based on the absence of features found in other headaches (Schoenen, 2006).

(1) Diagnostic criteria (ICHD-2) for all tension-type headaches
 (a) Headache lasts from 30 minutes to 7 days.
 (b) At least two of the following characteristics are present:
  (i) Pressing or tightening (nonpulsating) quality
  (ii) Mild or moderate intensity
  (iii) Bilateral location
  (iv) No aggravation by routine physical activity
 (c) Both of the following characteristics are present:
  (i) No nausea or vomiting
  (ii) Absence of photophobia, phonophobia, or both
 (d) Headache is not attributed to another disorder.

(2) Specific diagnostic criteria for an infrequent episodic tension-type headache
 (a) At least 10 episodes occur on less than 1 day per month (less than 12 days per year).

(3) Specific diagnostic criteria for frequent episodic tension-type headache
 (a) At least 10 episodes occur on more than 1 day but less than 15 days per month for at least 3 months (more than 12 days and less than 180 days per year).

(4) Specific diagnostic criteria for chronic tension-type headache
 (a) Headache occurs on more than 15 days per month on average for more than 3 months (more than 180 days per year).

(5) Specific diagnostic criteria for *probable tension-type headache*
 (a) Episodes fulfill all but one of the criteria for tension-type headache and do not fulfill criteria for migraine without aura.

(6) Diagnostic workup
 (a) Take a history.
 (b) Check vital signs: temperature, blood pressure, and pulse.
 (c) Examine motor function, cranial nerves, sensory response, and coordination.
 (d) Usually no diagnostic tests are needed. If symptoms are not consistent with aforementioned criteria, however, use a CT scan, MRI, magnetic resonance angiography, lumbar puncture, electroencephalography, and erythrocyte sedimentation rate to rule out temporal arteritis if it is part of the differential diagnosis.

(7) Treatment options are as follows:
 (a) NSAIDs
 (b) Acetaminophen-, aspirin-, and caffeine-containing products
 (c) Tricyclic antidepressants

(d) Botulinum toxin (Rollnik et al., 2000)
(e) Relaxation and biofeedback
(f) Cognitive-behavioral therapies (stress reduction)
(g) Physical therapy
(h) Oromandibular treatment

c. *Cluster headache and other trigeminal autonomic cephalgias* are a group of headaches characterized by unilateral trigeminal distribution pain that occurs in association with ipsilateral cranial autonomic features (Goadsby, 2006).

(1) Cluster headache has two forms:
(a) Episodic attacks in periods lasting 7 days to 1 year separated by pain-free periods lasting 1 month or more.
(b) Chronic attacks occur for more than 1 year without remission or with remissions lasting less than 1 month.

(2) Signs and symptoms
(a) Headache is unilateral.
(b) Excruciating pain occurs around the orbital and temporal regions.
(c) Headache lasts from 15 minutes to 3 hours.
(d) Pain is accompanied by autonomic symptoms, e.g., lacrimation, nasal congestion, miosis, ptosis, and facial flushing).

(3) Diagnostic criteria
(a) Severe unilateral orbital, supraorbital, temporal, or a combination of these types of pain last 15 to 180 minutes if untreated.
(b) Attack frequency is from one every other day to eight per day.
(c) At least one of the following signs must be present on the pain side:
(i) Conjunctival injection
(ii) Lacrimation
(iii) Nasal congestion
(iv) Rhinorrhea
(v) Forehead or facial sweating
(vi) Miosis
(vii) Ptosis
(viii) Eyelid edema
(ix) Sense of restlessness or agitation

(4) Diagnostic workup
(a) Check vital signs: temperature, blood pressure, and pulse.
(b) Examine motor function, sensory testing, and coordination.
(c) The patient may need a CT scan, MRI, magnetic resonance angiography, lumbar puncture, electroencephalogram, and erythrocyte sedimentation rate for a thorough workup if temporal arteritis is a part of the differential diagnosis.

(5) Treatment
(a) Acute treatment includes the following:
(i) Administration of oxygen for 15 minutes
(ii) Triptans
(iii) Intranasal lidocaine
(iv) Ergotamine
(b) Preventive measures (Goadsby, 2006) are as follows:
(i) Verapamil
(ii) Lithium
(iii) Ergotamine
(iv) Dihydroergotamine
(v) Corticosteroids
(vi) Melatonin (Goadsby, 2006)

(vii) Greater occipital nerve blockade (Peres et al., 2002)
(viii) Trigeminal sensory root rhizotomy (Jarrar, Black, Dodick, & Davis, 2003)
(ix) Radiofrequency trigeminal gangliorhizolysis (Mathew & Hurt, 1988)
(x) Microvascular decompression of the trigeminal nerve (Lovely, Kotsiakis, & Jannetta, 1998)
(xi) Neuromodulation (Franzini, Ferroli, Leone, & Broggi, 2003)

d. Other primary headaches
   (1) This category includes various headache disorders that are not associated with a structural lesion.
   (2) These may mimic secondary headaches, so they must be carefully evaluated.
   (3) Subcategories are as follows:
      (a) Primary stabbing headache
      (b) Primary cough headache
      (c) Primary exertional headache
      (d) Primary headache associated with sexual activity
      (e) Hypnic headache: dull headache that awakens a person from sleep, known as the "alarm clock" headache
      (f) Primary thunderclap headache: acute onset high-intensity headache resembles a ruptured cerebral aneurysm for which immediate emergent, emergency department, and neurology referral may be indicated
      (g) Hemicrania continua: persistent unilateral headache
      (h) New daily persistent headache
   (4) This category includes controversies in the classification of primary chronic daily headaches of long duration (Bigal & Lipton, 2006). Silberstein-Lipton criteria divide the primary chronic daily headache of long duration (more than 4 hours a day) into four main diagnoses (Silberstein et al., 1999):
      (a) Transformed migraine
      (b) Chronic tension-type headache
      (c) New daily persistent headache
      (d) Hemicrania continua

2. Secondary headaches have a causal relationship with a causative disorder. These headaches are greatly reduced or disappear within 3 months or after successful treatment or spontaneous remission of the causative disorder (Bigal & Lipton, 2006). They can be attributed to the following:
   a. Head and neck trauma
   b. Cranial or cervical vascular disorders
   c. Nonvascular intracranial disorders
   d. Substance or its withdrawal
   e. Infection
   f. Disorder of homeostasis
   g. Disorders of cranium, neck, eyes, ears, nose, sinuses, teeth, mouth, or other facial structures
   h. Psychiatric disorders
3. For cranial neuralgias and central causes of facial pain and headaches not classified elsewhere, pain in the head and neck is mediated by afferent fibers in the trigeminal, glossopharyngeal, nervus intermedius, and vagus nerves and the upper cervical roots via the occipital nerves. Stimulation of these nerves can cause pain in the innervated areas (ICHD-2), which include the following (International Headache Society, 2008):
   a. Trigeminal neuralgia
   b. Glossopharyngeal neuralgia
   c. Nervus intermedius neuralgia
   d. Superior laryngeal neuralgia

e. Nasociliary neuralgia (Charlin)
f. Supraorbital neuralgia
g. Neck-tongue syndrome
h. External compression headache
i. Cold stimulus headache
j. Constant pain caused by compression, irritation, or distortion of cranial nerves or upper cervical roots by structural lesions
k. Optic neuritis
l. Ocular diabetic neuropathy
m. Herpes zoster
n. Tolosa-Hunt syndrome
o. Ophthalmoplegic migraine
p. Central causes of facial pain

V. Musculoskeletal Pain

A. *Osteoarthritis* is a disease of the cartilage that progressively produces a local tissue response, mechanical change, and failure of function (APS, 2002). It is the most common noninflammatory arthritic condition, often termed *degenerative joint disease.*

1. Signs and symptoms
   a. Deep aching pain results from a degenerative process in a single or multiple joints.
   b. It typically affects the joints of the hand, feet, ankles, and spine, as well as weight-bearing joints (hips and knees).
   c. Severity is related to disease progression.
   d. Pain occurs at rest, with initiation of activity, and later in the disease process, at night.
   e. It is associated with stiffness after inactivity and in the morning.
   f. Incidence increases with age.
   g. Joint line tenderness and crepitus occur on active or passive joint motion.
   h. Noninflammatory effusions may be present.
   i. Later stages may show gross deformity, bony hypertrophy, and contracture.
2. Diagnostic workup (Tutuncu & Kavanaugh, 2005)
   a. There are no laboratory findings.
   b. There can be a discrepancy between radiological findings and clinical complaints.
   c. In later stages, radiological evidence shows joint space narrowing, sclerosis, cysts, and reactive osteophytes.
   d. Arthrocentesis may be therapeutic, as well as diagnostic.
3. Treatment
   a. NSAIDs and COX–2 inhibitors can be used.
   b. Acetaminophen can be given.
   c. Glucosamine can be helpful (Towheed et al., 2005).
   d. Reduce load through the use of a walking stick or weight loss.
   e. In early phases, intraarticular steroids may be helpful.
   f. Apply capsaicin cream.
   g. Apply a lidocaine patch over the affected joint.
   h. Use occupational therapy for fine motor function, splinting when necessary, and paraffin wax application.
   i. Use physical therapy for large motor function, pacing, adaptive equipment when necessary, myofascial release, TENS unit application, and ultrasound therapy.
   j. Intraarticular hyaluronic acid can be used.

B. *Rheumatoid arthritis* is a chronic autoimmune disorder characterized by symmetrical synovitis of the joints, usually involving diarthrodial joints, and leads to progressive destruction (APS, 2002).

1. Signs and symptoms

a. Aching and burning joint pain related to systemic inflammatory disease affects synovial joints, muscle, ligaments, and tendons. It is often associated with morning stiffness and chronic fatigue.
b. Pain is associated with tenderness, swelling, decreased range of motion, and occasionally subcutaneous nodules.
c. According to the 1987 American College of Rheumatology Diagnostic Criteria, rheumatoid arthritis is considered present when the first four of the following criteria have been present for at least 6 weeks (Scott, 2006):
   (1) Morning stiffness lasting longer than 1 hour before improvement
   (2) Arthritis involving three or more joint areas
   (3) Arthritis of the hand joints
   (4) Symmetrical arthritis
   (5) Rheumatoid nodules
   (6) Positive serum rheumatoid factor
   (7) Radiographic evidence of rheumatoid arthritis
d. Chronic destruction and joint deformity are common.
e. Occasionally, inflammation may affect eyes, heart, or lungs.

2. Diagnostic workup (APS, 2002) includes the following:
   a. Anemia or a falling serum albumin
   b. Elevated erythrocyte sedimentation rate or C-reactive protein
   c. Rheumatoid factor positive
   d. Thrombocytosis
   e. Radiographic changes
   f. Synovial histopathology consistent with rheumatoid arthritis
   g. Characteristic nodule pathology
3. Treatment options are as follows (Scott, 2006):
   a. Disease-modifying antirheumatic drugs
   b. NSAIDs or COX–2 inhibitors and acetaminophen
   c. Immunosuppressive drugs (methotrexate)
   d. Gold salts (sodium aurothiomalate)
   e. Corticosteroids
   f. Cytokine antagonist (e.g., Etanercept or Infliximab)
   g. Rheumatology referral
   h. Physical therapy (see earlier description under osteoarthritis)
   i. Occupational therapy (see earlier description under osteoarthritis)

C. *Sickle cell disease* is an inherited disease in which pain is a hallmark clinical manifestation. Pain is a result of vasoocclusive crisis; however, the timing, severity, and frequency of painful episodes vary greatly (Payne, 2005).
   1. Signs and symptoms
      a. Pain can be severe and is usually present in the bone, chest, and abdomen.
      b. Children may experience sickle cell dactylitis causing swelling in the dorsal surfaces of the hands and feet.
      c. There may be ischemic manifestations such as hemolytic crisis, priapism, renal failure, jaundice, hepatomegaly, ischemic leg ulceration, or stroke.
      d. Acute chest pain syndrome, with or without fever, can occur in association with a pulmonary infiltrate caused by lung or rib infarction.
      e. Refer to assessment recommendations by the APS panel (1999) (Box 18–3).
   2. Diagnostic workup
      a. Obtain a history, and perform a physical examination.
      b. The patient's report of pain is the gold standard.
      c. MRI may show infarct-related changes in bone and soft tissue in the lower extremities.
      d. Laboratory findings may show changes in coagulation and fibrinolytic systems.

Box 18-3 Pain Assessment in Sickle Cell Disease

Clinicians should ask about pain, and patients' self-reports should be the primary source of assessment, with the exception of infants, for whom behavioral observations are the primary source of assessment.

For rapid assessment of pain during an acute painful event, clinicians should select a simple measurement of pain intensity, reassess frequently, and record the measurement for treatment evaluation.

A comprehensive biopsychosocial clinical assessment should be done yearly and more often for patients with frequent pain.

To promote adequate pain management, patients should be reassessed frequently and asked how much their pain has been relieved after the first treatment and after subsequent treatment adjustments.

When clinicians consistently observe a disparity between patients' verbal self-report of their pain and their ability to function, further assessment should be performed to ascertain the reason for the disparity.

Clinicians should understand and describe the pain in sufficient detail so that therapy can be tailored to the individual needs of patients.

Developmental stage, chronologic age, functional status, cognitive abilities, and emotional status should be considered in the choice of assessment methods and tools.

Data from American Pain Society. (1999). *Principles of analgesic use in the treatment of acute pain and cancer pain* (4th ed.). Glenview, IL: Author.

3. Treatment
   a. Pharmacological treatment (opioids)
      (1) Severe and acute pain should be considered emergent, requiring aggressive treatment to ease pain and maintain function. Consider patient-controlled analgesia.
      (2) For mild-to-moderate pain, try NSAIDs or acetaminophen.
      (3) If pain unresponsive to NSAIDs or acetaminophen, add an opioid.
      (4) For short-term pain (less than 24 hours), give a short-acting opioid.
      (5) For pain requiring several days to resolve, give a sustained-release opioid for more consistent analgesia.
      (6) Avoid sedatives or anxiolytics for pain management.
      (7) When the patient is discharged from the hospital to home, equianalgesic should be used at home. Specific instructions should be given for tapering the dosage as pain level reduces while reducing the risk of withdrawal symptoms.
      (8) Tolerance to an opioid should not be confused with addiction.
   b. Preventive treatment with hydroxyurea is reserved for patients with severe disease: it reduces the number of
      (1) Vasoocclusive crisis episodes.
      (2) Acute chest syndromes.
      (3) Transfusions.
   c. Behavioral treatment includes
      (1) Exercise.
      (2) Relaxation, deep breathing, biofeedback, behavior and modification.
   d. Psychological treatment relies on
      (1) Social support.
      (2) Cognitive therapies, hypnotherapy, visual imagery, and distraction.
   e. Physical treatment includes
      (1) Hydration.
      (2) Oxygen.
      (3) Heat, massage, hydrotherapy, ultrasound, acupuncture, TENS, and physical therapy.

f. Education
(1) Teach the patient about the disease, signs and symptoms of acute episodes, treatment options, precipitating factors, exercise options, and psychological support systems
(2) Provide instructions on follow-up care.
(3) Give instructions on home pain management, including
(a) The importance of rest, hydration, and avoiding precipitating factors.
(b) The medication regimen (APS, 1999) and National Institutes of Health guidelines.

4. Emergency guidelines for sickle cell disease can be found at http://www.health.state.mn.us/divs/fh/mcshn/nbsprsickle2.htm (Minnesota Department of Health, 2005).

VI. Chronic Abdominal and Pelvic Pain Syndromes

A. The differential diagnosis of chronic abdominal and pelvic pain syndromes is hugh. Collaboration with physician colleagues is imperative.

B. *Chronic abdominal pain:* Functional gastrointestinal disorders make up the majority of chronic abdominal pain (Wong & Mayer, 2006).

1. Differential diagnosis is as follows:
a. Pancreatitis
b. Cholecystitis, cholelithiasis
c. Hepatomegaly
d. Splenomegaly
e. Peptic ulcer disease
f. Gastritis
g. Esophagitis
h. Irritable bowel syndrome
i. Neoplasms
j. Pelvic inflammatory disease
k. Endometriosis
l. Uterine obstruction
m. Ovarian cyst torsion
n. Ovulatory pain
o. Ruptured ovarian cyst
p. Dysfunction of pelvic floor muscles

2. Diagnostic workup includes the following:
a. History and physical examination
b. Psychological assessment
c. Physical and sexual abuse history
d. Manual pelvic and abdominal examination
e. Imaging studies, including abdominal ultrasound, CT scan, MRI, positron emission tomography scan, and bone scan
f. Laboratory tests, including carcinoembryonic antigen, liver function tests, complete blood count, and hepatitis screen
g. Laparoscopy
h. Laparotomy

3. Treatment
a. Appropriately treat the cause when identifiable.
b. Establish goals with the patient.
c. Evaluate the patient's activity and pain log.
d. Use a stepwise trial of the following medication:
(1) Salicylates and acetaminophen if no contraindicated (Perneger, Whelton, & Klag, 1994; Pickering, Esteve, Loriot, Eschalier, & Dubray, 2008)
(2) NSAIDs and COX-2 inhibitors (with careful consideration as to the cause of the pain before recommending these)

(3) Tricyclic antidepressants
(4) Anticonvulsants
(5) Antispasmodics (for reports of spasm type pain)
(6) Opioids if appropriate

e. Use diagnostic nerve blocks (celiac block or sympathetic block).
f. TENS is an option.
g. Neurolytic procedures can be used.
h. Psychological interventions include
   (1) Cognitive-behavioral therapy.
   (2) Relaxation modalities.
   (3) Stress management.
i. Use physical medicine interventions as appropriate (described later).
j. Complementary therapies may be useful, such as
   (1) Yoga.
   (2) Meditation.
   (3) Nutritional therapy.
   (4) Therapeutic touch.

B. *Chronic pelvic pain* is defined as 6 months or more of nonmenstrual pelvic pain that is severe enough to cause functional disability or to require medical or surgical treatment (Howard, 2003).
   1. Differential diagnosis includes the following:
      a. Irritable bowel syndrome
      b. Neoplasm
      c. Pelvic inflammatory disease
      d. Endometriosis
      e. Uterine obstruction
      f. Ovarian cyst torsion
      g. Ovulatory pain
      h. Ruptured ovarian cyst
      i. Dysfunction of pelvic floor muscles
   2. Diagnostic workup includes the following:
      a. History and physical examination
      b. Psychological assessment
      c. Physical and sexual abuse history
      d. Manual abdominal and pelvic examination
      e. Imaging studies, including pelvic ultrasound, transvaginal scanning, CT scan, MRI, positron emission tomography scan, and bone scan
      f. Laboratory tests; carcinoembryonic antigen (CEA), cancer antigen (CA-125), liver function tests, renal function tests, and complete blood count
      g. Laparoscopy and laparotomy
      h. Diagnostic nerve blocks
   3. Treatment
      a. Appropriately treat the cause when identifiable.
      b. Establish goals with the patient.
      c. Evaluate the patient's activity and pain log.
      d. Use a stepwise trial of the following medications:
         (1) Salicylates and acetaminophen (Perneger et al., 1994; Pickering et al., 2008)
         (2) NSAIDs and COX-2s
         (3) Tricyclic antidepressants
         (4) Anticonvulsant agents
         (5) Opioids, if appropriate
      e. Consider TENS.
      f. Neurolytic procedures can be used.

g. Psychological interventions include
   (1) Cognitive-behavioral therapy.
   (2) Relaxation modalities.
   (3) Stress management.
   (4) Anger management.
h. Use physical medicine interventions as appropriate (described later).
i. Complementary therapies may be useful, such as
   (1) Yoga.
   (2) Meditation.
   (3) Nutritional therapy.
   (4) Therapeutic touch.
   (5) Acupressure and acupuncture.

C. *Chronic pancreatitis* is characterized by progressive and irreversible pancreatic injury related to intermittent inflammatory flare (Abdel Aziz & Lehman, 2007; Gachago & Draganov, 2008; Warshaw, Banks, & Fernandez-Del Castillo, 1998).
1. Signs and symptoms
   a. Pain is the major disabling symptom.
      (1) Pain is highly variable among patients; it may be intermittent, frequent, or persistent, and it may be mild, moderate, severe, or absent.
      (2) Pain is located in the upper abdomen.
      (3) Gnawing pain radiates to the back; it is aggravated by food and alcohol.
   b. The patient may experience weight loss.
   c. Diabetes can be an indicator for chronic pancreatitis.
   d. Jaundice can be a symptom.
   e. The patient may have problems with digestion or malabsorption.
   f. Steatorrhea (foul-smelling, greasy stools) is a sign.
2. Diagnostic workup includes the following (National Guidelines Clearinghouse, 2004):
   a. Endoscopic retrograde pancreatography
   b. CT scan
   c. Ultrasound
   d. Magnetic resonance cholangiopancreatography
   e. Biopsy
   f. Laboratory tests, carbohydrate antigen 19-9, glucose tolerance test, and amylase, which may or may not be elevated
3. Cause
   a. Alcohol abuse is the most common cause in the United States.
   b. Other possible causes are
      (1) Tumors.
      (2) Strictures.
      (3) Hypercalcemia.
      (4) Hyperlipidemia.
      (5) Genetic mutations.
      (6) Drugs (e.g., anticonvulsants).
   d. Dietary or environment causes are possible.
   e. The cause may be unknown.
4. Treatment
   a. Discontinue alcohol consumption.
   b. Discontinue contributing medication
   c. Switch to a low-fat diet.
   d. Use opioids, if appropriate.
   e. Use antidepressants.

f. Suppress secretion of acid of pancreatic enzymes, such as
   (1) Proton-pump inhibitors.
   (2) H_2-blocking agents.
   (3) Pancreatic enzymes.
g. Use antioxidant therapy, such as
   (1) Selenium.
   (2) Beta-carotene.
   (3) Vitamin C.
   (4) Methionine.
   (5) Vitamin E.
h. Use octreotide.
i. Interventional medical texts continue to include nerve block—celiac plexus block—as an intervention (de Leon-Casasola, Molloy, & Lema, 2005; Waldman, 2004c). However, the American Gastroenterological Association speaks against it (Warshaw et al., 1998).
j. Endoscopic treatment to place stents may be beneficial.
k. Use surgical interventions (National Guidelines Clearinghouse, 2004).

D. ***Interstitial cystitis*** is a debilitating inflammatory condition of the urinary bladder characterized by excessive urinary frequency, urgency, nocturia, and pain. The only defining pathology is the presence of mucosal ulcers or glomerulations (Ness, 2006).
1. Signs and symptoms
   a. Mild burning to excruciating pain occurs in the bladder, lower abdomen, perineum, vagina, low back, and thighs.
   b. Pain often is associated with filling of the bladder.
   c. The patient may have a period of symptomatic flares and remissions.
   d. Pain may be aggravated by menstruation or sexual intercourse.
   e. It may be accompanied by psychological, social, and hygienic problems.
   f. Chronic pain and sleep loss contribute to depression.
2. Diagnostic workup
   a. Take a complete history.
   b. Make a gynecological (pelvic and rectal) examination.
   c. Take urine cultures for an antiproliferative factor.
   d. Use cystoscopy with bladder hydrodistention.
   e. Use cystometry.
   f. Perform a bladder biopsy.
   g. Hunner's patches (mucosal ulceration) may be present.
   h. The patient may have bladder petechial mucosal hemorrhages (glomerulations) in the absence of ulceration.
3. Treatment (Ness, 2006)
   a. The patient can be given the following:
      (1) Antihistamines
      (2) Tricyclic antidepressants
      (3) Pentosan polysulfate sodium (Elmiron)
      (4) Nifedipine and other calcium channel blockers
      (5) Opioids
   g. Intravesical (intrabladder) therapy can include the following (Moldwin, Evans, Stanford, & Rosenberg, 2007; Pontari, Hanno, & Wein, 1997):
      (1) Dimethyl sulfoxide
      (2) Dimethyl sulfoxide plus steroids, heparin, bicarbonate, or lidocaine
      (3) Silver nitrate
      (4) Clorpactin
      (5) Hyaluronic acid

(6) Bacille Calmette-Guérin vaccine (BCG)
(7) Botulinum toxin type A

i. Neural blockade has been shown to be effective in some patients, including the following:
(1) Hypogastric block
(2) Continuous epidural infusion
(3) Spinal opioid infusion
(4) Spinal cord stimulator

j. Cognitive-behavioral techniques can be used.

k. TENS is an option.

l. Surgery, supravesical diversions or cystectomy, is a last resort.

VII. Human Immunodeficiency Virus (HIV)—Related Pain

A. Pain incidence

1. Pain is related to the progression of disease or the medical treatment of the disease. Pain prevalence estimates range from 30% to 90% (Breitbart et al., 1996; O'Neill & Sherrard, 1993).
2. Patients had on average two or more types of pain at any given time (Breitbart et al., 1996; O'Neill & Sherrard, 1993).
3. Patients with this pain are more likely to have progressive disease, with low T4 cell counts, multiple opportunistic infections, and low Karnofsky performance scores (i.e., less able to function) (Singer et al., 1993).

B. Types of pain

1. Oral pain includes the following:
   a. Candidiasis
   b. Dental caries
2. Oral ulcerations include the following:
   a. Herpes simplex virus
   b. Cytomegalovirus (CMV)
   c. Epstein-Barr virus
   d. Mycobacterial infection
   e. Cryptococcal infection
   f. Histoplasmosis
   g. Kaposi sarcoma (Lebovits et al., 1989)
3. Esophageal pain includes the following:
   a. Candidiasis
   b. Other fungal infections
   c. CMV
   d. Herpes simplex virus
4. Abdominal pain includes the following:
   a. Cryptosporidial diarrhea
   b. *Shigella* infection
   c. *Salmonella* infection
   d. Campylobacter enteritis
   e. CMV ileitis and colitis
   f. Lymphoma
   g. Kaposi sarcoma (Barone, Gingold, Nealon, & Arvanitis, 1986)
5. Biliary and pancreatic pain includes the following:
   a. Coincidental cholelithiasis
   b. Acalculous cholecystitis related to cryptosporidium
   c. CMV
   d. Mycobacterial infection

   e. Kaposi sarcoma (KS)
   f. Sclerosing cholangitis related to CMV and cryptosporidium
   g. Pancreatitis associated with drug therapy, in particular pentamidine and antiretroviral agents
   h. Acute pancreatitis associated with CMV (Bonacini, 1992)
6. Anorectal pain includes the following:
   a. Perirectal abscesses
   b. Kaposi sarcoma
   c. CMV proctitis
   d. Fissures
   e. Herpes simplex virus (HSV)
   f. Cancer
   g. Genital warts (Goldberg, Orkin, & Smith, 1994; Penfold & Clark, 1992; Yuhan et al., 1998)
7. Neurological pain includes the following:
   a. Headaches related to primary HIV syndromes
   b. HIV encephalitis
   c. Atypical septic meningitis
   d. Viral and nonviral nervous system infections
   e. Acquired immunodeficiency syndrome (AIDS)—related neoplasm
   f. Common migraines
   g. Sinus infections (Brew & Miller, 1993; Goldstein, 1990; Singer et al., 1993)
8. Peripheral neuropathy
   a. Symmetrical sensory neuropathies constitute 15% to 50% of pain diagnoses (Breitbart et al., 1996; Dalakas & Pezeshkpour, 1988; Fuller, Jacobs, & Guiloff, 1993; Parry, 1988).
   b. Distal peripheral neuropathy is the most common neuropathy in HIV and occurs in approximately one-third of patients (Luciano, Pardo, & McArthur, 2003).
      (1) HIV neuropathies are characterized by burning, numbness, or pins and needles.
      (2) Several antiretroviral agents, such as didanosine, zalcitabine, stavudine, vincristine, phenytoin, and isoniazid, can cause painful peripheral neuropathies (Singer et al., 1993).
   c. Kaposi sarcoma results in lower extremity pain in 45% of patients.
   d. Demyelinating polyneuropathies are caused by
      (1) Guillain-Barré syndrome.
      (2) Chronic mononeuritis multiplex.
      (3) Progressive inflammatory polyradiculopathy of the lower limbs (Breitbart et al., 1996; Dalakas & Pezeshkpour, 1988; Fuller et al., 1993; Parry, 1988).
9. Rheumatological pain includes the following:
   a. Reactive arthritis
   b. Arthropathies
   c. Psoriatic arthritis
   d. Septic arthritis
   e. Myopathy and myositis, possibly related to drug therapy
   f. Sometimes an unknown cause (Berman et al., 1988; O'Neill & Sherrard, 1993)
10. Pain related to HIV therapy arises from the following:
   a. Drugs (many cause peripheral neuropathies) (McArthur, Brew, & Nath, 2005)
   b. Chemotherapy
   c. Radiation therapy
   d. Procedures
   e. Surgery (Portenoy, 2000; Singer et al., 1993)
11. Pain related to concomitant problems includes the following:
   a. Low back pain
   b. Diabetic neuropathy (Breitbart & Patt, 1994; Hewitt, Breitbart, & Rosenfeld, 1994)

C. Diagnostic workup
   1. The first move toward treating HIV pain is a thorough assessment that includes the following:
      a. Thorough history and physical examination
      b. Assessment of pain characteristics
      c. Laboratory results as indicated
      d. Imaging studies as indicated
      e. EMG and nerve conduction studies as indicated
      f. Psychosocial assessment
      g. Substance abuse history
D. Treatment
   1. Treat the cause of the pain when known. The same interventions are appropriate in the HIV population as in the non-HIV population.
   2. The choice of pain therapy depends on the type of pain.
      a. Opioids are one option.
      b. Use tricyclic antidepressants for neuropathic pain syndromes.
      c. Use anticonvulsants for neuropathic pain syndromes.
      d. Use NSAIDs and salicylates for inflammatory pain syndromes.
      e. Use steroids for inflammatory pain syndromes.
      f. Acetaminophen is an option (Perneger et al., 1994; Pickering et al., 2008).
      g. Use of the World Health Organization analgesic ladder applies in HIV disease and in cancer pain treatment (Breitbart & Patt, 1994; Hewitt et al., 1994; Lebovits et al., 1989; O'Neill & Sherrard, 1993; Singer et al., 1993).

PART TWO: MEDICATION MANAGEMENT FOR NONCANCER PAIN

I. General Guidelines for Medication Management

A. Take a thorough medication history.
   1. What has been tried?
   2. What were the doses?
   3. What were the side effects?
   4. Was it effective?
   5. Why was it stopped?
B. Diagnose and treat each pain as indicated.
   1. Somatosensory pain is
      a. Described as localized and sharp.
      b. Treated with NSAIDs, acetaminophen, topical medications, and local anesthetic injections.
   2. Visceral pain is
      a. Described as diffuse, generalized, tightness, pressure, and deep.
      b. Treated with nerve blocks, tricyclic antidepressants, and anticonvulsants.
   3. Neuropathic pain is
      a. Described as burning, prickling, tingling, and numbness.
      b. Treated with nerve blocks, tricyclic antidepressants, and anticonvulsants.
   4. Muscular pain is
      a. Described as sore, aching, and spasms.
      b. Treated with trigger point injections, NSAIDs, acetaminophen, and muscle relaxants.
   5. Psychogenic pain needs an evaluation with a psychologist or psychiatrist for the following:
      a. Passivity
      b. Unrealistic expectations
      c. Low motivation

d. Chemical dependency
e. Personality style
(1) Impulsive
(2) Obsessive-compulsive
(3) Nonconforming
f. Pain-related anxiety

C. Individualize drug, dose, interval, and route.
1. Dose *around the clock* for constant pain; reassess frequently.
2. Monitor at appropriate intervals.
3. Start low and go slow.
4. Anticipate and manage side effects.
5. Evaluate effectiveness.
6. If one drug does not work, consider another drug trial.

D. Analgesia selection depends on the balance between the medication's efficacy in relieving the particular symptom and the medication's side effects. The following are other things to consider:
1. Type of pain
2. Intensity of pain
3. Comorbid features
4. Allergies
5. Balance between medication's efficacy and side effects
6. Past side effects from trials at other times
7. Tolerance
8. Age of patient
9. Laboratory findings

E. Titrate analgesia medication (i.e., opioid, NSAIDs, tricyclic antidepressants, or anticonvulsants) to
1. Find the optimal dosage for an individual patient.
2. Reduce the level of pain; level of pain intensity may not be a good measurement of outcome in this population (see later under long-term opioid therapy) (Dworkin et al., 2005).
3. Minimize side effects.
4. Return the patient to optimal function.

F. Escalation depends on
1. Level of pain intensity.
2. Patient's age.
3. Other medications the patient is taking, including herbals.
4. Patient's mental status.
5. Patient's ability to function.
6. Presence of side effects (e.g., sedation, gastrointestinal effects, cardiac side effects, renal side effects, depression, or insomnia).
7. Evidence of a new pain syndrome.

II. Nonopioid Analgesics

A. NSAIDs (see the chapter on Overview of Pharmacology, referring to Appendix 14-8)
1. Indications include the following:
a. Inflammation
b. Headaches
c. Myalgias
d. Bone pain
e. Joint pain
f. Rheumatological conditions
2. Choice of NSAIDs
a. Run an empirical trial for 1 week or more.
b. If therapy is effective, continue unless toxicity occurs.

c. There is a large amount of individual variability even when NSAIDs are structurally similar in the same chemical family (Insel, 1996).

B. Steroids (see the chapter on Overview of Pharmacology, referring to Appendix 14-10A and 14-10B)
   1. Indications include the following:
      a. Rheumatological conditions
      b. Tumors
      c. Peripheral and spinal blocks
      d. Inflammatory reactions
      e. Headache related to increased intracranial pressure
      f. Sympathetically maintained pain syndromes (i.e., CRPS)

C. Acetaminophen (see the chapter on Overview of Pharmacology) (Perneger et al., 1994; Pickering et al., 2008)
   1. Indications for pain that is initiated in the peripheral nerve endings (e.g., headache, incisional, or burns) include the following:
      a. Rheumatological conditions
      b. Tumors
      c. Peripheral and spinal blocks
      d. Inflammatory reactions
      e. Headache related to increased intracranial pressure
   2. Use
      a. Dosage (refer to Appendix 14-12A)
         (1) Give 325 to 1,000 mg, not to exceed 4,000 mg in 24 hours in adults. With renal dysfunction, do not exceed 2,500 mg in 24 hours.
         (2) "The American Liver Foundation recommends that people not exceed three grams of acetaminophen a day for any prolonged period of time" (American Liver Foundation, 2008; Watkins et al., 2008).
         (3) See the chapter on pediatric pain management for appropriate dosing in children.
         (4) Check with a physician before using in patients with hepatic dysfunction.

D. Tricyclic antidepressants (see the chapter on Overview of Pharmacology, referring to Appendix 14-3)
   1. Indications are as follows:
      a. Neuropathic pain, including
         (1) Burning
         (2) Prickling
         (3) Tingling
      b. Myofascial pain
      c. Interstitial cystitis

E. Anticonvulsants (see the chapter on Overview or Pharmacology, referring to Appendix 14-2)
   1. Indications are as follows:
      a. Neuropathic pain syndromes
      b. RSD
      c. Central pain syndromes

F. Muscle relaxants (see the chapter on Overview of Pharmacology, referring to Appendix 14-7)
   1. Use
      a. The primary route is oral.
      b. Muscle relaxants are alternatives to NSAIDs and opioids.
      c. Cyclobenzaprine, carisoprodol, and methocarbamol should not be administered with the mistaken belief that they relieve muscle spasms.

G. Benzodiazepines (see the chapter on Overview of Pharmacology, referring to Appendix 14-5)

H. Local and topical analgesics and anesthetics (see the chapter on Overview of Pharmacology, referring to Table 14-1)
   1. Indications

a. Topical preparation of capsaicin may be useful in localized neuropathic pain and other localized conditions, such as arthritis and diabetic neuropathy. (Use caution when using with a heating pad because burns may occur.)
b. Topical preparation of antiinflammatory drugs may be useful in localized neuropathic pain, arthritis, and diabetic neuropathy.
c. Topical preparation of local anesthetics may be useful for intravenous punctures or other painful procedures, prolonged incisional pain after healing, and neuropathies.
d. Efficacy in long-term use is unknown (Rowbotham, 1994; Thiessen & Portenoy, 1997).

2. Availability
   a. Capsaicin cream
      (1) The mechanism of action depletes substance P in primary afferent neurons (Thiessen & Portenoy, 1997).
      (2) Use
         (a) Apply three to four times a day for a minimum of 4 weeks.
         (b) Avoid eye contact.
         (c) Wash hands immediately after use.
      (3) Side effects
         (a) Initial burning and redness can occur at the site of application.
         (b) At times, this burning is severe enough to discontinue therapy.
   b. EMLA® cream
      (1) Mechanism of action is a topical local anesthetic agent (lidocaine and prilocaine, 1:1) that inhibits depolarization of nerve and blocks neuronal firing
      (2) Indication
         (a) Use local anesthesia before skin puncture of any kind.
         (b) Consider sensitivity to the skin surface.
      (3) Use
         (a) Apply a thick coating and cover with an occlusive dressing for at least 1 hour. Absorption and depth of anesthesia may increase up to 3 hours.
         (b) Thin coating may be useful in some patients for analgesia (Thiessen & Portenoy, 1997).
   c. Lidocaine patch (Argoff, 2000)
      (1) Mechanism of action is a topical local anesthetic agent.
      (2) Indications are local neuropathic pain syndromes, including postherpetic neuralgia, diabetic neuropathy, postsurgical syndromes, phantom pain syndrome, plexopathies, and CRPS.
      (3) Use
         (a) Apply to localized area of pain, leaving the patch on for 12 hours and then removing it for 12 hours.
         (b) The patch may be cut to fit.
         (c) Use no more than three patches at one time.
         (d) Apply to intact skin.
      (4) Side effects
         (a) Local rash and irritation are possible.
         (b) A systemic response is rare.
   d. NSAIDs, aspirin cream, and menthol-impregnated patches (see the chapter on Overview of Pharmacology, Table 14-1)
      (1) The mechanism of action is not understood.
      (2) Indications: The use of topical antiinflammatory agents remains ***unproven*** for neuropathic pain and local tenderness.
      (3) Use
         (a) These are available over the counter.
         (b) Apply over the tender site.

III. Long-term Opioid Therapy for Persistent Noncancer Pain (Institute for Clinical Systems Improvement, 2007; McLennon, 2005; Veterans Health Administration, Department of Defense, 2003)

A. Goals of treatment
   1. Total pain relief may not be a reasonable or achievable goal; emphasis is on pain reduction versus pain elimination.
      a. The mean pain reduction is about 30% (Furlan, Sandoval, Mailis-Gagnon, & Tunks, 2006; Kalso, Edwards, Moore, & McQuay, 2004).
   2. Improvement in functional status is evaluated in defined outcomes of increased activity and function.
   3. Titrate doses to achieve optimal balance among pain relief, side effects, and function.

B. In persistent noncancer pain, different perspectives regarding opioid use exist.
   1. Positive outcomes: Improvements in sleep quality, compliance, functional status, and possibly quality of life have been shown (Nicholson & Passik, 2007). Patients may function better because comfort is improved.
   2. Negative outcomes: Some multidisciplinary pain centers report greater pain complaints, more functional impairment, neuropsychological toxicity, a tendency toward deception regarding drug use, and poor response to multimodal pain treatment in patients using opioids long term (Portenoy, 1994).
   3. Portenoy (1994) suggested that the two perspectives may be due to subgroup variations within the population of patients with chronic nonmalignant pain. Recognition of these variations is necessary to avoid generalizing from one subgroup to another. Available evidence suggests that functional status is enhanced in some patients and compromised in others with the use of opioids.
   4. One study of 416 patients found "that patients with longstanding CNCP [chronic noncancer pain] who choose to participate in an interdisciplinary rehabilitative program that incorporates opioid withdrawal experience significant improvement in pain severity, functioning, mood, and pain catastrophizing immediately posttreatment ($P < 0.001$) and six months following treatment ($P < 0.11$). Patients experienced significant improvements in treatment outcomes regardless of opioids use status (nonopioid, low- and high-dose opioids) at admission" (Townsend et al., 2008, p. 186).
   5. Several systematic reviews of the extant literature concerning the use of opioids for chronic nonmalignant pain conclude that there is good evidence that opioids are initially effective, but the evidence for long-term effectiveness is unclear. Many patients were found to discontinue opioid therapy due to adverse events or insufficient pain relief (Ballantyne & Shin, 2008; Furlan et al., 2006; Kalso et al., 2004; Martell et al., 2007; Moore & McQuay, 2005; Noble, Tregear, Treadwell, & Schoelles, 2008).

C. Improvement in functional status
   1. Return to work.
      a. Return to work is one method of documenting improvement in functional status.
      b. Increasing participation in societal roles may be a more comprehensive measure (Vallerand, 1998
   2. Decrease health care usage with higher functional status.
   3. Improve family dynamics.
      a. Measurement in this area is similar to that of functional status and may mirror the enhancement and compromise discussed in the two aforementioned subgroups.
      b. Patients and their families may be so focused on the alleviation of pain that the related problems go unaddressed.
      c. Assessment of family dynamics before beginning opioid therapy and periodically throughout therapy allows for the formulation and measurement of goals (i.e., decreasing family discord) (Turk & Nash, 1996).
      d. Involving the family as a part of the patient's team of caregivers may decrease the family's frustration with the chronicity of the pain and increase the sense of control. Periodic family conferences may be helpful in monitoring family dynamics and addressing concerns.
      e. Communication between the patient and the family regarding pain should be assessed and enhanced if necessary.

4. Close disability claims. An open disability claim may hamper the outcomes of treatment (i.e., secondary gain) (Atlas et al., 2000).
5. Written patient goals usually include
   a. Decrease in pain.
   b. Increase in activity and function.
   c. Improvement of quality of life.
6. Controlled substance agreement
   a. Content statements
      (1) The patient will not exceed the prescribed dosage without consulting the pain specialist.
      (2) The patient will not obtain opioid prescriptions from other sources.
      (3) The patient will not receive medication from more than one pharmacy.
      (4) The patient will not refuse a periodic random drug screening when requested.
   b. Benefits of an agreement
      (1) An agreement identifies expectations and mutual responsibilities of patient and clinician.
      (2) It shows that the decision to use opioids was considered seriously by all parties involved.
      (3) It acknowledges the validity of the patient's pain complaint.
      (4) The agreement obtains patient consent for opioid treatment, whereby the patient is explained the risk and benefits of long-term opioid treatment.
      (5) It may provide protection against medicolegal problems.
      (6) Adherence monitoring with controlled substance agreement was associated with a 50% reduction in opioid abuse (Manchikanti et al., 2006).
      (7) An agreement may be used as an education tool.
   c. Risks of an agreement
      (1) An agreement may be subject to abuse.
      (2) It may not be signed in a free and informed manner (i.e., a patient in severe pain may feel coerced) (Biller & Caudill, 1999).

IV. Guidelines for Long-term Opioid Therapy in Noncancer Pain

A. Comprehensive guidelines (Institute for Clinical Systems Improvement, 2007; McLennon, 2005; Portenoy, 1994, 1996; Trescot et al., 2006; Veterans Health Administration/Department of Defense, 2003)
   1. Consider opioid treatment after all other reasonable attempts at analgesia have failed.
   2. History of substance abuse, severe character pathology, and chaotic home environment should be viewed as relative contraindications.
   3. A single practitioner should take primary responsibility for treatment.
   4. The patient should give informed consent at the start of therapy. Consent should include
      a. Recognition of low risk of true addiction as an outcome.
      b. Potential for cognitive impairment with the drug alone and in combination with sedative or hypnotics, including risks with driving or using heavy machinery (Chapman, 2001; Vainio, Ollila, Matikainen, Rosenberg, & Kalso, 1995).
      c. Likelihood of physical dependence and what can be done about this.
      d. Understanding by female patients that children born when the mother is on opioid maintenance therapy may be physically dependent at birth and will need immediate treatment for withdrawal.
      e. Potential long-term effects of opioid use.
   5. After drug selection, doses should be given around the clock; several weeks should be used for dose titration, and although improvement in functional status is consistently stressed, at least partial analgesia should be the agreed-on goal of therapy.
   6. Failure to achieve at least partial analgesia in the nontolerant patient should raise questions about the responsiveness of pain to opioids and prompt reassessment.
   7. Improved analgesia should be enhanced by attempts at increased physical and social function; opioid therapy should be complementary to other analgesic and rehabilitative therapy.

8. The daily dose plus medication for breakthrough pain for days of increased pain should be provided.
9. Initially, patients must be seen and drugs should be prescribed at least monthly. When patients are stable, less frequent visits may be used.
10. Exacerbations that are not treated effectively by breakthrough medication may be managed best in the hospital, where dose escalation with close observation is available.
11. Evidence of aberrant behaviors must be assessed carefully. In some cases, tapering and discontinuation of therapy may be required. In other cases, therapy may be continued within more rigid guidelines. Consultation with an addiction medicine specialist may be considered.
12. Pain self-report instruments may be helpful but should not be required.
13. Each visit should include a complete assessment and documentation.

B. Documentation
   1. Intake assessment should include the following:
      a. Pain assessment
      b. History and physical examination
      c. Chemical use and abuse (past and present)
      d. Support systems and living situation
   2. Random urine drug screens should be made periodically throughout treatment; results should be part of medical record.
   3. Although diversion is difficult to determine, pill counts may help the practitioner to determine compliance with a controlled substance. Documentation would reflect pill counts routinely.
   4. Ongoing assessment
      a. At each visit, the following assessments are made and documented (4 "A"s) (Nicholson & Passik, 2007):
         (1) Analgesia: Is the patient gaining pain relief?
         (2) Activity: What are the physical and psychosocial functioning levels?
         (3) Adverse medication effects: What are the side effects?
         (4) Aberrant behavior

C. Patient behaviors (see the chapter on Coexisting Addiction and Pain)
   1. Aberrant drug-related behaviors are cause for concern.
      a. Assess carefully so as not to label the patient unfairly.
      b. Many behaviors classified as aberrant may be signs of pseudoaddiction (see definitions subsequently).
   2. Behaviors that are considered aberrant have been classified by Portenoy (1996) as those that are assumed to be relatively more predictive and those that are assumed to be relatively less predictive of addiction.
      a. More predictive behaviors include the following:
         (1) Selling prescription drugs
         (2) Prescription forgery
         (3) Stealing or borrowing drugs from others
         (4) Injecting oral formulations
         (5) Obtaining prescription drugs from nonmedical sources
         (6) Concurrent abuse of alcohol or illicit drugs
         (7) Multiple dose escalations or other noncompliance with therapy despite warnings
         (8) Multiple episodes of prescription loss
         (9) Repeatedly seeking prescriptions from other clinicians or from emergency departments without informing the prescriber or after warnings to desist
         (10) Evidence of deterioration in the ability to function at work, in the family, or socially that appear to be related to drug use
         (11) Repeated resistance to changes in therapy despite clear evidence of adverse physical or psychological effects from the drug

b. Less predictive behaviors include the following:
   (1) Aggressive complaining about the need for more drug
   (2) Drug hoarding during periods of reduced symptoms
   (3) Requesting specific drugs
   (4) Openly acquiring similar drugs from other medical sources
   (5) Unsanctioned dose escalation or other noncompliance with therapy on one or two occasions
   (6) Unapproved use of the drug to treat another symptom
   (7) Reporting psychological effects not intended by the clinician
   (8) Resistance to a change in therapy associated with tolerable adverse effects with expressions of anxiety related to return of severe symptoms

3. The Addiction Behaviors Checklist (ABC) may be useful in evaluating adverse behaviors (see Appendix 18-1)

D. Addiction: Clarifying terms related to addiction can decrease concerns regarding the existence of addiction and assist the clinician in identifying patients at risk (see the chapter on Taxonomy for Pain Management Nursing).

E. Controlled substance regulation

1. The Drug Enforcement Administration (DEA) of the U.S. government determines the schedule for drugs. Enforcement is focused on drug diversion. The use of opioids to treat pain is supported by the DEA.
2. Additional guidelines are set by individual states. Programs to regulate controlled substances differ from state to state.
3. Examples of programs strongly favored by those in regulatory and law enforcement include the following.
   a. *Triplicate prescription program:* This program requires prescribers to write prescriptions for Schedule II drugs on special state-issued triplicate prescription pads. A copy of the prescription stays with the prescribing physician, the patient's copy stays with the pharmacist, and one copy is sent to the state.
   b. *Official prescription program:* This program requires prescribers to write prescriptions for Schedule II drugs on a single state-issued prescription instead of the three-part form and for the electronic transmission of prescription information from the pharmacy to the program.
   c. *National All Schedules Prescription Electronic Reporting (NASPER) Act:* An organization obtained federal funds to set up databases nationwide to track prescribing patterns and allowed prescribers to have access to information about where and when patients received opioid prescriptions (Brumas & Shoemaker, 2005; Elliott, 2004; Miles & Souvall, 2005; NASPER.org, 2005a, 2005b; Wehrman, 2005.
      (1) The goal was to be able to identify the "doctor-shopper." The assumption was that doctor-shoppers only had the intention of diverting prescription opioids into an illegal realm.
      (2) This legislation was successful in 2005 but has no funding at the present time. It would prevent interstate doctor-shopping by people seeking multiple prescriptions of controlled substances.
         (a) Critics' state that this is a government form of meddling into the delivery of appropriate pain medicine and that it undermines medicine and the care of the dying (Elliott, 2004). The fear is that the DEA antidiversion efforts focus on physicians, making them criminals.
         (b) Proponents of this tracking mechanism state that it is designed to prevent doctors from becoming criminals by alerting prescribers when patients might be doctor-shopping.
         (c) The prescription drug monitoring bill was designed to ensure that health care practitioners have information they need to provide safe, timely, and effective treatment for pain and other medical conditions (Brumas & Shoemaker, 2005; Miles & Souvall, 2005).

(d) This monitor would be effective across state lines and would give the health care practitioner the capability to check a patient's prescription drug activity before writing a new prescription (Wehrman, 2005).

(e) The introduction of House file-1132 and Senate file-518 on March 3, 2005, to the 109th Congress was to provide a national databank called NASPER that would help establish or improve state-run prescription drug monitoring programs.

(f) Senate file-518 was written by Senators Jeff Sessions (R-AL) and Dick Durbin (D-IL) and cosponsored by Senators Edward Kennedy (D-MA) and Christopher Dodd (D-CT).

(g) Congressmen Ed Whitfield (R-KY) and Frank Pallone (D-NJ) wrote House file-1132. In August 2005, President George W. Bush signed the bills intended to improve quality patient care in pain management and provide accountability for prescription opioids (NASPER.org, 2005a, 2005b).

(h) On May 26, 2007, Governor Timothy Pallenty in Minnesota signed NASPER into law. This law intended to improve patient access and prevent doctor-shopping and drug diversion when patients receive prescriptions from multiple prescribers to treat the same pain problem. There would be access to patient records to show what controlled substances have already been prescribed.

4. Programs of this type were designed to address the diversion of Schedule II drugs to the street. In November, 2008, 38 states enacted legislation for prescription drug monitoring programs (DEA, 2008).
5. Despite the growing body of knowledge regarding the appropriateness of the use of opioids for the treatment of chronic nonmalignant pain, a reluctance remains on the part of many practitioners to prescribe opioids for chronic nonmalignant pain.

F. Model guidelines for the use of controlled substances for the treatment of chronic nonmalignant pain

1. The Federation of State Medical Boards of the United States (1998) initiated the development of model guidelines for state medical boards and other health care regulatory agencies to use in regulating the prescribing of controlled substances, such as opioids, in the management of chronic cancer and noncancer pain.
2. The efforts of the federation encourage the medical community to adopt consistent standards, promote public health by facilitating the provision of adequate and effective pain management, and increase the awareness and education of the medical community on the treatment of chronic pain within the boundaries of professional practice.
3. The intention is to protect legitimate medical uses of controlled substances while preventing diversion.
4. Opioid administration for noncancer chronic pain shows documentation of
   a. Selection of opioid.
   b. Type or origin of pain.
   c. History of trials of various agents and effects of these trials.
   d. Intensity of pain.
   e. History of tolerance.
   f. History of chemical dependency.
5. Escalation
   a. If one opioid is being changed to another, the equianalgesic charts offer the clinician guidelines for conversion.
   b. An updated equianalgesic chart can be found in the APS guidelines (2008).
6. Teaching issues for patients on opioid therapy include
   a. Necessity of bowel regimen.
   b. Signs and symptoms of opioid withdrawal.
   c. Signs and symptoms of opioid escalation (i.e., early refill requested or frequent requests for increases in dosage).
   d. Monitoring of side effects.

   e. Nonmedicine modalities for pain management to be used in parallel with opioid medicines.
   f. Location of local pharmacies carrying the medication.
7. Teaching issues for patients on transdermal fentanyl are as follows.
   a. Understand the necessity of a bowel program.
   b. Take the backing off of the patch to expose a sticky surface to apply to the skin.
   c. Rotate the patch placement site. The patient should be instructed not to shave or prepare the site with alcohol. Avoid heating pad over patch.
   d. Prepare the skin, keeping the skin dry and intact. The patient may need to use a transparent dressing over the patch to maintain contact of the patch with the skin.
   e. Hold a hand over the patch for a full minute immediately after placing on the skin. This aids in skin adherence.
   f. Do not cut off block areas of the patch. Instruct the patient in patch placement.
   g. Properly dispose of a used patch.
   h. Understand what to do if the patch falls off.
   i. Watch for signs and symptoms of withdrawal.
   j. Monitor side effects.
   k. Know the location of local pharmacies carrying the medication.
   l. Understand the cost of long-term medication and availability of patient assistance programs, use of generic forms, or both.
8. Nursing considerations before rectal administration of medication (see the chapter on Overview of Pharmacology).
   a. Administration is contraindicated with rectal irritation, rectal bleeding, diarrhea, hemorrhoids, or low platelets.
   b. Suppository as a vehicle
      (1) If a suppository softens, it must be hardened before insertion; this can be achieved by keeping it refrigerated or running it under cold water.
      (2) Insert the suppository above the internal anal sphincter (2 to 3 inches).
      (3) The dose of the suppository cannot be divided by cutting the suppository because the medicine may not be distributed evenly throughout the suppository.
      (4) Drug is released at a slow, steady rate.
      (5) An evacuant enema may be helpful to ensure rectal contents will not get in the way of absorption of the medication (McKenry & Salerno, 1998).
9. Patient-controlled analgesia may be used for acute pain episodes superimposed on chronic noncancer pain to determine requirements for dosing change in baseline pain management (see the chapter on Taxonomy for Pain Management Nursing).

PART THREE: INTERVENTIONAL THERAPIES

I. Intraspinal Infusions of Opioids Used for the Treatment of Persistent Pain (Gianino, York, & Paice, 1996; Markman & Philip, 2007)

A. Epidural and intrathecal opioid administration is an invasive and effective option for patients with pain that is refractory to conventional therapies.

B. Intraspinal anatomy and physiology

1. Epidural route
   a. Epidural space is potential space that surrounds the tissue of the spinal cord.
   b. The epidural space is surrounded by the ligamentum flavum and the dura mater.
   c. Contents of the epidural space are a vascular network of large-bore, thin-walled veins; nerve root; and fat that is directly proportional to the body fat in the individual.
   d. Catheter insertion into the epidural space necessitates penetrating through the ligamentum flavum with a technique that the interventional physician uses called *loss of resistance.*
   e. Medications that enter the epidural space diffuse through the dura, where there is uptake

by the CSF in the intrathecal space. The action of the opioid medication is at the spinal cord, specifically, the substantia gelatinosa.

2. Intrathecal route
   a. Intrathecal space contains CSF.
   b. The intrathecal space is surrounded by the arachnoid mater (lying next to the dura mater) and the pia mater (surrounding the spinal cord).
   c. The intrathecal space runs parallel to the epidural space and directly surrounds the spinal cord.
3. The term *intraspinal* encompasses both the epidural space and the intrathecal space.
   a. The term *spinal space* describes the intrathecal space.
   b. The terms *peridural* and *extradural* describe the epidural space.

C. Pharmacodynamics and pharmacokinetics of the intraspinal space
1. When medication instilled into the epidural space diffuses through the dura mater, the rate of diffusion depends on the lipid solubility of the medicine.
2. Examples of high-lipid-soluble medications are fentanyl, sufentanil citrate and hydromorphone. These diffuse through the dura, bind at the spinal cord at a rapid rate, and produce a narrow segment of analgesia.
3. An example of high-water-soluble medication is morphine sulfate. Morphine diffuses through the dura slowly and acts at the spinal cord. The CSF is water based. The water-soluble medication shows affinity to water-based CSF and spreads with the CSF flow.
4. *Rostral spread:* The water-soluble medicine spreads with the flow of the CSF.
5. All opioids in the intraspinal space bind with the opiate receptors at the substantia gelatinosa of the spinal cord.
6. The substantia gelatinosa lies at laminae 2 and 3 and contains opiate receptors.
7. When exogenous opioid binds at the opiate receptor at the substantia gelatinosa, analgesia occurs.
8. Opioids used in intraspinal analgesia need to be preservative free to avoid a toxic effect on the spinal cord.
9. Local anesthetic agents in the intraspinal space
   a. Local anesthetics are lipid soluble.
   b. Analgesia and anesthesia effects are dose related.
   c. Action occurs at the sympathetic chain ganglion (see the chapter on Overview of Pharmacology).

D. Types of infusion devices for spinal infusions (Du Pen, 2005; Staats & Luthardt, 2005)
1. Implantable epidural portal system
   a. The epidural catheter is threaded percutaneously around the flank to the front of the body.
   b. The epidural port is implanted over the lower ribs for stability.
   c. The catheter is connected to the port.
   d. The port allows easy access to the epidural space so that infusions can be connected to the port via a noncoring needle, or the medication can be injected into the port through a noncoring needle.
   e. The epidural port contains a filter to remove large particulate.
2. External percutaneous long-term epidural catheter
   a. The epidural catheter is threaded percutaneously around the flank to the front of the body, where it exits.
   b. An ambulatory external infusion pump is connected to this access.
   c. Dressing changes over the exit site are needed regularly.
      (1) Alcohol is contraindicated for preparing the site or accessing the catheter because of the potential for migration of alcohol into the epidural space, causing nerve destruction.
      (2) Povidone–iodine may be used.
      (3) A 0.22 micron filter without surfactant should be used for medication administration.
   d. The catheter stays in place by a percutaneous adhering cuff.

3. Implanted infusion pumps
   a. Devices that continually infuse concentrated medication into an intrathecal or epidural space may be used for spasms related to SCI (spinal cord injury), cancer pain, or chronic low back pain responsive to a test dose.
   b. A small pump placed in the abdomen delivers pain medication to the intrathecal or epidural space.
   c. Minimal amounts of opioid can provide substantial relief with minimal side effects.
   d. These pumps can be used to administer opioid, local anesthetic, γ-aminobutyric acid (GABA) agonist and other adjuvants, although preservative-free morphine, ziconotide, and baclofen (Lioresal®) are the only U.S. Food and Drug Administration-approved medications (Erdine & De Andres, 2006).
   e. Pumps are manufactured with varied flow rates, sizes, and volume capacities.
   f. Pumps can be programmed externally using telemetry.

E. Indications for use and criteria for patient selection for implantable devices (Staats & Luthardt, 2005)
   1. Pain is refractory to conventional therapy.
   2. Intolerable side effects from other routes of administration are present.
   3. Pain is responsive to test dosing.
   4. The patient is physiologically stable and able to tolerate insertion and implantation.
   5. No contraindication exists to epidural or intrathecal placement.
      a. There is no anticoagulant therapy or coagulation disorders.
      b. There is no intraspinal infection.
      c. Active or untreated bacterial infection is absent.
   6. Psychological evaluation indicates emotional stability.
   7. An adequate support system is in place to facilitate care and refills of pump.
   8. Life expectancy of months to years warrants the cost of inserting the device.
   9. Insertion and care are financially feasible (insurance or self-payment). Cost of the delivery system, drugs, needles, and supplies is discussed with patient before implantation.

F. Patient teaching preoperatively
   1. Intraspinal infusion requires implantation of the delivery system in the operating room.
   2. The patient will experience acute postoperative pain at the pump pocket site, back incision, or both.
   3. The patient should be instructed not to wear constrictive clothing or a seat belt over the pump pocket site.
      a. Teaching points
         (1) The patient should know the signs and symptoms of infections, including pump pocket site and back incision site infection signs and signs of meningitis.
         (2) The patient should understand the necessity of a bowel regimen.
         (3) Signs and symptoms of withdrawal should be noted.
         (4) The patient should monitor side effects.
         (5) The patient should carry identification and Medic-alert information at all times.
         (6) The patient should notify the clinician of pending air travel plans; pumps are altitude sensitive.
         (7) The patient should notify the clinician of fever and use a hot tub or heating pad with caution. Elevated body temperature may increase an intrathecal pump's rate of infusion.
         (8) Medtronic (Minneapolis, MN) and Arrow (Reading, PA) pumps are compatible with MRI use. The Medtronic pump must be reassessed after MRI with the programmer for verification of ordered infusion settings.
         (9) Discuss any activity restrictions with the patient.

G. Medication management
   1. All intraspinal solutions must be preservative free because of potential for neurotoxicity.
   2. *Caution:* If the patient has an older Medtronic SynchroMed pump, it may have a side port that can be accessed during a refill, and the patient could be overdosed accidentally.

3. Frequency of refill depends on the rate of infusion and the concentration of the medication.
4. Common intraspinal opioids through pump infusion include morphine, hydromorphone, and fentanyl.
5. A pump is often used in combination with systemic adjuvant analgesics.

H. Opioid infusions
1. Indication: Chronic pain patients are unresponsive to other therapeutic modalities.
2. Medications: Morphine, hydromorphone, fentanyl, and sufentanil citrate are options.
3. Dosing: Epidural opioid doses of hydrophilic opioid are significantly smaller than dosages by oral or parenteral route (APS, 2003)
   a. The relative dosage value is the dosage difference between various drug delivery routes. There is a 10-fold difference in the effective epidural dose of morphine compared to the effective intrathecal dose.
   b. Examples of morphine equivalent doses are 30 mg orally (when administered on a regular schedule), 10 mg intravenously, 1 mg of epidural, or approximately 0.1 mg of intrathecal (APS, 2003, p. 24)

I. Local anesthetic infusions
1. Indication: Chronic pain patients are unresponsive to other therapeutic modalities and have pain that is neuropathic.
2. Medications: Bupivacaine and ropivacaine can be used.
3. Dosing: With the initial dose, monitor continuous intravenous access, cardiac status, oxygen saturation, mental status, blood pressure, and pulse.
4. Side effects
   a. Nausea, tinnitus, metallic taste, lightheadedness, drowsiness, and agitation are typical side effects. Anxiety and psychosis are rare side effects.
   b. Moderate toxicity leads to vision difficulty, nystagmus, slurred speech, dysarthria, numbness of lips and tongue, and tingling or heavy feeling in the extremities.
   c. Late and central nervous system toxicity leads to hypotension or hypertension, seizures, anaphylaxis, and unconsciousness. Cardiac and respiratory failure, coma, and death may occur in the late stages of central nervous system toxicity.

J. γ-Aminobutyric acid (GABA) agonist infusion (baclofen)
1. Indications: Chronic spinal spasticity patients or patients with neuropathic pain should receive this infusion.
2. Medication: Baclofen can be used.
3. Dosage: Titrate to effect. With the initial dose, monitor continuous intravenous access, cardiac status, oxygen saturation, mentation monitoring, blood pressure, and pulse every 5 minutes.

K. Other additives with opioids
1. α_2-Agonists: clonidine, epinephrine, dexmedetomidine, tizanidine
2. *N*-methyl-D-aspartate receptor antagonist: ketamine
3. N-type (neuronal specific) calcium channel blocker: ziconotide (Prialt®)]

L. Outcome measures for persistent pain patients
1. Increase function.
2. Improve quality of life.
3. Improve pain control.

II. Peripheral Nerve Stimulation and Spinal Cord Stimulation

A. Electrical stimulation along a nerve or nerve root uses varying pulse width and amplitudes to decrease pain transmission.
1. Peripheral nerve stimulation limits paresthesias to the distribution of the nerve transmitting pain (Schon & Davies, 2005).
2. Spinal cord stimulation provides paresthesias to a large portion of the extremity.

B. The most common indication is failed back surgery syndrome. Others include CRPS-I and CRPS-II, direct nerve injury, intractable angina pectoris, multiple sclerosis, phantom limb pain, and lower extremity spasticity (North, 2005).

C. Considerations for implantation
   1. An established and specific diagnosis should exist for the pain.
   2. Other treatment modalities (pharmacological, surgical, physical, or psychological therapies) have been tried and do not prove satisfactory, have been judged unsuitable, or are contraindicated for the patient.
   3. The patient has undergone careful screening and diagnosis by a multidisciplinary team before implantation.
   4. All facilities, equipment, and professional support personnel required for the proper diagnosis, treatment, training, and follow-up of the patient are available.
   5. Demonstration of pain relief with a temporary implanted electrode precedes permanent implantation.

D. Contraindications
   1. The patient fails the screening.
   2. The patient is averse to electrical stimulation.
   3. The patient is averse to an implant as a modality.
   4. There is an active and uncontrolled coagulopathy.
   5. Localized or disseminated infection is found.
   6. The physician lacks the necessary experience or training.
   7. The patient has a demand cardiac pacemaker, defibrillator, or both.
   8. The patient needs MRI in the immediate foreseeable future.

E. Risks associated with spinal cord stimulation surgery include
   1. Bleeding.
   2. Headache and CSF leak.
   3. Hardware or equipment difficulties, generator failure, and electrode migration or malposition.
   4. Spinal cord or nerve injury.
   5. Infection.
   6. Allergic reactions.
   7. Exposure to electromagnetic fields (security systems).
   8. Failure to relieve pain.

F. Patient education
   1. Explain activity restrictions to prevent the lead from moving (10 to 12 hours after implantation of neurostimulator).
   2. Describe how to make computerized adjustments using a graphic input device.

III. Nursing Care for Patients with Intraspinal Analgesia (Gilfor & Viscusi, 2005)

A. Patient care requires careful monitoring.

B. Site care
   1. Inspect the site for swelling, redness, hematoma, and drainage.
   2. The dressing should be dry, intact, and sterile.
   3. The catheter should be intact with proper placement.
   4. Tubing and connections should be assessed for patency.

C. Response to analgesia
   1. With adequate analgesia, continue to monitor routinely.
   2. With inadequate pain relief, investigate further, looking for the following:
      a. Insufficient dosages of opioids and local anesthetics
         (1) Administer bolus or breakthrough medication.
         (2) Contact the prescriber for changes to medication orders.
      b. Undetermined surgical complication
      c. Advancing disease process
      d. Infection
         (1) Check for elevated temperature.
         (2) Look for redness, swelling, or drainage at the catheter insertion site.
         (3) Determine whether there is pain at the catheter insertion site.

e. Epidural catheter migration
    (1) Notify the anesthesiologist immediately for suspected catheter migration.
    (2) Placement needs to be assessed.

D. Side effects
1. Respiratory depression
    a. Apnea monitor may be ineffective if the patient is receiving supplemental oxygen.
    b. Capnography can be used.
2. Mental status changes such as confusion or sedation, possibly indicating that the patient is receiving too much opioid
    a. Reduce or stop the opioid.
    b. Administer naloxone.
3. Excessive somnolence or confusion
4. Nausea and vomiting
5. Urinary retention
6. Pruritus
7. Constipation
8. Numbness in the lower extremities with epidural administration
    a. Check bowel and bladder function.
    b. The patient may have difficulty or be unable to ambulate.

IV. Nonneuroablative Interventional Techniques

A. Trigger point injections
1. Injection of a trigger point (a palpably firm, tense band in a muscle) is with local anesthetic, steroid, or botulinum toxin. A twitch response, also known as ***hyperstimulation analgesia,*** helps identify the trigger point (Benzon, 1996). Dry needling is the injection of trigger points without instilling medication (Gunn, 2001; Molloy, 2005a).
2. Mechanisms for trigger point development
    a. Trauma locally tears the sarcoplasmic reticulum and releases calcium.
    b. The calcium and the available adenosine triphosphate continuously activate local contractile activity. The intense muscle metabolic activity produces substances that sensitize sensory nerve endings.
    c. Restricted stretch range of motion is produced; weakness and atrophy of muscle are seen with no neurological defect.
    d. Localized vasoconstriction reflex is stimulated to control runaway metabolic activity (Benzon, 1996; Travell & Simons, 1983).
3. Indications include the presence of myofascial trigger points (described earlier).
4. Procedure
    a. A trigger point is singled out.
    b. Skin is prepared with povidone-iodine (if not allergic).
    c. A 22-gauge (or smaller) needle is inserted into the trigger point.
    d. The syringe is aspirated and medication (steroid, local anesthetic, or combination of these or Botox®) is instilled. The amount instilled depends on the size of muscle and location of the trigger point in the body.
5. Advantages
    a. The procedure is simple.
    b. Deep infiltration of local anesthetic medication provides immediate relief of muscular pain.
    c. Physical therapy may perform myofascial release therapy immediately after the procedure to break up the trigger point.
    d. Numbness is present for the length of time the local anesthetic creates anesthesia.
    e. Botulinum toxin may produce longer effects than other medications (Molloy, 2005a). Of note, one reference states that there may be little difference in outcomes between saline placebo and Botox® for neck or low back pain (Lew, Lee, Castaneda, Klima, & Date, 2008).

6. Disadvantages and potential complications (Alvarez & Rockwell, 2002; Benzon, 1996)
   a. The procedure may need to be repeated several times to produce long-lasting effects (Benzon, 1996).
   b. It involves a needle, which some patients may not want.
   c. There is potential for pneumothorax with deep chest wall injections.
   d. Local scarring is possible after repeated injection.
   e. Vasovagal syncope is possible.
   f. Skin infection can occur.
   g. Hemothorax may occur.
   h. Needle breakage is possible.
7. Contraindications are as follows (Alvarez & Rockwell, 2002):
   a. Anticoagulation or bleeding disorders
   b. Aspirin ingestion within 3 days of injection
   c. The presence of local or systemic infection
   d. Allergy to anesthetic agents or Botox®
   e. Acute muscle trauma
   f. Extreme fear of needles
8. Nursing interventions include the following:
   a. Patient education
   b. Informed consent
   c. Administration of the procedure if allowed by the state nurse practice act
   d. Monitoring for side effects and complications

B. Joint and bursa injections (Cardone & Tallia, 2002)
   1. Intraarticular injections are made (into the joint) for either diagnostic or therapeutic reasons.
      a. Injection of steroid, local anesthetic, or both or one of the hyaluronates is into the cavity of the joint (Benzon, 1996; About.com, 2008).
      b. Mechanisms
         (1) Corticosteroids (e.g., betamethasone, methylprednisolone, triamcinolone) reduce inflammation. Low-solubility corticosteroid agents (e.g., dexamethasone) should not be used for soft tissue injection due to the increased risk of surrounding tissue atrophy.
         (2) Local anesthetics (e.g., bupivacaine or lidocaine) provide localized numbness to the joint.
         (3) Hyaluronates (e.g., Synvisc®) act as viscosupplementation. The injection of gellike substances (hyaluronates) into a joint supplements the viscous properties of synovial fluid.
      c. Indications include the following:
         (1) Crystalloid arthropathies
         (2) Synovitis
         (3) Inflammatory arthritis
         (4) Advanced osteoarthritis
         (5) Aspiration for diagnostic purposes (effusion of unknown origin or suspected infection)
      d. Procedure
         (1) Joint space is defined.
         (2) Skin is prepared with povidone-iodine.
         (3) The needle is inserted in the joint space.
         (4) Medication is instilled or aspiration is accomplished, and the needle is removed.
      e. Advantage: Analgesia is effective and at times improves mobility.
      f. Disadvantages
         (1) A skilled clinician is needed to perform the procedure because it is difficult to access the joint space.
         (2) The patient should be informed that the procedure may be painful and risk of infection is present.
         (3) Injection into tendon may cause rupture.

g. Contraindications
   (1) Absolute contraindications are as follows:
      (a) Local cellulitis
      (b) Septic arthritis
      (c) Acute fracture
      (d) Bacteremia
      (e) Joint prosthesis
      (f) Achilles or patella tendinopathies
      (g) History of allergy or anaphylaxis to injectable pharmaceuticals or constituents
   (2) Relative contraindications are as follows:
      (a) Minimal relief after two previous corticosteroid injections
      (b) Underlying coagulopathy
      (c) Anticoagulation therapy
      (d) Evidence of surrounding joint osteoporosis
      (e) Anatomically inaccessible joints
      (f) Uncontrolled diabetes mellitus

2. Extraarticular (bursa) injections (outside the joint)
   a. Injection of steroid or local anesthetic or both is outside the cavity of the joint.
   b. Mechanisms
      (1) The injection reduces inflammation and creates localized numbness to the muscular support of the joint.
      (2) Medications used are steroids with or without local anesthetics (without epinephrine).
   c. Indication
      (1) The patient has pain with palpation over the bursa or soft tissue conditions, including
         (a) Bursitis.
         (b) Tendonitis or tendinosis.
         (c) Trigger points.
         (d) Ganglion cysts.
         (e) Neuromas.
         (f) Entrapment syndromes.
         (g) Fasciitis.
   d. Procedure
      (1) The painful bursa site is palpated.
      (2) Skin is prepared with povidone-iodine.
      (3) A needle is inserted into bursa area only, not into the joint.
      (4) Medication (steroid, local anesthetic, or both) is instilled into the area. The amount depends on the bursae location.
   e. Advantages
      (1) The procedure is simple.
      (2) Short-term relief of pain is effective.
      (3) Physical therapy supports the procedure by increasing strength of the musculature surrounding the joint and enhancing range of motion.
   f. Disadvantages and potential complications include the following:
      (1) Short-term relief of pain
      (2) Small risk of infection
      (3) Soft tissue (fatty) atrophy
      (4) Depigmentation at site
      (5) Periarticular calcifications
      (6) Tendon rupture
      (7) Hyperglycemia in diabetic patients
   g. Contraindications are the same as those for joint injections, as described earlier.

h. Relief occurs within 10 to 15 minutes postinjection and lasts 8 to 12 hours (Bonica & Buckley, 1990).
i. Nursing interventions include the following:
(1) Patient education
(2) Informed consent
(3) Administration of the procedure if allowed by the state nurse practice act
(4) Monitoring for side effects and complications

C. Intercostal block (Molloy, 2005b)
1. A local anesthetic, steroid, phenol, or alcohol is injected into the intercostal space.
2. Mechanisms
a. Steroid reduces inflammation at the intercostal spaces and around the site of injection.
b. Local anesthetic creates localized numbness.
c. Phenol or alcohol kills nerve tissue, thereby interrupting pain transmission.
3. Patient selection for neurolytic blocks (Patt & Burton, 1999)
a. Pain is severe.
b. Pain is expected to persist.
c. Pain is not modified by less invasive means.
d. Pain is well localized (e.g., rib metastasis).
e. Pain is well characterized.
f. Pain is not multifocal.
g. Pain is of somatic or visceral origin.
h. Life expectancy is limited.
4. Indications are as follows:
a. Postherpetic neuralgia along the thoracic dermatome
b. Surgical incisions
c. Fractured ribs
d. Rib boney metastasis
e. Chest tubes
5. The procedure should be performed by a trained clinician.
6. The patient should be told to notify the physician about any difficulty breathing, shortness of breath, pain with breathing, and unusual chest pain
7. Advantages
a. The block provides localized analgesia to a painful area.
b. The patient has improved respiratory function (Narchi, Singelyn, & Paqueron, 2008).
8. Disadvantages
a. There is the risk of a needle penetrating through to the intrapleural space, creating a pneumothorax.
b. Systemic toxicity can occur from local anesthetic absorption and hypotension.
c. There is the potential for necrosis at skin level when phenol or alcohol is used.
9. Contraindications are as follows:
a. Allergy to medication instilled
b. Infection in the area
10. The effect of the block lasts 10 to 12 hours using local anesthetic (Bonica & Buckley, 1990).
11. The effect of the block may last 6 to 10 months if phenol or alcohol is used (Jain & Gupta, 2001).
12. Postprocedure nursing interventions specific to intercostal blocks are
a. Dyspnea possibly related to puncture of the lung.
b. Unusual chest pain.
13. The long-term potential for skin necrosis if phenol or alcohol is the injectant.

D. Epidural injections (Benzon, 1996; Waldman, 2004a, 2004b, 2004d, 2004e, 2004i, 2004j).
1. Medication is injected into the epidural space.
a. Medications may be steroid (betamethasone, methylprednisolone, or triamcinolone), local anesthetic (bupivacaine, ropivacaine, or lidocaine), opioid, or some combination of these.

- (1) Steroids medications
  - (a) The mechanism reduces inflammation of a specific location in the epidural space.
  - (b) Indications are as follows:
    - (i) Generalized spine pain
    - (ii) Spinal stenosis
    - (iii) Radicular pain
    - (iv) Disc herniations
- (2) Local anesthetics
  - (a) The mechanism is anesthesia for either diagnostic injections or ongoing pain relief.
  - (b) Indications are as follows:
    - (i) Identifying the site potentially causing pain that might warrant surgical intervention (assist surgeons in this)
    - (ii) Pain relief for site-specific pain (e.g., chest tubes, vertebral fractures, CRPS, or cancer pain syndromes)
    - (iii) Postsurgical pain relief
- (3) Opioids
  - (a) The mechanism is deposit of the opioid near the spinal cord or spinal nerves.
  - (b) Indications are as follows:
    - (i) Postsurgical pain relief
    - (ii) Cancer pain relief

2. Procedure
   - a. Fluoroscopy with contrast dye may be used to confirm needle placement.
   - b. All medications injected into the epidural space must be preservative free.
   - c. All contrast material injected into the epidural or intrathecal space must be nonionic.
   - d. Cervical, thoracic, or lumbar injection can be accomplished by one of three methods:
     - (1) Translaminar: The Tuohy needle is placed between two vertebrae and advanced into the epidural space using fluoroscopic guidance and a loss-of-resistance syringe.
       - (a) Medications with or without preservative-free saline are injected after confirmation of epidural space with the injection of contrast dye.
       - (b) This method of epidural administration is used best in patients with generalized spinal pain, spinal stenosis, multiple-level disc herniations and bulges, multiple-level disc degeneration, and posterior disc herniations.
     - (2) Transforaminal: The spinal needle is placed into the neural foramen of the affected nerve root using fluoroscopic guidance.
       - (a) The nerve root and epidural space are confirmed by the injection of contrast dye.
       - (b) Medications are injected into the epidural space. This method provides a medication covering of the affected nerve root.
       - (c) This method is preferred for patients with pain generating from one or two specific nerve roots verified on CT scan, myelography, or MRI and through physical assessment.
         - (i) These patients generally have unilateral pain (Finch & Taylor, 1996).
         - (ii) Due to the proximity of vascular structures, the use of cervical steroids using this technique carries the risk of cerebral vascular events.
         - (iii) For this reason, many clinicians do not prefer this method.
     - (3) Caudal: The Tuohy needle is inserted into the caudal canal using fluoroscopic guidance and the loss-of-resistance technique.
       - (a) Steroid and local anesthetic with or without preservative-free saline are injected after confirmation of epidural space with the injection of contrast dye.
       - (b) This method is useful in the presence of an extant scar from prior surgery, as an alternative to other approaches, and as assurance of steroid placement close to the sacral nerves (Candido & Nader, 2005).

3. Advantages
   a. These techniques are known to many practitioners and are widely available.
   b. The procedures can be done on an outpatient basis.
   c. The procedures are normally of low risk and can be done at all clinically necessary spinal levels.
   d. When the patient is given local anesthetics, steroids, opioids, or a combination of these, two or three active treatments may be simultaneously given.
   e. Positive results may change the patient's attitude about medication use, need for surgery, and participation in rehabilitation.
   f. Money can be saved if surgery, long convalescence, and work interruption are avoided.
4. Disadvantages
   a. There is the potential for reaction to the local anesthetic, the corticosteroid injected, the opioid, or the contrast dye.
   b. There is a risk of tissue trauma with the occurrence of bleeding, infection, or ligamentous pain. If the needle punctures the dura, there is risk of postdural puncture headache (also known as a positional headache).
   c. The treatment may not help the patient overcome discouragement and loss of hope.
   d. Few studies clearly define which patients are the most appropriate for this treatment (Benzon, 1996).
   e. Repeated use of steroids may cause epidural lipomatosis and a worsening of spinal symptoms (Burkhardt & Hamann, 2006; Sandberg & Lavyne, 1999).
5. Efficacy
   a. Studies vary in their reports of efficacy of epidural steroid injections (Abdi et al., 2007; Armon et al., 2007; Benzon, 1996, 2005; Erjavec, 2001; Molloy & Benzon, 2005).
   b. In a review of the extant literature from April 2003 through February 2005, a subcommittee of the American Academy of Neurology concluded that, in general, epidural steroid injections for radicular lumbosacral pain have shown no impact on average impairment of function, on need for surgery, or on long-term pain relief beyond 3 months (Armon et al., 2007).
6. Nursing interventions
   a. Educate the patient.
   b. Assure informed consent.
   c. Assure that sterile technique is maintained during the procedure.
   d. Administer the procedure if allowed by the state nurse practice act.
   e. Immediately postprocedure, monitor the following:
      (1) Vital signs as per conscious sedation policy
      (2) Local bleeding at the site of injection
      (3) Ability to stand alone, especially if local anesthetic is injected close to the lumbar nerve root

E. Facet blocks
   1. A steroid with or without local anesthetic is injected into the facet joints (true synovial joints that connect adjacent vertebrae posteriorly) or median branch block of the posterior primary ramus (Ashburn & Rice, 1998; Clemans & Benzon, 2005; Waldman, 2004f, 2004k).
      a. These patients complain of hip and buttock pain; pain with extension of the back, neck, or thorax and when the back is manipulated over the involved facet joint; cramping lower extremity pain that does not go below the knee; and morning low back stiffness.
      b. Pain is commonly aggravated by prolonged sitting or standing. Patients may experience paraspinous muscle spasms.
      c. Pain in the hip, buttock, or low back may be present with a straight-leg raise.
      d. Facet joint pain is described as a dull, deep aching pain in the back and hips with some radiation to the knee (Clemans & Benzon, 2005; Neumann & Raj, 2000).
   2. Mechanisms: The injection of local anesthetic and steroid surrounds the posterior ramus nerve, innervating the joint, which decreases inflammation and eliminates pain (Neumann & Raj, 2000).
   3. These injections may be diagnostic or therapeutic.

4. Therapeutic indications are as follows:
   a. Facet syndrome related to inflammation
   b. Arthritis or segmental instability
   c. Focal tenderness over the facet joint
   d. Chronic low back pain with or without radiation
   e. Back pain with evidence of disc disease
   f. Facet arthritis
   g. Postlaminectomy syndrome
   h. Recurrent disc disease
5. Procedure: The procedure is performed using fluoroscopy (Ashburn & Rice, 1998).
6. Advantage: Immediate relief of pain occurs after the block in 54% to 65% of patients (Neumann & Raj, 2000).
7. Disadvantage: The procedure may need to be repeated because 20% to 30% of patients have relief for only 6 months (Neumann & Raj, 2000).
8. Contraindications include the following:
   a. Infection in overlying soft tissues (Neumann & Raj, 2000)
   b. Coagulation problems
9. Efficacy: Pain relief is experienced in 54% to 65% of patients initially; 20% to 30% reported relief longer than 6 months (Neumann & Raj, 2000).
10. Nursing interventions
   a. Educate the patient.
   b. Assure informed consent.
   c. Assure that sterile technique is used during the procedure.
   d. Administer the procedure if allowed by the state nurse practice act.
   e. Immediately postprocedure, monitor the following:
      (1) Vital signs as per conscious sedation policy
      (2) Local bleeding at the site of injection
      (3) Ability to stand alone if a lumbar local anesthetic is injected

F. Intravenous regional block (Bier block)
1. A medication (e.g., bretylium, reserpine, lidocaine, or clonidine) is injected into an exsanguinated extremity (Reuben & Sklar, 2002; Williams, Neumann, Goel, & Wu, 2008).
2. Mechanisms: Injected medications bind to sympathetic nerve endings and block the sympathetic response (Buckley, 2001).
3. Indication: CRPS of the extremities is the indicator.
4. Procedure
   a. An intravenous catheter is inserted into the involved extremity, and a second intravenous catheter is inserted in another extremity to allow rapid intravenous access.
   b. A rubber wrap is applied tightly to the limb to exsanguinate the extremity
   c. A tourniquet is applied to the involved extremity, and the pressure is raised per protocol of the interventional physician.
   d. The wrap is removed
   e. The medication is injected into the intravenous catheter in the affected limb, and the tourniquet is left on 30 to 45 minutes.
   f. After this time, the pressure is released a few seconds, and the patient is observed for side effects.
   g. The tourniquet is inflated and released two to three times during the next 5 minutes, and the patient is observed for side effects.
5. Advantages
   a. The procedure provides longer exposure of the nerve endings to the injected drugs.
   b. It reduces systemic side effects (Williams et al., 2008).
6. Disadvantages
   a. Postural hypotension, flushing, and burning can occur on injection (Williams et al., 2008).
   b. Use of a tourniquet or rubber band device is uncomfortable on an already-painful extremity.
7. Pain relief lasts 4 to 7 days (Buckley, 2001).

G. Sympathetic blocks
   1. A local anesthetic is injected into a sympathetic ganglion.
   2. Mechanism: This blocks pain transmission at the sympathetic chain ganglion.
   3. Indication: Sympathetic blocks can be used to treat CRPSs or painful extremities, phantom limb pain, and vascular disease.
   4. The following procedures should be performed by an anesthesiologist.
      a. Stellate ganglion block
         (1) Intravenous access is established in case intravascular injection, seizure activity, or full spinal block occurs.
            (a) The patient lies or sits with the neck slightly hyperextended by placing a roll between the shoulder blades.
            (b) The clinician palpates for the anterior tubercle of C6.
            (c) A needle is inserted into the neck into the stellate ganglion, which lies near C6 and C7.
            (d) A test dose is injected, and the patient is watched for toxic effects. After repeat aspiration, the anesthetic is injected in divided doses.
            (e) This may be done with fluoroscopy and contrast material to confirm needle placement.
         (2) Sympathetic blockade to the head and affected arm elevates the temperature of the arm on the side of the block; causes myosis, ptosis, and enophthalmos on the side of the block; and leads to throat numbness. The arm on the injected side may be weak, and there may be venous engorgement on the hands and forearms (Molloy & Benzon, 2008).
         (3) Potential complications are spinal headaches, infection, bleeding, vascular injection of the local anesthetic causing hypotension or seizures, aspiration, or complete spinal block causing full respiratory arrest.
         (4) Advantage: The block may be repeated three to five times at future dates if pain relief is obtained. The patient is to keep track of how long pain relief lasted and report to the anesthesiologist.
         (5) Disadvantages
            (a) See the potential complications given earlier.
            (b) The patient's ability to swallow may be impaired for 2 to 4 hours after the block.
            (c) Practitioners must ensure that patient remains NPO (take nothing by mouth) for at least 4 hours after the block to prevent potential aspiration of fluid or food caused by the numb throat.
            (d) Hot liquids should be avoided for 12 hours post-block (Molloy & Benzon, 2008).
         (6) Nursing care specific to postprocedure care relates to ability to swallow.
         (7) Nursing care during the procedure includes
            (a) Intravenous catheter patency.
            (b) Continuous oxygen saturation.
            (c) Cardiac monitoring and verbal monitoring.
            (d) Monitoring of blood pressure, pulse, and respirations every 5 minutes.
            (e) Monitoring of the temperature of the extremity before the block, at the conclusion of the block, and during the immediate postprocedure period.
            (f) Continue monitoring until the patient is stable, usually 30 to 60 minutes, and patient assurance as to expected side effects of the block (described earlier).
      b. Lumbar sympathetic block
         (1) The patient is placed in the lateral decubitus position with the affected side up or in prone position, depending on the preference of the clinician. Using fluoroscopic assistance, the L2 and L3 vertebrae are identified, the needle placement is confirmed with radiopaque dye, and then local anesthetic are injected.
         (2) Mechanism: Blocking the sympathetic fibers that pass through the second and third lumbar ganglia can denervate the entire lower limb (Molloy & Benzon, 2008).

(3) Indications are as follows (Molloy & Benzon, 2008; Waldman, 2004l):
  (a) CRPSs of the lower limbs
  (b) Increased vascular flow in the legs
  (c) Vascular pain of the lower limbs
  (d) Phantom limb pain

(4) Potential complications are as follows:
  (a) Spinal headache
  (b) Infection
  (c) Bleeding
  (d) Hematuria
  (e) Vascular injection of the local anesthetic, causing hypotension or seizures
  (f) Orthostatic hypotension
  (g) Perforation of the abdominal viscera
  (h) Segmental nerve injury
  (i) Transient backache and stiffness
  (j) Complete spinal block, causing temporary paralysis after local anesthetic injection, and postblock neuralgia
  (k) Possible lasting paralysis after alcohol or phenol injection (Nader & Benzon, 2005)

(5) Some clinicians will use three or more blocks. Injections may be continued until symptoms are minimal or no additional response is seen.

(6) Nursing care during the procedure involves
  (a) Intravenous catheter patency.
  (b) Continuous oxygen saturation and cardiac monitoring.
  (c) Verbal monitoring.
  (d) Monitoring of blood pressure, pulse, and respirations every 5 minutes.
  (e) Monitoring of the temperature of the affected limb before and after the procedure, as temperature elevation assists the clinician in confirming a successful localization of the sympathetic ganglion (Molloy & Benzon, 2008).

(7) Patient teaching
  (a) Do not drive a car for 8 hours after the block.
  (b) Be careful with walking, especially on stairs. Patient is at risk for falls.

5. The effectiveness of these blocks is variable. Patients with CRPS who are diagnosed and treated early, experience good response rates. Success rates of 90% or more have been reported (Buckley, 2001). Other outcome studies as cited in Buckley (2001) are as follows:
   a. Rest pain and ischemic ulcers: 386 patients, 80% relieved
   b. Gangrene of lower extremity: 50 patients, 55% relieved
   c. RSD: 12 patients, 50% relieved
   d. Claudication: 12 patients, 50% relieved
6. Other systematic reviews of sympathetic nerve blocks indicate a lack of high-quality evidence and that further understanding is needed about the role of the efferent sympathetic system in neuropathic pain (Wu, Lin, & Maine, 2008).
7. Contraindications
   a. The patient may be allergic to the medication injected.
   b. Chronic hypotension needs to be discussed with anesthesiologist before the procedure.

H. Botulinum toxin type A injections
1. The Botox® purified neurotoxin complex is a sterile, vacuum-dried form of purified botulinum toxin type A, produced from a culture of the Hall strain of *Clostridium botulinum* grown in a medium containing NZ-amine and yeast extract (Freund & Schwartz, 2000).
2. Mechanism
   a. The injection blocks neuromuscular conduction by binding to receptor sites on motor nerve terminals, entering the nerve terminals, and inhibiting the release of acetylcholine.

b. When injected intramuscularly in therapeutic doses, it produces a localized chemical denervation muscle paralysis (Silberstein et al., 1999).

3. Indications are as follows:
   a. Strabismus and blepharospasm associated with dystonia
   b. Intractable dystonias, spasms, and tremors
   c. Limb dystonias (sports or writers' cramp)
   d. Spasticity regardless of cause (i.e., stroke or multiple sclerosis)
   e. Rigidity resulting from extrapyramidal disorders (Adams et al., 1997; Jain & Francisco, 1998; Miyamoto, 1997)
   f. Muscle tension-type, chronic cervical, and migraine headache (Freund & Schwartz., 2000; Jankovic et al., 2006; Rollnik et al., 2000; Silberstein et al., 1999); one reference shows little difference between the use of saline placebo and Botox® for neck and low back pain (Lew et al., 2008)
   g. Temporomandibular disorder, whiplash injury, hemifacial pain, low back pain, myofascial pain, and piriformis syndrome (Sitzman, Chen, Clemans, Fishman, & Benzon, 2005)
   h. Postlaminectomy syndrome or "failed back syndrome" (Edwards, 2005; Edwards, Rosenthal, & O'Connor, 2007)
4. Contraindications are as follows:
   a. Myasthenia gravis
   b. Other diseases of the neuromuscular junction
5. Dosage
   a. Dose depends on muscle size and the type and extent of relaxation required (Miyamoto, 1997).
   b. For strabismus and blepharospasm, 0.05 to 0.15 ml is used.
   c. The recommended maximal dose per session is 400 U depending on site of injection (Jain & Francisco, 1998).
6. Procedure
   a. Reconstitute with preservative-free saline.
   b. Injections are given intramuscularly.
   c. Injections are guided by surface anatomy, EMG, or electrical stimulation (Jain & Francisco, 1998).
   d. EMG analysis helps determine which muscles are tonically contracted (Adams et al., 1997).
7. Clinical benefit is seen in 1 to 3 days and peaks in 4 to 6 weeks, lasting about 3 to 5 months (Adams et al., 1997; Jain & Francisco, 1998; Miyamoto, 1997).
8. Adverse reactions include the following:
   a. Flulike symptoms
   b. Diplopia and irritation with blepharospasm
   c. Enhanced muscle weakness
   d. Dysphagia when used to treat torticollis, which can lead to aspiration and subsequent pneumonia
   e. *Tachyphylaxis,* or decreased response to the drug with repeated injections, which may occur when high doses are used (e.g., in torticollis)
9. Antibody formation (Dressler & Benecke, 2007; Hackett & Kam, 2007)
   a. In a study of 32 patients with spasmodic torticollis who received Botox A, 12.5% developed antibodies after 2 to 9 months (Racz, 1998).
   b. Antibody formation from Botox A is probably less than 5% when used in the treatment of cervical dystonia (Porta, Perretti, & Gamba, 1998).
   c. Cross-reactivity between Botox A and Botox B is thought to be quite small.
   d. The formation of antibodies that neutralize the action of the drug may be associated with higher doses and frequent injections (Lang, 1999).
10. Precautions
   a. The patient may be allergic to the drug.
   b. It may be potentiated by aminoglycoside antibiotics.
   c. It may be potentiated by any other drugs that interfere with neuromuscular transmission.
   d. Sedentary patients need to be advised to resume activity slowly and carefully.

11. Nursing intervention
    a. Educate the patient.
    b. Assure informed consent.
    c. Administer the procedure if allowed by the state nurse practice act.
    d. Immediately postprocedure,
        (1) Monitor for allergic reaction.
        (2) Assess for local bleeding.

I. Percutaneous vertebroplasty (Liu & Bendok, 2005; Luginbuhl, 2008; Waldman, 2004m)
1. Percutaneous vertebroplasty is a therapeutic radiologically guided procedure that consists of percutaneous injection of surgical cement into a fractured or neoplastic site at the vertebral body.
2. Indications are as follows:
    a. Weakened bone due to osteoporosis
    b. Compression fractures from either malignant or nonmalignant cause
    c. Symptomatic vertebral hemangiomas
3. Procedure
    a. Using conscious sedation, the vertebra is identified through CT scan or fluoroscopy.
    b. The patient is prepared for a sterile procedure. Patients who cannot tolerate the prone position may require general anesthesia or deep sedation.
    c. Local anesthetic is injected to the skin and deeper structures, including the periosteum of the bone at the intended site of entry.
    d. The needle is advanced under fluoroscopic guidance. Intraosseous venography is used to confirm needle location within the trabecular spaces. Contrast injection is used to determine whether there are abnormally large or dangerous communications with the epidural space or vertebral and paravertebral veins.
    e. The vertebra is injected with polymethyl methacrylate (PMMA) bone cement. Fluoroscopy is used to monitor flow of the cement into undesirable locations, such as the epidural space or the inferior vena cava.
    f. The patient is asked to lie flat for approximately 2 hours to let the cement cure.
4. Advantages
    a. The patient has relief of pain from vertebral body compression fractures.
    b. The procedure strengthens bone, increases mobility, decreases analgesic need, and improves quality of life (Liu & Bendok, 2005).
5. Disadvantages
    a. Complications include pneumothorax, neurological complications (e.g., radiculopathy or neuralgias) resulting from leakage of cement, collapse of adjacent vertebrae, and dysphagia if the injection is in the cervical area (Barr, Barr, Lemley, & McCann, 2000)
    b. Pleural injury or rib fracture is possible (Liu & Bendok, 2005).
6. Contraindications are as follows:
    a. Coagulopathies
    b. Local infection
    c. Back pain not related to disease
    d. Presence of spinal canal stenosis
    e. Required open internal stabilization
    f. Poor visibility of the vertebrae with fluoroscopy
7. Of patients who underwent the procedure, 73% to 95% reported moderate to complete pain relief (Liu & Bendok, 2005; Waldman, 2004m)
8. Nursing interventions
    a. Educate the patient.
    b. Assure informed consent.
    c. Immediately postprocedure, monitor the following:
        (1) Vital signs as per conscious sedation policy
        (2) Local bleeding at the site of injection

J. Kyphoplasty (Liu & Bendok, 2005)
  1. Similar to vertebroplasty, kyphoplasty is a therapeutic, radiologically guided procedure that consists of percutaneous injection of surgical cement into a fractured or neoplastic site at the vertebral body.
  2. It was developed to overcome some limitations of vertebroplasty.
  3. Indications are as follows:
     a. Painful or progressive vertebral fractures
     b. Pain or progressive compression fractures related to neoplasms
     c. Prevention of sequelae of immobility (decubitus ulcers, decreased lung function, deep vein thrombosis, or urinary tract infections).
  4. Contraindications are as follows:
     a. Infection
     b. Uncorrectable coagulopathy
     c. Pregnancy
     d. Contrast allergy
     e. Pain unrelated to vertebral collapse
     f. Fractured pedicles
     g. Burst fracture
     h. Young age
     i. Solid tissue or osteoblastic tumors
     j. Vertebra plana (with the body of the vertebra reduced to a sclerotic disc)
  5. Procedure
     a. In addition to the procedure for vertebroplasty, it introduces a balloon into the vertebra through a cannula, which is then inflated to reduce the fracture.
     b. After the balloon is deflated, it leaves a space that may then be filled with viscous PMMA.
  6. Advantages over vertebroplasty are as follows:
     a. Restoration of vertebral height
     b. Restoration of bone stiffness
     c. Lower rate of extravasation of PMMA
     d. Lower complication rate than vertebroplasty
     e. Possible correction of sagittal imbalance
     f. Use of more viscous cement
     g. Increased vertebral body strength and stability
  7. Disadvantages compared with vertebroplasty
     a. Kyphoplasty is more expensive.
     b. Procedure time is increased.
     c. The procedure requires general anesthesia.
     d. It requires a larger device.
     e. The patient needs to be prone longer.
     f. An overnight hospital stay may be needed.
     g. The procedure requires insertion of cannulas from both sides of the vertebra.
  8. Nursing interventions
     a. Educate the patient.
     b. Assure informed consent.
     c. Immediately postprocedure monitor the following:
        (1) Vital signs as per conscious sedation policy
        (2) Local bleeding at the site of injection

V. Neuroablative Techniques

A. When persistent pain stems from benign origins, ablative procedures are fraught with high failure rates and neurological complications, especially additional uncomfortable sensory phenomena, and are not recommended in general.

B. Until the taxonomy of these disorders is clarified and the origins of the disorders determined, ablative procedures of any kind should be avoided (Pawl, 1996).

C. Neurolytic blocks or neurectomy
   1. A nerve-killing substance is injected for the purpose of pain relief.
   2. Indications
      a. In people with pain refractory to other modalities and interventions and with limited life expectancy, such a procedure is indicated because of its potential long-term complications.
      b. Use in people in whom life expectancy is unknown is controversial (Abram, Haddox, & Lynch, 1997).
   3. Procedure
      a. Neurolytic agents used are ethyl alcohol 50% to 100% and phenol 6.6% to a maximum of 10% in glycerin (Heavner, 1996).
         (1) *Alcohol* (hypobaric) produces more pain on injection if no local anesthetic is used before alcohol is injected.
            (a) This produces neurolysis quickly.
            (b) The patient needs to be positioned with the affected nerve root up because the drug rises.
         (2) *Phenol* (hyperbaric) produces no pain on injection.
            (a) It takes about 15 minutes to exert its neurolytic effect.
            (b) The patient needs to be positioned with the affected nerve root down because the drug follows gravity.
   4. Late causalgia is common to most procedures.
   5. Motor deficit occurs when mixed nerves are ablated.
   6. There is potential for unintentional damage to nontargeted tissue (Molloy & Benzon, 2008).

D. Radiofrequency electrocoagulation
   1. The ablation of a nerve is by heat using a radiofrequency current applied by an electrode (Noe & Racz, 1996).
   2. Mechanism
      a. Tissue is heated by ionic movement.
      b. Cell death occurs by thermal coagulation necrosis (Clemans & Benzon, 2005).
   3. Indications are as follows:
      a. Zygapophyseal (facet) joint syndromes
      b. Pain related to sympathetic ganglion conditions
   4. Procedure
      a. This is a neurodestructive procedure. It has to be considered an end-of-the-line procedure when conservative therapeutic modalities have failed.
      b. Verification of location by fluoroscopy is obtained.
      c. This can be performed without general anesthetic on an outpatient procedure (Noe & Racz, 1996).
   5. Advantages over other neurodestructive procedures
      a. There is no intravascular injection of solution or spread to unwanted sites.
      b. Lesion size is well controlled.
      c. It can be repeated (Noe & Racz, 1996).
   6. Potential problems or complications (Waldman, 2004f, 2004g)
      a. Morbidity and mortality are low.
      b. A short-term increase of local pain can occur immediately after the procedure.
      c. Longer-term increase of pain is rare.
      d. Complications of numbness or motor paralysis occur rarely.
      e. If there is a break in the insulation of the needle probe, tissue damage can occur at the site of breakage.
   7. Outcomes (Boswell, Colson, Sehgal, Dunbar, & Epter, 2007; Carragee et al., 2008)
      a. Carragee et al. (2008) conducted an extensive literature review and concluded that radiofrequency neurotomy for neck pain is not supported by the evidence.

b. Boswell et al. (2007) also conducted a systematic review of therapeutic facet joint interventions and concluded that moderate evidence supports radiofrequency ablation for cervical and lumbar spine pain for short- and long-term pain relief. Efficacy for thoracic pain was unable to be determined by the evidence.
c. Kirpalani and Mitra (2007, p. 770) conducted a literature review of cervical facet joint dysfunction and concluded that the "literature provides very limited information regarding the treatment of this condition, with only radiofrequency neurotomy showing evidence of effectively reducing pain from cervical facet joint dysfunction."

8. Nursing interventions
   a. Educate the patient.
   b. Assure informed consent.
   c. Assure that sterile technique is maintained during the procedure.
   d. Monitor the following during the procedure:
      (1) Continuous intravenous access
      (2) Cardiac and oxygen saturation
      (3) Blood pressure and pulse every 5 minutes
      (4) Functioning of radiofrequency machine
   e. Immediately postprocedure monitor the following:
      (1) Vital signs as per conscious sedation policy
      (2) Local bleeding at the site of injection

E. Intradiscal electrothermal therapy and annuloplasty (IDET, IDA)
1. The use of heat seals cracks in the disc wall. It is likely that the high temperature destroys the small nerve fibers that have grown into cracks and invaded the degenerated disc, causing back pain (Yurth, 2004).
2. Indications
   a. Use for internally ruptured discs or those with limited disc herniation that have not responded to more conservative treatment (Waldman, 2004h).
   b. Insurance companies may vary in coverage of this procedure (Blue Cross Blue Shield, 2008).
3. Procedure
   a. Under local anesthetic, using mild sedation and fluoroscopy, a copper cannula is placed into the disc through an introducer needle.
   b. The cannula is manipulated so that it lies between the disc and annulus.
   c. The cannula is heated gradually to 90°C over 17 minutes (American Academy of Physical Medicine and Rehabilitation, 2008).
4. Monitor the following:
   a. Continuous intravenous access
   b. Cardiac and oxygen saturation
   c. Blood pressure and pulse every 5 minutes
5. Complications and side effects are as follows:
   a. Bleeding
   b. Infection
   c. Discitis
   d. Retention of a foreign body
   e. Nerve damage
   f. Increased pain
   g. Paralysis
   h. Shearing of the catheter

VI. General Principles of Nursing Practice for Procedural Interventions (Youmans, 2001)

A. Educate the patient.
B. Assure informed consent.
C. Preprocedure nursing care

1. Assess the following:
   a. Pertinent medical and anesthetic history
   b. NPO status
   c. Baseline vital signs
   d. Weight
   e. Medications (especially anticoagulants)
   f. Allergies
   g. Mental status
   h. History of tobacco, alcohol, and substance use or abuse
   i. Preprocedural lab studies
   j. Immediate availability of oxygen and oxygen delivery devices, resuscitative and intubation equipment, suction apparatus, noninvasive blood pressure device, electrocardiograph equipment, and pulse oximeter
   k. Immediate availability of potentially needed resuscitative and reversal medications

D. Periprocedure nursing care
   1. Determine intravenous access on a case-by-case basis per hospital policy.
   2. Use cardiac monitoring on a case-by-case basis based on preprocedure assessment.
   3. Monitor oxygen saturation.
   4. Note rate and volume of respirations.
   5. Note level of consciousness.
   6. Check skin condition.
   7. Physiological monitoring will depend on the amount of sedation or analgesia used:
      a. Minimal monitoring should be of baseline vital signs and vital signs at the end of the procedure.
      b. Potential monitoring can include the following:
         (1) Continuous intravenous access
         (2) Continuous cardiac and oxygen saturation
         (3) Blood pressure and pulse every 5 minutes
   8. Assure that sterile technique is maintained during the procedure.

E. Postprocedure nursing care
   1. Monitor vital signs as per hospital sedation policy.
   2. Assess for bleeding.
   3. Check level of consciousness, reflexes, and respiratory functioning.
   4. Monitor pain level.
   5. Note allergic reactions to medications given.
   6. Determine whether the patient has the ability to stand alone if a local anesthetic was given near a lumbar nerve root or epidural space. Consider the patient a falls risk until proven otherwise.
   7. Educate the patient.
      a. Explain what may be expected from the particular procedure.
      b. Describe side effects or complications for which to be alert.
      c. Tell the patient how to contact clinicians if problems arise.

PART FOUR: NONMEDICINE MODALITIES FOR THE TREATMENT OF PAIN

I. Prevention Measures

A. Lifestyle changes
   1. Diet
      a. Maintenance of ideal weight optimizes health, minimizing some chronic pain conditions (e.g., low back pain and diabetes).

   b. A dietary consultation for weight loss may be beneficial for overweight patients with low back or joint problems.
2. Exercise
   a. Moderate exercise prevents some chronic pain conditions by maintaining circulation, preventing muscle atrophy, optimizing muscle tone, and preventing osteoporosis.
   b. Pool therapy may be especially beneficial because it provides buoyancy to the body, taking weight off joints.
3. Correct posture and correct lifting technique
   a. These may prevent back, shoulder, and neck pain.
   b. They may decrease the occurrence of carpal tunnel syndrome and other repetitive motion injuries.
   c. Ergonomic evaluation should be made at the patient's work station either at home or at the office.
4. Smoking cessation
   a. Smoking contributes to the cause of many diseases; however, there is increasing evidence of the correlation between smoking and back pain (Goldberg, Scott, & Mayo, 2000).
   b. Smoking causes a decrease in peripheral circulation, which also contributes to painful neuropathies (i.e., Buerger disease or peripheral vascular disease).
   c. Incidence of back pain is higher in adults and adolescents who smoke (Feldman, Rossignol, Shrier, & Abenhaim, 1999).
5. Minimal alcohol consumption
   a. Alcoholic neuropathy is nonexistent in people who do not drink.
   b. Pancreatitis is less frequent in nondrinkers.
6. Decrease stress. High levels of stress can interfere with sleep, the healing process, and the patient's overall ability to cope with pain.

II. Physical Medicine and Physical Therapy Interventions

A. Physical agents may serve as useful adjunctive modalities in pain management geared toward resolution of movement impairments and restoration of physical function (Allen, 2006).

B. Indications
1. Using a multidisciplinary team approach to patients suffering from persistent pain syndromes allows various modalities to be used.
2. Particular disciplines involved may vary from institution to institution or by region of the United States.
3. The modalities described involve physical therapy, occupational therapy, psychological services, and nursing.
4. Patient involvement
   a. Involving the patient in the activity enhances an internal locus of control, which places the patient in active engagement in recovery.
   b. Allowing the patient to be passive enhances an external locus of control, which places the patient in a passive, nonactive role in recovery.
   c. Some modalities allow the patient first to be passive and then to be taught a more active role, allowing the individual needs of the patient to be met.

C. Modalities: psychological interventions
1. Evidence for the use of mind-body therapies for the management of pain is limited, yet there are sound recommendations for many medical conditions (Astin, 2004) (see the chapter on Theories on Pain).
2. Cognitive-behavioral intervention (Flor & Turk, 2006)
   a. This intervention assumes the individuals are active processors of information and not passive reactors.
   b. Thoughts can influence mood, affect physiological processes, have social consequences, and serve as impetus to behavior.

c. Behavior is determined reciprocally by the individual and environmental factors.
d. Individuals are able to learn more adaptive ways of thinking, feeling, and behaving.
e. Individuals should be active in changing their maladaptive thoughts, feelings, and behaviors.

3. Phases of cognitive-behavioral intervention are as follows (Flor & Turk, 2006):
   a. Initial assessment
   b. Reconceptualization (reorienting the patient from the belief that symptoms or physical impairments are overwhelming and unmanageable)
   c. Skills acquisition
   d. Skills consolidation and application of training or homework
   e. Generalization, maintenance, and relapse prevention
   f. Posttreatment assessment and follow-up
4. Treatment techniques: The benefits of exercise are enhanced when combined with self-management education (Rooks et al., 2007).
   a. Self-monitoring
      (1) The patient records important behaviors such as exercise, medication intake, rest, relaxation, and function.
   b. Self-reinforcement
      (1) Teach chronic pain patients to reward themselves for engaging in wellness behaviors, such as exercise, socializing, and returning to work.
      (2) Patients develop a list of pleasurable activities or events.
      (3) Training of self-reinforcement emphasizes the use of naturally occurring rewards.
   c. Relaxation skills can provide progressive muscle relaxation to decrease muscle tension and help patients generalize their skills to daily situations and body positions (Turk, Swanson, & Tunks, 2008).
      (1) Teach the patient to recognize and reduce excessive muscle tension that may contribute to the pain.
      (2) Use an individual therapist or audiotape to guide the patient through the exercises.
      (3) Relaxation skills for chronic pain management include imagery and visualization, autogenics, and deep breathing exercises, as well as muscle tense-relax exercises and passive muscle relaxation.
         (a) Visual imagery
            (i) Assist the individual to imagine a place that person would like to be.
            (ii) Involve all the senses so that the patient can visualize it, hear noises in the area, smell and taste the food or drink associated with this experience, and feel items in the scene imagined.
         (b) Autogenics
            (i) A specific mantra is repetitive and considered to be healing.
            (ii) Autogenics encourages repetitive thoughts of extremities being warm and heavy to decrease sympathetic activity and help the patient increase the temperature of hands and feet.
         (c) Breathing techniques
            (i) Focusing on breathing offers distraction and allows the patient to self-comfort.
            (ii) Breathing techniques can vary with counts; for example, breathe in for a count of 4, and breathe out for a count of 4.
            (iii) Instruct the patient that ***breathing in*** is through the nose and ***breathing out*** is through the mouth.
            (iv) The patient can imagine the ***breath in*** fills the abdomen and the ***breath out*** releases the pain.
5. Biofeedback techniques
   a. Biofeedback presents the individual with a sensory signal (visual or auditory) that changes in proportion to a biological process. Subjects receive instructions in relaxation techniques and receive immediate feedback on the level of relaxation.

(1) Common types of biofeedback are EMG, which measures muscle tension; thermography, for temperature biofeedback; electroencephalography, which measures brain wave activity; and electrodermography, which measures sweat gland activity in typically the hands and feet.
(2) Pneumography and plethysmography biofeedback may be helpful in teaching deep breathing relaxation skills.

b. Mechanism
   (1) Biofeedback disrupts the pain-anxiety-tension cycle.
   (2) It produces a generalized decrease in the sympathetic nervous system and metabolic activity.
c. Biofeedback may be beneficial for patients with migraine headache, myofascial pain, or other muscle tension problems.

6. Stress management
   a. The patient can learn to recognize and adapt new coping strategies with life stressors.
   b. Stress management decreases the physical reaction to these stressors.
   c. Refer the patient for psychiatry or counseling if unresolved.
7. Sleep hygiene
   a. Poor sleep can contribute to overall body pain.
   b. Chronic pain patients do experience sleep disturbance.
      (1) Refer the patient for psychiatry and counseling.
      (2) Teach the patient relaxation techniques.
      (3) Medications may be appropriate.
8. Depression and anxiety management
   a. Evaluation by psychology services for psychotherapy is advisable.
   b. The patient may need referral for psychiatry.
9. Hypnosis and self-hypnosis
   a. Hypnosis encourages a feeling of mental relaxation.
   b. It gives an absorbed and sustained focus on one or a few targets.
   c. Therapists require appropriate training.
   d. The technique has presuggestion and postsuggestion components.
      (1) Using the presuggestion phase, the participant focuses on relaxation and passively disregards intrusive thoughts.
      (2) The suggestion phase introduces specific goals; analgesia specifically may be suggested.
      (3) The postsuggestion phase involves suggesting continued use of the suggested behavior after the hypnosis.

D. Modalities: physical medicine (Allen, 2006)
   1. Goals are
      a. To regain function.
      b. To maintain support.
      c. To establish optimal home exercise for the individual.
   2. Modalities are as follows:
      a. Stretching and strengthening exercises as indicated
      b. Gait training
         (1) Instruct the patient in ambulation to improve balance and efficiency of gait and motor planning.
         (2) Reinforce if assistive device is used and distance ambulation is part of gait training.
      c. Hydrotherapy (i.e., whirlpool or pool therapy)
         (1) Whirlpool is a form of convecting energy using buoyancy, temperature, hydrostatic pressure, and turbulence.
         (2) Hydrotherapy can be used for heating or cooling.
      d. Braces and prosthetic devices as indicated
      e. Massage, or the use of hands to manipulate soft or bony tissues (Hurley & Bearne, 2008)

f. Myofascial release
g. Craniosacral manipulation
h. Ergonomic evaluations
i. TENS, or pulsed electrical activity over the skin on a painful area that activates large afferent fibers stimulating inhibitory dorsal horn neurons and releasing endorphins (Sharma, 2005)
j. Interferential stimulation
   (1) Using the ionization theory, interferential stimulation produces pain relief through reduction of edema and inflammation.
   (2) This affects all tissue layers, skin, muscles, and bone.
k. Iontophoresis
   (1) Either local anesthetics or steroids are moved through the skin into deeper tissues by electrically charged molecules.
   (2) Home units are available through physical therapy departments.
l. Heat application
   (1) Goals
      (a) Increase the extensibility of collagen tissues.
      (b) Decrease joint stiffness.
      (c) Produce pain relief.
      (d) Relieve muscle spasms.
      (e) Assist in resolution of inflammatory infiltrates, edema, and exudates.
      (f) Increase blood flow.
   (2) Superficial heat application (Chou & Huffman, 2007)
      (a) Conduction of heat can be through hot packs, paraffin, conversion using hot lamps, or convection hydrotherapy.
         (i) Hot packs are superficial forms of moist heat. Avoid insensate areas.
         (ii) Paraffin bath uses paraffin and mineral oil. The affected area is dipped in the paraffin and wrapped in towels after a layer is formed for about 20 minutes. It is helpful in treating rheumatoid arthritis and scleroderma.
         (iii) Conversion employing hot lamps uses long waves and short waves. Treatment is not localized but is more diffuse. It can be helpful in treating muscle spasms.
         (iv) Convection using hydrotherapy provides benefit through buoyancy, hydrostatic pressure, turbulence, and temperature. It is helpful with muscle spasms, CRPS, rheumatoid arthritis, myalgia, wounds, and burns.
      (b) Heat application elevates the temperature of tissue a few degrees at depths of a few centimeters.
      (c) Caution should be used with capsaicin cream on the skin during these therapies.
   (3) Deep heat application (Leung & Cheing, 2008)
      (a) Ultrasound (Cetin, Aytar, Atalay, & Akaman, 2008)
         (i) Ultrasound uses high-frequency sound waves capable of reflection, refraction, penetration, and absorption.
         (ii) Heat is greatest at tendon and ligaments and overlying muscle and bone.
      (b) Short-wave diathermy (Cetin et al., 2008)
         (i) Short-wave diathermy is beneficial for relieving muscle spasms. It can reach deeper tissues.
         (ii) It causes significant tissue temperature increase to a depth of 3 cm.
         (iii) Avoid over a pregnant uterus, growing bones, malignancies, infection, and metallic devices.
      (c) Microwave diathermy
         (i) Microwave diathermy heats superficial muscles and joints.
         (ii) It does not penetrate as deeply as ultrasound or short-wave diathermy.
      (d) Deep heat application is helpful in spasticity, muscle spasm, edema, sprains,

strains, and contusions. Caution should be used with skin areas that have decreased sensitivity.

m. Cold application uses ice massage.
    (1) Mechanisms are as follows:
        (a) Vasoconstriction through sympathetically mediated reflex mechanisms, stimulating smooth muscle contraction
        (b) Vasodilation resulting in decreased ischemic pain
        (c) Vasodilation resulting in enhancement and washout of pain mediators
        (d) Cutaneous counterirritation
        (e) Alteration or decrease of nerve conduction (Linchitz, Capulong, Battista, & Mizhiritsky, 1998)
        (f) Muscle relaxation
        (g) Reduced local and systemic metabolic activity
        (h) Endorphin-mediated response
        (i) Alteration of cell membrane permeability

n. Pacing instructions
    (1) Altering physical activity keeps the pain level from escalating to levels associated with dysfunction and distress.
    (2) It can be helpful with pain that is worsened by activity.
    (3) A pain diary can help determine time frames for activities, and a plan for pacing can be developed.

III. Patient Self-intervention of Pain

A. There are further techniques to empower the individual for self-help (St. Marie & Arnold, 2002).
   1. Music therapy uses music to address physical, emotional, cognitive, and social needs of an individual of any age.
      a. Principles
         (1) Music with a beat slower than the heartbeat relaxes.
         (2) Music with a beat faster than the heartbeat energizes.
         (3) Select music the individual enjoys.
      b. Selected benefits
         (1) Alleviate pain.
         (2) Promote wellness.
         (3) Manage stress.
         (4) Express feelings.
         (5) Promote physical rehabilitation.
   2. Acupressure
      a. This healing art uses fingers to press key points on the skin to stimulate the body's self-healing properties.
      b. It is an effective method for self-treatment of painful problems.
      c. It can be taught by a qualified acupressurist.
      d. There is a theoretical risk during pregnancy.
   3. Ball therapy
      a. Self-massage uses a tennis ball-size ball or any ball of various sizes over trigger points (tender points).
      b. A partner may use the ball to massage over trigger points.
      c. The ball can be used over acupressure points (use caution with pregnancy).

Conclusion

Numerous well-defined strategies are available today to assist patients in the management of persistent pain. As new techniques become available, nurses are vital in their outreach to patients. Nursing research and quality improvement strategies are needed to continue to care for patients with persistent pain. Medical research has taken us far, but with the persistent pain population, the nursing discipline is challenged with the task of enhancing and improving the outcome of patient care further.

References

Abdel Aziz, A. M., & Lehman, G. A. (2007). Current treatment options for chronic pancreatitis. *Current Treatment Options in Gastroenterology, 10*(5), 355–368.

Abdi, S., Datta, S., Trescot, A. M., Schultz, D. M., Adlaka, R., Atluri, S. L., Smith, H. S., & Manchikanti, L. (2007). Epidural steroids in the management of chronic spinal pain: A systematic review. *Pain Physician, 10*(1), 185–212.

Abram, S. E., Haddox, J. D., & Lynch, N. T. (1997). Chronic pain management. In P. G. Barash, B. F. Cullen, & R. K. Stoelting (Eds.), *Clinical anesthesia* (p. 1355). Philadelphia: Lippincott-Raven.

Abrams, B. (2000). Electromyography in the diagnosis and management of pain. In P. P. Raj (Ed.), *The practical management of pain* (3rd ed., p. 371). St. Louis: Mosby.

Adams, R. D., Victor, M., & Ropper, A. H. (1997). Diseases of the peripheral nerves. In R. D. Adams, M. Victor, & A. H. Ropper (Eds.), *Principles of neurology* (6th ed., pp. 1302–1369). New York: McGraw-Hill.

Allen, R. J. (2006). Physical agents used in the management of chronic pain by physical therapists. *Physical Medicine and Rehabilitation Clinics of North America, 17*(2), 315–345.

Alvarez, D. J., & Rockwell, P. G. (2002). Trigger points: Diagnosis and management. *American Family Physician, 65*(4), 653–660.

American Academy of Physical Medicine and Rehabilitation. (2008). *Intradiscal electrothermal therapy (IDET)*. Retrieved December 29, 2008, from http://www.aapmr.org/condtreat/pain/idet.htm.

American College of Occupational and Environmental Medicine. (2004). *Low back complaints*. Retrieved May 17, 2008, from http://www.guideline.gov/summary/summary.aspx?ss=15&doc_id=8546&nbr=4755.

American Liver Foundation. (2008). *The American Liver Foundation issues a warning on dangers of excess acetaminophen.* Retrieved November 22, 2008, from http://www.liverfoundation.org/about/news/33/.

American Pain Society. (1999). *Guideline for the management of acute and chronic pain in sickle cell disease.* Glenview, IL: Author.

American Pain Society. (2002). *Guideline for the management of pain in osteoarthritis, rheumatoid arthritis, and juvenile chronic arthritis* (2nd ed.). Glenview. IL: Author.

American Pain Society. (2003). *Principles of analgesic use in the treatment of acute pain and cancer pain* (5th ed.). Glenview, IL: Author.

American Pain Society. (2008). *Principles of analgesic use in the treatment of acute pain and cancer pain* (6th ed.). Glenview, IL: Author.

Argoff, C. E. (2000). New analgesics for neuropathic pain: The lidocaine patch. *Clinical Journal of Pain, 16,* S62–S66.

Armon, C., Argoff, C. E., Samuels, J., & Backonja, M. M. (2007). Use of epidural steroid injections to treat radicular lumbosacral pain: Report of the Therapeutics and Technology Assessment Subcommittee of the American Academy of Neurology. *Neurology, 68*(10), 723–729.

Arnett, F. C., Jr. (1998). Sacroiliitis, ankylosing spondylitis, and Reiter's syndrome. In L. R. Barker, J. R. Barton, & P. D. Zieve (Eds.), *Principles of ambulatory medicine* (5th ed., pp. 1010–1019). Baltimore: Williams & Wilkins.

Arnold, L. M. (2006). *Biology and therapy of fibromyalgia: New therapies in fibromyalgia. Arthritis research and therapy.* Retrieved May 7, 2008, from http://www.medscape.com/viewarticle/536239_1.

About.com. (2008). *Viscosupplementation: Hyaluronan injections. Joint fluid therapy.* Retrieved December 28, 2008, from http://arthritis.about.com/od/kneetreatments/Viscosupplementation_Hyaluronan_Injections_Joint_Fluid_Therapy.htm.

Ashburn, M. A., & Rice, L. J. (1998). *The management of pain.* New York: Churchill Livingstone.

Astin, J. A. (2004). Mind-body therapies for the management of pain. *Clinical Journal of Pain, 20*(1), 27–32.

Atlas, S. J., Chang, Y., Kammann, E., Keller, R. B., Deyo, R. A., & Singer, D. E. (2000). Long-term disability and return to work among patients who have a herniated lumbar disc: The effect of disability compensation. *Journal of Bone and Joint Surgery, 82*(1), 4–15.

Attal, N., Cruccu, G., Haanpaa, M., Hansson, P., Jensen, T. S., Nurmikko, T., Sampaio, C., Sindrup, S., Wiffen, P., & European Federation of Neurological Societies Task Force. (2006). EFNS guidelines on pharmacological treatment of neuropathic pain. *European Journal of Neurology, 13*(11), 1153–1169.

Ballantyne, J. C., & Shin, N. S. (2008). Efficacy of opioids for chronic pain: A review of the evidence. *Clinical Journal of Pain, 24*(6), 469–478.

Barlas, P., & Lundeberg, T. (2006). Transcutaneous electrical nerve stimulation and acupuncture. In S. B. McMahon & M. Koltzenburg (Eds.), *Textbook of pain* (5th ed., pp. 19–835). Philadelphia: Elsevier.

Barone, J. E., Gingold, B. S., Nealon, T. F., & Arvanitis, M. L. (1986). Abdominal pain in patients with acquired immunodeficiency syndrome. *Annals of Surgery, 204,* 619–623.

Barr, J. D., Barr, M., Lemley, T. J., & McCann, R. M. (2000). Percutaneous vertebroplasty for pain relief and spinal stabilization. *Spine, 25,* 923–928.

Benzon, H. T. (1996). Epidural steroids. In P. P. Raj (Ed.), *Pain medicine: A comprehensive review* (p. 260). St. Louis: Mosby-Year Book.

Benzon, H. T. (2005). Selective nerve root blocks and transforaminal epidural steroid injections for back pain and sciatica. In H. T. Benzon, S. N. Raja, R. E. Molloy, S. S. Liu, & S. M. Fishman (Eds.), *Essentials of pain medicine and regional anesthesia* (2nd ed., pp. 341–347). Philadelphia: Elsevier, Churchill Livingstone.

Berman, A., Espinoza, L. R., Diaz, J. D., Aguilar, T. R., Vasey, F. B., Germain, B. R., & Lockey, R. F. (1988). Rheumatic manifestations of human immunodeficiency virus infection. *American Journal of Medicine, 85,* 59–64.

Beth Israel University Hospital and Manhattan Campus for the Albert Einstein College of Medicine. (2008). *Phantom and stump pain.* Retrieved June 3, 2008, from http://www.stoppain.org/pain_medicine/content/chronicpain/phantom.asp.

Bigal, M. E., & Lipton, R. B. (2006). Headache. In S. B. McMahon & M. Koltzenburg (Eds.), *Textbook of pain* (5th ed., pp. 837–886). Philadelphia: Elsevier.

Bigal, M. E., Serrano, D., Buse, D., Scher, A., Stewart, W.F., & Lipton, R.B. (2008). Acute migraine medications and evolution from episodic to chronic migraine: A longitudinal population-based study. *Headache, 48*(8), 1157–1168.

Biller, N., & Caudill, M. A. (1999). Commentary: Contracts, opioids, and the management of chronic nonmalignant pain. *Journal of Pain and Symptom Management, 17,* 144–145.

Blue Cross Blue Shield. (2008). *Intradiscal electrothermal annuloplasty and percutaneous intradiscal radiofrequency thermocoagulation.* Retrieved December 29, 2008, from http://www.wellmark.com/e_business/provider/medical_policies/policies/Intradiscal_Therapy.htm.

Boden, S. D., & Wiesel, S. W. (1992). Chronic low-back pain: Avoiding common diagnostic and therapeutic error. In G. M. Aronoff (Ed.), *Evaluation and treatment of chronic pain* (2nd ed., pp. 243–244). Baltimore: Williams & Wilkins.

Bonacini, M. (1992). Hepatobiliary complications in patients with human immunodeficiency virus infection. *American Journal of Medicine, 92,* 404–411.

Bonica, J. J., & Buckley, F. B. (1990). Regional analgesia with local anesthetics. In J. J. Bonica (Ed.), *The management of pain* (pp. 1883–1966). Philadelphia: Lea & Febiger.

Borsook, D., LeBel, A., Stojanovic, M., & Fishman, S. (1998). Central pain syndromes. In M. A. Ashburn & L. J. Rice (Eds.), *The management of pain* (pp. 323–334). New York: Churchill Livingstone.

Boswell, M. V., Colson, J. D., Sehgal, N., Dunbar, E. E., & Epter, R. (2007). A systematic review of therapeutic facet joint interventions in chronic spinal pain. *Pain Physician, 10,* 229–253.

Breitbart, W., & Patt, R. B. (1994). Pain management in the patient with AIDS. *Hematology/Oncology Annals, 2,* 391–399.

Breitbart, W., McDonald, M. V., Rosenfeld, B., Passik, S. D., Hewitt, D., Thaler, H., & Portenoy, R. K. (1996). Pain in ambulatory AIDS patients: Pain characteristics and medical correlates. *Pain, 68,* 315–321.

Brew, B. J., & Miller, J. (1993). Human immunodeficiency virus-related headache. *Neurology, 43,* 1098–1100.

Brumas, M., & Shoemaker, J. (2005). *Senators' Jeff Sessions and Dick Durbin introduce prescription drug monitoring bill.* Retrieved October 5, 2007, from http://www.sessions.senate.gov.

Brummett, C. M., & Cohen, S. P. (2008). Facet joint pain. In H. T. Benzon, J. P. Rathmell, C. L. Wu, D. C. Turk, & C. E. Argoff (Eds.), *Raj's practical management of pain* (4th ed., pp. 1003–1037). Philadelphia: Mosby Elsevier.

Buckley, F. B. (2001). Regional anesthesia with local anesthesia. In J. D. Loeser (Ed.), *Bonica's management of pain* (3rd ed., pp. 1893–1952). Philadelphia: Lippincott Williams & Wilkins.

Burckhardt, C. S., Goldenberg, D., Crofford, L., Gerwin, R., Gowans, S., Jackson, K., Kugel., P., McCarberg, W., Rudin, N., Schanberg, L., Taylor, A. G., Taylor, J., & Turk, D. (2005). *Guideline for the management of fibromyalgia syndrome pain in adults and children.* APS Clinical Practice Guidelines series, No. 4. Glenview, IL: American Pain Society.

Burkhardt, N., & Hamann, G. F. (2006). Extradural lipomatosis after long-term treatment with steroids. *Nervenarzt, 77*(12), 1477–1479.

Candido, K. D., & Nader, A. (2005). Caudal anesthesia. In H. T. Benzon, S. N. Raja, R. E. Molloy, S. S. Liu, & S. M. Fishman (Eds.), *Essentials of pain medicine and regional anesthesia* (2nd ed., pp. 587–597). Philadelphia: Elsevier, Churchill Livingstone.

Cardone, D. A., & Tallia, A. F. (2002). Joint and soft tissue injection. *American Family Physician, 66*(2), 283–288.

Carragee, E. J., Hurwitx, E. L., Cheng, I., Carroll, L. J., Nordin, M., Guzman, J., Peloso, P., Holm, L. W., Cote, P., Hogg-Johnson, S., van der Velde, G., Cassidy, J. D., & Haldeman, S. (2008). Treatment of neck pain: Injections and surgical interventions. Results of the Bone and Joint Decade 2000–2010 Task Force on Neck Pain and Its Associated Disorders. *Spine, 33*(45), S153–S169.

Cavanaugh, J. M., & Weinstein, J. N. (1994). Low back pain: Epidemiology, anatomy and neurophysiology. In P. D. Wall & R. Melzack (Eds.), *Textbook of pain* (3rd ed., pp. 446–451). New York: Churchill Livingstone.

Cetin, N., Aytar, A., Atalay, A., & Akaman, M. N. (2008). Comparing hot pack, short-wave diathermy, ultrasound, and TENS on isokinetic strength, pain, and functional status of women with osteoarthritic knees: A single-blind, randomized, controlled trial. *American Journal of Physical Medicine and Rehabilitation, 87*(6), 443–451.

Challapalli, V., Tremont-Lukats, I. W., McNicol, E. D., Lau, J., & Carr, D. B. (2005). Systemic administration of local anesthetic agents to relieve neuropathic pain. *Cochrane Database of Systematic Reviews,* Issue 4. Retrieved May 24, 2009, from http://www.cochrane.org/reviews/en/ab003345.html.

Chan, B. L., Witt, R., Charrow, A. P., Magee, A., Howard, R., & Pasquina, P. F. (2007). Mirror therapy for phantom limb pain. *New England Journal of Medicine, 357*(21), 2206–2207.

Chapman, S. (2001). The effects of opioids on driving ability in patients with chronic pain. *APS Bulletin, 11*(1), 1, 5, 9.

Chou, R., & Huffman, L. H. (2007). Nonpharmacologic therapies for acute and chronic low back pain: A review of the evidence for an American Pain Society/American College of Physicians clinical practice guideline. *Annals of Internal Medicine, 147,* 492–504.

Chou, R., Qaseem, A., Snow, V., Casey, D., Cross, J. T., Shekelle, P., & Owens, D. K. (2007). Diagnosis and treatment of low back pain: A joint clinical practice guideline from the American College of Physicians and the American Pain Society. *Annals of Internal Medicine, 147*(7), 478–491.

Cimino, C. (1999). Painful neurological syndromes. In G. M. Aronoff (Ed.), *Evaluation and treatment of chronic pain* (2nd ed., pp. 59–60). Baltimore: Williams & Wilkins.

Clemans, R. R., & Benzon, H. T. (2005). Facet syndrome: Facet joint injections and facet nerve blocks. In H. T. Benzon, S. N. Raja, R. E. Molloy, S. S. Liu, & S. M. Fishman (Eds.), *Essentials of pain medicine and regional anesthesia* (2nd ed., pp. 348–355). Philadelphia: Elsevier, Churchill Livingstone.

Cruccu, G., Aziz, T. Z., Garcia-Larrea, L., Hansson, P., Jensen, T. S., Lefaucheur, J. P., Simpson, B. A., & Taylor, R. S. (2007). EFNS guidelines on neurostimulation therapy for neuropathic pain. *European Journal of Neurology, 14*(9), 952–970.

Dalakas, M. C., & Pezeshkpour, G. H. (1988). Neuromuscular diseases associated with human immunodeficiency virus infection. *Annals of Neurology, 23,* S38–S48.

Dawson, E. G. (2008). *Arachnoiditis.* Retrieved May 5, 2008, from http://www.spineuniverse.com/displayarticle.php/article 180.html.

de Leon-Casasola, O. (2007). Epidural steroid injections for pain therapy. *Revista Mexicana de Anestesiologia, 30* (Suppl. 1), S108–S113.

de Leon-Casasola, O., Molloy, R. E., & Lema, M. (2005). Neurolytic visceral sympathetic blocks. In H. Benzon, S. N. Raja, R. E. Molloy, S. S. Liu, & S M. Fishman (Eds.), *Essentials of pain medicine and regional anesthesia* (2nd ed., pp. 543–546). Philadelphia: Elsevier, Churchill Livingstone.

DEA (2008). State Prescription Drug Monitoring Programs. Retrieved on July 4, 2009 from http://www.deadiversion.usdoj.gov/faq/rx_monitor.htm.

Dionne, R. A., Kim, H., & Gordon, S. M. (2006). Acute and chronic dental and orofacial pain. In S. B. McMahon & M. Koltzenburg (Eds.), *Textbook of pain* (5th ed., pp. 19–835). Philadelphia: Elsevier.

Dressler, D., & Benecke, R. (2007). Pharmacology of therapeutic botulinum toxin preparations. *Disability and Rehabilitation, 29*(23), 1761–1798.

Dubinsky, R. M., Kabbani, H., El-Chami, Z., Boutwell, C., & Ali, H. (2004). Practice parameter: treatment of postherpetic neuralgia: an evidence-based report of the Quality Standards Subcommittee of the American Academy of Neurology. *Neurology, 63*(6), 959–965.

Dubuisson, D. (1994). Nerve root damage and arachnoiditis. In P. D. Wall & R. Melzack (Eds.), *Textbook of pain* (3rd ed., p. 725). New York: Churchill Livingstone.

Du Pen, S. (2005). Spinal drug delivery. In M. S. Wallace & P. S. Staats (Eds.), *Pain medicine & management just the facts* (pp. 341–343). New York: McGraw-Hill.

Dworkin, R. H., O'Connor, A. B., Backonja, M., Farrar, J. T., Finnerup, N. B., Jensen, T. S., Kalso, E. A., Loeser, J. D., Miaskowski, C., Nurmikko, T. J., Portenoy, R. K., Rice, A. S., Stacey, B. R., Treede, R. D., Turk, D. C., & Wallace, M. S. (2007). Pharmacologic management of neuropathic pain: Evidence-based recommendations. *Pain, 5;132*(3), 237–251.

Dworkin, R. H., Turk, D. C., Farrar, J. T., Haythornwaite, J. A., Jensen, M. P., Katz, N. P., Kerns, R. D., Stucki, G., Allen, R.R., Bellamy, N., Carr, D.B., Chandler, J., Chowen, P., Dionne, R.A., Rothman, M., Royal, M.A., & Simon, L. (2005). Core outcome measure for chronic pain clinical trials: IMMPACT recommendations. *Pain, 113*(1–2), 9–19.

Edwards, K. (2005). Botulinum toxin type A for filed back syndrome. *Journal of Pain, 6*(3 Suppl. 1), S30.

Edwards, K., Rosenthal, B., & O'Connor, J. (2007). Long term efficacy of botulinum toxin type A for post laminectomy syndrome. *Journal of Pain, 8*(4 Suppl. 1), S38.

Elliott, V. S. (2004). *Physicians spot significant substance abuse issues: Amednews.com.* Retrieved October 5, 2007, from http://www.ama-assn.org/amednews/2004/12/06/hlsc1206.htm.

Erdine, S., & De Andres, J. (2006). Drug delivery systems. *Pain Practice, 6*(1), 51–57.

Erjavec, M. (2001). Epidural steroids for low back pain. In J. D. Loeser (Ed.), *Bonica's management of pain* (3rd ed., pp. 1551–1564). Philadelphia: Lippincott Williams & Wilkins.

Fallin, T. W., Goble, E. M., Hoy, R. W., Justin, D. F., Chervitz, A., Paganelli, J. V., & Triplett, D. (2007). *Facet joint replacement: USPTO Application No. 20070270967.* Retrieved November 21, 2008, from http://www.freshpatents.com/Facet-joint-replacement-dt20071122ptan20070270967.php.

Federation of State Medical Boards of the United States. (1998). *House of Delegates, May, 1998.* Retrieved December 15, 2008, from http://www.fsmb.org/grpol_pain_policy_resource_center.html.

Feldman, D. E., Rossignol, M., Shrier, I., & Abenhaim, L. (1999). Smoking: a risk factor for development of low back pain in adolescents. *Spine, 24,* 2492–2496.

Finch, P. M., & Taylor, J. R. (1996). Functional anatomy of the spine. In S. D. Waldman & A. P. Winnie (Eds.), *Interventional pain management* (pp. 39–64). Philadelphia: W. B. Saunders.

Flor, H., & Turk, D. C. (2006). Cognitive and learning aspects. In S. B. McMahon & M. Koltzenburg (Eds.), *Textbook of pain* (5th ed., pp. 241–258). Philadelphia: Elsevier.

Foldi, M., & Strossenreuther, R. (2008). *Foundations of manual lymphatic drainage* (3rd edition). Philadelphia: Elsevier Press.

Franzini, A., Ferroli, P., Leone, M., & Broggi, G. (2003). Stimulation of the posterior hypothalamus for treatment of chronic intractable cluster headaches. *Neurosurgery, 52,* 1095–1101.

Freedman, K. B. (2006). *Herniated nucleus pulposus (slipped disk).* Retrieved May 15, 2008, from http://www.nlm.nih.gov/medlineplus/ency/article/000442.htm.

Freund, B. J., & Schwartz, M. (2000). Treatment of chronic cervical-associated headache with botulinum toxin A: A pilot study. *Headache, 40,* 231–236.

Fuller, G. N., Jacobs, J. N., & Guiloff, R. J. (1993). Nature and incidence of peripheral nerve syndromes in HIV infection. *Journal of Neurology, Neurosurgery, and Psychiatry, 56,* 372–381.

Furlan, A. D., Sandoval, J. A., Mailis-Gagnon, A., & Tunks, E. (2006). Opioids for chronic noncancer pain: a meta-analysis of effectiveness and side effects. *Canadian Medical Association Journal, 174*(11), 1589–1594.

Gachago, C., & Draganov, P. V. (2008). Pain management in chronic pancreatitis. *World Journal of Gastroenterology, 14*(20), 3137–3148.

Geisser, M. E., Roth, R. S., Bachman, J. E., & Eckert, T. A. (1996). The relationship between symptoms of post-traumatic stress disorder and pain, affective disturbance and disability among patients with accident and non-accident related pain. *Pain, 66*(2–3), 207–214.

Gellner, V., Kurschel, S., Krell, W., Holl, E. M., Ofner-Kopeinig, P., & Unger, R. (2008). Recurrent trigeminal neuralgia: Long term outcome of repeat gamma knife radiosurgery. *Journal of Neurology, Neurosurgery, and Psychiatry, 78,* 1405–1407.

Gerwin, R. D. (2005). Myofascial pain and fibromyalgia. In M. S. Wallace & P. S. Staats (Eds.), *Pain medicine & management just the facts* (pp. 204–210). New York: McGraw-Hill.

Gianino, J. M., York, M. M., & Paice, J. A. (1996). *Intrathecal drug therapy for spasticity and pain: Practical patient management.* New York: Springer-Verlag.

Gilfor, J. M., & Viscusi, E. R. (2005). Epidural analgesia. In M. S. Wallace & P. S. Staats (Eds.), *Pain medicine & management: Just the facts* (pp. 204–210). New York: McGraw-Hill.

Goadsby, P. J. (2006). Primary neurovascular headache. In S. B. McMahon & M. Koltzenburg (Eds.), *Textbook of pain* (5th ed., pp. 851–874). Philadelphia: Elsevier.

Goldberg, G. S., Orkin, B. A., & Smith, L. E. (1994). Microbiology of human immunodeficiency virus anorectal disease. *Diseases of the Colon and Rectum, 37,* 439–443.

Goldberg, M. S., Scott, S. C., & Mayo, N. E. (2000). A review of the association between cigarette smoking and the development of nonspecific back pain and related outcomes. *Spine, 2,* 995–1014.

Goldstein, J. (1990). Headache and acquired immunodeficiency syndrome. *Neurology Clinics, 8,* 947–960.

Graham, J. R., & Bana, D. S. (1992). Headache. In G. M. Aronoff (Ed.), *Evaluation and treatment of chronic pain* (2nd ed., p. 103). Baltimore: Williams & Wilkins.

Gunn, C. C. (2001). Neuropathic myofascial pain syndromes. In J. D. Loeser (Ed.), *Bonica's management of pain* (3rd ed., pp. 522–529). Philadelphia: Lippincott Williams & Wilkins.

Hackett, R., & Kam, P. C. (2007). Botulinum toxin: Pharmacology and clinical developments. A literature review. *Medicinal Chemistry, 3*(4), 333–345.

Hackworth, R. J., Tokarz, K. A., Fowler, I. M., Wallace, S. C., & Stedje-Larsen, E. T. (2008). Profound pain reduction after induction of memantine treatment in two patients with severe phantom limb pain. *Anesthesia & Analgesia, 107*(4), 1377–1379.

Haddox, J. D. (1996). Coanalgesic agents. In P. P. Raj (Ed.), *Pain medicine: A comprehensive review* (pp. 142–153). St. Louis: Mosby-Year Book.

Heavner, J. E. (1996). Neurolytic agents. In P. P. Raj (Ed.), *Pain medicine: A comprehensive review* (pp. 285–286). St. Louis: Mosby-Year Book.

Hewitt, D., Breitbart, W., & Rosenfeld, B. (1994). *Pain syndromes in the ambulatory AIDS patient.* Abstract No. 94746. Paper presented at the 13th Annual Meeting of the American Pain Society, Miami, FL.

Howard, F. M. (2003). Chronic pelvic pain. *Obstetrics and Gynecology, 101,* 594–611.

Hurley, M. V., & Bearne, L. M. (2008). Non-exercise physical therapies for musculoskeletal conditions: Best practice & research. *Clinical Rheumatology, 22*(3), 419–433.

Insel, P. A. (1996). Analgesic-antipyretic and antiinflammatory agents and drugs employed in the treatment of gout. In J. G. Hardman, L. E. Limbird, P. B. Molinoff, R. W. Ruddon, & A. G. Gilman (Eds.), *The pharmacological basis of therapeutics* (9th ed., p. 624). New York: McGraw-Hill.

Institute for Clinical Systems Improvement. (2007). *Assessment and management of chronic pain.* Retrieved November 8, 2008, from http://www.guideline.gov/summary/summary.aspx?ss=15&doc_id=10724&nbr=5586.

International Headache Society, Headache Classification Subcommittee. (2004). The international classification of headache disorders (2nd ed.). *Cephalalgia, 24*(Suppl. 1), 9–160.

International Headache Society. (2008). *IHS classification ICHD-II.* Retrieved June 7, 2009, from http://ihs-classification.org/en/.

International Research Foundation for RSD/CRPS. (2003). *Reflex sympathetic dystrophy/complex regional pain syndrome* (3rd ed.). Tampa, FL: Author. Retrieved May 17, 2008, http://www.guideline.gov/summary/summary.aspx?ss=15&doc_id=4117&nbr=3162.

Jain, S. S., & Francisco, G. E. (1998). Parkinson's disease and other movement disorders. In J. A. DeLisa & B. M. Gans (Eds.), *Rehabilitation medicine: principles and practice* (3rd ed.). Philadelphia: Lippincott-Raven.

Jain, S., & Gupta, R. (2001). Neurolytic agents in clinical practice. In SD Waldman (Ed.), *Interventional pain management* (2nd ed., pp. 220–225). Philadelphia: W. B. Saunders.

Jankovic, J., Hunter, C., Dolimek, B. Z., Dolimbek, G. S., Adler, C. H., Brashear, A., Comella, C. L., Gordon, M., Riley, D. E., Sethi, K., Singer, C., Stacy, M., Tarsy, D., & Atassi, M. Z. (2006). Clinico-immunologic aspects of botulinum toxin type B treatment of cervical dystonia. *Neurology, 67,* 2233–2235.

Jarrar, R. G., Black, D. F., Dodick, D. W., & Davis, D. H. (2003). Outcome of trigeminal nerve section in the treatment of chronic cluster headache. *Neurology, 60,* 1360–1362.

Jeynes, L. C., & Gauci, C. A. (2008). Evidence for the use of botulinum toxin in the chronic pain setting: A review of the literature. *Pain Practice, 8*(4), 269–236.

Johnson, B. W., Jr. (2000). Pain mechanisms: Anatomy, physiology, and neurochemistry. In P. P. Raj (Ed.), *Practical management of pain* (3rd ed., pp. 127–134). St. Louis: Mosby.

Kafiluddi, R., & Hahn, M. B. (2000). Epidural neural blockade. In P. P. Raj (Ed.), *Practical management of pain* (3rd ed., p. 649). St. Louis: Mosby.

Kalso, E., Edwards, J. E., Moore, R. A., & McQuay, H. J. (2004). Opioids in chronic non-cancer pain: systematic review of efficacy and safety. *Pain, 112,* 372–380.

Kirpalani, D., & Mitra, R. (2007). Cervical facet joint dysfunction: A review. *Archives of Physical Medicine and Rehabilitation, 89*(4), 770–774.

Lang, A. M. (1999). Botulinum toxin for myofascial pain. In *Advancement in the treatment of neuromuscular pain.* (syllabus, chapter 5. pp. 23–28). Baltimore, M.D.: Johns Hopkins University Office of Continuing Medical Educations.

Lebovits, A. H., Lefkowitz, M., McCarthy, D., Simon, R., Wilpon, H. L., Jung, R., & Fried, E. (1989). The prevalence and management of pain in patients with AIDS: A review. *Clinical Journal of Pain, 5,* 245–248.

Leung, A. Y. (2005). Acupuncture. In M. S. Wallace & P. S. Staats (Eds.), *Pain medicine & management: Just the facts* (pp. 260–266). New York: McGraw-Hill.

Leung, M. S., & Cheing, G. L. (2008). Effects of deep heat and superficial heating in the management of frozen shoulder. *Journal of Rehabilitation Medicine, 40*(2), 145–150.

Lew, H. W., Lee, E. H., Castaneda, A., Klima, R., & Date, E. (2008). Therapeutic use of botulinum toxin type A in treating neck and upper-back pain of myofascial origin: A pilot study. *Archives of Physical Medicine and Rehabilitation, 89*(1), 75–80.

Linchitz, R. M., Capulong, E., Battista, D. J., & Mizhiritsky, M. Y. (1998). Physical modalities for pain management. In M. A. Ashburn & L. J. Rice (Eds.), *The management of pain* (pp. 401–405). Philadelphia: Churchill Livingstone.

Lippit, A. B. (1984). The facet joint and its role in spine pain: Management with facet joint injections. *Spine, 9,* 746–750.

Liu, J. C., & Bendok, B. R. (2005). Osteoporosis and percutaneous vertebroplasty. In H. Benzon, S. N. Raja, R. E. Molloy, S. S. Liu, & S. M. Fishman (Eds.), *Essentials of pain medicine and regional anesthesia* (2nd ed., pp. 501–507). Philadelphia: Elsevier, Churchill Livingstone.

Lovely, T. J., Kotsiakis, X., & Jannetta, P. J. (1998). The surgical management of chronic cluster headache. *Headache, 38,* 590–594.

Luciano, C. A., Pardo, C. A., & McArthur, J. C. (2003). Recent developments in the HIV neuropathies. *Current Opinion in Neurology, 16*(3), 403–409.

Luginbuhl, M. (2008). Percutaneous vertebroplasty, kyphoplasty and lordoplasty: Implications for the anesthesiologist. *Current Opinions in Anesthesiology, 21,* 504–513.

MacIver, K., Lloyd, D. M., Kelly, S., Roberts, N., & Nurmikko, T. (2008). Phantom limb pain, cortical reorganization and the therapeutic effect of mental imagery. *Brain, 131*(8), 2181–2191.

Mailes, A., & Bennett, G. J. (1999). Painful neurological disorders: Clinical aspects. In G. M. Aronoff (Ed.), *Evaluation and treatment of chronic pain* (2nd ed., pp. 93–113). Baltimore: Williams & Wilkins.

Manchikanti, L., Manchukonda, R., Damron, K. S., Brandon, D., McManus, C. D., & Cash, K. (2006). Does adherence monitoring reduce controlled substance abuse in chronic pain patients? *Pain Physician, 9,* 57–60.

Markman, J. D., & Philip, A. (2007). Interventional approaches to pain management. *Anesthesiology Clinics, 25*(4), 883–898.

Martell, B. A., O'Connor, P. G., Kerns, R. D., Becker, W. C., Morales, K. H., Kosten, T. R., & Fiellin, D. A. (2007). Systematic review: Opioid treatment for chronic low back pain: prevalence, efficacy, and association with addiction. *Annals of Internal Medicine, 146*(2), 116–127.

Mathew, N. T., & Hurt, W. (1988). Percutaneous radiofrequency trigeminal gangliorhizolysis in intractable cluster headache. *Headache, 28,* 328–331.

Mayo Clinic. (2008a). *Phantom pain: Mayo Foundation for Medical Education and Research.* Retrieved May 17, 2008, from http://www.mayoclinic.com/health/phantom-pain/DS00444/DSECTION=2.

Mayo Clinic. (2008b). *Spinal stenosis: Mayo Foundation for Medical Education and Research.* Retrieved May 17, 2008, from http://www.mayoclinic.com/health/spinal-stenosis/DS00515/DSECTION=3.

Mayo Clinic. (2008c). *Trigeminal neuralgia: Mayo Foundation for Medical Education and Research.* Retrieved November 22, 2008, from http://www.mayoclinic.org/trigeminal-neuralgia/treatment.html.

McArthur, J. C., Brew, B. J., & Nath, A. (2005). Neurological complications of HIV infection. *Lancet Neurology, 4*(9), 543–555.

McKenry, L. M., & Salerno, E. (1998). Principles of drug action. In L. M. McKenry & E. Salerno (Eds.), *Mosby's pharmacology in nursing* (20th ed.). St. Louis: Mosby-Year Book.

McLennon, S. M. (2005). *Persistent pain management.* Iowa City, IA: University of Iowa Gerontological Nursing Interventions Research Center, Research Translation and Dissemination Core. Retrieved November 8, 2008, from http://www.guideline.gov/summary/summary.aspx?doc_id=8627.

MD Consult. (2007). *Ankylosing spondylitis.* Retrieved June 1, 2008, from http://www.mdconsult.com/das/pdxmd/body/94050489-2/0?type=med&eid=9-u1.0-_1_101_1014910.

Miles, J., & Souvall, A. (2005). *Congressman Whitfield and Pallone introduce prescription drug abuse legislation.* Retrieved October 6, 2007, from http://www/nasper.org.

Minnesota Department of Health. (2005). *Minnesota sickle cell disease emergency guidelines.* Retrieved June 7, 2009, from http://www.health.state.mn.us/news/pressrel/sicklecell091305.htm

Mitra, M. (2006). FDA approves shingles vaccine: Herpes zoster vaccine targets older adults. *Journal of the American Medical Society, 296*(2), 157–158.

Miyamoto, M. D. (1997). Agents affecting neuromuscular transmission. In C. R. Craig & R. E. Stitzel (Eds.), *Modern pharmacology with clinical applications* (5th ed., p. 358). Boston: Little, Brown.

Moldwin, R. M., Evans, R. J., Stanford, E. J., & Rosenberg, M. T. (2007). Rational approaches to the treatment of patients with interstitial cystitis. *Urology, 69*(Suppl. 4A), 73–81.

Molloy, R. E. (2005a). Myofascial pain syndrome. In H. T. Benzon, S. N. Raja, R. E. Molloy, S. S. Liu, & S. M. Fishman (Eds.), *Essentials of pain medicine and regional anesthesia* (2nd ed., pp. 367–368). Philadelphia: Elsevier, Churchill Livingstone.

Molloy, R. E. (2005b). Truncal blocks: Intercostal, paravertebral, interpleural, suprascapular, ilioinguinal, and iliohypogastric nerve blocks. In H. T. Benzon, S. N. Raja, R. E. Molloy, S. S. Liu, & S. M. Fishman (Eds.), *Essentials of pain medicine and regional anesthesia* (2nd ed., pp. 636–638). Philadelphia: Elsevier, Churchill Livingstone, pp. 636–644.

Molloy, R. E., & Benzon, H. T. (2005). Interlaminar epidural steroid injections for lumbosacral radiculopathy. In H. T. Benzon, S. N. Raja, R. E. Molloy, S. S. Liu, & S. M. Fishman (Eds.), *Essentials of pain medicine and regional anesthesia* (2nd ed., pp. 331–340). Philadelphia: Elsevier, Churchill Livingstone, pp. 636–644.

Molloy, R. E., & Benzon, H. T. (2008). Neurolytic blocking agents: Uses and complications. In H. T. Benzon, J. P. Rathmell, C. L. Wu, D. C. Turk, & C. E. Argoff (Eds.), *Raj's practical management of pain* (4th ed., pp. 839–850). Philadelphia: Mosby Elsevier.

Moore, R. A., & McQuay, H. J. (2005). Prevalence of opioid adverse events in chronic non-malignant pain: Systematic review of randomised trials of oral opioids. *Arthritis Research & Therapy, 7*(5), R1046-R1051.

Nader, A., & Benson, H. (2005). Peripheral sympathetic blocks. In H. T. Benzon, S. N. Raja, R. E. Molloy, S. S. Liu, & S. M. Fishman (Eds.), *Essentials of pain medicine and regional anesthesia* (2nd ed., pp. 636–638). Philadelphia: Elsevier, Churchill Livingstone. pp. 687–693.

Naja, Z. M., Al-Tannir, M. A., Zeidan, A., El-Rajab, M., Ziade, F., & Baraka, A. (2007). Nerve stimulator-guided repetitive paravertebral block for thoracic myofascial pain syndrome. *Pain Practice, 7*(4), 348–351.

Narchi, P., Singelyn, F., & Paqueron, X. (2008). Truncal blocks. In H. T. Benzon, J. P. Rathmell, C. L. Wu, D. C. Turk, & C. E. Argoff (Eds.), *Raj's practical management of pain* (4th ed., pp. 905–915). Philadelphia: Mosby Elsevier.

NASPER.org. (2005a). *Breaking News: NASPER Victory in Senate.* Retrieved October 6, 2007, from http://www.nasper.org/breaking_news.htm.

NASPER.org. (2005b). *Senate committee approves NASPER.* Retrieved October 6, 2007, from http://www.nasper.org/Documents/senate_committee_approves_nasper.htm.

National Guidelines Clearinghouse. (2004). Operative treatment for chronic pancreatitis. Retrieved May 22, 2008, from http://www.guideline.gov/summary/summary.aspx?doc_id=5506&nbr.

National Institute of Neurological Disorders and Stroke, National Institutes of Health. (2001). *Reflex sympathetic dystrophy/complex regional pain syndrome (CRPS): State of the science.* Retrieved May 17, 2008, from http://www.ninds.nih.gov/news_and_events/proceedings/reflex_sympathetic_dystrophy_2001.htm.

National Institute of Neurological Disorders and Stroke, National Institutes of Health. (2007). *Arachnoiditis.* Retrieved May 15, 2008, from http://www.ninds.nih.gov/disorders/arachnoiditis/arachnoiditis.htm?css=print.

National Institute of Neurological Disorders and Stroke, National Institutes of Health. (2008a). *NINDS central pain syndrome.* Retrieved May 18, 2008, from http://www.ninds.nih.gov/disorders/central_pain/central_pain.htm.

National Institute of Neurological Disorders and Stroke, National Institutes of Health. (2008b). *NINDS complex regional pain syndrome.* Retrieved May 17, 2008, from http://www.ninds.nih.gov/disorders/reflex_sympathetic_dystrophy/reflex_sympathetic_dystrophy.htm.

National Institute of Neurological Disorders and Stroke, National Institutes of Health. (2008c). *NINDS trigeminal neuralgia.* Retrieved May 17, 2008, from http://www.ninds.nih.gov/disorders/trigeminal_neuralgia/trigeminal_neuralgia.htm.

National Institute of Neurological Disorders and Stroke, National Institutes of Health. (2008d). *Peripheral neuropathy fact sheet.* Retrieved May 17, 2008, from http://www.ninds.nih.gov/disorders/peripheralneuropathy/detail_peripheral neuropathy.htm.

National Institute of Neurological Disorders and Stroke, National Institutes of Health. (2008e). *Syringomyelia fact sheet.* Retrieved June 7, 2008, from http://www.ninds.nih.gov/disorders/syringomyelia/detail_syringomyelia.htm.

National Institutes of Health. (1997). Acupuncture: Consensus statement. *NIH, 15,* 1–34.

Ness, T. J. (2006). Genitourinary pain. In S. B. McMahon & M. Koltzenburg (Eds.), *Textbook of pain* (5th ed., pp. 777–791). Philadelphia: Elsevier.

Neumann, M., & Raj, P. P. (2000). Facet syndromes and blocks. In P. P. Raj (Ed.), *Practical management of pain* (3rd ed., p. 745–751). St. Louis: Mosby.

Newham, D. J., Edwards, R. H. T., & Mills, K. R. (1994). Skeletal muscle pain. In P. D. Wall & R. Melzack (Eds.), *Textbook of pain* (3rd ed., p. 433). New York: Churchill Livingstone.

Nicholson, B., & Passik, S. D. (2007). Management of chronic noncancer pain in the primary care setting. *Southern Medical Journal, 100*(10), 1028–1036.

Noble, M., Tregear, S. J., Treadwell, J. R., & Schoelles, K. (2008). Long-term opioid therapy for chronic noncancer pain: A systematic review and meta-analysis of efficacy and safety. *Journal of Pain and Symptom Management, 35*(2), 214–228.

Noe, C. E., & Racz, G. B. (1996). Radiofrequency. In P. P. Raj (Ed.), *Pain medicine: A comprehensive review* (pp. 305–307). St. Louis: Mosby-Year Book.

North, R. B. (2005). Spinal cord stimulation. In M. S. Wallace & P. S. Staats (Eds.), *Pain medicine & management: Just the facts* (pp. 285–288). New York: McGraw-Hill.

O'Neill, W. M., & Sherrard, J. A. (1993). Pain in human immunodeficiency virus disease: A review. *Pain, 54,* 3–14.

Orthogate. (2006). *Internet Society of Orthopaedic Surgery and Trauma: Spondylolysis.* Retrieved June 3, 2008, from http://www.orthogate.org/patient-education/lumbar-spine/lumbar-spondylolysis.html.

Oxman, M. N., Levin, M. J., Johnson, G. R., Schmader, K. E., Straus, S. E., Gelb, L. D., Arbeit, R. D., Simberkoff, M. S., Gershon, A. A., Davis, L. E., Weinberg, A., Boardman, K. D., William, H. M., Hongyuan Zhang, J., Peduzzi, P. N., Beisel, C. E., Morrison, V. A., Guatelli, J. C., Brooks, P. A., Kauffman, C. A., Pachucki, C. T., Neuzil, K. M., Betts, R. F., Wright, P. F., Griffin, M. R., Brunell, P., Soto, D. E., Marques, A. R., Keay, S. K., Goodman, R. P., Cotton, D. J., Gnann, J. W., Loutit, J., Holodniy, M., Keitel, W. A., Crawford, G. E., Yeh, S. S., Lobo, Z., Toney, J. F., Greenberg, R. N., Keller, P. M., Harbecke, R., Hayward, A. R., Irwin, M. R., Kyriakides, T. C., Chan, C. Y., Chan, I. S. F., Wang, W. W. B., Annunziato, P. W., & Silber, J. L. (2005). A vaccine to prevent herpes zoster and postherpetic neuralgia in older adults. *New England Journal of Medicine, 353*(22), 2271–2284.

Parry, G. J. (1988). Peripheral neuropathies associated with human immunodeficiency virus infection. *Annals of Neurology, 23,* S49–S53.

Patt, R. B., & Burton, A. W. (1999). Pain associated with advanced malignancy, including adjuvant analgesic drugs in cancer pain management. In G. M. Aronoff (Ed.), *Evaluation and treatment of chronic pain* (3rd ed., pp. 362–366). Baltimore: Williams & Wilkins.

Pawl, R. P. (1996). Ablative techniques. In P. P. Raj (Ed.), *Pain medicine: A comprehensive review* (p. 323). St. Louis: Mosby-Year Book.

Payne, R. (2005). Sickle cell anemia. In M. S. Wallace & P. S. Staats (Eds.), *Pain medicine & management: Just the facts* (pp. 234–236). New York: McGraw-Hill.

Pediatric Orthopaedic Society of North America. (2007). *Spondylolysis.* Retrieved June 3, 2008, from http://www.posna.org/members/coreCurr/-spondylolysis.cfm?showreg=yes&showreg7=yes.

Penfold, J., & Clark, A. J. M. (1992). Pain syndromes in HIV infection. *Canadian Journal of Anaesthesia, 39,* 724–730.

Peres, M. F., Stiles, M. A., Siow, H. C., Rozen, T. D., Young, W. B., & Silberstein, S. D. (2002). Greater occipital nerve blockade for cluster headache. *Cephalalgia, 22,* 520–522.

Perneger, T. V., Whelton, P. K., & Klag, M. J. (1994). Risk of kidney failure associated with the use of acetaminophen, aspirin, and nonsteroidal antiinflammatory drugs. *New England Journal of Medicine, 331,* 1675–1679.

Pickering, G., Esteve, V., Loriot, M. A., Eschalier, A., & Dubray, C. (2008). Acetaminophen reinforces descending inhibitory pain pathways. *Clinical Pharmacology & Therapeutics, 84*(1), 47–51.

Pontari, M. A., Hanno, P. M., & Wein, A. J. (1997). Logical and systematic approach to the evaluation and management of patients suspected of having interstitial cystitis. *Urology, 49*(Suppl. 5A), 114–120.

Porta, M., Perretti, A., & Gamba,M. (1998). The rationale and results of treating muscle spasm and myofascial syndromes with botulinum toxin type A. *Pain Digest, 8,* 346–352.

Portenoy, R. K. (1994). Opioid therapy for chronic nonmalignant pain: Current status. In H. L. Fields & J. C. Liebeskind (Eds.), *Pharmacological approaches to the treatment of chronic pain: New concepts and critical issues* (pp. 247–287). Seattle: International Association for the Study of Pain Press.

Portenoy, R. K. (1996). Opioid therapy for chronic nonmalignant pain: A review of the critical issues. *Journal of Pain and Symptom Management, 11,* 203–217.

Portenoy, R. K. (2000). *Pain in oncologic and AIDS patients.* Newtown, PA: Handbooks in Health Care.

Racz, G. B. (1998). Botulinum toxin as a new approach for refractory pain syndromes. *Pain Digest, 8,* 353–356.

Reuben, S. (2006a). *Preventing postmastectomy pain syndrome: Mastectomy. International Research Foundation for RSD/CRPS.* Retrieved May 17, 2008, from http://www.rsdfoundation.org/en/Preventing_RSD_Mastectomy.html.

Reuben, S. (2006b). *Preventing postthoracotomy pain syndrome: Thoracotomy. International Research Foundation for RSD/CRPS.* Retrieved May 17, 2008, from http://www.rsdfoundation.org/en/Preventing_RSD_Thoracotomy.html.

Reuben, S. S., & Sklar, J. (2002). Intravenous regional anesthesia with clonidine in the management of complex regional pain syndrome of the knee. *Journal of Clinical Anesthesia, 14,* 87–91.

Rollnik, J. D., Hierner, R., Schubert, M., Shen, Z. L., Johannes, S., Troger, M., Wohlfarth, K. L., Berger, A. C., & Dengler, R. (2000). Botulinum toxin treatment of cocontractions after birth-related brachial plexus lesions. *Neurology, 55,* 112–114.

Rooks, D. S., Gautam, S., Romeling, M., Cross, M. L., Stratigakis, D., Evans, B., Goldenberg, D. L., Iversen, M. D., & Katz, J. N. (2007). Group exercise, education, and combination self-management in women with fibromyalgia. *Archives of Internal Medicine, 167*(20), 2192–2200.

Rowbotham, M. C. (1994). Topical analgesic agents. In H. L. Fields & J. C. Liebeskind (Eds.), *Progress in pain research and management* (Vol. 1, pp. 211–227). Seattle: IASP Press.

Royal College of Dental Surgeons of Ontario. (2006). *Guidelines diagnosis & management of temporomandibular disorders & related musculoskeletal disorders.* Ontario: Author.

Russell, I. J. (2008). Fibromyalgia syndrome: New developments in pathophysiology and management. *CNS Spectrums, 13*(3 Suppl. 5), 4–5.

Sandberg, D. I., & Lavyne, M. H. (1999). Symptomatic spinal epidural lipomatosis after local epidural corticosteroid injections: Case report. *Neurosurgery, 45*(1), 162–165.

Scadding, J. W. (1994). Peripheral neuropathies. In P. D. Wall & R. Melzack (Eds.), *Textbook of pain* (3rd ed., pp. 675–677). New York: Churchill Livingstone.

Schmader, K. E., & Dworkin, R. H. (2008). Natural history and treatment of herpes zoster. *Journal of Pain, 9*(1), S3–S9.

Schoenen, J. (2006). Tension-type headache. In S. B. McMahon & M. Koltzenburg (Eds.), *Textbook of pain* (5th ed., pp. 875–886). Philadelphia: Elsevier.

Schon, L. C., & Davies, P. W. (2005). Peripheral nerve stimulation. In M. S. Wallace & P. S. Staats (Eds.), *Pain medicine & management: Just the facts* (pp. 315–318). New York: McGraw-Hill.

Schreiber, S., & Galai-Gat, T. (1993). Uncontrolled pain following physical injury as the core-trauma in post-traumatic stress disorder. *Pain, 54*(1), 107–110.

Scott, D. L. (2006). Osteoarthritis and rheumatoid arthritis. In S. B. McMahon & M. Koltzenburg (Eds.), *Textbook of pain* (5th ed., pp. 653–667). Philadelphia: Elsevier.

Sharma, M. (2005). Complementary and alternative medicine. In M. S. Wallace & P. S. Staats (Eds.), *Pain medicine & management: Just the facts* (pp. 277–282). New York: McGraw-Hill.

Sharp, T. J., & Harvey, A. G. (2001). Chronic pain and posttraumatic stress disorder: Mutual maintenance? *Clinical Psychology Review, 21*(6), 857–877.

Siddall, P. J., Yezierski, R. P., & Loeser, J. D. (2000). Pain following spinal cord injury: Clinical features, prevalence, and taxonomy. *IASP Newsletter, 3,* 5–6.

Silberstein, S. D., Lipton, R. B., Goadsby, P. J., & Smith, R. T. (1999). *Headache in primary care* (pp. 83–84). Oxford: Isis Medical Media.

Silberstein, S., Mathew, N., Saper, J., & Jenkins, S. (2000). Botulinum toxin type A as a migraine preventive treatment. *Headache, 40,* 445–450.

Sindrup, S. H., & Jensen, T. S. (2002). Pharmacotherapy of trigeminal neuralgia. *Clinical Journal of Pain, 18*(1), 22–27.

Singer, E. J., Zorilla, C., Fahy-Chandon, B., Chi, S., Syndulko, I., & Tourtellotte, W. (1993). Painful symptoms reported by ambulatory HIV-infected men in a longitudinal study. *Pain, 54,* 15–19.

Sist, T., Miner, M., & Lema, M. (1999). Characteristics of postradical neck pain syndrome: A report of 25 cases. *Journal of Pain and Symptom Management, 18,* 95–102.

Sitzman, B. T., Chen, Y., Clemans, R. R., Fishman, S. M., & Benzon, H. (2005). Pharmacology for the interventional pain physician. In H. Benzon, S. N. Raja, R. E. Molloy, S. S. Liu, & S. M. Fishman (Eds.), *Essentials of pain medicine and regional anesthesia* (2nd ed., pp. 175–177). Philadelphia: Elsevier, Churchill Livingstone.

Smith, W. C. S., Bourne, D., Squair, J., Phillips, D. O., & Chambers, W. A. (1999). A retrospective cohort study of post mastectomy pain syndrome. *Pain, 83*(1), 91–95.

Spangfort, E. (1994). Disc surgery. In P. D. Wall & R. Melzack (Eds.), *Textbook of pain* (3rd ed., p. 1068). New York: Churchill Livingstone.

Staats, P. S., & Luthardt, F. W. (2005). Intrathecal therapy for cancer pain. In M. S. Wallace & P. S. Staats (Eds.), *Pain medicine & management: Just the facts* (pp. 90–99). New York: McGraw-Hill.

Stankus, S. J., Dlugopolski, M., & Packer, D. (2000). Management of herpes zoster (shingles) and postherpetic neuralgia. *American Family Physician, 61,* 2437–2448.

St. Marie, B. (2001). Management of cancer pain with epidural morphine. In A. DuPen (Ed.), *Independent study module.* St. Paul, MN: SIMS Deltec.

St. Marie, B. J., & Arnold, S. (2002). *When your pain flares up.* Minneapolis: Fairview Press.

Tasker, R. R. (1999). Spinal cord injury and central pain. In G. M. Aronoff (Ed.), *Evaluation and treatment of chronic pain* (pp. 131–146). Baltimore: Williams & Wilkins.

Thiessen, B., & Portenoy, R. K. (1997). Adjuvant analgesics. In R. Kanner (Ed.), *Pain management secrets.* Philadelphia: Hanley & Belfus.

Todor, D. R., Mu, H. T. M., & Milhorat, T. H. (2000). Pain and syringomyelia: A review. *Neurosurgery Focus, 8*(3), 1–6.

Towheed, T. E., Maxwell, L., Anastassiades, T. P., Shea, B., Houpt, J., Robinson, V., & Hochberg, M. C. (2005). Glucosamine therapy for treating osteoarthritis. *Cochrane Database Systematic Review.* Retrieved June 7, 2009 , from http://www.cochrane.org/reviews/en/ab002946.html

Townsend, C. O., Kerkvliet, J. L., Bruce, B. K., Rome, J. D., Hooten, W. M., Luedtke, C. A., & Hodgson, J. E. (2008). A longitudinal study of the efficacy of a comprehensive pain rehabilitation program with opioids withdrawal: Comparison of treatment outcomes based on opioid use status at admission. *Pain, 140,* 177–189.

Travell, J. G., & Simons, D. G. (1983). *Myofascial pain and dysfunction; The trigger point manual.* Baltimore: Williams & Wilkins.

Trescot, A. M., Boswell, M. V., Atluri, S. L., Hansen, N. C., Deer, T. R., Abdi, S., Jasper, J. F., Singh, V., Jordan, A. E., Johnson, B. W., Cicala, R. S., Dunbar, E. E., Helm, S., II, Varley, K. G., Suchdev, P. K., Swicegood, J. R., Calodney, A. K., Ogoke, B. A., Minore, W. S., & Manchikanti, L. (2006). Opioid guidelines in the management of chronic non-cancer pain. *Pain Physician, 9*(1), 1–39.

Turk, D. C., & Nash, J. M. (1996). Psychologic issues in chronic pain. In R. K. Portenoy & R. M. Kanner (Eds.), *Pain management: Theory and practice* (pp. 323–335). Philadelphia: F. A. Davis.

Turk, D. C., Swanson, K. S., & Tunks, E. R. (2008). Psychological approaches in the treatment of chronic pain patients: When pills, scalpels, and needles are not enough. *Canadian Journal of Psychiatry, 53*(4), 213–223.

Tutuncu, Z., & Kavanaugh, A. (2005). Arthritis. In M. S. Wallace & P. S. Staats (Eds.), *Pain medicine & management: Just the facts* (pp. 179–182). New York: McGraw-Hill.

Ullrich, P. M., Jensen, M. P., Loeser, J. D., & Cardenas, D. D. (2008). Pain intensity, pain interference and characteristics of spinal cord injury. *Spinal Cord, 46,* 451–455.

Vainio, A., Ollila, J., Matikainen, E., Rosenberg, P., & Kalso, E. (1995). Driving ability in cancer patients receiving long-term morphine analgesia. *Lancet, 346,* 667–670.

Vallerand, A.H. (1998). Development and testing of the inventory of functional status- chronic pain. *Journal of Pain and Symptom Management,* 15, 125-139.

Veterans Health Administration/Department of Defense. (2003). *VA/DoD clinical practice guideline for the management of opioid therapy for chronic pain.* Washington, DC: Author. Retrieved May 18, 2008, from http://www.guideline.gov/summary/summary.aspx?ss=15&doc_id=4812&nbr=3474.

Waldman, S. D. (2004a). Caudal epidural nerve block: Lateral position. In *Atlas of interventional pain management* (2nd ed., pp. 393–398). Philadelphia: Saunders.

Waldman, S. D. (2004b). Caudal epidural nerve block: Prone position. In *Atlas of interventional pain management* (2nd ed., pp. 380–392). Philadelphia: Saunders.

Waldman, S. D. (2004c). Celiac plexus block. In *Atlas of interventional pain management* (2nd ed., pp. 265–293). Philadelphia: Saunders.

Waldman, S. D. (2004d). Cervical epidural block: Foraminal approach. In *Atlas of interventional pain management* (2nd ed., pp. 136–142). Philadelphia: Saunders.

Waldman, S. D. (2004e). Cervical epidural block: Translaminar approach. In *Atlas of interventional pain management* (2nd ed., pp. 129–135). Philadelphia: Saunders.

Waldman, S. D. (2004f). Cervical facet neurolysis: Radiofrequency lesioning of the cervical medial branch. In *Atlas of interventional pain management* (2nd ed., pp. 326–332). Philadelphia: Saunders.

Waldman, S. D. (2004g). Cervical selective nerve root block. In *Atlas of interventional pain management* (2nd ed., pp. 142–147). Philadelphia: Saunders.

Waldman, S. D. (2004h). Intradiscal electrothermal annuloplasty. In *Atlas of interventional pain management* (2nd ed., pp. 573–579). Philadelphia: Saunders.

Waldman, S. D. (2004i). Lumbar epidural nerve root block. In *Atlas of interventional pain management* (2nd ed., pp. 340–349). Philadelphia: Saunders.

Waldman, S. D. (2004j). Lumbar epidural nerve root block: Transforaminal approach. In *Atlas of interventional pain management* (2nd ed., pp. 350–355). Philadelphia: Saunders.

Waldman, S. D. (2004k). Lumbar facet block: Radiofrequency lesioning of the medial branch of the primary posterior rami. In *Atlas of interventional pain management* (2nd ed., pp. 326–332). Philadelphia: Saunders.

Waldman, S. D. (2004l). Lumbar sympathetic ganglion block. In *Atlas of interventional pain management* (2nd ed., pp. 308–312). Philadelphia: Saunders.

Waldman, S. D. (2004m). Percutaneous vertebroplasty. In *Atlas of interventional pain management* (2nd ed., pp. 587–590). Philadelphia: Saunders.

Warshaw, A. L., Banks, P. A., & Fernandez-Del Castillo, C. (1998). American Gastroenterological Association Clinical Practice and Practice Economics Committee. AGA technical review: Treatment of pain in chronic pancreatitis. *Gastroenterology, 115,* 765–776.

Watkins, P. B., Kaplowitz, N., Slattery, J. T., Colonese, C. R., Colucci, S. V., Stewart, P. W., & Harris, S. C. (2008). Aminotransferase elevations in healthy adults receiving 4 grams of acetaminophen daily: A randomized controlled trial. *Journal of the American Medical Society, 296*(1), 87–93.

Wehrman, J. (2005). Bill targets painkiller abusers [Electronic version]. *Courier & Press Washington Bureau,* March 7, 2005. Retrieved October 5, 2007, from http://www.courierpress.com/ecp/local_news/article/0,1626,ECP_745_3600466,00.html.

Widerstrom-Noga, E., Biering-Sorensen, R., Bryce, R., Cardenas, S. S., Finnerup, N. B., Jensen, M. P., Richards, J. S., & Siddall, P. J. (2008). The international spinal cord injury pain basic data set. *Spinal Cord, 46,* 818–823.

Williams, B. A., Neumann, K. J., Goel, S. K., & Wu, C. L. (2008). Postoperative pain and other acute pain syndromes. In H. T. Benzon, J. P. Rathmell, C. L. Wu, D. C. Turk, & C. E. Argoff (Eds.), *Raj's practical management of pain* (4th ed., pp. 299–334). Philadelphia: Mosby Elsevier.

Wolfe, F., Smythe, H. A., Yunus, M. B., Bennett, R. M., Bombardier, C., Goldenberg, D. L., Tugwell, P., Campbell, S. M.,Abeles, M., Clark, P., Fam. A.G., Farber, S.J., Fiechtner, J.J., Franklin, C.M., Gatter, R.A., Hamaty, D., Lessard, J., Lichtbroun, A.S., Masi, A.T., McCain, G.A., Reynolds, W.J., Romano, R.J., Russell, I.J., & Sheon, R.P. (1990). The American College of Rheumatology 1990 criteria for the classification of fibromyalgia: Report of the Multicenter Criteria Committee. *Arthritis and Rheumatism, 33*(2), 160–165.

Wong, H. Y., & Mayer, E. A. (2006). A clinical perspective on abdominal pain. In S. B. McMahon & M. Koltzenburg (Eds.), *Textbook of pain* (5th ed., pp. 753–776). Philadelphia: Elsevier.

Wu, C. L., & Raja, S. N. (2008). An update on the treatment of postherpetic neuralgia. *Journal of Pain, 9*(1), S19–S30.

Wu, C. L., Lin, E. E., & Maine, D. N. (2008). Outcomes, efficacy, and complications of neuropathic pain. In H. T. Benzon, J. P. Rathmell, C. L. Wu, D. C. Turk, & C. E. Argoff (Eds.), *Raj's practical management of pain* (4th ed., pp. 1249–1260). Philadelphia: Mosby Elsevier.

Wu, S. M., Compton, P., Bolus, R., Schieffer, B., Pham, Q., Baria, A., Van Vort, W., Davis, R., Shekelle, P., & Haliboff, B. D. (2006). The Addiction Behaviors Checklist: Validation of a new clinician-based measure of inappropriate opioid use in chronic pain. *Journal of Pain and Symptom Management, 32*(4), 342–351.

Yaksi, A., Ozgonenel, L., & Ozgonenel, B. (2007). The efficiency of gabapentin therapy in patients with lumbar spinal stenosis. *Spine, 32*(9), 939–942.

Youmans, L. (2001). Conscious sedation. In Hankins, J., Lonsway, R. A. W., Hedrick, C., & Perdue, M. B. (Eds.), *The infusion nurses society infusion therapy in clinical practice* (pp. 604–614). St. Louis: W. B. Saunders.

Yuhan, R., Orsay, C., DelPino, A., Pearl, R., Pulvirenti, J., Kay, S., & Abcarian, H. (1998). Anorectal disease in HIV-infected patients. *Diseases of the Colon and Rectum, 11,* 1376–1370.

Yurth, E. F. (2004). *New technologies for treating low back pain.* Retrieved August 23, 2008, from http://www.mapletonhill.com/resources/a-yurth.html.

Ziger, J. (2005). *Facet technologies.* Retrieved November 21, 2008, from http://www.spine-health.com/treatment/artificial-disc-replacement/facet-technologies.

Suggested Readings

Abramson, S. (1991). Therapy with and mechanisms of nonsteroidal antiinflammatory drugs. *Current Opinion in Rheumatology, 3,* 336–340.

Taiwo, Y., & Levine, J. (1988). Prostaglandins inhibit endogenous pain control mechanisms by blocking transmission at spinal noradrenergic synapses. *Journal of Neuroscience, 8,* 1346–1349.

Zed, P. J., & Krenzelok, E. P. (1999). Treatment of acetaminophen overdose. *American Journal of Health-System Pharmacy, 56,* 1081–1091.

appendix

18-1

Addiction Behaviors Checklist

Instructions: Code only for patients prescribed opioid or sedative analgesics on behaviors exhibited "since last visit" and "within the current visit."

Addiction behaviors-since last visit			
1. Patient used illicit drugs or evidences problem drinking	Y	N	NA
2. Patient has hoarded medications	Y	N	NA
3. Patient used more narcotic than prescribed	Y	N	NA
4. Patient ran out of medications early	Y	N	NA
5. Patient has increased use of narcotics	Y	N	NA
6. Patient used analgesics PRN when prescription is for time-contingent use	Y	N	NA
7. Patient received narcotics from more than one provider	Y	N	NA
8. Patient bought medications on the streets	Y	N	NA
Addiction behaviors-within current visit			
1. Patient appears sedated or confused (e.g., slurred speech, unresponsive)	Y	N	NA
2. Patient expresses worries about addiction	Y	N	NA
3. Patient expresses a strong preference for a specific type of analgesic or a specific route of administration	Y	N	NA
4. Patient expresses concern about future availability of narcotic	Y	N	NA
5. Patient reports worsened relationships with family	Y	N	NA
6. Patient misrepresents analgesic prescription or use	Y	N	NA
7. Patient indicates she or he "needs" or "must have" analgesic medications	Y	N	NA
8. Discussion of analgesic medications is the predominant issue of visit	Y	N	NA
9. Patient exhibits lack of interest in rehab or self-management	Y	N	NA
10. Patient reports minimal or inadequate relief from narcotic analgesic	Y	N	NA
11. Patient indicates difficulty with using medication agreement	Y	N	NA
Other			
1. Significant others express concern over patient's use of analgesics	Y	N	NA

Y, yes; N, no; NA, not assessed; PRN, as needed.done.

From *Journal of Pain and Symptom Management*, Volume 32, 4. Reprinted by permission of Elsevier. Permission conveyed through Rightslink.

chapter

19

Cancer Pain Management

Linda Vanni, RN, MSN, ACNS-BC, NP
Marsha N. Rehm, MSN, RN-BC, FAAPM

Objectives

After studying this chapter, the reader should be able to:

1. Describe the causes of cancer pain.
2. Identify a class of adjuvant medication, including the mechanism of action and two adverse effects, used in the treatment of neuropathic pain syndromes.
3. Identify a clinical benefit and a quality-of-life issue in the use of palliative chemotherapy and radiation.
4. Describe a nonpharmacological management modality in each of the following categories: physical interventions and cognitive-behavioral interventions.
5. Identify a clinical indication for each of the following interventional approaches: neuraxial opioid therapy, regional analgesia, neuroaugmentation, and surgery.
6. Describe a caregiver and quality-of-life issue in home pain management.

I. Cause of Cancer Pain

A. Cancer pain results from three primary causes.
   1. Tumors are involved in 65% to 85% of cases.
   2. Cancer-related procedures and treatment affect 15% to 25% of patients.
   3. Causes unrelated to cancer or its treatment occur in 3% to 10% of patients (Garofalo, Gatchel, & Baum, 2007).

B. Cancer pain can be further categorized as acute or chronic in duration.
   1. Cancer-related acute pain syndromes most commonly are due to diagnostic or therapeutic interventions (Cherny, 1998).
   2. Most chronic cancer-related pain is caused directly by the tumor. Bone pain and compression of neural structures are the two most common causes (Garofalo et al., 2007).

C. Cancer-related pain syndromes can be characterized as nociceptive, neuropathic, or mixed.
   1. *Nociceptive* pain results from the activation of nociceptors in somatic and visceral structures. often relating to tissue damage, such as bone metastasis (Miaskowski, 2003).
   2. *Neuropathic* pain is sustained by abnormal processing of sensory input by the central or peripheral nervous system and can be caused by tumor itself or treatment (Fine, Miaskowski, & Paice, 2004; Fromer, 2003).

D. Multiple dimensions
   1. The *affective dimension* encompasses emotional responses to pain, including anxiety, depression, mood changes, anger, irritability, personality traits, and actual psychiatric diagnosis (Ahles & Martin, 1992; McGuire, 2004).
   2. The *cognitive dimension* consists of the manner in which pain influences the individual's thought processes, the way in which the individual views himself or herself, and the meaning of pain to the individual (Ahles & Martin, 1992; McGuire, 2004).
   3. The *behavioral dimension* includes two categories:
      a. Behaviors showing the presence and severity of pain: unconscious, reflexive, and deliberate
      b. Behaviors unconsciously or deliberately undertaken to control pain (Wilkie & Keefe, 1991)
   4. The *sociocultural dimension* consists of demographic characteristics, ethnic background, and other factors within pain sufferers and their caregivers (McGuire, 2004).

II. Cancer Pain Syndromes

A. Pain can be related to musculoskeletal tumor involvement: general bone involvement, acute pathological fracture, metastatic disease, osteosarcomas, or multiple myeloma.

B. Pain can be associated with tumor involvement of the viscera: intestinal obstruction, carcinomatosis, or advanced cancer of the pancreas, colon, uterus, or ovaries.

C. Pain can be associated with peripheral or central nervous system involvement: tumor infiltration of peripheral nerves; tumor infiltration of the brachial, lumbar, or sacral plexus; spinal cord compression; epidural metastases; peripheral neuropathies; or acute and postherpetic neuralgia.

D. Postsurgical pain can be associated with cancer treatment: postmastectomy syndrome, postthoracotomy syndrome, or phantom limb pain (Goldstein, 1999; McGuire, 2004).

E. Postradiation pain syndromes can be associated with cancer treatment: myelopathy, radiation burns, mucositis, or osteoradionecrosis (McGuire, 2004; Sonis, 2007).

III. Guidelines, Position Papers, and Consensus Statement

A. Guidelines are used to guide clinical practice. As the discipline matures, guidelines offer further details into various pain issues.
   1. The World Health Organization, using its analgesic ladder, has historically provided a strong foundation for educating health care providers on the sequence for treating cancer pain (Jacox et al., 1994; Mercadante, 1999).

2. The NCCN treatment algorithms incorporate an integrative approach to cancer pain management (Rainone, 2004). Please see the following URL for the specific algorithms on Adult Cancer Pain Guidelines: http://www.nccn.org/professionals/physician_gls/f_guidelines.asp.
3. The Agency for Healthcare Research and Quality (formerly the Agency for Healthcare Policy and Research) has its own guidelines (Jacox et al., 1994).
4. The National Comprehensive Cancer Network (2008) has issued cancer pain treatment guidelines for patients.
5. The American Pain Society (APS, 2005) has its own guidelines.

B. Position papers
1. Oncology Nursing Society (Spross, McGuire, & Schmitt, 1990)
2. American Society for Pain Management Nursing (2003)
3. American Society of Anesthesiologists (1996)

C. Consensus statement
1. American Society of Regional Anesthesia and Pain Medicine (Horlocker et al., 2003)

IV. Pharmacological Interventions

A. Opioids (see the chapter on Overview of Pharmacology)
1. The mechanism of action produces an analgesic effect through spinal and supraspinal mechanisms by binding to the μ, δ-, and κ-receptors. The type of opioid receptor and its location determine the effects an opioid drug produces (Pasternak, 2007; Reisine & Pasternak, 1996).
   a. Opioids are thought to activate endogenous pain-modulating systems mimicking the action of endogenous opioid compounds (Fine & Portenoy, 2004).
   b. Opioid receptors are located in the central nervous system, in the pituitary gland, in the gastrointestinal tract, in cells of the immune system, and on peripheral terminals of sensory nerves. They are particularly abundant in the periaqueductal gray and the dorsal horn of the spinal cord (Fine et al., 2004; Portenoy, 1996).
2. Indications for clinical use are mild-to-severe pain in acute, chronic, and postoperative pain states (see the chapter on Acute Pain Management).
   a. The oral route is the preferred route because it is convenient, well tolerated, and usually the least expensive. When patients are unable to take oral agents, other noninvasive routes, such as rectal or transdermal, should be tried (Grady, Severn, & Eldridge, 2007).
3. *Ceiling effect* is a dose above which further dose increments produce no change in effect.

B. Adjuvant medications (see the chapter on Overview of Pharmacology)
1. General principles
   a. Selection is usually suggested by a characteristic of pain or the existence of another concurrent symptom amenable to the nonanalgesic effect of the drug.
   b. The response to all adjuvant analgesics varies greatly, including within the same class. Sequential trials may be beneficial.
   c. Considerations
      (1) Select the adjuvant and dose based on careful assessment and evaluation of comorbid conditions.
      (2) Use specific adjuvants for specific indications.
      (3) Understand the pharmacology of the adjuvant.
      (4) Recognize interindividual and intraindividual variability.
      (5) Consider the risk and benefit of polypharmacy (Portenoy, 1993).
2. Types of adjuvant medications (see the chapter on Overview of Pharmacology)
   a. Acetaminophen and nonsteroidal antiinflammatory drugs (NSAIDs)
      (1) Acetaminophen works on a proposed mechanism of inhibition of a third isoform of cyclooxygenase (COX-3) found in the central nervous system (APS, 2003; Chandrasekharan et al., 2002). The result is analgesic and antipyretic. NSAIDs inhibit synthesis of COX-1 and COX-2 to prostaglandins, the primary neurosensitizer for peripheral and central nerves to painful stimulus.

(2) The indication for clinical use is inflammatory pain associated with surgery, trauma, arthritis, and cancer (APS, 2003).
(3) Adverse effects
(a) Acetaminophen
(i) Acute overdose (more than 4,000 mg/d) is associated with fatal hepatic necrosis.
(ii) Acetaminophen should be avoided in chronic ethanol use or liver disease.
(iii) Caution should be taken in patients who are fasting and those on warfarin therapy (APS, 2003).
(b) NSAIDs
(i) NSAIDs are contraindicated in those with coagulopathies, history of gastrointestinal bleeding, or renal insufficiency.
(ii) Occasionally, central nervous system symptoms may occur, including decreased attention span, short-term memory loss, and headache (Portenoy, 2000).

b. Tricyclic antidepressants
(1) Tricyclic antidepressants inhibit presynaptic neuronal reuptake of serotonin and norepinephrine.
(2) They are used to treat neuropathic pain from surgery, radiation, chemotherapy, and malignant nerve infiltration. Taken before bedtime, the sedative effects can improve sleep in some patients (APS, 2003; Portenoy, 2000).
(3) Adverse effects are dry mouth, urinary retention, constipation, delirium, sedation, and orthostatic hypotension. Use is contraindicated in patients with coronary disease associated with arrhythmias.

c. Anticonvulsants
(1) Anticonvulsants decrease the ectopic, spontaneous firing of central nervous system neurons associated with neuropathic pain (APS, 2003).
(2) They are used in neuropathic pain described as lancinating or with "stabbing" or paroxysmal properties (APS, 2003; Portenoy, 2000).
(3) Adverse effects of nausea, vomiting, rash, dizziness, edema, and confusion are most common. Other more potentially serious reactions include pancytopenia and depression.

d. Corticosteroids (see chapter on Overview of Pharmacology Appendices 14-10A and 14-10B)
(1) Corticosteroids have an unknown regarding analgesic mechanism.
(2) They have been shown to reduce the spontaneous discharge from injured nerves (Fine et al., 2004).
(3) It seems several processes are mediated: reduction of peritumoral edema, decrease of tumor mass, decreased concentration of inflammatory mediators, and decreased electrical activity in damaged nerves (Portenoy, 1993).
(4) Indications for clinical use are neuropathic pain, bone pain, headache resulting from increased intracranial pressure, obstruction of hollow viscera, arthralgias, and spinal cord compression (Watanabe & Bruera, 1994). Corticosteroids are also useful in brachial and lumbosacral plexus tumors, as well as improved appetite, decreased nausea, and enhanced mood (APS, 2003).
(5) Adverse effects
(a) Acute, short-term use is usually well tolerated. Changes in mood, perception, or cognitive functioning; hyperglycemia; fluid retention; and gastrointestinal disturbances may occur.
(b) Long-term effects include development of cushingoid appearance, weight gain, hypertension, severe osteoporosis, increased risk of infection, and increased risk of skin diseases and skin tears. Taper is needed to avoid a withdrawal syndrome of muscle and joint pain, malaise, headache, mood disturbances, and pain flare (APS, 2003; Haynes, 1990).

(6) Available agents
  (a) Dexamethasone (Decadron®) is usually selected because of its relatively low mineralocorticoid effects that result in less fluid retention and electrolyte disturbance.
  (b) Methylprednisolone (Medrol®) and prednisone are also used. A common conversion is 4 mg of prednisone, to 5 mg of methylprednisolone, to 0.75 mg of dexamethasone.

e. Benzodiazepines
  (1) Mechanism of action
    (a) Benzodiazepines influence γ-aminobutyric acid.
    (b) Mediated inhibition of impulses and ectopic nerve firing occurs.
    (c) Benzodiazepines produce effects on the emotional—motivational component but not on the sensory—discriminative or central component (Reddy & Patt, 1994).
  (2) Indications for clinical use are pain associated with anxiety, muscle spasm, and lancinating pain from nerve injury.
    (a) Except for pain related to muscle spasm, these agents are not effective analgesics. Some benefit is seen in cancer patients with recurrent anxiety in whom antidepressants are not indicated and for terminal dyspnea. Opioid titration should precede treatment with benzodiazepines (APS, 2003).
  (3) Adverse effects are sedation, respiratory depression, slurred vision and speech, and central nervous system excitation in the elderly.
    (a) Combining with opioids can potentiate side effects of both; reducing the dose of the benzodiazepine by one-third is recommended (Somerson, Husted, & Sicilia, 1995).
    (b) If it is necessary to reverse the sedative effect, give the antagonist, flumazenil (Romazicon®). This may precipitate seizures and other withdrawal symptoms in patients taking benzodiazepines long term (Hobbs, Rall, & Verfoorn, 1996).
  (4) Available agents (see the chapter on Overview of Pharmacology)

f. Local anesthetics
  (1) Mechanism of action
    (a) Local anesthetics block sodium ion channels, imposing a conduction block of the action potential
    (b) They may possibly inhibit synaptic transmission (Backonja, 1994).
  (2) Indications for clinical use are continuous dysesthetic neuropathic pain, complex regional pain syndrome types I and II, phantom pain, and trigeminal and postherpetic neuralgia.
    (a) Local anesthetics are considered the second line after tricyclic antidepressants and anticonvulsants.
    (b) They are used in three ways: for localized injection into the tissue, near major nerves or intraspinally; for localized analgesia by absorption of a topical application; and for generalized analgesia by systemic administration (McCaffery & Pasero, 1999).
  (3) Adverse effects consist of central nervous system and cardiac effects.
    (a) Information about long-term safety is limited.
    (b) Central nervous system effects
      (i) At lower concentrations, the patient may experience dizziness from orthostasis, circumoral anesthesia, other paresthesias, or tremor.
      (ii) At higher concentrations, the patient may have progressive encephalopathy or seizures.
    (c) Cardiac conduction disturbances and myocardial depression can occur. Use local anesthetics cautiously in patients with preexisting heart disease (Covina, 1993).

(d) High intraspinal concentrations can cause numbness in dermatomes covered by the local anesthetic.

(5) Available agents are described in the chapter on Overview of Pharmacology.

g. Antineoplastic therapies

(1) Types and rationale for chemotherapy are primary (curative), adjuvant, and palliative.

(a) Adjuvant is used as potentially curative therapy after all gross evidence of disease has been removed by surgery or radiation, but risk of recurrence is great.

(b) Palliative chemotherapy is the use of antineoplastic medications to reduce the adverse signs and symptoms directly or indirectly caused by the malignant disease process.

(c) Effect is usually described by response rate and the benefit-to-toxicity ratio.

(d) Giving subtherapeutic doses of chemotherapy to prevent the patient from believing the case is hopeless is discouraged.

(e) Prospective trials of treatment versus watch and wait do not permit a definite recommendation regarding when to treat the asymptomatic patient with incurable malignancy (Ellison, 1998).

(2) Prognostic factors

(a) Most important after tumor type is performance status or activity level. An Eastern Cooperative Oncology Group (ECOG) score of 3 or 4 and a Karnofsky score of less than 50% are more likely to show excessive chemotherapy toxicity than beneficial response.

(b) Cancers recurring within 6 months of cessation of adjuvant chemotherapy are less likely to respond.

(3) Quality-of-life (QOL) issues

(a) QOL and prolongation of life are important parameters in determining chemotherapy treatments. Treatment that does not alter survival but improves QOL usually is considered beneficial (Gough & Dalgleish, 1991).

(b) A patient's QOL often is underestimated by the health care provider and family when compared with the patient's self-report (Tsevat et al., 1995).

(i) For similar survival advantages, patients always would choose radiotherapy versus chemotherapy (Brundage, Davidson, & Maokillop, 1997).

(ii) Patients of any age living with children are more likely to accept aggressive chemotherapy, even with a low probability of success (Yella & Cella, 1995).

(iii) Patients who previously received chemotherapy are more likely to accept aggressive and more toxic treatment (Yella, Cella, & Leslie, 1994).

(iv) Patients tend overwhelmingly to accept the physician's advice (Siminoff & Fetting, 1991).

(v) Patients' attitudes change dramatically when they receive a diagnosis of cancer. The reality of the diagnosis means that more risks are taken, even for relatively low likelihood of benefit (Slevin et al., 1990).

V. Nonpharmacological Interventions

A. Invasive therapies

1. Radiation therapy (Aistars & Vehlow, 2007)

a. Benefits or radiation therapy are that it relieves pain, improves function and appearance, alleviates obstruction, and controls bleeding.

b. Patients diagnosed with lung cancer are most commonly referred, followed by patients with breast, prostate, kidney, gastrointestinal tract, and head and neck cancer; gynecological patients; non-Hodgkin lymphoma patients; and patients with melanoma.

c. The most common metastatic sites are brain, skeleton, lung, gastrointestinal tract, and genitourinary tract.

d. Treatment side effects are early, late, or both. Early side effects are influenced by fractional dose, total dose, and overall treatment time; late side effects are influenced primarily by fractional dose.
   (1) Bone metastases
      (a) Most solid tumors have similar patterns of spread, involving the vertebrae (69%), pelvis (41%), femur (25%), and skull (4%) (Malawer & Delaney, 1993).
      (b) Goals are to palliate pain, reduce the need for opioids, improve ambulation, and reduce complications of spinal cord compression and pathological fracture.
      (c) External-beam radiation is the standard, providing durable pain relief in 73% to 90% of patients. It does not improve survival (Trodella, 1984).
      (d) Approximately 25% to 30% of patients require retreatment, with 87% responding (Mithal, Needham, & Hoskins, 1994).
      (e) Systemic intravenous radiopharmaceuticals
         (i) Strontium-89 (Metastron®) has shown pain relief in patients with multiple skeletal metastases. The strontium-89 half-life is 50 days, with a 10-fold disposition in areas of increased bone metabolism; the nadir level is 4 to 8 weeks after dose at 50% to 60% of baseline (Silberstein, 1993).
         (ii) The samarium-153 (Quadramet®) half-life is 46 hours, and the dose delivery rate is fast. Pain flare may occur within 3 days of administration. Onset of pain relief usually 1 to 2 weeks. Duration of myelosuppression is shorter, and recovery is faster than with strontium-89 (Iuliano, Abruzzese, Peta, Toraldo, & Palerno, 2004).
   (2) Brain metastases
      (a) It has been found that 25% to 30% of all cancer patients experience metastatic spread to the central nervous system, with melanoma the highest, followed by breast and lung (Wright, Delaney, & Buckner, 1993).
      (b) The goal is to maintain the highest neurological function attainable.
      (c) Corticosteroids are also usually given to reduce cerebral edema.
      (d) Surgical resection with solitary brain metastases is controversial (Noordijk et al., 1994).
      (e) Cranial irradiation can improve the median survival 3 to 6 months (Coia, 1992).
      (f) Stereotactic radiosurgery (gamma knife) is likely to have an important role in multiple brain metastases or recurrent disease (Flickinger et al., 1994).
   (3) Thoracic symptoms
      (a) The symptoms are airway obstruction, hemoptysis, cough, dyspnea, chest pain.
      (b) The goal is to improve QOL; it does not extend survival (Slawson & Scott, 1979).
      (c) Radiation with or without chemotherapy is well established to relieve esophageal obstruction and swallowing symptoms (Burmeister et al., 1995).
   (4) Hepatic metastases
      (a) Up to 50% of patients with colorectal carcinoma develop liver disease.
      (b) Goals are to palliate pain and decrease opioid usage, nausea, and intraductal obstruction.
      (c) Radiation alone is indicated for painful hepatomegaly, with improvement in 55% to 95% of patients (Richter & Coia, 1985).
e. Acute treatment side effects (Murphy, 2007)
   (1) Radiation mucositis, chemotherapy mucositis, or both results in acute, pain difficult to treat. Systemic analgesics, topical anesthetics, effective oral care, dietary modifications, and topical mucosal protectants are used to control pain (Pico, Avila-Garavito, & Naccache, 1998).
   (2) Radiation dermatitis may result in the need to decrease the dosage of treatment. Hydrocolloid dressings may be used for pain relief (Hymes, Strom, & Fife, 2006). Calendula cream is also effective in decreasing painful areas (McQuestion, 2006).

2. Interventional approaches
   a. General principles
      (1) Perform a complete history and physical examination because diagnostic testing alone is never sufficient. Attempt to establish a diagnosis or mechanism; optimize the balance between efficacy and side effects.
      (2) Do not rely on high technology to replace the practical; in most cases, withhold interventional approaches until optimal oral analgesic regimens fail.
      (3) No singular approach is a panacea. Approaches should have enough flexibility to accommodate future change. The number of options increases as the patient becomes sicker and symptoms become more complex (APS, 2005).
   b. Neuraxial opioid therapy
      (1) Use neuraxial opioid therapy only when pain is refractory to less invasive treatments or there are intolerable or untreatable side effects.
      (2) This type of therapy is classified into five types:
         (a) Percutaneous epidural or intrathecal catheter
         (b) Percutaneous intrathecal or epidural catheter that is tunneled a few inches from the insertion site
         (c) Implanted epidural or intrathecal catheter tunneled across the flank and attached to an internal injection port
         (d) Manually activated pump
         (e) Completely implanted pump (White & Rajagopal, 2006)
      (3) Complete neurological examination should be performed. Magnetic resonance imaging (MRI) or computed tomography may be recommended to exclude tumor from the operative site.
      (4) Opioid selection is based on the lipophilic or hydrophilic properties of the opioid and the neuraxial spread required to cover the painful area.
      (5) Risks are of infection, bleeding, and complicated care after placement; resources are limited for following this technology.
      (6) Benefits are a lower opioid dose for improved analgesia, with fewer side effects and improved survival (Smith et al., 2004).
   c. Regional analgesia
      (1) Diagnostic and temporary blocks use local anesthetic, usually large volumes if peripheral, to ascertain the specific nociceptive pathway, define the mechanism of pain and the site of noxious stimuli, and relieve severe regional pain. Regional analgesia may be performed epidurally or intrathecally with smaller volumes of local anesthetic.
         (a) Risks arise from invasive needle procedures requiring high level of skill.
         (b) Benefits are a decrease in opioid requirements and blockage of the pain cycle (Hough, Goudas, & Carr, 2004).
      (2) Neurolytic, permanent, and neurodestructive blocks
         (a) The primary effect appears to be the denaturing of protein and nonselective damage to neural tissue (Politis, Schaumburg, & Spencer, 1980).
         (b) Chemical neurolysis occurs with injection of phenol or alcohol. Alcohol partially preserves the myelin sheath, which is thought helpful in preventing the formation of painful neuromas. Body positioning is key (Hough et al., 2004).
         (c) Pain relief is not permanent; duration may be days, weeks, or months (Auad, 2006).
         (d) Complications can occur due to systemic absorption.
         (e) Blocks may be subarachnoid, epidural, or peripheral.
         (f) Considerations
            (i) Neurolytic, permanent, and neurodestructive blocks should be considered for localized pain not responding to conservative techniques.
            (ii) They lack the specificity of diagnostic blocks.

(iii) They should not stand alone as therapeutic intervention.
(iv) These blocks rarely eliminate all painful sensation.
(v) They have a narrow risk-to-benefit ratio.

(3) Autonomic blockade entails either pure sympathetic fibers, as in the stellate ganglion, or visceral afferent fibers, as in celiac plexus, hypogastric block, and ganglion impar (Waldman, 2007). This is used to treat ischemic pain and sympathetically maintained neuropathic pain.
(a) Stellate ganglion is for neuropathic pain related to malignancy of the face, upper extremity, and chest wall at level C6 to C7 (see the dermatome map in the Taxonomy for Pain Management Nursing chapter).
(b) Celiac plexus block for pain is associated with malignancy of the liver, pancreas, or gastrointestinal tract at the level of L1, anterior to the aorta and the superior vena cava (Baheti, 2001; Stefaniak et al., 2005; Yan & Myers, 2007; Zhang et al., 2008).
(c) Hypogastric block is used for lower abdominal malignancy and pelvic pain.
(d) Ganglion impar block is for pain associated with malignancy of the perineum, rectum, and genitalia (Waldman, 2007).

(4) Cryoanalgesia is a technique in which low temperatures interrupt afferent flow, producing pain relief by inducing a reversible conduction block by complete immersion of the tissue in a cold environment. Pain relief lasts weeks to months (Saberski, 2007).
(a) Axons and myelin sheaths degenerate, but epineurium and perineurium remain intact and are thus unlikely to form painful neuromas.
(b) Cryoanalgesia is used for localized conditions originating from small, well-localized lesions on peripheral nerves, such as in postthoracotomy pain, craniofacial pain syndromes, and postherpetic neuropathies (Evans, 1981).

d. Neurosurgical approaches are appropriate for less than 5% of cancer pain cases (Waldman, 2007).
(1) Cordotomy is used in unilateral somatic pain from the torso to the lower extremities. Exclude patients with life expectancies greater than 2 years because of late-developing dysesthesias.
(2) Surgical rhizotomy is seldom performed because of required extensive laminectomies, and there may be failure due to regrowth of neurons from adjacent skin or within the spinal cord. The preferred method is percutaneous surgical or chemical rhizotomy.

e. Interventional radiological or pain medicine techniques
(1) Stereotactic radiosurgery image-guided neuroablative procedures include thalamotomy, cingulotomy, and rhizotomy. Procedures involve use of electrodes placed deeply into intracranial targets (Fenstermaker, 2006).
(a) A gamma knife, an MRI-targeted computer system, uses beams of radiation with a head frame for achievement of precise ablation. Minimally invasive, it requires no skull opening. The procedure is limited to head and neck lesions only. Pain relief is not immediate.
(b) CyberKnife uses precise beams of radiation without the need for frame attachment. It allows for a divided treatment schedule to preserve nonaffected tissue areas. It is not limited to head and neck lesions. Pain relief is also not immediate (Hoffelt, 2006).

(2) Vertebroplasty and kyphoplasty are minimally invasive techniques used for the treatment of painful vertebral compression fractures resulting from malignancy or osteoporosis (Alberico & Abdel-halim, 2007) (see the chapter on Persistent Pain Management).
(a) Vertebroplasty is the percutaneous fixation of a pathological vertebral compression fracture by injection of polymethyl methacrylate inserted into the vertebral body (Alberico, Abdel-halim, & Husain, 2006). Concerns with procedure include possible cement extravasation, which does not address the issue of deformity (Alberico & Abdel-halim, 2007).

(b) Kyphoplasty is a dual-needle approach with balloons inflated into the fractured vertebral body. Balloons are inflated to elevate the end plates, thus creating a cavity. The balloons are deflated and removed, and then the cavity is filled with bone cement (Alberico & Abdel-halim, 2007).

(3) Cryotherapy or cryoablation is the formation of ice crystals causing direct injury, including cellular damage, to cancerous areas that results in cell microcirculatory failure (Solomon et al., 2008). It is used for cancers refractory to conventional therapy (Beland, Dupuy, & Mayo-Smith, 2005).

(a) Percutaneous, image-guided insertion of a probe or probes produces a cytotoxic ice zone more than 1 cm beyond apparent tumor margins (Solomon et al., 2008). Pain relief results from defined ice ball formation, rapid cooling to −100°C within a few seconds, and active thawing at the defined cancerous lesion (Callstrom et al., 2006).

(b) Cryotherapy or cryoablation is used for treatment of painful conditions such as gynecological cancer metastases (Solomon et al., 2008), extraabdominal metastatic disease (Beland et al., 2005), and soft tissue and bone metastases (Tuncali et al., 2007).

f. Neuroaugmentation (Saberski, 1998)

(1) The mechanism may include inhibition of afferent nociceptive input via the gate control mechanism, stimulation of enkephalin release, activation of opioid receptors, or enhanced regional blood flow.

(2) The four types are transcutaneous electrical nerve stimulation, dorsal column stimulation, deep brain stimulation, and peripheral nerve stimulation (Burton & Hassenbusch, 2006).

(a) Dorsal column stimulation and deep brain stimulation are limited in cancer pain because they are inserted and adjusted to treat symptoms at the time of implantation and may not have flexibility to accommodate disease progression and sequential MRIs.

(b) Peripheral nerve stimulation is indicated for deafferentation pain confined to a single peripheral nerve.

g. Surgery

(1) The goal is relief of symptoms or complications associated with a tumor, with preservation or improvement in QOL.

(2) Indications are pain, gastrointestinal or biliary obstruction, hemorrhage, perforation, and malignant ascites. Surgery offers the only prospect of cure in pancreatic cancer (Whooley & Conlon, 1998).

(3) Principles

(a) First resection is the best opportunity for cure.

(b) Simple tumor debulking does not provide durable palliation.

(c) Local recurrence is not indicative of disseminated disease.

(d) Timing of surgery for pain control is important (Jacox et al., 1994).

(4) Side effects are postoperative pain and complications, postmastectomy, and postthoracotomy pain syndromes.

B. Complementary therapies: physical or cognitive-behavioral (see the chapter on Integrative Therapies Used in Pain Management Nursing)

1. General principles

a. Analgesics are the mainstay of pain relief. Most pain is treated with a combination of medication and nonmedication approaches (Anderson et al., 2006).

b. Outcomes for nonmedication therapies are unpredictable.

c. Benefits and rationale for use of analgesics are that they may diminish the emotional components of pain, they have strengthen-coping abilities, and they reduce perceived threat, give the patient and family a sense of control, change expectations, enhance comfort, contribute to pain relief, decrease fatigue, restore hope, promote sleep, and improve QOL (Spross & Wolfe, 1995; Stephenson, Swanson, Dalton, Keefe, & Engelke, 2007).

d. Relaxation techniques, chiropractic, and massage are most commonly used (Eisenberg et al., 1993). Reiki, reflexology, aromatherapy, guided imagery, and acupuncture have also been shown to be effective (Fellowes, Barnes, & Wilkinson, 2004; Kwekkeboom, Hau, Wanta, & Bumpus, 2008; Stephenson et al., 2007).

e. Active or passive treatments reducing pain directly involve the body. They may reduce pain through direct effects on the integumentary, musculoskeletal, and nervous systems (Fernandez, 1986).

2. Physical modalities
   a. Cutaneous stimulation
      (1) Historically, the gate-control theory has been used to explain effectiveness. It promotes superficial increases in circulation, counteracting decreased oxygenation and accumulation of metabolites (Abram & Raj, 1987).
      (2) Various sites other than the pain site may produce relief. In cancer pain, the most popular methods are heat and massage and vibration (Rhiner, Ferrell, Ferrell, & Grant, 1993).
   b. Superficial heating and cooling
      (1) The underlying mechanism of pain relief unknown. Both heating and cooling cause decreased sensitivity to pain and may progress to partial or complete anesthesia of the skin (Michlovitz, 1990).
      (2) Selection is based on trial and error. Heating and cooling probably work best for localized pain.
         (a) It is generally believed that heat relieves pain related to muscle tension by improving circulation to the area. Side effects include burns, bleeding, and swelling.
         (b) Cold relieves pain related to swelling by vasoconstriction. Cold relieves pain faster, and the relief lasts longer than that from heat (Michlovitz, 1990). Side effects include tissue ischemia and frostbite.
         (c) Alternating heat and cold is probably more effective than either alone.
   c. Vibration
      (1) Vibration works by stimulating inhibitory interneurons in the spinal cord, which reduces the pain signal transmission (Smith, Comite, Balasubramanian, Carver, & Liu, 2004).
      (2) A trial-and-error approach is necessary.
      (3) The longer the duration of vibration, the longer the relief afterward. High frequency tends to be the most effective.
   d. Massage
      (1) Massage works by interfering with pain transmission and perception at a peripheral level (Ferrell-Torrey & Glick, 1993).
      (2) It leads to improved self-reports of pain, anxiety, and depression (Ferrell-Torrey & Glick, 1993).
      (3) Patients have improved psychological well-being and less perceived distress (Currin & Meister, 2008; Fellowes et al., 2004).
      (4) Care should be used to avoid massage directly over the tumor (National Cancer Institute, 2008, p. 43).
   e. Acupressure and acupuncture
      (1) Application of pressure is to anatomical points that correspond to meridians. A likely correspondence exists between these Eastern techniques and Western use of trigger point massage (Simons & Travell, 1989).
      (2) In contrast to other strategies, acupressure and acupuncture reproduce the painful symptoms before eliciting relief.
   f. Transcutaneous electrical nerve stimulation
      (1) Electrical energy is transmitted across the skin to the nervous system.

(2) Some success is seen with postmastectomy and postthoracotomy pain (McCaffery & Pasero, 1999).

g. Positioning and movement

(1) Positioning is the deliberate placement of the body into postures that maintain or facilitate normal physiological function. Movement interventions are exercises designed to maintain or restore the integrity of muscles, ligaments, joints, bones, and nerves used in human locomotion (Wells & Lessard, 1989).

(2) Range of motion stimulates mechanisms that reduce pain by activating neurophysiological reflexes; the technique may be passive, active-assisted, or active (Spross & Wolfe, 1995).

h. Progressive muscle relaxation

(1) Combined with guided imagery, progressive muscle relaxation produces a relaxation response that may break the pain—muscle tension—anxiety cycle (Sloman, 1995).

i. Relaxation techniques with the most scientific evidence supporting their use

(1) Relaxation techniques have physical, cognitive, and behavioral effects.

(2) Theoretically, they may precipitate hypotension or psychotic break.

(3) Preintervention and postintervention pulse and blood pressure monitoring are recommended.

(4) Use these techniques with caution with bradycardia, heart block, or history of psychosis (Titlebaum, 1988).

(5) Proper breathing enhances any relaxation intervention. Maximal stress reduction is with a 20-minute technique used three times a day (Benson, Beary, & Carol, 1974).

(6) Patients tend to have a narrow focus with repetition of one thing; relaxation is more effective if the same technique is used each time.

3. Cognitive and behavioral interventions

a. Cognitive interventions influence pain through the medium of one's thoughts (cognitions), which are private events and self-initiated. Distraction sometimes referred to as *cognitive refocusing* (Johnson & Petrie, 1997; McCaffery & Pasero, 1999).

b. Behavioral interventions involve actions, behaviors, and situations that can be manipulated externally (Fernandez, 1986).

c. Based on models of stress and coping, cognitive interventions are unlikely to alter painful sensory input directly; however, they can alter the perception of the painful stimulus (Arathuzik, 1994).

d. Theoretically, a person's capacity for processing information is limited; the allocation of attention to one task limits the amount that may be given to another (Kahneman, 1973).

e. Strategies demanding the most patient involvement are the most effective and most appropriate for use over a brief period (McCaul & Malott, 1984).

(1) Imagery is a mental process that draws on any or all of the senses, creating mental representations of reality to reduce pain (Arathuzik, 1994; Stephens, 1992).

(2) Music may reduce pain perception by evoking emotions, releasing endogenous opiates; reducing muscle tension; competing effectively for neurological pathways, reducing transmission of pain messages; diminishing feelings of anxiety, helplessness, and powerlessness; and improving mood (Beck, 1991).

(3) Humor is a communication and coping mechanism, a cognitive and emotional process, often spontaneous and inducing a change of mind (Hunt, 1993). Humor has also been shown to increase pain tolerance and raise the pain threshold (Matz & Brown, 1998) (see the chapter on Integrative Therapies Used in Pain Management Nursing).

VI. Home Pain Management

A. Management is best viewed not as care to a single individual in the home but as a family experience in which every aspect of care affects the others (Musolf, 1991).

1. Benefits are improved physical comfort, psychological comfort of familiar surroundings, opportunity for healing relationships, compassion of giving and receiving comfort care, and shared transition from life to death (Hull, 1993).

2. Barriers are the patient's and family's fear of addiction, failure to report pain, limited access to needed services, and diminished choice for home care (Ferrell & Ferrell, 1991).
3. The profound experience of dying, or caring for someone dying, transcends all aspects of home care and is all-encompassing (Ferrell & Ferrell, 1991).

B. Caregiver issues
1. Care in 70% of cases is provided by elderly spouses; 20% of care is provided by daughters or daughters-in-law balancing full-time employment and family needs (Lubin, 1992).
2. Caregivers often lack the necessary knowledge to judge indications for administration or titration of medication. Education and support are mandatory for any pain management.
3. Costs are assumed by patients and family members (Ferrell, 1996).
4. The caregiver's health, attitudes, and knowledge have profound effect on the management of the patient's symptoms (Snelling, 1990).

C. QOL issues (Ferrell, 1998)
1. Domains are physical well-being and symptoms, psychological well-being, social well-being, and spiritual well-being, which presents the greatest challenge to home care.
2. Formal assessment screening instruments for functional and psychological impairments are helpful and minimize the possibility of missed problems.
3. Patients and families are eager to add nondrug interventions and have found them extremely helpful in reducing their sense of helplessness.
4. Family interventions often are recalled during bereavement as positive memories in providing greater comfort during terminal illness.

References

Abram, S., & Raj, P. (1987). Musculoskeletal pain. In R. P. Raj (Ed.), *Practical management of pain* (pp. 279–285). Chicago: Yearbook Medical Publishers.

Ahles, T. A., & Martin, J. B. (1992). Cancer pain: A multidimensional perspective. In D. C. Turk & C. S. Feldman (Eds.), *Noninvasive approaches to pain management in the terminally ill* (pp. 25–48). New York: Hayworth.

Aistars, J., & Vehlow, K. (2007). *A pilot study to evaluate the validity of skin care protocols followed by women with breast cancer receiving external radiation.* Retrieved May 31, 2009 from http://www.medscape.com/viewarticle/572310_2

Alberico, R. A., & Abdel-halim, A. N. (2007). Vertebroplasty and kyphoplasty. In S. D. Waldman (Ed.), *Pain management* (pp. 1475–1488). Philadelphia: Saunders Elsevier.

Alberico, R. A., Abdel-halim, A. N., & Husain, S. H. S. (2006). Vertebroplasty and kyphoplasty. In O. A. de Leon-Casasola (Ed.), *Cancer pain: Pharmacological, interventional, and palliative care approaches* (pp. 438–449). Philadelphia: Saunders Elsevier.

American Pain Society. (2002). Guideline for the Management of Pain in Osteoarthritis, Rheumatoid Arthritis, and Juvenile Chronic Arthritis. Retrieved on May 31, 2009, from http://www.ampainsoc.org/pub/arthritis.htm

American Pain Society. (2003). *Principles of analgesic use in the treatment of acute pain and cancer pain* (5th ed.). Glenview, IL: Author.

American Pain Society. (2005). *Guideline for the management of cancer pain in adults and children.* Glenview, IL: Author.

American Pain Society. (2005). Guideline for the management of Fibromyalgia Syndrome Pain in Adults and Children. Retrieved May 31, 2009, from http://www.ampainsoc.org/pub/fibromyalgia.htm

American Pain Society. (2006). *Pain: Current understanding of assessment, management, and treatments.* Reston, VA: National Pharmaceutical Council.

American Society for Pain Management Nursing. (2003). Pain management at the end of life: ASPMN position paper. Retrieved on May 31, 2009, from http://www.aspmn.org/Organization/documents/EndofLifeCare.pdf

American Society of Anesthesiologists. (1996). Pain management: Cancer pain section. *Anesthesiology, 84,* 1243–1257.

Anderson, K. O., Cohen, M. S., Mendoza, T. R., Guo, H., Harle, M. T., & Cleeland, C. S. (2006). Brief cognitive-behavioral audiotape interventions for cancer-related pain: Immediate but not long-term effectiveness. *Cancer, 107,* 207–214.

Arathuzik, D. (1994). Effects of cognitive-behavioral strategies on pain in cancer patients. *Cancer Nursing, 17*(3), 207–214.

Auad, O. (2006). Forgotten techniques in cancer pain management. In O.A. de Leon-Casasola (Ed.). *Cancer pain management: Pharmacological, interventional, and palliative care approaches* (pp. 529–541). Philadelphia: Saunders Elsevier.

Backonja, M. M. (1994). Local anesthetics as adjuvant analgesics. *Journal of Pain and Symptom Management, 9,* 491–499.

Baheti, D. K. (2001). Neurolytic celiac plexus block (NCPB): A ten year review of 212 cases (1991–2000). Retrieved May 31, 2009 from http://medind.nic.in/imvw/imvw3115.html

Beck, S. (1991). The therapeutic use of music for cancer-related pain. *Oncology Nursing Forum, 18,* 1327–1337.

Beland, M. D., Dupuy, D. E., & Mayo-Smith, W. W. (2005). Percutaneous cryoablation of symptomatic extraabdominal metastatic disease: Preliminary results. *American Journal of Radiology, 184,* 926–930.

Benson, H., Beary, J., & Carol, M. (1974). The relaxation response. *Psychiatry, 37,* 3746.

Brundage, M., Davidson, J., & Maokillop, W. (1997). Trading treatment toxicity for survival in locally advanced non-small cell lung cancer. *Journal of Clinical Oncology, 15,* 330–340.

Burmeister, B. H., Denham, J. W., O'Brien, M., Jamieson, G. G., Gill, P. G., Devitt, P., Yeoh, E., Hamilton, C. S., Ackland, S. P., & Lamb, D. S., Spry, N.A., Joseph, D.J., Atkinson, C., & Walker, Q.J. (1995). Combined modality therapy for esophageal carcinoma: Preliminary results from a large Australian multicenter study. *International Journal of Radiation Oncology Biology and Physics, 32,* 997.

Burton, A. W., & Hassenbusch, S. J. (2006). Spinal cord stimulation. In O. A. de Leon-Casasola (Ed.), *Cancer pain: Pharmacological, interventional, and palliative care approaches* (pp. 429-437). Philadelphia: Saunders Elsevier.

Callstrom, M. R., Atwell, T. D., Charboneau, J. W., Farrell, M. A., Goetz, M. P., Rubin, J., Sloan, J. A., Novotney, P. J., Welch, T. J., Maus, T. P., Wong, G. Y., & Caraceni, A. (2006). Clinical correlates of common cancer pain syndromes. *Hematology/Oncology Clinics of North America, 10,* 57–78.

Chandrasekharan, N., Dai, H., Roos, K., Evanson, N., Tomsik, J., Elton, T., & Simmons, D. (2002). Cox-3, a cyclooxygenase-1 variant inhibited by acetaminophen and other analgesic/antipyretic drugs: Cloning, structure, expression. *Proceedings of the National Academy of Sciences of the United States of America, 99,* 13926–13931.

Cherny, N. I. (1998). Cancer pain: Principles of assessment and syndromes. In A. M. Berger, R. K. Portenoy, & D. E. Weissman (Eds.), *Principles and practice of supportive oncology* (pp. 3–42). Philadelphia: Lippincott-Raven.

Coia, L. R. (1992). The role of radiation therapy in the treatment of brain metastases. *International Journal of Radiation Oncology, Biology, and Physics, 23,* 229.

Covina, B. G. (1993). Local anesthetics. In F. M. Ferrante & T. R. VadeBoncouer (Eds.), *Postoperative pain management* (pp. 211–253). New York: Churchill Livingstone.

Currin, J., & Meister, E. A. (2008). A hospital-based intervention using massage to reduce distress among oncology patients. *Cancer Nursing, 31,* 214–221.

Eisenberg, D. M., Kessler, R. C., Foster, C., Norlock, F. E., Calkins, D. R., & Delbanco, T. L. (1993). Unconventional medicine in the United States: Prevalence, costs, and patterns of use. *New England Journal of Medicine, 328,* 246–252.

Ellison, N. M. (1998). Palliative chemotherapy. In A. M. Berger, R. K. Portenoy, & D. E. Weissman (Eds.), *Principles and practice of supportive oncology* (pp. 667–679). Philadelphia: Lippincott-Raven.

Evans, P. (1981). Cryoanalgesia: The application of low temperatures to nerves to produce anesthesia or analgesia. *Anaesthesia, 36,* 1003.

Fellowes, D., Barnes, K., & Wilkinson, S. (2004). Aromatherapy and massage for symptom relief in patients with cancer. *Cochrane Database Systems Review,* Issue 2. Retrieved May 31, 2009 http://medschool.umaryland.edu/integrative/cochrane-reviews/cochrane-rev-cancer-se.asp

Fenstermaker, R. A. (2006). In O. A. de Leon-Casasola (Ed.), *Cancer pain: Pharmacological, interventional, and palliative care approaches* (pp. 531–533). Philadelphia: Saunders Elsevier.

Fernandez, E. (1986). A classification system of cognitive coping strategies for pain. *Pain, 26,* 141–151.

Ferrell, B. A., & Ferrell, B. R. (1991). Pain management at home. *Geriatric Home Care, 7,* 765–776.

Ferrell, B. R. (1996). Pain: How patients and families pay the price. In M. J. M. Cohen & J. N. Campbell (Eds.), *Pain treatment at the crossroads* (Vol. 7). Seattle: International Association for the Study of Pain.

Ferrell, B. R. (1998). Home care. In A. M. Berger, R. K. Portenoy, & D. E. Weissman (Eds.), *Principles and practice of supportive oncology* (pp. 709–715). Philadelphia: Lippincott-Raven.

Ferrell-Torrey, A. T., & Glick, O. J. (1993). The use of therapeutic massage as a nursing intervention to modify anxiety and the perception of cancer pain. *Cancer Nursing, 16*(2), 93–101.

Fine, P.G., & Portenoy, R.K. (2004). The endogenous opioid system. Retrieved May 31, 2009, from http://www.stoppain.org/pcd/_pdf/OpioidChapter2.pdf

Fine, P. G., Miaskowski, C., & Paice, J. A. (2004). Meeting the challenges in cancer pain management. *Journal of Supportive Oncology, 2*(4), 5–21.

Flickinger, J. C., Kondziolka, D., Lunsford, L. D., Coffey, R. J., Goodman, M. L., Shaw, E. G., Hudgins, W. R., Weiner, R., Harsh, G. R., IV, & Sneed, P. K. (1994). A multi-institutional experience with stereotactic radiosurgery for solitary brain metastases. *International Journal of Radiology Biology and Physics, 28,* 797.

Fromer, M. J. (2003). Managing cancer pain: New approaches, new alternatives. *Oncology Times, 25,* 9–15.

Garofalo, J. P., Gatchel, R. J., & Baum, A. (2007). Paradigm shift in cancer pain management. *Practical Pain Management, 7,* 14–22.

Goldstein, M. L. (1999). Cancer-related pain. In M. McCaffery & C. Pasero (Eds.), *Pain: Clinical manual* (2nd ed., pp. 531–543). St. Louis: Mosby.

Gough, I. R., & Dalgleish, L. I. (1991). What value is given to quality of life assessment by health professionals considering response to palliative chemotherapy for advanced cancer? *Cancer, 68,* 220.

Grady, K., Severn, A., & Eldridge, P. (2007). Cancer pain: Drugs. In *Key topics in pain medicine* (3rd ed., pp. 50–55). Abingdon, UK: Informa Healthcare.

Haynes, R. C. (1990). Adrenocorticotrophic hormone: Adrenocortical steroids and their synthetic analogs—Inhibitors of the synthesis and actions of adrenocortical hormones. In A. G. Gilman, T. W. Rall, & T. Nies (Eds.), *The pharmacological basis of therapeutics* (8th ed., pp. 1431–1462). New York: McGraw-Hill.

Hobbs, W. R., Rall, T. W., & Verfoorn, T. A. (1996). Hypnotics and sedatives: Ethanol. In J. G. Hardman & L. E. Limbird (Eds.), *Goodman and Gilman's the pharmacological basis of therapeutics* (9th ed., pp. 361–396). New York: McGraw-Hill.

Hoffelt, S. C. (2006). Gamma knife vs. CyberKnife. *Oncology Issues, September/October,* 18–20.

Horlocker, T. T., Wedel, D. J, Benzon, H., Brown, D. L., Enneking, F. K., Heit, J. A., Mulroy, M. F., Rosenquist, R. W., Rowlingson, J., Tryba, M., & Yuan, C. S. (2003). Regional anesthesia in the anticoagulated patient: Defining the risks. The second annual ASRA Consensus Conference on Neuraxial Anesthesia and Anticoagulation. *Regional Anesthesia and Pain Medicine, 28*(3), 172–197.

Hough, S. W., Goudas, L. C., & Carr, D. B. (2004). Anesthetic interventions in cancer pain. In C. A. Warfield & Z. H. Bajaw (Eds.), *Principles & practices of pain medicine* (2nd ed., pp. 477–491).

Hull, M. M. (1993). Coping strategies of family caregivers in hospice home care. *Caring, 12*(2), 78–88.

Hunt, A. (1993). Humor as a nursing intervention. *Cancer Nursing, 16,* 34–39.

Hymes, S. R., Strom, E. A., & Fife, C. (2006). Radiation dermatitis: Clinical presentation, pathophysiology, and treatment 2006. *Journal of the Academy of Dermatology, 54,* 28–46.

Iuliano, F., Abruzzese, E., Peta, A., Toraldo, A., & Palerno, S. (2004). Samarium & zoledronic acid present synergistic action and are able to control pain and significantly improve QOL in elderly patient with MM. *Journal of Clinical Oncology, 22*(14S), Abstract 6737.

Jacox, A., Carr, D. B., Payne, R., Berde, C.B., Breibart, W. Cain, J.M., Chapman, C.R., Cleeland, C.S., Ferrell, B.T., Finley, R.S., Hester, N.O., Stratton Hill, C., Leak, W.D., Lipman, A.G., Logan, C.L., McGarvey, C.L., Miaskowski, C.A., Mulder, D.S., Paice, J.A., Shapiro, B.S., Silberstein, E.B., Smith, R.S., Stover, J., Tsou, C.V., Vecchiarelli, L., & Weissman, D.E.et al. (1994). *Management of cancer pain.* Clinical Practice Guideline No. 9. (AHCPR Publication No. 94-0592). Rockville, MD: Agency for Health Care Policy and Research, Public Health Services, U.S. Department of Health and Human Services.

Johnson, M. H., & Petrie, S. M. (1997). The effects of distraction on exercise and coldpressor tolerance for chronic low back pain sufferers. *Pain, 69,* 43–48.

Kahneman, D. (1973). *Attention and effort.* Englewood Cliffs, NJ: Prentice-Hall.

Kwekkeboom, K. L., Hau, H., Wanta, B., & Bumpus, M. (2008). Patients' perceptions of the effectiveness of guided imagery and progressive muscle relaxation interventions used for cancer pain. *Complementary Therapy Clinical Practice, 14,* 185–194.

Lubin, S. (1992). Palliative care: Could your patient have been managed at home? *Journal of Palliative Care, 8,* 18–22.

Malawer, M. M., & Delaney, T. F. (1993). Treatment of metastatic cancer to the bone. In V. T. DeVita & S. A. Rosenberg (Eds.), *Cancer: Principles and practice of oncology* (p. 2225). Philadelphia: J. B. Lippincott.

Matz, A., & Brown, S. T. (1998). Humor and pain management: A review of current literature. *Journal of Holistic Nursing, 16*(1), 68–75.

McCaffery, M., & Pasero, C. (Eds.). (1999). *Pain: Clinical manual* (2nd ed.). St. Louis: Mosby.

McCaul, K. D., & Malott, J. M. (1984). Distraction and coping with pain. *Psychology Bulletin, 95,* 516–533.

McGuire, D. B. (2004). Occurrence of cancer pain. *Journal of the National Cancer Institute Monographs, 32,* 51–56.

McQuestion, M. (2006). Evidenced-based skin care management in radiation therapy. *Seminars in Oncology Nursing, 22*(3), 163–173.

Mercadante, S. (1999). World Health Organization guidelines: Problem areas in cancer pain management. *Cancer Control, 6,* 191–197.

Miaskowski, C. (2003). Pain assessment and evaluation of patient outcomes: When is relief from cancer pain good, fair, or poor? In *Oncology Nursing Society 2003 Annual Congress: Symposia highlights* (pp. 25–26). Oncology Nursing Society: San Antonio, Texas.

Michlovitz, S. L. (1990). Cryotherapy: The use of cold as a therapeutic agent. In S. L. Michlovitz (Ed.), *Thermal agents in rehabilitation* (pp. 63–87). Philadelphia: F. A. Davis.

Mithal, N. P., Needham, P. R., & Hoskins, P. J. (1994). Retreatment with radiotherapy for painful bone metastases. *International Journal of Radiation Oncology, Biology, and Physics, 29,* 1011.

Murphy, B. A. (2007). Clinical and economic consequences of mucositis induced by chemotherapy and/or radiation therapy. *Supportive Oncology, 5, 9*(4), 13–21.

Musolf, J. M. (1991). Easing the impact of the family caregiver role. *Rehabilitation Nursing, 16,* 82–84.

National Cancer Institute. (2008). *Pain (PDQ).* Retrieved May 28, 2008, from http://www.cancer.gov/cancertopics/pdq/supportivecare/pain/healthprofessional.

National Comprehensive Cancer Network. (2008). *Practice guidelines for cancer pain, version 1.* Rockledge, PA: Author.

Noordijk, E. M., Vecht, C. J., Haaxma-Reiche, H., Padberg, G. W., Voormolen, J. H., Hoekstra, F. H., Tans, J. T., Lambooij, N., Mesaars, J. A., & Wattendorff, A. R. (1994). The choice of treatment of single brain metastases should be based on extracranial tumor activity and age. *International Journal of Radiation Oncology, Biology, and Physics, 29,* 711.

Pasternak, G. W. (2007). Opioid receptors in pain control. In J. H. Von-Roenn (Ed.), *Journal of Supportive Oncology, 5,* 61.

Pico, J. L., Avila-Garavito, A., & Naccache, P. (1998). Mucositis: Its occurrence, consequences, and treatment in the oncology setting. *Oncologist, 3,* 446–451.

Pinover, W. H., & Coia, L. R. (1998). Palliative radiation therapy. In A. M. Berger, R. K. Politis, M. J., Schaumburg, H. H., & Spencer, P. S. (1980). Neurotoxicity of selected chemicals. In P. S. Spencer & H. H. Schaumburg (Eds.), *Experimental and chemical neurotoxicity.* Baltimore: Wilkins & Wilkins.

Portenoy, R. K. (1993). Adjuvant analgesics in pain management. In D. Doyle, G. Hanks, & N. MacDonald (Eds.), *Oxford textbook of palliative medicine* (pp. 187–203). Oxford, UK: Oxford University Press.

Portenoy, R. K. (1996). Basic mechanisms. In P. K. Portenoy & R. M. Kanner (Eds.), *Pain management: Theory and practice* (pp. 19–39). Philadelphia: F. A. Davis.

Portenoy, R. K. (2000). Nonopioid and adjuvant analgesics. In *Contemporary diagnosis and management of pain in the oncologic and AIDS patients* (3rd ed., pp. 143–182). Newtown, PA: Handbooks in Healthcare.

Rainone, F. (2004). Treating adult cancer pain in primary care. *Journal of the American Board of Family Practice, 17,* 48–56.

Reddy, S., & Patt, R. B. (1994). The benzodiazepines as adjuvant analgesics. *Journal of Pain and Symptom Management, 9,* 510–514.

Reisine, T., & Pasternak, G. (1996). Opioid analgesics and antagonists. In J. G. Hardman & L. M. Limbird (Eds.), *Goodman and Gilman's the pharmacological basis of therapeutics* (9th ed., pp. 521–555). New York: McGraw-Hill.

Rhiner, M., Ferrell, B. R., Ferrell, B. A., & Grant, M. M. (1993). A structured non-drug intervention program for cancer pain. *Cancer Practice, 1,* 137–143.

Richter, M. P., & Coia, L. R. (1985). Palliative radiation therapy. *Seminars in Oncology, 12,* 375.

Saberski, L. R. (1998). Interventional approaches in oncological pain management. In A. M. Berger, R. K. Portenoy, & D. E. Weissman (Eds.), *Principles and practice of supportive oncology* (pp. 93–108). Philadelphia: Lippincott-Raven.

Saberski, L. R. (2007). Cryoneurolysis. In S. D. Waldman (Ed.), *Pain management* (pp. 1460–1474). Philadelphia: Saunders Elsevier.

Silberstein, E. B. (1993). The treatment of painful osseous metastases with phosphorus-32-labeled phosphates. *Seminars in Oncology, 20,* 10.

Siminoff, L. A., & Fetting, J. H. (1991). Factors affecting treatment decisions for a life-threatening illness: The case of medical treatment of breast cancer. *Social Sciences of Medicine, 32,* 813.

Simons, D., & Travell, J. (1989). Myofascial pain syndromes. In P. D. Wall & R. Melzack (Eds.), *Textbook of pain* (pp. 368–385). Edinburgh: Churchill Livingstone.

Slawson, R., & Scott, R. (1979). Radiation therapy in bronchogenic carcinoma. *Radiology, 132,* 175.

Slevin, M. L., Stubbs, L., Plant, H. J., Wilson, P., Gregory, W. M., Armes, P. J., & Downer, S. M. (1990). Attitudes to chemotherapy: Comparing views of patients with those of doctors, nurses and general public. *British Medical Journal, 300,* 1458.

Sloman, R. (1995). Relaxation and the relief of cancer pain. *Nursing Clinics of North America, 30,* 697–709.

Smith, K. C., Comite, S. L., Balasubramanian, S., Carver, A., & Liu, J. F. (2004). Vibration anesthesia: A noninvasive method of reducing discomfort prior to dermatologic procedures. *Journal of Dermatology Online,* 10. Retrieved November 06, 2008, from http://arabmedmag.com/issue-15-01-2005/dermatology/main02.htm.

Smith, T. J., Staats, P. S., Deer, T., Stearns, L., Rauck, R. L., Boortz-Marx, R. L., Buchser, E., Catala, E., Bryce, D. A., Coyne, P. J., & Pool, G. E. (2004). Randomized clinical trial of an implantable drug delivery system compared with comprehensive medical management for refractory cancer pain: Impact on pain, drug-related toxicity, and survival. *Journal of Clinical Oncology, 20*(19), 4040–4049.

Snelling, J. (1990). The role of the family in relation to chronic pain: Review of the literature. *Journal of Advanced Nursing, 15,* 771.

Solomon, L. A., Munkarah, A. R., Vorugu, V. R., Deppe, G., Adam, B., Malone, J. M., & Littrup, P. J. (2008). Image-guided percutaneous cryotherapy for the management of gynecologic cancer metastases. *Gynecologic Oncology, 40, 10,* 1–6.

Somerson, S. J., Husted, C. W., & Sicilia, M. R. (1995). Insights into conscious sedation. *American Journal of Nursing, 95,* 26–33.

Sonis, S. T. (2007). Pathobiology of oral mucositis: Novel insights and opportunities. *Supportive Oncology, 5, 9*(4), 3–11.

Spross, J. A., & Wolfe, M. W. (1995). Nonpharmacological management of cancer pain. In D. B. McGuire, C. H. Yarbro, & B. R. Ferrell (Eds.), *Cancer pain management* (2nd ed., pp. 159–205). Boston: Jones & Bartlett.

Spross, J. A., McGuire, D. B., & Schmitt, R. M. (1990). Oncology nursing society position on cancer pain. *Oncology Nursing Forum, 17,* 595–614, 751–760, 943–955.

Stefaniak, T., Basinski, A., Vingerhoets, A., Makarewicz, W., Connor, S., Kaska, L., Stanek, A., Kwiecinska, B., Lachinski, A. J., & Sledzinski, Z. (2005). A comparison of two invasive techniques in the management of intractable pain due to inoperable pancreatic cancer: Neurolytic celiac plexus block and videothoracoscopy splanchnicectomy. *European Journal of Surgical Oncology, 31*(7), 768–773.

Stephens, R. (1992). Imagery as a means of coping. In J. F. Miller (Ed.), *Coping with chronic illness: Overcoming powerlessness* (2nd ed., pp. 353–375). Philadelphia: F. A. Davis.

Stephenson, N. L., Swanson, M., Dalton, J., Keefe, F. J., & Engelke, M. (2007). Partner-delivered reflexology: Effects on cancer pain and anxiety. *Oncology Nursing Forum, 34,* 127–132.

Titlebaum, H. (1988). Relaxation. In R. Zahourek (Ed.), *Relaxation and imagery: Tools for therapeutic communication and intervention* (pp. 28–52). Philadelphia: W. B. Saunders.

Trodella, L. (1984). Pain in osseous metastases: Results of radiotherapy. *Pain, 18,* 387.

Tsevat, J., Cook, F., Green, M. L., Matchar, D. B., Dawson, N. V., Broste, S. K., Wu, A. W., Phillips, R. S., Oye, R. K., & Goldman, L. (1995). Health values of the seriously ill. *Annals of Internal Medicine, 122,* 514.

Tuncali, K., Morrison, P. R., Winalski, C. S., Carrino, J. A., Shankar, S., Ready, J. E., vanSonnenberg, E., & Silverman, S. G. (2007). MRI-guided percutaneous cryotherapy for soft-tissue and bone metastases: Initial experience. *American Journal of Radiology, 189,* 232–239.

Waldman, S. D. (2007). *Pain management.* Philadelphia: W. B. Saunders.

Watanabe, S., & Bruera, E. (1994). Corticosteroids as adjuvant analgesics. *Journal of Pain and Symptom Management, 9,* 446–453.

Wells, P., & Lessard, E. (1989). Movement education and limitation of movement. In P. D. Wall & R. Melzack (Eds.), *Textbook of pain* (pp. 952–963). Edinburgh: Churchill Livingstone.

White, C., & Rajagopal, A. (2006). Intraspinal therapy. In O. A. de Leon-Casasola (Ed.), *Cancer pain: Pharmacological, interventional, and palliative care approaches* (pp. 329-428). Philadelphia: Saunders Elsevier.

Whooley, B. P., & Conlon, K. C. (1998). Palliative surgery. In A. M. Berger, R. K. Portenoy, & D. E. Weissman (Eds.), *Principles and practice of supportive oncology* (pp. 627–637). Philadelphia: Lippincott-Raven.

Wilkie, D. J., & Keefe, F. J. (1991). Strategies of patients with lung-cancer-related pain. *Clinical Journal of Pain, 7,* 292–299.

Wright, D. C., Delaney, T. F., & Buckner, J. C. (1993). Treatment of metastatic cancer to the brain. In V. T. DeVita, S. Hellman, & S. A. Rosenberg (Eds.), *Cancer principles and practice of oncology* (p. 2170). Philadelphia: J. B. Lippincott.

Yan, B. M., & Myers, R. P. (2007). Neurolytic celiac plexus block for pain control in unresectable pancreatic cancer. *American Journal of Gastroenterology, 102*(2), 430–438.

Yella, S. B., & Cella, D. F. (1995). Someone to live for: Social well-being, parenthood status and decision making in oncology. *Journal of Clinical Oncology, 13,* 1255.

Yella, S. B., Cella, D. F., & Leslie, W. T. (1994). Age and clinical decision making in oncology patients. *Journal of the National Cancer Institute, 86,* 1766.

Zhang, C. L., Zhang, T. J., Guo, Y. N., Yang, L. Q., He, H. W., Shi, J. Z., & Ni, J. X. (2008). Effect of neurolytic celiac plexus block guided by computerized tomography on pancreatic cancer pain. *Dig Dsi Science, 53*(3), 856–860.

Suggested Readings

American Pain Society. (1999). *Principles of analgesic use in the treatment of acute pain and cancer pain* (4th ed.). Glenview, IL: Author.

Basbaum, A. L., & Fields, H. L. (1984). Endogenous pain control systems: Brainstem spinal pathways and endorphin circuitry. *Annual Review of Neuroscience, 7*, 309–338.

Benjamin, L. J., Dampier, C. D., Jacox, A. K., Odesina, V., Phoenix, D., Shapiro, B. Stafford, M., & Treadwell, M. (1999). *Guideline for the management of acute and chronic pain in sickle-cell disease.* Clinical Practice Guideline Series, No. 1. Glenview, IL: American Pain Society.

Brown, K. J. (2006). Painful metastases involving bone: Percutaneous image-guided cryoablation—Prospective trial interim analysis. *Vascular and Interventional Radiology, 241*(2), 572–580.

Buckhardt CS, Goldenberg D, Crofford L, Gerwin R, Gowens S, Jackson K, Kugel P, McCarberg W, Rudin N, Schanberg L, Taylor AG, Taylor J, Turk D. (2005). Guideline for the management of fibromyalgia syndrome pain in adults and children. Glenview (IL): American Pain Society (APS).

Cornblath, D. R., & McArthur, J. C. (1988). Predominantly sensory neuropathy in patients with AIDS and AIDS-related complex. *Neurology, 38*, 794–796.

Ferrell, B. R., Rhiner, M., Cohen, M. Z., & Grant, M. (1991). Pain as a metaphor for illness. I. Impact of cancer pain on family caregivers. *Oncology Nursing Forum, 18*, 1303–1309.

Foley, K. M. (1993). Pain assessment and cancer pain syndromes. In D. Doyle, G. H. Hanks, & N. McDonald (Eds.), *Oxford textbook of palliative medicine* (pp. 148–165). Oxford, UK: Oxford University Press.

Lyness, W. H. (1989). Pharmacology of neurolytic agents. In G. B. Racz (Ed.), *Techniques of neurolysis* (pp. 13–25). Boston: Kluwer Academic.

McCaffery, M., & Portenoy, R. K. (1999). Nonopioids. In M. McCaffery & C. Pasero (Eds.), *Pain: Clinical manual* (2nd ed., pp. 129–160). St. Louis: Mosby.

McGuire, D. B. (1995). The multiple dimensions of cancer pain: A framework for assessment and management. In D. B. McGuire, C. H. Yarbro, & B. R. Ferrell (Eds.), *Cancer pain management* (2nd ed., pp. 1–17). Boston: Jones & Bartlett.

McQuay, H., Carroll, D., Jadad, A. R., Wiffen, P., & Moore, A. (1995). Anticonvulsant drugs for management of pain: A systematic review. *British Medical Journal, 311*, 1047–1052.

McQuay, H. J., Tramer, M., Nye, B. A., Carroll, D., Wiffen, P. J., & Moore, R. A. (1996). A systematic review of antidepressants in neuropathic pain. *Pain, 68*, 217–227.

Miaskowski C, Cleary J, Burney R, Coyne P, Finley R, Foster R, Grossman S, Janjan N, ay J, Syejala K, Weisman S, Zahrbock C. (2005). Guideline for the management of cancer pain in adults and children. Glenview (IL): American Pain Society (APS).

Moryl, N., Coyle, N., & Foley, K. M. (2008). Managing an acute pain crisis in a patient with advanced care: "This is as much of a crisis as a code." *Journal of the American Medical Association, 299*(12), 1457–1467.

Patt, R. B. (1993). *Cancer pain.* Philadelphia: Lippincott.

Portenoy, R. K. (1996). Opioid analgesics. In P. K. Portenoy & R. M. Kanner (Eds.), *Pain management: Theory and practice* (pp. 249–276). Philadelphia: F. A. Davis.

Portenoy, & D. E. Weissman (Eds.), *Principles and practice of supportive oncology* (pp. 603–626). Philadelphia: Lippincott-Raven.

Ripamonti, C., Groff, L., Brunelli, C., Polastri, D., Stavrakis, A., & DeConno, F. (1998). Switching from morphine to oral methadone in treating cancer pain: What is the equianalgesic dose ratio? *Journal of Clinical Oncology, 16*, 3216–3221.

Serafini, A. N. (1998). Palliation of pain associated with metastatic bone cancer using samarium-153 lexidronam: A double-blind, placebo-controlled clinical trial. *Journal of Clinical Oncology, 16*, 1574.

Simon, L.S., Lipman, A.G., Caudill-Slosberg, M., Gill, L.H., Keefe, F.J., Kerr, K.L., Minor, M.A., Sherry, D.D., Vallerand, A.H., Vasudevan, S. (2002). Guidelines for the Management of Osteoarthritis, Rheumatoid Arthritis and Juvenile Chronic Arthritis. Glenview (IL): American Pain Society (APS).

Sindrup, S. H., Gram, L. F., Brosen, K., Eshoj, O., & Mogensen, E. F. (1990). The selective serotonin reuptake inhibitor paroxetine is effective in the treatment of diabetic neuropathy symptoms. *Pain, 42,* 135–144.

Singh, G. (1998). Recent considerations in nonsteroidal anti-inflammatory drug gastropathy. *American Journal of Medicine, 105*(Suppl. 1B), 31S–38S.

Vogl, D., Rosenfeld, B., Breitbart, W., Thaler, M., Passik, S., McDonald, M., & Portenoy, P. K. (1999). Symptom prevalence, characteristics, and distress in AIDS outpatients. *Journal of Pain and Symptom Management, 18,* 253–262.

Waldman, S. D., & Coombs, D. W. (1989). Selection of implantable narcotic delivery systems. *Anesthesia and Analgesia, 68,* 377.

Weinberger, J., Nicklas, W. J., & Berl, S. (1976). Mechanism of action of anticonvulsants. *Neurology, 26,* 162–173.

Weinrich, S., & Weinrich, M. (1990). The effect of massage on pain in cancer patients. *Applied Nursing Research, 3,* 140–145.

Weissman, D. E., & Haddox, J. D. (1989). Opioid pseudoaddiction: An iatrogenic syndrome. *Pain, 36,* 363–366.

World Health Organization. (1990). *Cancer pain relief and palliative care: Report of a WHO expert committee.* Geneva, Switzerland: Author.

chapter

20

Pediatric Pain Management

Theresa J. Di Maggio, MSN, CRNP, PNP-BC
Lynn M. Clark, MS, RN-BC, CPNP-PC
Michelle L. Czarnecki, MSN, RN-BC, CPNP-PC

Objectives

After studying this chapter, the reader should be able to:

1. Discuss strategies for assessing pain in children.
2. State how the developmental levels of children influence pain assessment techniques and interventions for managing pain.
3. Describe specific pain measurement tools used in pediatrics.
4. Describe pharmacological interventions for managing acute and chronic pain in infants, children, and adolescents.
5. Discuss some strategies for managing procedural pain in pediatric patients.
6. Discuss regional analgesia techniques in the pediatric population, including epidural and peripheral nerve catheters.
7. Discuss pain management for specific disorders in pediatric patients.
8. Describe complementary techniques that may be used with traditional pain management methods in infants, children, and adolescents.

We will remember Donna Wong (1948-2008) and her devotion to nursing and patients that will always be her legacy. Her gentle compassion and dedication to assessment and management of pediatric pain reached children throughout the world. We thank Dr. Wong for the Pediatric textbooks, the Maternal-Child textbooks, and the Wong-Baker scale for assessing pain in children.

PART ONE: PEDIATRIC PAIN ASSESSMENT AND MEASUREMENT

I. Introduction

A. Children experience the same pain that adults with similar processes experience. It must be assumed that if it is painful to an adult, it is painful for a child.

B. Many children are not asked routinely about their pain, even when they suffer from a disease or condition with a known pain process (Fanurik, Koh, Schmitz, Harrison, & Conrad, 1999; Malviya et al., 2001).

C. Cultural differences and language barriers may make pediatric pain assessment more complex and should be considered during all phases of pediatric pain assessment and management.

D. Children require an age-appropriate explanation of pain. It should be reinforced that the pain is not a form of punishment.

E. Infants, young children, and children with developmental delay have varying levels of difficulty communicating their pain. This difficulty places them at risk that their pain may go unrecognized and untreated (American Pain Society [APS], 2003; Fanurik et al., 1999; Malviya et al., 2001; Oberlander, O'Donnell, & Montgomery, 1999).

F. Developmental issues make pain assessment in children more difficult than in adults. The typical exchange experienced when interacting with adults is not possible with children.

1. As infants cannot communicate verbally, they depend on clinicians to assess and interpret their pain. Behaviorally they may exhibit many pain behaviors, including crying, facial grimacing, eye squeeze, a quivering chin, limb withdrawal, hypertonicity, and touch aversion. The combination of facial grimacing with taut tongue may indicate greater pain. Facial expression combined with a short latency to onset of cry, and a cry with a long duration, typifies the common reaction to invasive procedures (Grunau, Johnston, & Craig, 1990).
2. Toddlers and many school-age children lack the cognitive ability to use standard adult self-report pain scoring tools. Typically, a toddler can say only whether pain is present or absent, although some may be able to localize the pain by pointing to the area (Kahn & Weisman, 2007). Displayed nonverbal cues are more important than language (Craig & Korol, 2008).
3. By the time children reach school age, they can provide a description of their pain.
4. Adolescents typically are able to use adult pain assessment tools. They may or may not be able to make independent decisions, and parents differ on their ability to accept the decisions of their children (Kline, 2004).
5. During times of stress or illness, children sometimes regress to earlier developmental stages. For hospitalized children, the threatening environment and fear of the unknown only compound the physical pain they experience.
6. Pain in infants and children should be relieved as quickly as possible while a complete evaluation is ongoing. For example, the treatment of abdominal pain should not be withheld while awaiting surgical evaluation (Kim, Strait, Sato, & Hennes, 2002).

II. Pain Assessment Techniques

A. Various pain assessment techniques can be used to evaluate the child in pain. One method is QUESTT (Baker & Wong, 1987):

1. Question
2. Use pain rating scales
3. Evaluate behavior
4. Secure parents' involvement
5. Take cause of pain into account
6. Take action

B. Another method to remember the components of any pain assessment is to use the mnemonic PAINED (Lynch, 2001):
   1. *Place:* Location of pain (may be more than one site)
   2. *Amount of pain:* Pain intensity score, duration of pain, pattern of onset (e.g., continuous or intermittent)
   3. *Intensifiers:* What makes the pain worse (e.g., position, movement, or time of day)
   4. *Nullifiers:* What makes the pain better (e.g., position, heat or cold, or medications)
   5. *Effects:* Consequences of pain medication (e.g., relief or side effects) and effects of pain on activities of daily living and quality of life
   6. *Description:* Quality of the pain (e.g., dull, sharp, aching, stabbing, or cramping)

C. An evaluation or reassessment should be integrated following interventions (APS, 2003; Sloman, Wruble, Rosen, & Rom, 2006).

III. Complexities of Pediatric Pain Assessment

A. A child's report of pain is limited by the child's cognitive ability to communicate thoughts.
   1. A young child may not know the meaning of the word *pain.* Frequently used terms include "owie," "boo-boo," or "it hurts."
   2. Ask how and to whom the child communicates pain.
   3. Preoperational children (2 to 7 years old)
      a. Preoperational children relate to pain as a physical experience. They do not understand cause and effect; they believe in the magical appearance and disappearance of pain and do not understand the connection between taking an analgesic and experiencing pain relief. They may see pain as a punishment. They may also hold someone responsible for their pain and may respond by physical aggression (Hurley & Whelan, 1988).
      b. Preoperational children need reassurance that pain is not a punishment.
   4. Concrete–operational children (7 to 12 years old)
      a. Concrete–operational children are acquiring new knowledge in school. They have an increased awareness of the body and internal organs and are particularly fearful of bodily harm (Hurley & Whelan, 1988).
      b. Concrete–operational children need reassurance about fears of bodily harm. These children should be given basic age-appropriate explanations about their pain and its treatment (Twycross, 1998).
   5. Transitional–formal children (10 to 12 years old)
      a. Transitional–formal children are not as literal as younger children and are beginning to understand "if–then." A nurse can say, "If you use ice, then the swelling will go down, and you will have less pain" (Hurley & Whelan, 1988).
   6. Formal–operational children (12 years and older)
      a. Formal–operational children are beginning to problem-solve, although they lack sufficient life experience to have the maturity level of an adult (Hurley & Whelan, 1988).
      b. Adolescents need information about their condition and treatment plan. They need support when under stress because they may decompensate and regress, and may forget to use resources available to them. Privacy, the ability to express comfort needs without feeling demeaned, and a sense of control are all important at this stage (Hurley & Whelan, 1988).

B. Behavioral and physiological changes must be taken into account when evaluating a child's pain. Physiological changes typically are seen only during the acute onset of pain and may occur for reasons other than pain.
   1. Specific behaviors besides crying and groaning that may indicate pain include lying on one's side with legs flexed, refusing to move or be moved, and turning the head from side to side. Changes in appetite or sleep pattern can be evidence of pain. Some behavioral cues that are seen more often in chronic pain include irritability, depression, apathy, and a flat affect.
   2. When taking a pain history, ask the parent about the child's behavior and previous response to pain. The parent knows the child best.

IV. Pain Characteristics

A. Somatic pain
   1. Pain originating from bone, joint, muscle, skin, or connective tissue can be related to
      a. Primary or metastatic bone disease.
      b. Postoperative pain.
   2. Somatic pain is typically described as aching or throbbing.
   3. Treat with opioids, nonopioids, and adjuvants, depending on pain severity (see the chapter on Overview of Pharmacology).

B. Visceral pain
   1. Pain originating from visceral organs can be related to
      a. Stretching of thoracic or abdominal viscera or both by tumor.
      b. Intestinal pain from a bowel obstruction.
   2. Visceral pain is typically described as aching.
   3. Treat with opioids, nonopioids, and adjuvants, depending on pain severity (see the chapter on Overview of Pharmacology).

C. Neuropathic pain
   1. Pain originating from the peripheral or central nervous system can be related to
      a. Phantom limb pain.
      b. Herpes zoster dermatomal pain, which may be present before rash, during rash, or both.
      c. Compression or infiltration of peripheral nerves or the spinal cord.
      d. Nerve injury related to radiation or chemotherapy (e.g., after vincristine administration).
   2. Neuropathic pain is typically described as numbness, burning, tingling, shooting, or electrical pain.
   3. Pharmacological treatment includes adjuvant medications such as tricyclic antidepressants or anticonvulsants, oral and local cutaneous anesthetics, corticosteroids, α_2-agonists, and *N*-methyl-D-aspartate (NMDA) antagonists (APS, 2003; Schecter, Berde, & Yaster, 2003) (see the chapter on Overview of Pharmacology).
      a. The use of opioids is controversial as they may not be effective (Schecter et al., 2003).
   4. Nonpharmacological treatment includes physical therapy, if indicated. Cognitive-behavioral therapy can be used for relaxation, stress reduction, or biofeedback (Schecter et al., 2003).

V. Pediatric Pain History

A. Cause
   1. Classify the type of pain as somatic, visceral, or neuropathic.
   2. Consider the anticipated course and duration of pain. Knowing the pathology or procedure to be done indicates the expected type, intensity, and duration of pain.

B. Location
   1. Ask the child where it hurts using age-appropriate language.
   2. It can be helpful to have the child give the location of the pain by marking the body part on a human figure drawing, or pointing to the area on the child's own body, a doll, or a stuffed toy.
      a. Children 4 years and older can use crayons or colored markers to locate pain on a body diagram (Eland, 1981). The precision of the location improves with the age of the child.

C. Pain quality
   1. Descriptive terms such as ***burning, sharp,*** or ***dull*** can assist in identifying the cause of the pain. Many young children are unable to describe their pain (see IV. Pain Characteristics for further information).

D. Pain intensity
   1. Pain scoring tools
      a. Because pain is subjective, it is measured best by self-report (APS, 2003).
      b. Levels of reliability and validity vary for the multitude of pain intensity scoring tools available for pediatric patients.
      c. Nurses need to be educated to recognize and quantify pain using age-appropriate ***validated*** pain scoring tools. This is particularly true when using observational scales.

d. The lower age limit for successful use of a self-report pain scale is generally 3 or 4 years old (Hicks et al., 2001; Wong & Baker, 1988).
e. When first introducing the child to a pain scale, explain that this is one way for children to let the nurse know how they hurt.
f. The same scale should be used to avoid confusing the child and to aid staff in following the trend of pain scores. To avoid confusion, clinicians are encouraged not to change from a self-report scale to an observational scale while a child is asleep.
g. The selection of an appropriate scale depends on the cognitive level of the individual child. A developmental progression occurs in a child's understanding of pain (Craig & Korol, 2008). Children express pain verbally and nonverbally according to their developmental level. It is advisable to use a scale that appeals to the child.
   (1) Children 2 to 7 years old are unable to abstract, quantify, or symbolize (Beyer & Wells, 1989).
      (a) Toddlers are able to localize pain (point to the area) (Kahn & Weisman, 2007). Displayed nonverbal cues are more important than language (Craig & Korol, 2008).
      (b) Preschoolers begin to understand explanations of causes of pain and alleviating factors. They may be more open during assessment when parents are present (Craig & Korol, 2008). Some can use easier self-report scales (i.e., Faces) (Schecter et al., 2003; von Baeyer, 2008). For those unable to use self-report scales, observational scales are needed (von Baeyer, 2008).
   (2) School-age children 7 to 12 years old begin to understand abstract thought. A verbal numerical rating scale (VNRS) and visual analogue scales (VAS) become increasingly appropriate as children become more comfortable with numbers. A child must understand rank and order (i.e., 9 is higher than 3) to use a numerical scale.
      (a) Self-report is more reliable at this age (Craig & Korol, 2008).
      (b) Behaviorally, they may display crying, stall tactics, oppositionality, anger, fear, or withdrawal (Kahn & Weisman, 2007).
   (3) Children 11 to 14 years old are able to abstract, quantify, and qualify the pain experience (Schecter et al., 2003).
   (4) Often, children do not answer questions verbally. This is especially true when they are anxious, depressed, or in severe pain. A scale that allows nonverbal responses (pointing) may be required (World Health Organization [WHO], 1998).
   (5) Selected self-report pain scoring tools are shown in Tables 20-1 and 20-2:
      (a) Faces Pain Scale, revised (Bieri Faces)
      (b) Faces Pain Rating Scale (Wong-Baker Faces)
      (c) Oucher
      (d) Poker Chip Tool
      (e) Color Tool

2. Factors that influence self-report of pain
   a. Children may modify their pain scores based on the specific situation (i.e., setting, person asking, or what they expect to happen as a result of their answer).
      (1) Children may underreport their pain if they are concerned a high pain score will result in an analgesic given by intramuscular injection, if they lack the knowledge that the pain can be treated, or if they do not want to disappoint or upset their parents.
      (2) Occasionally, some children may overstate their pain because this can result in increased attention.
      (3) If a discrepancy exists between the observed pain behaviors and a child's self-report of pain, further assessment by the clinician is required (Schecter, Berde, & Yaster, 1993).
      (4) Various factors can affect a child's report of pain, including nausea, anxiety, or fear. Research suggests that younger children may confuse fear with pain (Carr, Lemanek, & Armstrong, 1998).

Table 20-1 Self-Report Pain Rating Scales for Children

Pain Scale and Description	Instructions	Recommended Age and Comments
*Faces Pain Rating Scale** (Wong & Baker, 1988, 1999): The scale consists of six cartoon faces ranging from smiling face for "no pain" to tearful face for "worst pain."	*Original instructions:* Explain to the child that each face is for a person who feels happy because there is no pain (hurt) or sad because there is some or a lot of pain. Face 0 is happy because there is no hurt. Face 1 hurts just a little bit. Face 2 hurts a little more. Face 3 hurts even more. Face 4 hurts a whole lot, but Face 5 hurts as much as you can imagine, although you don't have to be crying to feel this bad. Ask the child to choose the face that best describes the child's own pain. Record the number under the chosen face on the pain assessment record. *Brief word instructions:* Point to each face using the words to describe the pain intensity. Ask the child to choose the face that best describes the child's own pain, and record the appropriate number.	Use for children as young as 3 years. Using original instructions without affect words, such as ***happy*** or ***sad,*** or brief words resulted in the same pain rating, probably reflecting the child's rating of pain intensity. For coding purposes, the numbers 0, 2, 4, 6, 8, and 10 can be substituted for the 0–5 system to accommodate the 0–10 system. The Faces system provides three scales in one: facial expressions, numbers, and words.

0	1	2	3	4	5
No hurt	Hurts little bit	Hurts little more	Hurts even more	Hurts whole lot	Hurts worst

Pain Scale and Description	Instructions	Recommended Age and Comments
Oucher† (Beyer, Denyes, & Villarruel, 1992): The scale consists of six photographs of a child's face representing "no hurt" to "biggest hurt you could ever have." It includes a vertical scale with the numbers 0–100. Scales for Black and Hispanic children have been developed (Villarruel & Denyes, 1991).	*Numerical scale:* Point to each section of the scale to explain variations in pain intensity: "0 means no hurt. This means little hurts" (pointing to the lower part of the scale, 1–9). "This means middle hurts" (pointing to the middle part of the scale, 30–69). "This means big hurts" (pointing to the upper part of the scale, 70–99). "100 means the biggest hurt you could ever have." The score is the actual number stated by the child. *Photographic scale:* Point to each photograph on Oucher and explain variations in pain intensity using the following language: "The first picture from the bottom is no hurt, the second is a little hurt, the third is a little more hurt, the fourth is even more hurt than that, the fifth is a lot of hurt, and the sixth is the biggest hurt you could ever have." Score pictures 0–5, with the bottom picture scored as 0. *General:* Practice using Oucher by recalling and rating previous pain experiences (e.g., falling off a bike). The child points to a number or photograph that describes the pain intensity associated with the experience. Obtain a current pain score from the child by asking, "How much hurt do you have right now?"	Use for children 3–13 years. Use the numerical scale if the child can count to 100 by ones and identify the larger of any two numbers, or can count by tens (Jordan-Marsh, Yoder, Hall, & Watson, 1994). Determine whether the child has the cognitive ability to use a photographic scale; the child should be able to seriate six geometric shapes from largest to smallest. Determine which ethnic version of Oucher to use. Allow the child to select a version of Oucher, or use the version that most closely matches the physical characteristics of the child.

Tool	Instructions	Recommended Age
Poker Chip Tool‡: This tool uses four red poker chips placed horizontally in front of the child (Hester et al., 1998).	Say to the child: "I want to talk with you about the hurt you may be having right now." Align the chips horizontally in front of the child on the bedside table, a clipboard, or other firm surface. Tell the child, "These are pieces of hurt." Beginning at the chip nearest the child's left side and ending at the one nearest the right side, point to the chips and say, "This (point to the first chip) is a little bit of hurt, and this (point to the fourth chip) is the most hurt you could ever have." For a young child or for any child who may not fully comprehend the instructions, clarify by saying, "That means this (point to chip 1) is just a little hurt, this (point to chip 2) is a little more hurt, this (point to chip 3) is more yet, and this (point to chip 4) is the most hurt you could ever have." Do not give children an option for zero hurt. Research with the Poker Chip Tool has verified that children without pain will indicate this by responses such as "I don't have any." Ask the child, "How many pieces of hurt do you have right now?" After initial use of the Poker Chip Tool, some children internalize the concept "pieces of hurt." If a child gives a response such as "I have one right now," ***before*** you ask or before you lay out the poker chips, record the number of chips on the pain flow sheet. Clarify the child's answer with words such as, "Oh, you have little hurt? Tell me about the hurt."	Use for children as young as 4 years
Color Tool: Uses crayons or markers for the child to construct a scale that is used with a body outline (Eland & Banner, 1999).	Present eight crayons or markers to the child in random order. Ask the child to "pick a crayon with a color that reminds you of the most hurt (or pain) that you could possibly have"; once that crayon is selected, separate it from the others. Next, ask the child to select a crayon with a color that "reminds you of pain that is a little less than the pain we just talked about"; once the second crayon is selected, separate it from the group and place it with the first crayon selected. Ask the child to select a third crayon with a color "that reminds you of only a little pain"; separate this crayon and move it to the selected group. Finally, ask the child to select a crayon with a color that "reminds you of no hurt (or pain)" and separate that fourth color. Show the four crayons selected to the child and arrange them in order of "worst hurt (or pain)" to "no hurt (or pain)." Ask the child to show on the body outline "where the hurt is." If the child offers any verbal comments, note them.	Use for children as young as 4 years, provided that they know their colors, are not color blind, and are able to construct the scale if in pain.

Note: Several variations of the Faces scale exist (Bieri et al., 1990; Kuttner & LePage, 1989; McGrath, de Veber, & Hearn, 1985).

*The *Wong-Baker Faces Pain Rating Scale Reference Manual* describing development and research of the scale is available from the Pain Resource Center, City of Hope National Medical Center, 1500 East Duarte Road, Duarte, CA 91010; (626) 359-8111, ext. 3829; fax: (626) 301-8941; e-mail: mayday_pain http://www.mosby.com/WOW/. A compilation of many pain scales, including Faces, is available free from Purdue Frederick, 100 Connecticut Avenue, Norwalk, CT 06850-3950; (800) 733-1333 or (203) 853-0123, ext. 7378 or 7314; website: http://www.partnersagainstpain.com. The use of Faces with children is demonstrated in *Whaley and Wong's Pediatric Nursing Video Series*, "Pain Assessment and Management," narrated by Donna Wong, PhD, RN. It is available from Mosby, 11830 Westline Industrial Drive, St. Louis, MO 63146; (800) 426-4545; fax: (800) 535-9935; website: http://www.mosby.com.

†Oucher is available for purchase from the Association for the Care of Children's Health, P.O. Box 25707, Alexandria, VA 22313; (703) 684-6179 or (800) 808-ACCH (2224); fax: (703) 684-1589; website: http://www.acch.org.

‡The Poker Chip Tool was developed in 1975 by N. O. Hester, University of Colorado Health Sciences Center, School of Nursing, Denver, CO 80262. It is also available in Spanish and French.

Wong, D. L., & Hess, C. S. (2000). *Wong and Whaley's clinical manual of pediatric nursing* (5th ed.). St. Louis: Mosby.

Table 20-2 Faces Pain Scale, Revised (Bieri Faces)

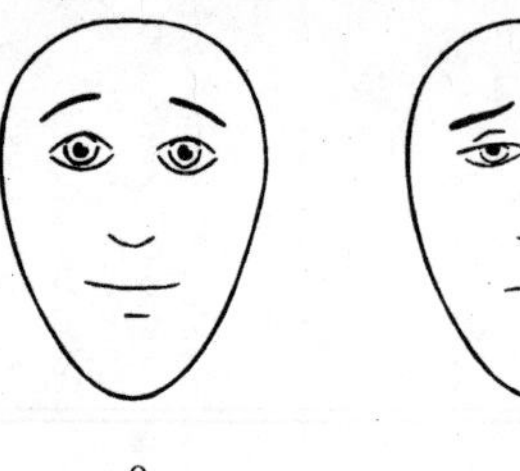
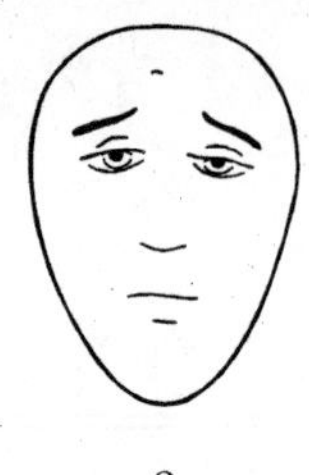
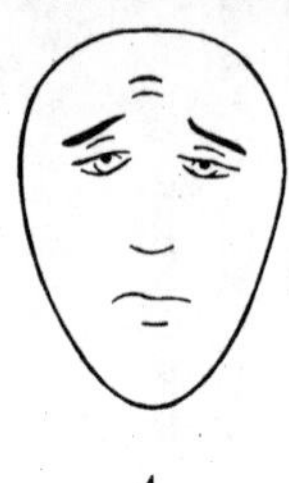
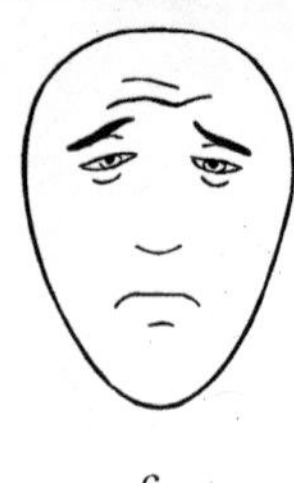
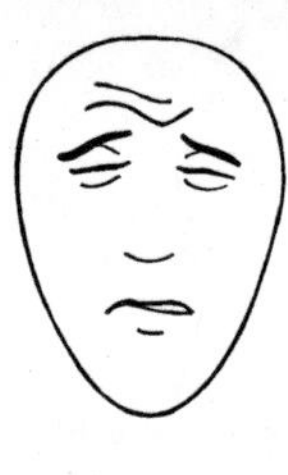
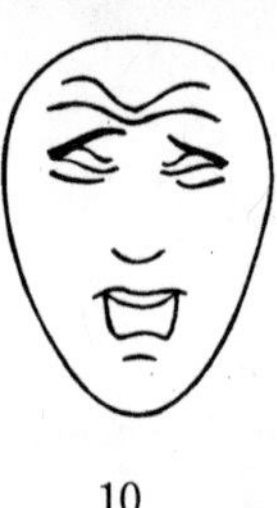

0	2	4	6	8	10

"These faces show how much something can hurt. This face (point to the leftmost face) shows no pain. The faces show more and more pain (point to each from left to right) up to this one (point to the rightmost face)—it shows very much pain. Point to the face that shows how much you hurt (right now)."

Hicks, C. L., von Baeyer, C. L., Spafford, P., van Korlaar, I., & Goodenough, G. (2001). The Faces Pain Scale, revised: Toward a common metric in pediatric pain measurement. *Pain, 93*(2), 173–183. Scale adapted from Bieri, D., Reeve, R., Champion, G. D., Addicoat, L., & Ziegler, J. (1990). The Faces Pain Scale for the self-assessment of the severity of pain experienced by children: Development, initial validation, and preliminary investigation for ratio scale properties. *Pain, 41*, 139–150.

3. Observational or behavioral pain scoring for children who are unable to self-report.
   a. Observational pain scoring tools can provide information in the overall pain assessment for children who have limited cognitive or language skills and are unable to self-report their pain.
   b. Most observational scales add the sum of the scores from several observed behaviors on the particular scale.
   c. Pain that is sharp and short in duration (procedural pain) has the highest reliability and validity for behavioral pain scoring tools (Schecter et al., 2003).
   d. It is difficult to differentiate among behaviors specific to pain and anxiety when using observational pain scoring tools.
   e. Factors other than pain can influence behavioral responses (i.e., loneliness or fear). If the nurse is uncertain whether a behavior indicates pain but has reason to suspect pain is present, an analgesic dose can be diagnostically helpful.
   f. Enlist the assistance of parents because they can recognize subtle changes in behavior in their child.
4. Children who are developmentally delayed have varying levels of difficulty self-reporting their pain or may be unable to do so. When self-report is not possible, careful observation of behaviors that suggest pain is crucial.
   a. No research supports that children with developmental delay are less sensitive to painful stimuli than children with normal development (Oberlander et al., 1999).
   b. A limited number of pain assessment tools are validated in children with developmental delay (Malviya, Voepel-Lewis, Burke, Merkel, & Tait, 2006).
      (1) The *revised* FLACC (face, legs, activity, cry, consolability) scale has been validated in children from 4 to 19 years of age with cognitive impairment (Malviya et al., 2006).
      (2) The Individualized Numeric Rating Scale (INRS) (Solodiuk & Curly, 2003) (see Table 20-6 for a clinical practice example)
         (a) The INRS is an adaptation of the numerical rating scale that asks parents, caregivers, or both to identify an individual patient's typical pain behavior and asks them to indicate what pain rating number that behavior correlates with on a scale from 0 to 10 (Solodiuk & Curly, 2003).
   c. For older children with mild delay, using a self-report scale may be appropriate and is more beneficial than using an observational scale (e.g., a 16 year old who is cognitively functioning

at 5 years of age may be able to self-report using the Faces scale but not a numerical rating scale). Tables 20-3 through 20-6 show select observational pain scoring tools for infants and children.

d. Intubated children
   (1) Few scales have been validated in intubated children.
   (2) The Distress Scale for Ventilated Newborns (Sparshott, 1996) has established validity and reliability for use in ventilated newborn infants for procedural pain.
   (3) The Comfort Scale (Ambuel, Hamlett, & Marx, 1990; Bear & Ward-Smith, 2006) has established validity and reliability for use in mechanically ventilated children. It combines six behavioral and two physiological measures.
   (4) Monitor physiological parameters such as dilation of pupils, flushing, pallor, muscle tension, hand sweating, increases in heart rate, blood pressure, respirations, and decreased oxygen saturation (Yaster, Krane, Kaplan, & Lappe, 1997).

Table 20-3 FLACC Behavioral Pain Assessment Scale

1. Categories	Scoring		
	0	1	2
Face	No particular expression or smile	Occasional grimace or frown; withdrawn, disinterested	Frequent to constant frown, clenched jaw, quivering chin
Legs	Normal position or relaxed	Uneasy, restless, tense	Kicking, legs drawn up
Activity	Lying quietly, normal position, moves easily	Squirming, shifting back and forth, tense	Arched, rigid, jerking
Cry	No cry (awake or asleep)	Moans or whimpers, occasional complaint	Crying steadily; screams, sobs; frequent complaints
Consolability	Content, relaxed	Reassured by occasional touching, hugging, being talked to; distractible	Difficult to console or comfort

Each of the five categories is scored 0–2, resulting in a total score between 0 and 10.

2. How to Use FLACC

In patients who are awake: Observe for 1 to 5 minutes or longer. Observe the legs and body uncovered. Reposition the patient or observe activity. Assess the body for tenseness and tone. Initiate consoling interventions if needed.

In patients who are asleep: Observe for 5 minutes or longer. Observe the body and legs uncovered. If possible, reposition the patient. Touch the body and assess for tenseness and tone.

3. Interpreting the behavioral score

A. Face

- Score 0 if the patient has a relaxed face, makes eye contact, or shows interest in surroundings.
- Score 1 if the patient has a worried facial expression, with eyebrows lowered, eyes partially closed, cheeks raised, or mouth pursed.
- Score 2 if the patient has deep furrows in the forehead, closed eyes, an open mouth, or deep lines around the nose and lips.

Table 20-3 FLACC Behavioral Pain Assessment Scale *(continued)*

B. Legs

- Score 0 if the muscle tone and motion in the limbs are normal.
- Score 1 if the patient has increased tone, rigidity, or tension or if intermittent flexion or extension of the limbs occurs.
- Score 2 if the patient has hypertonicity, the legs are pulled tight, exaggerated flexion or extension of the limbs is observed, or the patient has tremors.

C. Activity

- Score 0 if the patient moves easily and freely, with normal activity or restrictions.
- Score 1 if the patient shifts positions, appears hesitant to move, demonstrates guarding, has a tense torso, or puts pressure on a body part.
- Score 2 if the patient is in a fixed position, rocking, or demonstrates side-to-side head movement or rubbing of a body part.

D. Cry

- Score 0 if the patient has no cry or moan, awake or asleep.
- Score 1 if the patient has occasional moans, cries, whimpers, or sighs.
- Score 2 if the patient has frequent or continuous moans, cries, or grunts.

E. Consolability

- Score 0 if the patient is calm and does not require consoling.
- Score 1 if the patient responds to comfort by touching or talking in 30 seconds to 1 minute.
- Score 2 if the patient requires constant comforting or is inconsolable.

When self-report is not possible, interpretation of pain behaviors and decisions regarding treatment of pain require careful consideration of the context in which the pain behaviors are observed.

Each category is scored on the 0–2 scale, which results in a total score of 0–10.

4. Interpreting the behavioral score

0 = Relaxed and comfortable

1–3 = Mild discomfort

4–6 = Moderate pain

7–10 = Severe discomfort or pain

The FLACC scale was developed by Sandra Merkel, MS, RN; Terri Voepel-Lewis, MS, RN; and Shabha Malviya, MD at C. S. Mott Children's Hospital, University of Michigan Health System, Ann Arbor, MI). From Merkel, S., Voepel-Lewis, T., Shayevits, J., Malviya, S. (1997). The FLACC: A behavioral scale for scoring postoperative pain in young children. *Pediatric Nursing, 23*(3), 294–297.

Table 20-4 FLACC, Revised (for Cognitively Impaired Children)

Revised FLACC tool and a sample description of individual behavior provided by parents (*revisions noted in italics*)

	*Individual Behavior**
Face 0 = No particular expression or smile 1 = Occasional grimace or frown; withdrawn or disinterested; *appears sad or worried* 2 = Consistent grimace or frown; frequent or constant quivering chin, clenched jaw; *distressed-looking face, expression of fright or panic* Individualized behavior:________________	"Pouty" lip; clenched and grinding teeth; eyebrows furrowed; stressed looking; stern face; eyes wide open—looks surprised; blank expression; nonexpressive
Legs 0 = Normal position or relaxed; *usual tone and motion of limbs* 1 = Uneasy, restless, tense; *occasional tremors* 2 = Kicking, or legs drawn up; *marked increase in spasticity, constant tremors or jerking* Individualized behavior:________________	Legs and arms drawn to center of body; clonus in left leg with pain; very tense and still; legs tremble
Activity 0 = Lying quietly, normal position, moves easily; *regular, rhythmic respirations* 1 = Squirming, shifting back and forth, *tense or guarded movements; mildly agitated (e.g., head back and forth, aggression); shallow, splinting respirations, intermittent sighs* 2 = Arched, rigid or jerking; *severe agitation; head hanging; shivering (not rigors); breath holding, gasping or sharp intake of breaths, severe splinting* Individualized behavior:________________	Grabs at site of pain; nods head; clenches fists, draws up arms; arches neck; arms startle; turns side to side; head shaking; points to where it hurts; clenches fist to face, hits self, slapping; tense, guarded, posturing; thrashes arms; bites palm of hand; holds breath
Cry 0 = No cry or verbalization 1 = Moans or whimpers; occasional complaint; *occasional verbal outburst or grunt* 2 = Crying steadily, screams or sobs, frequent complaints; *repeated outbursts, constant grunting* Individualized behavior:________________	States, "I'm okay" or "All done"; mouth wide open and screaming; states "Owie" or "No"; gasping, screaming; grunts or short responses; whining, whimpering, wailing, shouting; asks for medicine; crying is rare
Consolability 0 = Content and relaxed 1 = Reassured by occasional touching, hugging or being talked to; distractible 2 = Difficult to console or comfort; *pushing away caregiver, resisting care or comfort measures* Individualized behavior:________________	Responds to cuddling, holding parent, stroking, kissing; distant and unresponsive when in pain

*Excerpts from the additional descriptions of the individuals child's pain behavior recorded by parents on the revised FLACC tool during the preoperative interview. Only 21 parents added such comments to the revised FLACC.

From *Pediatric Anesthesia*, Volume 16, issue 3, pages 260. Reprinted with permission of Blackwell Publishing Ltd.

Table 20-5 CRIES Scale

Indicator	Scoring 0	1	2
Crying	No	High pitched or consolable	Inconsolable
Requires oxygen to keep saturation greater than 95%	No	< or = 30% supplemental oxygen to keep oxygen saturation greater than 95%	>30% supplemental oxygen to keep oxygen saturation greater than 95%
Increased vital signs	Heart rate and blood pressure no higher than they were preoperatively	Heart rate or blood pressure increased < or = 20%	Heart rate or blood pressure increased more than 20%
Expression	None	Grimace	Grimace or grunt
Sleepless	No	Wakes at frequent intervals	Constantly awake

Coding tips for using CRIES

Indicator	Coding tips
Crying	The characteristic cry of pain is ***high pitched.*** If no cry or cry is not high pitched, score 0. If cry is high pitched but baby is easily consoled, score 1. If cry is high pitched and baby is inconsolable, score 2.
Requires oxygen for saturation greater than 95%	Look for *changes* in oxygenation. Pain is manifested by decreases in total carbon dioxide level or oxygen saturation. (Consider other causes of changes in oxygenation: atelectasis, level pneumothorax, oversedation, etc.) If no oxygen is required, score 0. If less than 30% oxygen is required, score 1. If more than 30% oxygen is required, score 2.
Increased vital signs	*Note:* Take blood pressure last. Use baseline preoperative parameters from a nonstressed period. Multiply baseline heart rate by 0.2, and then add this to the baseline heart rate to determine the heart rate that is 20% over baseline. Do likewise for blood pressure. Use mean blood pressure. If heart rate and blood pressure are both unchanged or less than baseline, score 0. If heart rate or blood pressure is increased but the increase is less than 20% of baseline, score 1. If either one is increased more than 20% over baseline, score 2.
Expression	The facial expression most often associated with pain is a grimace. This may be characterized by: brow lowering, eyes squeezed shut, deepening of the nasolabial furrow, and open lips and mouth. If no grimace is present, score 0. If grimace alone is present, score 1. If grimace and noncry vocalization grunt are present, score 2.
Sleepless	Sleeplessness is scored based on the infant's state during the hour preceding this recorded score. If the child has been continuously asleep, score 0. If the child has awakened at frequent intervals, score 1. If the child has been awake constantly, score 2.

From Krechel, S. W., & Bildner, J. (1995). CRIES: A new neonatal postoperative pain measurement score. Initial testing of validity and reliability. *Paediatric Anaesthesia, 5*, 53–61.

Table 20-6 INRS

The following scale will help us assess and manage your child's pain

Directions:

1. Think about your child's past painful events. How does your child act when in mild pain, moderate pain, or severe pain?
2. In the diagram below, write in your child's typical pain behaviors on the line that corresponds to pain intensity, where 0 = no pain and 10 = worst possible pain.
3. When describing your child's pain, think about changes in
   1. Facial expression
      Squinting eyes, frowning, distorted face, grinds teeth, thrusts tongue
   2. Leg or general body movements
      Tense, gestures (more or less) or touches part of body that hurts
   3. Activity, or social interaction
      Not cooperative, cranky, irritable, unhappy; not moving, less active, quiet or more active, fidgety,
   4. Cry or vocalization
      Moaning, whimpering, crying, yelling
   5. Consolability
      Less interaction, seeks comfort or physical closeness, difficult to distract/satisfy
   6. Other changes: Tears, sweating, holds breath, gasping

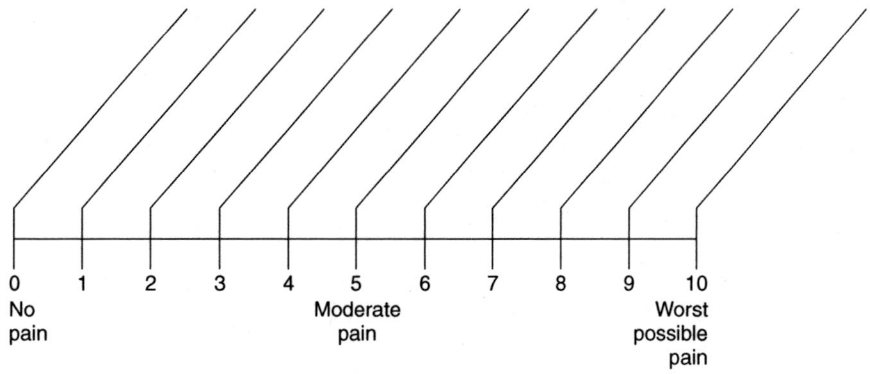

Example of INRS

Date 9 / 10 / 02 Completed by: BJ Relationship: mother

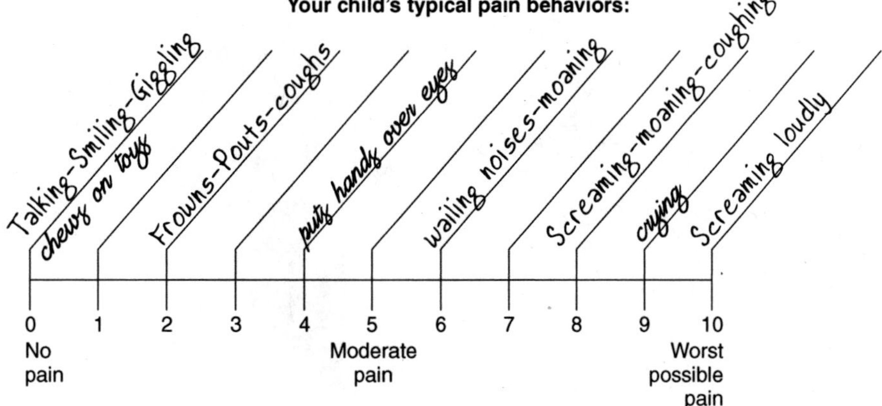

PART TWO: PEDIATRIC ACUTE PAIN

I. Introduction

A. An essential component of caring for a child is providing pain management. Adequate pain management must be provided regardless of whether the child is in a pediatric tertiary care center or a community hospital.

B. Knowledge of normal growth and development of children and assessment and management of sick children is necessary to treat pain optimally in children.

C. Nurses are well positioned to be advocates for infants and children of all ages, developmental levels, and cultures.

II. Pharmacological Interventions

Use of the WHO analgesic ladder is based on the child's level of pain. If pain control is inadequate, move to the next step up the ladder (WHO, 1998) (see Fig. 20-1).

1. Weak opioids and strong opioids are determined not only by the opioid selected but also by the dose.
2. For mild pain, use a nonopioid (e.g., acetaminophen) with or without an adjuvant.
3. For mild-to-moderate pain, use an opioid (e.g., codeine) and supplement analgesia with a nonopioid, adjuvant, or both as necessary.
4. For moderate-to-severe pain, use a μ-opioid agonist (e.g., morphine) and, if necessary, supplement analgesia with a nonopioid, adjuvant, or both.

A. Nonsteroidal antiinflammatory drugs (NSAIDs)

1. A reduction in opioid use and pain scores was found in children undergoing surgery when using NSAIDs (Morton & O'Brien, 1999; Vetter & Heiner, 1994). NSAIDs may trigger bronchospasm in patients with asthma. Use them with caution in patients with compromised gastric mucosa, thrombocytopenia, or renal insufficiency.
2. Ibuprofen
   a. Ibuprofen is used commonly in children. The product labeling is for infants greater than 6 months of age. Dose is 10 mg/kg orally every 6 hours.

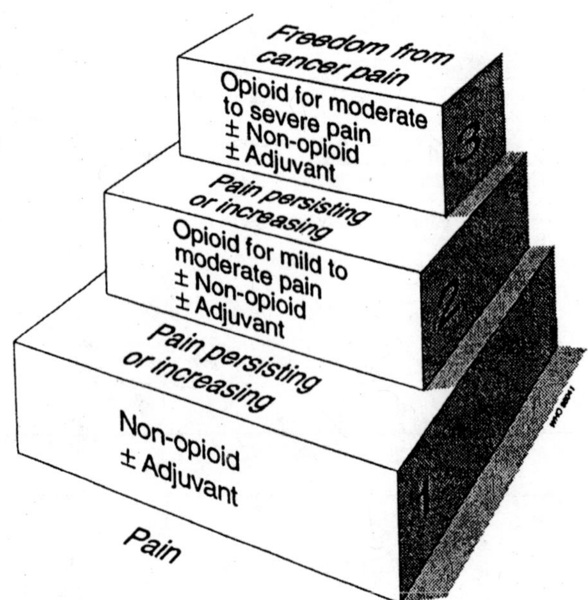

Figure 20-1 | The three-step analgesic ladder.

From World Health Organization (1998). *Cancer pain relief and palliative care in children* (p. 25). Geneva: Author.

3. Ketorolac (Toradol®)
   a. Dosing is 0.5 mg/kg intravenously every 6 hours, with a maximum dose of 15 mg. Ketorolac should not be used for more than 5 days. Some recommend 48 to 72 hours as the maximum duration of parenteral ketorolac (Deshpande & Anand, 1996). Decreasing the dose frequency or length of treatment may decrease the incidence and severity of side effects.
   b. The maintenance dose of ketorolac is similar in children, adolescents, and adults (Dsida et al., 2002; Hamunen, Maunuksela, Sarvela, Bullingham, & Olkkola, 1999). Only a single dose of ketorolac is approved by the U.S. Food and Drug Administration (FDA) for children 2 to 16 years of age (Taketomo, Hodding, & Kraus, 2007).
   c. Published studies are lacking on dosing pharmacokinetics or safety in infants less than 6 months of age. Retrospective chart review of 53 infants less than 6 months of age receiving at least one dose of ketorolac noted that blood urea nitrogen and serum creatinine levels increased from baseline following ketorolac administration in all infants but stayed within normal limits (Moffett, Wann, Carberry, & Mott, 2006; Papacci et al., 2004).
4. Acetaminophen (Tylenol®)
   a. Acetaminophen is the most widely administered analgesic in children. It is metabolized in infants by sulfonation pathway and is eliminated more slowly in newborns due to immature glomerular filtration rate and tubular secretion compared to children and adults. It is ***not*** appropriate to withhold use of acetaminophen in neonates.
   b. The oral pediatric dose is 10 to 15 mg/kg every 4 to 6 hours in children and every 6 to 8 hours in full-term infants 1 month old or less (Taketomo et al., 2007; Zagaria, 2008). The typical dose of 10 mg/kg may be inadequate for pain relief because this dose is based on antipyretic dose schedules. The safe maximal dosage generally is considered to be 90 mg/kg in 24 hours in children and 60 mg/kg in 24 hours in neonates and infants (Penna, Dawson, & Penna, 1993; Rowbotham & Macintyre, 2003; Schecter et al., 2003). Toxicity has been associated with maximum therapeutic doses administered for extended periods; therefore, some recommend acetaminophen not be administered at the maximum dose for longer than 5 days (Hynson & South, 1999; Rowbotham & Macintyre, 2003
   c. Rectal absorption varies greatly, from 24% to 98% (Rowbotham & Macintyre, 2003). In practice, the same dose is used rectally as orally despite the difference in bioavailability of the two routes (Dahl & Raeder, 2000).
5. Acetylsalicylic acid (Aspirin®)
   a. Pediatric use has declined since the early 1980s, when a possible link was found between the use of salicylates in children during respiratory or viral illness and the development of Reye syndrome. A decrease in the incidence of Reye syndrome has occurred since the use of salicylates has declined (Arrowsmith, Kennedy, Kuritsky, & Faich, 1987; Hurwitz, 1988).
   b. Children older than 1 year of age eliminate aspirin at approximately the same rate as adults.
   c. Standard dosing is 10 to 15 mg/kg every 4 to 6 hours. However, due to its association with Reye syndrome and the need to dose it three to four times per day, it is not typically used even in patients with juvenile rheumatoid arthritis. Standard dosing is 10 to 15 mg/kg every 4 to 6 hours. Other NSAIDs, such as naprosyn sodium, diclofenac or sulindac, or daily medications such as piroxicam are preferred for juvenile rheumatoid arthritis or in general.

B. Opioids
   1. Table 20-7 lists commonly used μ-agonist drugs.
   2. Opioids in general
      a. Weak opioid drugs
         (1) Manage mild-to-moderate pain with or without a nonopioid. Weak opioids include medications such as codeine and nalbuphine, a mixed agonist–antagonist.
         (2) If the child has inadequate pain control, change medication to a strong opioid and discontinue the weak opioid.

Table 20-7 Commonly Used μ-Agonist Drugs

Agonist	Equipotent IV Dose (mg/kg)	Duration (hours)	Bioavailability (%)	Comments
Morphine	0.1	3–4	20–40	Seizures in newborns; also in all patients at high doses. Histamine release, vasodilation. Avoid in asthmatics and in circulatory compromise. Morphine sulfate (MS Contin®) has a duration of 8–12 hours.
Meperidine	1.0	3–4	40–60	Catastrophic interactions with MAOIs. Tachycardia; negative inotrope. Metabolite produces seizures; not recommended for long-term use.
Methadone	0.1	6–24	70–100	Can be IV even though the package insert says SQ or IM.
Fentanyl	0.001	0.5–1		Bradycardia; minimal hemodynamic alterations. Chest wall rigidity (>5 μg/kg in rapid IV bolus). Prescribe naloxone or paralyze with succinylcholine or pancuronium.
Codeine	1.2	3–4	40–70	Oral route only. Prescribe with acetaminophen.
Hydromorphone (Dilaudid®)	0.015–0.02	3–4	40–60	< CNS depression than morphine; < itching, nausea than morphine; can be used in IV and epidural PCA.
Oxycodone (component opioid in Tylox®)	0.15	3–4	50	A third less than morphine but with better oral bioavailability; often used when weaning from IV to oral medication (one-third less potent).

CNS, central nervous system; IV, intravenous; IM, intramuscular; MAOI, monoamine oxidase inhibitor, PCA, patient-controlled analgesia; SQ, subcutaneous.

From Schecter, N. L., Berde, C. B., & Yaster, M. (Eds.). (2003). *Pain in infants, children, and adolescents* (p. 183). Baltimore: Lippincott Williams & Wilkins. Copyright 1997 by Lippincott Williams & Wilkins.

b. Strong opioid drugs
   (1) Strong opioids manage moderate-to-severe pain; the dose is limited only by side effects. There is no defined upper dose due to tolerance.
   (2) The half-life of morphine in children is 2 to 3 hours (Schecter et al., 2003).
   (3) Extended-release opioid medications (e.g., controlled-release morphine sulfate [MS Contin®] and oxycodone [OxyContin®]) reach steady state in 3 to 5 days. This requires slower increases in dose titration. A short-acting opioid may be needed for use as a rescue until the longer-acting opioid dose is titrated. Excretion is slow after drug has been stopped. Use long-acting opioids with extreme caution in children in rapidly changing clinical situations.
   (4) *Note:* Extreme care must be taken when using methadone because its half-life increases with repeated doses.

c. Use of opioids
   (1) Opioid side effects are well known and should be anticipated and treated. Side effects such as itching, nausea, and mild sedation may resolve within 1 week of opioid initiation. The exception is constipation, which does not resolve without intervention.

3. Morphine
   a. Morphine is the gold standard, widely studied in infants and children. The intravenous dose is 0.05 to 0.1 mg/kg every 3 to 4 hours as needed. There is a wide range of interpatient pharmacokinetic variability, particularly for infants. The dose should be adjusted based on age and condition. Careful titration of the dose and monitoring is required for infants less than 6 months old. Often, starting doses for infants less than 6 months of age is 25% of the usual pediatric dose on a per-kilogram basis relative to the standard pediatric dose for older children (Schecter et al., 2003). That is, morphine at 0.012 to 0.025 mg/kg/dose intravenously every 3 hours ***as needed*** can be used instead of 0.05 to 0.1 mg/kg/dose.
   b. Premature and full-term infants have immature responses to hypoxia and hypercarbia; they are at greater risk of respiratory depression. Use in infants younger than 2 months should be in a monitored intensive care unit setting (Schecter et al., 2003). Infants less than 2 months old have a decreased rate of elimination because of decreased renal clearance and the immaturity of the cytochrome P450 system in the liver. Hepatic function, specifically glucuronidation, which metabolizes morphine to active and inactive metabolites, develops to adult levels by 2 to 6 months of age. Chronological age (days postbirth) of the infant, not gestational age (number of weeks in utero), determines how an infant metabolizes opioids. Because of a reduced concentration of albumin and α_1-acid glycoproteins, unbound or free morphine increases, allowing an increased amount of active drug to reach the brain and resulting in increased sensitivity to opioid central nervous system depressant effects (Blackburn & Loper, 1992; Schecter et al., 2003).
   c. Continuous infusion when necessary avoids peaks and troughs. Dosage range is 0.01 to 0.05 mg/kg/hr intravenously. Rescue doses are given as needed. Rate should be adjusted every 12 to 24 hours based on pain and number of rescue doses needed.
   d. For patient-controlled analgesia (PCA) dosing, the initial demand dose of morphine is traditionally 0.02 mg/kg, allowing five PCA doses per hour with a lockout time of 6 to 8 minutes (Schecter et al., 2003). A rescue dose of 0.05 to 0.1 mg/kg every 3 to 4 hours should be available if needed to control the child's pain. Background infusion of 0.001 to 0.02 mg/kg/hr can be added (see III. Strategies for Pain Control for additional PCA information).
   e. Initial oral morphine (immediate release) dosing is 0.2 to 0.3 mg/kg every 4 to 6 hours as needed, and extended-release dosing, with the exception of Kadian® and Avinza®), is 0.3 to 0.6 mg/kg every 8 to 12 hours as needed.
4. Hydromorphone (Dilaudid®)
   a. Hydromorphone is approximately five times more potent than morphine. Hydromorphone is useful when the child experiences excessive side effects to morphine or when morphine use is complicated by renal impairment. The intravenous dose is 0.015 mg/kg every 3 to 4 hours as needed (Taketomo et al., 2007, p. 788). There is large interpatient variability. Hydromorphone can be used as a continuous infusion or by PCA.
   b. Initial oral hydromorphone dosing is 0.03 to 0.08 mg/kg every 3 to 4 hours as needed (Taketomo et al., 2007).
5. Fentanyl
   a. Fentanyl is 80 to 100 times more potent than morphine. It is an appropriate choice for short procedures. Initial dosage of fentanyl is 1 to 3 μg/kg given intravenously over 3 to 5 minutes. For continued pain relief, it is more appropriate to administer by continuous infusion, giving 1 to 3 μg/kg/hr.
   b. Infants 3 to 12 months old eliminate fentanyl more quickly than children older than 12 months, and the elimination half-life is longer (Singleton, Rosen, & Fisher, 1987). In practice, fentanyl dosing is determined by the specific circumstances and individual patient response. Use caution when administering a continuous infusion or repeated doses; drug may accumulate because of its lipophilic properties and drug interactions with inhibitors of cytochrome P450 3A4, the major substrate for fentanyl metabolism. Fentanyl has high lipid solubility with rapid entry into the brain.

c. Transdermal administration is limited severely by the weight of the patient: *The patch cannot be trimmed to obtain appropriate dosing for small children.* Opioid patches may be considered while being cognizant of the following warning. *Warning:* Use in a pediatric patient only if the patient is opioid tolerant, is receiving at least 60 mg/day morphine equivalent, and is greater than or equal to 2 years of age. Safety in children younger than 2 years has not been established (Taketomo et al., 2007, p. 645). No data are available in infants, in whom dermal differences (skin thickness) may affect dose.

d. The oral transmucosal form of fentanyl (Actiq®) is approved for patients 16 years and older experiencing breakthrough cancer pain who are opioid tolerant and taking at least 60 mg of morphine each day, at least 25 μg of transdermal fentanyl per hour, or an equianalgesic dose of another opioid each day (Cephalon, 2007) for 7 days (APS, 2005). There is a paucity of published studies in pediatric patients.

6. Meperidine (Demerol®)
   a. Meperidine is 10 times less potent than morphine. The intravenous dose is 1 mg/kg every 3 to 4 hours as needed for 48 hours or less. When the principal metabolite of meperidine, normeperidine, accumulates, it may cause central nervous system excitation, including tremors, hyperactive reflexes, and seizures. Meperidine has a half-life of 3 to 5 hours, while its metabolite has a long half-life of 8 to 21 hours in patients with normal renal function. Because of the accumulation of this metabolite, meperidine should not be used for an extended period, and it should not be used in patients with renal insufficiency or disease because normeperidine accumulates more quickly. *Other opioids should be considered because other opioids have the same analgesic effects but fewer disadvantages.*
   b. The oral form is not recommended.
7. Methadone
   a. Methadone is typically used when weaning children from long-term opioid use.
   b. Methadone can be effective treatment for severe pain in situations in which a PCA or continuous infusion is not desired. A single dose of methadone results in a high plasma level and can provide analgesia for an extended period (Schecter et al., 2003).
   c. Caution must be exercised because its respiratory depressant effect lasts longer than its analgesic effect. When a blood level is achieved, after a few doses, patients require less methadone because of its slow elimination and low clearance rate. Patients must be carefully monitored to avoid overmedication with repeated dosing (Manfredi & Houde, 2003). If a child is comfortable after initial doses, the dose should be reduced or the interval extended to avoid potential overdosage. If oversedation occurs with initial dosing, it is recommended to discontinue the methadone (Berde, Sethna, Holzman, Reidy, & Gondek, 1987; Berde, Beyer, Bournaki, Levin, & Sethna 1991).
8. Oxycodone
   a. The oral dose is 0.05 to 0.15 mg/kg every 4 to 6 hours as needed (Taketomo et al., 2007). When commercially prepared with acetaminophen (i.e., Percocet® [oxycodone with acetaminophen], Tylox®, Roxicodone® [plain oxycodone], or Roxicet® [oxycodone with acetaminophen]), dose is limited by the appropriate dose of oxycodone and acetaminophen.
   b. No injectable dosage form is available.
9. Codeine
   a. The parenteral form not recommended because of potential for apnea and hypotension (Deshpande & Anand, 1996). Codeine is not approved for intravenous administration (Taketomo et al., 2007).
   b. The oral dose is 0.5 to 1 mg/kg every 4 hours. Most pharmacies supply codeine with acetaminophen in set amounts (i.e., Tylenol® No. 2 has acetaminophen at 325 mg and codeine phosphate at 15 mg; Tylenol® No. 3 has acetaminophen at 325 mg and codeine phosphate at 30 mg; and Tylenol® with codeine elixir has acetaminophen at 120 mg and codeine phosphate at 12 mg/5 ml with 7% alcohol). The dose prescribed is limited by the appropriate dose of codeine and the safe dose of acetaminophen. Caution parents not to augment a prescription or administer any other medication containing acetaminophen because toxic levels of acetaminophen may be produced.

10. Hydrocodone bitartrate
    a. The oral dosage guideline from the Agency for Health Care Policy and Research is 0.2 mg/kg every 4 hours as needed. Commercially prepared with acetaminophen (i.e., Lorcet®, Lortab® [available as an elixir], or Vicodin®), the dose is limited by the appropriate dose of hydrocodone and acetaminophen.
    b. No injectable dosage form is available.
11. Nalbuphine (Nubain®)
    a. The intravenous dose for analgesia is 0.1 mg/kg every 3 to 4 hours as needed. The dose to counteract some side effects of pure agonist opioids is 0.01 to 0.05 mg/kg every 4 hours as needed. At the high end of the dosage range, mixed agonist–antagonist drugs may precipitate withdrawal when physical dependence on opioids is present. Nalbuphine may block agonist binding or have no clinically apparent effect on it.

C. General anesthetic
1. Ketamine
    a. Appropriate equipment (i.e., suction), monitoring, and a skilled professional with the ability to maintain an airway are required. Use with a prophylactic antisialagogue (anticholinergic agent that decreases flow of saliva), such as glycopyrrolate.
    b. The ketamine dose is 0.25 to 1.0 mg/kg intravenously every 3 minutes until desired level of anesthesia is achieved. Doses of less than 0.5 mg/kg generally preserve airway reflexes (gag reflex and airway tone). Doses of 1 mg/kg or greater produce anesthesia and can cause an incompetent gag reflex. The oral dose is 6 to 10 mg/kg for one dose given 30 minutes before procedure (Taketomo et al., 2007).
    c. The adverse effect seen most often is emergence delirium or hallucinations. When benzodiazepines are administered before ketamine, the occurrence of hallucinations is decreased.
    d. Ketamine's activity on the NMDA receptor suggests that it may decrease pain resulting from central sensitization and pathological pain states such as hyperalgesia or opioid tolerance, neuropathic pain, cancer pain, visceral pain, or severe acute pain (Hocking, Visser, Schug, & Cousins, 2007).

D. Sedatives
1. Demerol, Phenergan, and Thorazine (DPT) cocktail or pedicocktail
    a. *Black box warning:* Use with extreme caution in children, and avoid use in children less than 2 years of age due to the potential for severe and potentially fatal respiratory depression. A wide range of weight-based doses have resulted in respiratory depression. Excessively high doses have been associated with sudden death in children. Use the lowest effective dose in children more than 2 years of age, and avoid concomitant use with other medications that have respiratory depression effects (Takemoto et al., p. 1324).
    b. This cocktail consists of meperidine (Demerol®), promethazine hydrochloride (Phenergan®), and chlorpromazine hydrochloride (Thorazine®) administered by intramuscular injection. As discussed previously, the use of intramuscular injections for pain relief in children is inappropriate. The DPT cocktail causes excessive central nervous system depression, and sedation effects may last 7 hours or longer (Nahata, Clotz, & Krogg, 1985). Duration of pain relief is shorter, lasting 3 to 4 hours. Use of this cocktail is not recommended. Alternate agents with fewer risks should be used.
    c. The DPT cocktail potentiates the respiratory depressant effect of the meperidine. Phenothiazines also lower the seizure threshold, and seizures have been reported in children without risk factors after DPT cocktail administration (Snodgrass & Dodge, 1989).

E. Benzodiazepines
1. Midazolam (Versed®)
    a. Midazolam is commonly used as a preanesthetic agent or for sedation. For painful procedures, midazolam must be used with an analgesic. It should be administered in an observed setting; when it is administered intravenously, resuscitation equipment with skilled personnel to maintain an airway and support ventilation must be immediately available.

b. The oral dose before a procedure is typically 0.25 to 0.5 mg/kg with an onset of approximately 20 minutes. Patients 6 months to 6 years may require higher doses, up to 1 mg/kg (Taketomo et al., 2007, p. 1060). Patients with respiratory or cardiac compromise or concomitant central nervous system depressants may require decreased dosing, such as 0.25 mg/kg (Deshpande & Anand, 1996; Taketomo et al., 2007). Midazolam has a bitter taste and needs to be mixed with a flavored syrup; acetaminophen elixir is also a good vehicle to mix midazolam. The volume of diluent should be kept to a minimum.
c. The intranasal form is irritating to mucous membranes; use is limited by the volume of drug to be administered. The intranasal dose is 0.2 mg/kg (Taketomo et al., 2007, p. 1060). Large volumes drip down the throat, especially if the head is tilted back, and are absorbed orally, resulting in a slower onset.
d. The intravenous dose for sedation for a procedure is 0.05 to 0.15 mg/kg titrated to effect. Onset is rapid. Respiratory depression is a significant side effect, especially with concomitant use of other respiratory depressants. Apnea is dose related (Taketomo et al., 2007, p. 1060).

2. Diazepam (Valium®)
   a. Diazepam is commonly used to relieve muscle spasm. In addition, it has anxiolytic, hypnotic, and antiepileptic properties.
   b. The oral dose (0.2 to 0.3 mg/kg) is give 45 to 60 minutes before a procedure. The oral doses for muscle relaxation, sedation, and anxiety are 0.12 to 0.8 mg/kg/day in divided doses every 6 to 8 hours. Intravenous dosing is 0.04 to 0.3 mg/kg every 2 to 4 hours to a maximum of 0.6 mg/kg in 8 hours if needed for muscle relaxation, sedation, and anxiety (Taketomo et al., 2007, p. 483).
3. Lorazepam (Ativan®)
   a. Lorazepam is used to treat acute anxiety or insomnia for a brief period. Although often used in pediatrics, safety and effectiveness have not been established in children younger than 12 years of age. Typical dosing is 0.05 mg/kg every 4 to 8 hours, with a range of 0.02 to 0.1 mg/kg in infants and children. Intravenous and oral dosing are the same. In ill or very young children, it is prudent to start at very low doses to avoid oversedation. Newborns have a prolonged excretion of the drug (mean half-life is 40 hours) (Schecter et al., 2003). The diluent in the intravenous formulation contains propylene glycol, polyethylene glycol, and 2% benzyl alcohol, which may be toxic at higher doses and in the neonatal population (Taketomo et al., 2007; Tobias, 2005).
   b. The dose should be tapered to avoid potential withdrawal.

F. Local and topical anesthetics
1. Local anesthetics are designed to reduce pain sensation. Children should be told they may feel some sensation of pressure depending on the type of procedure being performed.
2. EMLA® (lidocaine 2.5% and prilocaine 2.5%)
   a. Apply a dollop of cream to the desired area; cover with an occlusive dressing for a minimum of 1 hour before a procedure. Longer application times of 2 to 4 hours provide deeper local anesthetic penetration. Prolonged application leads to increased absorption; this may lead to toxicity in infants.
   b. There is a risk of methemoglobinemia in very young children and children who are glucose-6-phosphate dehydrogenase deficient. Methemoglobinemia can result when hemoglobin is exposed to prilocaine. The hemoglobin can oxidize to form methemoglobin, which is not an effective carrier of oxygen. In infants younger than 3 months, there is a reduced level of the enzyme that converts methemoglobin back to hemoglobin. EMLA® should not be used in infants younger than 12 months who are receiving methemoglobinemia-inducing drugs (e.g., acetaminophen, sulfonamides, nitrates, phenytoin, and class I antiarrhythmics). Methemoglobinemia has been found to be rare in children with EMLA® use (Koren, 1993).
   c. EMLA® is approved for pediatric patients with a gestational age of 37 weeks or greater. EMLA® may be applied to more than one location on the child's body, but the total area of application should not exceed the recommended maximums. See Table 20-8 for the EMLA® cream maximal dose, application area, and application time by age and weight.

Table 20-8 EMLA® Cream Maximal Recommended Dose, Application Area, and Application Time by Age and Weight*

Age and Body Weight Requirements	Maximal Total Dose of EMLA® (g)	Maximal Application Area (cm²)	Maximal Application Time (hours)
0–3 months or <5 kg	1	10	1
3–12 months and >5 kg	2	20	4
1–6 years and >10 kg	10	100	4
7–12 years and >20 kg	20	200	4

*These maximums are for infants and children based on application to intact skin. If a patient greater than 3 months old does not meet the minimal weight requirement, the maximal total dose of EMLA® should be restricted to that which corresponds to the patient's weight.

From Astra Pharmaceuticals. (1999). EMLA package insert. AstraZeneca, Wayne, PA.

d. A study of 30 preterm neonates using a single EMLA® dose of 0.5 g applied for 1 hour resulted in no measurable changes in methemoglobin levels (Taddio et al., 1995).
e. In total, 85% of patients receiving EMLA® before venous access experience significant analgesic benefit (Zempsky, 2008).
f. Studies confirm the use of EMLA® in alleviating pain from venous cannulation, vaccination, lumbar puncture, and venous port access (Halperin et al., 1989; Miser et al., 1994; Taddio, Nulman, Goldbach, Ipp, & Koren, 1994). Anxiety is still an issue that needs behavioral intervention.

3. 2.4% liposomal lidocaine cream (LMX®) (previously called ELA-Max®)
   a. LMX® is available without a prescription. It is labeled for use in children 2 years of age and older. Lidocaine molecules encapsulated in a lipid layer, which allow rapid absorption into the skin. Dermal analgesia is attained after 20 to 30 minutes. More invasive procedures require 45 minutes occluded. Increasing application times may result in decreased local anesthesia as the drug dissipates quickly.
   b. One-third of the intended final dose should be rubbed into the skin for approximately 30 to 60 seconds, and then the remainder of the dose is applied in a thick layer. Occlusive dressing is optional but may prevent oral ingestion and help the cream stay in place on an active child. The time to onset of local anesthesia depends on whether an occlusive dressing is used.
   c. The advantages of LMX®4 over EMLA® are that it has a faster onset of anesthesia and that it is not associated with methemoglobinemia.
   d. Studies confirm that 30-minute application of LMX4® is as effective as a 60-minute application of EMLA® for pain relief during venipuncture (Eichenfield, Funk, Fallon-Friedlander, & Cunningham, 2002; Kleiber, Sorenson, Whiteside, Gronstal, & Tannous, 2002).
   e. A higher success rate for peripheral intravenous cannulation, shorter procedure time, and less reported pain for children who received liposomal lidocaine 4% than those who received placebo (Taddio, Soin, Schuh, Koren, & Scolnik, 2005).
   f. LMX4® provided similar pain reduction compared with buffered lidocaine in a randomized trial of children 4 to 17 years of age undergoing peripheral intravenous insertion (Luhmann, Hurt, Shootman, & Kennedy, 2004).
   g. Study compared the analgesic efficacy of LMX4® (application time 20 minutes), EMLA® (application time 30 minutes), and dorsal penile block for circumcision. LMX®4 was an effective analgesic for circumcision (Tutag et al., 2005).
4. Lidocaine, 70 mg, and tetracaine, 70 mg, topical anesthetic patch (Synera™)
   a. Synera™ is approved for children 3 years and older.
   b. The patch contains the local anesthetic mixture and an oxygen-activated heating pod to facilitate drug delivery. It should be applied for 20 to 30 minutes to provide dermal analgesia to intact skin for superficial venous access procedures.

c. Keeping a patch on longer can result in systemic toxicity. Simultaneous or sequential application of more than two Synera™ patches is not recommended (Endo Pharmaceuticals, 2006).
d. Significantly decreased pain during venipuncture with a 20-minute application time was found in 59% of children, compared to 20% of children in placebo patch group (Sethna et al., 2005).
e. The patch must be removed before magnetic resonance imaging procedures.

5. Buffered lidocaine
   a. A local anesthetic can be used by injecting 0.1 ml or less of buffered lidocaine intradermally over the intended puncture site using a 30-gauge needle. Buffered lidocaine (1 part 8.4% sodium bicarbonate to 10 parts 1% to 2% lidocaine [i.e., 0.1 ml of sodium bicarbonate to 1 ml of lidocaine]) can be used. The suggested maximum dose of lidocaine is 4.5 mg/kg (McKay, Morris, & Mushlin, 1987; Wong & Pasero, 1997). Its advantage is the speed of onset.
   b. Although the method requires two needlesticks, the self-reported pain from a lidocaine injection has been shown to be lower than that of intravenous catheter insertion in adults (Brown & Larson, 1999).
6. Saline wheal
   a. Inject 0.2 to 0.4 ml of normal saline (with 0.9% benzyl alcohol as a preservative, not bacteriostatic saline) with a small-gauge needle (30 gauge) intradermally to form a wheal. Cannula insertion is made into the wheal. A mild stinging sensation may be experienced when saline is injected.
7. Iontocaine (Numby Stuff™)
   a. Iontocaine is a topical solution of 2% lidocaine hydrochloride with epinephrine (1:100,000). The solution is delivered transdermally using iontophoresis. Iontophoresis uses a low electrical current to force water-soluble drugs across intact skin. Two electrodes are attached to the patient: One electrode contains a hydrogel-like material containing the lidocaine solution, and the other electrode is a ground that completes the circuit. The electrodes are connected to a small battery-powered unit that delivers a low level of current. Local anesthesia is provided to a depth of 10 mm in about 10 to 15 minutes.
   b. The advantage over topical local anesthetic creams is the shorter onset for local anesthesia. Some children are bothered by the tingling sensation when the current is applied.
8. Lidocaine, epinephrine, and tetracaine (LET)
   a. The local anesthetic mixture provides similar levels of anesthesia as tetracaine, adrenaline, and cocaine (TAC) with fewer adverse reactions when applied correctly (Ochsenreither, 1996). TAC is not recommended because life-threatening systemic toxicity has been reported (Yaster et al., 1997).
   b. LET decreases the pain associated with suturing of facial and scalp lacerations. LET solution is placed on the wound bed and around its edges for a minimum of 10 minutes and a maximum of 30 minutes. It has been studied in adults for various laceration locations (Gaufberg, Walta, & Workman, 2007).
   c. LET (or TAC) should not be applied to mucus membranes or end arterioles (i.e., pinna, end of nose, fingers, toes, or penis) because of vasoconstriction and possible ischemia to affected areas (Yaster et al., 1997).
9. Vapocoolants
   a. Some children feel spray is too cold and causes pain itself.
   b. Caution must be exercised to not spray the skin for longer than 10 seconds, as severe local hypothermia with cell death can occur (Farion, Splinter, Newhook, Gaboury, & Splinter, 2008).
   c. Vapocoolants have a short duration of action: less than 1 minute. It may be prudent to have two providers available, one to administer the spray and the other to perform the procedure (Zempsky, 2008).
   d. Vapocoolants are useful for immunizations.
   e. One study showed a reduction in pain with intravenous catheter insertion, and 18% more children reported no or minimal pain with Pain Ease vapocoolant spray compared to those who received placebo. A cannulation attempt occurred within 60 seconds. A secondary outcome

measure showed cannulation on the first attempt was more successful with the use of the vapocoolant spray (Farion et al., 2008).

f. *Caution:* Vapocoolant ethyl chloride is flammable.

10. J-Tip™

a. J-Tip™ delivers user-loaded lidocaine under the skin via a needle-free device with a jet of compressed carbon dioxide through a device placed tightly against the skin. Analgesia occurs in 1 to 3 minutes. Prepare the child for the noise made by the device.

b. Pain was rated significantly lower in a pediatric study comparing the J-Tip™ system to EMLA® cream. It was also noted that the visual analogue pain scores for J-Tip™ administration were lower than those associated with removing the occlusive dressing for the EMLA® group (Jimenez, Bradford, Seidel, Sousa, & Lynn, 2006).

III. Strategies for Pain Control

A. Medication selection

1. Selecting the delivery technique or techniques appropriate for the child is key.
2. Actual analgesic may be less important than the delivery technique.

B. Route

1. *Oral:* An oral route is ideal because of ease of administration. Many medications are available in multiple oral forms. Ask the child or the parent about the child's ability to swallow pills or preference for liquids or chewable tablets. For children unable to swallow pills, crush tablets except when contraindicated, such as time-released or enteric-coated preparations. Mix crushed tablets immediately before administration with a small amount of liquid, such as juice or syrup, or with soft food, such as applesauce or pudding. Avoid mixing medications with large amounts of food or drink to ensure the dose is received. When using liquid medications, consider the actual volume required (i.e., some medications are more concentrated than others, so less liquid is required).
2. *Sublingual:* Many children are not receptive to a sublingual method because of the bitter taste of the medication. A young child may not leave medication in the mouth for a substantial period.
3. *Intranasal:* The intranasal route has a limited number of medications available. Many are irritating to the nasal mucosa, causing a burning sensation, or have an unpleasant taste.
4. *Transdermal:* Only a few medications available by the transdermal method, and even fewer are in doses low enough for low weight children. This route should only be used for patients whose opioid tolerance is known. Oral opioids for breakthrough pain should be made available (APS, 2003).
5. *Rectal:* The rectal route is useful for children who are unable to take medication by mouth but is less reliable than oral route because the absorption varies. Older children and many toddlers dislike the use of suppositories. ***Cutting a suppository in half does not guarantee delivery of half the dose because the drug may not be distributed evenly throughout the suppository*** (Macintyre & Ready, 1996).
6. *Intramuscular:* This is an unacceptable method to deliver pain medication to a child. Most children would rather suffer in silence than receive an injection. Also, there is wide fluctuation in absorption from the muscle, relatively long onset time, and possible formation of sterile abscesses (APS, 2003).
7. Parenteral

a. *Intermittent:* This route works well only if serum levels not permitted to decrease before next dose. This route is labor intensive for the nurse and results in longer wait times for the patient. In the psychological context, the more demonstrative a child is in the expression of pain, the more likely the child will receive pain medication (Horbury, Henderson, & Bromley, 2005; McGrath & Craig, 1989).

b. *Continuous:* This route provides consistent drug levels without peaks and troughs. Extreme care must be exercised with infants because they have a prolonged elimination half-life.

c. PCA

(1) PCA is safe and effective in pediatric patients (Gaukroger, Tomkins, & Van Der Walk, 1989; Gureno & Reisinger, 1991; Monitto et al., 2000).

(2) Children 7 to 8 years old with normal cognitive development usually use PCA appropriately after instruction because they understand the principle of cause and effect. However, children less than 7 years of age may require additional instruction and reinforcement because the analgesic effect of the medication lags several minutes behind the actual button push. *Children in this age group and children with developmental delay need to be evaluated frequently to ensure they are receiving adequate pain relief.* Parents and the nurse should remind the younger children to push the button when they are experiencing pain.

(3) Advantages over other delivery techniques

(a) PCA allows the children to control their own pain medication within the built-in safety features of the pump (e.g., lockout interval between doses and hourly maximum of medication allowed).

(b) It has more timely administration than nurse-administered intermittent doses.

(c) PCA has high patient and parent satisfaction (Berde, Lehn, Yee, Sethna, & Russo, 1991; Gureno & Reisinger, 1991).

(4) PCA should only be initiated after adequate pain control has been established by titration to effect with initial rescue or loading doses.

(a) *Titration to effect* is accelerated dosing of an opioid using small doses frequently over a short period to reach a blood level for adequate analgesia. This titration is done before the patient is placed on steady-state analgesia.

(5) Basal or background infusions can be helpful when pain is most severe.

(a) Basal infusions can also be helpful for young children who may not understand the use of the PCA button completely, but they may result in decreased pulse oximetry reading (Doyle, Robinson, & Morton, 1993; McNeely & Trentadue, 1997).

(b) Studies report similar pain and sedation scores for children receiving only PCA demand doses compared with PCA with a basal or background infusion (McNeely & Trentadue, 1997).

(c) *Caution:* Basal infusions subject patients to opioids whether the child is asleep or awake, in pain or comfortable. This may increase the risk of opioid-induced sedation and respiratory depression. Practitioners are advised to weigh the risk-benefit ratio for individual patients.

d. Authorized agent-controlled analgesia (AACA) (see the chapter on Taxonomy of Pain Management Nursing)

(1) For children who are unable to activate a PCA button independently due to physical or cognitive disabilities, others (parents or nurses) may be *educated and authorized* to do so for the patient. Anyone who has not been educated and authorized should *not* be activating the PCA under any circumstances.

(2) This treatment modality has been referred to as Authorized Agent Controlled Analgesia (AACA) by the American Society for Pain Management Nursing (ASPMN) (Wuhrman et al., 2007). Parent- or nurse-controlled analgesia and has been studied in several pediatric populations, such as oncology patients and children with developmental delay (Anghelescu et al., 2005; Czarnecki et al., 2008; Malviya et al., 2001; Monitto et al., 2000; Voepel-Lewis, Marinkovic, Kostrezewa, Tait, & Malviya, 2008).

(3) Advantages include the following:

(a) Using AACA allows the parent or nurse to medicate the patient as soon as the presence of pain is determined. This approach avoids the time-consuming process of obtaining opioids from the medication cabinet for intermittent administration.

(b) For some parents, assisting with pain management provides them with a sense of control in a setting where they often experience a loss of control. It can provide parents with one way to participate in their child's care. It also provides immediate relief for the child's pain.

(4) Having anyone other than the patient activate a PCA button can be dangerous and is controversial (Institute for Safe Medication Practices, 2002; Joint Commission, 2004).
   (a) Studies show a 2.8% to 7.6% adverse event rate (Czarnecki et al., 2008; Monitto et al., 2000; Voepel-Lewis et al., 2008).

(5) Safety recommendations are based on studies, the Joint Commission sentinel event warning (2004), and the ASPMN position statement (Wuhrman et al., 2007).
   (a) AACA should only be used for children who are unable to operate conventional PCA independently.
   (b) Diligent patient monitoring and precise medication management are required. Concomitant medications have been associated with increased risk of respiratory depression (Czarnecki et al., 2008; Malviya et al., 2001; Monitto et al., 2000; Voepel-Lewis et al., 2008).
   (c) Institutions must develop clear policies directing the use of AACA, and staff must be held accountable for practicing such policies.
   (d) While AACA is more timely than intermittent administration, it removes the inherent safety factor that the child must be awake enough to push the PCA button, which places a child at increased risk. Parents and nurses must be cautioned not to press the PCA button for a sleeping child.
   (e) Parents who are not comfortable or reliable should not have AACA; strictly nurse-controlled analgesia would be more appropriate.
   (f) AACA should not require the parent to be continuously awake and alert, which would result in increased stress.
   (g) Only one parent in a time interval should be responsible for pushing the PCA button.
   (h) Documentation of the family member's level of understanding, as well as continual reinforcement, is essential.
   (i) Patients should be closely monitored, including pulse oximetry, capnography, or both (Maddox, Williams, Oglesby, Butler, & Colclasure, 2006); vital signs; level of sedation; and pain assessment.
   (j) Evaluation and documentation of hourly injections and attempts can provide valuable information regarding the amount of opioid administered and the effectiveness of AACA (Czarnecki et al., 2008).
   (k) *Caution:* Basal infusions increase the risk of opioid-induced sedation and respiratory depression. Practitioners are advised to weigh the risk-benefit ratio for individual patients.

8. See Appendix 20-1 for the position statement of the ASPMN regarding authorized and unauthorized dosing of analgesic infusion pumps.

IV. Procedural Pain

A. General concepts

1. Procedures are often times viewed worse than the condition initiating the need for the procedure (Schecter et al., 2003). It is imperative that procedural pain is optimally managed every time a procedure is performed.
2. Nonpharmacological techniques, topical anesthetics, procedural sedation, and general anesthesia are options to help control the procedure-related pain. No one method is better than another; the appropriate choice depends on the individual child, family, and physician. The use of psychological and pharmacological intervention should be based not only on the type of procedure but also on the child's age, temperament, coping style, and preference.
3. A child's room should be considered a *safe zone.* Painful procedures should be done in a designated treatment or procedure area unless the patient requests otherwise.
4. Prepare the environment.
   a. Ensure privacy.
   b. Adjust lighting.

c. Decrease noise.
d. Limit the number of people in the room to necessary personnel and a support individual or individuals for the patient.
e. Offer to provide a favorite toy or security object.
f. Ensure supplies for nonpharmacological techniques are readily available.
g. Monitor parent and staff behavior, and provide feedback to ensure the environment remains safe and relaxed for the patient.

2. Prepare the child.
   a. Children should not be lied to about painful procedures. They need to be able to trust their parents and the health care team.
   b. Explanations need to be tailored to the child. Some children want little information, others extensive information. Explanations need to be tailored to the individual child and parent.
   c. Only give choices when choices exist.
3. Prepare the parent.
   a. Most children feel more secure with their parent or parents present. Whenever possible, parents should be present to provide support for their child. Parents should never be pressured to remain with their child during a procedure, if they are not comfortable doing so; they should be allowed to step away.
   b. Parents should be prepared appropriately for what they will see and be given simple instructions for what they should do, such as handholding or talking in a soothing voice. Their role in a procedure is to comfort their child; a parent should not be asked to help restrain the child.
      (1) Encourage parents to
         (a) Talk to their child about what to expect.
         (b) Reassure their child that it is okay to be scared or nervous.
         (c) Praise their child for waiting patiently, holding still during an examination or procedure, talking about their feelings, etc.
         (d) Stay calm. The child will often follow the example set by the parent. Seeing a parent more relaxed may help the child be less nervous.
4. Nonpharmacological techniques are an essential component of managing procedural pain, but this should not preclude the use of appropriate analgesics (see Part 5. Nonpharmacological Pain Management for techniques used in children).
5. If sedation is to be administered for a procedure such as a bone marrow aspirate or biopsy, appropriate monitoring, equipment (pulse oximetry, suction, Ambu bag, supplemental oxygen), and a skilled professional with the ability to maintain a pediatric airway are required. (See Table 20-9 later in the chapter for specific recommendations for lumbar puncture and bone marrow aspiration.)
   a. The goal of procedural sedation is the prevention of pain. A child who is not afraid or not in pain will be more cooperative and more likely able to remain still for an extended period. When using sedation, a desired outcome is a rapid recovery with minimal medication side effects (Schecter et al., 2003).
   b. Summary of care to be provided during procedural sedation (Hertzog & Havidich, 2007; Joint Commission, 2008; Krauss & Green, 2000)
      (1) A plan must be developed for any procedure that involves the administration of procedural sedation and be agreed upon or developed by a licensed independent practitioner with appropriate clinical privileges (Joint Commission, 2008).
      (2) Consultation with specialists, anesthesiology, or both for more complicated cases is recommended (Hertzog & Havidich, 2007).
6. General anesthesia may be an appropriate choice for some children who are young or particularly fearful. General anesthesia may help decrease anxiety with painful procedures, such as bone marrow aspirates and biopsies or lumbar punctures. This method requires an anesthesiologist.
7. All procedures carry risk, but that risk is increased when sedation or anesthesia is administered.

B. Procedures often seen in the pediatric population

In addition to the general concepts above, consider the following:

1. Sucrose has been found to reduce the pain response of premature and young infants up to 6 months of age during immunizations, heel sticks, and nasogastric tube placement (Hatfield, Gusic, Dyer, & Polomano, 2008; McCullough, Halton, Mowbray, & Macfarlan, 2008; Morash & Fowler, 2004).
   a. Administer sucrose via syringe or pacifier (a pacifier may provide the added benefit of non-nutritive sucking) 2 minutes before the procedure (McCullough et al., 2008).
2. Circumcision
   a. Controversy remains whether circumcision is or is not beneficial (American Academy of Pediatrics [AAP], 1999; Geyer et al., 2002). If the decision is made to proceed with circumcision, procedural analgesia should be provided (AAP, 1999). Several interventions are available and are supported by the AAP and ASPMN (see Appendix 20-2).
   b. Oral sucrose is a simple, noninvasive intervention that studies show comforts infants during painful procedures Sucrose on a pacifier should not be used as a sole method of pain control for circumcision.
      (1) Combining sucrose with a dorsal penile nerve block decreases pain behavior in newborns undergoing neonatal circumcision (Geyer et al., 2002).
      (2) One study evaluated sucrose water as an analgesic during routine circumcisions. Control infants who were circumcised without intervention cried 67% of the time; infants who received a water-moistened pacifier cried 49% of the time; and infants who received a sucrose-flavored pacifier to suck cried 31% of the time (Blass & Hoffmeyer, 1991). It is possible that sucrose is effective partly because sucking activity is incompatible with crying behavior.
   c. EMLA®—has historically been shown to decrease cry time and reduce the increase seen in heart rate during circumcisions (AAP, 1999; Benini, Johnston, Faucher, & Aranda, 1993; Lander, Brady-Fryer, Metcalfe, Nazarali, & Muttitt, 1997; Taddio et al., 1997).
      (1) However, subcutaneous ring blocks are more effective (Benini et al., 1993; Lander et al., 1997).
      (2) EMLA® may not add any benefit when used with dorsal penile nerve block (Geyer et al., 2002).
   d. Dorsal penile nerve block is found to be effective for relieving pain experienced with neonatal circumcision when heart rate, pulse oximetry, crying time, and pain scores were used as outcomes. Glucose water was found to be ineffective (Kass & Holman, 2001).
      (1) Dorsal penile nerve block was more effective than LMX™4 at skin lysis using reoccurrence rate as the outcome. Using heart rate as the primary outcome, the sample size was too small to detect statistical significance (Tutag et al., 2005).
   e. Subcutaneous ring block is a simple and highly effective technique for pain control during a circumcision. Subcutaneous ring block was found to be more effective than either EMLA® or dorsal penile nerve block in one study (Geyer et al., 2002; Lander et al., 1997).
      (1) The AAP report states that subcutaneous ring block may provide the best analgesia (AAP, 1999).
   f. Other intervention recommended by Geyer and colleagues (2002) include
      (1) Acetaminophen before and around the clock for 24 hours after circumcision.
      (2) Swaddling and padding the restraint board or chair, which decreases movement and provides warmth and containment.
      (3) A peaceful environment with soft music.
3. Intravenous catheter insertion and venipuncture
   a. Strongly consider use of local anesthetics to decrease the pain associated with needle punctures (see the discussion of local and topical anesthetics under V. Pharmacological Interventions).
   b. Use personnel most skilled in intravenous insertion or venipuncture.
4. Lumbar puncture
   a. Pain experienced from the needle puncture is compounded by the additional distress caused by the body position required for a lumbar puncture. Table 20-9 lists recommendations for lumbar punctures.

5. Bone marrow aspirate and bone marrow biopsy
   a. Performing bone marrow aspirate and bone marrow biopsy without psychological or pharmacological intervention (or both) is not acceptable given the data on pain and distress in children resulting from this procedure.
   b. Psychological intervention, pharmacological management, and general anesthesia should be alternatives offered to children and their parents (Jay, Elliot, Fitzgibbons, Woody, & Siegal, 1995).
   c. Use of only an injection of lidocaine anesthetizes the skin and bone, however, does not affect the intense pain caused by suctioning and biopsying the bone marrow.
   d. Table 20-10 lists recommendations for bone marrow aspirations.

Table 20-9 Lumbar Punctures

Age	Recommendations
0–6 months	1. Perform the procedure on an infant who is warmed appropriately and settled (i.e., not on a crying infant immediately after another procedure). 2. Give local anesthesia using 1% lidocaine. 3. The use of opioids and sedatives in this age group for procedural sedation is difficult. Further studies need to be performed before firm recommendations can be made. If analgesics are deemed necessary, the use of small doses of single medications (not combined with other drugs) should be considered.
6–24 months	1. Preparation: A parent should carry the infant to the treatment room and maintain physical contact during the procedure. The parent can be instructed to talk soothingly to the child and to stroke or rub a part of the child's body. 2. Local anesthetic should be used. Administer 1% lidocaine intradermally and then subcutaneously, and wait 4–5 minutes before insertion of lumbar puncture needle. 3. If sedation and analgesia are deemed necessary, recommendations for pain assessment using behavioral measures are the same as for the age group in Table 20-2. 4. Attach flexible tubing (i.e., T-connector) to spinal needle to enable easier injection of intrathecal medications.
2–5 years	1. Preparation should be included for all children in this age group. In addition to the parent maintaining physical and verbal contact with the child throughout the procedure, the parent can be given specific instruction regarding the use of storytelling, popup books, bubbles, and dolls for distraction during the procedure. The 3- to 5-year-old child also can benefit from preprocedure preparation regarding what to expect. 2. For guidelines regarding the need for sedation, past behavior during other procedures and a rating (0–10 scale) by parents of how cooperative and manageable they expect their child to be should be used. 3. If sedation is used, preparation of midazolam, 0.2–0.4 mg/kg (IV solution) can be given orally 45 minutes before lumbar puncture. 4. Local anesthetic recommendation is same as for the 6- to 24-month age group. 5. If the preceding interventions are unsuccessful, consider deep sedation or general anesthesia under the supervision of an anesthesiologist.
5 years and older	1. Psychological preparation, behavioral intervention, and local anesthesia may be sufficient. 2. Psychological preparation includes giving the child information and a chance to practice the procedure. Behavioral intervention includes distraction methods such as counting, deep breathing, storytelling, and helping the child to engage in an imaginary fantasy based on something with which the child is familiar (e.g., TV show, pets, friends, or past experiences). The use of props (e.g., favorite doll) and parental physical and verbal presence (with specific instructions) should be dictated by the child's age and anxiety level. The adolescent should be given the choice regarding parental presence during the lumbar puncture. 3. If pharmacological intervention is deemed necessary, sedatives alone (with local anesthetic) should suffice.

V. Antagonizing Pain Management

A. Use of naloxone (Narcan®) for full or partial reversal of narcotic

1. For mild somnolence, give 0.001 to 0.01 mg/kg/dose by intravenous push or subcutaneously. Small, incremental doses may make it possible to reverse respiratory depression without reversing analgesia.
2. Postanesthesia opioid reversal in infants and children 0.01 mg/kg/dose may repeat every 2 to 3 minutes as needed based on response (Taketomo et al., 2204).
3. After administration, the child must be observed because the duration of naloxone is much shorter than the opioid duration.
4. For opioid-induced pruritus, nausea and vomiting, a recent double-blind, prospective, randomized, controlled study concludes that naloxone should be given at 0.25 μg/kg/hr (continuous infusion) (Maxwell et al., 2005).
5. Naloxone can precipitate withdrawal when given to children who are physically opioid dependent.

B. Use of flumazenil (Romazicon®) for reversal of benzodiazepines

1. The suggested dose is based on adult data. Flumazenil is not approved by the FDA for children. Give 0.01 or 0.02 mg/kg (maximum dose 0.2 mg) with repeat doses of 0.01 mg/kg (maximum dose 0.2 mg) every 5 minutes. The suggested maximum total dose is 1 mg (Deshpande & Anand, 1996).
2. After administration, the child must be observed because the duration of flumazenil is shorter than that of most benzodiazepines.
3. The manufacturer states the use of flumazenil has been associated with the occurrence of seizures. Seizures have been seen most often in patients with long-term benzodiazepine use or in overdose cases in which patients are showing signs of cyclic antidepressant overdose (Thomson PDR, 2007).

VI. Regional Analgesia Techniques

A. Regional analgesia techniques provide superior analgesia compared to systemic opioids (Liu & Wu, 2007).

B. Epidural analgesia (for additional information, see the chapter on Acute Pain Management)

1. Delivery of analgesic solution is typically a local anesthetic, opioid, or both into the epidural space. Occasionally Clonidine, an α_2-agonist, may be added to supplement analgesia. Epidural analgesia can be delivered by continuous infusion with an indwelling catheter or as a single injection. An anesthesiologist with expertise in pediatric regional anesthesia should be consulted if anesthetic techniques are being considered for a pediatric patient.
2. Continuous epidural analgesia is useful in children who are undergoing extensive abdominal surgical procedures, extensive lower extremity surgeries (including amputations), and thoracic procedures. Epidural analgesia may also provide profound relief for patients with cancer, sickle cell disease with lower extremity pain, pancreatitis, and complex regional pain syndrome (CRPS). Sucato, Duey-Holtz, Elerson, and Safavi (2005) reported that continuous epidural infusion in children provided significantly decreased pain scores, less fluctuation in pain, and lower maximum pain levels during the postoperative period after surgery for treatment of adolescent idiopathic scoliosis.
3. Patient-controlled epidural analgesia may be considered based on the developmental age of the child (Birmingham et al., 2003).
4. In infants and small children, the caudal space may be more accessible than lumbar or thoracic spaces. Introduction of a caudal catheter has a decreased risk of lumbar puncture or spinal cord trauma than a catheter placed in the thoracic area (Bubeck, Boos, Krause, & Thies, 2004; Seefelder, 2002).
   a. Caudal catheters may be advanced to a lumbar or thoracic level as needed. Confirmation of appropriate catheter tip placement with radiological technique is recommended.
   b. Single-shot caudal injections are appropriate for patient undergoing urological, general, and orthopedic surgery involving the lower abdomen and limbs. Single-shot caudals provide limited dermatomal distribution and short duration of analgesia (Tsui & Berde, 2005).

Table 20-10 Bone Marrow Aspirations*

Age	Recommendations
0–6 months	I. Perform the procedure on an infant who is warmed appropriately and settled (i.e., not on a crying infant immediately after another procedure). II. Use local anesthesia with 1% lidocaine. III. Use a lumbar puncture needle. IV. The use of opioids and sedatives in this age group for procedural sedation is difficult. Further studies need to be performed before firm recommendations can be made. If analgesics are deemed necessary, the use of small doses of single medications (not combined with other drugs) should be considered.
6–24 months	I. Preparation: The parent should carry the infant to the treatment room and maintain physical and eye contact during the procedure. The parent can be instructed to talk soothingly to child and to stroke or rub a part of the child's body. II. Establish IV access if an IV line is not already present. III. To provide adequate pain control, either general anesthesia or sedation using sedatives, opioids, and local anesthesia is necessary. A. Sedatives 1. Give midazolam, 0.2–0.4 mg/kg maximum to 15 mg (IV solution) orally, 30–45 minutes or 0.05 mg/kg intravenously 3 minutes before the procedure, or 2. Give diazepam, 0.2–0.3 mg/kg maximum of 10 mg orally, 45–60 minutes before the procedure (diazepam burns when given by an IV route). B. Opioids 1. Use IV morphine sulfate, 0.05–0.1 mg/kg over 1–2 minutes, given 5 minutes before the procedure (skin can be cleansed, draped during this time), or 2. Use IV fentanyl, 1–2 μg/kg, 3 minutes before procedure, or 3. Use IV meperidine (if morphine sulfate or fentanyl is not available), 0.5–1 mg/kg for 1–2 minutes, given 2–5 minutes before the procedure. 4. With the above preceding opioids, half of original dose can be repeated if the child does not appear adequately comfortable during the local anesthetic needle. C. Local anesthetics: 1% lidocaine is given slowly intradermally and then slowly subcutaneously to the periosteum. Wait 4–5 minutes. IV. After the procedure, the child should be placed on his or her side, observed, and discharged when fully conscious (see American Academy of Pediatrics guidelines); a nurse should monitor the child until he or she can be easily aroused. Oxygen saturation monitoring should be continued during the recovery period. Supplemental oxygen should be administered if the oxygen saturation is less than 95%. V. General anesthesia should be considered if procedural sedation efforts are inadequate.
2–5 years	I. Environment or psychological preparation A. See "6–24 months" regarding parent's physical presence. B. Preparation: Play preparation and practice with models, stuffed animals, and dolls can be used to let child know what to expect and what is expected of him or her. The child life worker, parent, or nurse can do this for many children with proper instruction.

	C. Enhance coping skills. Concrete objects are needed for distraction: popup books, bubbles, toys, or dolls. Children can use imagination (especially those 4–5 years old) to supplement the physical distractions. II. Suggest pharmacological measures for all BMAs and use of psychological measures as adjuncts. III. Use recommendations discussed earlier (6 months to 2 years) for pharmacological intervention. General anesthesia should be considered if psychological measures and attempts at procedural sedation fail.
5–12 years	I. First BMA: Use IV sedation and analgesia or general anesthesia. The doses recommended for sedatives and analgesics are mentioned earlier. With children entering adolescence, the lowest recommended dose should be used as the starting dose. Supplemental doses, if necessary, that titrate to effect are encouraged. II. Subsequent BMAs: An attempt should be made to individualize the treatment approach for each child. Some children will benefit from behavioral intervention alone (with local anesthetic), while others will require continued pharmacological support. III. If an oral sedative has not been given but sedation becomes necessary just before the procedure, the following can be administered intravenously: A. Midazolam, 0.05 mg/kg 3–4 minutes before BMA; repeat if necessary ∞ 2 B. Diazepam, 0.1 mg/kg 3–5 minutes before BMA (only give intravenously if there is a central line); repeat if necessary ∞2 C. Pentobarbital, 2 mg/kg (a maximum of 100 mg) 5–10 minutes before BMA
Adolescents (>12 years or pubertal)	I. Treat adolescents the same as school-age children, but the sedation and analgesia maximal doses should be limited to the following: A. Benzodiazepine 1. Diazepam, oral 10 mg, IV 5 mg; half-dose can be repeated 2. Midazolam, IV 0.5 mg every 3–4 minutes until effect achieved 3. Triazolam, 0.25-mg tablet orally B. Opioids 1. Morphine sulfate, IV 3–4 mg; repeat in 5 minutes if necessary 2. Fentanyl, IV 25–50 μg (0.5–1 ml or 50 μg/ml solution); full dose can be repeated in 5 minutes if necessary, and if needed, repeat four to five times with 25 μg at 5-minute intervals 3. Meperidine, IV 40 mg repeated one to two times at 5-minute intervals C. Barbiturates, IV 100 mg pentobarbital (Nembutal) or same dose orally if planning BMA with other procedures and need prolonged sedation II. Encourage more participation by the adolescent in the decision-making process regarding how to best manage pain during procedures and to provide an opportunity to learn behavioral procedures, including rehearsal.

BMA, bone marrow aspiration; IV, intravenous.

*The protocol also applies to other invasive procedures, such as Broviac catheter removal, incision, and drainage.

5. Medications that are commonly used in epidural analgesia in pediatrics include bupivacaine and ropivacaine. Ropivacaine causes less risk of cardiac toxicity and fewer cardiac changes than bupivacaine (Ecoffey, 2007). Ropivacaine at low concentrations may produce less motor block and allow patients to maintain more motor function than bupivacaine. Dosage guidelines for continuous infusion of local anesthetic are 0.2 mg/kg/hr for neonates and up to 0.4 mg/kg/hr in infants and children (Bosenberg, 2004).

C. Patient care and monitoring
1. Close monitoring with a cardiac-apnea monitor and pulse oximetry is important but does not replace regular assessment of the patient by a nurse.
2. Dermatome levels should be assessed on patients developmentally capable of providing the information (Pasero, Eksterowicz, Primeau, & Crowley, 2007). Dermatome levels of infants and toddlers cannot be reliably assessed. Instead, infants and toddlers should be assessed for abnormal vital signs, irritability (from pain or possible local anesthetic toxicity), and the ability to move all extremities (if appropriate).
3. Upon discontinuation of the epidural catheter, ensure that appropriate analgesics are ordered to maintain adequate pain control.

VII. Peripheral Nerve Blocks (for additional information see chapter on Acute Pain Management)

A. Local anesthetic solution is delivered to a peripheral nerve sheath. The target is the nerve or nerves that control pain to a specific region of the body. Peripheral nerve blocks provide analgesia to an extremity. Some common sites are infraclavicular for distal arm procedures, interscalene for shoulder procedures, femoral for lower extremity, sciatic for procedures involving the foot, and lumbar plexus for hip and lower extremity. The benefit is analgesia to the affected region without many of the unwanted side effects seen with opioid use (Evans, Steele, Nielsen, & Tucker, 2005).
1. Peripheral nerve blocks can be done as a single dose. A significant disadvantage of a single dose without catheter placement is that the duration of the pain often outlasts the block.
2. Peripheral nerve catheters can be placed to provide continuous analgesia for a set period, typically 2 days for postoperative pain. Catheters left in place greater than 2 days may be an independent risk factor for catheter colonization and local inflammation (Capdevila et al., 2005).
3. Additional systemic analgesia is often not required unless the surgical procedure is outside the distribution of the nerves.
4. Medications, either ropivacaine or bupivacaine, in varying concentrations and volumes depending on anesthesiologist preference and institutions protocols.

B. Patient care and monitoring
1. Do not use disinfectants on any tubing connections as nerves can be injured.
2. Protect the insensate extremity by preventing pressure or thermal injury (i.e., do not apply cold to the area affected by the nerve block; frostbite can occur).
3. Avoid placing any tension on the catheter itself to prevent catheter dislodgement.
4. Inspect the catheter entry site for any signs of infection.
5. Assess motor function.

C. Home management
1. Pediatric patients may be candidates for home management if their surgical procedure warrants and the patient or family have the cognitive ability to learn care of the catheter, appropriate monitoring, and emergency procedures (Ganesh et al., 2007).
2. Written home instructions must be provided, including signs of local anesthetic toxicity.
3 Support staff must be available 24 hours a day to answer any questions that arise. Daily follow-up telephone contact is necessary. a home care visit by a registered nurse familiar with peripheral nerve catheters is ideal (Ganesh et al., 2007). Whether caregivers should be responsible for catheter removal is an individual institution decision.

PART THREE: PEDIATRIC CANCER PAIN

I. Introduction

A. The comprehensive care of children with cancer includes curative therapies such as surgery, radiation, and chemotherapy and the treatment of symptoms and pain management.

B. Knowledge of the natural history and treatment of pediatric malignancies is beneficial to manage pediatric cancer pain effectively.

C. Greater than 75% of children diagnosed with cancer will achieve 5-year survival (American Cancer Society, 2007). All children with cancer are affected by pain at some point during their diagnosis or treatment.

D. Leukemias and lymphomas are the most common type of pediatric cancer in the United States (34%), followed by tumors of the central nervous system (Bleyer, 1990).

E. Major barriers to effective pain treatment in pediatric oncology patients are inadequate pain assessment and patient and family hesitancy to report the presence or increase of pain (Jacob, McCarthy, Sambuco, & Hockenberry, 2008).

F. In addition to the challenges faced by any patient with cancer, children's and adolescent's normal growth and development are affected. Hospitalization separates them from their peers, and peer interaction is vital to their social development (Kline, 2004).

II. Causes of Pediatric Cancer Pain

A. Cancer-related pain
   1. Cancer-related pain can be predicted by knowledge of natural history of tumor.
   2. It can be acute or chronic.
   3. Bone pain can be widespread or localized. In leukemia, a common presenting symptom is diffuse back or bilateral leg pain, but with a primary bone tumor the pain can be localized to one area.
   4. Tumor pain can result from central nervous system involvement.
      a. Headache can result from increased intracranial pressure from central nervous system leukemia, primary brain tumor, or brain metastases from a solid tumor.
      b. Back pain from spinal cord compression may be localized, radiating, or referred to a corresponding sensory dermatome.
      c. Pain of soft tissue or organ invasion is possible.
      d. Pain can be related to compression of a neural plexus or peripheral nerve (less common).

B. Procedure-related cancer pain (see Part Two. Pediatric Acute Pain for additional information)
   1. Procedure-related pain is experienced by all children with cancer. Many procedures must be repeated at frequent intervals. If procedural pain is managed poorly, distress and pain tend to intensify with subsequent procedures (Weisman, Bernstein, & Schecter, 1998; WHO, 1998). It is important to provide optimal pain relief with the first procedure.
   2. Many children find procedural pain more painful and distressing than the underlying malignancy (Miser & Miser, 1989). The younger the children, the more present-oriented they are; they tend to be more fearful of the procedure than the disease itself.
   3. In contrast to adults, most pain is treatment related rather than cancer related for the following reasons.
      a. There are an increased number of hematological cancers in children versus solid tumors in adults (Chapman & Foley, 1993; WHO, 1998).
      b. Pediatric cancers are highly responsive to initial therapies. Typically, an initial complete remission follows induction chemotherapy in most pediatric cancers; therapy-related pain is the major cause of pain once initial tumor control has been achieved (Chapman & Foley, 1993; Elliot et al., 1991).
   4. A child with cancer undergoes innumerable procedures. The most often experienced procedure-related pain is a result of needle punctures. The pain experienced from venipuncture, accessing an

implanted venous access device, lumbar puncture, bone marrow aspiration, and biopsy is a significant problem. Using a combination of pharmacological measures, cognitive-behavioral techniques, and developmentally supportive care is the best approach (Zempsky, 2008).

a. Centers caring for pediatric oncology patients should develop an algorithm with pain management techniques for bone marrow aspiration and biopsy to insure that the appropriate modality is selected for the individual child (Schecter et al., 2003).
b. There is also the possibility of postlumbar puncture headache (rare).

C. Cancer therapy–related pain

1. Cancer therapy–related pain is predicted by anticancer therapy used for particular tumor type. Precise knowledge of the anticancer regimen is extremely beneficial in the management of this type of pain.
   a. Therapy-related pain includes postoperative pain, mucositis from radiation or after administration of many chemotherapy agents, phantom limb pain, infection such as perirectal cellulitis, and typhlitis (inflammation in many areas of the colon) (Schecter et al., 2003). In addition, radiation-induced dermatitis and other forms of local inflammation cause aching or diffuse abdominal pain from generalized sepsis, graft-versus-host disease, gastrointestinal distress, gastritis, corticosteroid-induced bone changes (especially spine and femoral heads) (APS, 2005), drug-induced neuropathy or joint pain, phantom limb pain, and drug extravasation.
   b. Management of postoperative pain in a child with cancer is similar to management of surgical pain for a child without cancer (see Part Two. Pediatric Acute Pain). Children who have required opioids preoperatively typically require their usual medication in addition to standard postoperative pain medications.
2. Pain-related side effects of specific antineoplastic agents include the following:
   a. Colony-stimulating factors: aches and pain in the bones or muscles (Kline, 2004)
   b. Cytosine: flulike symptoms (aches)
   c. Dacarbazine: flulike symptoms (aches)
   d. Fluorouracil: tingling hands and feet
   e. L-Asparaginase: joint pain and drowsiness
   f. Leucovorin: localized pain at injection (Schecter et al., 2003)
   g. Mesna: abdominal pain (Kline, 2004)
   h. Methotrexate: headache (no NSAIDs within 72 hours of methotrexate; NSAIDs increase methotrexate toxicity by elevating serum methotrexate levels)
   i. Methylprednisolone, prednisone, and prednisolone: fractures with long-term use
   j. Procarbazine: headache and flulike symptoms (muscle and joint aches) (Kline, 2004)
   k. Retinoic acid or isotretinoin: headache
   l. Paclitaxel: muscle and joint pain and numbness and tingling of hands and feet (Kline, 2004; Ozdogan et al., 2004)
   m. Thiotepa: localized pain at injection (Schecter et al., 2003)
   n. Vinblastine: abdominal pain and nerve irritation causing tingling and numbness in hands or feet; rarely bone pain (Kline, 2004)
   o. Vincristine: abdominal pain, jaw pain, and nerve irritation causing numbness and tingling of fingers and toes (Kline, 2004; Ozdogan et al., 2004). Usually self-limiting condition

D. Other causes unrelated to cancer or its treatment

1. Children with cancer can be affected by common childhood illness and trauma similar to any other child.

III. Assessment of Pain (see Part One: Pediatric Pain Assessment and Measurement for further pediatric assessment issues)

A. Cause

1. Relieve pain as quickly as possible while complete evaluation is ongoing.
2. Classify as procedure related, cancer related, therapy related, or other cause.

B. Location
   1. Ask the child where it hurts using age-appropriate language.
   2. Exercise caution, realizing the possibility of radiating or referred pain. Consider using a body diagram.
C. Pain quality and intensity
   1. When having difficulty ascertaining the intensity of child's pain, compare current pain with a previous painful experience (e.g., laceration) to obtain potentially valuable information (Schecter et al., 1993).
   2. It may be difficult to obtain pain scores because of the severity of illness or fatigue (APS, 2005).
   3. A child with cancer may regress similar to any other acutely or chronically ill child. Use developmentally appropriate pain scoring tool.
   4. Intensity of pain is a possible indicator of what is occurring in the disease.
   5. If a child is unable to self-report pain, the child must be observed for behavioral signs of pain.
   6. Always question parents about their child's pain because they know their child best and can pick up on subtle clues.
D. Anticipated course and duration of pain based on primary cause
   1. Consider pain from a newly diagnosed tumor responsive to therapy versus pain from a therapy-resistant tumor.
E. Consider the child's response to previous pain medications and doses.
F. Assess for presence of opioid side effects. Children may not volunteer all side effects (e.g., constipation). Children may be embarrassed or fearful of what may be done as a result of information they may offer
G. Consider available routes of drug administration. Selecting the appropriate delivery technique is just as important as selecting the appropriate analgesic.
H. Consider the psychological state of the child, including degree of anxiety and depression and ability to sleep. The child can become exhausted from lack of sleep. Consider the need for a sedative or hypnotic at bedtime to assist with normal sleep patterns.
I. Assess the family's response to illness, pain, and stress because it greatly affects the child.
J. Assess the caregiver's ability to sleep. This is particularly important when chemotherapy intensifies (Kline, 2004).
K. Regularly evaluate the effectiveness of the pain interventions and modify the plan as necessary.

IV. Considerations in Selecting the Appropriate Route of Administration (see III. Strategies for Pain Control in Part Two: Pediatric Acute Pain for additional information)

A. *Intramuscular injections are not acceptable for pain relief in a child.* A child is likely to deny pain to avoid an injection. Typically, a long-term venous access device is available for use when initial therapies have begun.
B. Intermittent intravenous administration for rapid control of moderate-to-severe pain or management of rapidly changing pain. If pain is constant, continuous infusion may provide better pain relief.
C. PCA
   1. PCA is widely used successfully for children 7 years old or older with normal cognitive development.
   2. Some oncology patients 4 to 6 years old become medically sophisticated during their treatments and can use PCA successfully (Pizzo & Poplack, 1997).
   3. PCA is an ideal delivery technique to help control pain exacerbation. PCA option can enable children with oropharyngeal mucositis to time opioid use with routine mouth care and other periods of increased mouth pain (Mackie, Coda, & Hill, 1991) (Table 20-11). Other agents can be used as adjunctive treatment for mucositis.
   4. Use PCA with basal or continuous infusion to avoid continual awakening during the night.
D. AACA is more controversial (see the chapter on Taxonomy for Pain Management Nursing). The inherent safety of PCA is that the child must be awake enough to push the button. There are case reports of respiratory depression because of parents' pushing the PCA button for opioid-naïve patients (Pizzo & Poplack, 1997). Experience demonstrates AACA can be employed safely in pediatric oncology patients with appropriate education (see Part Two. Pediatric Acute Pain for information on AACA).

Table 20-11 Agents Used in the Treatment of Mucositis

Agent	Mechanism or Therapeutic Effect
Lip balm	Prevents cracking and bleeding of dried lips.
Toothbrush	Removes loose debris. Limit use with thrombocytopenia.
Toothette	Similar to the effect of a toothbrush but with less chance of trauma.
Normal saline rinse	Removes debris.
Sodium bicarbonate	Neutralizes intraoral pH. Loosens debris.
Chlorhexidine rinse	Potent antibacterial action. Decreases secondary infection of abraded mucosa.
Nystatin rinse	Treats secondary candidal infections.
Hydrogen peroxide	Not recommended. Delays healing by breakdown of proteins.
Mylanta	Increases oral pH. Coating action protects mucosa.
Sucralfate suspension	Increases oral pH. Coating action protects mucosa.
Commercial mouthwash	Not recommended. High alcohol content can be painful.
Benadryl elixir	Topical anesthetic action.
Viscous lidocaine	Topical anesthetic action. Repeated doses can lead to toxicity.
Dyclonine mouth wash	Topical anesthetic action. Repeated doses can lead to toxicity.
Oral capsaicin lozenges	Inhibits nociceptive activity of free nerve endings, perhaps related blockade of substance P release.

From Deshpande, J. K., & Tobias, J. (1996). *The pediatric pain handbook* (p. 171). St. Louis: Mosby. Copyright 1996 by Mosby.

E. Subcutaneous opioid infusion
   1. Use a 27-gauge needle placed under the skin in the thorax, abdomen, or thigh with attached microbore (thin, low volume) tubing; the site is changed every 3 to 5 days or longer. Generally, rates should not exceed 1 to 3 ml/hr (Pizzo & Poplack, 1997).
   2. Hydromorphone is a good choice when a potent, highly concentrated agent is needed to minimize fluid volumes because it can be prepared in concentrations of 50 mg/ml (Pizzo & Poplack, 1997).

F. Transdermal administration of medication (e.g., fentanyl) should not be used for patients with rapidly changing pain intensity (see Part Two. Pediatric Acute Pain for additional information).

G. Enteral administration of medication
   1. Assess the child's ability to tolerate oral medications, including the presence of mucositis, vomiting, impaired gastrointestinal tract absorption, or extreme lethargy that would place the child at risk for aspiration. Some younger children may refuse oral medications.

H. Rectal administration
   1. Rectal administration is contraindicated in child who is thrombocytopenic or immunosuppressed secondary to risk of perirectal abcess.
   2. It is not appropriate if rapid relief is required unless unable to obtain intravenous access.

V. Pharmacological Interventions

A. Major pain management modalities are
   1. Anticancer therapy (e.g., chemotherapy, radiation, and surgery).
   2. Analgesic medications. Pain medications are based on the child's weight, the child's age, and the severity of pain. For a detailed discussion of analgesic medications, see Part Two. Pediatric Acute Pain.

B. Classes of medication
   1. The following information is limited to information of significance for pediatric cancer pain. Pain medication selection for children with cancer is based on the WHO analgesic ladder. For a full discussion of medications and pediatric dosages, see II Pharmacological Interventions in Part 2 Pediatric Acute Pain.

2. NSAIDs (see the chapter on Overview of Pharmacology for further information).
   a. NSAIDs often contraindicated in oncology patients at risk for bleeding because of thrombocytopenia.
   b. Choline magnesium trisalicylate, 10 to 15 mg/kg orally every 8 to 12 hours, is a potential alternative, although, similar to aspirin, it is associated with Reye syndrome. Although it has been shown to have minimal effect on platelet function, its use is not recommended in children at risk for bleeding (WHO, 1998).
   c. Caution parents to report fever even when the fever is responsive to an NSAID; there is risk of infection in an immunocompromised patient.
3. Adjuvant drugs
   a. Tricyclic antidepressants
      (1) Use tricyclic antidepressants for phantom limb, peripheral neuropathy, radiation-induced nerve injury, or pain secondary to tumor-associated nerve damage.
      (2) Tricyclic antidepressants should be used with caution in children who have received doxorubicin because of cardiac side effects. An initial electrocardiogram should be done; follow-up monitoring is warranted.
   b. Anticonvulsants
      (1) Use anticonvulsants for chronic or neuropathic pain.
      (2) Most commonly used are carbamazepine and gabapentin. Monitor serum levels when using carbamazepine or to avoid toxicity, risk of bone marrow suppression, and alteration in liver function.
      (3) Use of anticonvulsants may not be appropriate for patients with compromised bone marrow function or for children receiving myelosuppressive chemotherapy.
   c. Corticosteroids
      (1) Use corticosteroids for spinal cord compression, cerebral edema, secondary tumor, or bone metastases.
      (2) Dosage is case specific. The optimal dose for various indications has not been studied sufficiently.
      (3) Dexamethasone is the steroid of choice because of its superior cerebrospinal fluid penetration (Balis, Lester, Chraisos, Heideman, & Poplack, 1987).
4. Topical anesthetics
   a. See Part Two: Pediatric Acute Pain for information on topical local anesthetics for needle puncture procedures.
   b. Viscous lidocaine
      (1) Mouthwashes containing viscous lidocaine or dyclonine should be used sparingly in children with mucositis because of rapid absorption through excoriated oral mucosa. This rapid absorption can result in an increased risk of systemic toxicity in the pediatric patient. Note recommended dosing guidelines based on the patient's weight. Consider once-per-day dosing perhaps at bedtime; maximum use is three or four times a day.
5. Anesthetic techniques (see VI. Pediatric Regional Analgesia Techniques for information)
   a. Epidural administration of a local anesthetic with or without an opioid can be beneficial for postoperative pain or for a child with continued localized pain below the nipple line not obtaining adequate pain relief from systemic opioids and adjuvants.
   b. Peripheral nerve blocks are rarely used in pediatric oncology because childhood cancers typically are not limited to one particular area (WHO, 1998).
6. Sleep aids
   a. Adequate sleep is essential. Caffeinated beverages and other stimulants (including medications) should be avoided whenever possible. Nonpharmacological methods should be tried, such as creating a nightly sleep ritual.
   b. Diphenhydramine hydrochloride (*FDA warning:* Do not use for patients under 4 years of age)
      (1) Dosage for children 4 to 11 years old is 1 mg/kg, with a maximum 50-mg dose. Dosage for children 12 years and older is 50 mg. Give 30 minutes before bedtime (Taketomo et al., 2007).

VI. Nonpharmacological Interventions (see Part FIVE. Nonpharmacological Pain Management for information)

A. Behavioral, cognitive, and supportive techniques can help reduce pain. Nonpharmacological interventions should not replace appropriate pharmacological treatment (APS, 2005).

PART FOUR: PEDIATRIC CHRONIC PAIN

I. Introduction

A. Chronic pain is typically defined as pain that continues for more than 3 to 6 months. It may be continuous or intermittent.

B. The pain can be a symptom of an illness or disease process or may exist without a cause.

C. Because chronic pain does not have a single cause, treatment strategies vary widely from nonpharmacological approaches to simple analgesics to opioids (American Academy of Pain Medicine & American Pain Society, 1997).

D. Chronic pain significantly affects the quality of life not only for the child with pain but also for the entire family (Logan, Guite, Sherry, & Rose, 2006). Depression and anxiety often accompany chronic pain and may lead to dysfunction and social isolation (Kashikar-Zuck, Goldschneider, Powers, Vaught, & Hershey, 2001).

E. Parents often have feelings of guilt that their child is experiencing chronic pain. This may lead to doctor-shopping. Pain often challenges their ability as parents because they are unable to solve the problem. Parents and children should be given an explanation so that they can understand the context of pain and realize that the pain is not signaling there is an injury in chronic nonmalignant pain. Parents must be encouraged to maintain boundaries and limits on child behaviors to avoid dysfunction and slipping into the sick role.

II. Pain Diagnoses

A. Postherpetic neuralgia

1. Postherpetic neuralgia typically is defined as pain that persists beyond 1 month after the onset of zoster or pain that persists after the skin lesions have crusted over. The pain is described as a constant aching and burning with intermittent sharp shooting pains. The pain is neuropathic.
2. Herpes zoster is seen mainly in children who are immunodeficient. Most children do not experience postherpetic neuralgia.
3. No treatment of herpes zoster prevents postherpetic neuralgia with certainty, but some may reduce its likelihood (Kost & Straus, 1996). The lack of predictable effective treatment for the pain of postherpetic neuralgia has resulted in the focus on prevention of postherpetic neuralgia.
   a. Acyclovir therapy during herpes zoster reduces the risk of postherpetic neuralgia. It is recommended that acyclovir administration begin within 72 hours of the rash appearance to decrease the acute pain associated with zoster most effectively (Kost & Straus, 1996).
   b. Treatment seems to be more effective when started early in the course of the disease.
   c. A lidocaine 5% topical patch is approved by the FDA for the treatment of postherpetic neuralgia (Taketomo et al., 2007).
   d. Tricyclic antidepressants, amitriptyline the most commonly studied, and membrane stabilizers, such as gabapentin, can be used to help manage the pain of postherpetic neuralgia (Wu & Raja, 2008).

B. Juvenile rheumatoid arthritis

1. Subtypes are systemic, polyarticular (involvement of five or more joints), and pauciarticular (involvement of four or fewer joints) juvenile rheumatoid arthritis. The severity of pain varies according to the subtype of juvenile rheumatoid arthritis and the individual patient.
2. Treatment is focused on reducing inflammation and pain.
   a. NSAIDs given to reduce inflammation and relieve pain are first-line therapy and are sufficient therapy for most children (DeWitt, Sherry, & Cron, 2005; Groh, 2003).

   b. When NSAIDs fail, disease-modifying antirheumatic drugs, glucocorticoids, biological agents, hydroxychloroquine, oral and injectable gold, D-penicillamine, and methotrexate can be initiated to help control the disease. These treatments are limited by their potential toxic side effects (Groh, 2003; Guthrie, Rouster-Stevens, & Reynolds, 2007).
   c. Physical and occupational therapy is important to assist in maintaining functionality of affected joints (Cakmak & Bolukbas, 2004). Physical therapy regimen may include aquatic exercises, positioning, passive range of motion exercises and isometric exercises. Heat, cold, and massage may also be beneficial.
   d. The child should remain in school as much as possible with appropriate accommodations to maintain attendance. These accommodations may include having two sets of textbooks so that the child does not need to carry heavy loads and allowing the child to leave the classroom early.
   e. Cognitive-behavioral treatments such as guided imagery and other relaxation techniques have been shown to reduce the subjective pain experience and to improve functioning and are an effective adjunct to pharmacological interventions (Walco, Varni, & Ilowite, 1992).

C. Complex regional pain syndrome (CRPS)
   1. CRPS Type I (previously known as reflex sympathetic dystrophy) occurs without a definable nerve lesion.
   2. CRPS Type II (previously known as causalgia) occurs with a definable nerve lesion.
   3. In children and adolescents, CRPS-I has a male-to-female ratio of 1:4. It is uncommon for CRPS-I to be seen in children younger than 9 years old. Its presentation differs from adults in that it occurs more often in the lower extremities and there are fewer dystrophic changes, although color changes are common (Olsson, 1999). CRPS-I occurs more often in the lower extremity than the upper, with a higher incidence in the Caucasian population (Low, Ward, & Wines, 2007; Wilder, 2006).
   4. CRPS-II is much less common in children. Low et al. (2007) reviewed medical records of children diagnosed with CRPS in one pain clinic over a 4-year period. Twenty patients were diagnosed with CRPS-I, and no patients were diagnosed with CRPS-II. Wilder (2006) stated that CRPS-II occurs equally as often in boys and girls.
   5. The syndrome often affects children and adolescents who place high demands on themselves (Olsson, 1999; Wilder et al., 1992). Stress and anxiety magnify the severity of the pain symptoms and affect the child's and family's ability to cope with the pain.
   6. It is important to explain to the child and parents that the pain is not an indication that something is *wrong;* rather, there is a problem with the pain signal transmission. This may be difficult if the child and family have not begun to trust the health care provider because this is an abstract concept.
   7. Participation in physical therapy is the mainstay of treatment for CRPS. With persuasion, reassurance and provision of adequate analgesia, children may show a greater willingness to actively participate in physical therapy (Sherry, Wallas, Kelley, Kidder, & Sapp, 1999; Wilder, 2006).
      a. Physical therapy can include desensitization, use of heat, whirlpools, transcutaneous electrical nerve stimulation (TENS), passive range of motion, and exercise. Wilder and colleagues (1992) reported that out of 70 children and adolescents, two-thirds judged physical therapy to be helpful in regaining function and reducing pain. This was true even though there was a transient initial increase in pain with therapy. Sherry et al. (1999) reported that intense physical therapy provided increased function.
   8. Conservative treatments, such as medication, TENS, cognitive-behavioral pain management techniques, and psychological intervention, are intended to minimize the pain to enable physical therapy.
   9. Medications that act on central transmission of pain are recommended. These include tricyclic antidepressants, NMDA blockers, α_2-agonists (e.g., clonidine), local anesthetics, and anticonvulsants (e.g., gabapentin).
      a. Tricyclic antidepressants probably are the most commonly administered drugs. Newer, more selective serotonin reuptake inhibitors have not proved to be of value (Olsson, 1999; Rowbotham & Macintyre, 2003).

   b. Harden (2005) reports that anticonvulsants are often used in the treatment of CRPS. The pharmacological action of gabapentin is not clear, however it is thought to enhance the endogenous γ-aminobutyric acid (GABA) system, altering pain modulation. Other anticonvulsants may be effective, but limited studies exist.

10. Invasive techniques, such as sympathetic blockade with local anesthetic, can be used in some patients who fail conservative therapy. Children who require invasive techniques require either sedation or general anesthesia for regional blocks (Tanelian, 1996).
    a. Sympathetic nerve blocks should not be used as a sole treatment but rather as a means to an end. Blocks can provide a period of analgesia during which physical therapy can be done (Harden, 2005; Wilder, 1996).
    b. Continuous lumbar epidural infusion may be preferred over single injections for pediatric patients. Potential benefits include a mandated hospitalization due to the presence of an epidural catheter, thereby allowing for more intense physical therapy and psychological support. Disadvantages include motor block, sensory block, or both that may limit participation in physical therapy sessions (Wilder, 2006). Removing the child from the home environment may or may not be beneficial.
    c. Single-shot blocks require the same anesthetic or sedation as an indwelling catheter but do not limit the patient's ability to participate fully in physical therapy due to preservation of muscle strength and maintenance of sensation (Berde, Sethna, & Micheli, 1988). Single injections may need to be repeated but are done as on an outpatient basis.
    d. Rarely, clonidine has been used epidurally for refractory cases of CRPS-I. A study by Rauck, Eisenach, Jackson, Young, and Southern (1993) showed a decrease in visual analogue scores for patients receiving epidural clonidine, although no assessment of extremity function was done. Other mediations, including nifedipine, bisphosphonates, and α-adrenergic antagonists, may be found to be effective, but more studies are needed (Harden, 2005).
11. NSAIDs may not provide complete relief but can be used to help decrease the intensity of the pain. The use of opioids to treat CRPS is controversial and rarely provides relief of pain symptoms. Opioids may be necessary short term while further interventions, such as physical therapy are initiated (Rowbotham & Macintyre, 2003; Stanton-Hicks et al., 1998).
12. The use of oral steroids has also been found to be useful in some patients, but more study is needed (Stanton-Hicks et al., 1998).
13. Surgical or chemical sympathectomy is rarely used in children and adolescents.
14. It remains uncertain whether early intervention can alter the course of CRPS-I (Tanelian, 1996).
15. Drug therapy is often necessary to overcome road blocks and continue to gain function with physical therapy (Harden, 2005; Wilder, 2006).
16. Olsson (1999) found, after evaluating the first 70 patients with CRPS-I, that the average child missed more than 40 days from a 180-day school year. Only 5 days on average were missed because of pain after treatment was begun (Wilder, 1996). Return to school or preventing school absenteeism should be a primary goal of treatment and a measurement of functionality. Home-bound tutoring is not an acceptable alternative to school attendance and offers only a short-term solution.
17. Psychological support and cognitive-behavioral therapy can help children and adolescents to develop coping strategies to deal not only with pain but also with other stressful situations in their lives.
    a. Due to the function-limiting symptoms of CRPS, there is a great deal of stress placed on the entire family. Individual psychological therapy and family therapy can be beneficial in some cases.
    b. It is important to obtain "buy in" from the caregivers, as well as the patient, to progress toward functionality.
    c. Encourage patients to trial biofeedback and guided imagery to cope with flare episodes.
    d. Cognitive-behavioral therapy was provided to 28 children, and frequency of physical therapy was randomized to once a week or three times a week. Function and pain relief were sustained in both groups (Lee et al., 2002).

e. The reoccurrence rate of CRPS in children is remarkably higher than in the adult population; however, the reoccurrence commonly responds well to physical therapy and treatment (Lee et al., 2002).
f. Because of the complexity of CRPS-I, a multidisciplinary team approach provides the best possible outcome (Harden, 2005).

D. Phantom pain
1. Phantom sensation and phantom pain occur often after amputation in children and adolescents. Onset typically is within the first week postoperatively.
2. The overall incidence of phantom sensation and phantom pain is higher for children who require an amputation as a result of trauma or infection compared with children having an amputation as the result of a congenital limb deformity.
   a. Wilkins, McGrath, Finley, and Katz (1998) retrospectively reported the presence of phantom sensation as 7% for children with a congenital limb deformity requiring amputation compared with 69% for children who required amputation after trauma. The prevalence for phantom pain was lower for the congenital group (4%) compared with the trauma group (49%).
   b. A retrospective study by Krane and Heller (1995) noted 100% of children requiring amputation as a result of cancer, trauma or infection, or congenital deformity reported phantom sensation. The overall incidence of phantom pain was 92%.
3. Some studies note the duration, not the intensity, of the pain is an indicator for the incidence of phantom pain. Phantom pain is lower for patients with pain of short duration before amputation and in patients who do not have pain in the limb before amputation (Bach, Noreng, & Tjellden, 1988; Krane & Heller, 1995).
   a. A prospective study demonstrated that the best indicator for phantom limb pain at 6 months and 1 year is acute phantom limb pain intensity soon after amputation, and preamputation pain not pain duration was the best predictor for chronic phantom limb pain at 2 years (Hanley et al., 2007). However, preamputation pain intensity and duration were the best indicators of residual limb pain 24 months postamputation (Hanley et al., 2007).
   b. It is suggested that preoperative use of an epidural block might reduce the incidence of phantom limb pain (Bach et al., 1988; Krane & Heller, 1995).
4. Children and adolescents tend to experience a decrease in the frequency and the intensity of phantom pain over time (Krane & Heller, 1995).
5. Remedies for phantom pain include removing the prostheses, warming the stump, massage, and cognitive-behavioral methods, such as distraction or relaxation. A review by Moseley, Gallace, and Spence (2008) found that mirror therapy is probably no better than motor imagery to decrease immediate acute pain.
6. The most common medical therapies include anticonvulsants, tricyclic antidepressants, β-blockers, and TENS.
7. Residual limb pain must be treated as needed.

E. Myofascial pain syndromes and fibromyalgia
1. Myofascial pain syndrome is a regional pain disorder that is accompanied by trigger points.
2. Fibromyalgia typically is a more chronic syndrome with generalized diffuse musculoskeletal pain and tenderness at 11 or more of 18 specified tender point sites. The American College of Rheumatology has published specific criteria for the classification of fibromyalgia (Wolfe et al., 1990). No diagnostic criteria for juvenile fibromyalgia have been published. Patients with fibromyalgia often have fatigue, sleep disturbances, and morning stiffness.
3. It is not known whether children with widespread pain a primary symptom of fibromyalgia will grow into adults with the same pain symptoms. A prospective 4-year follow-up study of 1,282 Finnish schoolchildren found that widespread pain is as common as in adults but children have a more favorable prognosis (Mikkelsson et al., 2008).
4. Physical therapy is a major component of the treatment. Physical therapy should include supervised stretching and exercise.

5. Primary pharmacological treatment when required by the severity of symptoms is tricyclic antidepressants (Waldman, 1998).
6. Sympathetically maintained pain may be present with myofascial pain.
7. Massage can be beneficial with patients who experience spasm in association with myofascial pain. The use of massage also provides desensitization that may reduce allodynia from sympathetically maintained pain (Waldman, 1998).
8. TENS is a safe, noninvasive adjunct treatment. In a comparative study of four modes of TENS and a control group, high-frequency, high-intensity TENS was found to be effective in treating myofascial pain, although it did not effect changes in local trigger point sensitivity.

F. Headaches
1. Headaches are a common complaint in schoolchildren and adolescents.
   a. Headache is noted in about 35% to 51% of children by age 7, and 57% to 82% of all children have experienced a headache by 15 years of age (Lipton, 1997).
   b. The prevalence of recurrent headaches in the pediatric population varies, greatly from 6.3% to 49% of pediatric patients (McGrath, 2001).
2. Headache is less common in younger children and often indicates an underlying organic cause.
3. Most common recurrent headaches in schoolchildren and adolescents are migraine, tension type, and chronic daily headaches.
   a. Migraines occur equally in males and females before puberty. After puberty, females have a greater percentage of headaches compared to males. Larsson and Sund (2005) stated the frequency of migraines was twice as high for teenage girls than boys, relating this to pubertal development and hormone changes.
      (1) Migraine with aura has been shown to have a genetic component.
      (2) In children and adolescents, migraines occur more often than they do in adults (two to eight times a month), although the migraines are shorter in duration. Migraines may also be seasonal, with fewer occurring in the summer. Migraines in children are more often bilateral when compared with adults (Spierings, 1996), and commonly frontal (Hershey et al., 2005). Children may exhibit fatigue, crying, and irritability along with nausea, vomiting, photophobia, phonophobia, and osmophobia. Complaints of abdominal pain and motion sickness are also common (Fleener & Holloway, 2004).
   b. Tension type headaches are often described as "squeezing" in the occipital area of the head without nausea, vomiting, phonophobia, or photophobia. Presentation may be difficult to determine as home treatment with analgesics may cause rebound headaches.
   c. Chronic daily headaches occur daily or near-daily (at least 15 each month lasting more than 4 hr/d) with varying intensity and duration (Wiendels, van der Geest, Neven, Ferrari, & Laan, 2005). Accompanying symptoms may vary based on analgesics used and treatments trialed at home (McGrath, 2001).
4. When obtaining a history, it is important to assess the implications of headaches or migraines on school attendance, peer relations, and participation in leisure time activities.
   a. The use of headache diaries is recommended because children can document new symptoms, varying headache frequency, and varying intensity when maintaining a headache diary more accurately. The headache diary should be kept only as long as it is providing new or helpful information. The diary should not be allowed to become a focus or an irritant to the child or family.
   b. A thorough evaluation of a patient with headache should include a detailed headache history, including impact on quality of life and functionality. Psychosocial and family history should be obtained to identify triggers, stressors, and genetic components that may be contributors. A neurological examination is a necessity to evaluate for the potential source of the headache.
5. The treatment plan should include a multilayer approach: acute therapy, preventative therapy, and biobehavioral therapy (Hershey, Winner, Kabbouche, & Powers, 2007).
   a. Acute therapy is used to rapidly abort a headache currently in progress.

(1) Many children and adolescents tend to wait until after the onset of a headache before taking analgesic medications; they must be educated to take pain-relieving medications such as acetaminophen or ibuprofen at the first sign of a headache for optimal pain relief.
(2) It is difficult for young children to recognize the early stage of headache or aura of a migraine; this makes it more difficult for ergot derivatives and sumatriptan, or other similar serotoninergic drugs to work effectively.
(3) A child's pain often is managed by the parent; it is important to educate parents not to wait until the pain is severe before administering analgesics to the child.

b. The treatment plan for tension-type headaches or migraines depends on headache frequency and degree of impairment.
(1) The National Clearinghouse Guidelines for treatment of pediatric migraines report that mild headaches should be treated with rest, a quiet environment, nonpharmacological measures, and a simple analgesic (National Headache Foundation, 2004).
(2) The National Clearinghouse Guidelines for treatment of pediatric migraines (National Headache Foundation, 2004) states that for more severe headaches beneficial medications include abortive headache treatment such as simple analgesics (e.g., acetaminophen), NSAIDs, isometheptene mucate (e.g., Midrin®), and selective serotonin agonists (e.g., sumatriptan).
(3) Hamalainen, Hoppu, and Valkeila (1997) reported more than 50% of children experiencing a migraine had decreased pain within 2 hours of treatment with either acetaminophen or ibuprofen (Larsson, 1999).
(4) When using abortive treatment for migraine, aspirin or aspirin-containing compounds should be avoided in children younger than 12 years because of the risk of Reye syndrome (Lewis et al., 2004a; Spierings, 1996).
(5) 5-Hydroxytryptamine receptor agonists ("triptan agents") can also be used. Nasal spray should be considered for adolescents (Lewis et al., 2004a).
(6) Children with migraines who do not respond to mild analgesics can be given dihydroergotamine (Larsson, 1999).
(7) Ergot derivatives are warranted when headaches are severe but are too uncommon to justify prophylactic treatment.

c. Frequent analgesic use is common in the treatment of chronic daily headaches. Medication-overuse headaches (also known as rebound headaches or drug-induced headaches) can occur when medication is used more than twice a day (Lewis et al., 2004b). When this type of headache is suspected there should be a trial period when all analgesics are withdrawn. Hering-Hanit, Cohen, and Horev (2001) reported stopping daily analgesic use resulted in complete resolution of chronic daily headaches in 20 of 26 adolescents and a decrease in frequency in 5 additional patients.

d. When determining medication for the treatment of headaches, evaluate for comorbid conditions, including depression, anxiety, and obsessive-compulsive disorder, and coexisting conditions, including reactive airway disease and hypertension, as these may influence medication choice (Lewis et al., 2004b).

e. Preventative therapy is used to decrease frequency of headaches and/or increase functionality.
(1) When headaches are frequent or when repeated use of medications leads to rebound headaches, prophylactic medication may be considered.
(2) Prophylactic medications include antidepressants, anticonvulsants, antiserotonergics, antihypertensives (including β-blockers and calcium channel blockers), and ergots.
(3) As migraines in children are almost always associated with nausea, an antiemetic should be considered. Children often respond to antiemetics with relief of the headache (Lewis et al., 2004b; Spierings, 1996).
(4) Serotoninergic medications tend to be associated with fewer side effects (particularly nausea and vomiting) than ergotamines.

(5) Sumatriptan and other similar serotoninergic medications should ***not*** be used within 24 hours of any ergot compound (Selman, 2000). Ergot alkaloids have been reported to cause prolonged vasospastic reactions, and evidence suggests that this may be additive to the vasoconstrictor effects of sumatriptan and similar serotoninergic drugs.

f. Significant disability often accompanies pediatric headaches, including poor school attendance, failing academics, and altered peer and family relations (Winner, 2008). Biobehavioral therapy is divided into three components.

(1) *Normalizing lifestyle* includes returning to functional lifestyle, including school attendance and return to physical activities, establishing long-term goals, and using medications appropriately.

(2) *Treatment adherence* includes compliance with treatment regimens and removal or barriers that may be preventing execution of the plan.

(3) *Lifestyle adjustments* include identification of possible precipitating triggers. These can be identified more easily when a headache diary is maintained.

(a) Connelly (2003) describes some potential triggers such as food (soda, chocolate, eggs, nuts, cheese, wheat, lactose, skipping meals, or MSG), environmental conditions (heat, humidity, or allergens), sensory stimuli (bright lights or loud noises), behaviors (school work, physical activity, menstruation or hormone changes in females, change in sleep cycle, or dehydration), and emotions (stress, anger, or depression).

(b) Regulation of sleep, diet, and exercise should be discussed with the patient and family. Resuming a "normal" circadian rhythm with a similar bedtime and a similar wake time may reduce the effect on the patient's headache cycle.

g. For school-age and older children with headaches that affect the quality of their life, nonpharmacological methods, including stress management and cognitive-behavioral pain management techniques like biofeedback and relaxation therapy, should be included as part of the pain control plan (Hershey et al., 2007).

G. Recurrent abdominal pain

1. Recurrent abdominal pain, an example of a functional gastrointestinal disorder, is typically defined as abdominal pain that is episodic or continuous occurring at least once per week for at least 2 consecutive months and is severe enough to interfere with a child's normal activities (Rasquin et al., 2006). The diagnosis of recurrent abdominal pain can be given in the absence of "alarm" features, which include blood in the stool, emesis, unintentional weight loss, chronic severe diarrhea, unexplained fever, organomegaly, family history, or an abnormal physical finding that makes the provider suspicious for a physiological cause of the pain (DiLorenzo et al., 2005).

2. The pain typically is recurrent rather than constant and may be accompanied by nausea, vomiting, pallor, and headaches. Management should reflect the proposed cause of the abdominal pain. Some researchers suggest that recurrent abdominal pain is a behavioral response to pain, and others suggest the patient's reaction to physical stimuli such as stress, dietary changes, hormone changes, or inflammation may be abnormal (McOmber & Shulman, 2007).

3. Children with recurrent abdominal pain are less confident about their ability to deal with stressors and have fewer coping strategies, so pain episodes tend to be precipitated by stressful situations (Walker, Smith, Garber, & Claar, 2007). Stress may be associated with family dynamics, performance related to school, sports, or social events or may be contributed to learned behavior from a highly anxious parent (Ramchandani, Stein, Hotopf, Wiles, & the ALSPAC Study Team, 2006). Children with recurrent abdominal pain tend to be overachievers and eager to please others, especially their parents.

a. Patients who present with multiple nongastrointestinal symptoms, such as headache, other pain and fatigue, should be screened for depressive symptoms as this may affect treatment decisions (Little, Williams, Puzanovova, Rudzinski, & Walker, 2007).

b. It is important for the health care providers not only to evaluate for "alarm" symptoms and rule out an organic cause of the pain but also to discuss how normal physiological processes and psychosocial stressors contribute to functional abdominal pain.

(1) Unnecessary extensive medical evaluations risk prolonging the child and family's concern that the child is sick (Walker, 1999).
(2) It should not be assumed that a child has emotional problems causing abdominal pain because an organic cause is not found.

4. The child, and ideally the family, should be taught coping strategies to help alleviate the stress (Kain & Rimar, 1995). Robins, Smith, Glutting, and Bishop (2005) reported that patients who were taught cognitive-behavioral therapies reported significantly less abdominal pain and had fewer school absences. Compared to children who were taught breathing exercises alone, patients who were also taught progressive muscle relaxation were found to be more likely to return to functionality (Weydert et al., 2006). Treatment with guided imagery and progressive relaxation safely and effectively reduced symptoms and increased functionality and school attendance (Youssef et al., 2004).
5. Treatment addresses symptom management rather than curative. Treatment may include medications, diet modification, and psychological, behavioral, and coping mechanisms. Medications may include antispasmodics; antidepressants, of which TCAs are the most common; and serotonergic agents (Hyams, 2005).
   a. It is important to prevent the child with recurrent abdominal pain from assuming the role of a chronically ill child with frequent somatic complaints, limited peer interaction, and dependence on parents beyond what is typical of their developmental age. Symptoms may be prolonged by parents continuing to seek a "cause," parental attention to the child's pain, ongoing stress, and sexual abuse (Berger, Gieteling, & Benninga, 2007).

H. Sickle cell disease

1. Sickle cell pain can be characterized as acute, chronic, intermittent, recurrent, or persistent (Ballas, 1998). The frequency, intensity, and quality of pain are highly variable among individual children. Painful episodes or crises can last hours to weeks.
2. When the child with sickle cell disease presents with pain, it is important to consider all disease complications in the differential diagnosis. These include acute chest syndrome, splenic sequestration, neurological event, priapism, osteomyelitis, cholelithiasis, avascular necrosis of the hip, or splenic infarction and vasoocclusive crises (Ellison & Shaw, 2007).
3. Pain from vasoocclusive crises may be limited to one body area or may involve many areas. The most commonly effected sites include lower back, femur, hips and knees. Pain tends to recur in a particular area but may vary by crisis (Ballas, 2005).
   a. With vasoocclusive crisis, there are minimal physical findings related to pain. It is important to recognize that pain is subjective and should be assessed using self-report scales when the patient is developmentally able. Functional disability should also be considered. A multidimensional scale may be more helpful in assessing pain from sickle cell disease.
   b. It is difficult for a child to cope with the lack of control experienced through frequent, unpredictable episodes of severe pain.
   c. Increased analgesics, including opioids, are appropriate for the acute episode. Use of the WHO analgesic ladder (Fig. 20-1) is applicable to acute painful episodes. Clinicians should monitor the amount of relief obtained from analgesics and titrate to achieve optimal control. Side effects may be the limiting factor of optimal pain control (Jacob et al., 2003).
   d. In the emergency room, the severity of pain and poor response to the initial dose of intravenous analgesic may predict the need for hospital admission, thereby avoiding premature discharge from the emergency room. Selection of the inpatient analgesic regimen should be based on the severity of pain and initial medication response (Frei-Jones, Baxter, Rogers, & Buchanan, 2008).
   e. Care should be taken to discuss with the child and family past pain regimens, their effectiveness, and the child and family's preferences (Ellison & Shaw, 2007). Any change in pain treatment plans should be discussed with the child and family, and preferably a course of action should be decided when the patient is not in acute pain.
   f. Despite use of PCA, Jacob et al. (2003) found that pediatric patients self-administered only 35% of the morphine that was prescribed, which may have contributed to minimal reduction

in pain scores. This is a good indicator that clinicians need to continually assess pain and titrate analgesics for optimal pain relief.

g. Oral opioids may provide appropriate relief, but nausea, vomiting, and inability to absorb oral opioids due to abdominal crisis may limit their effectiveness.

4. Appropriate pain management addresses acute and chronic pain. Because most sickle cell pain is dealt with at home, it is imperative that the health care provider's focus be on teaching the child and parents how to manage the pain pharmacologically and nonpharmacologically (Fuggle, Shand, Gill, & Davies, 1996). The use of a pain diary may assist the family and patient in assessing pain from sickle cell disease and determining treatment successes (Dampier, Ely, Brodecki, & O'Neal, 2002).
   a. Beyer and Simons (2004) interviewed families of patients with sickle cell disease about home regimens for treating pain. Treatment should
      (1) Maintain health through rest, fluids, and nutrition.
      (2) Encourage children to maintain functionality despite pain.
      (3) Treat symptoms of pain early in the cycle.
      (4) Use distraction to avoid focusing on the pain.
      (5) Provide nonpharmacological relaxation techniques.
      (6) Avoid hospitalization unless symptoms are unrelenting.
   b. Parents should be given guidelines regarding when they should seek the assistance of their primary care provider, sickle cell specialist, or emergency department.

III. Interventions

A. Chronic pain treatment using a multidisciplinary approach provides the best outcomes. It is not always possible to eradicate the pain; return of function often is the goal.

B. Family participation in care
   1. The child must be viewed in the context of the family.
   2. Plan and set realistic goals with the child and family.

C. Pharmacological interventions
   1. Opioids
      a. Before initiating opioid therapy for chronic nonmalignant pain, appropriate classes of nonopioid and adjuvant medications in adequate doses should be tried in conjunction with nonpharmacological methods.
      b. There is controversy about whether neuropathic pain responds to opioid therapy (Portenoy, Foley, & Inturrisi, 1990). Practitioners may be hesitant to prescribe opioids for neuropathic pain (Anderson & Palmer, 2006). Opioid therapy should improve not only the quality of the patient's life but also the patient's ability to function. Failure to achieve improved analgesia with reasonable opioid doses should prompt the practitioner to question whether opioids are the appropriate class of pain medication (see earlier for specific opioid medications and dosages).
   2. NSAIDs (see earlier for specific drugs and dosages)
   3. Tricyclic antidepressants
      a. Analgesia is thought to be provided by blocking the reuptake of neurotransmitters, which increases the body's endogenous pain-modulating pathway, and tricyclic antidepressants may be an NMDA inhibitor (Boyer, Skolnick, & Fossom, 1998).
      b. Amitriptyline is not approved for use in pediatric patients. The FDA Black Box warning states there is an increased risk of suicidal thoughts and behavior in children, adolescents, and young adults with major depressive and other psychiatric disorders. Patients treated with antidepressants for any reason in these age groups require close monitoring and observation for clinical worsening of depression, suicidality, and unusual behavior, especially during first few months of therapy or with dose adjustments. Family members must be educated to closely observe the patient and communicate the patient's condition frequently with the prescriber (Taketomo et al., 2007).

c. Use tricyclic antidepressants for phantom limb, peripheral neuropathy, radiation-induced nerve injury, or pain secondary to tumor-associated nerve damage.
d. Use of tricyclics is contraindicated in patients with cardiac conduction disturbances. It may be prudent to obtain baseline and follow-up electrocardiograms.
e. The analgesic dose is lower than that required to treat depression.
    (1) The initial dose of amitriptyline is 0.1 mg/kg orally at bedtime; this may be advanced as tolerated over 2 to 3 weeks to 0.5 to 2 mg/kg orally at bedtime (Taketomo et al., 2007). Amitriptyline not recommended in children less than 12 years of age.
    (2) Administration of the dose at bedtime can reduce daytime sedation and benefit children who are having difficulty sleeping.
    (3) Hershey, Powers, Bentti, and deGrauw (2000) reported that 80% of children with chronic headaches treated with 1 mg/kg/d had a significant reduction of headache frequency and intensity.
    (4) The intravenous route of administration is not approved by the FDA.
f. To determine the efficacy of tricyclics, they must be tried for a sufficient period, depending on the specific medication (e.g., 3 weeks for amitriptyline).
g. Tricyclics have significant adverse effects related to their anticholinergic properties, such as sedation, orthostatic hypotension, dry mouth, constipation, and urinary hesitancy. These side effects typically subside as the child develops tolerance to the medication. Appropriate patient education regarding side effects must be taught.
    (1) Nortriptyline or desipramine may be substituted if side effects are not tolerable with amitriptyline.
    (2) Nortriptyline is available as a solution; it is useful for children who are unable to take pills.

4. Selective serotonin reuptake inhibitors or serotonin and norepinephrine reuptake inhibitors may be used to treat neuropathic pain, as well as depression or anxiety that may accompany chronic pain, and allow patients to focus on cognitive-behavioral coping skills (Gallagher, 2005).
5. Anticonvulsants
    a. Gabapentin
        (1) Gabapentin is probably the anticonvulsant prescribed most often in the treatment of neuropathic pain (Mellegers & Furlan, 2001).
        (2) There are few adverse effects. Because of its good safety profile and lack of drug interactions, it often is considered a first-line therapy for neuropathic pain (Portenoy, 1999).
        (3) Case reports initially documented the benefits of gabapentin for adult patients with refractory reflex sympathetic dystrophy with administration of only one or two 300-mg gabapentin capsules. Adult patients were maintained on 900 to 2,400 mg/d (Mellick & Mellick, 1995).
        (4) The initial dose is 5 mg/kg at bedtime, day 2 is 5 mg/kg/dose twice daily, and then day 3 increases to 5 mg/kg/dose three times a day. Gradually increase dose titrating to effect. Usual dosage range is 8 to 35 mg/kg/d divided into three doses per day. Maximum dose is 3,600 mg/d in three divided doses (Taketomo et al., 2007).
    b. Carbamazepine
        (1) Analgesia is likely because of its ability to modify voltage-dependent sodium channels; it probably possesses additional mechanisms of action.
        (2) Dosage should be adjusted according to patient response.
            (a) The dose for children younger than 6 years is 10 to 20 mg/kg/d divided in two or three doses for tablets, or four doses per day for liquid form; the maximum dose is 35 mg/kg/d (Taketomo et al., 2007).
            (b) The initial dose for children 6 to 12 years is 100 mg twice a day, increased by 100 mg/d at weekly intervals. The maximum recommended dose is 1,000 mg/d (Taketomo et al., 2007).

(c) The initial dose for children older than 12 years is 200 mg twice a day, increased by 200 mg/d at weekly intervals. The maximum recommended dose is 1,000 mg/d for children 12 to 15 years old and 1,200 mg/d for children older than 15 years (Taketomo et al., 2007).

(3) Studies document pain relief for trigeminal neuralgia in adults with carbamazepine (Killian & Fromm, 1968; Nichol, 1969; Tomson, Tybring, Bertilsson, Ekbom, & Rane, 1980).

(4) Carbamazepine induces hepatic enzymes and may accelerate its own metabolism and that of other drugs given concomitantly.

(5) Side effects include drowsiness, dizziness, unsteady gait, and the potentially serious side effects of bone marrow depression and hepatic dysfunction.

(a) Baseline complete blood count and liver function tests should be performed before initiation of therapy, and subsequent monitoring should be individualized as necessary.

6. Abortive migraine treatment (see earlier for information on acetaminophen and ibuprofen)

a. Ergotamine and caffeine (ergotamine tartrate, 1 mg, and caffeine, 100 mg)

(1) For adolescents, give 2 mg orally at the onset of a migraine attack and then, if needed, 1 to 2 mg every 30 minutes as needed, to a maximum of 6 mg per attack. The maximum is 10 mg/wk (Taketomo et al., 2007).

b. Dihydroergotamine

(1) Safety and efficacy have not been established in children. Dihydroergotamine, in a 20- to 40-μg/kg oral dose, was better than placebo in a pilot study of 12 children, but the results did not achieve statistical significance (Hamalainen, Hoppu, & Santavuori, 1997a). Some patients may have irritability and agitation related to administration (Connelly, 2003).

c. Sumatriptan

(1) Safety and efficacy have not been established in children, although limited clinical evidence suggests that safety and efficacy in children 6 to 18 years old are comparable to in adults (e.g., 0.06 mg/kg subcutaneously) (Linder, 1996). An open-label prospective study showed 78% of children older than 6 years of age who received sumatriptan 60 μg/kg subcutaneously reduced their pain to mild or no pain (Linder, 1996).

(2) Sumatriptan nasal spray has also been shown to be effective (Winner et al., 2000).

(3) Oral sumatriptan tablets failed to stop migraine attacks in one randomized placebo-controlled crossover design study of 23 children between 8 and 16 years old (Hamalainen, Hoppu, & Santavuori, 1997b). This study suggests oral sumatriptan is not as effective in children and adolescents as it is in adults.

7. Prophylactic migraine treatment

a. Propranolol

(1) Dosing for propranolol is 0.6 to 1.5 mg/kg/d orally divided every 8 hours (maximum, 4 mg/kg/d).

(a) For children 35 kg or less, give 10 to 20 mg orally three times a day.

(b) For children greater than 35 kg, give 20 to 40 mg orally three times a day (Taketomo et al., 2007).

(2) Propranolol was studied in 32 children in a double-blind, placebo-controlled, crossover design trial. Migraine attacks decreased by 70% during treatment with propranolol and by 9% during treatment with a placebo (Ludvigsson, 1974). The dose of propranolol was 20 mg three times daily in children weighing less than 35 kg and 40 mg three times daily in children weighing more than 35 kg (Ludvigsson, 1974).

(3) A meta-analysis suggested that propranolol may be useful in the prevention of migraine in children and adolescents (Hermann, Kim, & Blanchard, 1995).

(4) Propranolol is contraindicated in children with asthma, congestive heart failure and diabetes.

b. Cyproheptadine (Periactin®)
   (1) The cyproheptadine dose for children is 4 mg two or three times per day (Taketomo et al., 2007).
   (2) Intensity and frequency decreased in 83% of children who received cyproheptadine for migraine (Lewis et al., 2004b). Side effects include sedation and increased appetite.

c. Amitriptyline (see Part Four. Pediatric Chronic Pain for information

7. Local and topical anesthetics
   a. Lidocaine patch 5% (Lidoderm®)
      (1) The Lidoderm® patch is a 10 cm by 14 cm patch that contains 700 mg of lidocaine in an aqueous base. The penetration of lidocaine into intact skin after patch application is sufficient to produce analgesia. The lidocaine acts on sodium channels to inhibit pain transmission in the periphery and central sensitization (Gallagher, 2005). The amount of lidocaine absorbed systemically is related directly to the duration of application and the surface area of the patch.
      (2) The peak blood concentration of 15 healthy volunteers after a 12-hour patch application was approximately 0.13 mg/ml. (Blood levels greater than 5 μg/ml can be expected to produce toxicity.) The lidocaine blood concentration did not increase with daily use.
      (3) The Lidoderm® patch is indicated for the relief of pain associated with postherpetic neuralgia. It should be applied to intact skin to cover the most painful area. The patch is applied once for 12 hours within a 24-hour period. Patches can be cut into smaller sizes as needed. Excessive dosing by longer application times or to larger areas can result in increased absorption and serious adverse effects.
      (4) Even a used Lidoderm® patch contains a large amount of lidocaine. The risk exists for a young child to suffer adverse effects as a result of chewing or ingesting the patch. It is important that this formulation be used only for older children and be disposed of properly (Endo Pharmaceuticals, 1999).
   b. Capsaicin is a medication extracted from hot chili peppers and is used as a topical cream. It selectively stimulates and depletes substance P, one of the primary neurotransmitters of painful stimuli from the periphery to the central nervous system. Children report stinging to burning at the application site followed by analgesia. Younger children typically do not tolerate the localized burning sensation.

PART FIVE: NONPHARMACOLOGICAL PAIN MANAGEMENT

I. Pediatric Management Techniques

A. Nonpharmacological techniques are useful in addition to medication in the acute setting and may be the cornerstone for the treatment of many types of chronic pain. The goal of cognitive-behavioral therapies is to increase feelings of control, to restructure negative thinking that can lead to pain-amplifying behaviors, and to assist the individual to cope with situations that magnify pain perception (Clark & Odell, 2000). Negative thinking and poor coping are linked to higher reports of pain in children (Schanberg, Lefebvre, Keefe, Kredich, & Gil, 1997). The need to assist children to learn strategies to cope is imperative because it may improve their overall quality of life.
   1. *Parental presence:* Most children feel more secure with their parents present and most parents desire to be present during procedures. Parents may require instruction on how best to help their child manage pain and anxiety (Young, 2005).
   2. *Relaxation:* The best method for young children to relax is by deep breathing using pinwheels, bubbles, or kazoos. If at first the child does not appear interested in the activity, the nurse should try blowing the pinwheel or bubbles to help pique the child's interest. Older children can breathe

in and out for a count of 3 or 4 or be instructed to take a deep breath and let it out making a hissing sound. Children can be told to blow the pain away or blow out imaginary birthday candles. Relaxation has been reported to induce physiological change (vessel dilation, change in sympathetic outflow), which may be beneficial in patients with headache and CRPS (Connelly, 2003).

3. *Rocking and swaddling:* These provide security, particularly for infants and toddlers. Gentle rocking is used successfully worldwide.
4. *Distraction:* Redirect the child's attention. The more involved a child is in an activity, the greater the distraction from pain. Young children like popup or sound books and magic wands. Older children may like to listen to their favorite music or play electronic handheld games. The younger the child, the shorter the attention span. Distraction is a proven effective psychological intervention (Kleiber & Harper, 1999).
5. *Guided imagery:* Imagery can help the child focus on pleasant experiences. Encourage the child to focus on a pleasurable event during a painful time (French, Painter, & Courty, 1994). For younger children, use imaginary things that are concrete, such as a music box or storybook. For older children, use stories, music, or relaxation tapes that appeal to them. Follow the child's lead (i.e., the child's story is silly but distracting). Children with recurrent abdominal pain who used guided imagery and relaxation reported less pain (Ball, Shaprio, Monheim, & Weydert, 2003).
6. *Music therapy:* Music that is soothing to an adult is not necessarily soothing to a child. Music therapy has been used in the perioperative setting, in instances of procedural pain, during acute hospitalization, and in the chronic setting for relaxation and anxiety relief (Gerik, 2005). Infants respond best to repetitive songs such as nursery rhymes; classical music is too dynamic and unstructured. Music can be a mother's lullaby, tape, or compact disc. Live music has been reported to reduce pain and distress related to venipuncture (Caprilli, Anastasi, Grotto, Abeti, & Messeri, 2007).
7. *Hypnosis:* An altered state of consciousness lets the patient have complete focus away from painful state (Gerik, 2005). Hypnosis can be used for both acute or procedural pain and chronic pain syndromes.
8. *Massage:* Tactile stimulation and manipulation of the body occurs in a specific pattern that promotes relaxation, decreases stress and anxiety, and promotes good sleep. Sick infants, particularly preterm infants may require modification of touch, or only the use of healing or therapeutic touch to ensure the therapy is beneficial rather than detrimental. Healing or therapeutic touch is the process of using the hands to intentionally direct good energy toward the patient (Ireland & Olson, 2000).
9. *Heat and cold:* Temperature should not be used with infants because of the risk of thermal injury. Heat and cold are effective for chronic musculoskeletal injury and headaches. Heat and cold may be applied on the contralateral side of the body to decrease pain. This will not affect swelling but has been shown to decrease pain. Cold should be avoided in sickle cell disease because it exacerbates vasoocclusion.
10. In addition to the preceding techniques, the following are useful in the chronic pain management setting:
    a. *TENS:* Stimulation gives children and adolescents the added advantage of providing them with some control over their pain. TENS usually is well tolerated by older children and adolescents. Younger children tend to dislike the sensation. It is safe and noninvasive. Positive effects can be seen using TENS in children with reflex sympathetic dystrophy (Kesler, Saulsbury, Miller, & Rowlingson, 1988).
    b. *Biofeedback:* The child is taught to modify physiological responses that contribute to pain. Biofeedback has been found to be useful in many clinical areas, including decreasing frequency, intensity, and duration of headaches (Gerik, 2005). Relaxation with biofeedback is an effective prophylactic treatment for recurrent headaches and nonorganic recurrent abdominal pain (Kain & Rimar, 1995). Relaxation with biofeedback also is effective in chronic musculoskeletal injury.
    c. *Acupuncture:* Acupuncture can provide an overall therapeutic benefit for acute and chronic pain, but controlled studies are lacking. Of pediatric patients receiving acupuncture as a com-

plementary therapy for migraine headache, endometriosis, or reflex, sympathetic, 70% felt the treatment helped their symptoms (Kemper et al., 2000). The use of acupuncture in young children is limited because many may be needle-phobic. One phase I study demonstrated that anxiety decreased with treatment sessions (Zeltzer, 2004).

d. *Physical therapy:* Many children with chronic pain become physically deconditioned as a result of activity restriction through guarding a painful area or following the recommendation of a health professional to limit activity. Physical therapy may be required to regain function. Progress toward goals should be monitored frequently (Gallagher, 2005). Simple exercise such as swimming can improve the child's body image and provide aerobic conditioning, improved muscle strength, and a general sense of well-being.

e. *Psychological therapy:* Many children need assistance to develop coping skills to manage their pain. This is also known as cognitive-behavioral training. This therapy has been effective in assisting children with chronic abdominal pain and headaches (Gerik, 2005). Children often can become socially isolated from their peers when they experience chronic pain, particularly when the pain limits or prevents school attendance. Family therapy is often helpful.

f. *Support group:* Families need assistance in locating support groups with pediatric patients. It is not helpful for children or adolescents to attend support groups with an adult focus because issues affecting children and adolescents, and their roles in life are different from adult issues and roles. Coping strategies vary greatly within different stages of childhood.

PART SIX: OPIOID DEPENDENCE AND ADDICTION (see the chapter on Coexisting Addiction and Pain for further information)

I. Opioid Misconceptions

A. Some parents fear their child will become addicted to narcotics. Parents should be reassured that data suggest addiction is rare. A retrospective adult study published as a letter to the editor revealed only four documented cases of subsequent addiction in 11,882 adult patients who received an opioid in their hospital treatment for acute pain management (Porter & Jick, 1980). Prospective studies in the pediatric population are lacking. Health care providers should be aware that adolescents in particular may not recognize the consequence of their actions and are highly influenced by their peers.

B. Parents should be educated that opioid tolerance and physiological dependence are a normal process.

1. Tolerance is a decrease in the pharmacological effects of a drug with its repeated administration, or an increase in dose requirement to attain the same clinical effect (Anand & Arnold, 1994). Tolerance is a physiological phenomenon and should not be considered addiction. The dose needed to control a child's pain should be given (Anand & Ingraham, 1996).
   a. Tolerance occurs to both analgesic effects and side effects (APS, 2001).
   b. Cross-tolerance between opioids is incomplete (WHO, 1998).
   c. Tolerance to an opioid is reversed quickly when a patient has a short opioid-free period. Standard opioid dose should be used initially with rapid dose titration (WHO, 1998).
2. Physical dependence is manifested by the physical need to continue the administration of a drug to prevent withdrawal symptoms (Anand & Arnold, 1994). It is the expected physiological response to continuous use of opioids (APS, 2001).
   a. Patients who have received repeated doses of opioids for more than 7 days require gradual tapering of opioids to avoid withdrawal symptoms (WHO, 1998).
   b. Decreased drug level in the blood may result in withdrawal symptoms. This does not in and of itself imply psychological addiction.
   c. Naloxone should be used with caution in opioid-tolerant patients. If respiratory depression occurs, the degree of treatment depends on the individual child and clinical situation. "If the child is terminally ill, for example, respiratory compromise is part of the dying process

and attempts to treat the problem may not always be appropriate if they would intensify or prolong suffering" (WHO, 1998, p. 41).

3. Addiction is psychological dependence in which an individual craves and is consumed overwhelmingly in the process of obtaining a substance because of its euphoric properties (Anand & Arnold, 1994).
   a. It is a disease with genetic, psychosocial, and environmental factors influencing its development (APS, 2001).
   b. Behavioral criteria includes the three Cs: preoccupation with use (craving), impaired control over use (compulsive use), continued use despite harm (adverse consequences) (APS, 2001; Savage, Kirsh, & Passik, 2008).

C. Pseudoaddiction can occur when pain management is suboptimal. This is characterized by a child's watching the clock and repeatedly asking for increased dosages. This behavior typically resolves when adequate pain medications are administered and relief is satisfactory (WHO, 1998).

II. Opioid Weaning

A. Wean 10% to 20% of the total daily dose. Initial decreases may be larger, but as the taper reaches the end, the taper may need to slow down to prevent withdrawal symptoms.

B. Weaning one class of drug at a time may be prudent. In the event of withdrawal symptoms, it will be easier to identify which medication resulted in withdrawal symptoms.

C. Various methods are used to wean children dependent on an opioid, benzodiazepine, or both. Most weaning methods are based on length of drug exposure, type of opioid, individual provider preference, and presence or absence of pain (Berens et al., 2006).

References

Ambuel, B., Hamlett, K. W., & Marx, C. (1990). COMFORT scale manual. Unpublished manual. Requests for copies should be addressed to Seleste Marx, Department of Pediatrics, Rainbow Babies & Children's Hospital, 2011 Adelbert Road, Cleveland, Ohio 44106 (cited in Bear, 2006).

American Academy of Pain Medicine & American Pain Society. (1997). *The use of opioids for the treatment of chronic pain: Consensus statement.* Glenview, IL: Author.

American Academy of Pediatrics. (1999). AAP circumcision policy statement. *Pediatrics, 103,* 686–693.

American Cancer Society. (2007). *Cancer facts and figures 2007.* Atlanta: Author.

American Pain Society. (2001). Definitions related to the use of opioids for the treatment of pain. Consensus document from American Academy Pain Medicine, American Pain Society, and American Society of Addiction Medicine.

American Pain Society. (2003). *Principles of analgesic use in the treatment of acute pain and cancer pain* (5th ed.). Glenview, IL: Author.

American Pain Society. (2005). *Guidelines for the management of cancer pain in adults and children.* Glenview, IL: Author.

Anand, K. J., & Arnold, J. H. (1994). Opioid tolerance and dependence in infants and children. *Critical Care Medicine, 22,* 334–342.

Anand, K. J., & Ingraham, J. (1996). Tolerance, dependence, and strategies for compassionate withdrawal of analgesics and anxiolytics in the pediatric ICU. *Critical Care Nurse, 16*(6), 87–93.

Anderson, B., & Palmer, G. (2006). Recent developments in the pharmacological management of pain in children. *Current Opinions in Anaesthesiology, 19,* 285–292.

Anghelescu, D. L., Burgoyne, L. L., Oakes, L. L., & Wallace, D. A. (2005). The safety of patient-controlled analgesia by proxy in pediatric oncology patients. *Anesthesia Analogue, 101,* 1623–1627.

Arrowsmith, J. B., Kennedy, D. L., Kuritsky, J. N., & Faich, G. A. (1987). National patterns of aspirin use and Reye syndrome reporting: U.S., 1980 to 1985. *Pediatrics, 79,* 858–863.

Astra Pharmaceuticals. (1999). EMLA package insert. AstraZeneca, Wayne, PA.

Bach, S., Noreng, M. F., & Tjellden, N. U. (1988). Phantom limb pain in amputees during the first 12 months following limb amputation, after preoperative lumbar epidural blockade. *Pain, 33,* 297–301.

Baker, C., & Wong, D. (1987). Q.U.E.S.T.T.: A process of pain assessment in children. *Orthopedic Nursing, 6,* 11–21.

Balis, F. M., Lester, C. M., Chraisos, G. P., Heideman, R. L., & Poplack, D. G. (1987). Differences in cerebrospinal fluid penetration of corticosteroids: Possible relationship to prevention of meningeal leukemia. *Journal of Clinical Oncology, 5,* 202–207.

Ball, T., Shaprio, D., Monheim, C., & Weydert, J. (2003). A pilot study of the use of guided imagery for the treatment of recurrent abdominal pain in children. *Clinical Pediatrics, 42,* 527–532.

Ballas, S. (Ed.). (1998). *Sickle cell pain.* Seattle: IASP Press.

Ballas, S. (2005). Pain management of sickle cell disease. *Hematology Oncology Clinics of North America, 19,* 785–802.

Bear, L. A., & Ward-Smith, P. (2006). Interrater reliability of the COMFORT scale. *Pediatric Nursing, 32*(5), 427–434.

Benini, F., Johnston, C., Faucher, D., & Aranda, J. V. (1993). Topical anesthesia during circumcision in newborn infants. *JAMA, 270,* 850–853.

Berde, C. B., Beyer, J. E., Bournaki, M. C., Levin, C. R., & Sethna, N. F. (1991). Comparison of morphine and methadone for prevention of postoperative pain in 3- to 7-year-old children. *Journal of Pediatrics, 119,* 136–141.

Berde, C. B., Lehn, B. M., Yee, J. D., Sethna, N. F., & Russo, D. (1991). Patient-controlled analgesia in children and adolescents: A randomized, prospective comparison with intramuscular administration of morphine for postoperative analgesia. *Journal of Pediatrics, 118*(3), 460–466.

Berde, C. B., Sethna, N. F., Holzman, R. S., Reidy, P., & Gondek, E. J. (1987). Pharmacokinetics of methadone in children and adolescents in the perioperative period. *Anesthesiology, 67,* A519.

Berde, C. B., Sethna, N. F., & Micheli, L. J. (1988). A technique for continuous lumbar sympathetic blockade for severe reflex sympathetic dystrophy in children and adolescents. *Anesthesia & Analgesia, 67,* S1–S266.

Berens, R. J., Meyer, M. T., Mikhailov, T. A., Colpaert, K. D., Czarnecki, M. L., Ghanayem, N. S., Hoffman, G. M., Soetenga, D. J., Nelson, T. J., & Weisman, S. J. (2006). A prospective evaluation of opioid-weaning in opioid-dependent pediatric critical care patients. *Anesthesia & Analgesia, 102,* 1045–1050.

Berger, M. Y., Gieteling, M. J., & Benninga, M. A. (2007). Chronic abdominal pain in children. *British Journal of Medicine, 334,* 997–1002.

Beyer, J. E., & Simmons, L. E. (2004). Home treatment of pain for children and adolescents with sickle cell disease. *Pain Management Nursing, 5*(3), 126–135.

Beyer, J. E., & Wells, N. (1989). The assessment of pain in children. *Pediatric Clinics of North America, 36,* 837–854.

Beyer, J. E., Denyes, M. J., & Villarruel, A. M. (1992). The creation, validation and continuing development of the Oucher: A measure of pain intensity in children. *Journal of Paediatric Nursing, 7,* 335–346.

Bieri, D., Reeve, R., Champion, G. D., Addicoat, L., & Ziegler, J. (1990). The Faces Pain Scale for the self-assessment of the severity of pain experienced by children: Development, initial validation, and preliminary investigation for ratio scale properties. *Pain, 41,* 139–150.

Birmingham, P. K., Wheller, M., Suresh, S., Dsida, R. M., Rae, B. R., Obrecht, J., Andreoi, V. A., Hall, S. C., & Cote, C. J. (2003). Patient-controlled epidural analgesia in children: Can they do it? *Anesthesia & Analgesia, 96,* 686–691.

Blackburn, S. T., & Loper, D. L. (Eds.). (1992). *Maternal, fetal and neonatal physiology: A clinical perspective* (p. 571). Philadelphia: W. B. Saunders.

Blass, E. M., & Hoffmeyer, L. B. (1991). Sucrose as an analgesic for newborn infants. *Pediatrics, 87,* 215–218.

Bleyer, W. A. (1990). The impact of childhood cancer on the United States and the world. *Cancer Journal for Clinicians, 40,* 355–367.

Boşenberg, A. (2004). Pediatric regional anesthesia update. *Paediatric Anaesthesia, 14,* 398–402.

Boswinkel, J. P., & Litman, R. S. (2005). The pharmacology of sedation. *Pediatric Annals, 34*(8), 607–613.

Boyer, P. A., Skolnick, P., & Fossom, L. H. (1998). Chronic administration of imipramine and citalopram alters the expression of NMDA receptor subunit mRNAs in mouse brain: A quantitative in situ hybridization. *Journal of Molecular Neuroscience, 10,* 219–233.

Brown, J., & Larson, M. (1999). Pain during insertion of peripheral intravenous catheters with and without intradermal lidocaine. *Clinical Nurse Specialist, 13*(6), 283–285.

Bubeck, J., Boos, K., Krause, H., & Thies, K. (2004). Subcutaneous tunneling of caudal catheters reduces the rate of bacterial colonization to that of lumbar epidural catheters. *Anesthesia & Analgesia, 99,* 689–693.

Cakmak, A., & Bolukbas, N. (2004). Juvenile rheumatoid arthritis: Physical therapy and rehabilitation. *Southern Medical Journal, 98*(2), 212–216.

Capdevila, X., Pirat, P., Bringuier, S., Gaertner, E., Singelyn, F., Bernard, N., Choquet, O., Bouaziz, H., & Bonnet, F. (2005). Continuous peripheral nerve blocks in hospital wards after orthopedic surgery: A multicenter prospective analysis of the quality of postoperative analgesia and complications in 1,416 patients. *Anesthesiology, 103,* 1035–1045.

Caprilli, S., Anastasi, F., Grotto, R., Abeti, M., & Messeri, A. (2007). Interactive music as a treatment for pain and stress in children during venipuncture: A randomized prospective study. *Journal of Developmental & Behavioral Pediatrics, 28,* 399–403.

Carr, T. D., Lemanek, K. L., & Armstrong, F. D. (1998). Pain and fear ratings: Clinical implications of age and gender differences. *Journal of Pain and Symptom Management, 15,* 305–313.

Cephalon. (2007). *ACTIQ prescribing information.* Salt Lake City: Cephalon.

Chapman, C. R., & Foley, K. M. (Eds.). (1993). *Current and emerging issues in cancer pain: Research and practice* (pp. 371–382). New York: Raven Press.

Clark, S., & Odell, L. (2000). Fibromyalgia syndrome: Common, real—and treatable. *Clinician Reviews, 10,* 57–83.

Connelly, M. (2003). Recurrent pediatric headache: A comprehensive review. *Children's Health Care, 32*(3), 153–189.

Craig, K. D., & Korol, C. T. (2008). Developmental issues in understanding, assessing and managing pediatric pain. In Walco, G. A., & Goldschneider, K. R. (Eds.), *Pain in children: A practical guide for primary care* (pp. 9–20). Totowa, NJ: Humana Press.

Czarnecki, M. L., Ferrise, A. S., Garwood, M. M., Sharp, M., Jastrowski Mano, K. E., Davies, H., & Weisman, S. J. (2008). Parent/nurse controlled analgesia in children with developmental delay. *Clinical Journal of Pain, 24*(9), 817–824.

Dahl, V., & Raeder, J. C. (2000). Non-opioid postoperative analgesia. *Acta Anaesthesiologica, 44,* 1191–1203.

Dampier, C., Ely, B., Brodecki, D., & O'Neal, P. (2002). Characteristics of pain managed at home in children with sickle cell disease by using diary self-reports. *Journal of Pain, 3*(6), 461–470.

Deshpande, J. K., & Anand, K. J. (1996). Basic aspects of acute pediatric pain and sedation. In J. Deshpande & J. Tobias (Eds.), *The pediatric pain handbook* (p. 21). St. Louis: Mosby.

DeWitt, E., Sherry, D., & Cron, R. (2005). Pediatric rheumatology for the adult rheumatologist. I. Therapy and dosing for pediatric rheumatic disorders. *JCR: Journal of Clinical Rheumatology, 11*(1), 21–33.

DiLorenzo, C., Colletti, R. B., Lehmann, H. P., Boyle, J.T., Gerson, W.T., Hyams, J.S., Squires, R.H., Jr., Walker, L.S., & Kanda, P.T.(2005). Chronic abdominal pain in children: A clinical report of the American Academy of Pediatrics and the North American Society for Pediatric Gastroenterology, Hepatology and Nutrition. *Journal of Pediatric Gastroenterology and Nutrition, 40,* 249–261.

Doyle, E., Robinson, D., & Morton, N. S. (1993). Comparison of patient-controlled analgesia with and without a background infusion after lower abdominal surgery in children. *British Journal of Anaesthesia, 71,* 670–673.

Dsida, R. M., Wheeler, M., Birmingham, P. K., Wang, Z., Heffner, C. L., Cote, C., & Avram, M. J. (2002). Age-stratified pharmacokinetics of ketorolac tromethamine in pediatric surgical patients, *Anesthesia & Analgesia, 94,* 266–270.

Ecoffey, C. (2007). Pediatric regional anesthesia: Update. *Current Opinions in Anaesthesiology, 20,* 232–235.Eichenfield, L. F., Funk, A., Fallon-Friedlander, S., & Cunningham, B. B. (2002). A Clinical Study to Evaluate the Efficacy of ELA-Max (4% Liposomal Lidocaine) as Compared With Eutectic Mixture of Local Anesthetics Cream for Pain Reduction of Venipuncture in Children. *Pediatrics, 109*(6), 1093–1099.

Eland, J. M. (1981). Minimizing pain associated with prekindergarten intramuscular injections. *Issues in Comprehensive Nursing, 5,* 361–373.

Eland, J. A., & Banner, W. (1999). Analgesia, sedation and neuromuscular blockage in pediatric critical care. In M. F. Hazinski (Ed.), *Manual of pediatric critical care.* St. Louis: Mosby.

Elliot, S. C., Miser, A. W., Dose, A. M., Betcher, D.L., O'Fallon, J.R., Ducos, R.S., Shah, N.R., Goh, T.S., Monzon, C.M., & Tscetter, L. (1991). Epidemiologic features of pain in pediatric cancer patients: A co-operative community-based study. *Clinical Journal of Pain, 7*(4), 263–268.

Ellison, A., & Shaw, K. (2007). Management of vasoocclusive pain events in sickle cell disease. *Pediatric Emergency Care, 23*(11), 832–841.

Endo Pharmaceuticals. (1999). Lidoderm package insert. Chadds Ford, PA: Author.

Endo Pharmaceuticals. (2006). Synera prescribing information. Chadds Ford, PA: Author.

Evans, H., Steele, S. M., Nielsen, K. C., & Tucker, M. S. (2005). Peripheral nerve blocks and continuous catheter techniques. *Anesthesiology Clinics of North America, 23,* 141–162.

Fanurik, D., Koh, J. L., Schmitz, M. L, Harrison, R. D., & Conrad, T. M. (1999). Children with cognitive impairment: Parent report of pain and coping. *Journal of Developmental & Behavioral Pediatrics, 20*(4), 228–234.

Farion, K. J., Splinter, K. L., Newhook, K., Gaboury, I., & Splinter, W. M. (2008). The effect of vapocoolant spray on pain due to intravenous cannulation: A randomized controlled trial. *Canadian Medical Association Journal, 179*(1), 31–36.

Fleener, V. S., & Holloway, B. (2004). Migraines: Not just an adult problem. *Nurse Practitioner, 29*(11), 26–39.

Frei-Jones, M., Baxter, A., Rogers, Z., & Buchanan, G. (2008). Vasoocclusive episodes in older children with sickle cell disease: Emergency department management and pain assessment. *Journal of Pediatrics, 152,* 218–285.

French, G. M., Painter, E. C., & Courty, D. L. (1994). Blowing away shot pain: A technique for pain management during immunization. *Pediatrics, 93,* 384–388.

Fuggle, P., Shand, P. A., Gill, L. J., & Davies, S. C. (1996). Pain, quality of life, and coping in sickle cell disease. *Archives of Disease in Childhood, 75,* 199–203.

Gallagher, R. M. (2005). Rational integration of pharmacological, behavioral, and rehabilitation strategies in the treatment of chronic pain. *American Journal of Physical Medicine and Rehabilitation, 84*(3), S64–S76.

Ganesh, A., Rose, J. B., Wells, L., Ganley, T., Gurnaney, H., Maxwell, L. G., Di Maggio, T., Milovcich, K., Scollon, M., Feldman, J. M., & Cucchiaro, G. (2007). Continuous peripheral nerve blockade for inpatient and outpatient postoperative analgesia in children. *Anesthesia & Analgesia, 105,* 5, 1234–1242.

Gaufberg, S. V., Walta, M. J., & Workman, T. P. (2007). Expanding the use of topical anesthesia in wound management: Sequential layered application of topical lidocaine with epinephrine. *American Journal of Emergency Medicine, 25,* 379–384.

Gaukroger, P. B., Tomkins, D. P., & Van Der Walk, J. H. (1989). Patient-controlled analgesia in children. *Anaesthesia and Intensive Care, 17*(3), 264–268.

Gerik, S. (2005). Pain management in children: Developmental considerations and mind–body therapies. *Southern Medical Journal, 98*(3), 295–302.

Geyer, J., Ellsbury, D., Kleiber, C., Litwiller, D., Hinton, A., & Yankowitz, J. (2002). An evidence-based multidisciplinary protocol for neonatal circumcision pain management. *JOGNN, 31*(4), 403–410.

Groh, B. (2003). Current concepts in pediatric rheumatology. *Current Opinion in Orthopaedics, 14,* 385–391.

Grunau, R. V., Johnston, C. C., & Craig, K. D. (1990). Neonatal facial and cry responses to invasive and non-invasive procedures. *Pain, 42*(3), 295–305.

Gureno, M. A., & Reisinger, C. L. (1991). Patient-controlled analgesia for the young pediatric patient. *Pediatric Nursing, 17*(3), 251–254.

Guthrie, B., Rouster-Stevens, K., & Reynolds, S. (2007). Review of medications used in juvenile rheumatoid arthritis. *Pediatric Emergency Care, 23*(1), 38–46.

Halperin, D. L., Koren, G., Attias, D., Pellegrini, E., Greenberg, M. L., & Wyss, M. (1989). Topical skin anesthesia for venous, subcutaneous drug reservoir and lumbar punctures in children. *Pediatrics, 84,* 281–284.

Hamalainen, M. L., Hoppu, K., & Santavuori, P. R. (1997a). Oral dihydroergotamine for therapy-resistant migraine attacks in children. *Pediatric Neurology, 16,* 114–117.

Hamalainen, M. L., Hoppu, K., & Santavuori, P. R. (1997b). Sumatriptan for migraine attacks in children: A randomized placebo-controlled study. Do children with migraine respond to oral sumatriptan differently from adults? *Neurology, 48,* 1100–1103.

Hamalainen, M. L., Hoppu, K., & Valkeila, E. (1997). Ibuprofen or acetaminophen for the acute treatment of migraine in children: A double-blind, randomized, placebo-controlled, crossover study. *Neurology, 48*(1), 103–107.

Hamunen, K., Maunuksela, E. L., Sarvela, J., Bullingham, S., & Olkkola, K. T. (1999). Stereoselective pharmacokinetics of ketorolac in children, adolescents and adults. *Acta Anaesthesiologica Scandinavia, 43,* 1041–1046.

Hanley, M. A., Jensen, M. P., Smith, D. G., Ehde, D. M., Edwards, W. T., & Robinson, L. R. (2007). Preamputation pain and acute pain predict chronic pain after lower extremity amputation. *Journal of Pain, 8*(2), 102–109.

Harden, R. (2005). Pharmacotherapy of complex regional pain syndrome. *American Journal of Physical Medicine and Rehabilitation, 84,* S17–S28.

Hatfield, L. A., Gusic, M. E., Dyer, A. M., & Polomano, R. C. (2008). Analgesic properties of oral sucrose during routine immunizations at 2 and 4 months of age. *Pediatrics, 121*(2), e327–e334.

Hering-Hanit, R., Cohen, A., & Horev, Z. (2001). Successful withdrawal from analgesic abuse in a group of youngsters with chronic daily headache. *Journal of Child Neurology, 16,* 448–449.

Hermann, C., Kim, M., & Blanchard, E. B. (1995). Behavioral and prophylactic pharmacologic intervention studies of pediatric migraine: An exploratory meta-analysis. *Pain, 60,* 239–255.

Hershey, A., Powers, S., Bentti, A., & deGrauw, T. (2000). Effectiveness of amitriptyline in the prophylactic management of childhood headaches. *Headache, 40,* 539–549.

Hershey, A. D., Winner, P., Kabbouche, M. A., Cladstein, J., Yonker, M., Lewis, D., Pearlman, E., Linder, S.L., Rothner, A.D., & Powers, S.W. (2005). Use of the ICHD-II criteria in the diagnosis of pediatric migraine. *Headache, 45,* 1288–1297.

Hershey, A. D., Winner, P., Kabbouche, M. A., & Powers, S. (2007). Headaches. *Current Opinion in Pediatrics, 19,* 663–669.

Hertzog, J., & Havidich, J. (2007). Non-anesthesiologist-provided pediatric procedural sedation: An update. *Current Opinion in Anesthesiology, 20,* 365–372.

Hester, N. O., Foster, R. L., Jordan-Marsh, M., Ely, E., Vojir, C. P., & Miller, K. L. (1998). Putting pain measurement into clinical practice. In G. A. Finley & P. J. McGrath (Eds.), *Measurement of pain in infants and children* (Vol. 10). Seattle: International Association for the Study of Pain Stress.

Hicks, C. L., von Baeyer, C. L., Spafford, P. A., van Korlaar, I., & Goodenough, B. (2001). The Faces Pain Scale, revised: Toward a common metric in pediatric pain measurement. *Pain, 93*(2), 173–183.

Hocking, G. H., Visser, E. J., Schug, S. A., & Cousins, M. J. (2007). Ketamine in chronic pain: an evidence-based review. *Pain clinical updates, XV*(3), 1–6.

Horbury, C., Henderson, A., & Bromley, B. (2005). Influences of patient behavior on clinical nurses' pain assessment: Implications for continuing education. *Journal of Continuing Education in Nursing, 36*(1), 18–24.

Hurley, A., & Whelan, E. G. (1988). Cognitive development and children's perception of pain. *Pediatric Nursing, 14,* 21–24.

Hurwitz, E. S. (1988). The changing epidemiology of Reye's syndrome in the United States: Further evidence for a public health success. *JAMA, 260,* 3178–3180.

Hyams, J. (2005). Treatment of functional gastrointestinal disorders associated with abdominal pain. *Journal of Pediatric Gastroenterology and Nutrition, 41,* S47–S48.

Hynson, J. L., & South, M. (1999). Childhood hepatotoxicity with paracetamol doses less than 150 mg/kg per day. *Medical Journal of Australia, 171,* 497.

Institute for Safe Medication Practices. (2002). *More on avoiding opiate toxicity with PCA by proxy: Medication safety alert.* Retrieved May 31, 2009, from http://www.ismp.org/newsletters/acutecare/articles/20020529.asp.

Ireland, M., & Olson, M. (2000). Massage therapy and therapeutic touch in children: State of the science. *Alternative Therapies, 6*(5), 54–63.

Jacob, E., McCarthy, K. S., Sambuco, G., & Hockenberry, M. (2008). Intensity, location, and quality of pain in Spanish speaking children with cancer. *Pediatric Nursing, 34*(1), 45–52.

Jacob, E., Miakowski, C., Savedra, M., Beyer, J., Treadwell, M., & Styles, L. (2003). Management of vasoocclusive pain in children with sickle cell disease. *Journal of Pediatric Hematology/Oncology, 25*(4), 307–311.

Jay, S., Elliot, C. H., Fitzgibbons, I., Woody, P., & Siegal, S. (1995). A comparative study of cognitive behavior therapy versus general anesthesia for painful medical procedures in children. *Pain, 62,* 3–9.

Jimenez, N., Bradford, H., Seidel, K. D., Sousa, M., & Lynn, A. M. (2006). A comparison of a needle-free injection system for local anesthesia versus EMLA for intravenous catheter insertion in the pediatric patient. *Anesthesia & Analgesia, 102*(2), 411–414.

Joint Commission. (2008). *Comprehensive accreditation manual for hospitals: Refreshed core.* Retrieved May 31, 2009, from http://www.jointcommission.org.

Joint Commission. (2004). *Patient controlled analgesia by proxy: Sentinel event alert,* Issue 33. Retrieved May 31, 2009, from http://www.jointcommission.org/SentinelEvents/SentinelEventAlert/sea_33.htm.

Jordan-Marsh, M., Yoder, L., Hall, D., & Watson, R. (1994). Alternate Oucher form testing: Gender, ethnicity, and age variations. *Research in Nursing and Health, 17*(2), 111–118.

Kahn, K.A.., & Weisman, S.J.. (2007). Nonpharmacologic pain management strategies in the pediatric emergency department. *Pediatric Emergency Medicine, 8*(4), 240–248.

Kain, Z. N., & Rimar, S. (1995). Management of chronic pain in children. *Pediatrics in Review, 16,* 218–222.

Kashikar-Zuck, S., Goldschneider, K., Powers, S., Vaught, M., & Hershey, A. (2001). Depression and functional disability in chronic pediatric pain. *Clinical Journal of Pain, 17*(4), 341–349.

Kass, F. C., & Holman, J. R. (2001). Oral glucose solution for analgesia in infant circumcision. *Journal of Family Practice, 50*(9), 785–788.

Kemper, K., Sarah, R., Silver-Highfield, E., Xiarhos, E., Barns, L., & Berde, C. (2000). On pins and needles? Pediatric pain patients' experience with acupuncture. *Pediatrics, 105*(4), S941–S947.

Kesler, R. W., Saulsbury, F. T., Miller, L. T., & Rowlingson, J. C. (1988). Reflex sympathetic dystrophy I children: Treatment with transcutaneous electrical nerve stimulation. *Pediatrics, 82,* 728–732.

Killian, J. M., & Fromm, A. H. (1968). Carbamazepine in the treatment of neuralgia. *Archives of Neurology, 19,* 129–136.

Kim, M. K., Strait, R. T., Sato, T. T., & Hennes, H. M. (2002). A randomized clinical trial of analgesia in children with acute abdominal pain. *Academic Emergency Medicine, 9*(4), 281–287.

Kleiber, C., & Harper, D. (1999). Effects of distraction on children's pain and distress during medical procedures: A meta-analysis. *Nursing Research, 48,* 44–49.

Kleiber, C., Sorenson, M., Whiteside, K., Gronstal, B., & Tannous, R. (2002). Topical anesthetics for intravenous insertion in children: A randomized equivalency study. *Pediatrics, 110*(4), 758–761.

Kline, N. E. (2004). *The pediatric chemotherapy and biotherapy curriculum* (pp. 35–61). Glenview, IL: Association of Pediatric Oncology Nurses.

Koren, G. (1993). Use of eutectic mixture of local anesthetics in young children for procedure-related pain. *Journal of Pediatrics, 122,* S30–S35.

Kost, R. G., & Straus, S. E. (1996). Postherpetic neuralgia: Pathogenesis, treatment, and prevention. *New England Journal of Medicine, 335,* 32–42.

Krane, E. J., & Heller, L. B. (1995). The prevalence of phantom sensation and pain in pediatric amputees. *Journal of Pain and Symptom Management, 10,* 21–29.

Krauss, B., & Green, S. M. (2000). Sedation and analgesia for procedures in children. *New England Journal of Medicine, 342*(13), 938–945. Retrieved May 31, 2009, from http://content.nejm.org/cgi/content/short/342/13/938

Krechel, S. W., & Bildner, J. (1995). CRIES: A new neonatal postoperative pain measurement score. Initial testing of validity and reliability. *Pediatric Anaesthesia, 5,* 53–61.

Kuttner, L., & LePage, T. (1989). Faces scales for the assessment of pediatric page: A critical review. *Canadian Journal of Behavioural Science, 21,* 198–209.

Lander, J., Brady-Fryer, B., Metcalfe, J., Nazarali, S., & Muttitt, S. (1997). Comparison of ring block, dorsal penile nerve block, and topical anesthesia for neonatal circumcision. *JAMA, 278,* 2157–2162.

Larsson, B. (1999). Recurrent headaches in children and adolescents. In P. J. McGrath & G. A. Finley (Eds.), *Chronic and recurrent pain in children and adolescents* (pp. 115–140). Seattle: IASP Press.

Larsson, B., & Sund, A. M. (2005). One year incidence, course and outcome predictors of frequent headaches among early adolescents. *Headache, 45,* 684–691.

Lee, B. H., Scharff, L., Sethna, N. F., McCarthy, C.F., Scott-Sutherland, J., Shea, A.M., Sullivan, P., & Berde, C.B. (2002). Physical therapy and cognitive-behavioral treatment for complex regional pain syndrome. *Journal of Pediatrics, 141,* 135–140.

Lewis, D., Ashwal, S., Hershey, A., Hirtz, D., Yonker, M., & Silberstein, S. (2004a). Practice parameter: Pharmacological treatment of migraine headache in children and adolescents. *Neurology, 63,* 2215–2224.

Lewis, D., Diamond, S., Scott, D., & Jones. V. (2004b). Prophylactic treatment of pediatric migraine. *Headache, 44,* 230–237.

Linder, S. L. (1996). Subcutaneous sumatriptan in the clinical setting: The first 50 consecutive patients with acute migraine in a pediatric neurology office practice. *Headache, 36,* 419–422.

Lipton, R. B. (1997). Diagnosis and epidemiology of pediatric migraine. *Current Opinion in Neurology, 10*(3), 231–236.

Little, C. A., Williams, S. E., Puzanovova, M., Rudzinski, E. R., & Walker, L. S. (2007). Multiple somatic symptoms linked to positive screen for depression in pediatric patients with chronic abdominal pain. *Journal of Pediatric Gastroenterology and Nutrition, 44,* 58–62.

Liu, S. S., & Wu, C. L. (2007). The effect of analgesic technique on postoperative patient-reported outcomes including analgesia: A systematic review. *Anesthesia & Analgesia, 105*(3), 789–808.

Logan, D., Guite, J., Sherry, D., & Rose, J. (2006). Adolescent–parent relationships in the context of adolescent chronic pain conditions. *Clinical Journal of Pain, 22*(6), 576–583.

Low, A. K., Ward, K., & Wines, A. P. (2007). Pediatric complex regional pain syndrome. *Journal of Pediatric Orthopedics, 27*(5), 567–572.

Ludvigsson, J. (1974). Propranolol used in prophylaxis of migraine in children. *Acta Neurologica Scandinavia, 50,* 108–115.

Luhmann, J., Hurt, S., Shootman, M., & Kennedy, R. (2004). A comparison of buffered lidocaine versus ELA-Max before peripheral intravenous catheter insertions in children. *Pediatrics, 113*(3), e217–e220.

Lynch, M. (2001). Pain as the fifth vital sign. *Journal of Intravenous Nursing, 24*(2), 85–94.

Macintyre, P. E., & Ready, L. B. (1996). *Acute pain management: A practical guide* (p. 73). London: W. B. Saunders.

Mackie, A. M., Coda, B. C., & Hill, H. F. (1991). Adolescents use patient-controlled analgesia effectively for relief from prolonged oropharyngeal mucositis pain. *Pain, 46,* 265.

Maddox, R. R., Williams, C. K., Oglesby, H., Butler, B., & Colclasure, B. (2006). Clinical experience with patient-controlled analgesia using continuous respiratory monitoring and a smart infusion system. *AJHP, 63*(2),157–164.

Malviya, S., Voepel-Lewis, T., Burke, C., Merkel, S., & Tait, A. R. (2006). The revised FLACC observational pain tool: Improved reliability and validity for pain assessment in children with cognitive impairment. *Pediatric Anesthesia, 16,* 258–265.

Malviya, S., Voepel-Lewis, T., Tait, A. R., Merkel, S., Lauer, A., Munro, H., & Farley, F. (2001). Pain management in children with and without cognitive impairment following spine fusion surgery. *Paediatric Anaesthesia, 11,* 453–458.

Manfredi, P. L., & Houde, R. W. (2003). Prescribing methadone, a unique analgesic. *Journal of Supportive Oncology, 1*(3), 216–220.

Maxwell, L. G., Kaufmann, S. C., Bitzer, S., Jackson, E. V., McGeady, J., Kost-Bylerly, S., Kozlowski, L., Rothman, S. K., & Yaster, M. (2005). The effects of a small-dose naloxone infusion on opioid-induced side effects and analgesia in children and adolescents treated with intravenous patient-controlled analgesia: A double-blind, prospective, randomized, controlled study. *Anesthesia & Analgesia, 100,* 953–958.

McCullough, S., Halton, T., Mowbray, D., & Macfarlan, P. I. (2008). Lingual sucrose reduces the pain response to nasogastric tube insertion: A randomized clinical trial. *Archives of Disease in Childhood: Fetal and Neonatal Edition, 93,* F100–F103.

McGrath, P. (2001). Chronic daily headache in children and adolescents. *Current Pain and Headache Reports, 5*(6), 557–566.

McGrath, P. J., & Craig, K. D. (1989). Developmental and psychological aspects of pain in children. *Pediatric Clinics of North America, 36,* 823–836.

McGrath, P., de Veber, L., & Hearn, M. (1985). Multidimensional pain assessment in children. In H. Fields, R. Dubner, & F. Cervero (Eds.), *Advances in pain research and therapy* (Vol. 9). New York: Raven Press.

McGrath, P. J., Johnson, G., Goodman, J. T., Schillinger, J., Dunn, J., & Chapman, J. (1985). CHEOPS: A behavioral scale for rating postoperative pain in children. *Advances in Pain Research and Therapy, 9,* 395–402.

McKay, W., Morris, R., & Mushlin, P. (1987). Sodium bicarbonate attenuates pain on skin infiltration with lidocaine, with or without epinephrine. *Anesthesia & Analgesia, 66,* 572–574.

McNeely, J. K., & Trentadue, N. C. (1997). Comparison of patient-controlled analgesia with and without nighttime morphine infusion following lower extremity surgery in children. *Journal of Pain and Symptom Management, 13,* 268–273.

McOmber, M. E., & Schulman, R. (2007). Recurrent abdominal pain and irritable bowel syndrome in children. *Current Opinion in Pediatrics, 19,* 581–585.

Mellegers, M., & Furlan, A. (2001). Gabapentin for neuropathic pain: Systematic review of controlled and uncontrolled literature. *Clinical Journal of Pain, 17*(4), 284–295.

Mellick, G. A., & Mellick, L. B. (1995). Gabapentin in the management of reflex sympathetic dystrophy [letter]. *Journal of Pain and Symptom Management, 10,* 265–266.

Merkel, S. I., & Voepel-Lewis, T. (1997). The FACC: A behavioral scale for scoring postoperative pain in young children. *Pediatric Nursing, 23,* 293–297.

Mickkelsson, M., El-Metwally, A., Kautiainen, H., Auvinen, A., Macfarlane, G. J., & Salminen, J. J. (2008). Onset, prognosis and risk factors for widespread pain in schoolchildren: A prospective 4-year follow-up study. *Pain, 138*(3), 681–687.

Miser, A. W., Goh, S., Dose, A. M., O'Fallon, J. R., Niedringhaus, R. D., Betcher, D. L., Simmons, P., MacKellar, D. J., Arnold, M., & Loprinzi, C. L. (1994). Trial of a topically administered local anesthetic (EMLA cream) for pain relief during central venous port accesses in children with cancer. *Journal of Pain and Symptom Management, 9,* 259–264.

Miser, M. W., & Miser, J. S. (1989). The treatment of cancer pain in children. *Pediatric Clinics of North America, 36,* 979–999.

Moffett, B. S., Wann, T. I., Carberry, K. E., & Mott, A. R. (2006). Safety of ketorolac in neonates and infants after cardiac surgery. *Pediatric Anesthesia, 16,* 424–428.

Monitto, C. L., Greenberg, R. S., Kost-Byerly, S., Wetzel, R., Billet, C., Lebet, R. M., & Yaster, M. (2000). The safety and efficacy of parent-/nurse-controlled analgesia in patients less than six years of age. *Anesthesia & Analgesia, 91,* 573–579.

Morash, D., & Fowler, K. (2004). An evidence-based approach to changing practice: Using sucrose for infant analgesia. *Journal of Pediatric Nursing, 19*(5), 366–370.

Morton, N. S., & O'Brien, K. (1999). Analgesic efficacy of paracetamol and diclofenac in children receiving PCA morphine. *British Journal of Anaesthesia, 82*(5), 715–717.

Moseley, G. L., Gallace, A., & Spence, C. (2008). Is mirror therapy all it is cracked up to be? Current evidence and future direction. *Pain, 138,* 7–10.

Nahata, M. C., Clotz, M. A., & Krogg, E. A. (1985). Adverse effects of meperidine, promethazine, and chlorpromazine for sedation in pediatric patients. *Clinical Pediatrics, 24,* 558–560.

National Headache Foundation. (2004). *Special treatment situations: Pediatric migraine, standards of care for headache diagnosis and treatment.* Retrieved May 31, 2009, from http://www.guideline.gov/summary/summary.aspx?ss=15&doc_id=6586&nbr=4146

Nichol, C. F. (1969). A four year double-blind study of Tegretol in facial pain. *Headache, 54,* 54–57.

Oberlander, T. F., O'Donnell, M. E., & Montgomery, C. J. (1999). Pain in children with significant neurological impairment. *Journal of Developmental & Behavioral Pediatrics, 20*(4), 235–243.

Ochsenreither, J. (1996). Better topical anesthetic. *American Journal of Nursing, 96,* 21–22.

Olsson, G. L. (1999). Neuropathic pain in children. In P. J. McGrath & G. A. Finley (Eds.), *Chronic and recurrent pain in children and adolescents* (pp. 75–98). Seattle: IASP Press.

Ozdogan, M., Mustafa, S., Bozcuk, H. S., Aydin, H., Coban, E., & Savas, B. (2004). Venlafaxine for treatment of chemotherapy-induced neuropathic pain. *Turkish Journal of Cancer, 34*(3), 110–113.

Papacci, P., DeFrancisci, G., Iacobucci, T., DeCarolis, M. P., Zecca, E., & Romagnoli, C. (2004). Use of intravenous ketorolac in the neonate and premature babies. *Pediatric Anesthesia, 14,* 487–492.

Pasero, C., Eksterowicz, N., Primeau, M., & Crowley, C. (2007). Registered nurse management and monitoring of analgesia by catheter techniques: Position statement. *Pain Management Nursing, 8*(2), 48–54.

Pasero, C., Portenoy, R.K., McCaffery, M. (1999). Opioid analgesics. In M. McCaffery & C. Pasero (Eds.), Pain: Clinical Manual (2nd Ed.), p. 161-299. Philadelphia: W.B. Saunders.

Penna, A. C., Dawson, K. P., & Penna, C. M. (1993). Is prescribing paracetamol *pro re nata* acceptable? *Journal of Paediatrics and Child Health, 29,* 84–87.

Pizzo, P. A., & Poplack, D. G. (Eds.). (1997). *Principles and practice of pediatric oncology* (pp. 1189–1190). Philadelphia: Lippincott-Raven.

Portenoy, R. K. (1999). Opioid and adjuvant analgesics. In M. Max (Ed.), *Pain 1999: An updated review* (pp. 3–18). Seattle: IASP Press.

Portenoy, R. K., Foley, K., & Inturrisi, C. E. (1990). The nature of opioid responsiveness and its implications for neuropathic pain: New hypotheses derived from studies of opioid infusions. *Pain, 43,* 273–286.

Porter, J., & Jick, J. (1980). Addiction is rare in patients treated with narcotics [letter]. *New England Journal of Medicine, 302,* 123.

Ramchandani, P. G., Stein, A., Hotopf, M., Wiles, N., & the ALSPAC Study Team. (2006). Early parental and child predictors of Recurrent Abdominal Pain

at school age: results of a large population based study . *Journal of American Academy of Child Adolescent Psychiatry, 45*(6), 729–736.

Rasquin, A., DiLorenzo, C., Forbes, D., Guiraldes, E., Hyams, L., Staiano, A., & Walker, L.S. (2006). Childhood functional gastrointestinal disorders: Child/adolescent. *Gastroenterology, 130,* 1527–1537.

Rauck, R. L., Eisenach, J. C., Jackson, K., Young, L. D., & Southern, J. (1993). Epidural clonidine treatment for refractory reflex sympathetic dystrophy. *Anesthesiology, 79,* 1163–1169.

Robins, P., Smith, S., Glutting, J., & Bishop, C. (2005). A randomized controlled trial of a cognitive-behavioral family intervention for pediatric recurrent abdominal pain. *Journal of Pediatric Psychology, 30*(5), 397–408.

Rowbotham, D. J., & Macintyre, P. E. (Eds.). (2003). *Clinical pain management: Acute pain.* London: Arnold.

Savage, S. R., Kirsh, K. L., & Passik, S. D. (2008). Challenges in using opioids to treat pain in persons with substance use disorders. *Addiction Science and Clinical Practice, June,* 4–25.

Schanberg, L. E., Lefebvre, J. C., Keefe, F. J., Kredich, D. W., & Gil, K. M. (1997). Pain coping and the pain experience in children with juvenile chronic arthritis. *Pain, 73,* 181–189.

Schecter, N. L., Berde, C. B., & Yaster, M. (Eds.). (1993). *Pain in infants, children, and adolescents.* Baltimore: Williams & Wilkins.

Schecter, N. L., Berde, C. B., & Yaster, M. (Eds.). (2003). *Pain in infants, children, and adolescents.* Baltimore: Lippincott Williams & Wilkins.

Seefelder, C. (2002). The caudal catheter in neonates: Where are the restrictions? *Current Opinion in Anaesthesiology, 15,* 343–348.

Selman, J. E. (2000). Contemporary diagnosis and management of headache. *Clinical Advisor, June,* 37–46.

Sethna, N. F., Verghese, S. T., Hannallah, R. S., Solodiuk, J. C., Zurakowski, D., & Berde, C. B. (2005). A randomized controlled trial to evaluate s-caine patch for reducing pain associated with the vascular access in children. *Anesthesiology, 102*(2), 403–408.

Sherry, D., Wallas, C., Kelley, C., Kidder, M., & Sapp, L. (1999). Short and long-term outcomes of children with complex regional pain syndrome type I treated with exercise therapy. *Clinical Journal of Pain, 15*(3), 218–223.

Singleton, M. A., Rosen, J. I., & Fisher, D. M. (1987). Plasma concentrations of fentanyl in infants, children, and adults. *Canadian Journal of Anesthesia, 34,* 152–155.

Sloman, R., Wruble, A. W., Rosen, G., & Rom, M. (2006). Determination of clinically meaningful levels of pain reduction in patients experiencing acute postoperative pain. *Pain Management Nursing, 7*(4), 153–158.

Snodgrass, W. R., & Dodge, W. F. (1989). Lytic/DPT cocktail: Time for rational and safe alternatives. *Pediatric Clinics of North America, 36,* 1285–1291.

Solodiuk, J., & Curly, M. A. (2003). Pain assessment in nonverbal children with severe cognitive impairments: The individualized numeric rating scale (INRS). *Journal of Pediatric Nursing, 18*(4), 295–299.

Sparshott, M. M. (1996). The development of a clinical distress scale for ventilated newborn infants: Identification of pain and distress based on validated behavioural scores. *Journal of Neonatal Nursing, 2*(2), 5–11.

Spierings, E. L. (1996). *Management of migraine.* Boston: Butterworth-Heinemann.

Stanton-Hicks, M., Baron, R., Boas, R., Gordh, T., Harden, M., Hendler, N., Kolzenburg, M., Raj, P., & Wilder, R. (1998). Complex regional pain syndromes: Guidelines for therapy. *Clinical Journal of Pain, 14*(2), 155–166.

Sucato, D. J., Duey-Holtz, A., Elerson, E., & Safavi, F. (2005). Postoperative analgesia following surgical correction for adolescent idiopathic scoliosis: A comparison of continuous epidural analgesia and patient-controlled analgesia. *Spine, 30*(2), 211–217.

Taddio, A., Nulman, I., Goldbach, M., Ipp, M., & Koren, G. (1994). Use of lidocaine–prilocaine cream for vaccination pain in infants. *Journal of Pediatrics, 124,* 643–648.

Taddio, A., Shennan, A. T., Stevens, B., Leeder, J.S., Koren, G. (1995). Safety of lidocaine–prilocaine cream in the treatment of preterm neonates. *Journal of Pediatrics, 127*(6), 1002–1005.

Taddio, A., Soin, H. K., Schuh, S., Koren, G., & Scolnik, D. (2005). Liposomal lidocaine to improve procedural success rates and reduce procedural pain among children: A randomized controlled trial. *Canadian Medical Association Journal, 172*(13), 1691–1695.

Taddio, A., Stevens, B., Craig, K., Rastogi, P., & Ben-David, S. (1997). Efficacy and safety of lidocaine–prilocaine cream for pain during circumcision: A randomized clinical trial. *JAMA, 278,* 2157–2162.

Taketomo, C. K., Hodding, J. H., & Kraus, D. M. (2007). *Pediatric dosage handbook.* Hudson, OH: Lexi-Comp.

Tanelian, D. L. (1996). Reflex sympathetic dystrophy: A reevaluation of the literature. *Pain Forum, 5,* 247–256.

Thomson PDR. (2007). *Physician's desk reference* (pp. 2804–2807). Montvale, NJ: Author.

Tobias, J. D. (2005). Sedation and analgesia in the pediatric intensive care unit. *Pediatric Annals, 34*(8), 636–645.

Tomson, T., Tybring, G., Bertilsson, L., Ekbom, K., & Rane, A. (1980). Carbamazepine therapy in trigeminal neuralgia: Clinical effects in relation to plasma concentration. *Archives of Neurology, 37,* 699–703.

Tsui, B., & Berde, C. B. (2005). Caudal analgesia and anesthesia techniques in children. *Current Opinion in Anesthesiology, 18*(3), 283–288.

Tutag, V., Cepeda, E., Frattarelli, D. A., Thomas, R., LaMothe, J., & Aranda, J. V. (2005). Lidocaine 4% cream compared with lidocaine 2.5% and prilocaine 2.5% or dorsal penile nerve block for circumcision. *American Journal of Perinatology, 22*(5), 231–237.

Twycross, A. (1998). Children's cognitive level and perception of pain. *Professional Nurse, 14,* 35–37.

Vetter, T. R., & Heiner, E. J. (1994). Intravenous ketorolac as an adjuvant to pediatric patient-controlled analgesia with morphine. *Journal of Clinical Anesthesia, 6,* 110–113.

Villarruel, A. M., & Denyes, M. J. (1991). Pain assessment in children: Theoretical and empirical validity: *Advances in Nursing Science, 14,* 32–41.

Voepel-Lewis, T., Marinkovic, A., Kostrezewa, A., Tait, A. R., & Malviya, S. (2008). The presence of and risk factors for adverse events in children receiving patient-controlled analgesia by proxy or patient-controlled analgesia after surgery. *Pediatric Anesthesiology, 107*(1), 70–75.

von Baeyer, C. L. (2008). Measurement and assessment of pediatric pain in primary care. In Walco, G. A., & Goldschneider, K. R. (Eds.), *Pain in children: A practical guide for primary care* (pp. 21–27). Totowa, NJ: Humana Press.

Walco, G. A., Varni, J. W., & Ilowite, N. T. (1992). Cognitive-behavioral pain management in children with juvenile rheumatoid arthritis. *Pediatrics, 89,* 1075–1079.

Waldman, S. D. (1998). *Recent advances in the treatment of myofascial pain.* San Antonio, TX: Dannemiller Memorial Educational Foundation.

Walker, L. S. (1999). The evolution of research on recurrent abdominal pain: History, assumptions, and a conceptual model. In P. J. McGrath & G. A. Finley (Eds.), *Chronic and recurrent pain in children and adolescents* (pp. 141–172). Seattle: IASP Press.

Walker, L. S., Smith, C. A., Garber, J., & Claar, R. L. (2007). Appraisal and coping with daily stressors by pediatric patients with chronic abdominal pain. *Journal of Pediatric Psychology, 32,* 206–216.

Weisman, S. J., Bernstein, B., & Schecter, N. L. (1998). Consequences of inadequate analgesia during painful procedures in children. *Archives of Pediatric and Adolescent Medicine, 152,* 147–149.

Weydert, J. A., Shapiro, D. E., Acra, S. A., Monheim, C.J., Chambers, A.S., & Ball, T.M. (2006). Evaluation of guided imagery as treatment for recurrent abdominal pain in children: A randomized controlled trial. *BMC Pediatrics, November 8,6*:29

Wiendels, N., van der Geest, M., Neven, A., Ferrari, M., & Laan, L. (2005). Chronic daily headache in children and adolescents. *Headache, 45,* 678–683.

Wilder, R. T. (1996). Reflex sympathetic dystrophy in children and adolescents: Differences from adults. In W. Janig & M. Stanton-Hicks (Eds.), *Reflex sympathetic dystrophy: A reappraisal* (pp. 67–75). Seattle: IASP Press.

Wilder, R. T. (2006). Management of pediatric patients with complex regional pain syndrome. *Clinical Journal of Pain, 22*(5), 443–448.

Wilder, R. T., Berder, C. B., Wolohan, M., Vieyra, M. A., Masek, B. J., & Micheli, L. J. (1992). Reflex sympathetic dystrophy in children. *Journal of Bone and Joint Surgery, American Volume, 74,* 910–919.

Wilkins, K. L., McGrath, P. J., Finley, G. A., & Katz, J. (1998). Phantom limb sensations and phantom limb pain in children and adolescent amputees. *Pain, 78,* 7–12.

Winner, P. (2008). Pediatric headache. *Current Opinions in Neurology, 21,* 316–332.

Winner, P., Rothner, A., Saper, J., Nett, R., Asgharnejad, M., & Laurenza, A. (2000). A randomized double-blind, placebo-controlled study of sumatriptan nasal spray in the treatment of acute migraine in adolescents. *Pediatrics, 106,* 989–997.

Wolfe, F., Smythe, H. A., Yunus, M. B. Bennett, R. M., Bombardier, C., Goldenberg, D. L., Tugwell, P., Campbell, S. M., Abeles, M., Clark, P., Fam, A. G., Farber, S. J., Fiechtner, J. J., Franklin, C. M., Gattner, R. A., Hamaty, D., Lessard, J., Lichtbroun, A. S., Masi, A. T., McCain, G. A., Reynolds, W. J., Romano, T. J., Russell, I. J., & Sheon, R. P. (1990). The American College of Rheumatology criteria for the classification of fibromyalgia: Report of the multicenter criteria committee. *Arthritis and Rheumatism, 33,* 160–172.

Wong, D. L., & Baker, C. M. (1988). Pain in children: Comparison of assessment scales. *Pediatric Nursing, 14,* 9–17.

Wong, D., & Baker, C. (1999). *Reference manual for the Wong-Baker Faces Pain Rating Scale.* Tulsa, OK: Wong & Baker.

Wong, D. L., & Hess, C. S. (2000). *Wong and Whaley's clinical manual of pediatric nursing* (5th ed.). St. Louis: Mosby.

Wong, D., & Pasero, C. L. (1997). Pain control: Reducing the pain of lidocaine. *American Journal of Nursing, 97,* 17–18.

World Health Organization. (1998). *Cancer pain relief and palliative care in children* (pp. 24–53). Geneva: Author.

Wu, C. L., & Raja, S. (2008). An update on the treatment of postherpetic neuralgia. *Journal of Pain, 9*(1), S19–S30.

Wuhrman, E., Cooney, M. F., Dunwoody, C. J., Eksterowicz, N., Merkel, S., & Oakes, L. L. (2007). Authorized and unauthorized ("PCA by proxy") dosing of analgesic infusion pumps: Position statement with clinical practice recommendations. *Pain Management Nursing, 8*(1), 4–11.

Yaster, M., Krane, E. J., Kaplan, R. F., Cote, C. J., & Lappe, D. G. (1997). *Pediatric pain management and sedation handbook.* St. Louis: Mosby.

Young, K. (2005). Pediatric procedural pain. *Annals of Emergency Medicine, 45*(2), 160–171.

Youssef, N. N., Rosh, J. R., Loughran, M., Schuckalo, S. G., Cotter, A. N., Verga, B. G., & Mones, R. L. (2004). Treatment of functional abdominal pain in children with cognitive behavioral strategies. *Journal of Pediatric Gastroenterology and Nutrition, 39*(2), 192–196.

Zagaria, M. E. (2008). Unintentional acetaminophen overdose. *American Journal for Nurse Practitioners, 12*(6), 47–51.

Zeltzer, L. (2004). Phase I study on the feasibility and acceptability of an acupuncture/hypnosis intervention for chronic pediatric pain. *Journal of Pain and Symptom Management, 24*(4), 437–446.

Zeltzer, L. K., Altman, A., Cohen, D., & Lebaron, S. (1990). Report of the Subcommittee on the Management of Pain Associated with Procedures in Children. American Academy of Pediatrics. *Pediatrics, 86,* 828–829.

Zempsky, W. T. (2008). Pharmacologic approaches for reducing venous access pain in children. *Pediatrics, 122 Suppl 3, S140-153.*

Suggested Readings

Acute Pain Management Guideline Panel. (1992). *Acute pain management in infants, children, and adolescents: Operative and medical procedures.* Quick Reference Guide for Clinicians. (AHCPR Publication No. 92-002). Rockville, MD: Agency for Health Care Policy and Research, Public Health Service, U.S. Department of Health and Human Services.

American Pain Society. (1999). *Guideline for the management of acute and chronic pain in sickle cell disease.* Glenview, IL: Author.

Coventry, D. M., Martin, C. S., & Burke, A. M. (1991). Sedation for pediatric computerized tomography: A double-blind assessment of rectal midazolam. *European Journal of Anesthesiology, 8,* 29–32.McGrath, P. J., & Finley, G. A. (Eds.). (1999). *Chronic and recurrent pain in children and adolescents.* Seattle: IASP Press.

Graff-Radford, S. B., Reeves, J. L., Baker, R. L., & Chiu, D. (1989). Effects of transcutaneous electrical stimulation on myofascial pain and trigger point sensitivity. *Pain, 37,* 1–5..

Merkel, S. I., Voepel-Lewis, T., Shayevitz, J. R., & Malviya, S. (1997). The FLACC: A behavioral scale for scoring postoperative pain in young children. *Pediatric Nursing, 23,* 293–297.

Ridings, H. & Amaya, M. (2007). Male neonatal circumcision: An evidence-based review. *Journal of the American Academy of Physician Assistants, 20*(2), 32–36.

Spear, R. M., Yaster, M., Berkowitz, M. B., Maxwell, L. G., Bender, K. S., Naclerio, R., Manolio, T. A., & Nichols, D. G. (1991). Preinduction of anesthesia in children with rectally administered midazolam. *Anesthesiology, 74,* 670–674.

appendix

20-1

Authorized and Unauthorized ("PCA by Proxy") Dosing of Analgesic Infusion Pumps

Position Statement

The ASPMN recognizes the need for prompt, safe, and effective pain relief for all and supports the use of AACA for the patient who is unable to self-administer analgesics using an analgesic infusion pump. The ASPMN does not support the use of "PCA by proxy" in which an unauthorized person activates the dosing mechanism of an analgesic infusion pump and delivers analgesic medication to the patient, thereby increasing the risk for potential patient harm.

The ASPMN further delineates that support for AACA is contingent upon a health care agency having in place clear guidelines outlining the conditions under which such practice may be implemented, including monitoring procedures that will insure safe use of the therapy.

Ethical Tenets

The ethical principles of beneficence (the duty to benefit another) and nonmaleficence (the duty to do no harm) oblige health care professionals to provide pain management and comfort to all patients, including those individuals who are vulnerable to the undertreatment of pain, unable to speak for themselves, and lack the ability to self-administer medications. In situations in which a person is unable to self-administer analgesics due to cognitive or physical limitations, a consistent care provider can be educated to assist or to administer analgesics.

Providing quality and comparable pain management to individuals who cannot self-administer analgesics is directed by the principle of justice (the equal or comparative treatment of individuals). Respect for human dignity, the first principle in the Code of Ethics for Nurses (ANA, 2001), directs nurses to provide and advocate for humane and appropriate care whether that care is for restoration of health, alleviation of suffering, or supportive care at the end of life. When analgesics are administered to alleviate suffering and to provide comfort at the end of life, the principle of "double effect" may occur. Double effect occurs when treatment may have the effect of both relieving suffering and hastening death (double effect). If an action, such as AACA, were to cause death at the end of life, provided the primary intention is to relieve pain and not to cause death, then, although the possibility of death can be foreseen, the action is ethically and legally correct and the authorized agent may feel comfortable. Most importantly, there must be a sense of proportionality between the pain and suffering and the action).

Patient safety and patient rights are considered in the third principle of the Code of Ethics for Nurses (ANA, 2001). The development of practice standards, policies, and guidelines that promote

Wuhrman, E., Cooney, M. F., Dunwoody, C. J., Eksterowicz, N., Merkel, S., & Oakes, L. L. (2007). Authorized and unauthorized ("PCA by proxy") dosing of analgesic infusion pumps: Position statement with clinical practice recommendations. *Pain Management Nursing, 8*(1), 4–11.

safety emphasize this principle, as well as the principle of nonmaleficence. Based on the principle of justice, this care is given with compassion and unrestricted by consideration of personal attributes, economic status, or the nature of the health problem.

Definitions

PCA is a method of pain control designed to allow *the patient* to administer preset doses of an analgesic on demand (APS, 2003). Although the medications may be delivered via any route, for the purpose of this position statement, the term refers to medications that are administered using an analgesic infusion pump.

An *analgesic infusion pump* (often referred to as *PCA pump*) is an electronic microprocessing machine that can be programmed to deliver a prescribed amount of medication on demand, at specified intervals, by activation (pressing) of a button. It also has the programming options to deliver patient boluses with a continuous infusion or a continuous infusion without patient boluses (thus contradicting the term *PCA pump*). It can also be used to deliver supplemental clinician "boluses" or "loading" doses of medication.

PCA by proxy is a term that describes activation of the analgesic infusion pump by *anyone other than the patient.* The term denotes various practices and has been used to describe both authorized (approved) and unauthorized activation of the device. In this position statement, the term describes unauthorized activation of the pump that the prescriber intended for PCA.

Authorized agent controlled analgesia (AACA) is a method of pain control in which a consistently available and competent individual is authorized by a prescriber and properly educated to activate the dosing button of an analgesic infusion pump when a patient is unable in response to that patient's pain. The following variants are common:

- *Nurse-controlled analgesia (NCA):* The authorized agent is the nurse responsible for the patient.
- *Caregiver-controlled analgesia (CCA):* The authorized agent is a nonprofessional individual (e.g., parent or significant other).

Background

I. PCA

PCA, which was first introduced in the 1970s (Forest, Smethhurst, & Kienitz, 1970; Sechzer, 1971), is a method of pain control designed to allow a patient to self-administer a dose of an analgesic, usually an opioid, within a prescribed time interval. The patient is able to self-administer these analgesic doses by activating the pump's dosing button. This method of analgesia allows the patient to find an acceptable balance between analgesia and side effects. PCA also affords patients the ability to treat pain safely in a timely and individualized manner.

PCA is considered a common pain management technique in today's health care arena. In many hospitals, it is a common modality for postoperative pain management (Ballantyne & Ryder, 2002). It has proven to be both safe and efficacious in adults, adolescents, and children (Allagretta, 2005; Anghelescu, Burgoyne, Oakes, & Wallace, 2005; Macintyre, 2001) when candidates are chosen appropriately. Many studies have also shown a patient preference for this method of analgesia over traditional intermittent injections (Macintyre, 2001).

A fundamental safeguard of PCA is the fact that excessively sedated patients are usually too sedated to activate the dosing button, thereby preventing delivery of further opioid and subsequent clinically significant opioid-induced respiratory depression (Ballantyne et al., 2002; Pasero & McCaffery, 2005). This safety feature, coupled with careful patient selection, promotes patient safety. Candidates for PCA should be evaluated for cognitive and physical ability to activate the dosing button. The patient must understand the relationships among pain, pressing (activating) the analgesic infusion pump dosing button, and the goal of pain relief (Pasero & McCaffery, 2005). Therefore, patients who are confused or have other cognitive limitations are not appropriate candidates for PCA therapy. Generally, children less than 5 years old do not have the developmental capacity to understand the relationship between pressing the dosing button and achieving pain relief (APS, 2003). However, children as young as 5 years may successfully use PCA (Yaster & Krane, 1997).

II. PCA by Proxy versus AACA: Clarifying the Issue

The term *PCA by proxy* has been used to describe both unsafe and safe pain management practices. It has been used to describe the unsafe practice whereby an unauthorized person activates the analgesic dosing button for a patient who is receiving PCA. The term has also been used to describe AACA, which is considered a safe and effective therapy. It is, therefore, necessary to clearly differentiate between these unsafe and safe practices.

One method to assist in this clarification is to use terminology that more accurately reflects the desired practice. See, under the Definitions section, the terms authorized agent controlled analgesia (AACA), nurse controlled analgesia (NCA) and caregiver controlled analgesia (CCA). Other terms that clearly define an individual who has been identified as the person responsible for activating the dosing button include designated agent and identified agent.

For this appendix, the terms AACA, NCA, CCA, and authorized agent are used.

III. Authorized-Agent Controlled Analgesia

Use of authorized agents to activate the dosing button on an analgesic infusion pump has been described since the early 1990s (Pasero & McCaffery, 1993). According to Pasero, Portenoy, and McCaffery (1999, p. 177), when discussing authorized agent dosing, "ways have been found to use PCA technology safely and effectively, such as family-controlled analgesia and nurse activated dosing." In addition, two studies, published in 1991 and 1993, demonstrated the efficacy and safety of NCA and family-controlled analgesia (Allegretta, 2005; Gureno & Reisinger, 1991; Weldon, Connor, & White, 1993).

In 2005, a voluntary, unpublished survey of the American Pain Society Nurses Special Interest Group (SIG) yielded the following results: 16 of 34 (47%) respondents reported that their hospital policies allowed nurse-activated dosing of analgesic infusion pumps in specific situations, and 9 of 34 respondents (26%) allowed some form of caregiver-activated dosing.

Expert practice and recent studies indicate that, under certain circumstances in which the patient and the authorized agent are carefully chosen and educated, AACA is a safe and effective means of providing analgesia to patients who are unable to provide it for themselves (Anghelescu et al., 2005; Berde & Solodiuk, 2003; Lehr & BeVier, 2003; Monitto et al., 2000; Pasero & McCaffery, 2005; Petterson, Kindskog, & Owall, 2000; Taylor, Voytovitch, & Kozol, 2003). The Society of Critical Care Medicine and the American Society of Health-System Pharmacists report that analgesic infusion (PCA) pumps can be used appropriately for nurse controlled analgesia (NCA) (Jacobi et al., 2002).

AACA is not a new concept. Nursing has a long history of providing medications to patients who cannot medicate themselves (Pasero et al., 1999). Advances in technology have allowed the use of an analgesic infusion pump to improve on this traditional practice. Furthermore, the feasibility of AACA, with the nonprofessional caregiver as the authorized agent (CCA), is supported by families that have been successfully taught to provide highly technological care, such as home infusion therapy (Cox & Oakes, 2005), and to provide complicated medical therapies, such as pain management, for adults and children (Beyer & Simmons, 2004). One study showed that parents could manage their child's pain in the home if provided with appropriate information and suitable analgesia upon discharge from day surgery (Jonas, 2003).

IV. Danger of Unauthorized Activation of the Dosing Button

As discussed, an inherent safety feature of PCA is that a patient must be awake to self-administer a dose of medication. The sedated or sleeping patient usually does not press the button, consequently avoiding an overdose. However, unauthorized activation of the dosing button during PCA by someone other than the patient (a loved one, friend, or even health care provider) can have significant deleterious effects. Reports in the literature (Pasero & McCaffery, 2005), as well as sentinel event alerts (Joint Commission, 2004; Nurse Advise, 2005a, 2005b), clearly indicate the potential danger of such unauthorized practice.

These warnings should not go unheeded. They underscore the need for education and instructions to health professionals and laypeople about the potentially life-threatening risks of unauthorized dosing.

V. Advantages of AACA

AACA offers numerous advantages over traditional nurse-administered, or other caregiver, intermittent dosing. It reduces the potential for various medication administration errors and delays in administering analgesia. In addition, it affords a closed system for the infusion of medication, thereby decreasing risk of infection to entry sites (e.g., intravenous). It also offers the financial benefits of "reducing waste created by partially used opioid doses and supplies such as syringes and can also save nursing time" (Noah, 2003, p. 17).

Perhaps the greatest advantage of authorized-agent dosing via a pump is the proximity of the medication to the patient. This results in ease of dose administration and titration and more prompt management of incident pain. AACA enables a patient to receive timely, effective opioid analgesia without loss of dignity, periods of uncontrolled pain, or the high side-effect burden (e.g., sedation or vomiting) that is more likely when other methods are used.

Recommendations

The health care agency will do the following:

- The health care agency will ensure the implementation of procedures developed with input of physicians, nurses, pharmacists, risk managers, and other appropriate personnel. These procedures shall outline the parameters of AACA use, including the following:
  - Guidelines promoting safe and effective management of pain, including frequency of sedation and respiratory status checks during therapy

Note: When providing and advocating for humane and supportive care along the entire health care continuum, the prescription and delivery of AACA must be patient specific. Otherwise, some safeguards normally used in the delivery of both PCA and AACA would only limit appropriate care to patients who are critically or terminally ill, who may be unresponsive, who are at the end of life, or who fit a combination of these descriptions. Parameters that would, under normal circumstances, preclude activating the dosing button, such as unresponsiveness or a slow respiratory rate, may require adjustment in certain circumstances. In the hospice setting especially, the doctrine of "double effect" needs to be both considered and discussed with the family and authorized agent or agents.

  - The stipulation that AACA will be administered only in settings where staff are already familiar with the use of PCA and other analgesic infusion therapies
  - The limitation of AACA to only patients who, because of cognitive or physical limitations, cannot safely self-administer analgesic doses via an analgesic infusion pump
  - The provision of a mechanism to readily communicate to all health care providers caring for the patient that the patient is receiving AACA, such as chart, bed, or analgesic infusion pump or button label or sign
  - The stipulation that the nonprofessional caregiver authorized agent or agents shall be an adult or adults who
    - Are consistently with the patient
    - Are willing and able to learn to provide AACA
    - Demonstrate the ability to perform the responsibilities as detailed in the later section labeled "Caregivers will"
  - The need to limit the number of authorized agents to one *at a given time;* alternative authorized agents may be designated to provide respite, coverage, or both
  - Provision of a prescribing mechanism specifically designed for AACA, such as a preprinted AACA order set

- When PCA or AACA is to be administered, the health care agency will provide educational materials for patients and families regarding the principles of PCA and the negative consequences of unauthorized activation of the analgesic infusion pump dosing button.
- When AACA is to be administered, the agency will provide educational materials for each authorized agent regarding the requirements of being an authorized agent and the policies and procedures that must be followed when AACA is used.
- The health care agency will provide a means for nurses and other staff members to record the following:
  - Identity of the authorized agent or agents
  - Caregiver authorized agent education and feedback
  - Amount of medication given over a specified period
  - Assessment and reassessment of effectiveness of therapy
- The agency will provide ongoing education for all patient-care staff, specifically emphasizing
  - The dangers of unauthorized caregiver doses.
  - The need to follow the institution's policy and procedure for AACA.
- The health care agency will assure that use of AACA (especially in the case of CCA) does not preclude appropriate nursing observation, assessment, and management customary for other patients receiving analgesic infusion therapies.
- It will provide ongoing evaluation of outcomes regarding AACA (e.g., quality improvement activities, trends in incident reports, adverse events, and medication errors), including
  - Appropriateness of AACA orders.
  - Documentation of caregiver education.
  - Adverse events related to AACA.
  - Interventions in response to the above.

Prescribers will do the following:

- Prescribers will collaborate with the nursing staff regarding the need for AACA, considering
  - The anticipated course of illness and associated pain requiring the need for opioid analgesia.
  - The need for prompt management of incident-related pain (e.g., need for immediate opioids for dressing changes, repositioning in bed, or ambulation).
- They will prescribe PCA if and as soon as the patient is able to self-administer analgesia.
- Prescribers will follow established policy for the care of patients receiving PCA and AACA.

Nurses will do the following:

- Nurses will follow established policy for the care of patients receiving PCA and AACA.
- They will educate patients, family members, and other visitors about the purpose and proper use of analgesic pumps, including pump safety features and the dangers of unauthorized activation of the dosing button.
- They will participate in the selection of authorized agents by assessing the willingness and abilities of the patient's caregiver or significant other to understand AACA and follow instructions.
- Nurses will provide and document that the authorized agent has received, reviewed, and applied verbal and written instructions, which include the following:
  - How to recognize specific patient behaviors or circumstances that may indicate the need for analgesia
  - How to activate the analgesic dosing button
  - How to recognize *patient-specific* indicators that would preclude activating the dosing button at a given time (e.g., sedation, shallow or irregular respirations); such indicators require definition by prescription for each particular patient
  - The appropriate actions to take in the event of pump malfunction, unrelieved pain, excessive side effects or other such medical emergencies, and any other conditions the health care agency or particular prescriber specifies
  - Information that activation of the dosing button should only occur if the patient is awake and the patient's words or behaviors indicate to the authorized agent that the patient is in pain or pain is

anticipated (incidental pain) *unless otherwise specified by the prescriber, such as in the case of the unresponsive or end-of-life patient*

- When *not* to activate the dosing button, such as
  - For purposes other than pain relief (e.g., not for the purposes of having the patient sleep or to become less anxious)
  - While the patient is sleeping
  - If the patient cannot be readily awakened to baseline
  - If the patient is having abnormal breathing, as defined by prescriber (shallow, slow, or noisy)
- How to recognize pain, sedation, and respiratory depression
- What to do if an emergency situation arises (e.g., stimulates the patient, notify nurse, or call 911 in the home setting) (include emergency numbers as appropriate)

- The nurse will continually assess the ability of the caregiver to provide AACA. If the nurse has any concerns regarding a caregiver's ability to administer AACA, the nurse must stop the caregiver from activating any further doses, inform the prescriber of the situation, and obtain an order for an alternative means of pain relief.
- The nurse will provide a complete report of the patient's tolerance of AACA, including the authorized agent's performance, when the care of the patient is being transferred to another nurse.
- Nurses will communicate to all other health care providers that the patient is receiving AACA (e.g., chart, bed, or analgesic infusion pump or button label or sign).

Caregivers will do the following:

- Caregivers will actively participate in learning the principles of PCA and AACA and verbalize an understanding of the need to provide AACA safely and effectively through the following:
  - Recognition of the need to activate the dosing button for the responsive patient only when the patient is awake and the patient's words or behaviors indicate the presence of pain and need for analgesia
  - Recognition of other situations in which the prescriber has authorized the activation of the dosing button for purposes such as incident-related pain
  - In the unresponsive and end-of-life patient, under what circumstances activation of the dosing button should occur
  - Knowledge of how and when to alert staff if there are any concerns about AACA, including the patient's pain, level of sedation, respiratory status, or any opioid-induced side effects
  - Knowledge that it is necessary to inform other family members and visitors who are *not* designated as authorized agents for the patient that they cannot activate the dosing button even in the absence of the authorized agent
  - Knowledge that only a designated health care provider may educate an authorized agent; that one nonprofessional caregiver authorized agent may *not* educate another authorized agent
  - Knowledge of when not to activate the dosing button, such as if the patient is asleep, does not awaken easily, has a depressed respiratory rate (as defined by prescriber for each individual patient), or for any reason other than pain relief (e.g., sleep or anxiety), *unless otherwise ordered by the prescriber*
  - Agreement not to attempt any reprogramming of the analgesic infusion pump or otherwise violate the infusion system's integrity

Summary

A primary goal of the ASPMN is to provide prompt, safe, and effective pain management to all individuals with pain. To that end, the organization supports the use of AACA in various patient care settings where patients are unable to self-administer analgesia. This position statement describes criteria for the use of AACA, guidelines for selection and education of the authorized agent, key prescription and monitoring recommendations during therapy, and quality improvement activities to insure safety and effectiveness.

appendix

20-2

ASPMN Position Statement on Neonatal Circumcision Pain Relief

The American Society of Pain Management Nurses (ASPMN) believes that neonates who are being circumcised should receive an anesthetic for the procedure.

Definition:

Neonatal circumcision involves the amputation of the foreskin. This procedure causes tissue damage and, therefore, is a painful procedure.

Background:

Pain is defined by the International Association for the Study of Pain as "An unpleasant sensory and emotional experience associated with actual or potential tissue damage, or described in terms of such damage" (IASP, 1979). Neonates have the anatomic and functional ability to experience pain at birth, even when their birth is premature (Anand & Hickey, 1987). Neonates are equally as sensitive to pain as older children and adults (Anand, 1995). Premature neonates have poorly-developed inhibitory mechanisms for pain, which may make them more sensitive to painful stimuli. While neonates are unable to provide a subjective report of pain intensity, healthcare providers can infer pain from the neonate's behavioral and physiologic response to noxious stimuli. Unrelieved pain during circumcision can result in adverse physiologic stress responses (such as breath holding, apnea, cyanosis, gagging, and vomiting) which are potentially dangerous to the neonate. Neonates cannot advocate for their own pain relief and are, therefore, a vulnerable population dependent on healthcare providers to recognize and manage their pain.

While scientific evidence demonstrates potential medical benefits of circumcising male neonates, the American Academy of Pediatrics no longer recommends routine neonatal circumcision (AAP, 1999). Yet, parents continue to request the procedure for religious and cultural reasons. Neonatal circumcision is commonly performed without anesthesia. When circumcision is performed after the neonatal period, general anesthesia is often used. This would suggest that an anesthetic is also appropriate for the pain of the procedure in neonates.

Ethical Tenets:

The ethical principle of beneficence—the duty to benefit another—obliges healthcare professionals to manage pain and provide humane care (Agency for Healthcare Policy and Research [AHCPR], 1992). Anaesthetized circumcision violates the ethical principle of non-malfeasance which is the duty to do no harm.

Adapted from American Society for Pain Management Nursing (2001). *ASPMN position statement: Neonatal circumcision pain relief.* Pensacola, FL: Author.

Recommendations:

ASPMN recognizes that neonatal circumcision is a painful procedure. The Society recognizes that the neonate has a right to an anesthetic to prevent the pain of the procedure. Therefore, as healthcare providers, we are obligated to provide an appropriate anesthetic for neonatal circumcision

Summary:

The American Society of Pain Management Nurses opposes the participation of nurses and other healthcare professionals in the performance of male neonatal circumcision without an anesthetic to treat the pain inherent in the procedure.

Research suggests that the following interventions are appropriate:

Anesthetic Techniques:

- A subcutaneous ring block prevents crying and increases in heart rate better than EMLA or a dorsal penile nerve block.
- A dorsal penile nerve block is effective in reducing the behavioral and physiologic indicators of pain throughout all stages of neonatal circumcision.
- EMLA, when applied for 60–90 minutes prior to neonatal circumcision, shortens cry time and results in smaller heart rate increases when compared to placebo. The anesthetic is insufficient in alleviating pain during phases of the procedure that are associated with extensive tissue trauma such as during lysis of adhesions and tightening of the clamp (American Academy of Pediatrics, 1999)

Comfort Techniques:

- In addition to an anesthetic, the awake neonate should be comforted during the procedure.
- Sucrose pacifiers decrease crying during circumcision.
- Positioning the infant is a semi-recumbent position on a padded surface decreases distress during the procedure.

Post-procedural Pain Control:

The neonate will experience post-procedural pain when the anesthetic wears off. Analgesics should be provided to treat this post-procedural discomfort. Ideally, the first dose should be administered before the post-procedural pain begins.

References

American Academy of Pediatrics Task Force on Circumcision. (1999). Circumcision policy statement. *Pediatrics, 103*(3), 686–693.

Agency for Healthcare Policy and Research. (1992). Acute pain management: Operative or medical procedures and trauma. Clinical practice guideline AHCPR Pub No. 92–0032. Rockville, MD: Author.

Anand, K.J.S. (1995). Analgesia and sedation in ventilated neonates. Neonatal Respiratory Disease, 5, 1–11.

Anand, K.J.S., & Hickey, P.R. (1987). Pain and its effects in the human neonate and fetus. *New England Journal of Medicine*, 317,1321.

International Association for the Study of Pain. (1979). Pain terms: A list with definitions and notes on usage. Pain, 6, 249.

chapter

21

Palliative Care

Patrick J. Coyne, MSN, APRN, ACHPN, FAAN, FPCN
Barton T. Bobb, MSN, FNP-BC, ACHPN
Debra J. Drew, MS, RN-BC, ACNS-BC

Objectives

After studying this chapter, the reader should be able to:

1. Compare and contrast the models of hospice care, palliative care, and curative care.
2. Distinguish the concepts of pain and suffering.
3. Identify the most common symptoms associated with end of life.

I. Introduction

A. *Palliative care* is a broad term that describes a model of care for the ill. It is the foundation of the hospice movement, but it is not the same as hospice.

B. *Hospice* in the United States is an established Medicare benefit and is a highly regulated program.

C. Armed with knowledge of pain management techniques and symptom control, the pain management nurse is well positioned to participate in the continuum of care of patients with life-limiting disease.

D. Because the course of some diseases makes it difficult to determine when the patient has entered the final stages of the disease, pain management nurses can provide palliative care to patients at any stage of their disease.

II. Definition

A. Palliative care specializes in the relief of the symptoms and stress of serious illness and pain relief. The goal is to improve quality of life for patients and their families. Palliative care is appropriate at any point in an illness. It can be provided at the same time as curative treatment. Palliative care programs are growing in response to patient need. They provide for assessment and treatment of pain and other symptoms; help with patient-centered communications and decision making; and coordinate care across the continuum of care settings (Center to Advance Palliative Care, 2008).

B. Palliative care
   1. Affirms life and regards dying as a normal process.
   2. Neither hastens nor postpones death.
   3. Provides relief from pain and other distressing symptoms.
   4. Integrates the psychological and the spiritual aspects of patient care.
   5. Offers a support system to help patients live as actively as possible until death.
   6. Offers a support system to help the family cope during the patient's illness and in their own bereavement.

C. Hospice care
   1. The focus of hospice care is the patient and family (loosely defined to include relatives, friends, neighbors, or extended family).
   2. The care team includes nurses, physicians, social workers, spiritual caregivers, grief counselors, home health aides, other therapists, and volunteers.
   3. Hospice services are paid for by Medicare, Medicaid, some commercial insurances, and private resources.
      a. Eligibility usually requires a physician and hospice medical director to certify that the patient has terminal illness with a life expectancy of 6 months or less.
      b. Medicare Hospice Benefit (Part A) pays for
         (1) Physician services.
         (2) Nursing care in the home.
         (3) Social work services.
         (4) Chaplain services.
         (5) Medical equipment and supplies.
         (6) Medications for pain and symptom relief.
         (7) Short-term inpatient care.
         (8) Respite care to give the family a rest.
         (9) Physical therapy, occupational therapy, speech therapy, home health aid, homemaker services, and dietary services.
         (10) Bereavement services for approximately 1 year after the death.
      c. Volunteers are essential members of the hospice team.

III. History

A. Earliest hospices
   1. The earliest recorded hospice dates back to AD 475 in Rome. It was established by Christians to aid travelers and pilgrims. It offered a place of refuge from the perils of travel. Clean water, food, and a place to rest were welcomed by the weary traveler.

2. During the Middle Ages, religious orders established a network of hospices. These hospices eventually came to be known as places for spiritual renewal and a source of comfort for the dying.

B. Modern hospices (National Hospice and Palliative Care Organization, 2008)
   1. The modern concept of hospice began in 1879 in Dublin, Ireland, with the founding by Sister Mary Aikenhead of Our Lady's Hospice for the Dying.
   2. In 1905, the Irish sisters founded another hospice called St. Joseph's. It was there that Dame Cicely Saunders developed her principles of modern hospice and palliative medicine.
   3. In 1967, Saunders opened St. Christopher's Hospice in London.
   4. Educated as a nurse, social worker, and physician, Saunders embraced the concept of interdisciplinary teams as essential for the care of the dying.

C. Hospice movement in the United States
   1. Hospice originated as an alternative to the perceived medicalization and institutionalization of dying and death. The first hospice in the United States opened in 1974 in New Haven, Connecticut.
   2. Elisabeth Kübler-Ross (1969) observed and interviewed patients at the University of Chicago Medical Center then described stages of grief (denial, anger, bargaining, depression, and acceptance). Patients do not predictably progress through these stages; rather, the process is complex and dynamic.
   3. "Palliative medicine came into existence because a purely biologic model of illness and therapy distorted the priorities of care for patients with chronic, ultimately fatal illnesses and often failed to relieve patient—family suffering" (MacDonald, 1993, p. 197).

D. Reaction to medicalization of death
   1. Paradigm shift
      a. The earliest proponents of hospice viewed medical science with cynicism and distrust.
      b. Therapies such as chemotherapy and radiation were thought to be incompatible with the goals of hospice. Intravenous fluids and medications were discouraged.
      c. In the 1980s and 1990s, the science and art of palliative care matured from those pioneering days. Particular interventions no longer are rejected as inappropriate for palliative care measures.
      d. "There are few, if any, technical procedures unique to palliative care. Impeccable understanding of drug use is stressed, the care of the family as well as the patient is emphasized, as are an interdisciplinary approach to care, the development of communication skills, and attention to the needs of dying patients" (MacDonald, 1993, p. 197).

E. Medicare hospice benefit (Connor, 2007–2008)
   1. In 1982, the United States established the Medicare Hospice Benefit, which became effective on November 1, 1983. This system provided money and created more regulations for hospices.
   2. The understanding of the term ***hospice*** has become more complex.
      a. For some, the term is understood as the program of providing services.
      b. For others, the term is synonymous with a palliative philosophy and quality-of-life focus.
      c. For others, the word connotes imminent death and giving in to the inevitable.
   3. Many patients and their families have a hard time making the perceived change from curative therapies to palliative measures. The course of some diseases is unpredictable, and it is difficult to determine when the end stage actually begins.
   4. Providers of hospice and palliative care would like to shift the culture's notion that hospice or palliative care is the opposite of curative care. Instead, it is a more integrated approach in which palliative services are provided along a continuum of an individual's life-limiting disease. This would accurately reflect patients' experiences.

IV. Psychological Assessment and Care

A. Psychosocial assessment is essential to the full understanding of the patient's experience of pain and suffering. Appropriate assessment is the basis of care.

B. Depression
   1. *Incidence:* Of terminally ill patients, 25% to 77% experience depression (Wilson, Chochinov, de Faye, & Breitbart, 2000).

2. Risk factors for depression are as follows:
   a. Pain and other symptoms
   b. Progressive physical impairment
   c. Advanced disease
   d. Medications, such as steroids and benzodiazepines
   e. Particular disease, such as pancreatic cancer and stroke
   f. Spiritual pain
   g. Brain radiation therapy (Pasacreta, Minarik, & Nield-Anderson, 2006)
   h. Preexisting risk factors, such as the following:
      (1) Prior history of depression
      (2) Family history of depression
      (3) Social stress
      (4) Suicide attempts
      (5) Substance use or abuse
3. Signs and symptoms of depression in advanced illness
   a. Somatic symptoms are always present.
   b. Pain is not responding as expected.
   c. The patient can have sad mood or flat affect and be anxious or irritable.
   d. The patient has feelings of worthlessness, hopelessness, helplessness, guilt, and despair.
   e. Anhedonia (lack of joy) is a symptom.
   f. Lost self-esteem is common.
   g. The patient may have suicidal ideation.
4. Treatment
   a. Use a combination of supportive psychotherapy, cognitive-behavioral techniques, and antidepressant medications (Watson, 2006).
   b. Psychotherapy involves individual or group counseling.
   c. Cognitive-behavioral techniques can be used to influence emotions, behaviors and cognition. Techniques include but are not limited to:
      (1) Relaxation.
      (2) Imagery.
      (3) Breathing techniques.
   d. Psychopharmacology includes selective serotonin reuptake inhibitors (SSRIs), atypical antidepressants, tricyclic antidepressants, psychostimulants, and others (e.g., corticosteroids).
      (1) In recent years, the SSRIs (e.g., fluoxetine, sertraline, and paroxetine) and atypical antidepressants (e.g., duloxetine and venlafaxine) have become used widely because of their efficacy and low risk of significant side effects (Watson, 2006).
      (2) The psychostimulants (methylphenidate and dextroamphetamine) may promote a sense of well-being, decrease fatigue, and stimulate appetite at low doses for cancer patients. Furthermore, the onset of benefit may be rapid compared with antidepressants (Watson, 2006).

C. Anxiety
1. *Incidence:* Of patients with terminal illness, 25% to 50% experience anxiety (Stoklosa, Patterson, Rosielle, & Arnold, 2007).
2. Risk factors are as follows (Pasacreta et al., 2006):
   a. Existential and psychological concerns
   b. Pain (inadequate analgesia)
   c. Dyspnea, palpitations, or nausea
   d. Abnormal metabolic states, such as hypoxia, sepsis, or delirium
   e. Drugs
      (1) Corticosteroids produce motor restlessness, agitation, and depression at high doses or rapid tapers.

(2) Prochlorperazine and metoclopramide can cause extrapyramidal side effects of motor restlessness, hyperactivity, and akathisia.
(3) Withdrawal from alcohol, benzodiazepines, and opioids can result in anxiety, agitation, delirium, and violent paranoid behaviors (Pasacreta et al., 2006).

f. Past history of psychiatric disorder

3. Signs and symptoms include the following (Pasacreta et al., 2006):
   a. Agitation and restlessness
   b. Insomnia
   c. Sweating
   d. Tachycardia
   e. Hyperventilation
   f. Panic attacks
   g. Worry or hypervigilance
   h. Increased tension
4. Treatment (Pasacreta et al., 2006; Watson, 2006)
   a. Differentiate anxiety from the following:
      (1) Delirium
      (2) Depression
      (3) Bipolar disorder
      (4) Medication effects
      (5) Insomnia
      (6) Effects of alcohol or caffeine
      (7) Uncontrolled symptoms (e.g., pain or dyspnea)
   b. Medications include the following (Kuebler, Heidrich, Vena, & English, 2006):
      (1) Benzodiazepines
         (a) Use short-acting benzodiazepines for acute or situational anxiety (e.g., lorazepam and alprazolam).
         (b) Use long-acting benzodiazepines for chronic or persistent anxiety (e.g., clonazepam and diazepam).
      (2) Antidepressants (e.g., SSRIs)
      (3) Neuroleptic agents (e.g., haloperidol)
   c. Nonpharmacological interventions (Kuebler et al., 2006; Watson, 2006)
      (1) Use behavioral approaches, such as the following:
         (a) Relaxation exercises
         (b) Imagery or self-hypnosis
         (c) Meditation
         (d) Biofeedback
      (2) Provide adequate information in a supportive manner.
      (3) Recommend counseling.

D. Delirium (see the chapter on Gerontology Pain Management)

1. *Incidence:* Delirium is highly prevalent at the end of life (Kuebler et al., 2006, Watson, 2006).
2. Causes
   a. Direct causes of delirium are primary brain tumor, metastatic spread of cancer to brain, and seizures.
   b. Indirect causes of delirium are metabolic encephalopathy, electrolyte imbalance, medications, infection, nutrition, hypoxia, and others.
3. Signs and symptoms of delirium are as follows:
   a. Rapid onset with fluctuating severity of symptoms
   b. Inability to maintain or shift attention properly
   c. Waxing and waning of consciousness
   d. Disturbance in the sleep-wake cycle

e. Disorientation to person, place, or time
f. Abnormal perceptions (e.g., visual or auditory hallucinations) (Watson, 2006)

4. Treatment (Coyne & Panke, 2006; Del Fabbro, Dalal, & Bruera, 2006)
   a. Correct the cause of delirium (e.g., treat infection).
   b. Pharmacotherapy with haloperidol is the widely accepted drug of choice in palliative care (Kuebler et al., 2006).
   c. A short-acting benzodiazepine may be added if haloperidol is not tolerated or rapid titration of haloperidol alone does not achieve adequate results.

E. Suffering
1. Definition
   a. "Suffering is a state of severe distress induced by the loss of the intactness of person, or by a threat that the person believes will result in the loss of his or her intactness" (Cassell, 1989, p. 63).
   b. "A patient who is experiencing severe pain, dyspnea, or agitated confusion must be considered a medical emergency. No less emergent is the suffering of a person whose physical symptoms are controlled, but whose agony derives from the sense of impending disintegration or the loss of meaning and purpose in life" (Byock, 1996, pp. 243–244).
   c. "For the dying patient, suffering comes in many packages: physical pain, unrelenting symptoms (nausea, pruritus, dyspnea, etc.), spiritual distress, dependency, multiple losses, and anticipatory grieving. Even the benefits of medical treatments given to provide hope or palliation can sometimes be outweighed by side effects (e.g., sedation and constipation from pain medication), inducing yet further suffering" (Kemp, 2006b, p. 607).
   d. "Victor Frankl emphasizes that the dimension of meaning is central to the human experience of suffering. Pain and privation are insufficient to explain suffering, Frankl asserts. Human suffering requires the felt loss of meaning and purpose in life. Pain and privation can be endured if it is for a purpose" (Byock, 1996, p. 242).
2. Treatment
   a. "[It] is the duty of all who care for patients to alleviate suffering and not just treat the physical dimensions of the illness. This is no small task, for first, professionals must be free from denial and the need to self-protect to see the suffering of another. Then, they must be able to attend to it without trying to fix it or simplify it. The suffering needs to be witnessed; in the midst of suffering, presence and compassion become the balm and hope for its relief" (Kemp, 2006b, p. 607).
   b. "The role of the clinical team is to stand by the patient, steadfastly providing meticulous physical care and psychosocial support, while people strive to discover their own answers" (Byock, 1996, p. 251).

V. Spiritual Assessment and Care

A. The top 10 spiritual and emotional concerns regarding end-of-life care are as follows (Astrow & Smith, 2006; Plotnikoff, 2000):
1. Not having the chance to say goodbye to someone
2. Thinking that your death will be the cause of inconvenience and stress for loved ones
3. Not being forgiven by God
4. Not reconciling with others
5. Dying when you are removed or cut off from God or a higher power
6. The possibility of continued emotional suffering
7. Not being forgiven by someone for something you did
8. The possibility of being alone when you are dying
9. Not having a blessing from a family member or clergy person
10. Wondering whether anyone will miss you or remember you over time

B. Method of assessment of spiritual suffering
1. Suspect spiritual pain.
2. Establish a conducive atmosphere.

3. Express interest; ask specific questions.
4. Listen for broader meanings.
5. Be aware of your own beliefs and biases.

C. Treatment of spiritual suffering
   1. Respect religious traditions of the patient and family.
      a. "Religious traditions strive to give symbolic access and concrete visibility to the deepest levels of human existence, especially at critical turning points like terminal illness and death, when the search for meaning becomes intense" (O'Connell, 1995, p. 232).
   2. Honor rites and rituals that are meaningful to the patient and family.
      a. "The creation of rites and rituals provides an organized and symbolically meaningful pathway through serious illness to death and beyond" (O'Connell, 1995, p. 234).
   3. Foster realistic hope.
      a. "Finding meaning is inherent in hope and spirituality" (Post-White et al., 1996).
      b. Components of hope are (Post-White et al., 1996, p. 1572)
         (1) Realistic expectations and goals.
         (2) Motivation to achieve goals.
         (3) Anticipation of outcomes.
         (4) Establishing trust and interpersonal relationships.
         (5) Relying on internal and external resources.
         (6) Determination to endure.
         (7) Being oriented to future.
      c. Interventions to foster hope are (Koopmeiners et al., 1997)
         (1) Being present by taking time to listen.
         (2) Giving appropriate information in understandable language.
         (3) Showing caring behaviors.

VI. Pain Management in End-stage Disease

A. Although pain management has been described extensively throughout this text, its management within the palliative care area is different. In applying pain management interventions, we must examine the benefits versus the risks to the patient. This is a population for whom time is of the essence, and a 2-week analgesic trial may mean a lifetime. Rapid titration is crucial. The benefits of comfort are paramount, and the risk may be low in the "big picture."

B. When managing pain in individuals with life limiting diseases pain management options may be considered including neurolytic blocks, ketamine, lidocaine, or midazolam infusions.

C. Although the patient or family unit must be aware of the issues associated with these treatments, the options need to be considered, presented, and available for selected individuals. In this patient population, innovation becomes the rule.

D. Patients experiencing intractable side effects of current treatment or intractable, intolerable pain need help immediately.

E. Approximately 85% to 90% of all cancer patients can achieve good analgesia by using the World Health Organization cancer pain ladder. Only a small percentage of clients with end-stage disease require unique interventional techniques, such as lidocaine or ketamine infusions (Coyne, 2003; Dupen, 2006).

F. Pain management
   1. As end-stage diseases progress, pain may change significantly and rapidly. These changes may include a decrease in pain, perhaps as the duration of analgesics is extended because of hepatic or renal function failure.
   2. Comorbidity factors, such as hypercalcemia, may decrease the sensation of pain.
   3. Pain also may increase rapidly because of disease progression and attempted treatments (e.g., surgery or chemotherapy).
   4. In evaluation of pain in this setting of end-stage disease, the cause may not be known or pursued. The cause may not be *fixable* within the current situation, or the test to prove a diagnosis may be unrealistic.

5. The nurse should always assess for the following causes of discomfort in late-stage diseases. Although not all of these causes are common, they usually can be palliated easily and missing them would result in increased discomfort.
   a. Constipation
   b. Urinary retention
   c. Myoclonus
   d. Bone metastasis or pathological fractures
   e. Withdrawal
   f. Infectious processes
   g. Other symptoms that are contributing to ongoing discomfort or suffering

G. The American Society for Pain Management Nursing (ASPMN) supports the position that nurses should advocate for health care environments that foster humane and dignified care. ASPMN promotes ethical and effective pain and symptom management as an integral part of palliative care (ASPMN, 2003).
1. Nurses individually and collectively have an obligation to provide comprehensive and compassionate end-of-life care. This includes the promotion of comfort and the relief of pain and, at times, foregoing life-sustaining treatments (American Nurses Association [ANA], 1998).
2. In the context of the caring relationship, nurses perform a primary role in the assessment and management of pain and other distressing symptoms in dying patients. Therefore, nurses must use effective doses of medications prescribed for symptom control. Nurses have a moral obligation to advocate on behalf of the patient when a prescribed medication is insufficiently managing pain and other distressing symptoms. The increasing titration of medication to achieve adequate symptom control is ethically justified (ANA, 2005).
3. "The duty to benefit through relief of pain is by itself adequate to support the use of increasing doses (of opioids) to alleviate pain, even if there might be life shortening and expected side effects" (Cain & Hannes, 1994, p. 161).

VII. Common Symptoms at End of Life

A. Constipation (Economou, 2006)
1. Cause
   a. Constipation is a common complaint in all patients receiving analgesic agents, but this problem becomes a more common issue in end-of-life care. Constipation may be caused by the following:
      (1) Medications (e.g., opioids, nonsteroidal antiinflammatory agents, or chemotherapeutic agents)
      (2) Disease processes (e.g., partial bowel obstruction or hypercalcemia)
      (3) Diabetes as a compounding factor
      (4) Decreased oral intake, including fluids and fiber
      (5) Inactivity
      (6) Ongoing pain, especially if associated with having a bowel movement
   b. Constipation is typically an avoidable complication, and good nursing assessment and interventions should alleviate or prevent this symptom in most cases (Coyne & Panke, 2006).
2. Assessment
   a. Assessment for constipation requires obtaining a thorough bowel history, including
      (1) Use of laxatives.
      (2) Frequency of laxative use.
      (3) Recent abdominal surgery.
      (4) The patient's previous regularity.
      (5) Pain on defecation.
      (6) Recent medication changes.
   b. The nurse must conduct an abdominal assessment noting tenderness, bowel sounds (frequency and pitch), and distention, and a rectal examination, assessing for impaction and painful hemorrhoids.

c. When assessing constipation, the nurse should consider the possibility of bowel obstruction. This is a common occurrence in the clinical course of certain cancers, especially mesothelioma and ovarian and gastrointestinal cancers.

3. Potential complications of constipation
   a. Constipation can increase pain, decrease activity, decrease food and fluid intake, and make patients fearful to take analgesic medications. These complications can affect the patient's and family's quality of life.
4. Treatment
   a. The first treatment of constipation is prevention. Patients automatically should start a bowel program with their opioid.
   b. The maintenance of the bowel regimen must include a stool softener and stimulant, with rare exceptions. Numerous bowel regimens exist, all with pros and cons, regional variations, and cultural variations.
   c. The preference should be to resolve the constipation using the oral route.
   d. All pain medications may need adjusting appropriately.
5. Evaluation of treatment
   a. A bowel regimen should ensure, as a minimum, a bowel movement every 72 hours, regardless of intake.

B. Dyspnea
   1. Dyspnea, an unpleasant awareness of breathing, is a common symptom in people with advanced disease (Coyne, 2003; Dudgeon, 2006).
   2. *Incidence:* Dyspnea may occur in 70% of cases of end-stage cancer.
   3. Cause
      a. The causes of dyspnea are extremely varied and may include disease process, treatments, a comorbidity process, or other conditions, as in the following:
         (1) Tumor infiltration
         (2) Pleural effusions
         (3) Pulmonary embolism
         (4) Pneumonia
         (5) Asthma
         (6) Congestive heart failure
         (7) Anxiety
         (8) Severe anemia
         (9) Neuromuscular disease or trauma
         (10) Ascites
         (11) Obesity
   3. Signs and symptoms (Coyne & Panke, 2006)
      a. Similar to pain, dyspnea is a subjective complaint. The complaint nonetheless requires excellent assessment skills to determine whether a reversible cause exists (e.g., congestive heart failure).
      b. The assessment of breathlessness should include
         (1) Auscultation of heart and lungs.
         (2) Functional status.
         (3) The patient's perception of potential provoking factors (e.g., activity, pain, or anxiety).
         (4) A pain assessment.
   4. Potential complications of untreated dyspnea
      a. With the complaint of breathlessness, patients are unable to perform activities of daily living.
      b. The anxiety of ongoing dyspnea affects the patient's overall health status and requires aggressive treatment for comfort.
      c. With ongoing complaints of dyspnea, the nurse also should assess for depression.
      d. Many patients perceive that this complaint is often ignored.

5. Treatment
   a. The treatments for this complaint, besides treating the underlying cause, may be divided into two groups: nonpharmacological and pharmacological.
      (1) Nonpharmacological treatments that have shown some effectiveness include the following:
         (a) Counseling
         (b) Relaxation
         (c) Breathing training
         (d) Fans
         (e) Imagery
         (f) Oxygen
      (2) Pharmacological interventions for dyspnea
         (a) Opioids are noted to be effective for dyspnea with some malignancies and with chronic obstructive airway disease (Coyne, Viswanathan, & Smith, 2002).
         (b) Bronchodilators are used often in asthma and chronic obstructive pulmonary disease.
         (c) Diuretics are used for congestive heart failure and fluid overload.
         (d) Benzodiazepines may be used as an adjuvant to opioids, particularly if there is a significant anxiety component or for refractory dyspnea at the end of life.
         (e) Steroids may be useful for inflammatory processes.
         (f) Antibiotics to treat infectious processes may be required.
         (g) Anticoagulants are used for pulmonary embolism.

C. Cachexia (Kemp, 2006a)
   1. Cause
      a. Cachexia is a common and devastating complication of terminal disease process, particularly cancer and acquired immunodeficiency syndrome.
      b. Cachexia is malnutrition and a general, declining ill health following a period of anorexia, when the loss of appetite or inability to eat has resulted in significant weight loss. Although the exact mechanisms causing cancer cachexia are not entirely understood, there is a "complex interaction between the host and the tumour. Tumour cells interact with host cells within the tumour mass resulting in the production of catabolic mediators" that weaken the tissue, but "patient factors, including age and levels of physical activity, and the specific mechanics of protein metabolism in cancer patients may also have a significant impact" (Skipworth, Stewart, Dejong, Preston, & Fearon, 2007, p. 667).
      c. Unanticipated weight loss may be an early indicator of terminal illness.
      d. Potential causes include
         (1) Oral or systemic infections.
         (2) Depression.
         (3) Difficulty or pain with eating.
         (4) Dyspnea.
         (5) Diarrhea.
         (6) Chronic nausea.
         (7) Constipation.
         (8) Metabolic abnormalities.
         (9) Poor integrity of oral mucosa.
   2. Signs and symptoms of cachexia
      a. The most obvious sign is the patient's lack of appetite with apparent weight loss. Increased weight can be noted in end-stage heart disease, however.
      b. Weakness and fatigue are present.
      c. Muscle wasting, decreased cognition, and depression may exist.
      d. A decline in serum albumin typically is noted as a late feature.
      e. The patient's and family's perception of this symptom needs to be explored thoroughly.

3. Potential complications of cachexia
   a. The loss of weight is a constant reminder to the patient and family of the evolving disease process. The impact on the patient and family can be significant.
   b. Because eating is a cultural, social, and sometimes religious occasion, this lack of intake may have many repercussions. Many families associate eating with a major forum for family interactions. As appetite decreases, the family may feel guilty or frustrated as family dynamics change.
   c. The family may fear that the patient is starving to death.
4. Treatment (Coyne, Lyne, & Watson, 2002)
   a. Because the goal of comfort exists in this population and the cause often is irreversible, the objectives of treatment need careful consideration. Aggressive nutritional treatment typically has not been shown to improve survival, and no studies have shown improved quality of life.
   b. Oral nutrition is the ideal. In some cases, enteral nutrition may be useful in patients who cannot swallow but still have an appetite (Miller, 2006).
   c. Appetite stimulants (particularly megestrol acetate [Megace]) may be useful in improving intake.
   d. Other agents may be beneficial (e.g., cannabinoids, steroids, methylphenidate, alcohol, or thalidomide). Further research is needed in this area.
   e. Counseling regarding intake, body image, and level of energy needs to be offered.
   f. Oral care is comforting, especially if the patient is not eating.
5. Evaluation of treatment
   a. Follow-up
      (1) Record the patient's report of appetite.
      (2) Look for evidence of improved nutrition, such as skin tone, weight gain, and observed oral intake, strength, or energy.
      (3) Encourage expression of feelings from the patient and family regarding the cachexia (Miller, 2006).

D. Fatigue (Anderson & Dean, 2006)
1. Cause
   a. Fatigue is one of the most commonly mentioned complaints of cancer patients. Fatigue decreases the quality of life of the patient.
   b. Although its exact cause is unclear, many factors may contribute:
      (1) Increasing tumor burden
      (2) Decreased nutrition
      (3) Prolonged illness
      (4) Anemia
      (5) Treatments (e.g., radiation or chemotherapy)
      (6) Renal or organ failure (e.g., heart, liver, or lung)
      (7) Uncontrolled pain
      (8) Sleep disorder or disturbances
2. Assessment
   a. Assessment relies on a subjective complaint. This symptom, similar to pain, is ever evolving.
   b. Patients should be queried regarding their activity levels, feelings of depression, and precipitating or relieving activities.
   c. Patients' nutritional intake should be evaluated.
   d. Vital signs should be evaluated to determine whether rapid heart rate or fevers exist.
   e. Muscle strength, endurance, and symmetry need careful assessment.
   f. Appropriate laboratory tests include complete blood count, thyroid function, vitamin B_{12} levels, and glucose.
3. Treatment
   a. Pharmacological treatments for fatigue are varied but may include
      (1) Psychostimulants.
      (2) Steroids.

(3) Antidepressants (particularly the SSRIs).
(4) Erythropoietin (Minton, Richardson, Sharpe, Hotopf, & Stone, 2008).

b. Nonpharmacological interventions include
(1) Improved nutrition.
(2) Education in energy conservation activities.
(3) Consolidation of tasks.
(4) Rescheduling tasks.
(5) Use of distraction.
(6) Blood transfusions (when anemic).
(7) Occupational therapy, which may prove beneficial in assisting with energy conservation training.
(8) Exercise in early stages of disease processes.

4. Evaluation of treatment
a. The evaluation of the treatment of this symptom is based on the patient's response to assessment.
(1) Has the fatigue improved?
(2) Has the patient's function been maintained or improved?
(3) Are the patient and family's expectations realistic?

E. Terminal distress and restlessness (Del Fabbro et al., 2006; Lawlor & Bruera, 2002).
1. Cause
a. This condition may occur in the last days or hours of life.
b. The patient displays agitation that may include thrashing, anxiety, impaired mental status, and perhaps myoclonus.
c. The cause of this restlessness may be one of the following:
(1) Increased pain
(2) Dyspnea
(3) Constipation
(4) Urinary retention
(5) Withdrawal from medications
(6) Medication side effect

2. Signs and symptoms
a. The signs and symptoms are subjective and defined by the patient or family. Patients who appear agitated, extremely restless, or distressed fall within this category.
b. Evaluation for reversible causes is always appropriate. Assessment of constipation, urinary retention, opioid withdrawal, and other causes should be made.
c. The patient's family should be assessed to determine their perception and how they are coping with this extremely difficult situation.
d. At the end of life, determining the etiology is often not indicated and treatment is simply initiated.

3. Treatment
a. The initial treatment of distress in end-stage disease typically is opioid titration.
b. If confusion becomes the chief issue, haloperidol at scheduled doses may dramatically relieve this problem.
c. The use of intravenous fluids in some situations helps decrease confusion. Their role is limited, however.
d. Certain situations require sedation for comfort:
(1) Agitated delirium
(2) Refractory depression
(3) Anxiety
(4) Existential distress

e. Sedating agents to consider are midazolam and lorazepam. If these two medications fail, barbiturates could be considered (Coyne, Lyne, & Watson, 2002).

f. The use of sedating medications in end-stage disease may cause discomfort among some health care professionals. The goal of this therapy is to improve comfort and to decrease suffering. A secondary effect may be that death is hastened. This is not the intent and should not be interpreted as euthanasia or physician-assisted suicide.
g. When considering any of these treatments, the family's input is a requirement. The family should be supported throughout this situation.

4. Evaluation of treatment
   a. The optimal outcomes include an apparent decrease in the patient's distress level and the family's perceived improvement in comfort. This symptom requires aggressive treatment. If this treatment is delayed, a family's final memory of their loved one may be tragic.

VIII. Communication Needs in Palliative Care (Boreale & Richardson, 2006)

A. In one study, nurses were asked, "What things do you wish you were taught in nursing school about caring for dying or terminally ill patients/families?" The number one response was "how to talk to patients/families about dying." This is never a comfortable situation and requires confidence, poise, empathy, and a view of the total illness picture (White, Coyne, & Patel, 2001).

B. The unit of care is the patient and the patient's family; this makes the communication process more complex and difficult in an already stressful time. Communication is essential to ensure the group's needs are met. This is a role for the nurse to fulfill as the advocate for this population. The following guidelines can help the nurse through this process.

C. Rules for caring for the patient-family unit of a patient with an end-stage disease
   1. You will be honest.
   2. You will not abandon them.
   3. You know their goals and will help them achieve these when possible.
   4. You will help them explore their realistic options.
   5. When making decisions, you will consider the overall situation (e.g., support systems, economics, locality, and technical aspects).
   6. You will respond to their questions within a reasonable time and invite additional questions.
   7. You will respect their wishes.
   8. You will ensure that the entire health care team understands and has input into the plan of care. Remember that the patient and family are a part of the team, with veto power.
   9. When you do not know what to do, you will seek help.
   10. You will care for the patient and the patient's family.
   11. You will ask,
       a. What would you like me to do?
       b. What are your expectations?
       c. What do you need?
   12. You will take the time to listen.
   13. Ask yourself: Would you do this to a member of your family?

D. When the patient asks for death, the nurse needs to work to achieve a better level of comfort, offer realistic hope, and attempt to help the patient find a meaning to his or her life. The role of a team becomes imperative in helping support the patient and staff and ensuring all the patient's needs are being met. The following are questions to address:
   1. Is the pain adequately controlled?
   2. Is the patient experiencing unrelenting symptoms (e.g., nausea or dyspnea)?
   3. What does the patient fear?
   4. Is the patient's physical functioning deteriorating rapidly?
   5. Does the patient perceive that he or she is a physical or financial burden to the family?
   6. Is the patient depressed?
   7. Is the patient competent? Has a mini-mental status been conducted?
   8. Can the patient and family afford the care?

9. Are there spiritual issues that have not been addressed? Why?
10. Who else should be involved in the discussion (e.g., significant others or potential survivors)?

IX. Quality of Life of the Dying

A. Different criteria for the dying (Super, 2005)
   1. People confronting death and their loved ones may define quality of life differently than do people not facing imminent death. Traditionally, quality-of-life studies focus on functional ability and psychological well-being.
   2. Meaningful quality-of-life variables include the following:
      a. Dignity (sense of being valued as a person and of not being a burden)
      b. Resilience (ability to withstand stress and maintain emotional equilibrium and the extent of physiological reserve)
      c. Malaise (not feeling well)
      d. Sense of connection (not feeling alone and having the presence of individuals the patient wants there)
      e. Sense of closure (sense of having said and done all important things)
      f. Spiritual well-being and meaningfulness of life (finding meaning in the current life and satisfaction with the life lived)
      g. Transcendence (ability to prepare for the loss of the physical self and to find meaning beyond the life span)
      h. Suffering (anguish, terror, or hopelessness)
      i. Overall quality of dying from perspective of patient, family, and loved ones
         (1) The patient is dying free of avoidable distress and suffering for patients, families, and loved ones.
         (2) The patient is dying in accord with his or her own and the family's wishes.
         (3) The process is reasonably consistent with clinical, cultural, and ethical standards.

X. Advance Directives

A. Definitions
   1. *Advisory documents* are documents that represent the patient's views and wishes as fully and accurately as possible. In many cases, these documents review possible situations that would require decisions be made without the patient's input, such as if the patient is unconscious or not able to speak for self.
      a. Most *advance directive forms* are advisory documents. If a formal advance directive is not used, notes the doctor writes in a patient's medical chart are also recognized as advisory. Both of these documents are binding under common law if the patient is unable to act for self.
      b. *Advance directives* are also known as living wills. These are formal legal documents specifically authorized by state laws that allow patients to continue their personal autonomy and that provide instructions for care in case they become incapacitated and cannot make decisions. An advance directive may also be a durable power of attorney (Agency for Healthcare Research and Quality [AHRQ], 2003).
   2. Statutory documents such as living wills and durable power attorney for health care (designating a proxy) are designed to fit the language of state laws or statutes.
      a. *Living wills* provide general instructions regarding the medical care a patient would like to receive if decision-making capacity is lost. The language in these documents is generally broad and conceptual rather than specific, although many forms for living wills allow the patient to add specific information or requests not covered in the form (American Medical Association [AMA], 2001).
      b. A *durable power of attorney* is also known as a *health care proxy.* "This document allows the patient to designate a surrogate, a person who will make treatment decisions for the patient if the patient becomes too incapacitated to make such decisions" (AHRQ, 2003).

(1) If the decisions relate to medical treatment, then the agent appointed is known as a health care proxy. The health care proxy has, in essence, the same rights to request or refuse treatment that the individual would have if capable of making and communicating decisions (Mayo Clinic, 2008).
(2) A durable power of attorney may also apply to financial matters. In this case, the agent makes financial transactions on behalf of the agent while the principal is incapacitated (Mayo Clinic, 2008).
(3) The durable power of attorney does not take effect until the patient becomes incapable of making decisions (AMA, 2001). This is determined by the health care professional when decision-making capacity is jeopardized or when an individual does not have the insight to make decisions. This determination may vary by state (Nelson-Marten & Braaten, 2006).
(4) In August 1998, Minnesota combined the living will and durable power of attorney for health care into one form called the health care directive (Fairview Health Services, 2008).

B. History of the development of advance directives and health care directives
   1. Changes in how we die
      a. "Just a few generations ago, most people died suddenly, at any age. Now, most die of serious chronic disease, after a substantial period of disability" (Lynn et al., 2000, p. 255).
      b. "Disability is slowly progressive over years, with periodic bouts of severe symptoms. Once a terminal phase of failing health is apparent, death becomes reasonably predictable" (Lynn et al., 2000, p. 256).
      c. "With a chronic illness course, the timing of death is much less predictable, until perhaps the last day or two" (Lynn et al., 2000, p. 256).
      d. "For the past few decades, our society has conceived of the end of life as being a category that is discernable [sic], tied to high likelihood of death within six months, and congruent with the category of being 'terminally ill'" (Lynn et al., 2000, p. 259).
   2. Patient Self-Determination Act of 1990 (American Bar Association, 2008)
      a. Development of advance directives law and policies was based on the ethical tenets of autonomy and patient self-determination.
      b. The act included the assumption that enhanced patient-level decision making is the key to quality end-of-life care.
   3. The Physician Orders for Life-Sustaining Treatment (POLST) paradigm initiative began in Oregon in 1991.
      a. The initiative created portable medical orders based on the patient's values for life-sustaining treatments.
      b. Medical ethics leaders recognized that patient wishes for life-sustaining treatments were not being consistently honored despite the availability of advance directives.
      c. Growing number of other states and communities are implementing their own POLST paradigm programs.
      d. "The number of states in the U.S. authorizing these out-of-hospital do not resuscitate orders has increased from 11 states in 1992 to 42 states in 1999" (Schmidt, Hickman, Tolle, & Brooks, 2004, p. 1430).
      e. "When advance directives are turned into medical orders, most EMTs [emergency medical technicians] will follow them" (Schmidt et al., 2004, p.1434).
      f. Categories addressed are as follows:
         (1) Cardiopulmonary resuscitation (CPR)
         (2) Medical interventions (comfort measures only, limited additional interventions, or full treatment)
         (3) Antibiotics
         (4) Artificially administered nutrition
         (5) Summary of goals and signatures

g. The POLST should be reviewed and revised periodically when
   (1) The person is transferred from one care setting or care level to another.
   (2) A substantial change in the person's health status has occurred.
   (3) The person's treatment preferences change.

4. Studies funded by the Agency for Healthcare Research and Quality (AHRQ) indicate that many patients have not participated in effective advance care planning. Despite patients' rights to determine their future care, AHRQ research reveals the following:
   a. Less than 50% of the severely or terminally ill patients studied had an advance directive in their medical record (Bradley & Rizzo, 1999; Teno, Licks, et al., 1997; Teno, Lynn, et al., 1997; Virmani, Schneiderman, & Kaplan, 1994). Only 12% of patients with an advance directive had received input from their physician in its development (Teno, Lynn, et al., 1997).
   b. Between 65% and 76% of physicians whose patients had an advance directive were not aware that it existed (Teno, Lynn, et al., 1997; Virmani et al., 1994).
   c. Having an advance directive did not increase documentation in the medical chart regarding patient preferences (Teno et al., 1994; Teno, Licks, et al., 1997).
   d. Advance directives helped make end-of-life decisions in less than half of the cases in which a directive existed (Teno, Lynn, et al., 1997).
   e. Advance directives usually were not applicable until the patient became incapacitated (Schneiderman et al., 1992) and "absolutely, hopelessly ill" (Teno et al., 1998).
   f. Providers and patient surrogates had difficulty knowing when to stop treatment and often waited until the patient had crossed a threshold over to actively dying before the advance directive was invoked (Teno et al., 1998).
   g. Language in advance directives was usually too nonspecific and general to provide clear instruction (Teno, Licks, et al., 1997).
   h. Surrogates named in the advance directive often were not present to make decisions or were too emotionally overwrought to offer guidance (Teno et al., 1998).
   i. Physicians were only about 65% accurate in predicting patient preferences and tended to make errors of undertreatment, even after reviewing the patient's advance directive (Coppola et al., 2001).
   j. Care at the end of life sometimes appears to be inconsistent with the patients' preferences to forgo life-sustaining treatment, and patients may receive care they do not want (Teno, Lynn, et al., 1997).
   k. Another study found that patients received life-sustaining treatment at the same rate regardless of their desire to limit treatment (AHRQ, 2003; Danis et al., 1996).

5. In 1995, the Study to Understand Prognoses and Preferences for Outcomes and Risk of Treatments (SUPPORT) of 9,105 cases found prolonged intensive care unit stays were expensive and were often followed by death or disability.
   a. "Patients were more likely to receive care consistent with their preferences if they had discussed their care preferences with their physicians" (Teno et al., 2000, p. S70).
   b. Patients often completed directives containing little or no clinically useful information (Teno et al., 2000).

6. Inaccuracy of physicians and surrogates to predict patient's wishes
   a. A study was made of 24 primary physicians of 82 elderly patients, 17 emergency department and critical care physicians, and a baseline group of family surrogates.
      (1) "Family surrogates' judgments were more accurate than physicians'" even when the physician had patient's value-based advance directive or patient's scenario-based advance directive (Coppola et al., 2001, p. 431).
      (2) Advance directives increased the accuracy of hospital-based physicians, which may be important with the rise in hospitalists rather than the patient's private physician taking care of hospitalized patients.
      (3) Physicians were only about 65% accurate in predicting patient preferences and tended to make errors of undertreatment, even after reviewing the patient's advance directive (Coppola et al., 2001).

b. Surrogates who were family members tended to make prediction errors of overtreatment, even if they had reviewed or discussed the advance directive with the patient or assisted in its development (Ditto et al., 2001).

c. A study of 401 outpatients and self-designated surrogate decision makers randomized to one of five experimental conditions. "None of the interventions produced significant improvements in the accuracy of surrogate substituted judgment in any illness scenario or for any medical treatment" (Ditto et al., 2001, p. 421).

d. Study of factors considered important at the end of life found broad variation within and across all groups of patients, family members, physicians, and other care providers.

(1) "There is no one definition of a good death; quality end-of-life care is a dynamic process that is negotiated and renegotiated among patients, families, and health care professionals, a process moderated by individual values, knowledge, and preferences for care" (Steinhauser et al., 2000, p. 2481).

7. Patient satisfaction with care at end of life

a. Greater satisfaction with physician care came from patients with chronic illnesses when advance directives were discussed (n = 686 patients more than 75 years of age). This study should encourage physicians to initiate conversations about advance directives (Tierney et al., 2001).

b. A study was made of 475 family members of patients who had died 2 to 5 months before the interview.

(1) Pain was a problem in one-third of the sample.

(2) Other barriers included physician availability.

(3) "Remarkably, despite reports of moderate and severe pain for a significant proportion of decedents, there was generally a high level of satisfaction with clinicians' efforts to manage pain . . . which may be attributable in part to low expectations about pain management" (Tolle, Tilden, Rosenfeld, & Hickman, 2000, p. 315).

c. "A majority (94%) of family members reported that their loved one suffered at the end of life, but only worries about loss of quality of life were predictive of reports of suffering" (Hickman, Tilden, & Tolle, 2004, p. 20).

(1) Common worries included loss of bodily function, being dependent, being a burden (Hickman et al., 2004).

C. Need for more effective advance care planning

1. AHRQ (2003) research indicates that patients choose treatment based on the quality of the prospective health state, the invasiveness and length of treatment, and possible outcomes.

2. Researchers sponsored by AHRQ have suggested a five-part process that physicians and other health care providers can use to structure discussions on end-of-life care.

a. Initiate a guided discussion.

(1) AHRQ research indicates that most patients have not participated in advance care planning, yet many are willing to discuss end-of-life care.

b. Introduce the subject of advance care planning and offer information.

(1) One way to determine patients' preferences for end-of-life care is to discuss hypothetical situations and find out their opinions on certain treatment patterns.

(2) Patients do not always understand their realistic chances for a positive outcome (Moore et al., 1994).

(3) Other research indicates that patients significantly overestimate their probability of survival after receiving CPR and have little or no understanding of mechanical ventilation (Fischer et al., 1998).

(4) In one study, after patients were told their probability of survival, over half changed their treatment preference from wanting CPR to refusing CPR (Murphy et al., 1994).

c. Prepare and complete advance care planning documents.

(1) Advance care planning documents should contain specific instructions. Terms such as "no advanced life support" are too vague to offer guidance on specific treatments (Teno, Licks, et al., 1997).

d. Review the patient's preferences regularly and update documentation.
   (1) Patients should be reminded that advance directives can be revised at any time. It is difficult for people to fully imagine what a prospective health state might be like. Once they experience that health state, they may find it more or less tolerable than they imagined (Emanuel et al., 1995).
   (2) Preferences that change indicate that the physician needs to investigate the basis for the change (Emanuel et al., 1995).
   (3) A study linked changes in depression to changes in preferences for CPR. Increased depression was associated with patients' changing their initial preference for CPR to refusal of CPR, while less depression was associated with patients' changing their preference from refusal of CPR to acceptance of CPR (Rosenfeld et al., 1996).
e. Apply the patient's desires to actual circumstances.
   (1) AHRQ-sponsored research indicates that if patients desired nonbeneficial treatments or refused beneficial treatments, most physicians stated that they would negotiate with them, trying to educate and convince them either to forgo a nonbeneficial treatment or to accept a beneficial treatment.
   (2) Many patients do not lose their decision-making capacity at the end of life.
   (3) Physicians and families may encounter the difficulty of knowing when an advance directive should become applicable for patients who are extremely sick and have lost their decision-making capacity but are not necessarily dying (Teno et al., 1998).
   (4) Even if patients require a decision for a situation that was not anticipated and addressed in their advance directive, physicians and surrogates still can make an educated determination based on the knowledge they have about the patients' values, goals, and thresholds for treatment (Emanuel et al., 1995).

XI. Oncology Nurses Society (1999, revised 2003) and Association of Oncology Social Work Joint Position on End-of-Life Care (Oncology Nursing Society, 2007)

A. Despite the clear benefits of hospice care, too many patients die in settings that do not support an optimal death experience (Teno et al., 2004). Technical advances in health care have, in some cases, prolonged suffering.

B. The National Quality Forum (2008) affirmed the necessity of integrating timely and appropriate palliative care practices across the illness trajectory. That care involves addressing physical, intellectual, emotional, social, and spiritual needs and facilitating patient autonomy, access to information, and choice. Highlights include the following:
   1. Patients and families understand and evaluate the benefits and burdens of potential treatment options, as well as the accompanying financial costs.
   2. Patients and families consider hospice care when patients are likely to die within a year or reintroduction of hospice as patients decline.
   3. Assistance in adapting to altered goals of treatment and role responsibilities, as well as other difficult decision-making circumstances, is provided to patients and families.
   4. Families and significant others are included in the unit of care as evidenced by patient and family care conferences with appropriate members of the interdisciplinary team.
   5. Patients and families have access to ethics committees or ethics consultation across care settings.
   6. A timely care plan is based on a comprehensive interdisciplinary assessment of values, preferences, goals, and needs of patients and families.
   7. Psychological symptoms, including anxiety, depression, delirium, and behavioral disturbances, are measured comprehensively and documented using available standardized scales.
   8. Pain, dyspnea, constipation, and other symptoms are measured comprehensively and documented using available standardized scales.
   9. Physical and psychological symptoms are assessed, managed, and reassessed in a timely, safe, and effective manner to a level that is acceptable to patients and families.

10. Therapies traditionally considered part of active care are provided if they improve patients' symptoms and enhance quality of life.

C. A proactive and integrated approach to palliative and end-of-life care will improve quality of life across the care continuum.

References

Agency for Healthcare Research and Quality. (2003). *Advance care planning: Preferences for care at the end of life.* Research in Action, issue 12. (AHRQ Publication No. 03-0018). Rockville, MD: Author. Retrieved November 22, 2008, from http://www.ahrq.gov/research/endliferia/endria.htm.

American Medical Association. (2001). *AMA guide for patients, 2001.* Retrieved November 22, 2008, from http://www.ama-assn.org/ama/pub/category/14894.html.

American Bar Association. (2008). *Patient Self-Determination Act of 1990.* Retrieved November 22, 2008, from http://www.abanet.org/publiced/practical/patient_self_determination_act.html.

American Nurses Association (ANA) (1998). Position Statement: Assisted Suicide. Washington, D.C.: Author.

American Nurses Association. (2005). *Standards of nursing practice.* Kansas City, MO: Author.

American Society for Pain Management Nursing (2003). ASPMN Position Statement on Pain Management at the End of Life. Retrieved May 29, 2009 from http://www.aspmn.org/Organization/documents/EndofLifeCare.pdf.

Anderson, P., & Dean, G. (2006). Fatigue. In B. R. Ferrell & N. Coyle (Eds.), *Textbook of palliative nursing* (2nd ed., pp. 155–168). New York: Oxford University Press.

Astrow, A., & Smith, E. (2006). Spirituality. In J. Panke & P. Coyne (Eds.), *Conversations in palliative care* (2nd ed.). Dubuque, IA: Kendall/Hunt.

Boreale, K., & Richardson, B. (2006). Communication. In J. Panke & P. Coyne (Eds.), *Conversations in palliative care* (2nd ed.). Dubuque, IA: Kendall/Hunt.

Bradley, E. H., & Rizzo, J. A. (1999). Public information and private search: Evaluating the patient self-determination. *Journal of Health Politics, Policy and Law, 24*(2), 239–273.

Byock, I. R. (1996). The nature of suffering and the opportunity at the end of life. *Clinics in Geriatric Medicine, 12,* 237–252.

Cain, J.M. & Hammes, B.L. (1994). Ethics and pain management: Respecting patient wishes. *Journal of Pain and Symptom Management, 9,* 160–165.

Cassell, E. J. (1989). The relationship between pain and suffering. *Advances in Pain Research and Therapy, 11,* 61–70.

Center to Advance Palliative Care. (2008). *Making the case for hospital-based palliative care.* Retrieved May 29, 2008, from http://www.capc.org/building-a-hospital-based-palliative-care-program/case/index_html.

Connor, S. R. (2007–2008). Development of hospice and palliative care in the United States. *Omega (Westport), 56*(1), 89–99.

Coppola, K. H., Ditto, P. H., Danks, J. H., Smucker, J.H. (2001). Accuracy of primary care and hospital-based physicians' predictions of elderly outpatients' treatment preferences with and without advance directives. *Archives of Internal Medicine, 161,* 431–440.

Coyne, P. J. (2003). When the World Health Organization analgesic ladder fails: The role of invasive analgesic therapies. *Oncology Nursing Forum, 30*(5), 777–783.

Coyne, P. J., Lyne, M., & Watson, A. (2002). Symptom management in people with AIDS. *American Journal of Nursing, 102*(9), 48–56.

Coyne, P. J., & Panke, J. (2006). Symptom management. In J. Panke & P. Coyne (Eds.), *Conversations in palliative care* (2nd ed.). Dubuque, IA: Kendall/Hunt.

Coyne, P., J., Viswanathan, R., & Smith, T. (2002). Nebulized fentanyl citrate improves patients perception of breathing, respiratory rate, and oxygen saturation in dyspnea. *Journal of Pain and Symptom Management, 23*(2), 157–160.

Danis, M., Mutran, E., Garrett, J. M., Stearns, S.C., Slifkin, R.T., Hanson, L., Williams, J.F., Churchill, L.R. (1996). A prospective study of the impact of patient preferences on life-sustaining treatment and hospital cost. *Critical Care Medicine, 24,* 1811–1817.

Del Fabbro, E., Dalal, S., & Bruera, E. (2006). Symptom control in palliative care. III. Dyspnea and delirium. *Journal of Palliative Medicine, 9*(2), 422–436.

Ditto, P. H., Danks, J. H., Smucker, W. D., Bookwala, J., Coppola, K.M., Dresser, R., Fagerlin, A., Gready, R.M., Houts, R.M., Lockhard, L.K., Zyzanski, S.(2001). Advance directives as acts of communication. *Archives of Internal Medicine, 161,* 431–440.

Dudgeon, D. (2006). Dyspnea, death rattle, and cough. In B. R. Ferrell & N. Coyle (Eds.), *Textbook of palliative nursing* (2nd ed., pp. 249–264). New York: Oxford University Press.

Dupen, A. (2006). High tech pain management. In Panke, J., & Coyne, P. (Eds.), *Conversations in palliative care* (2nd ed.). Dubuque, IA: Kendall/Hunt.

Economou, D. (2006). Bowel management: Constipation, diarrhea, obstruction, and ascites. In B. R. Ferrell & N. Coyle (Eds.), *Textbook of palliative nursing* (2nd ed., pp. 401–420). New York: Oxford University Press.

Emanuel, L. L., Danis, M., Pearlman, R. A., Singer, P.A. (1995). Advance care planning as a process: Structuring discussions in practice. *Journal of the American Geriatric Society, 43*(4), 440–446.

Fairview Health Services. (2008). *Advanced directive.* Retrieved November 22, 2008, from http://www.fairview.org/news/Advance_Directive.pdf.

Fischer, G. S., Tulsky, J. A., Rose, M. R., Siminoff, L.A., Arnold, R.M. (1998). Patient knowledge and physician predictions of treatment preferences after discussion of advance directives. *Journal of General Internal Medicine, 13,* 447–454.

Hickman, S. E., Tilden, V. P., & Tolle, S. W. (2004). Family perceptions of worry, symptoms, and suffering in the dying. *Journal of Palliative Care, 20*(1), 20–27.

Kemp, C. (2006a). Anorexia and cachexia. In B. R. Ferrell & N. Coyle (Eds.), *Textbook of palliative nursing* (2nd ed., pp. 401–420). New York: Oxford University Press.

Kemp, C. (2006b). Meaning in illness. In B. R. Ferrell & N. Coyle (Eds.), *Textbook of palliative nursing.*

Koopmeiners, L., Post-White, J., Gutknecht, S., Ceronsky, C., Nickelson, K., Drew, D., Watrud

Kübler-Ross, E. (1969). *On death and dying.* New York: Macmillan.

Kuebler, K. K., Heidrich, D. E., Vena, C., & English, N. (2006). Delirium, confusion, agitation, and restlessness. In B. R. Ferrell & N. Coyle (Eds.), *Textbook of palliative nursing* (2nd ed., pp. 401–420). New York: Oxford University Press.

Lawlor, P. G., & Bruera, E. D. (2002). Delirium in patients with advanced cancer. *Hematology Oncology Clinics of North America, 16*(3), 701–714.

Lynn, J., Schall, M. W., Milne, C., Nolan, K.M., Kabcenell, A. (2000). Quality improvements in end of life care: Insights from two collaboratives. *Joint Commission Journal of Quality Improvement, 26*(5), 254–267.

MacDonald, N. (1993). The Canadian palliative care undergraduate curriculum. *Journal of Cancer Education, 8,* 197–201.

Mayo Clinic. (2008). *Resources on death and dying.* Retrieved November 22, 2008, from http://www.mayoclinic.org/support-groups/other-resources.html.

Miller, E. (2006). *Nutrition in conversations in palliative care* (2nd ed.). Dubuque, IA: Kendall/Hunt.

Minton, O., Richardson, A., Sharpe, M., Hotopf, M., & Stone, P. (2008). A systematic review and meta-analysis of the pharmacological treatment of cancer-related fatigue. *Journal of the National Cancer Institute, 100, 16,* 1155-1166.

Moore, K. A., Danks, J. H., Ditto, P. H., Druley, J.A., Townsend, A., Smucker, W.D. (1994). Elderly outpatients' understanding of a physician-initiated advance directive discussion. *Archives of Family Medicine, 3,* 1057–1063.

Murphy, D. J., Burrows, D., Santilli, S., Kemp, A.W., Tenner, S., Kreling, B., Teno, J. (1994). The influence of the probability of survival on patients' preferences regarding cardiopulmonary resuscitation. *New England Journal of Medicine, 330*(8), 545–549.

National Hospice and Palliative Care Organization. (2008). *History of hospice.* Retrieved November 23, 2008, from http://www.nhpco.org/i4a/pages/index.cfm?pageid=3285.

National Quality Forum (2008). Priority Area: Palliative Care. Retrieved on May 30, 2009 from http://www.qualityforum.org/pdf/about/priorities-partners/EOL%20Draft%20Goals%2006%2011%2008%20mtg.pdf

Nelson-Marten, P. & Braaten, J. (2006). Advance directives and legal issues. In J. Panke & P. Coyne (Eds.), *Conversations in palliative care* (2nd ed.). Dubuque, IA: Kendall/Hunt.

O'Connell, L. J. (1995). Religious dimensions of dying and death. *Western Journal of Medicine, 163,* 231–235.

Oncology Nursing Society (2007). Oncology Nursing Society and Association of Oncology Social Work Joint Position on Palliative Care and End-of-Life Care. Oncology Nursing Forum, 34,6.2007. Retrieved May 30, 2009 from http://www.ons.org/publications/positions/EndOfLifeCare.shtml

Pasacreta, J., Minarik, P., & Nield-Anderson, L. (2006). Anxiety and depression. In B. R. Ferrell & N. Coyle (Eds.), *Textbook of palliative nursing* (2nd ed., pp. 375–400). New York: Oxford University Press.

Plotnikoff, G. (2000). In search of a good death: The spiritual dimension. *Minnesota Medicine, 83,* 50–51.

Post-White, J., Ceronsky, C., Kreitzer, M. J., Nickelson, K., Drew, D., Watrud Mackey, K., Koopmeiners, L., & Gutknecht, S. (1996). Hope, spirituality, sense of coherence, and quality of life in patients with cancer. *Oncology Nursing Forum, 23,* 1571–1579.

Rosenfeld, K. E., Wenger, N. S., Phillips, R. S., Connors, A.F., Dawson, N.V., Layde, P., Califf, R.M., Liu, H., Lynn, J., Oye, R.K.(1996). Factors associated with change in resuscitation preference of seriously ill patients. *Archives of Internal Medicine, 156*(14), 1558–1564.

Schmidt, T. A., Hickman, S. E., Tolle, S. W., & Brooks, H. S. (2004). The physician orders for life-sustaining treatment program: Oregon emergency medical technicians' practical experiences and attitudes. *Journal of the American Geriatrics Society, 52*(9), 1430–1434.

Schneiderman, L. J., Kronick, R., Kaplan, R. M., Anderson, J.P., Langer, R.D. (1992). Effects of offering advance directives on medical treatment and costs. *Annals of Internal Medicine, 117*(7), 599–606.

Skipworth, R. J., Stewart, G. D., Dejong, C. H., Preston, T., & Fearon, K. C. (2007). Pathophysiology of cancer cachexia: much more than host-tumour interaction? *Clinical Nutrition, 26*(6), 667–676.

Steinhauser, K. E., Christakis, N. A., Clipp, E. C., McNeilly, M., McIntyre, L., Tulsky, J.A. (2000). Factors considered important at the end of life by patients, family, physicians, and other care providers. *Journal of the American Medical Association, 284,* 2476–2482.

Stoklosa, J., Patterson, K., Rosielle, D., & Arnold, R. (2007). *Anxiety in palliative care: Causes and diagnosis.* Fast Fact and Concept No. 186. End-of-Life/Palliative Education Resource Center. Retrieved November 22, 2008, from http://www.eperc.mcw.edu/.

Super, A. (2005). The context of palliative care in progressive illness. In B. Ferrell & N. Coyle (Eds.), *Textbook of palliative nursing* (2nd ed.). Oxford: Oxford University Press.

Teno, J. M., Fisher, E., Hamel, M. B., Wu, A.W., Murphy, D.J., Wenger, N.S., Lynn, J., & Harrell, F.E., Jr. (2000). Decision-making and outcomes of prolonged ICU stays in seriously ill patients. *Journal of the American Geriatric Society, 48,* S70–S74.

Teno, J. M., Licks, S., Lynn, J., Wenger, N., Connors, A.F., Phillips, R.S., O'Connor, M.A., & Murphy, D.P. (1997). Do advance directives provide instructions that direct care? *Journal of the American Geriatric Society, 45,* 508–512.

Teno, J. M., Lynn, J., Phillips, R. S., Murphy, D., Youngner, S.J., & Bellamy, P. (1994). Do formal advance directives affect resuscitation decisions and the use of resources for seriously ill patients? *Journal of Clinical Ethics, 5*(1), 23–30.

Teno, J., Lynn, J., Wenger, N., Phillips, R.S., Murphy, D.P., Connors, A.F., Desbiens, N., Fulkerson, W., Bellamy, P., & Knaus, W.A. (1997). Advance directives for seriously ill hospitalized patients: effectiveness with the Patient Self-Determination Act and the SUPPORT intervention. *Journal of the American Geriatric Society, 45,* 500–507.

Teno, J. M., Stevens, M., Spernak, S., & Lynn, J. (1998). Role of written advance directives in decision making. *Journal of General Internal Medicine, 13,* 439–446.

Tierney, W. M., Dexter, P. R., Gramelspacher, G. P., Perkins, A.J., Zhou, X.H., & Wolinsky, F.D. (2001). The effect of discussions about advance directives on patients' satisfaction with primary care. *Journal of General Internal Medicine, 16,* 32–40.

Tolle, S. W., Tilden, V. P., Rosenfeld, A. G., & Hickman, S. E. (2000). Family reports of barriers to optimal care of the dying. *Nursing Research, 49*(6), 310–317.

Virmani, J., Schneiderman, L. J., & Kaplan, R. M. (1994). Relationship of advance directives to physician-patient communication. *Archives of Internal Medicine, 154,* 909–913.

Watson, A. (2006). *Psychosocial issues in conversations in palliative care* (2nd ed.). Dubuque, IA: Kendall/Hunt.

White, K., Coyne, P., & Patel, U. (2001). Are nurses adequately prepared for end of life care? *Journal of Nursing Scholarship, 33,* 147–151.

Wilson, K. G., Chochinov, H. M., de Faye, B. J., & Breitbart, W. (2000). Diagnosis and management of depression in palliative care. In H. Chochinov & W. Breitbart (Eds.), *Handbook of psychiatry in palliative medicine* (pp. 25–49). Oxford, UK: Oxford University Press.

Websites

American Association of Colleges of Nursing, End-of-life care page
http://www.aacn.nche.edu/ELNEC/
End of Life/Palliative Education Resource Center, Medical College of Wisconsin
http://www.eperc.mcw.edu/
Hospice and Palliative Nurses Association
http://www.hpna.org

Suggested Readings

Ferrell, B., & Coyle, N. (Eds.). (2005). *Textbook of palliative nursing* (2nd ed.). Oxford, UK: Oxford University Press.

Ferrell, B., & Coyle, N. (2008). *The nature of suffering and the goals of nursing.* New York: Oxford University Press.

Fine, P. (1999). *Palliative medicine primer: Management of symptoms in advanced and terminal disease* (2nd ed.). Scottsdale, AZ: VistaCare Hospice.

Haas, B. K. (1999). Clarification and integration of similar quality of life concepts. *Image: Journal of Nursing Scholarship, 31,* 215–220.

Mackey, K., & Kreitzer, M. J. (1997). How healthcare professionals contribute to hope in patients with cancer. *Oncology Nursing Forum, 24,* 1507–1513.

Norlander, L. (2001). *To comfort always: A nurse's guide to end of life care.* Washington, DC: American Nurses Association.

Panke, J., & Coyne, P. (Eds.). (2006). *Conversations in palliative care* (2nd ed.). Dubuque, IA: Kendall/Hunt.

Vainio, A., & Auvinen, A. (1996). Prevalence symptoms among patients with advanced cancer: An international collaborative study. *Journal of Pain and Symptom Management, 12,* 3–10.

chapter

22

Gerontology Pain Management

Anne Marie Kelly, BSN, RN-BC, CHPN

Objectives

After studying this chapter, the reader should be able to:

1. Identify barriers to effective pain management in older adults.
2. Describe age-related factors that influence the assessment and management of pain in older adults.
3. Discuss how to assess pain in cognitively impaired and nonverbal older adults.

I. Demographics of Older Adults

A. Between 1990 and 2020, the population age 65 to 74 is expected to increase 74%, whereas the population younger than 65 years is expected to increase only 24%.

B. In 1999, people 65 years or older numbered 34.5 million and represented 12.7% of the U.S. population (Administration on Aging, 2000).

C. The elderly population explosion is expected to occur between 2010 and 2030 as the baby-boomer generation (people born between 1946 and 1964) reaches the age of 65 years.

D. One in five U.S. citizens will be elderly by 2030. The projection of 70 million older people by that year is more than twice their number in 1999 (Administration on Aging, 2000).

E. The elderly population numbered 30 million in 1988, is projected to reach 40 million by 2011, and is projected to reach 50 million by 2019 (U.S. Census Bureau, 2004).

F. Since 1900, the percentage of Americans 65 years or older has more than tripled, representing the fastest-growing segment of the U.S. population. This group will account for 20% of the country's total populace (U.S. Census Bureau, 2004).

1. In 1995, there were more than 1.5 million frail elderly people residing in 20,000 nursing homes in the United States (Ferrell, Ferrell, & Rivera, 1995). The elderly population can be subdivided into the following age groups:
   a. *Younger old:* 65 to 75 years old. The percentage of Americans 65 to 74 years old in 1994 was eight times larger than in 1900.
   b. *Older old:* 75 to 84 years old. The 75- to 84-year-old age group in 1994 was 14 times larger than in 1900.
   c. *Elite old:* 85 years old and older. The 2000 U.S. census reported 4.2 billion citizens older than 85 years (U.S. Government Census, 2000).
      (1) This group is growing faster than any other age group (U.S. Census Bureau, 2004).
      (2) The elite old group in 1994 had 3.5 million people, or 1% of the U.S. population.
      (3) By 2020, the population in the elite old group is projected to double to 7 million.
      (4) By 2040, the elite old group will double again to 14 million.
      (5) It has been predicted that by 2050, approximately 1.2 million people will be alive at 100 years of age (Brant & Wickham, 2001).

II. Barriers to Effective Pain Management in Older Adults

A. Myths and misconceptions (McCaffery & Pasero, 1999)

1. Pain is a normal consequence of aging.
2. Cognitively impaired older adults are less sensitive to pain (Benedetti, Arduino, Vighetti, Asteggiano, & Tarenzi, 2004; Ferrell, 1991).
3. Older adults cannot tolerate opioids.
4. If pain is not reported, it does not exist.
5. Pain prevents sleep (Brant & Wickham, 2001).
6. If a person can be distracted from pain, it does not exist.

B. Patient- or family-related barriers (McCaffery & Pasero, 1999; Nijmeh, 2008)

1. A fear of addiction is common.
2. The desire is to please the health care provider.
3. Pain is viewed as punishment.
4. Pain is considered normal and expected.
5. Concerns exist about unmanageable side effects.
6. Financial concerns include cost of medication, hospitalization, and lost wages.
7. Lack of knowledge about assistance programs or reluctance to apply creates a barrier to effective pain management.
8. There is poor adherence to a prescribed analgesic regimen (Miaskowski, Dodd, & West, 2001).
9. Pain is associated with worsening disease.
10. Poor communication creates a barrier.

C. Clinician barriers
   1. The clinician has inadequate knowledge about pain management.
   2. There is fear of addiction (Anderson & Richman, 2002).
   3. The clinician is unable discern among pain, suffering, and depression.
   4. Polypharmacy creates a clinical barrier
   5. Pain is poorly assessed (Bruera, Wiley, & Euert, 2005).
   6. Regulatory concerns arise.
   7. Reimbursement is inadequate.
   8. Cultural differences exist between clinicians and patients.

D. Health care system barriers (Survey, 2000)
   1. Regulations of controlled substances are restrictive.
   2. Treatment may not be reimbursed or may be too costly for the patient.
   3. Treatment protocols are inadequate.
   4. Treatment access problems arise.
   5. Care is fragmented.
   6. Gaps appear in knowledge about addiction, tolerance, and physical dependence.
   7. There is fear of regulatory scrutiny.
   8. Opiate availability in pharmacies is inadequate.

III. Consequences of Untreated Pain in Older Adults (American Geriatrics Society [AGS], 2002; Ferrell & Ferrell, 1990)

A. Untreated pain in older adults can lead to
   1. A decline in socialization and enjoyable activities (54%).
   2. Impaired gait (53%).
   3. Impaired posture (49%).
   4. Impaired sleep (45%).
   5. Depression (32%).
   6. Anxiety (26%).
   7. Alteration in nutrition (14%).
   8. Impaired cognition (12%).

IV. Common Causes of Pain in Older Adults (Boswell & Cole, 2006; Davis & Srivastava, 2003)

A. Pain can be caused by the following:
   1. Osteoarthritis or rheumatoid arthritis
   2. Polymyalgia rheumatica
   3. Fractures
   4. Osteoporosis
   5. Shingles or postherpetic neuralgia
   6. Spinal stenosis
   7. Diabetic neuropathy
   8. Peripheral vascular disease
   9. Temporal arteritis
   10. Degenerative joint disease
   11. Cervical and lumbar spondylosis
   12. Trigeminal neuralgia

V. Age-related Changes in Older Adults (Boswell & Cole, 2006; Vogel & Carter, 1998)

A. *Absorption* is the process by which drugs move from the site of administration to the circulatory system; this is slowed in the elderly because of
   1. Increased acidity or decreased pH (which may cause drugs to be poorly absorbed).
   2. Decreased intestinal blood flow.

3. Increased gastric emptying.
4. Decreased motility of the gastrointestinal tract (which may cause problems in absorption and increased gastrointestinal bleeding).

B. *Distribution* depends on the ratio of lean body tissue, which is determined by the amount of total body water and plasma proteins available to transport the drug. The drug remains longer in the tissues and acts for a longer time in older adults. The elderly have
1. Decreased lean body mass.
2. Increased body fat (which increases the volume of distribution of lipid-soluble drugs).
3. Decreased total body water volume (decreased volume of distribution for water-soluble drugs leads to higher peak plasma concentration).
4. Decreased muscle and soft tissue mass.
5. Increased plasma protein.
   a. In the elderly, lipid solubility factors and protein-binding potential of medications need to be understood because these change distribution of the medications.
      (1) Lipid-soluble medications deposit and accumulate in the subcutaneous fat, which is increased in older adults.
      (2) Protein-binding capacity of medications is influenced by the nutritional status of the older adult.

C. *Metabolism* is influenced by hepatic blood flow and other functions of the liver. In older adults, there is
1. Decreased liver mass.
2. Decreased microsomal enzyme activity.
3. Decreased hepatic blood flow.
   a. Clearance or elimination of medication is decreased in older adults because of reduction of hepatic blood flow and function of medication-metabolizing enzymes.
   b. Elimination half-life of medications is increased as a result of reduction of metabolic clearance.
   c. A decline occurs in the capacity of the liver to break down and convert drugs and their metabolites.

D. *Excretion and elimination* of most medications are through the kidneys. In older adults, there is
1. Decreased glomerular filtration and tubular reabsorption rates, which may result in prolonged analgesic effects.
2. Decreased creatinine clearance.
3. Decreased renal mass and blood flow.
   a. Clearance or elimination of medications is decreased in older adults because of reduced renal function.
   b. Decreased clearance of medications can lead to longer elimination of half-life (the time it takes for the plasma concentration of a drug in the body to be reduced from the bloodstream by 50%).

E. *Creatinine clearance* may decrease in the elderly even though serum creatinine may not change.
1. After age 40, the creatinine clearance decreases 10% every 10 years.
2. If creatinine clearance decreases to less than 30 mg/min, the excretion of the drug decreases significantly.
3. The formula for calculating the creatinine clearance is as follows (U.S. Pharmacopeial Convention, 1996):

$$\frac{\text{Male } (140 - \text{age}) \times \text{Ideal body weight in kilograms}}{72 \times \text{Serum creatinine (mg/dl)}}$$

Females use this formula and multiply by 0.85 (the estimated creatinine clearance for a female is 85% of that of a male).

Note: Nurses must understand the formula used in their respective facilities, as some formulas use ideal body weight while others use absolute body weight. Calculators on personal digital assistants and the Internet use the Cockroft-Gault formula, as seen at http://www.clinicalculator.com/english/nephrology/cockroft/cc.htm.

4. The ideal weight calculation is as follows:
    a. Males: 50 kg + (2.3 kg inches over 5 feet)
    b. Females: 45 kg + (2.3 kg inches over 5 feet)

VI. How to Assess Pain in Older Adults

A. Evaluation of physical, functional, psychological, spiritual, and cultural domains should be combined to ensure accurate assessment (Boswell & Cole, 2006; Ferrell, 2000; Herr & Garand, 2001).

B. A comprehensive assessment includes the following components.
1. A detailed history should be made that includes the following:
    a. Evaluation of pain report
    b. Medical diagnoses, pertinent laboratory, and diagnostic tests
    c. Analgesic history (prescription and over-the-counter medications, herbal remedies, vitamins, and alcohol use)
    d. Complementary therapies
    e. Functional ability (evaluation of activities of daily living)
    f. Psychological function (mood, anxiety, and depression)
    g. Spiritual and cultural beliefs and attitudes of patients and family
2. Perform a physical examination.
    a. Pay attention to the musculoskeletal and neurological systems.
        (1) Examine for trigger points and inflammation.
        (2) Use specific maneuvers, such as straight-leg raises and joint motion.
        (3) A neurological evaluation looks for autonomic, sensory, and motor deficits suggestive of neuropathic conditions and nerve injuries.
        (4) Thoroughly examine all painful sites.
    b. Any history of trauma should be evaluated.
    c. Any sudden change in character of pain may indicate deterioration or new injury and needs evaluation.
    d. Assess for sensory impairments.
    e. Observe current functional ability to determine mobility and independence (the importance of the family and caregiver as a source of information must not be overlooked).
    f. Evaluate for cognitive impairment. This evaluation can be done with a mini-mental state examination (simple) or the Minnesota Multiphasic Personality Inventory (extensive).
    g. Pain assessment scales can be used for qualitative and quantitative assessments (see the chapter on Pain Assessment).
3. A psychological evaluation is necessary as pain and emotions are closely linked.
4. Spiritual and cultural assessments are important as these can be a source of either pain or comfort to the patient and family.

VII. Factors to Consider When Assessing Older Adults

A. The following recommendations will assist with assessment of the elderly:
1. Prepare for a limited attention span.
2. Recognize that the patient may be easily distracted.
3. Speak slowly and clearly.
4. Keep the interview brief.
5. Repeat and reword questions.
6. Allow ample time to assimilate questions.
7. Supply good ambient lighting.
8. Give visual cues in large print.
9. Use amplified hearing devices.
10. Face the person directly.

IX. How to Assess Pain in Cognitively Impaired or Nonverbal Older Adults (AGS, 2002; American Society for Pain Management Nursing, 2006; Bjoro & Herr, 2008; Herr & Decker, 2004)

A. Attempt to illicit a self-report whenever possible. If inappropriate, document the reason.

B. Search for potential causes of pain:
   1. Acute pain (e.g., fractures, falls, bruises, surgery, or open wounds)
   2. Chronic pain (e.g., arthritis, constipation, back pain, degenerative joint disease, or postherpetic neuralgia)
   3. Environment (e.g., too hot, cold, or noisy)
   4. Unmet comfort needs (e.g., hunger, thirst, fatigue, or need for toileting)
   5. Mood (e.g., angry, sad, anxious, or depressed)

C. Seek surrogate reports of pain. Caregivers who know the person best can help by describing patterns and behaviors that are related to pain.

D. Observe behaviors that may be indicative of pain. Knowledge of the person's baseline behaviors is helpful in differentiating pain from other causes. Some common behaviors that may indicate discomfort in the cognitively impaired or nonverbal older adult may include the following (Herr, 2002):
   1. Noisy breathing
      a. The patient makes a negative-sounding noise on inspiration or expiration.
      b. Breathing looks strenuous or labored.
      c. Respirations sound loud, harsh, and gasping.
      d. The patient has episodic bursts of rapid breaths or hyperventilation.
   2. Negative vocalization
      a. Noise or speech has a negative or disapproving quality.
      b. There is constant muttering with a guttural tone.
      c. The patient makes noise with a definite unpleasant sound.
      d. The patient's speech is at a faster rate than a conversation or is drawn out, as in a moan or groan.
      e. The patient repeats the same words with a mournful tone expressing hurt or pain.
   3. Sad facial expression
      a. The patient has a troubled-looking face.
      b. The patient looks hurt, worried, lost, or lonesome.
      c. There is a distressed or sunken appearance.
      d. The patient has tears or is crying.
   4. Frightened facial expression
      a. A scared, concerned-looking face is seen.
      b. The patient looks bothered, fearful, or troubled.
      c. There is an alarmed appearance with open eyes and a pleading face.
   5. Frown
      a. The face looks strained.
      b. The patient has a stern or scowling expression.
      c. The face has a displeased look with a wrinkled brow and creases in the forehead.
      d. The corners of the mouth are turned down.
   6. Tense body language
      a. Extremities show tension.
      b. The body language includes wringing hands, clenched fists, or knees pulled up tightly.
      c. The patient appears to be in a strained and inflexible position.
   7. Activity pattern changes
      a. The patient has difficulty sleeping.
      b. A change in appetite occurs.
      c. There is cessation of normal routine activities.
      d. More rest periods than usual are needed.
   8. Changes in socialization
      a. Disruptive behavior occurs.
      b. The patient is resistive to care.

c. The patient is withdrawn.
d. The patient becomes isolated.
9. Fidgeting
a. Restless, impatient motion occurs.
b. The patient acts squirming or jittery.
c. There is the appearance of trying to get away from a hurt area.
d. Forceful touching, tugging, or rubbing body parts is seen (Feldt, 2000; Hurley, Volicer, & Hanrahan, 1992).

E. Attempt an analgesic trial. Assume pain is present unless proven otherwise, and initiate an analgesic trial. Select an appropriate analgesic according to the estimated intensity of pain derived from information, and titrate to effect (AGS, 2002).

X. Assessment Tools for Cognitively Impaired or Nonverbal Older Adults

A. Behavioral assessment tools may be used to identify the presence of pain; however, it is important to note that a behavioral score is not equivalent to a pain intensity rating when there is no self-report (Pasero & McCaffery, 2005).
B. The assessment tool should be appropriate to the person's condition and cognitive ability.
C. Some pain behavioral tools that have been reviewed and have strong conceptual support include the following (Herr, Decker, & Bjoro, 2003; Herr, Bjoro, & Decker, 2006):
1. Assessment of Discomfort in Dementia Protocol (Kovach, Noonan, Griffie, Muchka, & Weissman, 2002)
a. This is a systematic tool used by nurses to assess and treat physical and affective discomfort in people with dementia.
b. The five-step process includes a physical assessment, review of medical history, assessment of environmental stressors and needs, and the administration of analgesics.
c. It is a useful tool in clinical practice to improve the recognition and treatment of physical and affective discomfort.
d. It requires education and considerable time to implement.
2. CNPI: Checklist of Nonverbal Pain Indicators (Feldt, 2000) (see the chapter on Pain Assessment)
3. Doloplus 2 (Lefebre-Chapiro, 2001)
a. This behavioral assessment scale consists of 10 items divided into three subgroups proportional to the observed frequency (5 somatic items, 2 psychomotor items, and 3 psychological items)
b. Each item is scored from 0 to 3, with an overall score from 0 to 30.
c. This is a French tool, and several items in the English translation appear unclear.
4. Nursing Assistant-Administered Instrument to Assess Pain in Demented Individuals (Horgas, Nichols, Schapson, & Vietes, 2007; Snow et al., 2003)
a. This nursing assistant-administered tool focuses on observation of specific pain behaviors observed during movement and at rest.
b. It has four main sections:
(1) Pain behaviors observed during care
(2) Presence or absence of pain behaviors (pain faces, words, or rubbing)
(3) Pain behavior intensity
(4) Pain thermometer for rating overall pain
c. The tool is clinically useful and easy to use; however, scoring procedures are unclear and the scope of practice for nursing assistants in screening pain must be considered.
5. Pain Assessment Scale for Seniors with Severe Dementia (Fuchs-Lacelle & Hadjistavropoulos, 2004)
a. This is an observational tool of both common and subtle pain behaviors.
b. It is a checklist with four subscales and a total of 60 items, including facial expressions, activity and body movements, and social or mood and psychological items.
c. Scores can range from 0 to 60.

   d. It is clinically useful as a behavioral checklist, is simple to use, and is comprehensive; however, no interpretation of the total score is currently available.
6. Pain Assessment in Advanced Dementia Scale (PAINAD) (Hutchinson, Tucker, Kim, & Gilder, 2006; Warden, Hurley, & Volicer, 2003) (see the chapter on Pain Assessment)

XI. Nonopioid and Adjuvant Drugs in Older Adults

A. Nonsteroidal antiinflammatory drugs (NSAIDs) (e.g., ibuprofen®, naproxen®, and celecoxib®)
   1. NSAIDs have a multitude of drug interactions (Beyth & Shorr, 1999).
   2. Adverse effects can occur with prolonged use (Argoff & Cranmer, 2003; Kuo, 2006).
      a. *Gastrointestinal symptoms:* Dyspepsia, nausea, vomiting, diarrhea, constipation, and reflux are possible symptoms. Ulcerations can occur in the gastrointestinal tract, which can cause bleeding. Signs and symptoms in older adults may be insidious: the patient may feel light-headed, dizzy, tired all the time, fall, or become confused. Black tarry stools may be present. Statistics show that older adults given NSAIDs are four times more likely to develop peptic ulcer and five times more likely to die from gastrointestinal bleeding.
      b. *Renal symptoms:* A person could have subclinical symptoms. Signs of renal dysfunction could range from an increase in creatinine clearance to acute renal failure. Sodium and water retention could occur, leading to bilateral lower extremity edema. When lower extremity edema occurs in older adults, renal and cardiac function should be evaluated.
      c. *Hematological symptoms:* NSAIDs decrease platelet aggregation for the life of the NSAIDs in the bloodstream; this increases bleeding time. Aspirin binds with the platelet for the life of the platelet and can increase bleeding time for 2 to 3 weeks. Bone marrow depression from NSAIDs may occur, but it is rare.
      d. *Central nervous system symptoms:* NSAIDs can produce sedation, confusion, headache, depression, or psychosis. Aspirin can produce tinnitus.
      e. *Hepatic symptoms:* NSAIDs may elevate hepatic laboratory values. It is uncommon for NSAIDs to produce hepatitis or hepatic failure.
      f. *Pulmonary symptoms:* As with any age group, NSAIDs may enhance symptoms of asthma (Conaway, 1995).

B. Acetaminophen (American Pain Society [APS], 2003; DaCosta, 2006) (See the chapter on Overview of Pharmacology).
   1. Among potential hepatic effects, severe hepatotoxicity can develop in people with chronic alcoholism, those with liver disease, or those who are fasting.
   2. The American Liver Foundation recommends that people not exceed three grams of acetaminophen a day for any prolonged period of time (American Liver Foundation, 2008; Watkins et al., 2008).
   3. Acetaminophen may mask infection.
   4. Potential for drug interactions includes an elevation in the international normalized ratio (INR) with patients taking warfarin (Coumadin®) (Hylek, Heiman, Skates, Sheehan, & Singer, 1998).
   5. Overdoses are common because acetaminophen is present in many nonprescription and prescription medications.

C. Antidepressants (e.g., amitriptyline®, nortriptyline®, desipramine®, and duloxetine®) (APS, 2003; DaCosta, 2006)
   1. Antidepressants are adjuvant drugs for treatment of neuropathic pain.
   2. They may cause potent anticholinergic side effects, such as dry mouth (creating discomfort and risk of choking), constipation (creating discomfort and obstruction from fecal impaction), urinary retention, delirium, sedation, and orthostatic hypotension.
   3. An electrocardiogram may be required before start of therapy if a patient has a prolonged QT interval (more than 4 mm), and a cardiologist may need to be consulted.
   4. Duloxetine has been approved for the treatment of diabetic peripheral neuropathy and fibromyalgia.

D. Anticonvulsants (e.g., gabapentin®, pregabalin®, and valproic acid®) (APS, 2003; DaCosta, 2006)
   1. Anticonvulsants are adjuvant drugs for the treatment of neuropathic pain. Side effects may

include
    a. Dizziness.
    b. Sedation.
    c. Drowsiness.
2. Pregabalin has been approved for the treatment of postherpetic neuralgia.

E. Corticosteroids (e.g., dexamethasone®)
1. Corticosteroids are adjuvant drugs for the treatment of neuropathic pain, bone pain, cancer pain, and other pain syndromes (APS, 2003). Side effects may include
    a. Hyperglycemia.
    b. Weight gain.
    c. Neuropsychiatric symptoms (dysphoria, euphoria, or delirium).
    d. Osteoporosis with long-term use.
    e. Myopathy.

XII. Opioids (morphine®, oxycodone®, hydromorphone®, fentanyl®, hydrocodone®, and methadone®) (AGS, 2002; APS, 2003; Fuse, 2001) (see the chapter on Overview of Pharmacology)

A. The following are important considerations to remember when using opioids in older adults:
1. Start low and go slow.
2. Choose drugs with short half-lives and fewer side effects.
3. Assess and reassess at regular intervals.
4. Assess carefully for both effectiveness and presence of adverse effects.
5. Initiate bowel regimen at the *start* of opioid therapy to prevent constipation.
6. Assess for drug interactions.
7. Monitor for side effects from analgesics.
8. Assess for any renal and hepatic impairment.
9. Avoid intramuscular injections, which may cause tissue damage in frail elderly and create absorption changes.
10. Titrate to effect using short-acting medications. Consider long-acting analgesics for persistent pain.
11. Use around the clock dosing instead of as-needed dosing.
12. Use nonpharmacological modalities, along with analgesics.

XIII. Drugs to Avoid in Older Adults (APS, 2003; APS, 2008; Beers et al., 1991; Fick, Mion, & Beers, 2008; Wilcox, Himmelstein, & Woolhandler, 1994)

A. Meperidine (Demerol®)
1. The neurotoxic metabolite, normeperidine, can cause tremors, myoclonus, and generalized seizures especially, when renal impairment is present (not unique to elderly).
2. Intramuscular injections are painful, irritating to tissue, and should be avoided.
3. Oral meperidine has decreased analgesic efficacy due to first-pass metabolism.
4. Meperidine may cause delirium and agitation postoperatively in older adults.
5. Meperidine has a short duration of action (2.5 to 3.5 hours).
6. It should not be used for more than 48 hours in patients with renal and central nervous system disease.

B. Propoxyphene (Darvon®, Darvocet®)
1. The metabolite, norpropoxyphene, has a long half-life (30 to 36 hours), which accumulates with repeated doses and may cause seizures and cardiotoxicity.
2. Avoid use in older adults with renal insufficiency, as the drug is excreted by the kidneys.

C. Amitriptyline (Elavil®)
1. Potent anticholinergic side effects make this drug less well tolerated in older adults.
2. Nortriptyline and desipramine have fewer side effects and are better tolerated in the elderly (Maletta, Mattox, & Kysken, 2000)

D. Methadone (Dolophine®)
1. A long and variable half-life (12 to 150 hours) makes titration difficult.

2. Methadone takes longer to reach steady state.
3. Careful titration is critical in older adults to prevent drug toxicity.
4. Methadone should be prescribed and monitored by licensed professionals knowledgeable of the drug's pharmacokinetics and pharmacodynamics in relation to older adults.

E. Pentazocine (Talwin®)
1. Pentazocine is no better than aspirin in analgesic properties.
2. It can cause renal injury.
3. Use may lead to seizures and arrhythmias.
4. Pentazocine causes delirium and agitation in older adults (Ferrell, 1991).
5. Pentazocine has a short duration of action and high side-effect profile.

F. Sedatives and hypnotics (e.g., diazepam®, flurazepam®, meprobamate®, and chlordiazepoxide®)
1. Sedatives and hypnotics have a long duration of action.
2. Sedative effects can increase potential for falls and delirium in older adults.

G. Antihistamines (e.g., cimetidine®, ranitidine®, and diphenhydramine®)
1. Avoid use beyond 12 weeks, and avoid higher dose ranges.
2. Antihistamines increase the action of benzodiazepines.

H. Antiemetics (e.g., promethazine® and hydroxyzine®)
1. Antiemetics have sedative effects.
2. They can be irritating given as intramuscular injections.
3. Antiemetics have a long duration of action.
4. They can cause respiratory depression.

XIV. Local Topical Anesthetics (APS, 2003, APS, 2008)

A. *Lidoderm patch* (lidocaine® 5%): Lidocaine is used to relieve the pain of postherpetic neuralgia. Apply one to three patches on intact skin for up to 12 hours at the site or sites of pain.

B. *Capsaicin cream* (active ingredient in chili peppers): When applied to skin, capsaicin cream depletes substance P, a neurochemical that transmits pain. The recommended starting dose is 0.025%, applied four times a day. Avoid contact with the eyes.

C. *EMLA cream* (lidocaine® 2.5% and prilocaine® 2.5%): EMLA cream is used as a local anesthetic for venipuncture, accessing ports or arteriovenous fistulas. Apply the cream over the site, and cover with Tegaderm for 1 hour before accessing the site; remove Tegaderm and wipe off the cream before insertion.

XV. Delirium

A. Delirium is common in older adults, but too often it goes unrecognized and untreated.

B. Delirium is a significant problem that can accompany illness and hospitalization and is associated with morbidity and mortality rates (Marcantonio, Kiely, & Simon, 2005).

C. Establishing a baseline cognitive status is essential, especially in those who have dementia (Fick, 2007).

D. Incidence (Kiely, 2007; McCusker, Cole, Abrahamowicz, Primeau, & Betzile, 2002)
1. Delirium has been found in 10% to 22% of hospitalized older adults (Curyto et al., 2001)
2. At time of admission, 14% to 56% of these patients have delirium.
3. Of patients with delirium, 40% are in intensive care units.
4. After orthopedic surgery, 40% to 50% of older adults have been found to have delirium.
5. Delirium has been found in 80% of older adults near the end of life.

E. While the symptoms of delirium are varied and numerous, the main symptoms include (Inouye, 2006)
1. Mental status altered from baseline (acute onset or fluctuating).
2. Inattention (inability to focus and maintain attention).
3. Disorganized thinking.
4. Altered level of consciousness (hypoactivity, hyperactivity, or mixed).

F. Precipitating factors of delirium are (Alagiakrishnan & Wiens, 2004)
1. Metabolic disorders or imbalance.
2. Infections.

3. Medications.
4. Pain.
5. Acute illness (Bruce, 2007).
6. Dehydration.
7. Hypoglycemia.
8. Hypoxia.

G. Differences between delirium and dementia (Fick, 2002, 2007; Justic, 2000) (Table 22-1)

Table 22-1 Differences between Delirium and Dementia

	Delirium	Dementia
1.	Sudden onset	Insidious onset
2.	Lasts days to weeks	Lasts months to years
3.	Usually reversible	Usually irreversible
4.	Fluctuating course	Progressive course
5.	Cognitive and social inaccessibility	Flat affect
6.	Disoriented	Trouble executing motor function
7.	Decreased cooperativeness	Reduced ability to reason

H. Treatment
1. Identify the cause or causes early and treat promptly.
2. Interventions should be used to maintain safety.
3. Frequent reorientation restores prior cognitive function.
4. Monitor nutrition and hydration.
5. Modify environmental stimuli.
6. Address pain management.
7. Use nonpharmacological interventions (music, massage, etc.).
8. Review all medications.
9. Remove urinary catheters early.
10. Research shows that early identification of delirium and its source, and prompt treatment, result in
    a. Improved outcomes.
    b. Decreased mortality rates.
    c. Shorter hospital stays (Naughton, 2005).

I. Adverse physical consequences of delirium include the following (Fick & Mion, 2008):
1. Malnutrition
2. Falls
3. Skin breakdown
4. Aspiration
5. Increase in functional disability
6. Mortality and morbidity

J. Ongoing research is needed in providing optimal, evidence-based guidelines for the assessment, prevention, and management of delirium in older adults (Fick & Mion, 2008; Inouye, 2006).

XVI. Recommendations in Clinical Practice (AGS, 2002; American Medical Directors Association, 2003; APS, 2003; American Society for Pain Management Nursing, 2006)

1. Accept the person's report of pain.
2. Use the least invasive route. The oral route is the preferred route if appropriate and effective.
3. Start low and go slow.

4. Assess, anticipate, and mange side effects aggressively.
5. Use NSAIDs with caution and for short periods.
6. Treat severe pain with opioids. Use long-acting opioids for persistent pain, along with a short-acting analgesic for breakthrough pain.
7. Educate clinicians regarding the physiological changes in metabolism, absorption, and excretion of drugs in the elderly.
8. Encourage patients to be active participants in their care.
9. Promote coping behaviors (distraction, relaxation, imagery, massage, group support, etc.).
10. Discuss goals and treatment plans with the patient and family, and provide education to ensure compliance.
11. Educate patients, families, and clinicians about tolerance, physical dependence, and addiction. Provide ongoing education to patients, families, and clinicians.
12. Assess and reassess pain often.
13. Assess for the degree of renal and hepatic impairment.
14. Use consistent pain rating scales to assess pain intensity appropriate to the person's condition and cognitive level.
15. Implement safety measures for people with delirium or dementia.
16. Use multimodal approaches, including nonpharmacological interventions (cognitive-behavioral therapy, exercise, rehabilitation, etc.), for more favorable outcomes in the treatment of pain (Malan, Marsh, Grossman, Traylor, & Hubbard, 2003).
17. Choose medications with the least noxious side-effect profile and dose appropriately, considering the older adult's physiological parameters.
18. Implement policies and procedures to ensure that pain is being adequately addressed and monitored.

References

Administration on Aging. (2000). *Profile of older Americans.* U.S. Department of Health and Human Services. Retrieved May 30,2009, from http://www.aoa.gov/AoAroot/Aging_Statistics/Profile/2000/profile2000.pdf.

Alagiakrishnan, K., & Wiens, C. A. (2004). An approach to drug induced delirium in the elderly. *Postgraduate Medical Journal, 80*(945), 388–393.

American Geriatrics Society. (2002). The management of persistent pain in older persons. *Journal of the American Geriatrics Society, 50*(6), S205–S224.

American Liver Foundation. (2008). *The American Liver Foundation issues a warning on dangers of excess acetaminophen.* Retrieved November 22, 2008, from http://www.liverfoundation.org/about/news/33/.

American Medical Directors Association. (2003). *Chronic pain management in the long term care setting.* Clinical Practice Guidelines. Columbia, Maryland: Author.

American Pain Society. (2003). *Principles of analgesic use in the treatment of acute pain and cancer pain* (5th ed.). Glenview, IL: Author.

American Pain Society. (2008). *Principles of analgesic use in the treatment of acute pain and cancer pain* (6th ed.). Glenview, IL: Author.

American Society for Pain Management Nursing. (2006). *Position statement: Pain assessment in the non-verbal patient.* Lenexa, Kansas: Author.

Anderson, K. O., & Richman, J. (2002). Cancer pain management among undeserved minority out-patients: Perceived needs and barriers to optimal control. *Cancer, 94*(8), 2295–2304.

Argoff, C., & Cranmer, K. (2003). The pharmacological management of chronic pain in long-term care settings: Balancing efficacy and safety. *Consultant Pharmacist, 18*(Suppl. C), 4–18.

Beers, M. H., Ouslander, J. G., Rollingher, I., Reuben, D., Brooks, J., & Beck, J. C. (1991). Explicit criteria for determining inappropriate medication use in nursing home residents. *Archives of Internal Medicine, 151,* 1825–1832.

Benedetti, F., Arduino, C., Vighetti, S., Asteggiano, G., & Tarenzi, L. (2004). Pain reactivity in Alzheimer patients with different degrees of cognitive and brain activity deterioration. *Pain, 111,* 22–29.

Beyth, R. J., & Shorr, R. I. (1999). Epidemiology of adverse drug reactions in the elderly by drug class. *Drugs and Aging, 14,* 231–239.

Bjoro, K., & Herr, K. (2008). Assessment of pain in nonverbal or cognitively impaired older adults. *Clinics in Geriatric Medicine, 24*(2), 237–262.

Boswell, M., & Cole, E. (Eds.). (2006). *Weiner's pain management: A practical guide for clinicians* (7th ed.). Boca Raton, FL: CRC Press.

Brant, J. M., & Wickham, R. (2001). The challenge of pain assessment and management in the elderly: Look before you leap. Discussion Session. *Program and Abstracts of the 26th Congress of the Oncology Nursing Society,* May 17–20, San Diego, CA.

Bruce, A. J. (2007). The incidence of delirium associated with orthopedic surgery: A meta-analytic review. *International Psychogeriatrics, 19*(2), 197–214.

Bruera, E., Wiley, J. S., & Euert, P. A. (2005). Pain intensity assessment by bedside nurses and palliative care consultants: A retrospective study. *Support Care Cancer, 13*(40), 228–231.

Conaway, D. C. (1995). Using NSAIDs safely in the elderly. *Hospital Medicine, May 31,* 23.

Curyto, K. J., Johnson, J., TenHave, T., Mossey, J., Knott, K., & Katz, R. (2001). Survival of hospitalized elderly patients with delirium: A prospective study. *American Journal of Geriatric Psychiatry,* 141–147.

DaCosta, J. (2006). Pain management and geriatrics. In M. Boswell & E. Cole (Eds.), *Weiner's pain management: A practical guide for clinicians* (7th ed., pp. 1319–1325). Boca Raton, FL: CRC Press.

Davis, M. P., & Srivastava, M. (2003). Demographics, assessment and management of pain in the elderly. *Drug Aging, 20*(1), 23–67.

Feldt, K. (2000). Checklist of nonverbal pain indicators. *Pain Management Nursing, 1,* 13–21.

Ferrell, B. A. (1991). Pain management in elderly people. *Journal of the American Geriatrics Society, 39,* 64–73.

Ferrell, B. A. (2000). Comprehensive geriatric assessment. In D. Osterwll, K. Brummell-Smith, & J. C. Beck (eds.), *Pain* (pp. 381–397). New York: McGraw-Hill.

Ferrell, B. A., & Ferrell, B. R. (1990). Easing the pain. *Geriatric Nursing, 11,* 175–178.

Ferrell, B. A., Ferrell, B. R., & Rivera, L. (1995). Pain in cognitively impaired nursing home patients. *Journal of Pain and Symptom Management, 10,* 591–598.

Fick, D. M. (2002). Delirium superimposed on dementia: a systematic review. *Journal American Geriatric Society, 50*(10), 1723–1732.

Fick, D. M. (2007). Recognizing delirium superimposed on dementia: Assessing nurses' knowledge case vignettes. *Journal of Gerontological Nursing, 33*(2), 40–47.

Fick, D. M., & Mion, L. C. (2008). How to try this: Delirium superimposed on dementia. *American Journal of Nursing, 108*(1), 52–60.

Fick, D. M., Mion, L. C., & Beers, M. H. (2008). Health outcomes associated with potentially inappropriate medication use in older adults. *Research in Nursing & Health, 31*(1), 42–51.

Fuchs-Lacelle, S., & Hadjistavropoulos, T. (2004). Development and preliminary validation of the pain assessment checklist for seniors with limited ability to communicate. *Pain Management Nursing, 5*(2), 37–49.

Fuse, P. G. (2001). Opioid analgesic drugs in older people. *Clinics in Geriatric Medicine, 17,* 479–485.

Herr, K. (2002). Pain assessment in cognitively impaired older adults. *American Journal of Nursing, 102*(12), 65–67.

Herr, K., Bjoro, K., & Decker, S. (2006). Tools for assessment of pain in nonverbal older adults with dementia: A state-of-the-science review [Abstract]. *Journal of Pain & Symptom Management, 31,* 170–192.

Herr, K., & Decker, S. (2004). Assessment of pain in older adults with severe cognitive impairment. *Annals of Long Term Care, 12*(4), 45–52.

Herr, K., Decker, S., & Bjoro, K. (2003). *State of the art review of tools for assessment of pain in nonverbal adults.* Retrieved May 30, 2009, from http://prc.coh.org/pain-noa.htm.

Herr, K., & Garand, L. (2001). Assessment and measurement of pain in older adults. *Clinics Geriatric Medicine, 17,* 173–179.

Horgas, A. L., Nichols, A. L., Schapson, C. A., & Vietes, K. (2007). Assessing pain in persons with dementia: Relationships among the non-communicative patient's pain assessment instrument, self-report, and behavioral observations. *Pain Management Nursing, 8*(2), 77–85.

Hurley, A. C., Volicer, B. J., & Hanrahan, P. A. (1992). Assessment of discomfort in advanced Alzheimer's patients. *Research in Nursing and Health, 15,* 369–377.

Hutchinson, R. W., Tucker, W. F., Kim, S., & Gilder, R. (2006). Evaluation of a behavioral assessment tool for the individual unable to self-report pain. *American Journal of Hospice & Palliative Medicine, 23*(4), 328–331.

Hylek, E., Heiman, H., Skates, S. J., Sheehan, M. A., & Singer, D. E. (1998). Acetaminophen and other risk factors for excessive warfarin anticoagulation. *Journal of the American Medical Association, 279,* 657–662.

Inouye, S. K. (2006). Delirium in older persons. *New England Journal of Medicine, 354*(11), 1157–1165.

Justic, M. (2000). Does "ICU psychosis" really exist? *Critical Care Nursing, June,* 28–39.

Kiely, D. K. (2007). Association between psychomotor activity delirium subtypes and mortality among newly admitted post-acute facility patients. *Journals of Gerontology: Series A, Biological Sciences and Medical Sciences, 62*(2), 174–179.

Kovach, C. R., Noonan, P. E., Griffie, J., Muchka, S., & Weissman, D. E. (2002). The assessment of discomfort in dementia protocol. *Pain Management Nursing, 3*(10), 16–27.

Kuo, G. (2006). Nonsteroidal anti-inflammatory drugs. In M. Boswell & E. Cole (Eds.), *Weiner's pain management: A practical guide for clinicians* (7th ed., pp. 773–785). Boca Raton, FL: CRC Press.

Lefebre-Chapiro, S. (2001). The Doloplus 2 scale: Evaluating pain in the elderly. *European Journal of Palliative Care, 8*(5), 191–194.

Malan, T., Marsh, G., Grossman, E., Traylor, L., & Hubbard, R. (2003). Parecoxib sodium, a parenteral cyclooxygenase 2 selective inhibitor, improves morphine analgesia and is opioid-sparing following total hip arthroplasty. *Anesthesiology, 98,* 950–956.

Maletta, G., Mattox, K. M., & Kysken, M. (2000). Guidelines for prescribing psychotropic drugs. *Geriatrics, 56,* 65–79.

Marcantonio, E. R., Kiely, D. K., & Simon, S. E. (2005). Outcomes of older people admitted to post acute facilities with delirium. *Journal of American Geriatrics Society, 53*(6), 963–969.

McCaffery, M., & Pasero, C. (1999). Pain in the elderly. In *Pain: Clinical manual* (2nd ed., pp. 674–706). St. Louis: Mosby.

McCusker, J., Cole, M., Abrahamowicz, M., Primeau, F., & Betzile, E. (2002). Delirium predicts 12-month mortality. *Archives Internal Medicine, 162*(4), 457–463.

Miaskowski, C., Dodd, M. J., & West, C. (2001). Lack of adherence with the analgesic regimen: A significant barrier to effective cancer pain management. *Journal of Clinical Oncology, 19*(230), 4275–4279.

Naughton, B. J. (2005). A multifactorial intervention to reduce prevalence of delirium and shorten hospital stay. *Journal of American Geriatrics Society, 53*(1), 18–23.

Nijmeh, M. (2008). Patient-related barriers to effective cancer pain management. *Journal of Hospice & Palliative Nursing, 10*(4), 198–204.

Pasero, C., & McCaffery, M. (2005). No self-report means no pain-intensity rating. *American Journal of Nursing, 105*(3), 50–55.

Snow, A. L., Weber, J. B., O'Malley, K. J., Cody, M., Beck, C., & Bruera, E. (2003). NOPPAIN: A nursing assistant-administered pain assessment instrument for use in dementia. *Dementia and Geriatric Cognitive Disorders, 921,* 1–8.

Survey, Conducted for American Pain Society, American Academy of Pain Medicine, & Janssen Pharmaceutica. (2000). *Chronic pain in America.* Hanson, NY: Roper Starch Worldwide.

U.S. Census Bureau. (2004). *Projected population of the United States by age and sex, race, and Hispanic origin: 1995 to 2050, Washington, DC.* Retrieved May 30, 2009 from http://www.census.gov/prod/1/pop/p25-1130/p251130a.pdf.

U.S. Government Census. (2000). Census 2000 Special Tabulation on Aging. Retrieved May 30, 2009, from http://www.census.gov/mp/www/cat/decennial_census_2000/005977.html

U.S. Pharmacopeial Convention. (1996). *USP DI: Drug information for the health care professional* (16th ed.). Rockville, MD: Author.

Vogel, D., & Carter, P. B. (1998). Pharmacology and the older person: Effects on communication. *Topics in Geriatric Rehabilitation, 14,* 76–86.

Warden, V., Hurley, A. C., & Volicer, L. (2003). Development and psychometric evaluation of the pain assessment in advanced dementia (PAINAD) scale. *Journal of the American Medical Directors Association, 4*(1), 9–15.

Watkins, P. B., Kaplowitz, N., Slattery, J. T., Colonese, C. R., Colucci, S. V., Stewart, P. W., & Harris, S. C. (2008). Aminotransferase elevations in healthy adults receiving 4 grams of acetaminophen daily: A randomized controlled trial. *Journal of the American Medical Society, 296*(1), 87–93.

Wilcox, S. M., Himmelstein, D. U., & Woolhandler, S. (1994). Inappropriate prescribing for the community dwelling elderly. *Journal of the American Medical Association, 272,* 292–296.

Suggested Readings

Balducci, L. (2003). Management of cancer pain in geriatric patients. *Journal of Supportive Oncology, 1*(3), 175–188.

Ferrell, B. A., & Ferrell, B. R. (1991). Principles of pain management in older people. *Comprehensive Therapy, 17,* 53–58.

subsection

3

State of the Science

chapter

23

Gender or Sex Differences in Pain and Analgesia

Cathy D. Trame, RN-BC, MS, CNS
Cheryl Rawe, RN, MS, CNS, BC

Objectives

After studying this chapter, the reader should be able to:

1. Understand gender differences in nociception
2. Understand how gender may influence treatment of pain

Key points

- A comprehensive consensus report was formulated to direct future studies of sex and gender differences in pain and analgesia and should be referenced before conducting further research (Greenspan et al., 2007). "Sex" defines biological differences while "gender" defines psychosocial differences; the terms are not interchangeable (Greenspan et al., 2007).

I. Pathophysiological Differences

Key Points

- Genetic differences in nociception can be identified between males and females.
- Hormones and hormonal cycles influence pain thresholds in females but not in males.
- Attenuated adrenocortical response in females may alter physiological response; no elevation in blood pressure or heart rate may be identified with acute pain in females.
- Males show a greater propensity for the release of endogenous μ-opioids to mitigate acute pain, but studies conflict on gender-specific opioid requirements to relieve acute pain.

A. Animal studies
   1. No influence by sex was shown in response to incision pain on the paw of rats (Banik, Woo, Park, & Brennan, 2006; Kroin, Buvanendran, Nagalla, & Tuman, 2003).
   2. Male rats showed greater paw flinching than females related to induction of pain with endothelin-1 (vasoactive peptide), which is normally released into circulation after stress and cold pain and locally released in response to injury or disease (McKelvy, Mark, & Sweitzer, 2007).
   3. A literature review of biological studies from 1980 to 2004 found female rodents are more sensitive than males to noxious stimuli and produce less endogenous analgesia (Mogil & Chanda, 2005; Wiesenfeld-Hallin, 2005).

B. Human studies
   1. No genetic influences were identified by gender on study of twins with chronic widespread pain; however, findings indicate that environmental influences played a role (Kato, Sullivan, Evengard, & Pedersen, 2006). No sex-specific genetic influence on neck pain was identified in dizygotic twins; however, women had a much higher reported prevalence (Fejer, Hartvigsen, & Kyvik, 2006).
   2. Small, nonsignificant differences between women and men in nociceptive transmission and neuronal sensitization were found by measurement of Frey hair stimulation after application of thermal source of pain (Jensen & Petersen, 2006).
   3. A literature review from 1887 to 2005 regarding modulation of pain by emotion suggests gender differences in how pain is processed; that is, males have reduced pain in combination with sexual or erotic stimuli, and women have increased pain with fear, threat, or high emotional arousal. No differences in gender were found with low to moderate arousal, such as anxiety. This suggests the need for further well-controlled research (Rhudy & Williams, 2005).
   4. A literature review of biological studies from 1980 to 2004 found pain tolerance, sensitivity, and pain threshold in women varies with the stage of menstrual cycle (Becker et al., 2005; Wiesenfeld-Hallin, 2005).
      a. Capsaicin-induced trigeminal sensitization showed increased allodynic area during the menstrual phase versus the luteal phase in women; women revealed increased allodynic area overall as compared to men, despite the phase of the woman's menstrual cycle (Gazerani, Andersen, & Arendt-Nielsen, 2005).
      b. Significant differences in visceral pain sensitivity are found during different phases of the menstrual cycle (Arendt-Nielsen, Bajaj, & Drewes, 2004).

c. In a meta-analysis of 16 studies, pain related to pressure stimulation, cold pressor pain, thermal heat stimulation, and ischemic muscle pain revealed higher pain thresholds during the follicular phase of menstruation versus the luteal phase (Miaskowski & Levine, 2004).

5. Delayed muscle pain measured by induction of eccentric contractions 24 to 48 hours after exercise revealed no significant differences in pain ratings between men and women (Dannecker, Hausenblas, Kaminski, & Robinson, 2005).
6. Men demonstrated increased magnitudes of μ-opioid endogenous system activation traced by positron emission tomography in the anterior thalamus, ventral basal ganglia, and amygdala when exposed to deep tissue pain, as compared to women (Zubieta et al., 2002).
7. Correlation of pain perception to elevated heart rate was present in men, but not women, when pain was experimentally induced by immersion of a hand in hot water (Tousignant-Laflamme, Rainville, & Marchand, 2005).
8. Systolic blood pressure and stroke volume related to attenuated adrenocortical activity revealed a negative correlation to increased pain in women versus men with an experimentally induced hand cold pressor test (al'Absi, Petersen, & Wittmers, 2002).
9. The female sex hormone, estrogen, alters excitability of sensory neurons and trigeminal afferent fibers, causing noxious stimulation of craniofacial tissues (Cairns, 2007). Women of a reproductive age are more likely to seek treatment for orofacial pain conditions than are men (Shinal & Fillingim, 2007).
10. Macrophage migration inhibitory factor (neuroendocrine mediator) was positively correlated with testosterone and negatively correlated with estradiol. This was thought to contribute to the sex differences in a chronic pain report (Aloisi et al., 2005).
11. A comprehensive review of the literature regarding response to analgesics found opioid analgesics to be more effective in women than in men. Men needed higher doses of opioids to achieve pain relief (24% to 40% more), and κ-opioid receptor analgesics were more effective in women than in men (Miaskowski & Levine, 2004). Conflicting data by Ji, Murphy, and Traub (2006) found morphine to be more effective in male animals in experimentally induced pain, a higher requirement for morphine for postoperative pain in women versus men, and the disappearance of gender variance in patients older than 75 years (Aubrun, Salvi, Coriat, & Riou, 2005).
12. Vibratory stimulation experimentally applied to mitigate pain produced by electrocutaneous sensory detection increased pain thresholds for women but not men (Dahlin, Lund, Lundeberg, & Molander, 2006).
13. Overall, some biological differences in pain perception exist; however, the differences are more significantly influenced by psychosocial variables (Main & Spanswick, 2000). Response to analgesics in animal studies with rodents may be skewed since male rodents have more body fat than female rodents and the opposite is true in humans; therefore, lipophilic analgesics may be distributed differently (Greenspan et al., 2007).

II. Sex Differences in Types or Disease Sources

Key Point

Sex differences are clear in the prevalence of certain types of pain. Women have a higher prevalence of fibromyalgia, myofascial pain syndromes, migraine headaches, irritable bowel syndrome, osteoarthritis, rheumatoid arthritis, generalized pain, hip pain, neck pain, and facial pain.

A. *Sickle cell disease:* In a study of 226 adults with sickle cell disease, no sex differences were found in the number of days subjects experience pain or the number of pain episodes experienced in the prior 6 months. Opioid usage and pain ratings had no significant differences; men with sickle cell genotype were more likely to use health care resources (5.1% versus 2.7%) (McClish et al., 2006).

B. *Irritable bowel syndrome:* More North American women than males are affected by irritable bowel syndrome with resulting abdominal pain (Frissora & Koch, 2005).

C. *Neck pain:* A literature review of the prevalence of neck pain found women report neck pain more often than men (Fejer, Kyvik, & Hartvigsen, 2006).
D. *Chronic back pain:* Back pain was more prevalent in elderly females, age 70 to 77 years, than in males (Jacobs, Hammerman-Rozenberg, Cohen, & Stressman, 2006). No difference was seen in prevalence of sick days related to back pain in nonpregnant females versus males age 16 to 44 years (Sydsjo, Alexanderson, Dastserri, & Sydsjo, 2003).
E. *Laparoscopic cholecystectomy:* Higher visual analogue scale scores, increased analgesic use, and significantly higher body temperatures were recorded in females after laparoscopic cholecystectomy than in males (Uchiyama et al., 2006).
F. *Arthroscopic knee surgery:* Women reported more pain in a study of postoperative pain after arthroscopic knee surgery. On a visual analogue scale with a 0 to 100 range, the average pain score was for women 84 versus 57 for men (Rosseland & Stubhaug, 2004).
G. *Hip arthroplasty:* Women enrolled in Medicare report more severe pain with walking and are more disabled than men after elective total hip arthroplasty (Holtzman, Saleh, & Kane, 2002).
H. *Headaches:* Cluster headaches are five times more prevalent in men than in women (Cairns, 2007). Migraines and other types of headaches are more prevalent in women (Main & Spanswick, 2000; Miaskowski & Levine, 2004).
I. *Myofascial pain syndromes (fibromyalgia, musculoskeletal pain, joint pain, arthritis):* A higher prevalence of musculoskeletal pain, fibromyalgia, osteoarthritis, and rheumatoid arthritis has been identified in women than in men (Main & Spanswick, 2000; Miaskowski & Levine, 2004).
J. *Lung cancer:* No relationship was found in the existence of lung cancer pain between men and women (Hoffman, Given, von Eye, Gift, & Given, 2007).

III. Gender Differences in Pain Treatment

Key Point

Sex discrimination related to the treatment of chest pain has been repeatedly documented in the literature. Women are alarmingly less likely to have timely diagnostic testing, undergo invasive interventions, or be prescribed medications for chest pain, even with documented coronary disease. Since coronary artery disease is the leading cause of mortality in U.S. women, outcomes related to this discrimination should be examined further.

A. *Lumbosacral pain:* A retrospective review of patients with degenerative lumbosacral pathologies (n = 5,690) revealed women were more likely to have imaging tests ordered; however, men were more likely to have surgery recommended (Taylor et al., 2005).
B. *Cancer and acquired immunodeficiency syndrome (AIDS):* Women with cancer and with AIDS-related pain were less likely to have adequate pain management than were men with the same diagnoses (Miaskowski & Levine, 2004).
C. Chest pain
   1. Women experienced longer intervals than men for initial electrocardiogram (EKG) when presenting with chest pain that was ultimately found to be noncardiac (Takakuwa, Shofer, & Hollander, 2007).
   2. Women with stable angina were less likely to receive an exercise EKG, undergo a coronary angiography, or be prescribed antiplatelet and statin therapies even with confirmed coronary disease. Women were also less likely to be revascularized but were twice as likely to have nonfatal myocardial infarction or death within 1 year (Daly et al., 2006). Women with acute coronary syndrome were less likely to undergo coronary angiography, angioplasty, and coronary artery bypass graft surgery than were men. No higher incidence of death, recurrent myocardial infarction, or stroke was identified; however, women suffered an increased rate of refractory ischemia and rehospitalization as compared to men (Anand et al., 2005). A recent study identified that women were less

likely to receive angiography for angina pectoris, resulting in a higher risk of a coronary event (Sekhri et al., 2008).

3. Men with angina pectoris were more likely to undergo exercise EKG, have surgical revascularization, receive daily aspirin, and be prescribed triple antianginal medications than were women. Men were also more likely than women to receive care by a cardiologist versus a general practitioner and be prescribed a β-blocker after myocardial infarction (Crilly & Bundred, 2005).
4. In patients with high-risk angina, women were less likely than men to receive statins or antilipidemic medication or to have current cholesterol measurements (Hendrix, Mayhan, & Egan, 2005).
5. Women with acute coronary syndrome and underlying chronic kidney disease were less likely to receive angiotensin-converting enzyme inhibitors, aspirin, and coronary angiography than men (Sonson, Lum, Madison, Seto, & Spies, 2004).
6. Younger women have significantly higher mortality rates than men following myocardial infarction and coronary artery bypass surgery (Wenger, Shaw, & Vaccarino, 2008).
7. African American females who presented to the emergency room with chest pain received cardiac monitoring 37.5% of the time, compared to 54.5% of non-African American males (Pezzin, Keyl, & Green, 2007).

IV. Pain Description, Expression, and Behavior

Key Points

- Women show more behavioral expressions of pain and have a lower pain threshold than that of men.
- A higher incidence of chronic pain with related depression is seen in women; however, men report more interference with daily quality of life.

A. Studies have shown differences in pain description between men and women.

B. In a study testing pain drawings and pain severity, no significant differences were found in pain severity between men and women; however, differences were found in pain drawing areas, hypochondriasis, and coping by ignoring pain. The study sample consisted of 68 females and 58 males. All patients completed a pain drawing, the Multidimensional Pain Inventory, the Coping Strategies Questionnaire (CSR-Q), and the Minnesota Multiphasic Personality Inventory (MMPI-2).

1. Women were found to have a larger pain drawing area, which was positively correlated with the anatomical location of pain and hypochondriasis.
    a. The pain drawing area was measured using a quantitative scoring system, which assessed total area and included correlation and regression analysis.
    b. Individuals were instructed to mark the area of pain on the provided diagram. These were then scored manually, with one point corresponding to a square containing any marking (score range 0 to 240).
    c. Hypochondriasis for this study was determined by the use of the MMPI-2. Hypochondriasis is a scale on this inventory designed to measure awareness and preoccupation with physical symptoms.
    d. The final regression model accounted for 39% ($P < 0.001$) of the variance in the pain drawing area, and hypochondriasis ($P = 0.005$) was the only unique predictor.
2. Men had a smaller pain drawing area on a body chart and were correlated with pain severity and a coping style of ignoring pain.
    a. Pain drawing was negatively correlated with the coping style of ignoring pain. Coping strategies were measured using the CSR-Q.
    b. The final regression model for men accounted for 27% ($P = 0.003$) of the variance in pain drawing area, with pain severity ($P = 0.021$) and a coping style of ignoring pain ($P = 0.018$) as the only unique predictors.

3. The authors of this study conclude that clinicians interpreting pain diagram area should consider the gender of the individual when using the drawings to assist in clinical decisions of classification and treatment of pain (George, Bialosky, Wittmer, & Robinson, 2007).

C. Researchers investigated 20 males and 20 females for their subjective and facial responses to toxic heat stimulation at both painful and nonpainful levels. A higher correlation between pain and facial expression was exhibited by women (Kunz, Gruber, & Lautenbacher, 2006).

D. Compared to men, women displayed a lower threshold and tolerance for pressure and pain (Chesterton, Barlas, Foster, Baxter, & Wright, 2003; Garcia, Godoy-Izquierdo, Godoy, Perez, & Lopez-Chicheri, 2007; Soetanto, Chung, & Wong, 2006).

E. Women have a lower reflex threshold and pain threshold to cutaneous electrical stimulation than do men (Komiyama, Wang, Svensson, Arendt-Nielsen, & DeLaat, 2005).

F. In a longitudinal study of both male and female participants, age 70 to 77, with chronic back pain, the back pain was positively correlated with being female, economic difficulties, loneliness, and obesity (Jacobs et al., 2006).

G. In a large study of chronic pain, nearly one-third of the sample reported one of four chronic pain conditions (fibromyalgia, arthritis or rheumatism, back problems, and migraine headaches). The prevalence of depression in women was reported twice as often as the reports of depression in men (Munce & Stewart, 2007).

1. In another study on chronic pain among Norwegian citizens, women reported more chronic pain and significantly higher pain intensity, although men reported a poorer quality of life than women did (Rustoen et al., 2004).
2. In yet another study of gender differences in chronic pain, males reported greater mean severity scores and higher levels of disability and pain, with reduced physical and psychological quality of life, as compared with females (Marcus, 2003).

H. In a study of osteoarthritis knee pain, the quality of life was more negatively affected and at an earlier age in women than in men.

1. Women report more knee-related complications, higher pain scores, decreased activities of daily living function, and increased pain in the 55-to-74 age group. These complaints were not noted with men until age 75 to 84 (Paradowski, Bergman, Suden-Lundius, Lohmander, & Roos, 2006).
2. In another study of osteoarthritis knee pain, women were more likely to show an increase in knee pain over the course of a day and men were more likely to show an increase in coping efficacy over the course of the day (Keefe et al., 2004).

I. In an epidemiology study in Uppland, Sweden, the overall prevalence of pain conditions, especially headaches, was higher among women. Women also reported a higher severity of pain (Bingefors & Isacson, 2004).

J. Among patients with spinal cord injuries, women had a higher prevalence of nociceptive pain than men and a higher use of analgesics. No gender differences were seen regarding pain localization, pain descriptors, pain intensity ratings, and life satisfaction (Norrbrink, Budh et al., 2003).

K. Women with acute coronary syndromes were more likely than men to report chest "discomfort" than chest "pain," to identify body areas other than the chest as painful, and to identify unexplained anxiety (Chen, Woods, Wilkie, & Puntillo, 2005).

V. Psychosocial Aspects

Key Points

- Response to and reporting of pain are mediated by learned, modeled behavior.
- Masculine features exhibit restraint of pain reporting and expression.
- Feminine features exhibit outward expression and a higher incidence of pain reporting.
- Anxiety is more likely to influence and increase pain reporting in men.
- Depression influences pain reporting more in women than in men.
- Variable results were found in response to coping strategies and influence of interpersonal interactions.

A. Elderly females tend to report higher pain scores as well as higher overall pain intensity than elderly males. Elderly females also tended to have greater depressive tendency than males (Tsai, 2007).
B. Women displayed stronger relationships among mood, pain, and strength of disability, whereas in men mood was found to only partially mediate the relationship between pain and overall disability (Hirsh, Waxenberg, Atchison, Gremillion, & Robinson, 2006).
C. A study was done to determine differential effects of types of coping on the pain experience between healthy males ($N = 31$) and females ($N = 31$).
   1. In a cold pressor-induced pain study, participants were divided into two groups.
      a. One group was given acceptance instructions telling participants to be aware of their thoughts and accept their pain but not to change or control their thoughts.
      b. The other group was given control instructions in various strategies such as distraction or positive thinking.
   2. Females were found to have a lower pain tolerance; however, they benefit from acceptance coping as compared to males. No differences between genders were found with control-based coping (Keogh, Bond, Hanmer, & Tilston, 2004).
D. Higher trait anxiety scores revealed a correlation with higher pain scores in men (Elklit & Jones, 2006; Soetanto et al., 2006).
E. Whiplash pain was found to be modified by coping strategies; specifically, emotion-focused coping strategies were related significantly to decreased whiplash-related symptoms in men compared to women (Jones & Elklit, 2007).
F. The typical man is masculine, and the typical woman is feminine. If a female sees herself as more masculine than feminine, or if a male sees himself as more feminine than masculine, then that person is a low-identifying female or male, respectively.
   1. Two studies addressing identification with gender group social norms were conducted to investigate whether gender group identification moderates expected tolerance of a hypothetical painful stimulus.
      a. Men who highly identified with the male gender were found to tolerate a more painful stimulation than were high-identifying females.
      b. High-identifying males tolerated more painful stimuli than did low-identifying males.
      c. No differences existed between low-identifying men and women (Pool, Schwegler, Theodore, & Fuchs, 2007).
G. In a study involving 240 adolescents, masculinity correlated with lower heat pain ratings in boys but not girls (Myers et al., 2006).
H. In patients with chronic back pain, the women using opioids showed lower affective distress, whereas use of opioids among males was associated with greater affective distress. Opioid use was not associated with pain severity, although women reported greater pain than men (Fillingim, Doleys, Edwards, & Lowery, 2003).
I. Evidence suggests that women are more sensitive than men to threatening stimuli (physical, emotional, and verbal) and thus experience more negative effects than do men, including enhanced pain. Evidence also suggests that men may be more sensitive to positive events such as sexual or erotic stimuli than are women, which may lead to reduction of pain in men (Rhudy & Williams, 2005).
J. In patients with chronic pain, anxiety and depression were found to be positive predictors of pain and disability. When depression was high, greater disability was reported with women than with men. In the male population, a correlation was found between depression and number of medications used (Keogh, McCracken, & Eccleston, 2006).
K. The nature of interpersonal transactions exerts a greater influence on women's responses to noxious stimulation than those of men. In one experiment, subjects were randomly assigned to either a no transaction condition in which they coped alone with the cold pressor test or a transaction opportunity condition in which they also had the option of interacting with an empathetic, reflecting experimenter. Women had lower pain tolerance and reported more pain. Of those who chose to have a transaction opportunity, females were more pain focused than males and had lower coping abilities (Jackson, Iezzi, Chen, Ebnet, & Eglitis, 2005).

L. Smokers showed evidence for blunted hypothalamic—pituitary—adrenal axis function at rest and with stress, resulting in decreased β-endorphin and cortisol. This pathophysiological variance might explain why smokers have higher pain tolerances.
   1. In a study examining gender differences in smoking-related analgesia and stress-induced analgesia, women smokers had greater threshold and tolerance times to ischemic pain than did women nonsmokers.
   2. Women (both smokers and nonsmokers) also showed lower heat pain thresholds and pain tolerance levels than did males.
   3. Male smokers had greater tolerance to cold pressor pain than did male nonsmokers (Girdler et al., 2005).

M. A study examining gender differences that may exist in response to interdisciplinary pain management interventions aimed at improving function revealed improvements across a range of domains of outcomes for both men and women. Women did not show a reduction in distress or pain 3 months following treatment, whereas men did show a significant reduction (Keogh et al., 2005).

N. In a large prevalence study of 4,506 respondents from Uppland, Sweden, the comorbidity between pain conditions and psychiatric and somatic problems was higher among women than among men.
   1. Health-related quality of life differed by gender and type of pain condition.
      a. Quality-of-life scores were affected for men who reported headache complaints.
      b. Quality-of-life scores were affected in women who reported psychological issues.
   2. Among both men and women, pain conditions were correlated with poorer socioeconomic conditions and lifestyle factors.
      a. Education and unemployment were important variables among men that contributed to higher pain reports.
      b. Economic difficulties, half-time work and being married were associated with higher reports of pain among women (Bingefors & Isacson, 2004).

O. Data from a prospective randomized trial during interventional procedures showed a significant interaction between group attribution and sex with regard to drug request and pain and anxiety ratings of patients.
   1. Patients were divided into two groups; 76 patients were male, and 83 three were female.
      a. One group received standard care for the institution
      b. The other group received additional empathetic care throughout their procedure.
   2. All patients were asked to rate their pain and anxiety on a 0-to-10 self-rating scale.
      a. Men asked for more drugs than women under standard care but asked for fewer drugs in the attention, empathetic group.
      b. Pain and anxiety ratings for women were significantly lower in the attention group compared with standard treatment.
      c. For men, no significant difference was seen in pain and anxiety scores.
      d. The group receiving empathetic attention requested significantly fewer drugs than patients in the standard group (Stinshoff et al., 2004).

P. Gender was found to moderate the relationship between anticipatory distress and postoperative pain in girls but not boys. For this study, 102 boys and girls age 12 to 18 were recruited. Measures of anxiety and anticipated pain were obtained preoperatively. Postoperatively, coping skills, anxiety, and pain were measured, as well as patient-controlled analgesia usage.
   1. Preoperatively, girls reported higher anxiety scores and anticipated more pain than boys.
   2. Higher anticipatory distress predicted higher postoperative pain scores for girls but not for boys.
   3. Patient-controlled analgesia usage on postoperative days 0 to 1 did not vary between males and females (Logan & Rose, 2004).

Q. A meta-analysis review showed that emotion appears to influence pain. Gender differences in the experience of pain may arise from differences in the experience and processing of emotion, which in turn differentially alter pain processing (Rhudy & Williams, 2005).

References

al'Absi, M., Petersen, K. L., & Wittmers, L. E. (2002). Adrenocortical and hemodynamic predictors of pain perception in men and women. *Pain, 96*(1–2), 197–204.

Aloisi, A. M., Pari, G., Ceccarelli, I., Vecchi, I., Ietta, F., Lodi, L., & Paulesu, L. (2005). Gender-related effects of chronic non-malignant pain and opioid therapy on plasma levels of macrophage migration inhibitory factor (MIF). *Pain, 115*(1–2), 142–145.

Anand, S. S., Xie, C. C., Mehta, S., Franzosi, M. G., Joyner, C., Chrolavicius, S., Fox, K. A., & Yusuf, S.; CURE Investigators. (2005). Differences in the management and prognosis of women and men who suffer from acute coronary syndromes. *Journal of American College of Cardiologists, 46*(10), 1845–1851.

Arendt-Nielsen, L., Bajaj, P., & Drewes, A. M. (2004). Visceral pain: Gender differences in response to experimental and clinical pain. *European Journal of Pain, 8*(5), 465–472.

Aubrun, F., Salvi, N., Coriat, P., & Riou, B. (2005). Sex and age-related differences in morphine requirements for postoperative pain relief. *Anesthesiology, 103*(1), 156–160.

Banik, R. K., Woo, Y. C., Park, S. S., & Brennan, T. J. (2006). Strain and sex influence on pain sensitivity after plantar incision in the mouse. *Anesthesiology, 105*(6), 1246–1253.

Becker, J. B., Arnold, A. P., Berkley, K. J., Blaustein, J. D., Eckel, L. A., Hampson, E., Herman, J. P., Marts, S., Sadee, W., Steiner, M., Taylor, J., & Young, E. (2005). Strategies and methods for research on sex differences in brain and behavior. *Endocrinology, 146,* 1650–1673.

Bingefors, K., & Isacson, D. (2004). Epidemiology, co-morbidity, and impact on health-related quality of life of self-reported headache and musculoskeletal pain: A gender perspective. *Pain, 8*(5), 435–450.

Cairns, B. E. (2007). The influence of gender and sex steroids on craniofacial nociception. *Headache, 47*(2), 319–324.

Chen, W., Woods, S. L., Wilkie, D. J., & Puntillo, K. A. (2005). Gender differences in symptom experiences of patients with acute coronary syndromes. *Journal of Pain and Symptom Management, 30*(6), 553–562.

Chesterton, L. S., Barlas, P., Foster, N. E., Baxter, G. D., & Wright, C. C. (2003). Gender differences in pressure pain threshold in health humans. *Pain, 101*(3), 259–266.

Crilly, M. A., & Bundred, P. E. (2005). Gender inequalities in the management of angina pectoris: cross-sectional survey in primary care. *Scott Medical Journal, 50*(4), 154–158.

Dahlin, L., Lund, I., Lundeberg, T., & Molander, C. (2006). Vibratory stimulation increase the electro-cutaneous sensory detection and pain thresholds in women but not men. *BMC Complementary and Alternative Medicine, 6*(20), 1–6.

Daly, C., Clemens, F., Lopez Sendon, J. L., Tavazzi, L., Boersma, E., Danchin, N., Delahaye, F., Gitt, A., Julian, D., Mulcahy, D., Ruzyllo, W., Thygesen, K., Verheugt, F., & Fox, K. M.; Euro Heart Survey Investigators. (2006). Gender differences in the management and clinical outcome of stable angina. *Circulation, 113*(4), 467–469. Dannecker, E. A., Hausenblas, H. A., Kaminski, T. W., & Robinson, M. E. (2005). Sex differences in delayed onset muscle pain. *Clinical Journal of Pain, 21*(2), 120–126.

Elklit, A., & Jones, A. (2006). The association between anxiety and chronic pain after whiplash injury: Gender specific effects. *Clinical Journal of Pain, 22*(5), 487–490.

Fejer, R., Hartvigsen, J., & Kyvik, K. O. (2006). Sex differences in heritability of neck pain. *Twin Resource Human Genetics, 9*(2), 198–204.

Fejer, R., Kyvik, K. O., & Hartvigsen, J. (2006). The prevalence of neck pain in the world population: A systemic critical review of the literature. *European Spine Journal, 15*(6), 834–848.

Fillingim, R. B., Doleys, D. M., Edwards, R. R., & Lowery, D. (2003). Clinical characteristics of chronic back pain as a function of gender and oral opioid use. *Spine, 28*(2), 143–150.

Frissora, C. L., & Koch, K. L. (2005). The role of gender and biological sex in irritable bowel syndrome. *Current Gastroenterology Reports, 7*(4), 257–263.

Garcia, E., Godoy-Izquierdo, D., Godoy, J. F., Perez, M., & Lopez-Chicheri, I. (2007). Gender differences in pressure pain threshold in a repeated measures assessment. *Psychology Health Medicine, 12*(5), 567–579.

Gazerani, P., Andersen, O. K., & Arendt-Nielsen, L. (2005). A human experimental capsaicin model for trigeminal sensitization: Gender-specific differences. *Pain, 118*(1–2), 155–163.

George, S. Z., Bialosky, J. E., Wittmer, V. T., & Robinson, M. E. (2007). Sex differences in pain drawing area for individuals with chronic musculoskeletal pain. *Journal of Orthopedic & Sports Physical Therapy, 37*(3), 115–121.

Girdler, S. S., Maixner, W., Nafter, H. A., Stewart, P. W., Moretz, R. L., & Light, K. C. (2005). Cigarette smoking, stress-induced analgesia and pain perception in men and women. *Pain, 114*(3), 372–385.

Greenspan, J. D., Craft, R. M., LeResche, L., Arendt-Nielsen, L., Berkley, K. J., Fillingim, R. B., Gold, M. S., Holdcroft, A., Lautenbacher, S., Mayer, E. A., Mogil, J. S., Murphy, A. Z., & Traub, R. J.; the Consensus Working Group of the Sex Gender, and Pain Special Interest Group of the International Association for the Study of Pain. (2007). Studying sex and gender differences in pain and analgesia: A consensus report. *Pain, 132*(Suppl. 1), S26–S45.

Hendrix, K. H., Mayhan, S., & Egan, B. M. (2005). Gender and age-related differences in treatment and control of cardiovascular risk factors among high-risk patients with angina. *Journal of Clinical Hypertension, 7*(7), 386–394.

Hirsh, A. T., Waxenberg, L. B., Atchison, J. W., Gremillion, H. A., & Robinson, M. E. (2006). Evidence for sex differences in the relationships of pain, mood, and disability. *Journal of Pain, 7*(8), 592–601.

Hoffman, A. J., Given, B. A., von Eye, A., Gift, A. G., & Given, C. W. (2007). Relationships among pain, fatigue, insomnia, and gender in persons with lung cancer. *Oncology Nursing Forum, 34*(4), 785–792.

Holtzman, J., Saleh, K., & Kane, R. (2002). Gender differences in functional status and pain in a Medicare population undergoing elective total hip arthroplasty. *Medical Care, 40*(6), 447–450.

Jackson, T., Iezzi, T., Chen, H., Ebnet, S., & Eglitis, K. (2005). Gender, interpersonal transactions and the perception of pain: An experimental analysis. *Journal of Pain, 6*(4), 228–236.

Jacobs, J. M., Hammerman-Rozenberg, R., Cohen, A., & Stressman, J. (2006). Chronic back pain among the elderly: Prevalence, associations and predictors. *Spine, 31*(7), E203–E207.

Jensen, M. T., & Petersen, K. L. (2006). Gender differences in pain and secondary hyperalgesia after heat/capsaicin sensitization in healthy volunteers. *Journal of Pain, 7*(3), 211–217.

Ji, Y., Murphy, A. Z., & Traub, R. J. (2006). Sex differences in morphine induced analgesia of visceral pain are supraspinally and peripherally mediated. *American Journal of Physiology, 291*(2), R307–R314.

Jones, A., & Eklit, A. (2007). The association between gender, coping style and whiplash related symptoms in suffers of whiplash associated disorder. *Scandinavian Psychology, 48*(1), 75–80.

Kato, K., Sullivan, P. F., Evengard, B., & Pedersen, N. L. (2006). Importance of genetic influences on chronic widespread pain. *Arthritis and Rheumatism, 54*(5), 1682–1686.

Keefe, F. J., Affleck, G., France, C. R., Emery, C. F., Waters, S., Caldwell, D. S., Stainbrook, D., Hackshaw, K. V., Fox, L. C., & Wilson, K. (2004). Gender differences in pain, coping, and mood in individuals having osteoarthritic knee pain: A within-day analysis. *Pain, 110*(3), 571–577.

Keogh, E., Bond, F. W., Hanmer, R., & Tilston, J. (2004). Comparing acceptance- and control-based coping instructions on the cold-pressor pain experiences of healthy men and women. *European Journal of Pain, 9*(2005), 591–598.

Keogh, E., McCracken, L. M., & Eccleston, C. (2005). Do men and women differ in their response to interdisciplinary chronic pain management? *Pain, 114*(1–2), 37–46.

Komiyama, O., Wang, K., Svensson, P., Arendt-Nielsen, L., & DeLaat, A. (2005). Gender difference in masseteric exteroceptive suppression period and pain perception. *Clinical Neurophysiology, 116*(11), 2599–2605.

Kroin, J. S., Buvanendran, A., Nagalla, S. K. S., & Tuman, K. J. (2003). Magnesium sulfate potentiates antinociception at the spinal level. *Canadian Journal of Anesthesia, 50*(9), 904–908.

Kunz, M., Gruber, A., & Lautenbacher, S. (2006). Sex differences in facial encoding of pain. *Journal of Pain, 7*(12), 915–928.

Logan, D. E., & Rose, J. B., (2004). Gender differences in post-operative pain and patient controlled analgesia use among adolescent surgical patients. *Pain, 109*(3), 481–487.

Main, C. J., & Spanswick, C. C. (2000). Introduction to pain management. In *Pain management: An interdisciplinary approach* (pp. 48–51). Philadelphia: Churchill Livingstone.

Marcus, D. A. (2003). Gender differences in chronic pain in a treatment-seeking population. *Journal of Gender Specific Medicine, 6*(4), 19–24.

McClish, D. K., Levenson, J. L., Penberthy, L. T., Roseff, S. D., Bovbjerg, V. E., Roberts, J. D., Aisiku, I. P., & Smith, W. R. (2006). Gender differences in pain and healthcare utilization for adult sickle cell patients: The PiSCES project. *Journal of Women's Health, 15*(2), 146–154.

McKelvy, A. D., Mark, T. R. M., & Sweitzer, S. M. (2007). Age and sex-specific nociceptive response to endothelin-1. *Journal of Pain, 8*(8), 657–666.

Miaskowski, C., & Levine, J. D. (2004). Sex differences in pain perceptions, responses to treatment, and clinical management. In R. H. Dworkin & W. S. Breitbart (Eds.), *Psychosocial aspects of pain: A handbook for health care providers* (pp. 607–621). Seattle: IASP Press.

Mogil, J. S., & Chanda, M. L. (2005). The case for inclusion of female subjects in basic science studies of pain. *Pain, 117,* 1–5.

Munce, S. E., & Stewart, D. E. (2007). Gender differences in depression and chronic pain conditions in a national epidemiologic survey. *Psychomatics, 48*(5), 394–399.

Myers, C. D., Tsao, J. C., Glover, D. A., Kim, S. C., Turk, N., & Zeltzer, L. K. (2006). Sex, gender, and age: contributions to laboratory pain responding in children and adolescents. *Journal of Pain, 7*(8), 556–564.

Norrbrink Budh, C., Lund, I., Hultling, C., Levi, R., Werhagen, L., Ertzgaard, P., & Lundeberg, T. (2003). Gender related differences in pain in spinal cord injured individuals. *Spinal Cord, 41*(2), 122–128.

Paradowski, P. T., Bergman, S., Suden-Lundius, A., Lohmander, L. S., & Roos, E. M. (2006). Knee complaints vary with age and gender in the adult population: Population based reference data for the knee injury and osteoarthritis outcome score. *BMC Musculoskeletal Disorders, 7,* 38.

Pezzin, L. E., Keyl, P. M., & Green, G. B. (2007). Disparities in the emergency department evaluation of chest pain patients. *Academy of Emergency Medicine, 14*(2), 149–156.

Pool, G. J., Schwegler, A. F., Theodore, B. R., & Fuchs, P. N. (2007). Role of gender norms and group identification on hypothetical and experimental pain tolerance. *Pain, 129*(1–2), 122–129.

Rhudy, J. L., & Williams, A. E. (2005). Gender differences in pain: Do emotions play a role? *Gender Medicine, 2*(4), 208–226.

Rosseland, L. A., & Stubhaug, A. (2004). Gender is a confounding factor in pain trials: Women report more pain than men after arthroscopic surgery. *Pain, 112*(3), 248–253.

Rustoen, T., Wahl, A. K., Hanestad, B. R., Lerdal, A., Pail, S., & Miaskowski, C. (2004). Gender differences in chronic pain: Findings from a population-based study of Norwegian adults. *Pain Management Nursing, 5*(3), 105–117.

Sekhri, N., Timmis, A., Chen, R., Junghans, C., Walsh, N., Zaman, J., Eldridge, S., Hemingway, H., & Feder, G. (2008). Inequity of access to investigation and effect on clinical outcomes: Prognostic study of coronary angiography for suspected angina pectoris. *British Medical Journal, 10*(336), 1058–1061.

Shinal, R. M., & Fillingim, R. B. (2007). Overview of orofacial pain: Epidemiology and gender differences in orofacial pain. *Dental Clinics of North America, 51*(1), 1–18.

Soetanto, A. L. F., Chung, J. W. Y., & Wong, T. K. S. (2006). Are there gender differences in pain perception? *Journal of Neuroscience Nursing, 38*(3), 172–176.

Sonson, J. M., Lum, J. J., Madison, J. R., Seto, T. B., & Spies, C. (2004). Gender differences in therapy for patients admitted for unstable angina and myocardial infarction with underlying chronic kidney disease. *Hawaii Medical Journal, 63*(11), 337–340.

Stinshoff, V. J., Lang, E. V., Berbaum, K. S., Lutgendorf, S., Logan, H., & Berbaum, M. (2004). Effect of sex and gender on drug-seeking behavior during invasive medical procedures. *Academy of Radiology, 11*(4), 390–397.

Sydsjo, A., Alexanderson, K., Dastserri, M., & Sydsjo, G. (2003). Gender differences in sick leave related to back pain diagnoses: Influence of pregnancy. *Spine, 28*(4), 385–389.

Takakuwa, K. M., Shofer, F. S., & Hollander, J. E. (2007). The influence of race and gender on time to initial electrocardiogram for patients with chest pain. *Academic Emergency Medicine, 13*(8), 867–872.

Taylor, B. A., Casas-Ganem, J., Vaccaro, A. R., Hilibrand, A. S., Hanscom, B. S., & Albert, T. J. (2005). Differences in the work-up and treatment conditions associated with low back pain by patient gender and ethnic background. *Spine, 30*(3), 359–364.

Tousignant-Laflamme, Y., Rainville, P., & Marchand, S. (2005). Establishing a link between heart rate and pain in healthy subjects: A gender effect. *Journal of Pain, 6*(6), 341–347.

Tsai, Y. E. (2007). Gender differences in pain and depressive tendency among Chinese elders with knee osteoarthritis. *Pain, 130*(1–2), 6–7.

Uchiyama, K., Kawai, M., Tani, M., Ueno, M., Hama, T., & Yamaue, H. (2006). Gender differences in postoperative pain after laparoscopic cholecystectomy. *Surgical Endoscopy, 20*(3), 448–451.

Wenger, N. K., Shaw, L. J., & Vaccarino, V. (2008). Coronary heart disease in women: Update, 2008. *Clinical Pharmacologic Therapy, 83*(1), 37–51.

Wiesenfeld-Hallin, Z. (2005). Sex differences in pain perception. *Gender Medicine, 2*(3), 137–145.

Zubieta, J. K., Smith, Y. R., Bueller, J. A., Xu, Y., Kilbourn, M. R., Jewett, D. M., Meyer, C. R., Koeppe, R. A., & Stohler, C. S. (2002). μ-Opioid receptor-mediated antinociceptive responses differ in men and women. *Journal of Neuroscience, 22*(12), 5100–5107.

Suggested Readings

Cardenas, D. D., Bryce, T. N., Shem, K., Richards, J. S., & Elhefni, H. (2004). Gender and minority differences in the pain experience of people with spinal cord injury. *Archives of Physical Medicine and Rehabilitation, 85*(11), 1774–1781.

Unrod, M., Kassel, J. D., & Robinson, M. (2004). Effects of smoking, distraction, and gender on pain perception. *Behavior Medicine, 30*(3), 133–139.

chapter

24

Immunity and Pain

Christine Peltier, BSN, RN-BC
Barbara St. Marie, ANP, GNP, RN-BC, PhD Candidate

Objectives

After studying this chapter, the reader should be able to:

1. Understand the science in the neuroimmune activation system and how it is evolving and falls within the realm of a neuroscientist.
2. Identify the future importance of knowledge of immunity to nursing in how we treat pain: Does pain suppress the immune system? Do opioids suppress the immune system?
3. Explain the bidirectional communications of the central nervous system and the immune system.
4. Describe the role of cytokines in the immune process.
5. Explain the role of the hypothalamic-pituitary-adrenal (HPA) axis in the immune process.

The science of the neuroimmune activation system is evolving and falls within the realm of the neuroscientist. This chapter addresses these complex processes, thereby providing a basic understanding of the interactions of pain, immunity, and treatment of pain.

I. Function of Immune System

A. The immune system is the body's defense system (Watkins, Maier, & Goehler, 1995)

B. It is how the body protects itself from disease and injury (Chapman, Tuckett, & Song, 2008). It is also involved with tissue repair after injury (Watkins et al., 1995)

C. The immune system consists of physical and chemical barriers and inflammatory and immune responses (Corwin, 2006)

II. Definition of Terms

A. Macrophages
   1. Engulf and destroy infective agents.
   2. Produce and release proinflammatory cytokines.

B. Lymphocytes (immune cells)
   1. Include the B and T lymphocytes and natural killer (NK) cells.
   2. Are produced in the bone marrow.
   3. Mature there and in other lymphoid tissues.

C. Glia
   1. Provide silent support to nerve cells.
   2. Play an important role in proper functioning of neurons and in many chronic disease states, such as Alzheimer's disease, chronic pain (persistent pain), and spinal cord injury.
   3. Function to provide a stable internal environment around neurons and to take part in communication between neurons (Chapman et al., 2008, p. 129)
   4. Normally absorb glutamate at the postsynaptic neurons (Bleakman, Alt, & Nisenbaum, 2006) (see the chapter on Neurophysiology of Pain).
   5. Release cytokines, the *N*-methyl-D-aspartate (NMDA) agonist, nitric oxide, and arachidonic acid (Watkins et al., 1995)

D. Microglia
   1. Are a type of glial cell closely related to macrophages.
   2. Are activated by virtually any kind of disturbance in the nervous system.
   3. Laboratory studies demonstrate that spinal microglia and astrocytes are activated following nerve injury.
   4. Are the smallest and first glial cell to respond to stressors.
   5. Release substances that activate astrocytes (DeLeo, Tanga, & Tawfik, 2004).

E. Astrocytes
   1. Have been shown to gradually replace microglia on the neuronal surface and enwrap the injured neurons with a glial scar.
   2. Play an important role in maintaining central sensitization in laboratory studies, as with certain stimulation astrocytes release glutamate (Starkweather, Witek-Janusek, Nockels, Peterson, & Mathews, 2006).

F. NK cells
   1. Have an important role in the activation of adaptive antigen-specific immune responses (Starkweather et al., 2006).
   2. Decrease levels in acute physiological stress in both animals and humans (Starkweather et al., 2006, p. E641).
   3. Are crucial in controlling metastatic development (Page, 2005b).

G. Chemokines
   1. Promote an inflammatory response (DeLeo et al., 2004).
   2. Are responsible for cell trafficking and recruitment of leukocytes to the site of damage (DeLeo et al., 2004).
   3. Are involved in the perpetuation of pain states (DeLeo et al., 2004).

H. Cytokines
   1. Are small low molecular-weight proteins secreted by the immune system (Munden, 2006, p. 414).
   2. Are immunomodulating agents involved in communication between cells (Munden, 2006, p. 414).
   3. Induce or regulate various local and systemic inflammatory responses (Munden, 2006, p. 414).
   4. Impaired cytokine production or regulation may lead to certain disorders (Munden, 2006; Starkweather, Witek-Janusek, & Mathews, 2005).
      a. Cytokines have been strongly linked to generation of chronic pain states at both peripheral and central nervous system sites (DeLeo et al., 2004).
   5. Fall into two categories: proinflammatory and antiinflammatory.
      a. Proinflammatory cytokines are
         (1) Interleukin-1 (IL-1).
         (2) Interleukin-2 (IL-2).
         (3) Interleukin-6 (IL-6).
         (4) Tumor necrosis factor (TNF).
         (5) Interferon-γ (gamma).
      b. Antiinflammatory cytokines are
         (1) Interleukin-4 (IL-4).
         (2) Interleukin-10 (IL-10).
      c. Antiinflammatory cytokines decrease the secretion of the proinflammatory cytokines and stimulate activation of B cells (Corwin, 2006, p. 140). B cells are responsible for making antibodies against antigens.

I. Tumor necrosis factor
   1. Is primarily responsible for initiating the cascade of other cytokines regulating immune cells.
   2. Is implicated in multiple sclerosis, cerebral ischemia, experimental autoimmune encephalomyelitis, and exaggerated pain states (DeLeo et al., 2004).
   3. May produce systemic inflammation.

J. Interleukins
   1. Are a group of cytokines expressed by white blood cells and are key to the function of the immune system.
      a. IL-6 plays an important role in directing leukocyte trafficking. It facilitates transition between innate and acquired immune responses (Starkweather et al., 2005).
      b. IL-1 is involved in cartilage homeostasis. It may activate NK cells. It has the ability to change chondrocytes from anabolism (i.e., requires energy to promote growth and differentiation of cells) to catabolism (i.e., breaks down cells and releases energy) (Starkweather et al., 2005).

III. The Brain in Pain and the Immune System

A. An emerging concept in pain research is the "bidirectional communication between the immune system and the brain and the implications of this communication" (Starkweather et al., 2005, p. 196).

B. Recent evidence in pain research suggests that interactions between immune system and the nervous system result in the generation and maintenance of pathological pain (DeLeo, 2006).
   1. Through a neural route, products such as proinflammatory cytokines (IL-1, IL-6) that are released by activated immune cells communicate injury-related events and tissue pathology to the brain (Chapman, 2001, p. 470).
      a. Once the peripheral inflammation has occurred, immune cells are activated and cause a release of proinflammatory cytokines. These cytokines release substances that in turn stimulate the peripheral nerves that signal the spinal cord and the brain that inflammation has occurred (Watkins & Maier, 2005).
      b. In addition to bloodborne signaling, evidence indicates that neural pathways via the vagus and glossopharyngeal nerves relay information to the brain about inflammation and infection. The brain region where the afferent nerves project is implicated in sickness responses (Watkins & Maier, 2005, pp. 140–141).

2. The brain controls and challenges immune cells via the actions of the sympathetic nervous system and the hypothalamic secretion of releasing factors into the bloodstream, which in turn activates the anterior pituitary via the hypothalamic-pituitary-adrenal (HPA) axis (Chapman, 2001, p. 470).
    a. The cells and organs of the immune system express receptors to the hormones the pituitary body releases so that they respond to the messenger molecules.
3. Sickness responses include fever, increased sleep, depressed mood, less exploration interest, loss of libido, and diminished cognitive abilities. These responses, while negative, are aimed at conserving energy, which promotes host recovery (Chapman, 2001; Watkins & Maier, 2005).
4. A stressor such as tissue trauma activates this pathway, and then adaptive behaviors and physiological changes that are the sickness response occur (Chapman, 2001).

C. With recent advances in the field of pain, it is now recognized that there is a neuroimmune interaction and that the immune system plays a key role in the development of peripheral neuropathic pain (Thacker, Clark, Marchand, & McMahon, 2007).

D. Any nociceptive event provokes autonomic, endocrine, and immune processes, as well as sensory signaling (Chapman et al., 2008).

E. Defensive response to injury or disease
1. Inflammation activates the immune response.
2. A stimulated peripheral nerve signals to the spinal cord and brain that inflammation has occurred (Chapman et al., 2008).

F. It has been postulated that nociception and proinflammatory cytokines may play a mutual up-regulatory role. The proinflammatory cytokines IL-1β and IL-6 are considered mediators of hyperalgesia.
1. IL-1β contributes by causing up-regulating of cyclooxygenase-2 and by increasing production of substance P and nerve growth factor.
2. Both IL-1β and IL-6 are involved in mechanisms of allodynia and probably in the development of postoperative pain and chronic pain (Beilin et al., 2003).

IV. Does Pain Affect the Immune Function?

A. Based on research studies, pain results not only in suffering but also in suppressed immune function (Kremer, 1999)
1. It is important to recognize that pain suppresses the immune function (Ballantyne, 2006).
2. A stressful stimulus pain leads to a complex immune system response (Tsai, Won, & Lin, 2000, p. 158)

B. Acute pain
1. In response to acute pain (this study used a cold pressor test), there are changes in lymphocyte trafficking and lymphocyte function in human immunodeficiency virus (HIV)-positive and HIV-negative patients (Eller, 1998). No differences in immune response were found between the HIV-positive and the HIV-negative groups.
2. Increases in lymphocyte production lead to increases in cytokines that then mobilize additional immune reactions (Eller, 1998). This may be sympathetically related, and no differences have been found between physical and psychological threat.
3. The immune response to acute pain was the doubling of NK cell activity, which remained elevated for 1 hour. The author of this study theorized that with acute pain there is a natural body defense that would initially enhance NK cell activity. However, lymphocytic numbers returned to baseline within 1 hour. It is unclear whether lymphocytic numbers continue to drop below baseline and how long NK cell activity remained above baseline, as there were no measurements beyond the hour (Eller, 1998, pp. 209–210).
4. Pain is a stressor that is immunosuppressive and tumor enhancing (Page, 2005a, p. S29).
5. Immune-altering factors released from injured tissue substantially contribute to the immune consequences of undergoing and recovering from surgery (Page, 2005a, p. S27).
6. Animal studies with experimental abdominal surgery were found to have decreased lymphocyte and splenocyte proliferative responses to mitogen and NK cell activity. The more extensive the surgery, the greater the decrease in immune function (Page, 2005b, p. 303).

7. Human studies have shown decreased cell-mediated immunity as demonstrated by diminished lymphocyte proliferative responses to mitogens (begins cell division) and suppression of NK cell activity (Page, 2005b, p. 303).

C. The HPA axis and sympathetic nervous system are activated during surgical stress. As a result, immune responses are altered (Sacerdote et al., 2000).
   1. NK cell activity is suppressed with surgery and anesthesia (Akural et al., 2004).
   2. Pain with surgery and its recovery is a mediator for surgery-induced immunosuppression (Page, 2005b).
   3. Research in animals supports evidence that adequate pain control improves surgery-induced immunosuppression and creates host resistance against metastatic development (Page, 2005b).
   4. Human studies have shown a higher level and a longer duration of immunosuppression in surgery that result in severe pain and extensive tissue disruption (Kremer, 1999).
   5. Surgical experience creates tissue trauma and results in nociceptive pain.
      a. In the absence of anesthesia and analgesia, hormonal and metabolic stress responses are activated (Watkins & Maier, 2005).
      b. Surgery tissue trauma results in HPA axis stimulation, which in turn results in increased cortisol and corticosterone (a steroid hormone of corticosteroid). In addition to these stress hormones from the adrenal cortex, the hypothalamus activates the sympathetic nervous system, resulting in secretion of epinephrine from the adrenal medulla and norepinephrine from sympathetic terminals. These changes contribute to alterations in glucagon secretion and insulin levels, leading to a hypermetabolic state that has been shown to affect immunity (Page & Ben-Eliyahu, 1997, pp. 10–11).
   6. Studies with surgery and anesthesia have provided knowledge about the effects on immune functions, including suppression of NK cell activity (Akural et al., 2004).
      a. IL-6 is a key proinflammatory cytokine in anesthesia and surgery.
         (1) IL-6 is responsible for inducing the systemic changes known as the acute phase response (Akural et al., 2004, p. 253).
         (2) Production during injury or infection is a major signal and coordinator of the activity of different immune cells.

V. Do Opioids Affect Immune Function?

A. Opioid-immune interaction has important clinical implications.

B. A considerable amount of data suggests that acute administration of μ-agonist opioid analgesics are immunosuppressive (Page, 2005a).

C. Preclinical research has shown that opioid receptors are found on immune cells and that opioids do affect the development, differentiation, and function of immune cells (Ballantyne, 2006).

D. In HIV patients, opioids have been implicated in exacerbation of immunosuppression, suggesting that prolonged opioid use may impair immune function in these patients (Ballantyne, 2006, p. 1249).
   1. A single dose of morphine in the absence of pain suppresses immune function, but the results of this suppression are not well known (Page, 2005a).
   2. Repeated or chronic administration of opioids in the absence of pain appears to have quite significant negative consequences, including infectious disease (Page, 2005a).
      a. Individuals with opioid agonist addiction (e.g., heroin) show a high incidence of immunosuppression-related illnesses (Page, 2005a).

E. Opioids share many properties and actions with cytokines.
   1. Endogenous opioids enhance some immune functions.
   2. Exogenous opioids may suppress the immune function.
      a. One study shows that μ- and δ-receptors are immunosuppressive, whereas κ-receptors enhance immunity (Zakharova & Vasilenko, 2001).
   3. Opioid receptors in the central nervous system, in peripheral neurons, and on immune cells mediate immunosuppression (Vallejo, Leon-Casasola, & Benyamin, 2004).
   4. Acute versus long-term opioid administration may alter immune response in different ways.

a. Acute morphine administration is largely independent of the HPA axis response.
b. Long-term morphine administration may modify the μ-opioid receptor via activation of the HPA axis and produce a decrease in lymphocyte proliferation and NK cell activity (Vallejo et al., 2004, p. 361).

F. In one study of 10 patients with chronic pain syndrome receiving oral sustained-release morphine, it was observed that the humoral immune response that was already attenuated was further suppressed after receiving morphine in doses between 30 and 240 mg/d (Palm et al., 1998).

G. Another investigation studied of the effects of morphine and its active metabolites on both humoral and cellular immunity in individuals with advanced cancer needing pain management.
1. Morphine-derived metabolites morphine-3-glucuronide and morphine-6-glucuronide significantly modulated (regulated or adapted) the immune system in the early phase of morphine administration to patients with cancer pain (Hashiguchi, Morisaki, Kotake, & Takeda, 2005).

H. Previous studies with morphine administered intraspinally reported a lack of immunosuppressive effect (Tsai, et al., 2000), but also immunosuppressive effects mediated by brain opioid receptors (Beilin et al., 2003).
1. In rat studies, morphine suppressed lymphocyte proliferative response to mitogens when given systemically but not when given intrathecally (Beilin et al., 2003).

I. Another study compared postsurgical epidural analgesia with fentanyl and bupivacaine to intramuscular pethidine and patient-controlled analgesia morphine. The results demonstrated that the epidural group experienced the least suppression of lymphocyte proliferation response to mitogens and attenuated proinflammatory cytokine response to surgery (Beilin et al., 2003).
1. The reduced postoperative inflammatory response may be partly due to local anesthetic use in the epidural.
   a. Local anesthetic agents block neural transmission at the site of tissue injury and thus may diminish neurogenic inflammation.
   b. Local anesthetic agents have their own systemic antiinflammatory properties (Beilin et al., 2003).

J. Yet another study was made of preemptive use of epidural sufentanil before gynecological surgery. IL-1 and IL-6 responses were inhibited, which was a beneficial response. NK cell activity was increased (Akural et al., 2004).

K. In a study by Volk et al. (2004), epidural analgesia influenced lymphocyte distribution.
1. "Consistent immunological changes after stress (e.g., surgery) include a decrease in the CD4/CD8 ratio and an increase in NK cells and CD8" (Volk et al., 2004, p. 1091).
2. The decrease in CD4-to-CD8 ratio was prevented with epidural analgesia.
3. Surgical stress and pain may induce an accelerated lymphocyte depletion, resulting in postoperative infection. Epidural analgesia may improve resistance to postoperative infections.

VI. How Does This Affect the Future of Pain Management Nursing?

A. The knowledge that pain is immunosuppressive with potentially significant consequences if undertreated, especially in immunocompromised individuals and people with metastatic disease, makes it imperative that we incorporate appropriate pain management strategies that are preemptive and multimodal.

B. The knowledge that the use of long-term opioids may also inhibit the immune system and contribute to an increase in illnesses related to immunosuppression may also bolster the use of appropriate multimodal pain therapies for the persistent pain population.

C. Addressing and targeting mechanisms of pain transmission, including the immune system, allows the clinician the opportunity to use multimodal pain therapy in an effort to provide efficacious pain management and diminish side effects.

D. Recognizing the potential that the immune system has a role in pain may lead to new ideas for potential therapeutic treatment approaches (Starkweather et al., 2005).

E. The Pain Management Nurse who begins to gain a fundamental understanding of immunity and pain will be well positioned to provide further pain management opportunities to their patients as the research evolves.

References

Akural, E. I., Salomaki, T. E., Bloigu, A. H., Ryhanen, P., Tekay, A. H., Alahuhta, S. M., & Surcel, H. M. (2004). The effects of pre-emptive epidural sufentanil on human immune function. *Acta Anaesthesiologica Scandinavica, 48,* 750–755.

Ballantyne, J. C. (2006). Opioids for chronic nonterminal pain. *Southern Medical Journal, 99*(11), 1245–1255.

Beilin, B., Shavit, Y., Trabekin, E., Mordashev, B., Mayburd, E., Zeidel, A., & Bessler, H. (2003). The effects of postoperative pain management on immune response to surgery. *Anesthesia and Analgesia, 97,* 822–827.

Bleakman, D., Alt, A., & Nisenbaum, E. S. (2006). Glutamate receptors and pain. *Seminars in Cell Developmental Biology, 17,* 592–604.

Chapman, C. R. (2001). The psychophysiology of pain. In J. D. Loeser (Ed.), *Bonica's management of pain* (3rd ed.). Philadelphia: Lippincott Williams & Wilkins.

Chapman, C. R., Tuckett, R. P., & Song, C. W. (2008). Pain and stress in a systems perspective: Reciprocal neural, endocrine and immune interactions. *Journal of Pain, 9*(2), 122–145.

Corwin, E. (Ed.). 2006. *Handbook of pathophysiology.* Philadelphia: Lippincott Williams & Wilkins.

DeLeo, J. A., Tanga, F. Y., & Tawfik, V. L. (2004). Neuroimmune activation and neuroinflammation in chronic pain and opioid tolerance/hyperalgesia. *Neuroscientist, 10*(1), 40–52.

DeLeo, J. A. (2006). Basic science of pain. *Journal of Bone and Joint Surgery, 88* (A Suppl. 2). Retrieved August 3, 2008, from http://www.ejbjs.org.

Eller, L. S. (1998). Testing a model: Effects of pain on immunity in HIV+ and HIV(participants. *Scholarly Inquiry for Nursing Practice, 12*(3), 191–214.

Hashiguchi, S., Morisaki, H., Kotake, Y., & Takeda, J. (2005). Effects of morphine and its metabolites on immune function in advanced cancer patients. *Journal of Clinical Anesthesia, 17,* 575–580.

Kremer, M. J. (1999). Surgery, pain, and immune function. *Clinical Forum for Nurse Anesthetists, 10*(3), 94–100.

Munden, J. (Ed.). 2006. *Diseases: A nursing process approach to excellent care.* Philadelphia: Lippincott Williams & Wilkins.

Page, G. G. (2005a). Immunologic effects of opioids in the presence or absence of pain. *Journal of Pain and Symptom Management, 29*(5S), S25–S31.

Page, G. G. (2005b) Surgery induced immunosuppression. *AACN Clinical Issues, 16*(3), 302–309.

Page, G. G., & Ben-Eliyahu, S. (1997). The immune-suppressive nature of pain. *Seminars in Oncology Nursing, 13*(1), 10–15.

Palm, S., Lehzen, S., Mignat, C., Steinmann, J., Leimenstoll, G., & Maier, C. (1998). Does prolonged oral treatment with sustained-release morphine tablets influence immune function? *Anesthesia and Analgesia, 86,* 166–172.

Sacerdote, P., Bianchi, M., Gaspani, L., Manfredi, B., Maucione, A., Terno, G., Ammatuna, M., & Panerai, A. E. (2000). The effects of tramadol and morphine on immune responses and pain after surgery in cancer patients. *Anesthesia and Analgesia, 90,* 1411–1414.

Starkweather, A. R., Witek-Janusek, L., & Mathews, H. L. (2005). Neural-immune interactions: Implications for pain management in patients with low-back pain and sciatica. *Biological Research for Nursing, 6*(3), 196–206.

Starkweather, A. R., Witek-Janusek, L., Nockels, R. P., Peterson, J., & Mathews, H. L. (2006). Immune function, pain, and psychological stress in patients undergoing spinal surgery. *Spine, 31*(18), E641–E647.

Thacker, M. A., Clark, A. K., Marchand, F., & McMahon, S. B., (2007). Pathophysiology of peripheral neuropathic pain: Immune cells and molecules. *International Anesthesia Research Society, 105*(3), 838–847.

Tsai, Y., Won, S., & Lin, M. (2000). Effects of morphine on immune response in rats with sciatic constriction injury. *Pain, 88,* 155–160.

Vallejo, R., Leon-Casasola, O., & Benyamin, R. (2004). Opioid therapy and immunosuppression. *American Journal of Therapeutics, 11,* 354–365.

Volk, T., Schenk, M., Voigt, K., Tohtz, S., Putzier, M., & Kox, W. J. (2004). Postoperative epidural anesthesia preserves lymphocyte, but not monocyte, immune function after major spine surgery. *Anesthesia and Analgesia, 98,* 1086–1092.

Watkins, L. R., & Maier, S. F. (2005). Immune regulation of central nervous system functions: From sickness responses to pathological pain. *Journal of Internal Medicine, 257,* 139–155.

Watkins, L. R., Maier, S. F., & Goehler, L. E. (1995). Immune activation: The role of pro-inflammatory cytokines in inflammation, illness responses and pathological pain states. *Pain, 63,* 289–302.

Zakharova, L. A., & Vasilenko, A. M. (2001). The opioidergic system in the combined regulation of pain and immunity. *Biology Bulletin, 28*(3), 280–292.

Suggested Readings

Cabot, P. J. (2001). Immune-derived opioids and peripheral antinociception. *Clinical and Experimental Pharmacology and Physiology, 28,* 230–232.

Homburger, J. A., & Meiler, S. (2006). Anesthesia drugs, immunity and long-term outcome. *Current Opinion in Anaesthesiology, 19,* 423–428.

Leckband, S. G. (2001). Systemic opioid analgesics. In J. D. Loeser (Ed.), *Bonica's management of pain* (3rd ed.). Philadelphia: Lippincott Williams & Wilkins.

Machelska, H., & Stein, C. (2000). Pain control by immune-derived opioids. *Clinical and Experimental Pharmacology and Physiology, 27,* 533–536.

Palmer, S. N., Glesecke, M., Body, S. C., Shernan, S. K., Fox, A. A., & Collard, C. D. (March 2005). Pharmacogenetics of anesthetic and analgesic agents. *Anesthesiology, 102*(3), 663–671.

Puehler, W., & Stein, C. (2005). Controlling pain by influencing neurogenic pathways. *Rheumatic Disease Clinics of North America, 31,* 103–113.

Rittner, H. L., Brack, A., & Stein, C. (2008). Pain and the immune system. *British Journal of Anaesthesia,101*(1), 40–44.

Roy, S., & Loh, H. H., (1996). Effects of opioids on the immune system. *Neurochemical Research, 21*(11), 1375–1386.

Sacerdote, P. (2008). Opioid-induced immunosuppression. *Current Opinion in Supportive and Palliative Care, 2,* 14–18.

Starkweather, A. R., Witek-Janusek, L., Nockels, R. P., Peterson, J., & Mathews, H. L. (2008). The multiple benefits of minimally invasive spinal surgery: Results comparing transforaminal lumbar interbody fusion and posterior lumbar fusion. *Journal of Neuroscience Nursing, 40*(1), 32–39.

Uhlig, T., & Kallus, K. W. (2005). The brain: a psychoneuroimmunological approach. *Current Opinion in Anaesthesiology, 18,* 147–150.

Welters, I. D. (2003). Is immunomodulation by opioid drugs of clinical relevance? *Current Opinion in Anaesthesiology, 16,* 509–513.

Wu, C. L., Cohen, S. R., Richman, J. M., Rowlingson, A. J., Courpas, G. E., Cheung, K., Lin, E. E., & Liu, S. S. (November 2005). Efficacy of postoperative patient-controlled and continuous infusion epidural analgesia versus intravenous patient-controlled analgesia with opioids. *Anesthesiology, 103*(5), 1079–1088.

Zhang, J., & Huang, Y. (2006). The immune system: A new look at pain. *Chinese Medical Journal, 119*(11), 930–938.

chapter

25

Depression and Pain

Janette E. Elliott, RN-BC, MSN, AOCN
Barbara St. Marie, ANP, GNP, RN-BC, PhD Candidate

Objectives

After studying this chapter, the reader should be able to:

1. Discuss the neurophysiology overlap of pain and depression.
2. Describe the assessment of patients for depression.
3. State the symptoms of depression.
4. Understand the treatment of depression as it relates to patients with pain.
5. Describe collaborative practice with mental health clinicians.

Pain and depression often occur together. The suffering of pain and the suffering of depression are not always apparent in nursing practices. This chapter delves into this overlap that complicates pain, whether it is acute or persistent. As we strive to help relieve the suffering of individuals, we become cognizant of the reciprocal impact of the biological and the psychological.

I. Neuroanatomy of Depression in the Brain

A. Neuroimaging (Drevets et al., 1992).

1. Brain structure and functional changes are identified in patients with depression by using neuroimaging.
2. Neuroimaging visualizes hyperactivity and increased blood flow in brain structures of people with depression.
3. Neuroimaging of patients suffering from depression compared to people without depression looks significantly different in the prefrontal cortex, extending from the left ventrolateral prefrontal cortex to the medial prefrontal cortex surface.
4. Increased blood flow in the left amygdala is also seen in the patient with depression.
5. Neuroimaging shows that depressed people have a 32% smaller volume in the medial orbitofrontal cortex than that of the control group (Bremner et al., 2002; Drevets et al., 1997).

B. Neurobiology of the brain

1. The area of the subgenual prefrontal cortex has been implicated with mediation of emotional and autonomic response to socially significant stimuli and modulation of neurotransmitter systems (Drevets et al., 1997).
2. The hippocampus has connections to the amygdala and prefrontal cortex, which is involved in emotion and cognition. In depressed individuals, the hippocampus has a decrease in volume as compared to its volume in control groups (Bremner et al., 2000).
3. Brain-derived neurotrophic factor (BDNF)
   a. BDNF is thought to be a component of neuronal health and neurogenesis.
   b. It may also influence mood.
   c. The correlation of decreased BDNF and depression may exist (Maletic et al., 2007).
   d. Successful antidepressant therapy may increase levels of BDNF.
   e. Serotonin and norepinephrine play roles in modulating BDNF.
   f. The use of antidepressant medications may increase BDNF. This leads to enhanced neuroplasticity and cellular resilience (Malberg, Eisch, Nestler, & Duman, 2000).
4. Antidepressant medication targets neurogenesis in the hippocampus and may restore neuronal connections.
   a. After 8 weeks of treatment, BDNF levels are shown to increase in the hippocampi of rats (Malberg et al., 2000).
   b. With long-term treatment, antidepressant treatment (medication and electroconvulsive shock therapy) increases neurogenesis in the hippocampus (Malberg et al., 2000).
   c. Antidepressant medications increase BDNF expression of hippocampal neurons (Malberg et al., 2000).
5. Stress and BDNF (Duman & Monteggia, 2006).
   a. The hypothalamic-pituitary-adrenal axis has increased neural activity with stress.
   b. With stress, an increase appears in the production of glucocorticoids, catecholamines, inflammatory cytokines, and other excitatory neurotransmitters.
   c. The stress response results in decreased levels of BDNF and negative-impact on neuronal health.
   d. In the hypothalamic-pituitary-adrenal axis, a decreased level of BDNF is seen with stress (Duman & Monteggia, 2006).
   e. Prolonged stress and prolonged elevation of glucocorticoids may result in damage of the hippocampal neurons and reduction of neurogenesis (Sapolsky, 2000).
   f. Chronic mood disorders may impair neuroplasticity and cellular resilience (Manji et al., 2003).

6. Depressed patients have a dysfunctional pain-processing network (Strigo, Simmons, Matthews, Craig, & Paulus, 2008).
   a. Anticipation of painful stimuli resulted in increased activation in the right anterior insular region, dorsal anterior cingulated, and right amygdala in depressed patients.
   b. During pain stimulation, depressed patients showed increased activation in the right amygdala and decreased activation in periaqueductal gray matter and in the rostral anterior cingulated and prefrontal cortices.
   c. Depressed patients showed greater activation in the right amygdala during anticipation of pain, which was associated with greater levels of perceived helplessness.

II. Depression Symptomatology

A. Major symptoms of depression can be recalled using the mnemonic SIG-E-CAPS (American Psychiatric Association [APA], 2000; Veterans Health Administration/Department of Defense [VHA/DOD], 2000):
   1. *S*leep disorder (either increased or decreased sleep)
   2. *I*nterest deficit (anhedonia)
   3. *G*uilt (worthlessness, hopelessness, or regret)
   4. *E*nergy deficit
   5. *C*oncentration deficit
   6. *A*ppetite disorder (either decreased or increased)
   7. *P*sychomotor retardation or agitation
   8. *S*uicidality

B. To meet the diagnosis of major depression, a patient must have five of the preceding symptoms ***plus*** depressed mood or anhedonia for at least 2 weeks.

C. Patients may have passive thoughts of death or dying, suicidal ideation, or suicide attempts.

D. Other symptoms may accompany depression, such as anxiety, irritability, or body aches and pains.
   1. These other symptoms cause functional impairment and distress.

E. Depression warning signs include the following (VHA/DOD, 2000):
   1. Medically unexplained physical symptoms (including pain)
   2. A chronic, debilitating medical condition (e.g., any chronically painful condition)
   3. Current substance misuse
   4. Medically unexplained functional status changes
   5. A history of or current physical or sexual abuse or emotional neglect
   6. Loss of significant relationship, primary support system, or economic status
   7. A protracted caregiving role for a family member with a chronic, disabling condition
   8. Bereavement or widowhood
   9. Symptoms or signs of posttraumatic stress disorder

III. Screening for Depression

A. Several tools have been shown to be valid and reliable for use in the primary care setting to screen for depression (Sharp & Lipsky, 2002).
   1. Beck Depression Inventory (Beck & Steer, 1984; Beck, Rial, & Rickets, 1974; Beck, Ward, Mendelson, Mock, & Erbaugh, 1961)
      a. This inventory has been used for 35 years.
      b. It is highly reliable.
      c. It consists of 21 items completed in 5 to 10 minutes by the patient.
   2. Center for Epidemiological Studies Depression Scale (CES-D) (Radloff, 1977)
      a. This scale has been used for more than 40 years.
      b. It is highly reliable.
      c. It comprises 20 items completed in 5 to 10 minutes by the patient.
   3. Geriatric Depression Scale (GDS) (Sheikh & Yesavage, 1986; Yesavage et al., 1983)
      a. The GDS is consistent and externally valid.
      b. The long form is 30 items, completed in 10 to 15 minutes.

c. The short form is 15 items, completed in 5 to 10 minutes.
d. Ease of administration for the easily confused, elderly patient is one advantage of GDS.
e. GDS is completed by the patient.
f. This is the preferred instrument in cognitively intact elderly patients (Geesey, 2006).

4. Zung Self-Rating Depression Scale (Zung, 1965)
   a. This scale is not assessed in minorities or the elderly.
   b. It consists of 20 items, completed in 5 to 10 minutes.
5. Cornell Scale for Depression in Dementia (CSDD) (Alexopoulos, Abrams, Young, & Shamoian, 1988)
   a. This scale is valid and reliable.
   b. It comprises 19 items, which take 10 minutes to complete with the patient and 20 minutes to complete with the caregiver.
   c. It is clinician administered.

B. The simple question, "Do you often feel sad or depressed?" may screen as well as the GDS and save time (Geesy, 2006).
C. Depression screening questionnaires are more effective when administered by the clinician (Kanter et al., 2003).
D. "Widespread screening without adequate follow-up care may be harmful, not just merely unhelpful, Coye argues. He says patients who screen positive for depression on these tests may be prescribed unnecessary medications and put extra financial and work burdens on the health care system" (Center for the Advancement of Health, 2005, p. 3).

IV. Suicidality

A. Prevalence of suicidality in patients with persistent pain (Tang & Crane, 2006)
   1. Prevalence appears to be at least doubled relative to controls.
   2. Suicide ideation (thinking about suicide) was approximately 20%.
   3. Suicide attempts were between 5% and 14%.
B. Suicide risk factors
   1. SAD PERSONS (VHA/DOD, 2000)
      a. *S*ex: Males kill themselves three times more often than females.
      b. *A*ge: Older rather than younger patients, especially males, commit suicide.
      c. *D*epression: Depression precedes suicide in up to 70% of cases.
      d. *P*revious attempts: Most people who die from suicide do so on their first or second attempt. People who make multiple attempts (four or more) have increased risk for future attempts rather than completions.
      e. *E*thanol use: Patients who abuse substances are at increased risk for suicide completion.
      f. *R*ational thinking loss: Profound cognitive slowing, distorted perceptions, psychotic depression, and preexisting brain damage increase the risk.
      g. *S*ocial support deficit: This deficit may be a result of illness, which can cause social withdrawal, loss of job, loss of relationship, and legal difficulties.
      h. *O*rganized plan: Always ask about the presence of a suicide plan.
      i. *N*o spouse: Unmarried status may be a result or cause of a depression disorder.
      j. *S*ickness: An intercurrent medical illness is an illness that begins when the patient is already depressed.
C. Ask the patient the following: (APA, 2000)
   1. "Have you ever felt like life wasn't worth living?" Other variants might be "Have you ever felt like hurting yourself?" or "Have you ever felt suicidal?"
   2. If yes, ask, "Have you thought of acting on those feelings?" or "Do you have a plan on how to do this?"
   3. If the patient acknowledges a plan, explore this. What is it? How realistic is it? Have they acted on this? If yes, then ask, "Do you have a way of carrying this out?"
      a. A conclusive example: the patient states he would shoot himself and has a gun at home.

   b. A nonconclusive example: the patient states she plans to drive over a cliff but has no access to a vehicle.
4. If you deem the person to be suicidal, consider emergency referral to a mental health professional.
5. Asking patients about suicidality does not increase the likelihood of their killing themselves.

V. Pain and Depression

A. The prevalence of depression among patients with pain based on clinical location is as follows (Sansone & Sansone, 2008):
   1. Psychiatric clinics: 35%
   2. Pain clinics: 38%
   3. Rheumatology clinics: 52%
   4. Dental clinics: 78%

B. Arrow and colleagues (2006) found 41% of patients with major depression reported disabling persistent pain and 25% reported nondisabling persistent pain.

C. Arrow and colleagues (2006) also report that, of those meeting the criteria for major depression, approximately two-thirds also report persistent pain and those with chronic pain had a significantly higher rate of major depression.

D. VHA/DOD clinical practice guidelines include a listing of diagnoses related to depression. In these clinical practice guidelines, chronic pain syndrome is a subsection of depression. Included under chronic pain syndrome are fibromyalgia, reflex sympathetic dystrophy, low back pain, chronic pelvic pain, and medical disease-related pain. Among other subsections of depression are additional painful conditions such as systemic inflammatory response syndrome, diabetes, and neoplasms.

E. Relationship of depression and pain occurrences
   1. Depression can precede pain.
   2. Pain can precede depression.
   3. Prior depression can heighten the risk of subsequent depression with new-onset pain.
   4. Pain and depression can occur independently of each other.

F. The comorbidity of pain and depression makes antidepressant therapy a rational choice.

G. Treatment of the underlying cause of depression may alleviate anxiety, irritability, pain, or all of these.

VI. Treatment of Depression in the Patients with Pain (APA, 2000)

A. Pharmacological treatment with antidepressants (see the chapter on Overview of Pharmacology)
   1. General psychopharmacology principles (APA, 2000)
      a. No one agent has been shown to be superior to another.
      b. Use what has previously worked for the patient.
      c. An inadequate medication trial is the most common cause of treatment failure.
      d. Consider switching, combining, or increasing the medication if there is no response at 4 to 6 weeks.
      e. First drug choices are selective serotonin reuptake inhibitors due to ease of use, safety in overdose, and better side-effect profile.
      f. Potential risks and benefits need to be considered if treating pregnant women or those considering becoming pregnant.

B. Psychotherapy (VHA/DOD, 2000)
   1. Psychotherapy is as effective as antidepressants medications for most patients.
   2. It may be considered first line of therapy in most cases.
   3. Psychotherapy is brief, focused on current concerns and helping the patient learn new skills or change behavior patterns. Types of psychotherapy are
      a. Interpersonal psychotherapy.
      b. Behavior therapy.
      c. Cognitive therapy.
      d. Cognitive-behavioral therapy.

e. Short-term psychodynamic therapy.
f. Couples therapy.
4. The patient must be actively involved—attend sessions regularly and complete "homework."
5. Consider medications in addition or as an alternative to psychotherapy if the patient is not engaged in the therapy or is worse after 6 weeks.
6. If the patient remains unchanged after 12 weeks of psychotherapy, medication should be added.
7. Combine psychotherapy with medications for patients who have not responded to either single approach or for patients who have responded well to the combination in the past.

C. Ongoing clinical assessment (VHA/DOD, 2000)
1. Initially, reassess the patient every 1 to 2 weeks for 4 to 6 weeks.
a. Monitor for compliance and response to intervention.
b. Monitor for suicidality.
c. Rule out comorbidities.
d. Answer questions.
e. Assess side effects and provide reassurance; adjust doses of medications if needed.
f. Adapt psychotherapy as needed.
2. Maintain therapeutic medication doses for 4 to 9 months.
3. Maintain monthly office visits for 6 months.
4. Lifetime medications are recommended if the patient has experienced three or more episodes of major depression.
5. If psychotherapy is maintained, consider intermittent reevaluation.

VII. Outcomes

A. Reengineering Systems for Primary Care Treatment of Depression trial (Kroenke, Shen, Oxman, Williams, & Dietrich, 2007)
1. At baseline, 42% of depressed patients reported pain severe enough to moderately interfere with daily activities.
2. Severe pain at baseline is a risk factor for worse response to depression therapy.
3. Identifying comorbid pain and optimizing its management may be important in enhancing response and remission rates for patients with depression.
4. Treating pain may enhance treatment of comorbid depression, and treating depression may enhance treatment of comorbid pain.
5. Neglecting to treat one may impede the effective treatment of the other.

B. A literature review by Bair, Robinson, Katon, and Kroenke (2003) determined the following:
1. The presence of pain negatively affects the recognition and treatment of depression.
2. Comorbid pain is associated with more depressive symptoms and worse outcomes of treatment for depression.
3. Depression in patients with pain is associated with increased pain complaints and more functional impairment.
4. Pain is reported more often as depression increases.
5. Multiple sites of pain complaints are associated with the greater probability of comorbid depression (Bair et al., 2003, 2004; Von Korff, Ormel, Katon, & Lin, 1992).
6. "If all primary care patients presenting with a variety of pain conditions (e.g., abdominal pain, headache, joint pain, and back pain) were evaluated for possible depression, 60% of previously undetected depressions cases could have been recognized" (Bair et al., 2003, p. 2436).
7. "Providers frequently assess for physical causes for pain and treat medically instead of exploring the pain symptoms in a broader, biopsychosocial context" (Bair et al., 2003, p. 2436).
8. Comorbid pain and depression are associated with worse outcomes than either condition alone. Therefore, simultaneously treating both seems necessary for optimal outcomes.

VIII. Collaboration with Mental Health Clinicians

A. Given the extensive overlap of pain, depression, and suicidality, nurses are to be aware of the psychological resources available to their practice.

B. It is common practice for pain clinics to employ pain psychologists.
C. Pain psychologists may assist with patient assessment for depression and suicidality and with treatment of depression and persistent pain.
D. Pain psychologists may also conduct groups with persistent-pain patients that provide education about persistent pain and psychotherapy.

Summary

Pain and depression often occur together. Higher pain severity results in depression that responds less well to therapy. When patients present with reports of pain at multiple sites, the presence of depression needs to be assessed; these patients tend to be medically evaluated but not psychologically assessed, thereby overlooking the possibility of the diagnosis of major depression. To optimally alleviate either, both may need to be treated. May we as nurses act as advocates for our patients to ensure best possible treatment of both.

References

Alexopoulos, G. S., Abrams, R. C., Young, R. C., & Shamoian, C. A. (1988). Cornell scale for depression in dementia. *Biological Psychiatry, 23,* 271–284.

American Psychiatric Association. (2000). *Diagnostic and statistical manual of mental disorders* (4th ed., text rev., pp. 352–356) (DSM-IV-TR). Washington, DC: Author.

Arrow, B. A., Hunkeler, E. M., Blasey, C. M., Lee, J., Constantino, M. J., Fireman, B., Kraemer, H. C., Dea, R., Robinson, R., & Hayward, C. (2006). Comorbid depression, chronic pain, and disability in primary care. *Psychosomatic Medicine, 68,* 262–268.

Bair, M. J., Robinson, R. L., Eckert, G. J., Stang, P. E., Croghan, T. W., & Kroenke, K. (2004). Impact of pain on depression treatment response in primary care. *Psychosomatic Medicine, 66,* 17–22.

Bair, M. J., Robinson, R. L., Katon, W., & Kroenke, K. (2003). Depression and pain comorbidity: A literature review. *Archives of Internal Medicine, 163*(10), 2433–2445.

Beck, A. T., & Steer, R. A. (1984). Internal consistencies of the original and revised Beck Depression Inventory. *Journal of Clinical Psychology, 40*(6), 1365–1367.

Beck, A. T., Rial, W. Y., & Rickets, K. (1974). Short form of depression inventory: Cross-validation. *Psychological Reports, 34*(3), 1184–1186.

Beck, A. T., Ward, C. H., Mendelson, M., Mock, J., & Erbaugh, J. (1961). An inventory for measuring depression. *Archives of General Psychiatry, 4,* 561–571.

Bremner, J. D., Narayan, M., Anderson, E. R., Staib, L. H., Miller, H. L., & Charney, D. S. (2000). Hippocampal volume reduction in major depression. *American Journal of Psychiatry, 157,* 115–118.

Bremner, J. D., Vythilingam, M., Vermetten, E., Nazeer, A., Adil, J., Khan, S., Staib, L. H., & Charney, D. S. (2002). Reduced volume of orbitofrontal cortex in major depression. *Biological Psychiatry, 51,* 273–279.

Center for the Advancement of Health. (2005). Screening for depression. *Facts of Life: Issue Briefings for Health Reporters, 10*(12). Retrieved January 9, 2009, from http://www.cfah.org/factsoflife/vol10no12.cfm.

Drevets, W. C., Videen, T. O., Price, J. L., Preskorn, S. H., Carmichael, S. T., & Raichle, M. E. (1992). A functional anatomical study of unipolar depression. *Journal of Neuroscience, 12,* 3628–3641.

Drevets, W. C., Price, J. L., Simpson, J. R., Todd, R.D., Vannier, M., & Raichle, M.E. (1997). Subgenual prefrontal cortex abnormalities in mood disorders. *Nature, 386,* 824–827.

Duman, R. S., & Monteggia, L. M. (2006). A neurotrophic model for stress-related mood disorders. *Biological Psychiatry, 59,* 925–935.

Geesey, M. (2006). *RCMAR measurement tools: Depression assessment tools.* Retrieved January 9, 2009, from http://musc.edu/dfm/RCMAR/DepressionTools.html.

Kanter, J. W., Epler, A. J., Chaney, E. F., Liu, C., Heagerty, P., Lin, P., Felker, B., & Hedrick, S. C. (2003). Effectiveness of team treatment of depression in primary care. *Primary Care Companion Journal of Clinical Psychiatry, 5*(6), 245–250.

Kroenke, K., Shen, J., Oxman, T. E., Williams, J. W., & Dietrich, A. J. (2007). Impact of pain on the outcomes of depression treatment: Results from the RESPECT trial. *Pain, 135*(1–2), 209–215.

Malberg, J. E., Eisch, A. J., Nestler, E. J., & Duman, R. S. (2000). Chronic antidepressant treatment increases neurogenesis in adult rat hippocampus. *Journal of Neuroscience, 20,* 9104–9110.

Maletic, V., Robinson, M., Oakes, T., Iyengar, S., Ball, S. G., & Russell, J. (2007). Neurobiology of depression: An integrated view of key findings. *Integrative Journal of Clinical Practice, 61,* 2030–2040.

Manji, H. K., Quiroz, J. A., Sporn, J., Payne, J. L., Denicoff, K., Gray, N. A., Zarate, C. A., & Charney, D. S. (2003). Enhancing neuronal plasticity and cellular resilience to develop novel, improved therapeutics for difficult-to-treat depression. *Biological Psychiatry, 53,* 707–742.

Radloff, L. S. (1977). The CES-D scale: A self-report depression scale for research in the general population. *Applied Psychological Measurement, 1,* 284–401.

Sansone, R. A., & Sansone, L. A. (2008). Pain, pain, go away: Antidepressants and pain management. *Psychiatry, 5*(12), 16–19.

Sapolsky, R. M. (2000). Glucocorticoids and hippocampal atrophy in neuropsychiatric disorders. *Archives of General Psychiatry, 34,* 13–25.

Sharp, L. K., & Lipsky, M. S. (2002). Screening for depression across the lifespan: A review of measures for use in primary care settings. *American Family Physician, 66*(6), 1001–1008.

Sheikh, J. I., & Yesavage, J. A. (1986). Geriatric depression scale (GDS): Recent evidence and development of a shorter version. In T. L. Brink (Ed.), *Clinical gerontology: A guide to assessment and intervention* (pp. 165–173). New York: Haworth.

Strigo, I. A., Simmons, A. N., Matthews, S. D., Craig, A. D., & Paulus, M. P. (2008). Association of major depressive disorder with altered functional brain response during anticipation and processing of heat pain. *Archives of General Psychiatry, 65*(11), 1275–1284.

Tang, N. K. Y., & Crane, C. (2006). Suicidality in chronic pain: A review of the prevalence, risk factors and psychological links. *Psychological Medicine, 36*(5), 575–586.

Veterans Health Administration/Department of Defense (VA/DOD). (2000). *Management of major depressive disorder in adults in the primary care setting.* (Office of Quality and Performance Publication No. 10Q-CPG/MDD-00). Retrieved January 9, 2009, from http://www.oqp.med.va.gov/cpg/MDD/G/MDD-about.htm.

Von Korff, J., Ormel, J., Katon, W., & Lin, E. H. (1992). Disability and depression among high utilizers of health care: a longitudinal analysis. *Archives of General Psychiatry, 49,* 91–100.

Yesavage, J. A., Brink, T. L., Rose, T. L., Lum, O., Huang, V., Adey, M. B., & Leirer, V. O. (1983). Development and validation of a geriatric depression screening scale: A preliminary report. *Journal of Psychiatric Research, 17,* 37–49.

Zung, W. W. (1965). A self-rating depression scale. *Archives of General Psychiatry, 12,* 63–70.

chapter

26

Coexisting Addiction and Pain

Barbara St. Marie, ANP, GNP, RN-BC, PhD Candidate

Objectives

After studying this chapter, the reader should be able to:

1. Understand the significance of stigmatizing terms in clinical care.
2. Determine how to manage risk of coexisting addiction and pain.
3. Identify tools used to determine risk for opioid therapy.

Ethical concerns on how we care for individuals with coexisting addiction and pain are great. The literature provides us with ethical perspectives of clinical experts and nursing organizations (American Academy of Pain Medicine, American Pain Society, & American Society of Addiction Medicine, 2001; American Society for Pain Management Nursing, 2002; Cohen, Jasser, Herron, & Margolis, 2002; Swope, Amero, Kujawski, Miller, & St. Marie, 2009). These ethical concerns are driving the state of the science in coexisting addiction and pain.

I. Caring for Patients with Coexisting Addiction and Pain

A. As nurses, we must look beyond clinical and personal bias and instead look to the research to learn how best to care for patients with coexisting addiction and pain. Addiction is not a character flaw; it is a brain disease. In this patient population, we must balance the approach of appropriate pain management by using the scientific knowledge while assuring that opioid pain medications are used rationally, ethically, and legally.

B. The definitions found for addiction, physical dependence, and tolerance in the Taxonomy for Pain Management Nursing chapter are foundations for definitions of coexisting addiction and pain. However, they present ambiguity for clinicians treating patients experiencing this phenomenon.

1. The literature defines coexisting addiction and pain not as a unique phenomenon, but rather as separate entities that exist within one person (Kirsh, Whitcomb, Donaghy, & Passik, 2002; Michna et al., 2004; Passik & Kirsh, 2004; Savage et al., 2003; Schnoll & Weaver, 2003).
2. Schnoll and Finch (1994) differentiate characteristics found between the chronic pain patient and the addicted patient.
   a. The attributes of the chronic pain patient are
      (1) Being in control of medications.
      (2) Using medications to improve the quality of their life and function.
      (3) Being aware of the side effects.
      (4) Being concerned about medical problems.
      (5) Following the agreed-upon treatment plan.
      (6) Having medications left over from previous prescriptions.
   b. The attributes of the patient with addictive disease are
      (1) Out of control behaviors with medications.
      (2) Decreased quality of life and function due to medication.
      (3) Wanting medications to continue or increase despite side effects.
      (4) Being in denial about medical problems.
      (5) Not following the treatment plan.
      (6) Not having medications left over, losing prescriptions, and always having a "story" (Schnoll & Finch, 1994).

C. Identification of addiction behaviors in patients receiving chronic opioid therapy to treat their chronic pain has been studied (Wu et al., 2006).

1. A tool called the Addiction Behaviors Checklist was developed to track behaviors that are characteristic of addiction while participants are receiving opioid medication for chronic pain.
2. Wu et al. (2006) provide a detailed account of tool development.
3. This checklist tool is used in interviews in which the participant's answers are recorded.
4. The participant records the observations of behaviors on the tool during session and pertinent information from a medical chart review.
   a. The items are classified into two categories:
      (1) Addictive behaviors noted between visits
      (2) Addictive behaviors noted within the visit
   b. If the patient's family members or significant other was present in the session, their expressed concerns over the participant's use of analgesics were also recorded.
   c. The instrument includes 20 items, with dichotomous response scoring.

5. Primary behaviors of addiction are significant (Wu et al., 2006).
   a. Rapid identification through the use of this tool can facilitate early treatment.
   b. Aberrant behavior needs reassessment and possible referral.

D. To treat patients' pain, we may need to look beyond behaviors to know more. Different meanings to the sets of behaviors need to be understood.
   1. In a qualitative study using grounded theory, Morgan (2006) developed a model based on the experiences of participants with a history of drug abuse who were hospitalized and in pain.
      a. The model titled, Knowing How to Play the Game, was developed from the following research questions (Morgan, 2006, p. 33):
         (1) How do participants with substance abuse problems manage painful medical conditions during hospitalization?
         (2) What difficulties do they encounter in getting adequate help with pain while hospitalized?
         (3) How do participants with substance abuse problems understand their interactions with nurses around issues of pain?
      b. In this study, participants described strategies used to get their pain managed and the barriers they encountered to have their pain acknowledged and treated.
         (1) The participants perceived a lack of respect from staff and a lack of belief in their needs, fears, feelings, and pain.
         (2) The participants pointed out a lack of knowledge of staff about pain management and about addictions.
         (3) The model consisted of two core action categories identified by the participants (Morgan, 2006, p. 36):
            (a) "Feeling respected/not respected"
            (b) "Strategizing to get pain relief"
         (4) Knowing How to Play the Game was a necessary strategy for substance abusers to achieve respect and treatment of their pain in the hospital setting.
   2. This research can guide future qualitative and quantitative research with patients who experience the coexistence of addiction and pain. Subsequent qualitative studies may replicate similar phenomena.

II. Stigmatizing Terms

A. A derogatory term often used by nurses is ***drug seeking.*** McCaffery, Grimm, Pasero, Ferrell, and Uman (2005) surveyed nurses on their meaning of the term and how nurses regarded the use of the term in health care. Similarities were identified among three groups of nurses: emergency room nurses, general nurses, and pain management nurses.
   1. All three groups of nurses view the term in the same manner. These nurses listed attributes of patients labeled as "drug seeking." These attributes were
      a. Accessing different emergency departments to get opioids.
      b. Telling inconsistent stories about pain or medical history.
      c. Asking for a refill because the prescription was lost or stolen.
   2. All three groups of nurses felt the term ***drug seeking*** meant the patient was addicted to opioids, abusing prescription opioids, or manipulative.

B. The use of stigmatizing terms for individuals with coexisting pain and addiction can create huge barriers for those seeking pain relief with opioids. From Morgan's study (2006), we also saw that these derogatory terms are not hidden from our patients. Our patients hear us through either verbal or nonverbal communication.

C. Further study of the neurophysiology and the human experiences of coexisting addiction and pain perhaps can help us adjust our attitudes away from blaming the victim.

III. Having Useful Terminology

A. Proponents for the use of the term ***addiction*** believe the word would
   1. Convey the appropriate meaning of the compulsive drug-taking condition.
   2. Distinguish it from "physical" dependence, which is normal and can occur in anyone who takes medications that affect the central nervous system.

B. The proponents of the term *dependence* believe the word would
   1. Be a more neutral term that could easily apply to all drugs, including alcohol and nicotine.
   2. Replace the word *addiction,* which was viewed as a pejorative term that would add to the stigmatization of people with substance use disorder (personal communication with Charles O'Brien, chairman of the *Diagnostic and Statistical Manual of Mental Disorders,* 5th edition [DSM-V], revision).
C. DSM-III and the DSM-IV contain the term *dependence.*
   1. O'Brien writes, "We are now in the planning stages for DSM-V. There will be careful reviews of the criteria, but in the case of substance use disorders, the medical world drastically needs a change in the label. Addiction is a perfectly acceptable word. It is used by the American Society of Addiction Medicine (ASAM), the American Association of Addiction Psychiatrists (AAAP), the American Journal on Addictions, and the oldest journal in the field, simply known as *Addiction.* It is clear that any harm that might occur due to the pejorative connotation of the word *addiction* would be completely outweighed by the tremendous harm that is now being done to those patients who have had needed medication withheld because their doctors believe that they are addicted simply because they are dependent" (email communication, December 17, 2008).
   2. No decision has been made related to the use of *dependence* versus *addiction* for DSM-V.

IV. Prevalence Reports of Prescription-type Psychotherapeutic Drug Abuse

A. The Substance Abuse and Mental Health Services Administration (SAMHSA) conducts the National Survey on Drug Use and Health, providing the primary source on prevalence, patterns, and consequences of drug and alcohol use and abuse in the civilian population age 12 and over in the United States (SAMHSA, 2006).
B. The National Survey on Drug Use and Health (NSDUH) examines civilian, noninstitutionalized individual use of alcohol and illicit drugs during the past month. In 2005, 22.2 million individuals (9.1%) were classified with substance dependence or abuse in the past year.
   1. Substance dependence or abuse criteria were specified by DSM-IV (SAMHSA, 2006).
   2. Pain relievers, tranquilizers, stimulants, and sedatives are the four categories of prescription-type drug, referred to as *psychotherapeutics.* These drugs are available either through prescription or through illegal manufacturing.
      a. There were 6.4 million (2.6%) who used psychotherapeutics for nonmedical use. Of these, 4.7 million used pain medications, 1.8 used tranquilizers, 1.1 million used stimulants, and 272,000 used sedatives.
      b. In this survey, methamphetamine falls into the stimulant category. In 2005, use was 0.2%, showing no significant change since 2002.
      c. In 2005, the 59.8% of nonmedical users of psychotherapeutics obtained their drugs from a friend or relative for free, 16.8% received the drugs from one doctor, 4.3% obtained them from a drug dealer or stranger, and 0.8% received them over the Internet (SAMHSA, 2006).
   3. This survey indicates a growing national problem of prescription drug abuse in this country.
      a. In response to this survey, the National Institutes of Health, a department of the U.S. Department of Health and Human Services (DHHS), is initiating the first large-scale national study to treat addiction to prescription pain medications (DHHS, 2007).
      b. This study will recruit 648 participants in 11 sites across the country. The model that will be tested will include the use of buprenorphine and naloxone (Suboxone®) and different models of drug counseling for patients addicted to prescription opioids for chronic pain and those who abuse painkillers for nonmedical reasons.
      c. The clinical director of McLean's Alcohol and Drug Abuse Treatment Center and lead investigator for the study states, "This study is important because most of the research to date has been done on treatment for those addicted to heroin not prescription pain medications" (DHHS, 2007, p. 1).
      d. "It also isn't clear whether people who started taking these medications for legitimate reasons will respond to the same treatment in the same way as those who use pain medications solely on an illicit basis" (DHHS, 2007, p. 1).

C. In a study using the computerized patient record system through the U.S. Department of Veterans Affairs hospital system, a randomly selected group of patient charts was reviewed for details of pain complaints and analgesic prescribed by care providers (Clark, 2002).
   1. The purpose of the study was to determine how often chronic pain complaints were documented in the patient's chart, along with the management of prescription analgesics.
   2. This model of record keeping indicated pain complaint, anatomical location, presence or absence of side effects, goals of therapy, pain relief, and functional improvement.
   3. The average daily dose of morphine equivalents was 33 mg/d, with a range of 5 to 180 mg/d (Clark, 2002, p. 134).
   4. In the review, 21% of patients had documented substance abuse history and 40% had at least one psychiatric diagnosis.
   5. The presence of chronic pain in this U.S. Department of Veterans Affairs system general medical clinic was 48%.
   6. The computerized record system was a useful databank from which future studies, including prevalence studies, may be conducted.

V. Assessment and Screening Tools for Addiction and Pain

A. In recent years, the addictions and the pain literature have inspired tool development to identify patients who are at risk for abusing prescription pain medications used to treat their pain.

B. Several pain and addiction specialists have criticized DSM-IV as inappropriate for identifying opioid misuse in pain patients (Savage, 1999; Sees & Clark, 1993).

C. Tools have been designed to assist in identifying potential opioid misuse in pain patients. These tools are designed to screen for risk of prescription opioid abuse.
   1. Screening Tool for Addiction Risk (STAR) (Friedman, Li, & Mehrotra, 2003; Li, Katragadda, Mehrotra, Mosuro, & Friedman, 2001)
      a. There are 14 yes-or-no questions addressing
         (1) Prior treatment in chemical dependency rehabilitation.
         (2) Prior treatment in another pain clinic.
         (3) Use of nicotine, alcohol, and drugs.
         (4) Family and household members with drug or alcohol abuse.
         (5) Feelings of depression, anxiety, and altered mood.
      b. It is brief and used in chronic pain patients.
      c. The tool needs further study to determine prediction capability.
   2. Opioid Risk Tool (ORT) (Kirsh, 2007) (see the chapter on Pain Assessment)
   3. Pain Medication Questionnaire (PMQ) (Adams et al., 2004)
      a. This 26-item self-report screening tool measures risk of opioid medication misuse in the chronic pain population.
         (1) The 26 items reflect potential dysfunction of attitudes and aberrant behaviors while using pain medications.
         (2) The items have a 5-point Likert format and use verbal anchors. The higher the overall scores, the greater the presence of behaviors associated with risk for opioid misuse.
         (3) The Physician Risk Assessment (PRA) was designed for this study to provide another means of validating the Pain Medication Questionnaire (PMQ). It quantified the physicians' independent assessments of the patient's risk for opioid misuse as determined during their encounters.
      b. With further work and refinement, this questionnaire holds promise for measuring risk of opioid misuse (Adams et al., 2004).
   4. Screening Instrument for Substance Abuse Potential (SISAP) (Kirsh, 2007)
      a. This is a physician-administered tool.
      b. Five questions related to
         (1) Number of alcohol drinks in a typical day and week.
         (2) Past year use of marijuana.

(3) History of cigarette smoking.
(4) Age.

c. It can be used in primary care setting with chronic pain sufferers.
d. Further study is needed to determine its predictive value.

5. Leeds Dependence Questionnaire (LDQ) (Ferrari et al., 2005)
   a. This tool was previously validated for use in alcohol and opiate consumers (Raistrick et al., 1994).
   b. Items in this tool can decipher between a patient taking prescription opioids to manage pain and those using prescription opioids to maintain an addiction (Ferrari et al., 2005).
   c. Utilization of this tool is described later.
6. Screener and Opioid Assessment for Patients in Pain (SOAPP) (Butler, Budman, Fernandez, & Jamison, 2004) (see the chapter on Pain Assessment)
7. Diagnosis, Intractability, Risk, and Efficacy (DIRE) score (Belgrade, Schamber, & Lindgren, 2006)
   a. DIRE is a clinician-rated scale from 1 to 3, with higher scores indicating a better chance of opioid treatment efficacy and compliance.
   b. It uses four categories:
      (1) Diagnosis
      (2) Intractability
      (3) Risk
      (4) Efficacy
   c. DIRE explores psychological health, chemical health, reliability, and social support.
   d. Validation is in its preliminary phase.
   e. For clinicians who prefer an observer-based, clinician-rated assessment, DIRE has potential.

VI. Use of an Assessment Tool in a Specific Patient Population

A. In a study using the Leeds Dependence Questionaire (LDQ), a comparison was made between the need of headache groups for analgesics and the need of addicts for their abused drugs (Ferrari et al., 2005).
   1. The LDQ, a self-administered 10-item instrument, uses a rating scale of 0 to 3 for frequency (0 = never, 1 = sometimes, 2 = often, 3 = nearly always) and measures severity of dependence on various substances.
   2. Three groups of subjects were recruited. These groups were the chronic daily headache group, the episodic headache group, and the drug addict group.
      a. There were 122 chronic daily headache subjects, 71 episodic headache subjects, and 115 drug-addicted subjects. They were asked to think about their main substance or analgesic over the last week.
         (1) The results showed that the drug addict group and the chronic daily headache group were similar in mean total LDQ score.
         (2) When the drug addict group and the chronic daily headache group were compared with the episodic headache group, the differences were statistically significant in the mean total LDQ score.
         (3) No significant differences were seen in mean scores of the drug addict group and the chronic daily headache group in items related to thinking about the substances or analgesics, planning their day around the substances or analgesics, and taking substances or analgesics in a manner that increased the effect.
         (4) The drug addict group scored higher than the chronic daily headache group in items related to feeling compulsion for substances or analgesics that was too strong to control, compulsion to continue to take substances or analgesics once started, and a need to maintain the effect.
         (5) The chronic daily headache group scored higher than the drug addict group in items pertaining to frequency of consumption of analgesics, the effect as more important than the particular analgesic used, and difficulty with coping with life without analgesics.

B. The LDQ helped researchers find that patients with episodic headaches were cautious about their analgesic use. This tool also helped determine that when patients with chronic daily headache overused it was because of pain. The results of this study showed that the link between patients with chronic daily headache and their analgesics was strong and that they used their analgesics to cope with life despite their daily headaches.

VII. Clinical Issues in Treating Patients with Coexisting Addiction and Pain

A. Patients who experience either addiction or pain have historically shared being misunderstood, underdiagnosed, and undertreated. When individuals experience coexisting chemical dependency and pain, this experience is amplified (Trafton, Oliva, Horst, Minkel, & Humphreys, 2004).

B. Trafton et al. (2004) compared health care utilization of 228 Veterans Health Administration patients with substance use disorders with and without pain.
   1. Their results showed that patients with substance use disorders with pain had higher health care utilization and more severe behavior around seeking relief and using illicit drugs.
   2. Patients with substance use disorder with pain also demonstrated an increase in medical and psychiatric problems.

C. Currie, Hodgins, Crabtree, Jacobi, and Armstrong (2003) evaluated an intervention with concurrent use of techniques of pain management and relapse prevention to treat patients with coexisting chronic pain and addiction.
   1. The treatment program was held once a week for 90 minutes for 10 weeks.
   2. Measurement outcomes were determined with the Addiction Severity Indices, the McGill Questionnaire, and the Self-Control Scale.
      a. Measurements were taken pretreatment, 3 months posttreatment, and 12 months posttreatment.
      b. The Addiction Severity Indices indicated significant improvement.
         (1) Significant improvement was also seen in the patient's pain severity, emotional functioning, and reduced medication reliance.
         (2) The patients reported less pain at the posttreatment follow-up intervals, which also coincided with a reduction in medication and other substance use.
      c. The Self-Control Scale reflected a shift toward greater utilization of self-management and internal coping strategies.
      d. The study lacked a control group and did not account for extraneous variables such as participants' access to Alcoholics Anonymous or Narcotics Anonymous groups.

D. In a study of iatrogenic opioid addiction among chronic pain patients, a methadone program was structure for patients in pain and maintained on methadone (Rhodin, Gronbladh, Nilsson, & Gordh, 2006).
   1. For 60 patients who were started on methadone, a 34-month follow-up interview asked about pain relief, quality of life, and side effects on 48 patients.
   2. Doses ranged from 10 to 350 mg/d for patients of whom 40% experienced low back and musculoskeletal pain, 68% reported psychiatric disease, and 32% had a substance use disorder.
      a. Pain relief was rated good by 75% and moderate by 25% of the patients.
      b. The index of global quality of life was favorable, and the side effects were recorded as sedation, low energy, weakness, weight increase, sweating, and sexual dysfunction in between 40% and 60% of the patients (Rhodin et al., 2006).
   3. This study showed that a structured methadone program can be used for treating chronic pain patients with opioid dependence while improving their quality of life and pain relief.

E. Wiedemer, Harden, Arndt, and Gallagher (2007), studied nurse practitioner- and clinical pharmacist-run opioid renewal clinic in a primary care setting.
   1. Primary care physicians in a primary care clinic were trained on opioid-prescribing guidelines, using opioid treatment agreements, and interpreting random urine drug testing.
   2. The clinical pharmacist worked with a nurse practitioner on prescription management within the clinic.

3. A multispecialty pain team supported this treatment dyad.
    a. The opioid renewal program was managed by a nurse practitioner and clinical pharmacists.
    b. Primary care physicians referred patients via a consult.
    c. Documentation included urine drug screening, an opioid treatment agreement, and the "4 As": analgesia, activity, adverse events (side effects), and aberrant behaviors.
    d. The multidisciplinary pain team consisted of an addiction psychiatrist, a rheumatologist, an orthopedist, a neurologist, and a physiatrist. They met biweekly with the nurse practitioner and clinical pharmacist to review cases and advise on treatment plans.
    e. Outcome measures were on provider behaviors, pharmacy budget, and patient behaviors.
4. Results of this study
    a. Provider behaviors
        (1) The number of opioid treatment agreements more than doubled from their baseline.
        (2) Urine drug screening rose from 74 per month to an average of 200 per month over 6 months.
        (3) Provider satisfaction showed most primary care providers found the program helpful.
    b. Pharmacy budget
        (1) Pharmacy budget goals were met by reducing costs from $129,793 to $5,236.
        (2) This is attributed to the shift from expensive pharmaceutical intervention to less expensive pharmaceutical interventions.
    c. Patient behaviors
        (1) Of the patients referred for aberrant drug-taking behavior, 45% adhered to the opioid treatment agreement, 38% self-discharged from the practice, 22% required referral for addiction treatment, 4% were weaned from opioids due to consistently negative urine drug tests, and 49% had no documented aberrant behaviors.
        (2) The average number of monthly emergency department visits declined per patient by 72.7%, and unscheduled primary care visits declined by 59.6%.

F. Opioid withdrawal in a comprehensive pain rehabilitation program was studied at the Mayo Clinic (Townsend et al., 2008).
1. The hypothesis was that chronic pain patients on long-standing opioid use who undergo opioid withdrawal in the course of rehabilitative treatment will experience significant and sustained improvement in pain and functioning similar to patients who were not taking opioids.
2. The longitudinal study design measured admission, discharge, and 6-month posttreatment by opioid status by admission.
    a. Measurements included pain severity, depression psychosocial functioning, health status, and pain catastrophizing.
    b. Treatment was involvement in a 3-week interdisciplinary pain rehabilitation program focused on functional restoration.
3. Results
    a. Medication use on admission
        (1) Mean daily morphine equivalent was 99 mg, ranging from 1 to 1,060 mg. Median dose was 45 mg.
        (2) Over half the patients were taking opioids on admission.
    b. Patients who were on chronic opioid therapy on admission and completed rehabilitative treatment that incorporated opioid withdrawal improved to the same extent as those who were not using opioids upon admission.
        (1) "There were no significant differences between the opioid and nonopioid groups in the proportion of patients taking benzodiazepines, NSAIDs [nonsteroidal antiinflammatory drugs], muscle relaxants, tricyclic antidepressants, SSRI [selective serotonin reuptake inhibitor] antidepressants, and other antidepressants" (Townsend et al., 2008, p. 183).
        (2) "Although significantly reduced from admission, a significantly greater proportion of patients in the opioid group, compared to nonopioid group, were still taking opioids and anticonvulsant medications" (Townsend et al., 2008, p. 183).

c. The proportion of patients who chose to not complete the program due to illness, family stressors, or chemical dependency was similar between the opioid group and the nonopioid group. "There were no differences in sex, age, education, marital status, state of residence, opioid use status, pain duration, variables of psychosocial functioning, depression, and pain catastrophizing" (Townsend et al., 2008, p. 184).

d. The patients who did not complete the program were taking significantly higher daily doses of morphine equivalent on admission to the program.

e. Of the 91% of the patients who returned their questionnaire, 9% began taking opioids 6 months after participating in the treatment program.
   (1) The mean daily opioid equivalent was 67.6 mg.
   (2) Patients who completed the treatment program experienced significant improvement regardless of opioid use status at admission. ". . . study patients in the opioid cohort who completed rehabilitation that incorporates opioid withdrawal were able to maintain treatment gains comparable to those in the non-opioid cohort" (Townsend et al., 2008, p. 184).
   (3) Possible explanations of the results
      (a) Opioid-induced hyperalgesia may result from high doses of opioids that contribute to pain sensitization, decreasing pain thresholds and potentially masking resolution of the preexisting pain condition (Townsend et al., 2008, p. 187).
      (b) The comparable distress and disability experienced by both opioid and nonopioid groups upon admission raises the question of whether patients should be maintained on high or low doses of chronic opioid therapy.
      (c) Polypharmacy, including benzodiazepine, muscle relaxants, and anticonvulsants, along with opioids, was not associated with higher functioning when compared to the nonopioid group. Significant improvement in mood and functioning occurred when these medications were tapered, with comparable findings to opioid withdrawal (Townsend et al., 2008, p. 187).

G. Heit (2001, 2003) states that a better understanding of addiction medicine will allow health care professionals to better treat the patient in pain.
   1. The purpose of his statement was twofold:
      a. To ensure that people with moderate to severe chronic pain be properly treated
      b. To reduce the fear of addiction by educating the health care professional on the proper definitions of addiction, physical dependence, and tolerance
   2. He called for "universal" understanding of the definitions by the American Academy of Pain Medicine, American Pain Society, and American Society of Addiction Medicine.

H. Universal precautions in pain medicine treatments were developed.
   1. The use of opioids necessitates risk stratification and monitoring.
      a. It facilitates identification.
      b. It facilitates management of the treatable and potentially fatal disease of addiction, including
         (1) Endogenous potential risk for addiction.
         (2) Current drug use that is nonprescription.
         (3) Problematic use of prescription opioids (Gourlay, 2008).
   2. These precautions are applied to individuals with or without a personal or family history of substance abuse and to individuals with currently active substance use (Gourlay, Heit, & Amahregi, 2005; Stanley & Safford, 2004).
      a. Endogenous addiction risk hierarchy is listed from low risk to higher risk as follows:
         (1) No personal or family history
         (2) Family history of addiction
         (3) Personal history of nonopioid addiction
         (4) Personal history of opioid addiction
   3. Universal precautions format the following 10 steps to pain management:
      a. Diagnosis
      b. Psychological assessment

c. Informed consent
d. Treatment agreement
e. Intervention reassessment
f. Trial of opioid therapy
g. Reassessment of pain score and level of function
h. Routinely assessment of the 4 As: analgesia, activity, adverse effects, and aberrant behaviors
i. Periodically reevaluation of pain diagnosis and addiction diagnosis
j. Documentation of initial evaluation and follow-up visits using a standard approach, that is, the 4 As (Passik & Weinreb, 2000)

I. Clinical considerations
1. Determine the nature of the problem.
   a. Is this a pain problem alone?
   b. Is this acute, chronic, or acute on chronic pain?
   c. Is this an addiction disorder?
   d. Is this both pain and addiction? And which is worse?
   e. What about the pharmacotherapy used? Is it rational? What is it doing "to" the patient? What is it doing "for" the patient?
      (1) Retry past prescribed and ineffective medications while using a multimodal approach to pain.
      (2) Evaluate for utility of nonopioid therapies.
      (3) Avoid previous drugs of abuse.
2. Review your fitness to assist the patient.
   a. What is your expertise to help this patient? Do you have the training? Credentials? Experience?
   b. What resources are at your disposal to help this patient? How available are these resources?
3. Determine the boundaries from the beginning of care. It is difficult to do this later in the care process.
4. Make limits flexible and reasonable.
   a. If the patient runs out of opioid early and reports that being underdosed, consider increasing the dose within tighter parameters (i.e., weekly dispensing).
   b. Tighter prescribing intervals may allow you to understand the difficulties the patient is having.
   c. If patient has acute pain in the context of a persistent pain problem (i.e., pain flare), the patient will need more opioid than the usual daily dose.
   d. Treat the pain in a patient with substance use disorder, being aware that aberrant behavior may be due to pain or may represent a primary substance use disorder (Gourlay, 2008).
5. Assess the continuum of risk for the patient.
   a. Risk is dynamic.
      (1) As with other disease processes, time and trust may clarify how to best to care for the patient.
      (2) "The diagnosis of addiction is made prospectively, over time" (Gourlay, 2008).
      (3) "The diagnosis of pseudoaddiction is made retrospectively. Abnormal behavior that normalizes with rational treatment supports this diagnosis" (Gourlay, 2008).
      (4) Use tools of assessment to help with this determination (described previously).
6. Monitor the patient.
   a. Urine toxicology
      (1) Use knowledge and care when interpreting urine drug tests.
      (2) The presence of an unprescribed drug may indicate a problem such as misuse or addiction.
      (3) False positives, or negatives may occur; know the urine testing sensitivity and specificity.
      (4) A urine test is used to benefit the patient, not to create an adversarial relationship between the prescriber or health care team and the patient.
      (5) The dose of drug and urine levels do not always correlate (Gourlay, 2008).

b. Pill counts
   (1) Review the opioid supply at each visit.
   (2) Midprescription pill counts may reveal an absence of the appropriate amount. Further discussion is needed with the patient to determine binge taking, sharing, or diversion.

c. Frequent follow-up
   (1) Regular follow-up establishes a rapport with the patient.
   (2) It helps you pay attention to details.
   (3) The goal is to optimize pain treatment and identify and address concerns early.

d. Contingency or interval dispensing
   (1) Weekly to monthly dispensing is typical for initiation of opioids.
   (2) Some patients may require tighter control, such as more frequent dispensing and smaller quantities or dispensed to the patient by a trusted individual.
   (3) Opioids must be locked up to protect family and visitors from access to opioids that may be diverted or are potentially dangerous to them, (e.g., when small children are in the home).

Summary

A. Both acute and chronic pain problems create challenges for patients who are chemically dependent.
   1. Acute pain is due to acute tissue damage and has a definite pattern of onset. It will subside as the tissue damage heals.
      a. Reassure patient that they will continue to have their acute pain managed without withholding opioids.
      b. Reassure health care team that dosage requirements of multimodal analgesia will be greater.
   2. Chronic pain may or may not be associated with a distinct onset or specific cause and persists beyond apparent tissue healing. It can be associated with a chronic disease that causes pain to be continuous or recurring over months or years.
      a. Chronic opioid therapy for individuals with chemical dependency needs to be attended to, taking into consideration the suffering of pain and the suffering of addiction.
      b. Advocacy for patients with coexisting addiction and pain must occur within the realm of the patient's health care team, their families, and their support systems.
      c. Educating patients about side effects of medications, risks of relapse, precautions used in health care to optimize therapy, phone numbers to call for support, and nonmedicine ways of managing their pain is important.
   3. Pain must continue to be treated when chemically dependency exists, regardless of whether the individual is in recovery or has relapsed.
   4. Support of chemical dependency needs to occur through Alcoholics Anonymous, Narcotics Anonymous, family support, spiritual support, or a support system that is individualized by the person to meet that patient's needs.
   5. Pain management may include opioids and must be balanced with a multimodal approach to pain that includes nonopioids and nonpharmacological approaches (see the chapters on Overview of Pharmacology and Persistent Pain Management).

B. Compassionate care in the context of defined expectations of both the health care team and the patient will avoid causing harm to individuals with coexisting addiction and pain.
   1. We know from caring for patients that a person can experience pain and addiction, experience no pain and still experience addiction, experience pain with no addiction, or experience no pain and no addiction.
   2. We do not know why these experiences occur in some people and not others, nor do we know how the different experiences are acquired.
   3. People who experience coexisting addiction and pain share unique experiences.
   4. Each individual experience is different based on the complex influences by culture, environment, anticipation, previous experience, and various emotional and cognitive factors.

References

Adams, L. L., Gatchel, R. J., Robinson, R. C., Polatin, P., Gajraj, N., Deschner, M., & Noe, C. (2004). Development of a self-report screening instrument for assessing potential opioid medication misuse in chronic pain patients. *Journal of Pain and Symptom Management, 27*(5), 440–459.

American Academy of Pain Medicine, American Pain Society, & American Society of Addiction Medicine. (2001). *Definitions related to the use of opioids for the treatment of pain.* Retrieved October 22, 2007, from http://www.painmed.org/productpub/statements/pdfs/definition.pdf.

American Society for Pain Management Nursing. (2002). *Pain management in patients with addictive disease.* Retrieved October 5, 2005, from http://www.aspmn.org.

Belgrade, M. J., Schamber, C. D., & Lindgren, B. R. (2006). The DIRE score: Predicting outcomes of opioid prescribing for chronic pain. *Journal of Pain, 7*(9), 671–681.

Butler, S. F., Budman, S. H., Fernandez, K., & Jamison, R. N. (2004). Validation of a screener and opioid assessment measure for patients with chronic pain. *Pain, 112,* 65–75.

Clark, J. D. (2002). Chronic pain prevalence and analgesic prescribing in a general medical population. *Journal of Pain and Symptom Management, 23*(2), 131–137.

Cohen, M. M., Jasser, S., Herron, P. D., & Margolis, C. G. (2002). Ethical perspectives: Opioid treatment of chronic pain in the context of addiction. *Clinical Journal of Pain, 18,* S99–S107.

Currie, S. R., Hodgins, D. C., Crabtree, A., Jacobi, J., & Armstrong, S. (2003). Outcome from integrated pain management treatment for recovering substance abusers. *Journal of Pain, 4*(2), 91–100.

Ferrari, A., Cicero, A. F. G., Bertolini, A., Leone, S., Pasciullo, G., & Sternieri, E. (2005). Need for analgesics/drugs of abuse: A comparison between headache patients and addicts by the Leeds Dependence Questionnaire (LDQ). *Cephalalgia, 26,* 187–193.

Friedman, R., Li, V., & Mehrotra, D. (2003). Treating pain patients at risk: Evaluation of a screening tool in opioid-treated pain patients with and without addiction. *Pain Medicine, 4*(2), 182–185.

Gourlay, D. L. (2008). *Update on universal precautions in 2008: Clinical pearls in stratifying and monitoring risk.* Lecture given October 30, 2008, at the 8th International Conference on Pain and Chemical Dependency, Philadelphia.

Gourlay, D. L., Heit, A. A., & Amahregi, A. (2005). Universal precautions in pain medicine: A rational approach to the treatment of chronic pain. *Pain Medicine, 6,* 107–112.

Heit, H. A. (2001). The truth about pain management: The difference between a pain patient and an addicted patient. *European Journal of Pain, 5*(Suppl. A), 27–29.

Heit, H. A. (2003). Addiction, physical dependence, and tolerance: Precise definitions to help clinicians evaluate and treat chronic pain patients. *Journal of Pain & Palliative Care Pharmacotherapy, 17*(1), 15–27.

Kirsh, K. L. (2007). Disease management tools for chronic pain. *Managed Care, 16*(2 Suppl. 3), 10–15.

Kirsh, K. L., Whitcomb, L. A., Donaghy, K., & Passik, S. D. (2002). Abuse and addiction issues in medically ill patients with pain: Attempts at clarification of terms and empirical study. *Clinical Journal of Pain, 18,* S52–S60.

Li, V., Katragadda, R., Mehrotra, D., Mosuro, Y., & Friedman, R. (2001). Pain and addiction: Screening patients at risk. *Pain Medicine, 2*(3), 245.

McCaffery, M., Grimm, M. A., Pasero, C., Ferrell, B., & Uman, G. C. (2005). On the meaning of "drug seeking." *Pain Management Nursing, 6*(4), 122–136.

Michna, E., Ross, E. L., Hynes, W. L., Nedeljkovic, S. S., Soumekh, S., Janfaza, D., Palombi, D., & Jamison, R.N. (2004). Predicting aberrant drug behavior in patients treated for chronic pain: Importance of abuse history. *Journal of Pain and Symptom Management, 8*(3), 250–258.

Morgan, B. D. (2006). Knowing how to play the game: Hospitalized substance abusers' strategies for obtaining pain relief. *Pain Management Nursing, 7*(1), 31–41.

O'Brien, C. (2008). Email communication with Dr. Charles O'Brien, Chair of the DSM-V revision, December 17, 2008.

Passik, S. D., & Kirsh, K. L. (2004). Opioid therapy in patients with a history of substance abuse. *CNS Drugs, 18*(1), 13–25.

Passik, S. D., & Weinreb, H. J. (2000). Managing chronic nonmalignant pain: Overcoming obstacles to the use of opioids. *Advanced Therapeutics, 17,* 70–83.

Raistrick, D., Bradshaw, J., Rober, G., Weiner, J., Allison, J., & Healey, C. (1994). Development of the Leeds Dependence Questionnaire (LDQ): A questionnaire to measure alcohol and opiate dependence in the context of a treatment evaluation package. *Addiction, 89,* 563–572.

Rhodin, A., Gronbladh, L., Nilsson, L. H., & Gordh, T. (2006). Methadone treatment of chronic non-malignant pain and opioid dependence: A long-term follow-up. *European Journal of Pain, 10,* 271–278.

Savage, S. R. (1999). Opioid therapy of chronic pain: Assessment of consequences. *Acta Anaesthesiologica of Scandinavica, 43,* 909–917.

Savage, S. R., Joranson, D. E., Covington, E. D., Schnoll, S. H., Heit, H. A., & Gilson, A. M. (2003). Definitions related to the medical use of opioids: Evolution towards universal agreement. *Journal of Pain and Symptom Management, 26*(1), 655–667.

Schnoll, S. H., & Finch, J. (1994). Medication education for pain and addiction: Making progress toward answering a need. *Journal of Law, Medicine & Ethics, 22*(3), 252–256.

Schnoll, S. H., & Weaver, M. F. (2003). Addiction and pain. *American Academy of Addiction Psychiatry, 12,* S27–S35.

Sees, K. L., & Clark, H. W. (1993). Opioid use in the treatment of chronic pain: Assessment of addiction. *Journal of Pain and Symptom Management, 8,* 257–264.

Stanley, A. H., & Safford, M. M. (2004). Treating chronic pain in the presence of substance abuse. *Journal of the National Medical Association, 96*(8), 1102–1104.

Substance Abuse and Mental Health Services Administration. (2006). *Results from the 2005 National Survey on Drugs Use and Health: National Findings.* Office of Applied Studies, NSDUH Series H-30. (DHHS Publication No. SMA 06-4194). Rockville, MD: Author. Retrieved September 5, 2007, from http://oas.samhsa.gov/nsduhLatest.htm.

Swope, E., Amero, L., Kujawski, T., Miller, K., & St. Marie, B. J. (2009). American Society for Pain Management Nursing: Urine drug testing self-directed learning module. Lenexa, Kansas: American Society for Pain Management Nursing.

Townsend, C. O., Kerkvliet, J. L., Bruce, B. K., Rome, J. D., Hooten, W. M., Luedtke, C. A., & Hodgson, J. E. (2008). A longitudinal study of the efficacy of a comprehensive pain rehabilitation program with opioid withdrawal: Comparison of treatment outcomes based on opioid use status at admission. *Pain, 140,* 177–189.

Trafton, J., Oliva, E. M., Horst, D. A., Minkel, J. D., & Humphreys, K. (2004). Treatment needs associated with pain in substance use disorder patients: Implications for concurrent treatment. *Drug and Alcohol Dependence, 73,* 23–31.

U.S. Department of Health and Human Services. (2007). *NIDA launches first large-scale national study to treat addiction to prescription pain medications: NIH news.* Retrieved August, 5, 2007, from http://www.nih.gov/news/pr/mar2007/nida-07b.htm.

Wiedemer, N. L., Harden, P. S., Arndt, I. O., & Gallagher, R. M. (2007). The opioid renewal clinic: A primary care, managed approach to opioid therapy in chronic pain patients at risk for substance abuse. *Pain Medicine, 8*(7), 573–584.

Wu, S. M., Compton, P., Bolus, R., Schieffer, B., Pham, Q., Baria, A., VanVort, W., Davis, F., Shekelle, P., & Naliboff, B. D. (2006). The Addiction Behaviors Checklist: Validation of a new clinician-based measure of inappropriate opioid use in chronic pain. *Journal of Pain and Symptom Management, 32*(4), 342–351.

Suggested Readings

Erickson, C. K. (2007). *The science of addiction: From neurobiology to treatment.* New York: W. W. Norton.

Woodward, J. J. (2003). The pharmacology of alcohol. In A.W. Graham, T.K. Schultz, M.F. Mayo-Smith, R.K. Ries, & B.B. Wilford (Eds.), *Principles of addiction medicine* (3rd ed.). Chevy Chase, MD: American Society of Addiction Medicine.

section

4

Support for the Practice Roles of Pain Management Nursing

chapter

27

The Pain Management Nurse as a Change Agent

Theresa Grimes, MN, RN-BC, FNP-BC, CCRN

Objectives

After studying this chapter, the reader should be able to:

1. Explore theories of planned change to apply to nursing practice for outcome improvement.
2. Describe how combined concepts for change allow the formation of models to improve practice within systems and patient populations.
3. Examine a method using Lewin's change theory and Roger's adoption innovation curve to approach systems or organizational change in practice.
4. Examine a method using behavioral health theories, including the health belief model, Prochaska and DiClemente's transformational stages of change, and the theory of reasoned action, to promote a patient or client change in health behavior.
5. Identify sources and reasons for resistance.
6. Define the skills needed to manage change effectively.
7. Discuss the use of outcome measures for evaluating the effectiveness of change processes.

The decade of pain fostered new research-based evidence and standards for practice to promote the appropriate treatment of people with pain. This growing body of knowledge comprises national guidelines such as those published by the Agency for Healthcare Research and Quality (AHRQ), the American Pain Society (APS), the American Geriatrics Society (AGS) and the Joint Commission (JC). The scope and standards for pain management nursing and position statements published by the American Society for Pain Management Nursing (ASPMN) provide further direction for evidenced-based practice. Best practices begin with knowledge; however, education alone is not adequate to institute and sustain them. An organized, scientific approach developed through the efforts of a multidisciplinary team is needed to produce and "hardwire" changed practices at the individual, organizational, state, and national levels. Several theories drive change in practice; however, some may be better adapted to systems change, while others focus on behavior and may be better adapted to patient or client change processes. The pain management nurse embraces this act of *planned* change to improve organizational and patient outcomes. This chapter provides information to create planned change.

I. Glossary of Terms

A. *Change* is "the process which leads to alteration in individual or institutional patterns of behavior" (Kozier & Erb, 1988, p. 452).

B. *Planned change* is "a deliberate and collaborative process involving change-agent and client-systems. These systems are brought together to solve a problem or, more generally, to plan and attain an improved state of functioning in the client-system by utilizing and applying valid knowledge" (Bennis, Benne, & Chin, 1961, p. 11).

C. A *change agent* is "a person or group who initiates changes or who assists others in making modifications in themselves or the system" (Kozier & Erb, 1988, p. 452).

D. *Driving forces* are those forces compelling an essential change in practice.

E. *Resistance* is "behavior intended to maintain the status quo" (Kozier & Erb, 1988, p. 454).

F. *Restraining forces* are those forces that tend to maintain the status quo, preventing change (Lewin, 1942/1951).

G. *Innovation* is "the means by which an organization capitalizes upon its unique knowledge and capabilities, which in turn form the basis of product or service offerings" (Gilmartin, 1998, p. 72).

H. An *innovator* is an individual who introduces a way of approaching a problem or task.

I. *Entrepreneurship* is "a drive and direction that has an internal locus of control, high energy level, and some degree of risk taking" (White & Begun, 1998, p. 42).

J. *Interdependence* occurs when "a change in one part of the system affects other parts of the system" (Kozier & Erb, 1988, p. 453).

K. *Empowerment* is "provision of knowledge and information that will encourage self-direction" (Blanchard, Carlos, & Randolph, 1996, p. 5).

L. The stage of *unfreezing* is the act of overcoming the status quo (restraining forces) to effect needed change (driving forces) and thus to establish the best practice within a system.

M. The stage of *moving* shifts the system to a new state of equilibrium.

N. The stage of *refreezing* integrates the changes into the system and formalizes changes with policies. Individuals integrate new changes into their value systems as positive additions (Sullivan & Decker, 1988). This is the hardwiring of change.

II. Change Theory

A. Kurt Lewin's force field theory (Lewin, 1942/1951) forms the basis for a model of systems' change and organizational development. Opposing forces are manipulated to direct and hardwire a new practice.

1. *Unfreezing stage:* Identify a system practice, attitude, value, pattern, or structure that is in conflict with the best practice.
    a. Research-based evidence, position papers, guidelines, and expert practices support or drive the change from current "status quo" practice.
    b. Identify the driving and the restraining forces within the system.

(1) Driving forces support change.
(2) Restraining forces resist change to maintain the status quo.

c. Offer alternatives to established practices from multidisciplinary resources.
(1) This allows a reduction in restraining forces and an increase in consensus to drive through multidisciplinary practice frameworks.

2. *Moving stage:* The change agent petitions participants from all disciplines to seek collective perspectives for the proposed change and helps others see the need or value of the proposed change.
   a. Multidisciplinary teamwork with institutional support is essential to bring a clear vision, goals, and plan for successful change.
   b. The plan for change is endorsed, operationalized, and measured for outcome throughout the moving process.
3. *Freezing (or refreezing) stage:* The new practice becomes the norm or standard of practice.
   a. Integrated standards for practice, protocols, order sets, policies, and procedures define the expected practice.

B. Lawrence Lippitt's phases of change (Lippitt, Watson, & Westley, 1958) expands Lewin's steps to guide team interaction.
1. Diagnose the problem.
   a. This involves data gathering.
   b. Identify key people to collect pertinent data.
2. Assess the motivation and capacity for change.
   a. Analyze the organization for resources and constraints.
3. Determine the agent's motivation and resources.
   a. Seek commitment to change, energy, and future.
   b. Determine whether the change agent can sustain the change process and bring it to completion.
4. Develop objectives, an action plan, evaluation criteria, and specific strategies.
   a. The formal process of implementing the change is developed with *institutional support.*
   b. The change agent coordinates the team through clear communication, supportive of all levels of the organization and its goals.
   c. The agent is willing to take risks, able to maintain relationships, and able to meet resistance and handle it effectively.
5. The change agent role is adapted to the needs of the team.
   a. This role may be cheerleader, expert, consultant, or group facilitator.
   b. All participants in the change process identify and accept the specific *function* of the change agent.
   c. The change agent is able to develop or organize educational programs focusing on all levels of the system and patient populations. The agent believes in continuous learning and adaptability (Crow, 1998).
6. Maintain the change.
   a. There is willingness to work with interdisciplinary teams to facilitate and maintain changes.
   b. The change agent does not need to maintain sole control of the change process. Empowerment of the staff is key for the change to be maintained.
   c. All participants in the change process accept the change and offer feedback for revisions.
   d. Communication lines remain open for discussion (White & Begun, 1998).
7. Believe in *empowerment of staff* so that changes can be maintained.
   a. Control of the change process passes into the hands of the participants (Sullivan & Decker, 1988).

C. Diffusion of innovations (Rogers, 1995) describes dynamic characteristics that individual team members bring to influence the likelihood of adaptation of change and the processes of how innovations become known and are spread throughout a social system.
1. Diffusion is the process by which an innovation is communicated through communication channels, over time, among the members of a social system.

2. An innovation is an idea perceived as new by an individual or an organization.
   a. Every new idea comes into society over time (months or years).
   b. An individual's cognitive style (Kirton, 2003) determines the likelihood of team problem solving.
      (1) Adaptors prefer to think within the confines of current practices and to know internal challenges. Adaptors provide transactional and evolutionary change, such as changing current patient records to produce better compliance to reassessment of pain.
      (2) Innovators prefer to think outside the confines of current practice and to use external solutions. Innovators provide transformational and revolutionary change, preferring to create a new idea, such as introducing a neuraxial analgesia protocol for joint replacement where it did not previously exist.
      (3) Both styles are necessary to introduce and sustain an innovation.
3. *Critical mass* is the point at which enough individuals have adopted the innovation to make it self-sustaining.
   a. Traditionally, 15% of a population constitutes a critical mass.
4. Some innovations diffuse more rapidly than others.
   a. New ideas must have
      (1) Relative advantage.
      (2) Compatibility with prior beliefs or values.
      (3) Perceived simplicity.
      (4) Positive trialability if they are to be a pilot project.
      (5) Positive observability.
      (6) Strategic priority within the organization.
   b. Cost and resources are reasonable.
   c. Risk is low.
   d. Legal ramifications are present to drive the innovation or are absent to decrease resistance.
5. Characteristics of adopters of innovation
   a. Innovators are the first 2.5% who come up with new ideas. They are venturesome.
   b. Early adopters are 13.5% of the population. They are the opinion leaders who tell others. They are most influential to the critical mass.
   c. Early majority is formed by 34% of the population. These individuals are the first half of the mass.
   d. Late majority is formed by 34% of the population. These individuals are the last half of the mass.
   e. Laggards may never adopt the new ideas.
6. Stages of the innovation decision process
   a. *Knowledge:* Innovation is introduced. The change agent presents an idea or identifies a need and introduces the idea of change into the system.
      (1) Research-based evidence, position papers, guidelines, and expert practices for pain management are important for this knowledge stage.
      (2) Use of mass media is important.
      (3) Educational courses meet predetermined knowledge deficits.
   b. *Persuasion:* Favorable or obstructive attitudes to the proposed change are formed.
      (1) Person-to-person discussion facilitates attitude adjustments toward a new idea.
   c. *Decision:* The choice is made to proceed with or cancel change.
      (1) The decision is made to try a new plan.
   d. *Implementation:* Innovation is put into use.
      (1) Alterations or revisions of the proposed change take place based on measurement outcomes.
   e. *Confirmation:* Reinforcement ensures that the decision was correct, or the decision may be reversed.
      (1) Conflicting attitudes obstruct change, the decision supporting the change may be reversed, or the change may be put on hold for a later date.

(2) Confirm whether the organization wants to go forward with this innovation.
(3) Confirm that adequate stakeholders are part of the team with clear measurable mutual objectives.

f. Rogers' theory (1995) focuses on the individual experiencing the change. It introduces the idea that the change that has been implemented is not permanent and may be reversed in the future.

D. The health belief model of change forms a basis for individual, group, or population motivation to change based on perceived risk.
   1. In the value-expectancy framework, the person takes specific actions with the belief that there is risk for continuing current behavior. Coaching strategies are based on the specific unhealthy activity and potential change.
      a. *The person is at significant risk to develop a disease:* Provide risk information based on the individual.
      b. *The disease is severe enough to have life-threatening outcomes if left untreated:* Identify specific consequences of the disease and specific steps for action.
      c. *Taking action will outweigh the risks:* Specify healthy actions, provide support, and emphasize potential healthy outcomes.
      d. *External cues provide impetus to act:* Provide reminders of healthy outcomes, and enlist support groups.
      e. *The person believes he or she has the capability to create the change (self-efficacy)* (Bandura, 1994): Incorporate objective setting, education, and effective learning strategies.
   2. *Example:* Ms. Jones experiences chronic pain from fibromyalgia. At first presentation, she does not participate in an exercise program, believing that it will increase her pain. She believes that her prescription opioid is the only modality to reduce her pain.
      a. Using the health belief model, apply the following strategies to initiate and maintain healthy behaviors:
         (1) Explore the barriers to Ms. Jones initiating exercise. Is she knowledgeable about exercise and fibromyalgia? Does she plan activity when she is least tired? Does she have problems sleeping?
         (2) Provide information about the benefits of exercise, discuss the Arthritis Foundation's fibromyalgia self-help course, and provide information on support groups. Discuss the value of prescriptions indicated for fibromyalgia and those that are not. Provide studies in which exercise and information resulted in significant reduction in pain.
         (3) Set mutual objectives where exercise, self-help, and support will begin. Emphasize success of healthy actions, and promote self-efficacy toward choices to further reduce pain and sleep disorder.
      b. After 3 months of coaching, ongoing exercise, and support group activities, Ms. Jones elects to begin a more strenuous exercise program to promote pain control.

E. The transtheoretical model of change (Prochaska & DiClemente, 1986) recognizes the complexity of behavioral change through defined stages, allowing for individual variation to relapse and progress toward healthy lifestyle maintenance with final termination from the initial behavior.
   1. Distinct stages allow strategically planned motivational interventions to modify cognitive learning, beliefs, and behavior for lifestyle change.
      a. *Precontemplation:* The person has no desire to change behavior within the next 6 months. The individual is resistant, lacking adequate knowledge or confidence. Techniques may include nonjudgmental individualized information regarding the consequences of continuing behavior to allow expression of the person's thoughts about the disease and the impact on family.
      b. *Contemplation:* The person expresses a desire to make a change within the next 6 months. This intent may not provoke action. Techniques to begin preparation may include reflection on the desire to change and the benefits of acting. Coping skills are evaluated.
      c. *Preparation:* The person plans to start the action or actions within 30 days. Reinforce initial steps and request continued verbal commitment to change.

d. *Action:* Specific actions have been taken within the last 6 months. Predetermined rewards for achieving healthy goals may reinforce actions.
e. *Maintenance:* The individual successfully maintains healthy lifestyle change.

2. *Example:* Mr. Smith reports that he has experienced lumbar pain for 10 years following 20 years as a construction worker. He tells you that "I've been to several doctors who haven't helped me. I think surgery or another medication will take my pain away." He spends most of his day on the couch. Use the transtheoretical model of change to promote healthy behavior and self-management.
   a. Consciousness-raising discussions relate to how inactivity negatively affects pain and quality of life while planned activity and rest with successive frequency in activity promote pain control.
   b. Mr. Smith returns and states, "Even if the pain doesn't totally go away, I need to change what I'm doing." Reinforce the benefits of beginning activity on quality of life while emphasizing coping skills (pros) and discussing the chronic pain and life quality without change (cons).
   c. He next says that he is planning to attend a YMCA arthritis pool program in the next month. Reinforce his decision; include family members to initiate action. Continue to point out the reduction in pain and quality of life as Mr. Smith continues to increase his exercise program and social activities.

F. The theory of reasoned action expands the individual's (behavioral) beliefs to include normative beliefs.
   1. The individual values the opinions of others, and willingness to conform is fostered by those opinions. These values may be therapeutically incorporated to influence the individual's intention and outcome.

III. Process of Change

A. Types of change
   1. A *planned change* is a change that is part of an institutional program of development.
      a. The Joint Commission, among other regulating organizations, provides guidelines for practice based on evidence from pain management experts, organizations, guidelines, and position statements that institutions are compelled to integrate into policy, protocol, and procedure and to demonstrate in practice.
      b. Recognizing these standards as basic tenets of professional practice, the institution's multidisciplinary staff is charged with identifying and trending measurable outcomes to determine and maintain best practices. The pain management nurse coaches the team in best practice.
   2. An *unplanned change* is a change that is driven by an identified need; unplanned changes are not part of the institutional plan but are identified as necessary, and resources are devoted to exploring means of facilitating change (Sullivan & Decker, 1988).
      a. The pain management nurse coaches the multidisciplinary team to identify systems issues using the processes of planned change to bring the organization to an improved quality of practice with improved system outcomes.

B. Levels of change
   1. *System or grassroots* change processes start from the bottom of the system upward. Those identifying the need for change develop and submit the proposal for change. Institutional support for the proposed change must be solicited.
      a. *Example:* The pain management nurse, critical care nurses, oncology nurses, and hospitalists identify that patients with cancer are often transferred to the intensive care unit at the end of life to provide extensive services when supportive services are identified that promote symptom management and quality of life for the patient and family.
      b. Comply with Joint Commission standards by taking the following actions:
         (1) Develop and maintain an interdisciplinary work plan. This facilitates bridge-building between departments, disciplines, and customers.
         (2) Analyze the current pain management practices in the care setting. Concentrate on systems barriers.

(3) Develop an inpatient and outpatient standard for documentation of pain intensity and pain relief that fosters development and regular review by staff from all areas.

2. *System or organizational* change occurs from the top down in an organization. Institutional commitment to change is guaranteed because the change originates at the higher level. Those lower down in the organization need to be convinced of the need for change (Galpin, 1996). As discussed earlier, changes may be supported or motivated by innovators, such as the pain management nurse, who incorporate external influences to introduce the change.
   a. *Example:* The administration sees the initiative as beneficial to the organization because it is good customer service and can reduce costs by optimizing services while respecting the wishes of the patient and family. The administration supports a process to start the pain and symptom management initiative systemwide.
3. *Individual* change occurs through the belief that there is risk to continue unhealthy or maladaptive behaviors. Change is managed through a progression of stages that provides a framework to plan interventions based on the person's readiness for action.
   a. Individual behavior is the integral factor in group and population behavior.

IV. Effecting Systems Change

A. Strategies for change (Benne & Chin, 1961)
   1. *Power (coercive):* Change is imposed by managers or governments (authority). Sanctions may exist.
   2. *Rational (empirical):* Staff is persuaded through communication and incentive that change is beneficial to their status.
   3. *Normative (reeducative):* The change agent provides education; has administrative support, resources, pilot areas, and clinical leaders who facilitate staff; and uses a "leader as servant" for empowering staff (Wright, 1996). Norms and values are redefined and reinterpreted to new ones.

B. Managing the change
   1. Identify the issue that requires change, the symptoms that are evident to indicate a need for change, and the barriers to begin a plan for change.
   2. Diagnose the problem. Review the symptoms, barriers, and opportunities. Gather additional data that are needed.
   3. Explore options and consider alternative measures. Evaluate risks and benefits, driving and restraining forces, advantages and disadvantages, and possible outcomes.
   4. Select a course of action and establish accountability for pain management.
      a. Develop policies for ongoing assessment of pain management practices and outcomes.
      b. Develop a resource team of specialists.
   5. Plan the change.
      a. Write the objectives.
      b. Determine a timetable.
      c. Plan a budget.
      d. Recruit personnel to help implement the change.
      e. Determine the ability of the change agent to work with the system.
      f. Assess driving and restraining forces.
      g. Develop an evaluation process for specific expected outcomes.
      h. Determine what is needed to refreeze the system after the change (Lewin, 1942/1951).
   6. Implement the change.
      a. Pilot the idea on a small scale.
      b. Provide information about pharmacological, nonpharmacological, and interventional modalities to facilitate writing, interpretation, and implementation of orders.
      c. Place medication suggestions and starting doses or dosage ranges on standing orders.
      d. Use the bill of rights, mission statement, and patient education tools to instruct patients to report their pain level before and after treatments, particularly in relation to their comfort goal and quality of life. Provide a reasonable goal of the type of response patients will receive.

e. Provide education to the staff. Cognitive skill is the beginning point toward psychomotor and affective learning. To improve outcomes, pain management assessment, planning, implementation, and evaluation have to be straightforward.
   (1) Revised documentation sheets should simplify documentation of pain intensity and mental status.

7. Evaluate the outcome. Listen to feedback from those affected by the change.
   a. Continually improve quality of pain management through process improvement (see the chapter on Quality Evaluation and Improvement).
8. Identify measures needed to refreeze the system.

C. Resistance to change
   1. *Threatened self-interest:* Personal costs are seen as greater than benefit. For example, when pain medication orders are questioned, a misdirected anger response may occur.
   2. Inaccurate perceptions are caused by rumors, incomplete information, and gossip. For example, the nurses in general surgery believe that short-acting opioids provided as needed postoperatively will suffice to relieve chronic or persistent pain.
   3. *Objective disagreement:* More informed members of staff believe change will not have the planned effect. For example, the nurses in the recovery room are observing that patients with local anesthetic in their epidural infusion are hypotensive and need to spend a longer time in the recovery room before their blood pressure stabilizes.
   4. *Psychological reactance:* Attempts are made to maintain previous behaviors because the behaviors are seen as too important to change. For example, a nurse-physician team has attempted to remove propoxyphene from the hospital formulary. This attempt has met resistance from members of the pharmacy and therapeutics committee and the medical staff despite evidence from several research-based expert resources.
   5. *Low tolerance for change:* There may be an inability to accept change emotionally ("if it's not broken, don't fix it") (Kozier & Erb, 1988).

D. Acceptance of change
   1. The closer the individual is to the change process, the easier it is for the change to be accepted.
   2. The change process
      a. Individual becomes aware of the change.
         (1) Through a quality improvement monitor, the nurses have an increased awareness of documentation of pain.
      b. The change agent gathers information.
         (1) The nursing staff forms a task force to identify ways to improve documentation.
      c. The change agent evaluates and relates information to current situation.
         (1) The task force reports its literature research results during a staff meeting. The report provides nurses with examples of how other institutions document pain rating.
         (2) The task force defines the goal: make pain documentation easy. The group sets a goal to improve documentation by 50%.
      d. The change agent mentally tries out the proposed change.
         (1) The nurse task force charts a process for improving pain rating documentation that includes education, mentoring, and sample sheets posted with demonstration samples.
      e. The change agent makes a trial of the proposed change.
         (1) The nurse task force redesigns the vital sign sheet to incorporate pain rating.
         (2) Permission is received to try this new documentation sheet for 2 months on one floor.
         (3) Nurses are educated on the use of this new form.
      f. The change is adopted and integrated (Rogers, 1995).
         (1) The new vital sign sheet that incorporates pain rating is monitored through quality improvement monitor sheets.
         (2) The results show 60% improvement in documentation of pain rating after 2-week trial.
         (3) Management decides to continue with routine monitoring and teaching until there is 90% improvement over the next 6 months.

E. Skills for the pain management nurse to be a successful change agent
   1. The nurse should be clinically competent in pain management practice and demonstrate a research-based practice.
   2. It is important to be aware of personal behaviors and attitudes. Reflect on actions and their effect on others, and be able to identify personal barriers to actualizing proposed change (Sullivan & Decker, 1988).
   3. Use creative and innovative thinking. Use entrepreneurship, have the high energy level needed to sustain change, possess an emotional commitment to the change and a willingness to try new methods to facilitate the change (White & Begun, 1998). Constantly stimulate new initiatives.
   4. Have the clarity of vision to see where the organization's idea of pain management can be developed effectively, and have an accurate understanding of organizational practice. Effectively translate the vision for use within the system's current model (Sullivan & Decker, 1988).
   5. Show strong clinical leadership skills, perceived by the system as able to facilitate the change. It is important to be well respected by peers and able to lead and sustain the change initiative. Identify the institutional paradigm and work within the system to change the paradigm, appear self-confident, and possess the ability of self-reflection (Crow, 1998).
   6. The nurse should have intact organizational relationships and excellent communication skills, be willing to take risks, be able to maintain relationships, and be able to meet resistance and handle it effectively. This helps with building a coalition of supporters (Skelton-Green, 1995).
   7. The nurse should be able to develop education programs and place continuing focus on educating all levels of the system and patient populations. Belief in continuous learning and adaptability is important (Crow, 1998).
   8. Willingness to work with interdisciplinary teams to facilitate and maintain changes is key. The nurse does not need to maintain sole control of change processes (White & Begun, 1998).
   9. Believe in empowerment of staff to foster and maintain change.

F. Methods for evaluating change
   1. Standardize clinical practice through the use of clinical order sets and guidelines or protocols.
   2. Develop clinical practice standards and the monitoring of compliance to written policy.
   3. Use pilot studies.
   4. Implement quality assurance measures.
   5. Use surveys and needs assessments.
   6. Incorporate focus groups.
   7. Undertake chart review (Barnason, Merboth, Pozehl, & Tietjen, 1998).
   8. Plan-do-study-act educational opportunities using specific system problems can be coupled with education. Reflection on the change follows the education, which gives power and credence to the proposed change (Berwick & Nolan, 1998).

G. Data collecting instruments include the following:
   1. *Nursing Knowledge and Attitudes Regarding Pain Management* (City of Hope, 2008).
   2. Nursing cognitive assessment of pain management (NCAPM) (Barnason et al., 1998).
   3. Chart review (McCaffery & Pasero, 1999).
   4. Quality assurance and teaching quality information audits (McCaffery & Pasero, 1999) (see the chapter on Quality Evaluation and Improvement).

V. Effecting Individual Behavioral Change

A. Evaluate the level of commitment to change—from precontemplation, to contemplation, to action and maintenance—formulating interventions based on the stage of commitment and desire for healthy behavior.

B. Apply specific interventions to produce self-awareness, intentional action to change, and continued motivation to sustain healthy behavior.

C. *Example:* Ms. Adams, a 42-year-old nurse, sustained a low back injury while lifting a 400-pound patient in the intensive care unit. She initially rested for 2 days using ice therapy and nonsteroidal antiinflammatory oral medication followed by physical therapy evaluation and conservative ultrasound therapy to reduce inflammation.

1. Her magnetic resonance imaging scan demonstrates bulging discs at L1 to L2 and L4 to L5 without herniation or extrusion, osteophyte formation, and desiccation of discs consistent with chronic degenerative disease. There is evidence on the magnetic resonance imaging scan of vertebral angulation consistent with muscle spasm.
2. On examination, she has increased paraspinal tone and tenderness to palpation in the lumbar region bilaterally.
3. Despite conservative treatment of rest and ice with nonsteroidal antiinflammatory drug treatment she is admitted for continued severe pain on activity, unable to ambulate.
4. She has not attended physical therapy, stating that "It just makes the pain worse" and that "I need something stronger to make the pain go away because nothing else works. Someone needs to make my pain better."
5. Conclusions
   a. The patient is exhibiting precontemplation to modify behavior in which she does not recognize the value of physical therapy or other modalities for pain relief other than medication. Your actions are as follows:
      (1) Convey compassion, and accumulate information about the patient's feelings regarding the injury and the effect on family and lifestyle.
      (2) Provide evidence regarding the basis of myofascial pain and activities or actions that provide effective treatment, such as physical therapy passive to active modalities.
      (3) Allow dramatic relief: Have other nurses who have successfully controlled pain while returning to work and social obligations dialogue their successes while recognizing the patient's current problems.
      (4) Discuss factors that require the patient's attention to avoid further injury and pain.
      (5) Allow the patient to review the pros and cons of motivation and readiness to act, that is, to pursue a multimodality plan to reduce pain.
   b. The patient exhibits contemplation of behavior change. Ms. Adams recognizes that she cannot prevent pain and further injury with medication alone. She acknowledges that she needs to involve herself in a multimodality treatment program.
      (1) Facilitate goal setting based on her pros and cons for change. Select one cognitive-behavioral intervention to test; use a pain relief diary to identify flares and reductions in pain related to activity.
      (2) Reinforce knowledge and attitudes to reduce cons, such as continued inactivity with medication alone does not sustain pain relief.
   c. The patient exhibits preparation toward behavior modification. Ms. Adams intends to act within 1 month.
      (1) Assist her to develop specific objectives, such as attend physical therapy three times a week; do daily home stretching exercises; and continue the daily diary keeping with biweekly review to establish a concrete plan for specific pain-reducing activities.
      (2) Assist her to reflect on specific self-generated barriers to change behavior. Provide evidence-based information regarding a modified-duty return-to-work program to reduce painful activity while healing and strengthen progresses.
   d. The patient exhibits action toward behavior modification. Change is implemented for less than 6 months.
      (1) Continue to motivate the patient based on successes that reduce pain and increase desired activities.
      (2) Continue to reflect on actions that deter desired or continued prevention of pain.
      (3) Continue to set desired social and personal objectives with rewards.
         (a) Plan a desired car trip vacation to another state, with strategic stops to visit valued areas with the intent to break up prolonged inactivity.

(b) Praise the patient for a sustained home exercise program and scheduled activities to reduce stress and fatigue.

e. The patient exhibits maintenance. The modified behavior is sustained for more than 6 months.
   (1) Reinforce activities that reduce physical and mental stressors for continued pain control.
   (2) Reinforce the belief that the patient is capable of the continued desire and performance toward lifestyle change.

References

Bandura, A. (1994). Self-efficacy. In V. S. Ramachaudran (Ed.), *Encyclopedia of human behavior* (Vol. 4, pp. 71–81). New York: Academic Press. (Reprinted in H. Friedman [Ed.], *Encyclopedia of mental health.* San Diego: Academic Press, 1998).

Barnason, S., Merboth, M., Pozehl, B., & Tietjen, M. J. (1998). Utilizing an outcomes approach to improve pain management by nurses: A pilot study. *Clinical Nurse Specialist, 12*(1), 28–36.

Benne, K. D., & Chin, R. (1961). General strategies for effecting change in human systems. In Bennis, W. G., Benne, K. D., & Chin, R. (Eds.), *The planning of change* (pp. 32–59). London: Holt, Rinehart, & Winston.

Bennis, W. G., Benne, K. D., & Chin, R. (Eds.). (1961). *The planning of change.* London: Holt, Rinehart, & Winston.

Berwick, D., & Nolan, T. (1998). Developing and testing changes in the delivery of care. *Annals of Internal Medicine, 128,* 651–656.

Blanchard, K., Carlos, J. P., & Randolph, A. (1996). *Empowerment takes more than a minute.* San Francisco: Berrett-Koehler.

City of Hope. (2008). *Nursing knowledge and attitudes regarding pain management.* Retrieved December 18, 2008, from http://www.cityofhope.org/Search/default.aspx?k=knowledge+and+attitudes+survey.

Crow, G. (1998). The entrepreneurial personality: Building a sustainable future for self and the profession. *Nursing Administration Quarterly, 22,* 30–35.

Galpin, T. J. (1996). *The human side of change.* San Francisco: Jossey-Bass.

Gilmartin, M. (1998). The nursing organization and the transformation of health care delivery for the 21st century. *Nursing Administration Quarterly, 22,* 70–86.

Kirton, M. J. (2003). *Adaption-innovation: In the context of diversity and change.* London: Routledge.

Kozier, B., & Erb, G. (1998). *The process of change: Concepts and issues in nursing practice.* Reading, MA: Addison-Wesley.

Lewin, K. (1942/1951). Field theory and learning. In D. Cartwright (Ed.), *Field theory in social science* (pp. 60–86). New York: Harper & Row.

Lippitt, R., Watson, J., & Westley, B. (1958). *The dynamics of planned change.* New York: Harcourt, Brace and World.

McCaffery, M., & Pasero, C. (1999). *Pain: A clinical manual.* St. Louis: Mosby.

Prochaska, J. O., & DiClemente, C. C. (1986). Towards a comprehensive model of change. In: Miller, W. R., & Heather, N. (Eds.), *Treating addictive behaviours: Processes of change.* New York: Plenum Press.

Rogers, E. M. (1995). Lessons for guidelines from the diffusion of innovations. *Joint Commission Journal on Quality Improvement, 21,* 324–328.

Skelton-Green, J. M. (1995). How a better understanding of change theory can help improve your practice as a nurse administrator. *Canadian Journal of Nursing Administration, 8,* 7–22.

Sullivan, E. J., & Decker, P. J. (1988). Managing and initiating change. In *Effective management in nursing* (2nd ed., pp. 93–119). Menlo Park, CA: Addison-Wesley.

White, K. R., & Begun, J. W. (1998). Nursing entrepreneurship in an era of chaos and complexity. *Journal of Nursing Administration, 22,* 40–47.

Wright, S. G. (1996). The need to develop nursing practice through innovation and practice change. *International Journal of Nursing Practice, 2,* 142–148.

Suggested Readings

Bridges, W. (1991). *Managing transitions: Making the most of change.* Reading, MA: Addison-Wesley.

Covey, S. (1994). *The interdependent reality in first things first.* New York: Simon & Schuster.

Hazzard, M. E. (1971). An overview of systems theory. *Nursing Clinics of North America, 6,* 385–393.

Kirton, M. J. (1989). A theory of cognitive style. In M. Kirton (Ed.), *Adaptors and innovators: Styles of creativity and problem solving* (pp. 1–33). London: Routledge.

Neuman, B. (1989). *The Neuman systems model.* Norwalk, CT: Appleton & Lange.

Siefert, M. (1990). Quality control. In J. C. McCloskey & H. K. Grace (Eds.), *Current issues in nursing* (3rd ed., pp. 234–248). Boston: Blackwell.

Sparacino, P. (1998). An outcomes approach to pain management. *Clinical Nurse Specialist, 12*(1), 27.

Sweeney, S. S., & Witt, K. E. (1990). Does nursing have the power to change the health care system? In J. C. McCloskey & H. K. Grace (Eds.), *Current issues in nursing* (3rd ed., pp. 283–297). Boston: Blackwell.

Tiffany, C. R. (1994). Analysis of planned change theories. *Nursing Management, 25,* 60–62.

Suggested Readings

Joint Commission. (2001). *Accreditation manual for hospitals.* Oakbrook Terrace, IL: Author..

Kanter, R. M. (1985). Innovation: The only hope for times ahead? *Nursing Economist, 3,* 178–182.

Kirton, M. J. (2006). *Adaption-innovation: In the context of diversity and change* (rev. ed.). London: Routledge.

chapter

28

Quality Evaluation and Improvement

Debra B. Gordon, RN-BC, MS, ACNS-BC, FAAN

Objectives

After studying this chapter, the reader should be able to:

1. List attributes of quality health care.
2. Define high-quality pain management and measures that can be used to evaluate it.
3. Discuss methods used to improve the quality of pain management.
4. Outline the American Society for Pain Management Nursing and the American Nurses Association's pain management nursing scope and standards of practice.
5. Describe the American Pain Society's recommendations for improving the quality of acute and cancer pain.

I. Definitions

A. Health care quality is generally defined in terms of the attributes and outcomes of care provided by practitioners and received by patients (Blumenthal, 1996a).

B. Donabedian (1968) defined quality health care as the kind of care that is expected to maximize an inclusive measure of patient welfare after taking account of the balance of expected gains and losses that accompany the process of care in all its parts.

C. The Institute of Medicine (IOM) defined quality health care in 1990 as "the degree to which health services for individuals and populations increase the likelihood of desired health outcomes and are consistent with current professional knowledge" (Lohr, 1990, p. 21).

   1. The Institute of Medicine revisited this statement in 1998, redefining the phrase "desired health outcomes" to specifically include the health outcomes that patients desire (Chassin & Galvin, 1998).
   2. Thus, patient satisfaction is a recommended measure in most evaluations of quality.

D. Terminology, measurement, and improvement approaches continue to evolve and become ever more complex.

E. The definition of quality depends on both the purpose of measurement and the perspective of the measurer. For example, in any given instance of health care delivery, the patient, the provider, and the insurer may have different perceptions of the quality of care.

II. Historical Influences on Quality (Luce, Bindman, & Lee, 1994)

A. Origin of quality debate

   1. More than 100 years ago, a surgeon, Ernest Codman, first proposed standardized outcomes data collection to determine whether care was effective (Codman, 1920).
   2. Codman's ideas convinced the American College of Surgeons to establish a Committee on the Standardization of Hospital Care. This ultimately led to the formation of the Joint Commission (Katz & Sangha, 1997).

B. Medicare and Medicaid affect quality assessment and management

   1. Medicare and Medicaid were established in the 1960s at a time accompanied by steep inflation in health care costs.
   2. To keep costs down and maintain quality, both public and private health insurers turned to the development of standards of care as the basis for better, and presumably more cost-effective (and defensible), coverage policies and quality measurement.
   3. Of particular interest was how care standards could be used as tools to shape policy, assess utilization of services, and define and identify inappropriate medical care (Kinney, 2001).
   4. To help address these needs and ensure delivery of health care in a manner consistent with available standards, accreditation programs such as the Joint Commission and the Commission on Accreditation of Rehabilitation Facilities (CARF) became prerequisites for participation in the Medicare program.
   5. Following the lead of these accreditation bodies, many third-party payers adopted quality assessment and management requirements linking strong economic incentives to the development of quality programs.

C. Recent influences

   1. Competition developed in the marketplace.
   2. The cost of health care continued to rise.
   3. The development of clinical epidemiology first identified wide variation in the practice and outcome of care among patients treated for the same health care problems in different places and health care settings (Blumenthal, 1996b).
   4. Awareness of practice variations led to the need to better understand their effect on outcomes.
   5. Outcomes research and new techniques have made it faster, cheaper, and easier to accumulate and analyze multiple types of data.
   6. Information technology, including the Internet, online health information, and the spread of computer technology to offices and homes, has provided consumers, payers, and health care

professionals with a wealth of information about available clinical choices and new opportunities to examine quality.

7. The application of outcomes research has resulted in new measures of quality to help improve clinical practice, especially in the treatment of chronic illnesses such as back pain, where improved function is a primary objective (Deyo et al., 1998; Malmivaara et al., 1995).

III. Attributes of Health Care Quality

A. If quality is to be managed, it must be defined in terms of specific measurable attributes (Kritchevsky & Simmons, 1991).
   1. Several formulations and approaches to the management of quality are possible and legitimate, depending on the circumstances and purposes involved.
   2. Donabedian (1992) defined six important attributes of health care quality (Table 28-1).
   3. The degree of attention given to any given attribute will vary depending on the aspect of quality being assessed.
      a. Technical quality consists of "doing the right thing right" (Blumenthal, 1996b, p. 892), that is, performing the right tests or providing the right services to accomplish the desired result.
      b. Attributes of the provider–patient interaction include communication, trust, empathy, sensitivity, and honesty.

B. The structure–process–outcome model, first developed by Donabedian (1968), is a useful framework for conceptualizing quality.
   1. According to this model, any examination of quality should include measurements in all three of these dimensions (Litwin, 2008).
      a. *Structure* is defined as the physical and organizational properties of the setting in which care is provided.
         (1) Examples include training, organizational resources, time allotted per patient, and staffing levels.
      b. *Process* is defined as what is done for patients.
         (1) Examples include clinical activities (e.g., test ordering, drug prescribing, and referral patterns), as well as interpersonal activities, such as teaching and other aspects of patient–provider communication.
         (2) Process measures are widely used by purchasers and Medicare peer review organizations to evaluate quality, create practice guidelines, and stimulate quality improvement (QI) activities.

Table 28-1 Attributes of Health Care Quality

Attribute	Definition
1. Effectiveness	The ability to attain the greatest improvements in health now achievable by the best care
2. Efficiency	The ability to lower the cost of care without diminishing attainable improvements in health
3. Optimality	The balancing of costs against the effects of care on health (or on the benefits of health care, meaning the monetary value of improvements in health) so as to attain the most advantageous balance
4. Acceptability	Conformity to the wishes, desires, and expectations of patients and responsible members of their families
5. Legitimacy	Conformity to social preferences as expressed in ethical principles, values, norms, laws, and regulations
6. Equity	Conformity to a principle that determines what is just or fair in the distribution of health care and of its benefits among the members of a population

From Donabedian, A. (1992). The role of outcomes in quality assessment and assurance. *Quality Review Bulletin, 18*(11), 356–360.

c. *Outcome* is defined as what is accomplished for patients.
   (1) It refers to the patient's health status (e.g., changes in pain, physical function, affect, and social roles) after treatment concludes.
   (2) Variables in pain management may include changes in pain intensity, frequency, and location; changes in the disease process causing pain; changes in physical function and quality of life (mobility, activities of daily living, and household or work tasks); and indicators of patient satisfaction.

C. It is widely recognized that health care is laden with quality problems related to underuse, overuse, and misuse of services (Berwick, Calkins, McCannon, & Hackbarth, 2006).

IV. Approaches to Improving Quality

A. Certification and accreditation
   1. *Certification* establishes that individual providers have the credentials and training necessary to deliver the care they provide.
   2. *Accreditation* produces summary information about a health system's processes, capabilities, and control over activities in the context of delivering high-quality care (Sennett, 1998).
   3. Both are obtained through comprehensive peer review processes that determine the nurse's ability to meet standards of care developed by the particular field.
   4. Certification and accreditation review processes are thought to stimulate QI through education and the development of new or improved structures, processes, and assessment.
   5. The most notable pain management accreditation standards are the Joint Commission pain assessment and management standards developed in 1999 (Joint Commission, 2008).
      a. Recognize the right of patients to appropriate assessment and management of pain (Standard R1.2.10).
      b. Assess pain in all patients (Standard PC.8.10).
      c. Record the assessment in a way that facilitates regular reassessment and follow-up.
      d. Educate patients, families, and providers (Standard PC.6.10).
      e. Establish policies that support appropriate prescription or ordering of (pain) medicines (Standard MM3.20).
      f. Collect data to monitor the appropriateness and effectiveness of pain management (Standard P1.1.10).

B. Quality assurance
   1. Quality assurance (QA) is a broad-based form of audit and feedback in which outcomes such as percentages of satisfied patients, referral rates, or adverse events are used for comparison by administrative authorities.
   2. Standards of care are used as yardsticks, with a focus on reducing provider errors in the care of individual patients.
   3. The conventional QA paradigm popular in the 1970s and 1980s focused on identifying adverse outcomes and censuring responsible parties.
   4. A major limitation of QA is that feedback comes too late in the process and does little to explain differences in practice or outcomes.
   5. A primary source of QA review data is medical records that are notoriously incomplete and are often missing information important in evaluating the quality of pain management (Solomon et al., 2000).
   6. In 1990, Mitchell Max, then chairman of the American Pain Society's (APS) Quality of Care Committee, suggested that the traditional formula of education and QA was insufficient to improve pain management and treatment outcomes (Max, 1990).

C. Quality improvement
   1. QI is the broader and more comprehensive evolutionary descendant of QA focused on systems improvement.
   2. It has been used for years in the manufacturing industry.

3. QI focuses on reducing variation in a production process, standardization, and continuous improvement in outcomes rather than on the identification and elimination of defects.
4. QI theory states that data can be collected to help understand a system's processes and uncover the root causes of any inconsistencies or variations that contribute to quality problems.
   a. A system is a group of related processes or a sequence of tasks necessary to achieve a particular outcome.
   b. Organizations are systems designed to serve customers (patients).
   c. Unlike QA, there is no predetermined or final yardstick of quality; instead, the goal is continuous improvement.
5. QI is a compilation of methods adapted from psychology, statistics, and operations research to avert predictable human errors, eliminate unnecessary and harmful variations in practice, and improve the production of goods and services (Blumenthal, 1993).
6. QI depends on the development and implementation of care standards in the health care environment and the generation of data for performance measurement.
   a. To make care consistent and to reduce statistical errors, data must be generated and compared against an established standard (Kinney, 2001).
   b. The use of data to track trends has been shown to be a critical factor in successful hospital-based QI initiatives (Bradley et al., 2001).
7. QI involves enlisting an entire organization to work toward a goal of continuous improvement in quality by carefully studying the process one is attempting to improve and changes the responsibilities and power of frontline workers (Kritchevsky & Simmons, 1991; Nelson et al., 2000).
8. Numerous approaches to QI exist, such as those that follow, but the general principles are similar:
   a. Deming (Walton, 1986)
   b. Juran (1994)
   c. Six Sigma (Black & Revere, 2006)
   d. Lean thinking (Toyota) (Kim, Spahlinger, Kin, & Billi, 2006)
9. Various tools are used in QI to help outline a process, including flowcharts, workflow diagrams, deployment charts, Pareto charts, and Ishikawa or fishbone (cause and effect) diagrams (Fig. 28-1).

D. Clinical practice guidelines and evidence-based practice (Dijkstra et al., 2006)
1. Guidelines are systematically developed statements based on evidence designed to help practitioners and patients make appropriate health care decisions for specific clinical conditions.
2. In a randomized, controlled trial of community-based oncology clinics, implementation of pain management practice guidelines has been shown to enhance patient outcomes (Du Pen et al., 1999).
3. Limited evidence exists on the most effective approach to guideline dissemination and implementation (Grimshaw et al., 2004).

E. Public accountability (performance indicators)
1. Performance measures are rate based and reported as fractions or percentages of a total number of eligible events.
   a. For example, of all health plan members carrying a diagnosis of arthritis, how many are screened regularly for the presence of pain?
2. These measures are used to facilitate QI activities, as well as for purposes of external accountability and public reporting.
3. Health care purchasers use accountability measures, or performance indicators, to compare services.
4. Performance indicators should measure variations and improvements in performance and reflect the concerns of patients, providers, regulators, accreditation bodies, and other stakeholders (Joint Commission & National Pharmaceutical Council, 2003).
5. Performance indicators are reported back to the health care purchaser or consumer and can be powerful drivers of health care choice.
   a. The theory is that comparing performance among health care systems will create a market demand for the systems with the best performance scores.

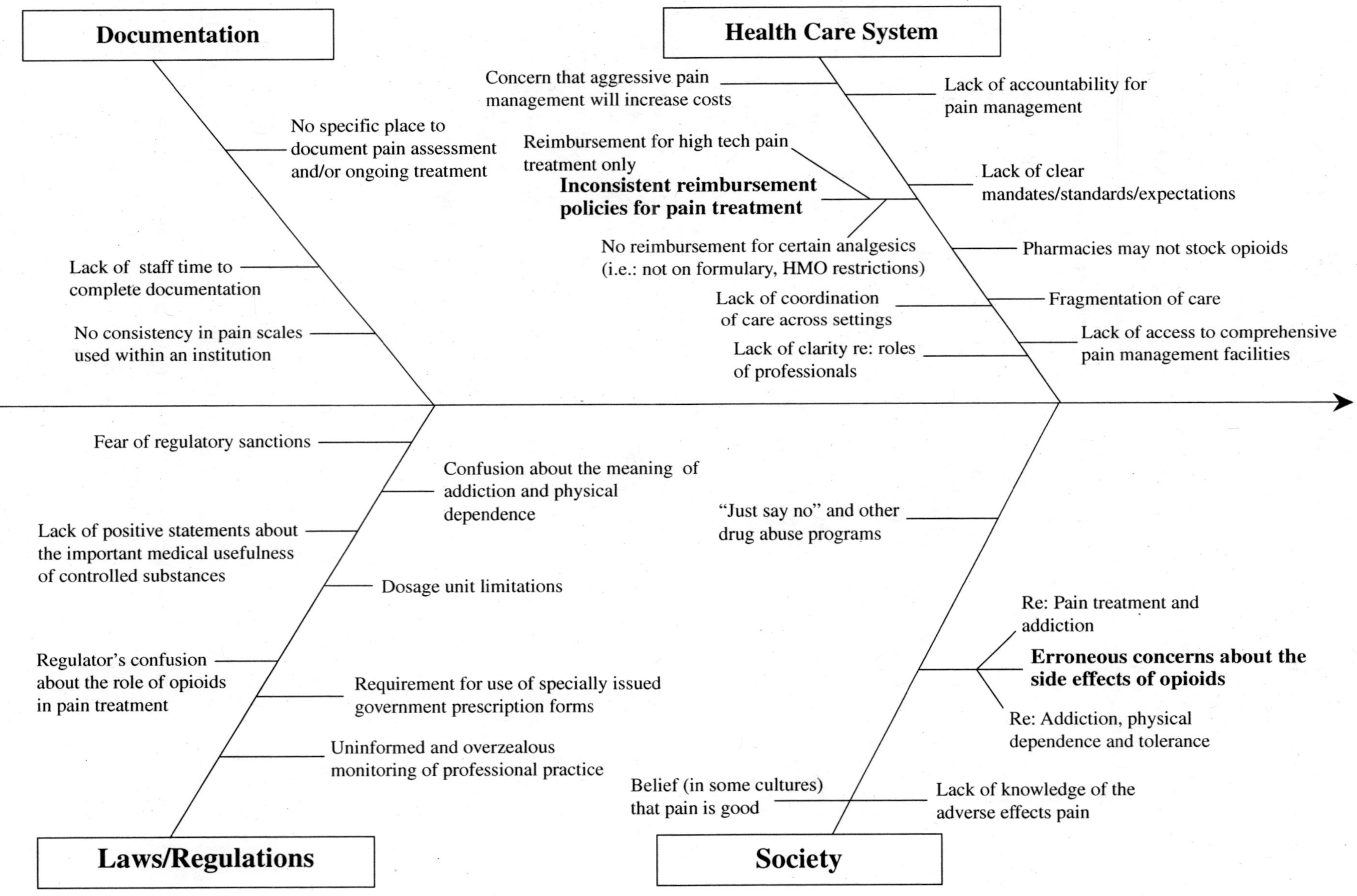

Documentation
No specific place to document pain assessment and/or ongoing treatment
Lack of staff time to complete documentation
No consistency in pain scales used within an institution
Health Care System
Concern that aggressive pain management will increase costs
Lack of accountability for pain management
Reimbursement for high tech pain treatment only
Inconsistent reimbursement policies for pain treatment
No reimbursement for certain analgesics (i.e.: not on formulary, HMO restrictions)
Lack of clear mandates/standards/expectations
Pharmacies may not stock opioids
Lack of coordination of care across settings
Fragmentation of care
Lack of clarity re: roles of professionals
Lack of access to comprehensive pain management facilities
Fear of regulatory sanctions
Confusion about the meaning of addiction and physical dependence
Lack of positive statements about the important medical usefulness of controlled substances
Dosage unit limitations
Regulator's confusion about the role of opioids in pain treatment
Requirement for use of specially issued government prescription forms
Uninformed and overzealous monitoring of professional practice
Laws/Regulations
"Just say no" and other drug abuse programs
Re: Pain treatment and addiction
Erroneous concerns about the side effects of opioids
Re: Addiction, physical dependence and tolerance
Belief (in some cultures) that pain is good
Lack of knowledge of the adverse effects pain
Society

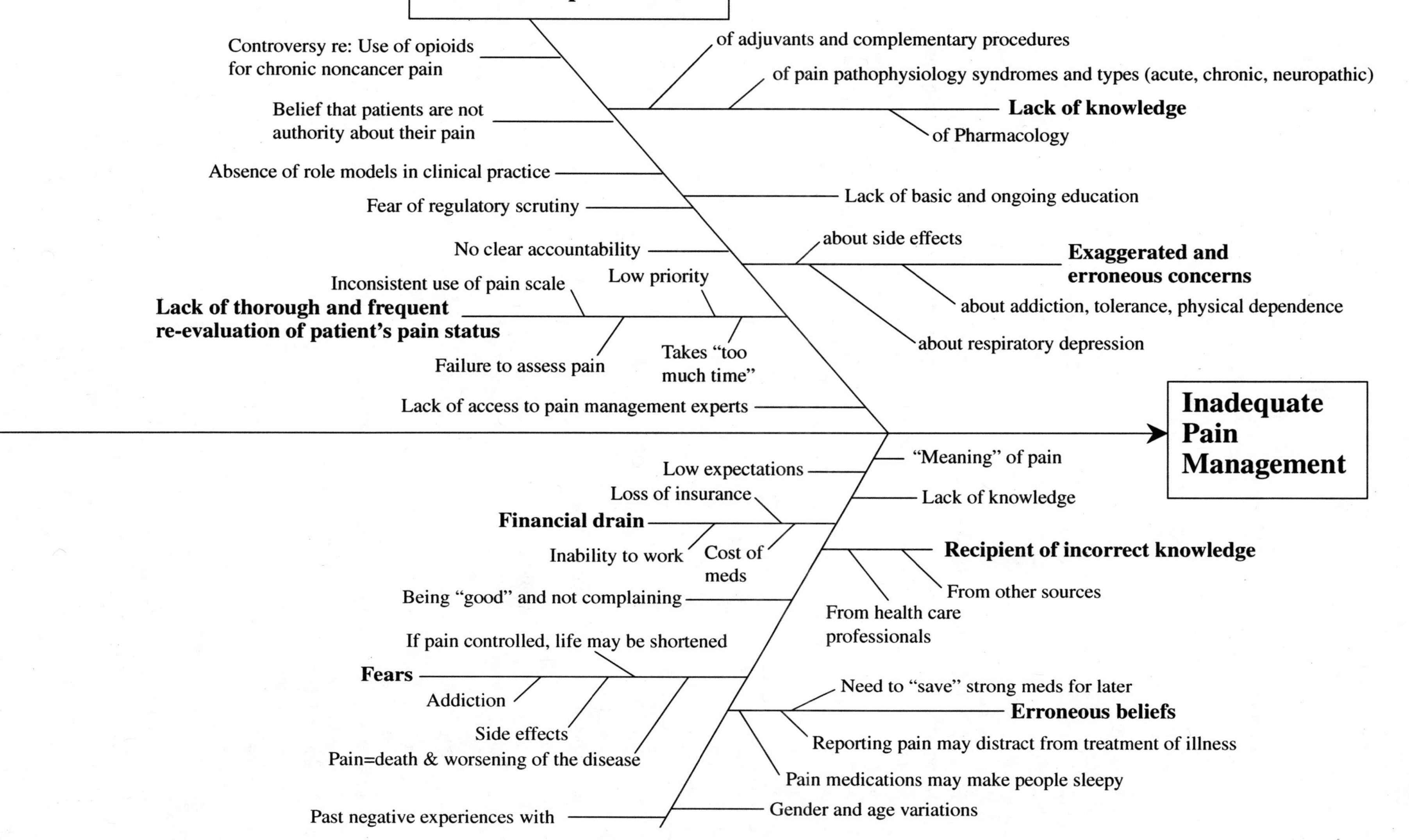

Figure 28-1 | Barriers to adequate pain management: an Ishikawa (fishbone) diagram. HMO, health maintenance organization.

From *Building an Institutional Commitment to Pain Management*, 2nd edition. Reprinted by permission of Outreach Program Manager.

b. This creates competition in the marketplace, which ostensibly leads to improvements in health care quality and service.
6. Several leaders in the development of broad-based national performance data sets include
   a. National Committee on Quality Assurance (NCQA).
   b. Foundation for Accountability (FACCT).
   c. Commission on Accreditation of Rehabilitation Facilities. (CARF)
   d. Joint Commission.
   e. National Quality Forum (NQF).

V. American Nurses Association (ANA) Nursing-sensitive Quality Indicators for Acute Care Settings (Alexander, 2007; Kurtzman & Corrigan, 2007)

A. Quality indicators were launched by the American Nurses Association (ANA) in 1994 as a multiphase initiative to investigate the impact of health care restructuring on the safety and quality of patient care, as well as on nursing (ANA, 2008).
B. ANA's safety and quality initiative
   1. Focuses on educating registered nurses about quality measurement.
   2. Informs the public and purchasing and regulating constituencies about safe, quality health care.
   3. Investigates research methods and data sources to evaluate safety and quality patient care.
C. The initiative led to identification and definition of 10 nursing-sensitive quality indicators and the National Database of Nursing-Sensitive Quality Indicators (NDNQI) in 1998. These indicators are as follows:
   1. A mix of registered nurses, licensed practical nurses, and unlicensed staff caring for patients in acute care settings
   2. Total nursing care hours provided per patient day
   3. Pressure ulcers
   4. Patient falls
   5. Patient satisfaction with pain management
      a. A persistent paradoxical finding in hospital pain QI studies has been that, despite high pain intensity ratings, most patients surveyed report extremely high satisfaction ratings (Gordon et al., 2002).
      b. The Institute of Medicine recommends including consumer satisfaction indices in any evaluation of quality.
      c. Patient satisfaction with pain management may be more representative of the quality of the interpersonal relationship between patient and caregiver than of the quality of the actual services or their outcomes.
      d. When evaluating the quality of pain management, questions about the adequacy of pain-related information provided to patients or their ability to participate in decisions about care may provide a better measure than general patient satisfaction questions.
   6. Patient satisfaction with educational information
   7. Patient satisfaction with overall care
   8. Patient satisfaction with nursing care
   9. Nosocomial infections
   10. Nurse staff satisfaction

VI. ANA and the American Society for Pain Management Nursing (2005) Scope and Standards of Practice

A. Standards of pain management nursing practice
   1. Standard I, Assessment: collects comprehensive data pertinent to the pain problem.
   2. Standard II, Diagnosis: analyzes the assessment data to determine pain diagnoses or problems.
   3. Standard III, Outcomes Identification: identifies expected pain management outcomes for a plan individualized to the patient with pain.
   4. Standard IV, Planning: develops a pain management plan that prescribes strategies and alternatives to attain expected outcomes.

5. Standard V, Implementation: implements the identified pain management plan.
    a. Standard 5a Coordinates the pain management plan.
    b. Standard 5b Employs strategies to promote, maintain, and restore pain-relieving behaviors (health teaching and promotion).
    c. Standard 5c The advanced practice registered nurse should provide consultation to influence the identified pain management plan, enhance the abilities of others, and effect change.
    d. Standard 5d The advanced practice registered nurse use prescriptive authority, procedures, referrals, treatments, and therapies in accordance with state and federal laws and regulations.
6. Standard VI, Evaluation: evaluates progress toward attainment of acceptable pain management outcomes.

B. Standards of professional performance
1. Standard VII, Quality of practice: systematically evaluates the quality and effectiveness of pain management practice.
2. Standard VIII, Education: attains knowledge and competency that reflects current pain management nursing practice.
3. Standard IX, Professional practice evaluation: evaluates a nursing practice in relation to professional pain practice standards and guidelines, relevant statues, rules, and regulations.
4. Standard X, Collegiality: interacts with and contributes to the professional development of peers and colleagues.
5. Standard XI, Collaboration: collaborates with the patient, family, and others in the conduct of pain management practice.
6. Standard XII, Ethics: integrates ethical provisions to guide pain management practices.
    a. This standard uses the ANA *Code of Ethics for Nurses with Interpretive Statements* (ANA, 2001).
    b. It protects patient confidentiality, autonomy, dignity, and rights.
7. Standard XIII, Research: integrates pain research findings into clinical practice.
8. Standard XIV, Resource utilization: considers factors related to safety, effectiveness, cost, and impact on practice in the planning and delivery of pain management.
9. Standard XV, Leadership: provides leadership in professional pain management.

VII. APS Quality Improvement Guidelines (Gordon et al., 2005)

A. High-quality pain management includes elements of structure, process, and outcome.
1. Appropriate assessment includes screening for the presence of pain, completion of a comprehensive initial assessment when pain is present, and frequent reassessments of patient responses to treatment.
2. Interdisciplinary, collaborative care planning includes patient input.
3. Appropriate treatment is efficacious, cost-conscious, culturally and developmentally appropriate, and safe.
4. Access to specialty care is provided as needed.

B. Factors complicating the discussion of quality pain management
1. The quality of pain treatment is difficult to define or measure partly because pain is highly subjective and hence difficult to reproducibly quantify.
2. The experience of pain is intertwined with its emotional impact (suffering), which is even more difficult to quantify and compare among individuals.

C. APS QI guidelines were first developed as QA standards in 1991 (Max, 1991) as a response to failure of traditional educational approaches to improve quality.

D. They were followed by QI guidelines in 1995 for acute and cancer pain recognizing the promise of QI in health care (APS Quality of Care Committee, 1995).

E. The guidelines were updated in 2005 to move beyond mere assessment and communication of pain to implementation and evaluation of improvements in pain treatment that are timely, safe, evidence based, and multimodal.

Table 28-2 Key Structural Elements of a Quality Improvement Approach to Pain

1. An interdisciplinary workgroup
2. Analysis of current pain management practices in the care setting
3. A written standard of practice for pain assessment and documentation
4. Explicit policies and procedures to guide the use of specialized techniques for analgesic administration
5. Clearly defined accountability for pain management
6. Information about pharmacological and nonpharmacological interventions for clinicians to facilitate order writing and interpretation and implementation of orders
7. Patient and family education programs and materials
8. Orientation and continuing education opportunities for staff
9. An ongoing process that evaluates the outcomes and works to improve the quality of pain management

F. Each institution is encouraged to develop an interdisciplinary QI team and use a structured approach (Table 28-2) to assess guideline implementation.

G. The APS QI guidelines emphasize five key elements to improve pain management as a starting point for institutional responsibility (Table 28-3).

1. Recognize and treat pain promptly.
   a. Avoid focusing on unidimensional aspects of pain such as simple pain intensity ratings to the detriment of patient safety.
   b. Move beyond simple screening and pain intensity ratings to comprehensive assessment appropriate to population and setting.
   c. Treatment needs to be more timely, more proactive, more preemptive, and more multimodal.
2. Involve patients in the pain management plan.
   a. Promote collaborative, shared decision making with patients.
   b. Patients need to know more than how to report pain and that pain management is a "right." They need to know pain control options, how to use them, and what their responsibilities are for participation in pain management.
   c. Treatment and goals should be customized to individual needs, desires, and circumstances.
3. Improve treatment patterns.
   a. Move from old routines, such as from as-needed dosing only to more preemptive, around-the-clock scheduled dosing when appropriate.
   b. For a most situations, use a multimodal approach that includes rational combinations of analgesics (with differing mechanisms of actions), along with nonpharmacological interventions.
   c. Ensure treatments are safe.
   d. Implement evidence-based advancements for regimens that are sensitive to the type of pain and treatment setting.
4. Reassess and adjust the pain management plan as needed.
   a. Establish realistic goals that focus not only on pain relief but also improve (or maintain) function and quality of life for both acute and chronic pain.
   b. Consider the burden of treatment on quality of life and resources.
5. Monitor processes and outcomes of pain management.
   a. Use questions to frame QI evaluations.
      (1) Why do we do what we do?
      (2) How do we know it works?
      (3) How can we do it better?
   b. Where possible, use standardized measures that have validity and reliability.

Table 28-3 Comparison of 1995 and 2005 American Pain Society (APS) Quality Improvement (QI) Guidelines for the Treatment of Acute and Cancer Pain

1995 APS QI Guidelines	2005 Updated and Expanded Recommendations
1. Recognize and treat pain promptly (emphasis on routine assessment and documentation of pain intensity).	1. Recognize and treat pain promptly (emphasis on comprehensive assessment and importance of preventive and prompt treatment based on evidence for neuroplasticity).
2. Make information about analgesics readily available.	2. Involve patients in the pain management plan (emphasis on customization of care and participation of patient in treatment plan).
3. Promise patients attentive analgesic care (emphasis on urging patients to report pain).	3. Improve treatment patterns (least evidence but most important new recommendation).
4. Define explicit policies for use of analgesic technologies.	4. Reassess and adjust pain management plan as needed (respond not only to pain intensity but also to functional status and side effects).
5. Examine the process and outcomes of pain management with the goal of continuous improvement.	5. Monitor processes and outcomes of pain management (new standardized QI indicators and comments about forthcoming national performance indicators).

c. A meta-analysis of 20 pain QI studies (Gordon et al., 2002) performed at eight large U.S. hospitals that used the APS QI guidelines led to six revised quality indicators for hospital-based pain management.
   (1) The intensity of pain is documented with a numerical (e.g., 0 to 10 or 0 to 5) or descriptive (e.g., mild–moderate–severe) rating scale.
   (2) Pain intensity is documented at frequent intervals.
   (3) Pain is treated by a route other than intramuscular.
   (4) Pain is treated with regularly administered analgesics, and when possible a multimodal approach is used (e.g., combinations of regional or local techniques, with nonopioid, opioid, adjuvant analgesics, and nonpharmacological methods).
   (5) Pain is prevented and controlled to a degree that facilitates function and quality of life.
   (6) Patients are adequately informed and knowledgeable about pain management.

H. Implementation of APS QI guidelines has been noted to result in improvements in
   1. Assessment of pain (Arbour, 2003; Duggleby & Alden, 1998; Erdek & Pronovost, 2004; Gordon et al., 2008; Rittenmeyer, Dolezal, & Vogel, 1997)
   2. Prescribing practices (Berger, Messenger, & Roth, 1999; Gordon, Jones, Goshman, Foley, & Bland, 2000; Illgen, Pellino, Gordon, Butts, & Heiner, 2006; Sayers et al., 2000)
   3. Patient outcomes (Cleeland et al., 2003; Fortner et al., 2003; Holzheimer, McMillan, & Weitzner, 1999; Oakes, Anghelescu, Windsor, & Barnhill, 2008).

Summary

Nurses play a critical role in advancing the quality of care and science of systems improvement. As we move forward in pain management nursing, it is more important than ever that we follow the Institute of Medicine's guiding principles for health care reform: knowledge-based, patient-centered, and system-minded care.

References

Alexander, G. R. (2007). Nursing sensitive databases: Their existence, challenges, and importance. *Medical Care Research and Review, 64*(2), 44S–63S.

American Nurses Association. (2001). *Code of ethics for nurses with interpretive statements.* Washington, DC: American Nurses Publishing.

American Nurses Association. (2008). *National Database of Nursing Quality Indicators (NDNQI).* Retrieved October 29, 2008, from http://www.nursingworld.org/MainMenuCategories/ThePracticeofProfessionalNursing/PatientSafety-Quality/NDNQI/NDNQI_1.aspx.

American Pain Society Quality of Care Committee. (1995). Quality improvement guidelines for the treatment of acute pain and cancer pain. *Journal of the American Medical Association, 274,* 1874–1880.

American Nurses Association & American Society for Pain Management Nursing. (2005). *Pain management nursing scope & standards of practice.* Silver Spring, MD: ANA nursesbooks.org.

Arbour, R. (2003). A continuous quality improvement approach to improving clinical practice in the areas of sedation, analgesia, and neuromuscular blockade. *Journal of Continuing Education in Nursing, 34*(2), 64–71, 90–91.

Berger, D., Messenger, F., & Roth, S. (1999). Self-administered medication packet for patients experiencing vaginal birth. *Journal of Nursing Care Quality, 13*(4), 47–59.

Berwick, D. M., Calkins, D. R., McCannon, C. J., & Hackbarth, A. D. (2006). The 100 000 lives campaign; Setting a goal and a deadline for improving health care quality. *Journal of the American Medical Association, 295*(3), 324–327.

Black, K., & Revere, L. (2006). Six Sigma arises from the ashes of TQM with a twist. *International Journal of Health Care Quality Assurance, 19*(3), 259–266.

Blumenthal, D. (1993). Total quality management and physicians' clinical decisions. *Journal of the American Medical Association, 269,* 2775–2778.

Blumenthal, D. (1996a). The origins of the quality-of-care debate, part 4. *New England Journal of Medicine, 335,* 1146–1148.

Blumenthal, D. (1996b). Quality of health care. I. What is it? *New England Journal of Medicine, 335*(12), 891–893.

Bradley, E. H., Holmboe, E. S., Mattera, J. A., Roumanis, S.A., Radford, M.J., & Krumholz, H.M., et al. (2001). A qualitative study of increasing β-blocker use after myocardial infarction. Why do some hospitals succeed? *Journal of the American Medical Association, 285,* 2604–2611.

Chassin, M. R., & Galvin, R. W. (1998). National roundtable on health care quality: The urgent need to improve health care quality. *Journal of the American Medical Association, 280,* 1000–1005.

Cleeland, C. S., Reyes-Gibby, C. C., Schall, M., Nolan, K., Paice, J., Rosenberg, J. M., Tollett, J. H., & Kerns, R. D. (2003). Rapid improvement in pain management: The Veterans Health Administration and the Institute for Healthcare Improvement collaborative. *Clinical Journal of Pain, 19*(5), 298–305.

Codman, E. (1920). *A study in hospital efficiency.* Boston: Thomas Todd.

Deyo, R., Battie, M., Beurskens, A. J., Bombardier, C., Croft, P., Koes, B., Malmivaara, A., Roland, M., VonKorff, M., & Waddell, G. (1998). Outcome measures for low back pain research: A proposal for standardized use. *Spine, 23*(18), 2002–2013.

Dijkstra, R., Wensing, M., Thomas, R., Reiner, A., Braspenning, J., & Grinshaw, J. (2006). The relationship between organisational characteristics and the effects of clinical guidelines on medical performance in hospitals, a meta-analysis. *BMC Health Services Research, 6*(53), 1–10.

Donabedian A. (1992). The role of outcomes in quality assessment and assurance. *Quality Review Bulletin, 18*(11), 356-360.

Donabedian, A. (1968). Promoting quality through evaluation of the process of patient care. *Medical Care, 6,* 181–202.

Donabedian, A. (1980). *Explorations in quality assessment and monitoring: Vol. 1. The definition of quality and approaches to its assessment.* Ann Arbor, MI: Health Administration Press.

Duggleby, W., & Alden, C. (1998). Implementation and evaluation of a quality improvement process to improve pain management in a hospice setting. *American Journal of Hospice and Palliative Care, 15*(4), 209–216.

Du Pen, S. L., Du Pen, A. R., Polissar, N., Hansberry, J., Kraybill, B.M., Stillman, M., Panke, J., Everly, R., & Syrjala, K. (1999). Implementing guidelines for cancer pain management: Results of a randomized controlled trial. *Journal of Clinical Oncology, 17*(1), 361–370.

Erdek, M. A., & Pronovost, P. J. (2004). Improving assessment and treatment in the critically ill. *International Journal on Quality Health Care, 16*(1), 59–64.

Fortner, B. V., Okon, T. A., Ashley, J., Kepler, G., Chavez, J., Tauer, K., Clements-Thompson, M., Schwartzberg, L., Demarco, G., & Houtse, A. C. (2003). The zero acceptance of pain (ZAP) quality improvement project: Evaluation of pain severity, pain interference, global quality of life, and pain-related costs. *Journal of Pain & Symptom Management, 25*(4), 334–343.

Gordon, D. B., Dahl, J. L., Miaskowski, C., et al. (2005). American Pain Society recommendations for improving the quality of acute and cancer pain management. *Archive of Internal Medicine, 165,* 1574–1580.

Gordon, D. B., Jones, H. D., Goshman, L. M., Foley, D. K., & Bland, S. E. (2000). A quality improvement approach to reducing the use of meperidine. *Joint Commission Journal on Quality Improvement, 26*(12), 686–699.

Gordon, D. B., Pellino, T. A., Miaskowski, C., McNeill, J.A., Paice, J.A., Laferriere, D., & Bookbinder, M. (2002). A ten-year review of quality improvement monitoring in pain management and recommendations for standardized measures. *Pain Management Nursing, 3*(4), 116–130.

Gordon, D. B., Rees, S. M., McCausland, M. P., Pellino, T.A., Sanford-Ring, S., Smith-Helmenstine, J., & Danis, D.M. (2008). Improving reassessment and documentation of pain management. *Joint Commission Journal on Quality and Patient Safety, 34*(9), 509–517.

Grimshaw, J. M., Thomas, R. E., MacLennan, G., Fraser, C., Ramsay, C., Vale, R., Whitty, P., & Hutchinson, A.et al. (2004). Effectiveness and efficiency of guideline dissemination and implementation strategies. *Health Technology Assessment, 8*(6), iii–iv, 1–72.

Holzheimer, A., McMillan, S. C., & Weitzner, M. (1999). Improving pain outcomes of hospice patients with cancer. *Oncology Nursing Forum, 26*(9), 1499–1504.

Illgen, R., Pellino, T. A., Gordon, D. B., Butts, S., & Heiner, J. P. (2006). Prospective analysis of a novel long-acting oral opioid analgesic regimen for pain control after total hip and knee replacement. *Journal of Arthroplasty, 21*(6), 814–820.

Joint Commission. (2008). *Accreditation manual for hospitals.* Oakbrook Terrace, IL: Author.

Joint Commission & National Pharmaceutical Council. (2003). *Improving the quality of pain management through measurement and action.* Oakbrook Terrace, IL: Joint Commission Resources.

Juran, D. (1994). Achieving sustained quantifiable results in an interdepartmental quality improvement project. *Joint Commission Journal on Quality Improvement, 20*(3), 105–119.

Katz, J. N., & Sangha, O. (1997). Assessment of the quality of care. *Arthritis Care and Research, 10*(6), 359–369.

Kim, C. S., Spahlinger, D. A., Kin, J. M., & Billi, J. E. (2006). Lean health care: What can hospitals learn from a world-class automaker? *Journal of Hospital Medicine, 1*(3), 191–199.

Kinney, E. D. (2001). The brave new world of medical standards of care. *Journal of Law, Medicine & Ethics, 29,* 323–334.

Kritchevsky, S. B., & Simmons, B. P. (1991). Continuous quality improvement: Concepts and applications for physician care. *Journal of the American Medical Association, 261,* 1817–1823.

Kurtzman, E. T., & Corrigan, J. M. (2007). Measuring the contribution of nursing to quality, patient safety, and health care outcomes. *Policy, Politics & Nursing Practice, 8*(1), 20–36.

Litwin, M. S. (2008). Health services research. *Seminars in Radiation Oncology, 18,* 152–160.

Lohr, K. N. (1990). *Medicare: A strategy for quality assurance.* Washington, DC: National Academy Press.

Luce, L. M., Bindman, A. B., & Lee, P. R. (1994). A brief history of health care quality assessment and improvement in the United States. *Western Journal of Medicine, 160,* 263–268.

Malmivaara, A., Hakkinen, U., Aro, T., et al. (1995). The treatment of acute low back pain: Bedrest, exercises, or ordinary activity? *New England Journal of Medicine, 332*(6), 351–335.

Max, M. (1991). American Pain Society quality assurance standards for relief of acute pain and cancer pain. In M. R. Bond, J. E. Charlton, & C. J. Woolf (Eds.), *Proceedings of the 6th World Congress on Pain.* Amsterdam: Elsevier Science.

Max, M. B. (1990). Improving outcomes of analgesic treatment: Is education enough? *Annals of Internal Medicine, 11*(1), 885–889.

Nelson, E. C., Splaine, M. E., Godfrey, M. M., Kahn, V., Hess, A. M., Batalden, P., & Plume, S. K. (2000). Using data to improve medical practice by measuring process and outcomes of care. *Joint Commission Journal on Quality Improvement, 26*(12), 667–685.

Oakes, L. L., Anghelescu, D. L., Windsor, K. B., & Barnhill, P. D. (2008). An institutional quality improvement initiative for pain management for pediatric cancer inpatients. *Journal of Pain & Symptom Management, 35*(6), 656–669.

Rittenmeyer, H., Dolezal, D., & Vogel, E. (1997). Pain management: A quality improvement project. *Journal of PeriAnesthesia Nursing, 12*(5), 329–335.

Sayers, M., Maradno, R., Fisher, S., Aquila, A., Morrison, B., & Dailey, T. (2000). No need for pain. *Journal of Healthcare Quality, 22*(3), 10–15.

Sennett, C. (1998). An introduction to the National Committee for Quality Assurance. *Pediatric Annals, 27*(4), 210–214.

Solomon, D. H., Schaffer, J. L., Katz, J. N., Horsky, J., Burdick, E., Nadler, E., & Bates, D.W. (2000). Can history and physical examination be used as markers of quality? An analysis of the initial visit note in musculoskeletal care. *Medical Care, 38*(4), 383–391.

Walton, M. (1986). *The Deming management method.* New York: Putnam.

chapter 29

The Pain Management Nurse as an Educator

Carol P. Curtiss, MSN, RN-BC

Objectives

After studying this chapter, the reader should be able to:

1. Discuss models of motivation and learning.
2. Explain methods of teaching pain management to patients and families, the public, and health care professionals.
3. Identify barriers to pain management education.

I. Patient Rights and Scope and Standards of Nursing Practice

A. The following guidelines relate to standards of nursing and patient rights:
   1. *Bill of Rights for People with Cancer Pain* (Alliance of State Pain Initiatives Board of Directors, 1998)
   2. Standards of practice and patient education
      a. The pain management nurse "provides patient/family education, . . . teaches ancillary personnel specific and appropriate aspects of pain management, mentors or serves as a resource for nurses with limited pain management knowledge, and continually stays up to date" (American Nurses Association [ANA] & American Society for Pain Management Nursing [ASPMN], 2005).
      b. The registered nurse "provides health teaching on such topics as pain prevention lifestyles, pain-reducing behaviors, developmental needs, activities of daily living, and self-care within the context of the patient's co-morbid features" (ANA & ASPMN, 2005).
      c. The registered nurse "uses health promotion and health teaching methods appropriate to the situation and the patient's developmental needs, readiness, ability to learn, language preferences and culture" (ANA & ASPMN, 2005).
   3. Arthritis and musculoskeletal patient education standards (Burckhardt et al., 1994)
   4. The Joint Commission accreditation requirements (2008)

B. Organizational statements regarding pain management
   1. ASPMN posts many pain-related position papers at http://aspmn.org/Organization/position_papers.htm.
   2. The American Pain Society (APS) posts many pain-related position papers at http://ampainsoc.org/advocacy/statements.htm.
   3. The Oncology Nursing Society position on cancer pain management is found at http://ons.org/publications/positions/CancerPainManagement.shtml.

II. Teaching and Learning

A. Andragogy and pedagogy
   1. *Andragogy* is the art and science of teaching ***adults*** (Knowles, 1980; Long & Morgan, 2008; Redman, 2007)
      a. Adults are self-directed.
      b. Adults incorporate life's experience and knowledge when learning.
      c. Adults are goal-oriented.
      d. Adults seek relevant, practical knowledge for immediate application.
      e. Adult learning shifts from subject-centeredness to problem-centeredness.
      f. Adults need to be shown respect throughout the learning process.
      g. Adults prefer interactive activities.
      h. With adults, the teacher becomes facilitator, establishes learning climate, plans a learning process with input from the learners, and structures learning experiences.
   2. *Pedagogy* is the art and science of teaching ***children and youth*** (Redman, 2007)
      a. Ability to learn ranges from concrete to abstract depending on age and level of maturation.
      b. The parent or teacher assumes responsibility for what the child should learn.
      c. Knowledge acquired is for application when appropriate.
      d. "Hands-on" approaches are encouraged, especially for younger children.

B. Motivation, learning, and adherence
   1. Health belief model (Redman, 2007)
      a. Health action depends on the following:
         (1) Individual's belief of susceptibility to the ill-health condition in question.
         (2) Individual's belief that the problem will have a serious effect on the individual's life.
         (3) Individual's belief that the benefit of action outweighs the barriers to action.
         (4) Individual's confidence in ability to perform the action.

2. Transtheoretical model (Prochaska & Farkas, 1996) (see the chapter on the Pain Management Nurse as a Change Agent)
   a. Intentional change requires nonlinear movement through discrete motivational stages over time, with relapse and return to earlier stages before eventually succeeding. These stages are as follows:
      (1) Precontemplation (unaware of need for change)
      (2) Contemplation (thinking about change)
      (3) Preparation (actively considering change)
      (4) Action (engaged in behavior change efforts)
      (5) Maintenance (maintaining already changed behavior)
      (6) Relapse (return of old behaviors)
   b. Active use of different processes of change occurs at different stages.
   c. Modifications of cognition, affect, and behaviors occur (Redman, 2007).
3. Pain stages of change model (Kerns, Rosenberg, Jamison, Caudill, & Haythornthwaite, 1997)
   a. This model predicts self-management participation using four distinct scales (see the chapter on the Pain Management Nurse as a Change Agent)
4. Representational approach to patient education (Donovan & Ward, 2001)
   a. Individuals have a set of thoughts about a health problem that include ideas about
      (1) Identity or labels associated with the illness.
      (2) Beliefs about origin or cause of the problem.
      (3) Ideas about the timeline: acute, chronic, or cyclic.
      (4) Consequences.
      (5) Beliefs about the possibilities of cure or control of the problem.
5. Motivational interviewing model (Jensen, Nielson, & Kerns, 2003)
   a. This model is designed to help clients address and resolve ambivalence about positive behavior change.
   b. Critical components are motivation, importance, confidence, and readiness.
   c. Steps are to express empathy, identify the discrepancies between current behavior and personal goals, avoid arguing, and support self-efficacy.
6. Patient-centered counseling model (Jensen et al., 2003)
   a. This brief intervention is designed to motivate positive health-related behavioral change.
   b. Thorough assessment is made of a patient's knowledge and concerns about a health problem.
   c. The counselor should provide specific and personalized advice to encourage self-management.
   d. The nurse should provide stage-specific information and feedback.
   e. A behavioral contract is developed with the patient.
   f. Patient self-efficacy increases.
7. Principles of motivation and readiness to learn
   a. Environment can be used to focus the patient's attention on what needs to be learned.
   b. Internal motivation is longer lasting and more self-directed than external motivation.
   c. Learning is most effective when an individual is ready to learn.
   d. Motivation is enhanced by the way instructional material is organized.
   e. Learning normally produces a mild level of anxiety, which is motivating; however, severe anxiety is incapacitating.
   f. Realistic goals sustain motivation.
   g. Affiliation and approval are strong motivators (Redman, 2007).
8. Promoting adherence with education
   a. Attitudinal barriers about pain and pain treatment can interfere with adherence to the plan and result in ineffective pain management (Fahey et al., 2008; Miaskowski et al., 2001).
   b. Low literacy and greater number of medications are associated with misunderstanding the instructions on prescription medicine labels (Davis et al., 2006).

C. Learning behavior categories and teaching methods (Table 29-1)

Table 29-1 Types of Learning and Appropriate Teaching Methods

Types of Learning	Steps and Related Behaviors	Teaching Methods
Cognitive:		
Intellectual abilities, knowledge, information	1. Knowledge: Remembering information (e.g., defines, describes, labels) 2. Comprehension: Lowest level of understanding; ability to grasp information (e.g., converts, defends, explains, predicts) 3. Application: Use of abstractions in concrete situations (e.g., changes, computes, demonstrates, solves) 4. Analysis: Ability to breakdown material into component parts so that structure is understood (e.g., diagrams, illustrates, outlines, relates) 5. Synthesis: Putting elements together to make a whole (e.g., categorizes, designs, modifies, organizes) 6. Evaluation: Judgment about extent to which criteria are met (e.g., appraises, summarizes, criticizes)	Lecture, case method, games, group discussion, clinical rounds, self-learning modules, concept mapping, critical incidents, role playing
Affective:		
Attitudes, values, expression of feelings	1. Receiving: Awareness, willingness to receive, controlled attention 2. Responding: Acquiescence, willingness to respond, satisfaction in responding 3. Valuing: Accepting, preferences, commitment to a value 4. Organization: Conceptualizing a value, relating complex values 5. Characterization by a value or value system: Attitude cluster	Discussion, questioning, role playing, role modeling, games, debates, simulation, case studies
Psychomotor:		
Motor skills performance	1. Perception: Becoming aware by use of sense organs 2. Set: Preparatory adjustment, readiness 3. Guided response: Overt act, imitation, trial and error 4. Mechanism (implementation): Habitual learned process 5. Complex overt response: High degree of skill with minimal expenditure of time and energy 6. Adaptation: Altered motor activities to meet demands of new problem 7. Origination: Creation of new motor skills out of understanding, abilities, skills (Rankin & Duffy Stallings, 1996)	Demonstration and return demonstration, simulation, checklists, observation, coaching

D. Evaluation of teaching or learning
   1. Sequential evaluation can be made of education or training programs (Kirkpatrick, 1994).
      a. Level 1 evaluation
         (1) Reactions: participant satisfaction, relevance of the education
         (2) Strategies: surveys, questionnaires, interview
      b. Level 2 evaluation
         (1) Learning: participants' progress in knowledge, skills, attitudes
         (2) Strategies: post-test, discussion, demonstration
      c. Level 3 evaluation
         (1) Transfer: participants' behavior change due to program
         (2) Strategies: periodic follow-up, observation, assess adherence to plans
      d. Level 4 evaluation
         (1) Results: any effect of change on the larger community, improved overall quality, costs
         (2) Strategies: quality improvement indicators, follow-up community needs assessment
   2. Competency-based evaluation tools are in development in nursing, medicine, and social work (Bogo, Regehr, Hughes, Power, & Globerman, 2002; Kligler et al., 2007). See an example of a pain management competency from the University of Wisconsin Hospitals and Clinics, Madison, Wisconsin, at http://prc.coh.org/pdf/UW_Competency.pdf.
      a. Competency areas (Gordon, Dahl, & Stevenson, 2000)
         (1) Knowledge of basic principles
            (a) Self-report.
            (b) Understand the complexity of the pain experience.
            (c) Know the differences among acute, chronic, noncancer, and cancer pain.
            (d) Recognize the major types of pain.
            (e) Understand the impact of inadequately treated pain.
            (f) Recognize major barriers to adequate pain management.
         (2) Assessment
            (a) Use a standard assessment tool and documentation of responses.
            (b) Perform and document regularly scheduled assessment.
         (3) Interventions
            (a) Recognize major classes of analgesic drugs and their appropriate use.
            (b) Use an equianalgesic chart accurately.
            (c) Know routes of administration and rationale for use.
            (d) Demonstrate and apply selected nonpharmacological interventions.
         (4) Side effect and risk management
            (a) Describe basic approaches to managing potential side effects of opioids.
            (b) Define tolerance, physical dependence, and addiction and articulate the differences.
            (c) Know major risks associated with nonsteroidal anti-inflammatory drugs and acetaminophen and their impact on the elderly.

III. Professional Education

A. The core content of a professional education curriculum is as follows (Charlton, 2005; St. Marie, 2002):
   1. Neurophysiology and pathophysiology of pain
   2. Assessment of pain
   3. Psychosocial aspects of care
   4. Cultural aspects of care
   5. Spiritual aspects of pain
   6. Pharmacological interventions
   7. Nonpharmacological interventions
   8. Taxonomy and common pain syndromes

9. Special populations, including infants and children, older adults, those with limited ability to communicate, those with substance dependency and abuse, those undergoing end-of-life care, and those in countries where deprivation and conflict are issues
10. Advocacy and legal and ethical aspects of care
11. Barriers to pain assessment and management

B. Resources for curriculum development include the following:
1. *American Society for Pain Management Nursing Core Curriculum for Pain Management Nursing* (St. Marie, 2002)
2. *Competency Guidelines for Cancer Pain Management in Nursing Education and Practice* (Wisconsin Cancer Pain Initiative Nursing Education Committee, 1995)
3. *Core Curriculum for Professional Education in Pain,* 3rd edition (Charlton, 2005)
4. *ASCO Core Curriculum Outline* (Muss et al., 2005)
5. *NCCN Clinical Practice Guideline: Adult Cancer Pain* (NCCN, 2008)
6. *NCCN Clinical Practice Guideline: Pediatric Cancer Pain* (NCCN, 2007)
7. *Management of Acute Pain: A Practical Guide* (International Association for the Study of Pain, 1992)
8. *Curriculum on Pain for Students in Psychology* (International Association for the Study of Pain, 1997)
9. "End of Life Nursing Education Consortium (ELNEC) Curriculum: An Introduction to Palliative Care" (Sherman, Matzo, Panke, Grant, & Rhome, 2003)
10. "Education for Physicians in End-of-life Care" (Emanuel, Ferris, & von Gunten, 2002)
11. *Acute Pain Management in Adults: Operative or Medical Procedures and Trauma* (Agency for Public Healthcare Policy and Research, 1992)
12. *Guideline for the Management of Cancer Pain in Adults and Children* (Miaskowski et al., 2005)
13. *Principles of Analgesic Use in the Treatment of Acute Pain and Chronic Cancer Pain* (APS, 2003)
14. *Pain: Clinical Manual* (McCaffery & Pasero, 1999)
15. American Geriatrics Society (2002) clinical practice guidelines
16. *Management of Opioid Therapy for Chronic Pain in Primary Care: Clinical Practice Guideline* (U.S. Veterans Administration & Department of Defense, 2003)
17. *Post Operative Pain: Clinical Practice Guideline* (U.S. Veterans Administration & Department of Defense, 2002)
18. *Guideline for the Management of Acute and Chronic Pain in Sickle Cell Disease* (APS, 1999)
19. *Guideline for the Management of Fibromyalgia Syndrome Pain in Adults and Children* (APS, 2005)
20. *Guideline for the Management of Pain in Osteoarthritis, Rheumatoid Arthritis, and Juvenile Chronic Arthritis* (APS, 2002)
21. "ASPAN Pain & Comfort Guidelines" (American Society for PeriAnesthesia Nurses, 2003)
22. *National Standards for Culturally and Linguistically Appropriate Health Care: Executive Summary* (Office of Minority Health, 2001).
23. *Essentials of Pediatric Oncology Nursing: A Core Curriculum* (Kline, 2004)

C. Methods of teaching health care providers (Table 29-2)

IV. Patient Education

A. Patient education is a combination of learning experiences designed to facilitate voluntary adaptations of behavior conducive to a patient's health (Green, Kreuter, Deeds, & Partridge, 1980; Redman, 2007).

B. Goals for patient education about pain are:
1. Improve pain relief.
2. Increase knowledge and awareness.
3. Decrease misconceptions.
4. Increase adherence to pain control regimens.

Table 29-2 Methods and Strategies for Teaching Health Care Professionals

Teaching Methods	Strategies
Didactic	Lecture with assistance of computer presentations, slides or overheads, video, teleconference, handouts, Web-based education
Case studies	Real, simulated, interactive, or developed scenarios for discussion
Discussion group	Journal club, support group, role playing, study groups
Laboratory experience	Simulated experiences (e.g., programming pumps in classroom setting)
Self-learning modules	CD-ROM, interactive learning, Internet, Web seminars, booklets, concepts mapping (Coffey, Hoffman, Canas, & Ford, 2002; Novak & Gowin, 1984)
Clinical practicum teams	1. Pain resource nurse model a. Interactive program of training for staff nurses to increase knowledge of pain management; nurses then are mentors for colleagues and advocates for patients (Ferrell, Grant, Ritchey, Ropchan, & Rivera, 1993) b. Benefits include improving pain management, increasing general awareness of pain, and dealing with barriers to pain management (Koss, Kearns, McCann-Jones, & Pelligrino, 1998, p. 990) c. Limitations include the degree of dependence of other staff if a pain resource nurse is not available 24 hours a day (Ferrell, Grant, et al., 1993) 2. Grand rounds 3. Closed-circuit television workshops and seminars

5. Facilitate effective communication between provider and patient.
6. Develop patient skills in pain control techniques (Rimer, Kedziera, & Levy, 1992).
7. Family-centered care (Ferrell & Rivera, 1997).

C. Process of patient and family education (Long & Morgan, 2008; Redman, 2007)
   1. Assess readiness to learn (see the needs assessment section that follows).
   2. Assess motivation to learn.
   3. Begin with a clear plan.
      a. Make a diagnostic statement.
      b. Set goals and objectives with the patient.
   4. Create an atmosphere conducive to learning.
   5. Let the teaching or learning episode occur.
   6. Document pertinent information from the session.
   7. Evaluate and reteach as needed.

D. Needs assessment (patient and caregivers) focuses on the following:
   1. Physical condition and present pain intensity.
   2. Current knowledge and understanding of disease and therapy.
   3. Readiness to learn and motivation.
   4. Informational preferences.
   5. Potential barriers to learning include the following:
      a. Ability to read, understand, and use information (literacy).
      b. Access to health care and pain management resources.
      c. Potential language barriers.
      d. Myths and misperceptions.
      e. Sensory or cognitive deficits.

6. Demographics include the following:
   a. Age.
   b. Family status.
   c. Past and present employment.
   d. Formal education.
7. Stage of life development.
8. Means of social support.
9. Emotional response to disease.
10. Meaning of pain.
11. Cultural values and beliefs (Office of Minority Health, 2001).
12. Educational preferences.
13. Spiritual beliefs.

E. Planning
1. Goal setting
   a. Develop goals collaboratively with the patient.
2. Content
   a. Content should be individualized based on the needs assessment.
   b. The following guidelines can be used:
      (1) Agency for Public Healthcare Policy and Research (1992) and APS (1999, 2002, 2003, 2005) guidelines
      (2) Commission on Accreditation of Rehabilitation Facilities (2001) guidelines
      (3) Guidelines for cancer pain education (Ferrell & Juarez, 2002; National Comprehensive Cancer Network [NCCN], 2007, 2008; Rimer et al., 1992)
         (a) Key concepts
            (i) Pain can be relieved and there is no benefit to suffering with pain.
            (ii) Patients can learn how to measure and describe their pain.
            (iii) Pain can usually be controlled with a multimodal approach and medication taken by mouth.
            (iv) Many options are available in addition to medications.
            (v) Morphine and morphine-like medications are often used.
            (vi) Medications should be stored in safe places at home.
            (vii) Effective communication with doctors and nurses is critical.
            (viii) Patients should know the names of each medication, its indication, and instructions of how and when to take each one.
            (ix) Patients should know the possible side effects and strategies to manage each.
            (x) Teach patients about the use of noninvasive therapies.
            (xi) Supply contact information for help with problems, pain, and side effects.
            (xii) Explain the plan for follow-up.
         (b) In addition,
            (i) Examine each patient's personal meaning of pain.
            (ii) Correct misconceptions about addiction and tolerance.
            (iii) Stress that the goal of cancer pain therapy is not only pain relief but also pain prevention (APS, 2005; Ferrell, Rhiner, & Rivera, 1993).
            (iv) Adapt teaching and educational materials to cultural preferences (Office of Minority Health, 2001).
      (4) Themes regarding what cancer patients want to know about pain include the following (Bender et al., 2008):
         (a) Understanding pain
         (b) Knowing what to expect
         (c) Options for pain control
         (d) Coping with pain
         (e) Talking with others about pain

(f) Finding help managing pain
(g) Describing pain

F. Implementation
1. The teaching session
a. Select a comfortable and quiet environment for the individual.
b. Provide accurate and current information.
c. Teach the smallest amount possible rather than overload the individual with information.
d. Use a combination of educational methods.
e. Keep each session brief with breaks as needed.
f. Present the most important materials first and last.
g. Use materials that are clear, concise, and culturally appropriate.
h. Avoid medical jargon.
i. Involve the family and significant others.
j. Use repetition and encourage questions.
k. Evaluate the individual's comprehension of the material.
l. Promote ongoing communication with the health care provider and family (Ferrell & Juarez, 2002; Ferrell, Rhiner, & Rivera, 1993).
2. Instructional methods
a. The following strategies depend on individual needs assessment and learning style:
(1) Individual (one-on-one) didactic sessions, discussion, lecture, concept mapping, motivational interviewing (e.g., return demonstration of preparing medication, lecture or discussion on managing chronic pain, or concept map of the effects of pain on an individual)
(2) Self-directed learning modules (e.g., DVDs or videos on back exercises)
(3) Group discussion or didactic sessions (e.g., exercise session to demonstrate stretching)
3. Teaching tools
a. The purposes of teaching tools are to retain, compare, visualize, and reinforce learning.
b. Evaluate readability of materials and tools based on the individual's literacy:
(1) Printed materials (e.g., pamphlets, articles, pictures, and posters)
(2) DVDs, videotape
(3) Audiotape
(4) Computer-assisted instruction
(5) Checklists
(6) Models
(7) Handouts
(8) Concept mapping (Coffey et al., 2002; Novak & Gowin, 1984)
c. Provide a script for communicating with health care providers.
4. Evaluation of learning includes
a. Test and retest.
b. Return demonstration.
c. Repetition of content.
d. Quality-of-life or other surveys.
e. Participants' written evaluation of content, presentation, and environment.
5. Documentation focuses on the following:
a. Content presented in session
b. Outcomes of education
(1) The patient independently understands the information or can demonstrate a skill.
(2) The patient partially understands the information or can partially demonstrate a skill.
(3) The patient needs complete reinforcement of information or skills.
c. Next steps in the education plan

G. Teaching individuals with low literacy (Doak, Doak, & Root, 1996; Kutner, Greenberg, Jin, & Paulsen, 2006; Mayer & Villaire, 2007).
1. Literacy is the ability to read, understand, and use information effectively.

2. Literacy has little to do with intelligence.
3. Adults with low health literacy
    a. Are often less likely to comply with instructions.
    b. Make more medication and treatment errors.
    c. Fail to seek preventative care.
    d. Lack skills needed to negotiate the health care system.
    e. Are more likely to misunderstand medication labels.
4. Strategies for teaching individuals with low literacy
    a. Simplify content to address these essential questions (Partnership for Clear Health Communication, 2008):
        (1) What is my problem?
        (2) What do I need to do?
        (3) Why is it important for me to do it?
    b. Prepare materials (Davis et al., 2006; Doak et al., 1996; Mayer & Villaire, 2007).
        (1) Calculate the reading level of materials using readability formulas.
        (2) Add pictures, diagrams, and white space.
        (3) Use short words and sentences.
        (4) Use visual cues.
        (5) Involve the reader or viewer.
        (6) Give clear action messages.
        (7) Place the most important messages first and last.

H. Special populations
1. *Children:* Adapt for maturity level, cognitive development, language development, learning level, reading ability, motor function, and concrete thinking.
2. *Adolescents:* Adapt for maturity level, learning level, reading ability, and ability to think in the abstract.
3. *Elderly:* Adapt for cognitive, sensory, and psychomotor changes; consider response time, energy and fatigue level.
4. *Ethnic or cultural groups:* Adapt language, content, and format to individual needs and preferences.

V. Public Education

A. The goals of public education include the following:
1. Increase awareness and knowledge.
2. Decrease misconceptions.
3. Facilitate access to appropriate health care.

B. Planning
1. Needs assessment
    a. Involve community leaders in planning and implementation.
    b. Identify the target audience.
    c. Identify the target audience's level of knowledge.
    d. Identify goals for education.
    e. Determine the overall message.
    f. Assess available resources.
    g. Select the type of education activity.
    h. Use culturally sensitive teaching strategies.
    i. Appeal to various learning styles.
    j. Implement the program using
        (1) Lectures.
        (2) Health fairs.
        (3) Demonstrations.

C. Evaluation can take the following forms:
1. Written evaluation of participants

2. Focus group feedback
3. Surveys
4. Debriefing of planners
5. Return demonstrations

VI. Barriers to Education

A. Professional and systems barriers
   1. Such barriers include the following:
      a. Lack of priority and accountability given to pain management.
      b. Time restrictions in practice settings.
      c. Lack of knowledge and skills of practitioner (Ferrell, Grant, et al., 1993; McCaffery & Ferrell, 1997).
      d. Misconceptions, concerns, and beliefs of health care providers (Berry & Ward, 1995; Thomason et al., 1998; Ward & Gatwood, 1994).
      e. Inadequate assessment (Ferrell & Juarez, 2002).
      f. Inconsistency of educational content (Syrjala et al., 2008).
      g. Ineffective treatment planning or lack of follow-up.
   2. Studies are inconclusive regarding evidence that education results in reduction of pain severity.
   3. Studies need to address costs of patient education.
   4. Studies of pain are limited in culturally diverse populations (Redman, 2007)

B. Patient and family barriers
   1. Knowledge does not equal behavior—see the health belief model given earlier (Rosenstock, 1990).
   2. Unrelieved pain, fear, anxiety, or sleeplessness interferes with the ability to concentrate or learn.
   3. Motivation and readiness to learn must be present.
   4. Other barriers include the following:
      a. Age, sex, socioeconomic status, and educational level
      b. Literacy
      c. Cultural differences (see the chapter on Historical and Cultural Influences on Pain Perceptions and Barriers to Treatment)
      d. Language differences
      e. Emotion (anxiety, grief, anger)
      f. External locus of control, that is, a belief that personal behavior is driven by chance, external factors, or others (Coughlin, Badura, Fleischer, & Guck, 2000)
      g. Mental illness, cognitive function, or personality disorders
      h. Myths and misperceptions of the patient or family, such as "pain should be tolerated," "fear of addiction," and "fear of not being able to control pain" (Ferrell & Juarez, 2002; Lin, Chou, Wu, Chang, & Lai, 2006; Sun et al., 2007; Thomason et al., 1998)
      i. Fatalism, or the belief that analgesics lead to adverse outcomes, dependence, tolerance, or addiction (Ward & Gatwood, 1994)
      j. Environmental factors including light, temperature, noise, timing, and distractions such as other people or activity in room
      k. Unacceptable or unmanaged side effects that prevent adherence
      l. Inability to purchase or access medications or other treatments

C. Common errors in teaching
   1. The needs assessment is not completed.
   2. Too much information is given at one time.
   3. Information is too complex.
   4. The timing is wrong.
   5. No interaction occurs with the learner.
   6. No feedback is given for comprehension.
   7. Information is not culturally sensitive.

References

Agency for Public Healthcare Policy and Research. (1992). *Acute pain management in adults: Operative or medical procedures and trauma.* Clinical Practice Guideline (Publication No. 92-0018). Rockville, MD: Author.

Alliance of State Pain Initiatives Board of Directors. (1998). *Bill of rights for people with cancer pain.* Retrieved May 27, 2008, from http://aspi.wisc.edu/documents/pdf/BOR.pdf.

American Geriatrics Society Panel on Chronic Pain in Older Persons. (2002). The management of chronic pain in older persons. *Journal of the American Geriatrics Society, 50,* 1–20.

American Nurses Association & American Society for Pain Management Nursing. (2005). *Pain management nursing: Scope and standards of practice.* Silver Springs, MD: American Nurses Association.

American Pain Society. (1999). *Guideline for the management of acute and chronic pain in sickle cell disease.* Glenview IL: Author.

American Pain Society. (2002). *Guideline for the management of pain in osteoarthritis, rheumatoid arthritis, and juvenile chronic arthritis.* Glenview IL: Author.

American Pain Society. (2003). *Principles of analgesic use in the treatment of acute pain and chronic cancer pain* (5th ed.). Skokie, IL: Author.

American Pain Society. (2005). *Guideline for the management of fibromyalgia syndrome pain in adults and children.* Glenview IL: Author.

American Pain Society. (2008). *Position papers.* Retrieved November 18, 2008, from http://ampainsoc.org/advocacy/statements.htm.

American Society for PeriAnesthesia Nurses. (2003). ASPAN pain & comfort guidelines. *Journal of PeriAnesthesia Nursing, 18,* 232–236.

Bender, J. L., Hohenadel, J., Wong, J., Katz, J., Ferris, L., & Shobbrook, C. (2008). What patients with cancer want to know about pain: A qualitative study. *Journal of Pain and Symptom Management, 35,* 177–187.

Berry, E. P., & Ward, S. (1995). Barriers to pain management in hospice: A study of family caregivers. *Hospice Journal, 10,* 19–33.

Bogo, M., Regehr, C., Hughes, J., Power, R., & Globerman, J. (2002). Evaluating a measure of student field performance in direct service: Testing reliability and validity of explicit criteria. *Journal of Social Work Education, 38,* 385–401.

Burckhardt, C. S., Lorig, K., Monceir, C., Melvin, J., Beardmore, T., Boyd, M., & Boutaugh, M. (1994). Arthritis and musculoskeletal patient education standards. *Arthritis Care Research, 7,* 1–4.

Charlton, J. E. (Ed.). (2005). *Core curriculum for professional education in pain* (3rd ed.). Seattle: IASP Press.

Coffey, J. W., Hoffman, R. R., Canas, A. J., & Ford, K. M. (2002). *A concept map-based knowledge modeling approach to expert knowledge.* Pensacola, FL: Florida Institute for Human and Machine Cognition. Retrieved May 28, 2008, from http://www.ihmc.us/users/acanas/Publications/IKS2002/IKS.htm.

Commission on Accreditation of Rehabilitation Facilities. (2001). *Standards of care.* Tucson, AZ: Author.

Coughlin, A. M., Badura, A. S., Fleischer, T. D., & Guck, T. P. (2000). Multidisciplinary treatment of chronic pain patients: Its efficacy in changing patient locus of control. *Archives of Physical Medicine and Rehabilitation, 81,* 739–740.

Davis, T. C., Wolf, S., Bass, P. F., Thompson, J. A., Tilson, H. H., Neuberger, M., & Parker, R. (2006). Literacy and misunderstanding prescription drug labels. *Annals of Internal Medicine, 145,* 887–894.

Doak, C. C., Doak, L. G., & Root, J. H. (1996). *Teaching patients with low literacy skills* (2nd ed.). Philadelphia: Lippincott.

Donovan, H. S., & Ward, S. (2001). A representational approach to patient education. *Journal of Nursing Scholarship, 33,* 211–216.

Emanuel, L. L., Ferris, F. D., & von Gunten, C. (2002). EPEC: Education for physicians in end-of-life care. *American Journal of Hospice and Palliative Care, 19*(1), 17.

Fahey, K. F., Rao, S. M., Douglas, M. K., Thomas, M. L., Elliott, J. E., & Miaskowski, C. (2008). Nurse coaching to explore and modify barriers interfering with effective cancer pain management. *Oncology Nursing Forum, 35,* 233–240.

Ferrell, B. R., Grant, M., Ritchey, K. J., Ropchan, R., & Rivera, L. (1993). The pain resource nurse training program: A unique approach to pain management. *Journal of Pain and Symptom Management, 8,* 549–556.

Ferrell, B. R., & Juarez, G. (2002). Cancer pain education for patients and the public. *Journal of Pain and Symptom Management, 23,* 329–336.

Ferrell, B. R., Rhiner, M., & Rivera, L. M. (1993). Empowering patients to control pain. *Current Issues in Cancer Nursing Practice Updates, 2,* 1–9.

Ferrell, B. R., & Rivera, L. M. (1997). Cancer pain education for patients. *Seminars in Oncology Nursing, 13,* 42–48.

Gordon, D. B., Dahl, J. L., & Stevenson, K. K. (2000). Wisconsin Cancer Pain Initiative, 1995. In *Building an institutional commitment of pain management.* Madison, WI: University of Wisconsin Board of Regents.

Green, L. W., Kreuter, M. W., Deeds, S. G., & Partridge, K. D. (1980). *Health education planning.* Mountain View, CA: Mayfield.

International Association for the Study of Pain. (1992). *Management of acute pain: A practical guide.* Task Force on Acute Pain. Seattle: IASP Press.

International Association for the Study of Pain. (1997). *Curriculum on pain for students in psychology.* Seattle: IASP Press.

Jensen, M. P., Nielson, W. R., & Kerns, R. D. (2003). Toward the development of a motivational model of pain self-management. *Journal of Pain, 4,* 477–492.

Joint Commission. (2008). *2009 Accreditation requirements chapters: Pre-publication preview.* Retrieved July 15, 2008, from http://www.jointcommission.org/Standards/SII/.

Kerns, R. D., Rosenberg, R., Jamison, R. N., Caudill, M. A., & Haythornthwaite, J. (1997). Readiness to adopt a self management approach to chronic pain: The stages of change questionnaire (PSOCQ). *Pain, 72,* 227–234.

Kirkpatrick, D. L. (1994). *Evaluating training programs: The four levels.* San Francisco: Berrett-Koehler.

Kligler, B., Koithan, M., Maizes, V., Hayes, M., Schneider, C., Lebensohn, P., & Hadley, S. (2007). Competency-based evaluation tools for integrative medicine training in family medicine residency: A pilot study. *BMC Medical Education.* Retrieved November 12, 2008, from http://www.biomedcentral.com/1472-6920/7/7.

Kline, N. E. (2004). *Essentials of pediatric oncology nursing* (2nd ed.). Toronto, ON: Association of Pediatric Oncology Nurses.

Knowles, M. S. (1980). *The modern practice of adult education.* New York: Associated Press.

Koss, J., Kearns, M., McCann-Jones, E., & Pelligrino, A. (1998). Pain resource nurses make education painless. *Oncology Nursing Forum, 25,* 990.

Kutner, M., Greenberg, E., Jin, Y., & Paulsen, C. (2006). *The health literacy of America's adults: Results from the 2003 National Assessment of Adult Literacy* (NCES 2006–483). Washington, DC: U.S. Department of Education, National Center for Education Statistics. Retrieved May 8, 2008, from http://nces.ed.gov/pubs2006/2006483.pdf.

Lin, C. C., Chou, P. L., Wu, S. L., Chang, Y. C., & Lai, Y. L. (2006). Long-term effectiveness of a patient and family patient education program on overcoming barriers to management of cancer pain. *Pain, 122,* 271–281.

Long, C. O., & Morgan, B. M. (2008). *Pain management: The resource guide for home health and hospice nurses.* Baltimore: Hopkins Medical Products.

Mayer, G. G., & Villaire, M. (2007). *Health literacy in primary care: A clinician's guide.* New York: Springer.

McCaffery, M., & Ferrell, B. R. (1997). Nurses' knowledge of pain assessment and management: How much progress have we made? *Journal of Pain and Symptom Management, 14,* 175–188.

McCaffery, M., & Pasero, C. (1999). *Pain: Clinical manual* (2nd ed.). St. Louis: Mosby.

Miaskowski, C., Cleary, J., Burney, R., Coyne, P., Finley, R., Foster, R., Grossman, S., Janjan, N., Ray, J., Syejala, K., Weisman, M., & Zahrbock, C. (2005). *Guideline for the management of cancer pain in adults and children.* APS Clinical Practice Guideline Series, No. 3. Glenview, IL: American Pain Society.

Miaskowski, C., Dodd, M. J., West, C., Paul, S. M., Tripathy, D., Koo, P., & Schumacher, K. (2001). Lack of adherence with the analgesic regimen: A significant barrier to effective cancer pain management. *Journal of Clinical Oncology, 19*(23), 4275–4279.

Muss, H. B., Von Roenn, J., Damon, L. E., Deangeles, L. M., Flaherty, L. E., Harari, P. M., Kelly, K., Kosty, M.P., Loscalzo, M.J., Pisters, P.W.T., Saltz, L., Schapira, L., & Sparano, J. (2005). ASCO core curriculum outline. *Journal of Clinical Oncology, 23*(9), 2049–2077.

National Comprehensive Cancer Network. (V.I. 2008). *NCCN clinical practice guideline: Adult cancer pain.* Retrieved May 30, 2008, from http://www.nccn.org/professionals/physician_gls/PDF/pain.pdf.

National Comprehensive Cancer Network. (V.I. 2007). *NCCN clinical practice guideline: Pediatric cancer pain.* Retrieved May 30, 2008, from http://www.nccn.org/professionals/physician_gls/PDF/pediatric_pain.pdf.

Novak, J. D., & Gowin, D. B. (1984). *Learning how to learn.* Ithaca, NY: Cornell University Press.

Office of Minority Health. (2001). *National standards for culturally and linguistically appropriate health care: Executive summary.* Rockville MD: U.S. Department of Health and Human Services.

Partnership for Clear Health Communication. (2008). *Ask me 3: What can providers do?* National Patient Safety Foundation. Retrieved May 27, 2008, from http://www.npsf.org/askme3/PCHC/what_can_provid.php.

Prochaska, J., & Farkas, A. (1996). *The transtheoretical approach: Crossing traditional boundaries of therapy.* Homewood, IL: Dow Jones-Irwin.

Rankin, S. H., & Duffy Stallings, K. (1996). *Patient education: Issues, principles, practices* (3rd ed.). Philadelphia: Lippincott.

Redman, B. (2007). *The practice of patient education: A case study approach* (10th ed.). St. Louis: Mosby/Elsevier.

Rimer, B., Kedziera, P., & Levy, M. H. (1992). The role of patient education in cancer pain control. *Hospice Journal, 8,* 171–191.

Rosenstock, I. M. (1990). The health belief model: Exploring health behavior through expectancies. In K. Glanz, F. M. Lewis, & B. K. Rimer (Eds.), *Health behavior and health education: Theory, research and practical* (pp. 39–62). San Francisco: Jossey-Bass.

Sherman, D., Matzo, M., Panke, J., Grant, M., & Rhone, A. (2003). End of Life Nursing Education Consortium (ELNEC) curriculum: An introduction to palliative care. *Nurse Educator, 28,* 111–120.

St. Marie, B. (2002). *American Society for Pain Management Nursing core curriculum for pain management nursing.* Philadelphia: W. B. Saunders.

Sun, V., Bordeman, T., Ferrell, B. R., Piper, B., Koczwash, M., & Choi, K. (2007). Overcoming barriers to cancer pain management: An institutional change model. *Journal of Pain and Symptom Management, 34,* 359–364.

Syrjala, K. L., Abrams, J. R., Polissar, N. L., Hansberry, J., Robison, J., DuPen, S., Stillman, M., Fredrickson, M., Rivkin, S., Feldman, E., Gralow, J., Rieke, J.W., Raish, R.J., Lee, D.J., Cleeland, C.S., DuPen, A. (2008). Patient training in cancer pain management using integrated print and video materials: A multisite randomized controlled trial. *Pain, 135,* 175–186.

Thomason, T. E., McCune, J. S., Bernard, S. A., Winer, E. P., Tremont, S., & Lindley, C. M. (1998). Cancer pain survey: Patient centered issues in control. *Journal of Pain and Symptom Management, 15,* 275–284.

U.S. Veterans Administration & U.S. Department of Defense. (2002). *Post operative pain: Clinical practice guideline.* Retrieved May 25, 2008, from http://www.oqp.med.va.gov/cpg/PAIN/PAIN_Base.htm.

U.S. Veterans Administration & U.S. Department of Defense. (2003). *Management of opioid therapy for chronic pain in primary care: Clinical practice guideline.* Retrieved May 25, 2008, from http://www.oqp.med.va.gov/cpg/cot/cot_cpg/frameset.htm.

Ward, S., & Gatwood, J. (1994). Concerns about reporting pain and using analgesics: A comparison of persons with and without cancer. *Cancer Nursing, 17,* 200–206.

Wisconsin Cancer Pain Initiative Nursing Education Committee. (1995). *Competency guidelines for cancer pain management in nursing education and practice.* Madison, WI: Wisconsin Cancer Pain Initiative.

Suggested Reading

American Society for Pain Management Nursing. (2008). *Position papers.* Retrieved November 18, 2008, from http://aspmn.org/Organization/position_papers.htm.

chapter

30

The Role of the Clinical Nurse Specialist in Pain Management

Mary Zaccagnini, DNP, RN, ACNS-BC, AOCN

Objectives

After studying this chapter, the reader should be able to:

1. Define the major components of practice for the pain management clinical nurse specialist.
2. Define the subroles within the major components of practice for the pain management clinical nurse specialist.
3. Discuss the variations in pain management practice between the nurse practitioner and the clinical nurse specialist.
4. Describe the differences between direct and indirect advanced practice care.
5. Discuss the scope of practice for the pain management clinical nurse specialist.
6. Discuss the future of the role of the pain management clinical nurse specialist.

I. History

A. In 1910, nurses were designated as specialists. Frances Reiter first used the title ***nurse clinician*** in 1943 to describe a nurse with advanced knowledge and clinical expertise (LaSala, Connors, Pedro, & Phipps, 2007). Anne Norris stated that the actual concept of a clinical nurse specialist was advanced in 1944 by the National League for Nursing Education (Hamric & Spross, 1989). Hildegard Peplau noted that the title *clinical nurse specialist* was created in 1938; however, Peplau, in her 1965 article outlining the role, was the first to actually title this group of specialty practitioners as *Clinical Nurse Specialist* (National Association of Clinical Nurse Specialists [NACNS], 2004).

B. Whether the title or the intent of the title began with Peplau or with the inception of the first formal curriculum developed for the role of the clinical nurse specialist, the clinical nurse specialist role as we know it today is a more recent development within the nursing profession.

C. In 1995 the NACNS was formed; in 1996 NACNS identified clinical nurse specialist core competencies; and in 1998 NACNS issued the *Statement on Clinical Nurse Specialist Practice and Education* (LaSala et al., 2007).

II. Education

A. In 1949, the University of Minnesota advanced the concept of graduate classes for a nursing clinical specialty in a formal setting. Before this, postgraduate classes were conducted as on-the-job training courses held within specialty hospitals. Clinical nurse specialists were the first advanced practice nursing group to require a graduate degree for practice and therefore to be a model for other advanced practice roles (Rose, All, & Gresham, 2008).

B. The psychiatric nursing specialty was the first to develop clinical experiences at the graduate level. In 1954, Peplau developed the first master's program at Rutgers University that focused exclusively on the development of a clinical nurse specialist role in psychiatric nursing (Hamric & Spross, 1989).

C. Oncology is credited with developing specialized education early in its evolution. In 1947, Nelson developed the first graduate course in cancer nursing. Today, the curriculum guide and role definition for an oncology clinical nurse specialist by the American Cancer Society states the criterion as a master's degree with a specialty in oncology nursing (LaSala et al., 2007).

D. The role of the clinical nurse specialist is defined by the criterion of graduate preparation in nursing. A master's or doctorate degree, with a clinical specialty, is the minimum level of education required throughout the United States.

E. The American Nurses Credentialing Center provides national credentialing for clinical nurse specialists in the areas of pediatrics, adult health, and gerontology. Some specialties, such as critical care and oncology, also provide testing for advanced practice within the specialty.

F. During formal education, the clinical nurse specialist develops a specialty focus, primarily through clinical experiences within the chosen specialty.

G. Although only minimal formal education in pain management exists for the advanced practice nurse, clinical nurse specialists receive components of pain management theory and clinical practice within the auspices of symptom management for their specialty population.
   1. Many local and national pain conferences are available.
   2. The Joint Commission has said that pain education must be part of the overall pain management plan within hospitals.

III. Definitions

A. According to the NACNS, the clinical nurse specialist is a licensed registered nurse who has graduate preparation (a master's or a doctorate degree) in nursing as a clinical nurse specialist. The clinical nurse specialist is a clinical expert in theory-based, research-based, or both types of nursing practice within a specialty area who integrates knowledge; designs, implements, and evaluates programs; is a leader, consultant, and change agent; and leads multidisciplinary groups (NACNS, 2004).

B. The definition from the American Nurses Association (2004) cites the clinical nurse specialist as an expert clinician and patient advocate in a particular specialty or subspecialty of nursing practice.

IV. Evaluation of the Current Role of the Advanced Practice Nurse in Pain Management

A. Various associations, organizations, and publications have proclaimed or proposed a singular title of *advanced practice nurse* that would include the nurse practitioner, the clinical nurse specialist, the nurse anesthetists, and nurse midwives. Although some merging has occurred, to date the roles remain different in practice and setting.

B. The clinical nurse specialist role in pain management
   1. The clinical nurse specialist in pain management practices primarily in an inpatient setting. Often, the primary focus is on a specialized patient population, the given health care system, and teaching and mentoring other health care professionals.
   2. Although the clinical nurse specialist may provide direct and indirect patient care in pain management, this role rarely is exclusive to individual direct patient assessment and management in an outpatient or primary care setting. The clinical nurse specialist role in pain management generally includes other activities, such as program development, research, change facilitation, and quality management.

C. Merging the roles of clinical nurse specialist and nurse practitioner
   1. As both roles evolve and as credentialing, reimbursement criteria, and laws change, it is clear that the roles are merging and blending. Education and practice are often similar; however, to date differences remain in practice and credentialing. It is also noteworthy that the two practitioner groups, through individual national organizations, remain clear in the desire for role preservation.
   2. In many settings, clinical nurse specialists and nurse practitioners integrate skills to provide a comprehensive pain management program that includes direct patient care, population management, education for patients and health care professionals, and improved continuum of care and care management practices.
   3. As the roles progress in merging education and practice, we see distinction of roles remaining. In most instances, the nurse practitioner remains the direct care practitioner whereas the clinical nurse specialist generally facilitates and manages the pain team and program. According to Zuzelo (2003), the clinical nurse specialist focuses on the larger picture of patient care rather than regular intervention in direct care to individual patients. Zuzelo also notes that the clinical nurse specialist has expertise in systems theory, program evaluation, evidence-based practice, and outcome management.

V. Components and Scope of Practice of the Clinical Nurse Specialist Role in Pain Management

A. Past literature described the major components of practice for the clinical nurse specialist as expert or advanced practitioner, educator, consultant, and researcher. Within these major categories lie various subroles, such as change agent, project manager, program development and manager, quality manager, and administrative leader.

B. The 2004 revision of the *Statement on Clinical Nurse Specialist Practice and Education* developed a framework or conceptual model to describe clinical nurse specialist practice. This practice description and the competencies that followed were framed as three spheres of influence:
   1. Patient/client
   2. Nursing and nursing practice
   3. Organization and system

C. According to the current draft of the *Consensus Model for APRN Regulation: Licensure, Accreditation, Certification & Education* (NACNS, 2004), the primary goal of the clinical nurse specialist is continuous improvement of nursing care and outcomes within and throughout each sphere.

D. Spheres of influence
   1. The three spheres (patient/client, nursing and nursing practice, and organization and system) of clinical nurse specialist influence provide an organizing framework to describe core clinical nurse specialist competencies (NACNS, 2004).
   2. The clinical nurse specialist employs clinical expertise to improve outcomes across all three spheres of influence. This model integrates clinical nurse specialist practice and focuses on practice rather than roles (Darmody, 2005).

3. Patient/client
   a. The patient sphere is the fundamental sphere of the clinical nurse specialist practice (Zuzelo, 2003).
   b. *Direct patient care* generally occurs within an inpatient acute care setting and often for a specialty population.
      (1) A clinical nurse specialist may practice the direct patient care component autonomously or as a member of an interdisciplinary pain team.
      (2) As a member of a team, the clinical nurse specialist in pain management is often the first line of triage.
      (3) The pain management clinical nurse specialist
         (a) Conducts a complete pain assessment, which incorporates location, intensity, quality, onset, duration, and causative and relieving factors (McCaffery & Pasero, 1999).
         (b) Uses pain rating tools and scales that are valid and reliable and that are selected for differences in culture and language and for developmental and cognitive differences.
         (c) Incorporates preexisting and coexisting pain conditions (e.g., peripheral neuropathies secondary to diabetes) as part of the total pain assessment of the current acute condition.
         (d) Collaborates with the health care team if applicable to develop the most appropriate plan of care.
         (e) Sets goals that are mutually acceptable to the patient (e.g., pain is acceptable at a level of 4 on a 0-to-10 scale) and the health care team.
         (f) Recommends pharmacological interventions. These recommendations incorporate the knowledge of the anatomy and physiology of pain mechanisms and pathways, pain classes or categories (such as visceral, somatic, and neuropathic), drug classifications with optimal dosing ranges and toxicity profiles, and complete knowledge of the use of adjuvant drugs for pain management. The clinical nurse specialist incorporates the variances for age and culture in all applicable recommendations and interventions.
         (g) May prescribe treatments within the guidelines of the state in which the license is obtained.
         (h) Recommends nonpharmacological therapies, such as relaxation and massage.
         (i) Provides education, which includes the modalities and plan of treatment, the pathophysiology of the pain, and any potential side effects, to the patient, family, and other caregivers.
         (j) Develops an evaluation and plan of care that includes the efficacy of treatment and is compared against the toxicity of treatment.
         (k) Performs continuous and regular reassessment of pain and interventions, including appropriate adjustments within the goal of the patient.
   c. *Indirect patient care:* Indirect patient care performed by the pain management clinical nurse specialist can affect an individual patient and entire patient populations.
      (1) The pain management clinical nurse specialist's responsibilities in this role may extend to the inpatient setting, community and outpatient services.
      (2) The pain management clinical nurse specialist
         (a) Is instrumental in the development of pain protocols, standards, guidelines, and policies. This role may be accomplished autonomously or in collaboration with additional disciplines.
         (b) Develops educational materials for staff, patients, families, and the community.
         (c) Will integrate evidence-based practice to assure safety in practice and to translate research into practice (Goudreau, Clark, Lyon, & Rust, 2007).
         (d) Will publish new clinical pain phenomena and share specific effectiveness to new interventions (Goudreau et al., 2007).

4. Nursing and nursing practice
   a. The clinical nurse specialist is responsible for identifying the pain management learning needs of health care professionals in the health care system and maintaining clinical competence and ongoing skill development within standards of practice.
   b. Education of nurses and other health care professionals, which includes the development and presentation of curricula with special focus on pain assessment and management, is a core component of this sphere of influence. These presentations should include the pathophysiology and pathways of pain, appropriate assessment and documentation, and the development of plans that include the patient and other members of the team.
   c. The clinical nurse specialist is often involved in a formal teaching setting. This area includes presentation of pain management curriculum to undergraduate and postgraduate nursing students (Chuk, 1997).
      (1) The pain management clinical nurse specialist may be invited as a guest speaker for a university department, such as nursing and pharmacy.
      (2) The pain management clinical nurse specialist may act as a preceptor or mentor for nursing students in a clinical rotation, as well as act as a mentor to nursing staff. This role is especially important in an environment in which nurses had minimal coursework in pain management nursing.
   d. Within this sphere, the pain management consultation is a large component of practice. The literature notes the clinical nurse specialist consultant as the most valued role of the clinical nurse specialist.
      (1) In the consultative role, the pain management clinical nurse specialist may be called on to deliver direct patient assessment followed by recommendations for care.
      (2) Indirect consultation by the clinical nurse specialist involves assisting in the development of the plan of care for the patient in pain.
      (3) Complex pain issues are probably the most common consultative activity of the pain management clinical nurse specialist (Chuk, 1997).
         (a) *Example:* Assist with the management of a complex pain patient who recently has undergone surgery and has a history of concurrent and additional pain issues, such as osteoarthritis, or peripheral neuropathy.
      (4) Consultation may involve indirect patient care by assisting nurses in the management of difficult pain patients.
         (a) *Example:* Biases may influence nurses in managing the postoperative pain of a chemically dependent patient. The clinical nurse specialist could educate staff with respect to the research on this patient population and then help them to develop an appropriate plan.
      (5) The pain management clinical nurse specialist is expected to develop an evaluation process as a part of the consultative role. This evaluation may involve the nurse's reporting the identified outcomes back to the clinical nurse specialist. A reevaluation would be done to determine whether the outcomes were met or whether the plan requires modification.
   e. The clinical nurse specialist is responsible for following up-to-date literature and sharing research findings to promote evidence-based practice (Darmody, 2005).
      (1) The review of pain management literature involves gathering, reviewing, and evaluating the quality and applicability of the articles. The clinical nurse specialist communicates these findings to the staff.
         (a) *Example:* Introduce a medication or class of medications used in pain management or a process for evaluation that has proved useful in other settings.
      (2) Research use would include the application of significant findings to patient care.
         (a) *Example:* Develop a guideline or protocol that would include the use of preemptive pain management before surgery.

5. Organization and system
   a. The pain management clinical nurse specialist would articulate clinical problems within the context of the organization (NACNS, 2004).
      (1) *Example:* A change in a current pain practice could benefit fiscal outcomes of the organization.
      (2) *Example:* Changing practice would decrease length of stay.
   b. The pain management clinical nurse specialist provides a pain program and role evaluation that would include the understanding of a cost-benefit analysis to assure retention of a current pain program or practitioner role.
   c. The pain management clinical nurse specialist identifies outcomes that address processes, strategies, initiatives, and programs in the larger context of the organization (Zuzelo, 2007).
   d. The clinical nurse specialist analyzes the cost-effectiveness and cost-benefits of new products for the organization (Goudreau et al., 2007).
   e. The clinical nurse specialist provides leadership in multidisciplinary task forces, system committees, and the development of programs directly related to pain management.

E. Additional dimensions of the pain management clinical nurse specialist role
   1. *Change agent:* The pain management clinical nurse specialist uses theories of change within an organization to implement a change.
      a. *Example:* Introduce a procedure or develop a new policy and procedure related to the care of an epidural catheter.
      b. *Example:* Use research findings regarding the inappropriate use of naloxone to implement a change in practice within an institution.
   2. *Project manager:* The pain management clinical nurse specialist is called on to develop or lead projects related to pain management.
      a. *Example:* Develop processes and systems to ensure implementation of Agency for Health Care Policy and Research guidelines or Joint Commission standards for pain management.
      b. *Example:* Facilitate the development of an institutional pain model, program, or interdisciplinary team.
   3. *Quality manager:* The pain management clinical nurse specialist exemplifies quality at the core of practice.
      a. Quality assessment and monitoring are intertwined within all categories and subcategories of the role of pain management clinical nurse specialist.
      b. On a larger scale, the pain management clinical nurse specialist often is called on to manage all quality management processes related to pain management and to develop initiatives for the larger pain program, department, or institution.
         (1) A study done in 1999 showed the role of the clinical nurse specialist as an influence on nursing practice and pain management outcomes in the acute care setting. This study, a descriptive study of interventions including new routes of postoperative analgesia and a focused educational program, involved assessment of postoperative pain and baseline audit of nursing documentation. Evaluations at 3 months and 2 years indicated improvement in documentation and management of pain (White, 1999).
   4. *Administrative leader:* The pain management clinical nurse specialist may be hired as a nursing or administrative leader for an institutional pain program or an independent pain clinic to perform the following functions:
      a. Coordinate, hire, and schedule staff to ensure optimal pain personnel coverage.
      b. Hold responsibility for developing and understanding reimbursement and billing strategies to ensure appropriate growth and income potential.
      c. Evaluate systems, products, and processes that will ensure cost containment without a decrease in the quality of patient care and clinical pain practices.
      d. Hold responsibility for the management and evaluation of pain management personnel.

5. *Researcher:* The pain management clinical nurse specialist is involved in either partnering on or conducting pain management research. This involvement would include the identification and investigation of problems within the clinical setting.
6. *Educator:* It is well established that clinical nurse specialists are educators for patients or clients and nurses within hospitals and hospital systems. Clinical nurse specialists are often also clinical educators within schools of nursing in colleges and universities.

VI. Vision of the Future for Clinical Nurse Specialist Practice

A. Clinical nurse specialist practice
   1. As hospitals strive to attain Magnet status, it is imperative and is well documented that the clinical nurse specialist plays an integral role in this process as an institutional leader in evidence and outcome-based nursing care.
   2. As more clinical nurse specialists obtain prescriptive authority, the role may include providing more direct inpatient care, ordering tests, ordering durable medical supplies, and prescribing of pharmacological agents (Goudreau et al., 2007). As a pain practitioner, this could include a greater focus on direct patient care, as well as continued work as a consultant and program leader.
   3. With the development of new care delivery systems that include length-of-stay initiatives, the clinical nurse specialist has the educational background to assure patient safety and efficacious practice within a cost-effective program.
   4. As health care costs increase, the expertise of the clinical nurse specialist will be used to analyze the cost-benefit ratio of new products, interventions, and programs (Goudreau et al., 2007).
   5. With an increase in the aging population, it will be imperative to include the clinical nurse specialist in the planning of programs and therapies that are effective, safe, and cost-effective for the elderly. This includes the clinical nurse specialist understanding insurance and Medicare and Medicaid payment systems and benefits.

B. Education
   1. In October 2004, the American Association of Colleges of Nursing (AACN, 2004) endorsed the *Position Statement on the Practice Doctorate in Nursing* and decided that the level of education for all advanced practice nursing roles should be moved from a master's degree to a doctoral degree by 2015 (AACN, 2008). This decision was based on
      a. The changing demands of the nation's complex health care environment.
      b. The rapid expansion of knowledge that underlies practice.
      c. Shortages of doctorally prepared nursing faculty.
      d. Increasing complexity of care.
      e. National concerns about safety of care.
      f. An increase in the need for clinical and administrative leadership in patient care areas.
      g. An increase in the need for leadership in the discipline of nursing.
   2. The doctor of nursing practice (DNP)
      a. Focus is normally evidence-based practice versus research.
      b. A movement is occurring in the direction of other health professionals such as medicine, pharmacy, dentistry, physical therapy, and audiology (AACN, 2008).
      c. Current nursing master's degree programs often carry a credit load equivalent to doctoral degrees in other health professionals (AACN, 2008).
      d. The doctor of nursing practice degree will share rigorous and demanding expectations: a scholarly approach to the discipline of nursing and a commitment to nursing practice (AACN, 2007a).
      e. *The Essentials of Doctoral Education for Advanced Practice Nursing* as stated by AACN (2007b) are
         (1) Scientific underpinnings for practice.
         (2) Organization and system leadership and management, quality improvement, and systems thinking.

(3) Clinical scholarship and analytical methods for evidence-based practice.
(4) Information systems and technology and patient care technology for the improvement and transformation of health care.
(5) Health policy for advocacy in health care.
(6) Interprofessional collaboration for improving patient and population health care outcomes.
(7) Clinical prevention and population health for improving the nation's health.
(8) Advanced nursing practice.

Summary

Attainment of the doctor of nursing practice degree would prepare the pain practitioner to influence not only health care outcomes in the three spheres of influence but also pain care practice at the local, state, national, and international levels (Goudreau et al., 2007). According to AACN (2007b) it would also prepare the practitioner to do the following:

1. Use science-based theories to determine the significance of health care phenomena and to describe the actions required to enhance, alleviate, and ameliorate health care phenomena.
2. Eliminate health care disparities and evaluate approaches to meet the needs of this population.
3. Use analytical methods to evaluate literature and evidence for practice.
4. Design and direct quality improvement methodologies.
5. Evaluate health care information systems and patient care technology.
6. Demonstrate the conceptual ability and technical skills to develop and execute a plan involving data extraction from information systems and databases.
7. Design, influence, and implement health care policies that frame health care financing, practice regulation, access, safety, quality, and efficacy.
8. Synthesize concepts, including psychosocial dimensions and cultural diversity, related to clinical prevention and population health in developing, implementing, and evaluating interventions to address health promotion, improve health status, and address gaps in the care of individuals, aggregates, or population.
9. Practice at the aggregate, systems, and organization level.

References

American Association of Colleges of Nursing. (2004). *Nurse practitioner and clinical nurse specialist competencies for older adult care.* Washington, DC: Author.

American Association of Colleges of Nursing. (2007a). *The essentials of master's education for the advanced practice nursing.* Washington, DC: Author.

American Association of Colleges of Nursing. (2007b). *The essentials of doctoral education for the advanced practice nursing.* Washington, DC: Author.

American Association of Colleges of Nursing. (2008). *Doctor of nursing practice (DNP) talking points.* Washington, DC: Author.

American Nurses Association. (2004). *Nursing scope and standards of practice.* Washington, DC: ANA nursesbooks.org.

Chuk, P. K. (1997). Clinical nurse specialists and quality patient care. *Journal of Advanced Nursing, 26,* 501–506.

Darmody, J. V. (2005). Observing the work of the clinical nurse specialist: A pilot study. *Clinical Nurse Specialist, 19*(5), 260–268.

Goudreau, K. A., Clark, A., Lyon, B., & Rust, J. (2007). A vision of the future for clinical nurse specialists. *Clinical Nurse Specialist, 21*(6), 310–320.

Hamric, A. B., & Spross, A. (1989). *The clinical nurse specialist in theory and practice* (classic ed.). Philadelphia: W. B. Saunders.

LaSala, C. A., Connors, P. M., Pedro, J. T., & Phipps, M. (2007). The role of the clinical nurse specialist in promoting evidence-based practice and effecting positive patient outcomes. *Journal of Continuing Education in Nursing, 38*(6), 262–270.

McCaffery, M., & Pasero, C. (1999). *Pain: Clinical manual* (2nd ed.). St. Louis: Mosby.

National Association of Clinical Nurse Specialists. (2004). *Model rules and regulations for CNS title protection and scope of practice. Statement on clinical nurse specialist practice and education.* Harrisburg, PA: Author.

Rose, S. B., All, A. C., & Gresham, D., (2008). Role preservation of the clinical nurse specialist practitioner. *Internet Journal of Advanced Nursing Practice, ISSN* 1523-6064.

White, C. L. (1999). Changing pain management practice and impacting on patient outcomes. *Clinical Nurse Specialist, 13*(4), 169–179.

Zuzelo, P. R. (2003). Clinical nurse specialist practice: Spheres of influence. *AORN, 77*(2), 361–364, 366, 369–372.

Zuzelo, P. R. (2007). *The clinical nurse specialist handbook.* Sudbury, MA: Jones and Bartlett.

Suggested Readings

Baldwin, K. M., Lyon, B. L., Clark, A. P., Fulton, J., & Dayhoff, N. (2007). Developing clinical nurse specialist practice competencies. *Clinical Nurse Specialist, 21*(6).

Barker, A. M. (Ed.). (2009). *Advanced practice nursing: Essential knowledge for the profession.* Sudbury, MA: Jones and Bartlett.

Chase, S. K., & Pruitt, R. H. (2006). The practice doctorate: Innovation or disruption? *Journal of Nursing Education, 45*(5), 155–161.

Hamric, A. B., Spross, J. A., & Hanson, C. M. (Eds.). (2005). *Advanced practice nursing: An integrative approach* (3rd ed.). St. Louis: Elsevier Saunders.

Michaels, T. K., Hubbartt, E., Carroll, S., A., & Hudson-Barr, D. (2007). Evaluating an educational approach to improve pain assessment in hospitalized patients. *Journal of Nursing Care Quality, 22*(3), 260–265.

Musclow, S., Monakshi, M., & Watt-Watson, J. (2002). The emerging role of advanced nursing practice in acute pain management throughout Canada. *Clinical Nurse Specialist, 16*(2), 63–62.

Nelson, P. J., Holland, D. E., Derscheid, D., & Tucker, S. J. (2007). Clinical nurse specialist influence in the conduct of research in a clinical agency. *Clinical Nurse Specialist, 21*(2), 95–100.

Pipe, T. (2006). Optimizing nursing care by integrating theory-driven evidence-based practice. *Journal of Nursing Care Quality, 22*(3), 234–238.

Sievers, B., & Wolf, S. (2006). Achieving clinical nurse specialist competencies and outcomes through interdisciplinary education. *Clinical Nurse Specialist, 20*(2), 75–80.

chapter

31

The Role of the Nurse Practitioner in Pain Management Nursing

Michelle L. Witkop, FNP-BC, ACHPN

Objectives

After studying this chapter, the reader should be able to:

1. Define the role of the nurse practitioner.
2. Differentiate among sources of licensure and certification for nurse practitioners.
3. Differentiate among levels of certification for licensure versus specialty.
4. Identify four components of an evaluation for pain.
5. Identify four types of treatment options that nurse practitioners can use to treat pain based on goal setting.
6. Describe prescriptive authority for nurse practitioners.

I. History of Nurse Practitioners

A. Nurse practitioners originated through the vision and efforts of Loretta C. Ford and Henry Silver at the University of Colorado Medical Center in 1965 (Ford, 1997). The role began as a demonstration project to develop the pediatric nurse practitioner role with two goals:
   1. Test the expansion of the scope of practice of nurses for well-child care in community-based settings.
   2. Have findings integrated into collegiate nursing curricula (Ford, 1997).

B. The project expanded the role of nursing assessment and clinical judgment while remaining grounded in prevention and promotion of the health of individuals and families.

C. Barriers at the time included lack of leadership and interest by nursing educators, leading to insufficient curricula standards and controls, multiple specialties, and eventual issues with political support and financing (Ford, 1997).

D. Monies for training and establishment of nurse practitioner programs were first obtained through the Nurse Training Act of 1964, Title II of the 1968 Health Manpower Act, and the Nurse Training Act of 1975 (Hawkins & Thibodeau, 1993).

E. In 1974, the American Nurses Association congress of nursing practice published definitions of the advanced practice role that included scope of practice issues and required skills.

F. The National Organization of Nurse Practitioner Faculties was organized in 1974 as a small group of educators who developed the nurse practitioner core competencies and domains for curricula guidelines. The first guidelines were developed in 1990, with updated versions released in 1995, 2000, 2002, and 2006 (National Organization of Nurse Practitioner Faculties, 2006).

G. In 1976, the American Nurses Association implemented the first nurse practitioner certification.

II. Definitions

A. The American College of Nurse Practitioners (ACNP, 2008e; AANP, 2002) defines nurse practitioners as registered nurses who are prepared, through advanced education and clinical training, to provide a range of preventive and acute health care services to individuals of all ages.
   1. Nurse practitioners complete graduate-level education preparation that leads to a master's degree.
   2. Responsibilities include compiling health histories, completing physical examinations, diagnosing and treating many common acute and chronic problems, interpreting laboratory results and X-rays, prescribing and managing medications and other therapies, providing health teaching and supportive counseling with an emphasis on prevention of illness and health maintenance, and referring patients to other health professionals as needed.
   3. Nurse practitioners are authorized to practice across the nation and have prescriptive privileges, of varying degrees, in all 50 states.

B. Today, the pain management nurse practitioner role encompasses many areas of practice along the health care continuum.
   1. New education programs encourage the development of nurse practitioners in many specialty areas of practice, including oncology, palliative care, chronic pain management, acute pain management, intensive care, and cardiac care. Specialties emerge based on the health care needs of the population.
   2. Research supports positive patient outcomes by nurse practitioners, patient education being the number one reason for those outcomes (Holcomb, 2000).

III. Practice and Education

A. According to the Health Resources and Services Administration (2004), the combination of the nurse practitioners' clinical knowledge and experience as registered nurses with their advanced clinical training enables them to work with patients on a range of clinical tasks.
   1. Growing numbers of specialties and settings have found acceptance of the nurse practitioner's ability to manage patients in both inpatient and outpatient settings.
   2. The current number of practicing nurse practitioners is smaller than the number of practicing physicians, so they are employed in only a fraction of the sites where physicians work.

B. Licensure of nurse practitioners is done by each state board of nursing or other state-designated agencies, with the board of nursing regulating advance practice according to each state's nurse practice act.
   1. Nurse practitioners are licensed independent practitioners who may specialize but are not licensed at their specialty. It is expected that nurse practitioners practice within standards established or recognized by a licensing body.
      a. Each nurse practitioner is accountable to patients, the nursing profession, and the licensing board to comply with the requirements of the state nurse practice act for the quality of the advance nursing practice rendered, for recognizing their limits of knowledge and experience, and for consulting with and referring patients to other health care providers as appropriate.
      b. Specialties provide depth in a nurse's practice within the established population foci (AANP, 2007a through 2007e).
   2. Phillips (2007) discusses the legislative atmosphere of the nation for advance practice nursing.
   3. Graphs show which states regulate nurse practitioners through the nursing board versus a combined effort with the state nursing board and the board of medicine (AANP, 2008b).

C. Demographics
   1. The 2004 Health Resources and Services Administration sample survey report shows 141,209 nurse practitioners in the United States, an increase of more than 27% over 2000 data. The actual number of nurse practitioners in 2006 was estimated to be at least 145,000 (ACNP, 2008a).
   2. Certification is available for nurse practitioners through the American Nurses Credentialing Center (ANCC) and the American Academy of Nurse Practitioners (AANP) (ACNP, 2008b) and through the Pediatric Nursing Certification Board.
      a. The ANCC (2008) offers eight certifications for nurse practitioners:
         (1) Acute care
         (2) Adult
         (3) Family
         (4) Gerontological
         (5) Pediatric
         (6) Adult psychiatric or mental health
         (7) Family psychiatric or mental health
         (8) Advanced diabetic management
      b. The AANP (2008a, 2008c) offers three specialty certifications:
         (1) Adult
         (2) Gerontological
         (3) Family nurse practitioner
      c. The Pediatric Nursing Certification Board offers certification to primary care and acute care pediatric nurse practitioners.
      d. Once certified as a nurse practitioner, additional specialty certification can be obtained.
         (1) Certification can be obtained through the ANCC (2008) specifically for pain management nursing.
            (a) This certification informs the public of the specialization of nurses and their advanced study beyond their licensure.
            (b) This certification is not for licensure.
         (2) The Hospice and Palliative Nurses Association offers certification for nurse practitioners who specialize in end-of-life care, including pain and symptom management (Hospice and Palliative Nurses Association, 2008).

D. Education
   1. Advance practice registered nurses are described as nurse practitioners, clinical nurse specialists, nurse anesthetists, and certified nurse midwives (American Association of Colleges of Nursing, 2004).
   2. Historically, most nurse practitioner programs were post-registered nurse certificate programs focusing heavily on clinical training. Currently, the nurse practitioner education programs in the United States confer a master's degree based on the criteria set by the *Criteria for Evaluation of*

Nurse Practitioner Programs and endorsed by the ACNP (2008d). The document containing the criteria for evaluating nurse practitioner programs is available at http://www.nonpf.com/criteria.htm (National Organization of Nurse Practitioner Faculties, 2006).

3. In 2004, the ANCC developed a position statement paper regarding the research-focused doctorate and the practice-focused doctorate. The recommendations included the following:
   a. Using the term *practice doctorate* instead of *clinical doctorate.*
   b. Using only one degree title, *doctorate of nursing practice,* which should represent this terminal degree, and phasing out other titles.
   c. Planning a transition period to allow master's prepared nurse practitioners to obtain additional education.
   d. Having the doctorate of nursing practice be the terminal degree for nurse practitioners beginning in 2015.

E. Pain management
   1. The role of the nurse practitioner in pain management is emerging and growing.
   2. The level of independence, level of collaboration, and scope of practice vary according to geographical location, state regulations and guidelines, institutional policies, and the expertise and comfort level of the involved practitioners (Schneider, 2008).
   3. The ASPMN reports that 154 (almost 10%) of its 1,596 members are nurse practitioners.

IV. Merging the Pain Specialist and Nurse Practitioner Roles

A. The role of the pain management nurse practitioner is to provide pain management along a continuum of care that is supported by the licensure. It encompasses many areas of practice, including acute, chronic, and long-term care.
   1. As with many physicians, on-the-job training is the norm, with many job descriptions developing progressively as the role expands.
   2. More formalized general training programs are being offered across the nation, but little is offered specifically for the nurse practitioner.
   3. A clinical preceptorship with a pain management nurse practitioner is the ideal educational forum. But as Schneider (2008) noted, the role expands as the confidence and experience of nurse practitioners increase within their setting. As the role expands, more nurse practitioners are being recruited for employment in pain management settings.

B. The following are basic competencies for practice.
   1. Evaluation
      a. The history and physical examination are the basis for diagnosis and treatment. Proceeding in an orderly, systematic fashion limits the possibility of overlooking a key issue. Developing a partnership with the patient through open communication allows integration of all physical and psychological features that will affect the outcome of any evaluation.
      b. In this age of ever increasing technology, excellent communication and interviewing skills that focus on the patient as a whole will lead to enhanced differential diagnosis and outcomes (Seidel, Ball, Dains, & Benedict, 1991) (see the chapter on Pain Assessment).
      c. Differential diagnosis
         (1) A sequential comprehensive physical examination coupled with a thorough history defines the potential differential diagnosis. Techniques in the interview should include facilitation, reflection, clarification, and empathetic responses.
         (2) It is important to integrate primary disease management with analgesic therapy. The process must facilitate pharmacological, nonpharmacological, cognitive, and complementary and integrative modalities, with the ultimate goal being quality patient outcomes and pain disease management. Goals and measurable benchmarks need to be identified for each patient.
         (3) The application of differential diagnosis in the pain management process includes identification of possible diagnoses (e.g., radiculopathy versus stenosis) and integration of primary disease treatment with analgesic therapy (e.g., diabetic peripheral neuropathy).

Consideration is given to comorbidities (e.g., ulcer disease, liver disease, and kidney disease) in determining appropriate medications to use.

(4) The pain management nurse practitioner is often the initial pain specialist that the patient encounters for first-line evaluation. Pain as an indicator of disease remains the tenet of the physical evaluation.

d. Initial treatment planning

(1) The pain management nurse practitioner identifies emergency pain treatment scenarios, assesses quickly, intervenes promptly, and begins the treatment plan.

(2) The initial treatment plan should flow logically from the pain assessment. Whenever possible, the patient and, if appropriate, family or significant other is included in this planning.

(3) Frequent reevaluation and assessment drive the adjustments to the plan.

(4) Thorough planning incorporates several options or contingency plan when first options fail.

(5) The pain management nurse practitioner should look at a multimodal approach to pain management, which includes rational combinations of analgesics with different mechanisms of actions.

(a) Pharmacological mechanisms are nonsteroidal anti-inflammatory drugs, acetaminophen, opioids, antidepressants, and anticonvulsants, etc.

(b) Nonpharmacological mechanisms include physical therapy, transcutaneous electrical nerve stimulation, interferential stimulators, blocks, neural blockade, implanted nerve stimulators, and implanted pain pumps.

(c) Cognitive modalities are biofeedback, cognitive-behavioral therapy, counseling, distraction, guided imagery, etc.

(d) Complementary and integrative modalities are massage, hypnosis, acupuncture, acupressure, etc.

(e) A multimodal approach is driven by patient demand: active integration of complementary and traditional techniques is becoming more standard. The nurse practitioner must question the patient on use of these mechanisms during the initial history taking.

e. Initial goal setting

(1) Mutual goals of the nurse practitioner, the patient, and when appropriate, the family are set, defining outcomes for evaluation.

(2) Pain levels, functionality, psychosocial status, and quality of life that are consistent with the disease and pain state measure outcomes for the pain patient.

(3) Medication agreements should be used to develop a clear understanding of the guidelines that need to be followed when certain medications are used.

f. Multidisciplinary interface

(1) Recognition of the inherent value of ongoing collaborative treatment with other disciplines and specialists is imperative.

(2) This contrasts with referring a patient to another specialized provider and then not continuing to follow the patient or with seeking a one-time consultation with a specialty provider.

g. Merged role

(1) Despite the expansion of advance nursing practice to incorporate parts of the medical model into the nurse practitioner role, it is essential to maintain the timeless and enduring nature of nursing.

(2) Nursing is "caring for and about others, helping them to optimize their health strengths through education, forming partnerships to accomplish the goals of primary, secondary, and tertiary prevention, and health promotion" (Ford, 1997, p. 4).

(3) "Pain is not a homogenous sensation; rather, the intensity, quality, and duration of pain can vary according to the stimuli, pathological condition, and molecular mechanisms involved" (Carr, 2004, p. 16).

(4) Schneider (2008) recognizes that nurse practitioners are important in pain management and to the multidisciplinary team. The role varies depending on the environment, but nurse practitioner outcomes in general have been shown to be positive for the patient (Holcomb, 2000). While pain is not homogenous, neither is pain management nor the team that evaluates and treats pain. Nurse practitioners play a vital role on that team.

h. Barriers to treatment include the following (Schneider, 2008).
   (1) Fear of addiction
   (2) Fear of regulatory scrutiny
   (3) Lack of knowledge by providers, as well as by patients
   (4) Lack of sufficient numbers of pain specialists
   (5) Reluctance of primary care providers to take back patients and continue treatment plans started by pain specialists

2. Patient and family education
   a. Preventive teaching for chronic disease management
      (1) Nurse practitioners incorporate preventive teaching as a fundamental part of chronic disease management (e.g., back health through appropriate body mechanics). They also use disease-based education as a part of the global treatment planning.
   b. Education
      (1) Education is important for the patient and the family.
         (a) This should include the pathophysiology and basic concepts of pain (transduction, transmission, perception, modulation, and the various places in the pain pathway where therapies interrupt the pain cycle).
         (b) Emphasize the importance of accurate and consistent pain assessment.
         (c) Explain pharmacological, nonpharmacological, and cognitive pain treatment rationale.
         (d) Teach the patient and family the importance of adherence to optimize control of constant pain, as well as to quickly or preemptively control episodic pain.
         (e) Explain the need to communicate continually and effectively with health care providers.
      (2) The merged role of the nurse practitioner integrates preventive and disease-based education with pain-specific teaching for the patient and family.
         (a) This education covers episodic, acute, and chronic pain along the continuum of living with lifelong pain.
         (b) The concept of pain as a symptom of a bigger disease process and a complex symptom requiring focused planning and treatment should be discussed.
         (c) The nurse practitioner should show the knowledge base, interpersonal skills, and awareness of the learning needs for patient and family education.
      (3) Functional goal setting and limitations, implications of stress, and quality of life goals should all be addressed.
         (a) The goals should reflect a realistic view of the underlying pathology.
         (b) Goal setting should be done with a focus on what is achievable within defined time frames.
      (4) Chronic pain coping skills
         (a) Physical limit setting and pacing of activity are based on the pain complaint.
         (b) Stress reduction and management and their implication in ongoing pain complaints and relief are key skills.
         (c) This type of education and support should be initiated early and repeated often by the nurse practitioner.

3. Comprehensive treatment planning
   a. For the nurse practitioner, treatment planning flows from the differential diagnosis process. A diagnosis of diabetic peripheral neuropathy leads to a comprehensive treatment plan that incorporates nutritional education, dietary planning, exercise and weight loss, self-monitoring

of blood glucose, routine monitoring of kidney function, medication management, and a multitude of other health issues.
  b. Pain management nurse practitioners analyze assessment data and analgesic history to plan pharmacological and nonpharmacological therapies. These therapies facilitate improved pain outcomes that may or may not be associated with improved disease outcomes.
  c. The ideal merged role integrates both the nursing and the medical model. The nurse practitioner incorporates the differential diagnosis process, with a focus on comorbidities, as well as pain and symptom management, while pulling the best of both approaches into a comprehensive treatment-planning domain.
4. Evaluation of treatment efficacy
  a. Expected frequencies of reassessment are defined in the treatment plan.
  b. Efficacy is measured against the planned goals.
  c. Efficacy always must be measured against the toxicity associated with the prescribed therapy.
  d. Controlled pain is defined within the domains of the specific disease state and based on previously stated goals.
  e. In chronic pain populations, goals are defined in the context of function, pain perception, and quality of life.
  f. Psychological indicators of success include reduction in anxiety or depression, reengagement with work or family dynamics, or active use of coping techniques as a part of an integrated strategy.

V. Scope of Practice of the Pain Management Nurse Practitioner

A. Professional role
  1. Specialty focused
    a. The nurse practitioner is a unique health care provider within the constellation of the four roles of the advanced practice nurses: nurse practitioners, certified nurse midwives, nurse anesthetists, and clinical nurse specialists.
    b. Nurse practitioners practice according to their specialty, providing medical and nursing services to individuals, families, and groups.
    c. Services from a pain management nurse practitioner include history taking, physical examination, imaging and laboratory diagnostic testing with interpretation, prescribing of pharmacological agents, and nonpharmacological therapies. Counseling, education, and advocacy are key components of the role, along with research and pain consultation.
  2. Responsibility
    a. The pain management nurse practitioner's clinical practice is autonomous, with accountability for outcomes. High-quality care in pain management is ensured by periodic peer review, patient outcomes, maintenance of clinical skills, and continued certification and development. Research, leadership in the field, and improved clinical outcomes define quality practice.
    b. The role of the pain management nurse practitioner continually evolves in response to pain health care needs and societal changes.
    c. Leadership in pain management combines the role of clinician, researcher, mentor, educator, and administrator to provide quality pain management for the patient.
    d. National, state, and local participation in pain health care policy and involvement in professional organizations is crucial.
    e. Advancement of the pain management nurse practitioner role must be maintained through standards of practice (AANP, 2007c, 2007e; ACNP, 2008c).
  3. Legislative
    a. All nursing organizations have legislative arms to monitor and influence legislation pertinent to nursing and health care.
    b. As a patient advocate, nurse practitioners are encouraged to be involved with all levels of political platforms.

c. Ford (1997) encouraged nurses to promote and develop political careers. Ford felt a nurse should be a "leader and statesperson" (p. 5) to influence national and global health care. In a keynote address at the Children's Hospital of Philadelphia's advanced practice nurse conference on May 7, 2009, Loretta Ford stated, "... [the] new doctorate ... is necessary and very appropriate ... to advance their knowledge" (Ford, 2009).

d. Advancement of the pain management nurse practitioner role is the responsibility of the nurse practitioner (AANP, 2007e). The recent increased use of the Internet to promote legislative issues simplifies personal involvement with local, state, and national political leaders.

4. Research
   a. The AANP (2007e, p. 4) states in its standards of practice document that "nurse practitioners support research by developing clinical research questions, conducting or participating in studies, and disseminating and incorporating findings into [evidence-based] practice."
5. Professional associations
   a. Active participation in professional associations encourages networking, advocacy, and specialty awareness.

VI. Clinical Practice Considerations for the Pain Management Nurse Practitioner

A. Practice styles and settings (Schneider, 2008)

1. The nurse practitioner may be employed in the following settings:
   a. Hospital
      (1) Inpatient or outpatient
         (a) Increasing numbers of hospitals are employing nurse practitioner to see patients either in outpatient clinics or on inpatient consult teams (acute pain, chronic pain, palliative care, and oncology).
      (2) Privileges
         (a) Privileges are based on each individual institution's credentialing process and policies.
         (b) They are approved by the hospital's credentialing body.
   b. Long-term care
      (1) Extended-care facilities
      (2) Assisted living
      (3) Transitional care
      (4) Residential care
   c. Hospice and home health agencies
   d. Medical group
2. Independent private practice may employ a nurse practitioner based on state guidelines and regulatory atmosphere.
3. Certain states require a collaborative practice agreement for practice, prescriptive authority, or both (Phillips, 2007).
   a. Prescriptive authority (Phillips, 2007)
      (1) Prescriptive authority is state dictated.
      (2) The ability for pain management nurse practitioners to prescribe independently is defined as plenary prescriptive authority. As of 2006, all 50 states have some type of prescriptive authority for nurse practitioners.
   b. Collaborative authority
      (1) Collaborative authority requires physician oversight of prescribing and a collaborative agreement between the nurse practitioner and the physician that indicates the parameters of the prescription authority.
4. Scheduled drugs
   a. Limitations on certain drug prescriptions (schedule II to V) are defined by the federal government.
   b. Each state determines the nurse practitioners ability to prescribe scheduled drugs. As of 2007, only three states did not allow some type of scheduled drug prescriptive authority for

nurse practitioners. Each nurse practitioner must investigate the laws or guidelines within his or her own state to determine the optimal method of providing best practice when scheduled drugs are indicated.

B. Reimbursement (Phillips, 2007)
   1. Medicare
      a. Medicare is a federally regulated program.
      b. The Balanced Budget Act of 1997 was a major turning point for nurse practitioners. It allowed for the direct reimbursement of nurse practitioners in urban practice sites, where previously only nurse practitioners working in rural health care settings could receive Medicare reimbursement.
      c. Nurse practitioners, regardless of geographical location, should apply for the National Provider Information number that is required for billing.
      d. Nurse practitioners are traditionally reimbursed at 85% of the Medicare physician rate.
   2. Medicaid
      a. Medicaid is a state regulated program.
      b. Each state determines the ability of nurse practitioners to receive reimbursement, as well as the level of reimbursement.
   3. Third-party payers
      a. Nurse practitioners must apply for and be approved for inclusion into various preferred provider groups and managed care organizations, in the same manner as physicians, to bill fee-for-service.
   4. State and national nurse association groups continue to actively work on legislation to improve the reimbursement atmosphere for all nurse practitioners.

C. Where clinical nurse specialists and nurse practitioners meet
   1. The pain management nurse practitioner role combines the specialty expertise and critical thinking with the evaluation and management training of the nurse practitioner to provide effective patient care.
   2. The practice is evidence based.
   3. Counseling, education, advocacy, research, and pain consultations are key components to the role of the pain management nurse practitioner.
   4. As time goes on, we have seen that the roles of the clinical nurse specialists and the nurse practitioners are not far apart.
   5. With the reinforcement of the nursing organizations, the value of merging the education and practice of the clinical nurse specialist and the nurse practitioner will be realized. The doctorate of nursing practice is a step in this direction (American Association of Colleges of Nursing, 2004).
   6. The roles continue to evolve, and it is the patients who will benefit.

Summary

The role of nurse practitioner provides a system-wide clinical pain management approach with seamless standards of care. In the past, most education was through on-the-job training. In the future, it is hoped that more advanced practice nurse level of pain management courses will be developed and standardized. Specialty graduate programs are expected to be developed. The pain management nurse practitioner is rapidly becoming an integral part of rehabilitation, surgical, oncology, pediatric, and other department programs. The pain management nurse practitioner role has and will continue to affect pain outcomes and patient outcomes positively and will provide a community resource for pain management knowledge.

References

American Academy of Nurse Practitioners. (2002). *Nurse practitioners as an advance practice nurse role position statement.* Retrieved November 18, 2008, from http://www.npfinder.com/faq.pdf.

American Academy of Nurse Practitioners. (2007a). *Discussion paper: Doctor of nursing practice.* Retrieved November 18, 2008, from http://aanp.org/NR/rdonlyres/9DC9390F-145D-4768-995C-1C1FD12AC77C/0/DiscussionPaperDoctor_of_NursingPrac.pdf.

American Academy of Nurse Practitioners. (2007b). *Position statement on nurse practitioner prescriptive authority.* Retrieved November 18, 2008, from http://aanp.org/NR/rdonlyres/CFCFB108-1215-4BCF-93B2-1174CA9C4413/0/PrescriptivePrivileges.pdf.

American Academy of Nurse Practitioners. (2007c). *Quality of nurse practitioner practice.* Retrieved November 18, 2008, from http://aanp.org/NR/rdonlyres/34E7FF57-E071-4014-B554-FF02B82FF2F2/0/Quality_of_NP_Prac112907.pdf.

American Academy of Nurse Practitioners. (2007d). *Scope of practice for nurse practitioners.* Retrieved November 18, 2008, from http://aanp.org/NR/rdonlyres/FCA07860-3DA1-46F9-80E6-E93A0972FB0D/0/Scope_of_Practice.pdf.

American Academy of Nurse Practitioners. (2007e). *Standards of practice for nurse practitioners.* Retrieved November 18, 2008, from http://aanp.org/NR/rdonlyres/FE00E81B-FA96-4779-972B-6162F04C309F/0/Standards_of_Practice112907.pdf.

American Academy of Nurse Practitioners. (2008a). *Certification exam: Program description.* Retrieved November 18, 2008, from http://aanpcertification.org/.

American Academy of Nurse Practitioners. (2008b). *Nurse practitioner regulatory authority map.* Retrieved November 18, 2008, from http://www.capwiz.com/aanp/home/.

American Academy of Nurse Practitioners. (2008c). *Purpose of certification exam.* Retrieved November 18, 2008, from http://aanpcertification.org/.

American Association of Colleges of Nursing. (2004). *Position statement on the practice doctorate in nursing.* Retrieved November 18, 2008, from http://www.acnpweb.org/files/public/DNP_GROUP_LETTER_6-08_w_copyright.pdf.

American College of Nurse Practitioners. (2008a). *Number of nurse practitioners in U.S.* Retrieved May 30, 2008, from http://www.acnpweb.org/i4a/pages/Index.cfm?pageID=3353.

American College of Nurse Practitioners. (2008b). *Nurse practitioner certification.* Retrieved November 18, 2008, from http://www.acnpweb.org/i4a/pages/index.cfm?pageid=3324.

American College of Nurse Practitioners. (2008c). *Nurse practitioners scope of practice.* Retrieved November 18, 2008, from http://www.acnpweb.org/i4a/pages/index.cfm?pageid=3465.

American College of Nurse Practitioners. (2008d). *Position paper: Nurse practitioner education.* Retrieved May 24, 2008, from http://www.acnpweb.org.

American College of Nurse Practitioners. (2008e). *What is a nurse practitioner?* Retrieved May 29, 2008, from http://www.acnpweb.org/i4a/pages/index.cfm?pageid=3479#top.

American Nurses Credentialing Center. (2008). *Certification.* Retrieved November 17, 2008, from http://www.nursecredentialing.org/certification.aspx.

Carr, D. B. (2004). *The spectrum of pain.* New York: McMahon.

Ford, L. C. (1997). A voice from the past: 30 fascinating years as a nurse practitioner. *Clinical Excellence for Nurse Practitioners, 1*(1), 3–6.

Ford, J. (2009). Disruptive Innovator. *Advance for Nurse Practitioners.* Retrieved from http://nurse-practitioners.advanceweb.com/Editorial/Content/Editorial.aspx?CC=199510, on May 31, 2009.

Hawkins, J. W., & Thibodeau, J. A. (1993). *The advanced practitioner: Current practice issues.* New York: Tiresias Press.

Health Resources and Services Administration. (2004). *A comparison of changes in the professional practice of nurse practitioners, physician assistants, and certified nurse midwives: 1992 and 2000.* Retrieved May 24, 2008, from http://www.bhpr.hrsa.gov/healthworkforce/reports/nursing/changeinpractice/chapter4.htm.

Holcomb, L. (2000). A Delphi survey to identify activities of nurse practitioners in primary care. *Clinical Excellence for Nurse Practitioners, 4,* 163–172.

Hospice and Palliative Nurses Association. (1980). *Certification.* Retrieved November, 19, 2008, from http://www.nbchpn.org/DisplayPage.aspx?Title=Why%20Certification?.

National Organization of Nurse Practitioner Faculties. (2006). *Welcome to NONPF.* Retrieved August 23, 2008, from http://www.nonpf.com/index.htm.

Phillips, S. J. (2007). A comprehensive look at the legislative issues affecting advance nursing practice. *Nurse Practitioner, 32*(1), 14–16.

Schneider, J. (2008). Emerging role of NPs and PAs in pain management. *Practical Pain Management, June,* 22–27.

Seidel, H. M., Ball, J. W., Dains, J. E., & Benedict, G. W. (1991). *Mosby's guide to physical examination* (3rd ed.). St. Louis: Mosby.

Suggested Readings

Bates, B. (1991). *A guide to physical examination and history taking* (5th ed.). Philadelphia: J. B. Lippincott.

Bickley, L. S., Bates, B., & Szilagyi, P. G. (2005). *Bates guide to physical examination and history taking.* Philadelphia: Lippincott Williams & Wilkins.

McCaffery, M., & Pasero, C. (1999). *Pain: A clinical manual* (2nd ed.). St. Louis: Mosby.

Suggested Reading

National Task Force on Quality Nurse Practitioner Education. (2002). *Criteria for evaluation of nurse practitioner programs.* Washington, DC: Author.

chapter

32

Future of Pain Management Nursing

Paul Arnstein, PhD, RN, CS

Objectives

After studying this chapter, the reader should be able to:

1. Understand the contribution of pain management nursing to the nursing profession as a whole.
2. Develop a vision for the future of the clinical practice in pain management nursing.

On a train ride en route to his last International Association for the Study of Pain (IASP) plenary speech in Vienna, Austria, Patrick Wall, co-founder of the Melzack-Wall Gate Theory, was engaged in a conversation with this author to clarify a point for the first edition of the American Society for Pain Management Nursing's core curriculum chapter on pain theories. He validated the interpretation before explaining his change in thinking. His view of pain modulation as a dorsal horn "gate" (akin to an on-off switch) was updated with a "gain" (volume dial-like) mechanism. This gain system is likened to a series of pain signal amplifiers and dampeners extending beyond the dorsal horn, throughout the nervous system, as various environmental, social, and cultural factors influence the perception of pain (Wall, 1999). He also found it useful to view pain as a drive, like hunger, and saw the need for "an awareness of an action plan to be rid of it" (Wall, 1999).

In his 1999 book *Pain: The Science of Suffering,* Wall reflected on the nature of pain from his perspective as a neuroscientist and person living with a painful life-limiting disease. Despite the scathing critique of most health professionals, he believed that physical therapists or nurses were in the best position to solve the mysteries of pain (Wall, 1999). Physical therapists were singled out because of their understanding of "action systems." Nurses were favored by Wall to solve the mysteries of pain given their patient-centered focus and broad knowledge base, including an understanding of human responses, environmental influences, and the context of pain to the person's everyday life (personal communication, August 24, 1999). A prerequisite for nursing success is the need to shed "their own social stereotypes" that may bias care based on gender or other factors (Wall, 1999).

Wall's high opinion of nurses was likely shaped by the contributions of Margo McCaffery (1968), who established the foundation of pain management nursing by publishing, articulating, and defending her definition: "Pain is whatever the experiencing person says it is, existing whenever he [the experiencing person] says it does" (McCaffery & Pasero, 1999). Given that pain is the epitome of subjectivity, it requires nurses to ask patients to describe it and then believe their reports of discomfort. McCaffery explained that her definition challenges nurses to cross the line that separates the subjective experience from the objective display of pain, thereby understanding the experience from the patient's perspective (personal communication, September 4, 2008). An understanding of this personal viewpoint is an essential component of effective pain management nursing. This lays the foundation for providing individualized care, educating the patient and family, collaborating with the interdisciplinary team, and advocating for better pain management.

Opportunities to Improve the Current State of Pain Management Nursing

Practice-Based Opportunities for Improving the Quality of Pain Management

Despite an abundance of position papers and evidence-based guidelines detailing clinical approaches that make it possible to prevent or effectively relieve pain in almost all cases, about half of patients with those pain types remain undertreated or untreated. This is true for newborns enduring painful procedures (Maclean, Obispo, & Young, 2007), millions of Americans each year who undergo surgery (American Academy of Pediatrics & Canadian Paediatric Society, 2006), and millions more with chronic diseases like cancer and arthritis. Patients who are very young (Simons et al., 2003), very old (Bernabei et al., 1998), female (Hurley & Adams, 2008), Black, or Hispanic (Pletcher, Kertesz, Kohn, & Gonzales, 2008) are most likely to have their pain go untreated or to receive substandard treatment.

Failures to effectively prevent and control pain have a host of undesired consequences. Transient, but potentially problematic, dysfunctions within the cardiovascular, pulmonary, endocrine, psychological, neurological, metabolic, and immune systems are known to occur with high pain levels, in addition to interferences with eating, sleeping, and activities of daily living. The prolonged impact pain can have on a person's life has generally been underestimated. Almost 5 million Americans develop a pain-related disability each year following surgery or trauma (Rivara et al., 2008). A disturbing proportion of patients who undergo hernia repair, mastectomy, spinal surgery, thoracotomy, or amputation endure persistent pain for months and years after their recovery is complete (Macrae, 2001; Perkins & Kehlet, 2000). Providing preemptive and multimodal approaches, early and often, until pain subsides appears to be a promising strategy to lower the incidence of subsequent pain (Reuben & Buvanendran, 2007; Kehlet & Dahl 1993; Maheshwari, Boutary, Yun, Sirianni, & Dorr, 2006). Having the resources in place to consistently do this remains a challenging opportunity for improvement.

Practice-Based Opportunities for Improving the Safety of Pain Management

In some settings, aggressive efforts to prevent and treat pain have produced a new set of problems. The rise in toxicity and deaths has been noted from even the safest, nonprescription forms of pain relievers. A concerning rise in cases of opioid-induced respiratory depression has resulted in a call to put systems in place capable of identifying and communicating risks, as well as initiating risk-reduction strategies (American Society of Anesthesiologists, 2006). Despite the importance of this challenge, such systems have not been widely implemented (American Society of Anesthesiologists, 2006). All prescription analgesics have U.S. Food and Drug Administration (2007) warnings of potential harm and have a narrow margin for errors.

The Institute for Safe Medication Practices (2008) has identified a host of practice-based opportunities to reduce the risk of harm from these "high alert" drugs. In addition to putting generic safeguards in place, the Joint Commission, formerly known as the Joint Commission on Accreditation of Healthcare Organizations, urges organizations to examine their own practices for their unique problem-prone areas and take measures to eliminate the root causes of errors that harm patients. Although the nurse at the bed space may feel responsible if a patient was harmed by a pain treatment, root causes almost always deal with system errors (including leadership or communication failures) rather than human errors. Most errors that harm patients are really the result of two or more lapses involving different people; thus, the challenge for the future is to continue to refine systems that prevent inevitable errors from reaching the patient.

Education-Based Opportunities for Improvement

Although health care information available to nurse educators is much better than it was a decade ago, nursing and pharmacy textbooks used to educate tomorrow's cohort of professionals continue to be outdated or contain errant information. A study conducted in 2005 of nursing student knowledge and attitudes about pain revealed that the students were no more knowledgeable than previous student cohorts despite substantial advances in the field (Charlton, 2005; Joint Commission, 2008; Plaisance & Logan, 2005). This study, like many that preceded it, consistently showed that students were inadequately prepared to reliably assess and manage pain. Deficiencies were not improved as students progressed from one year of training to the next. Students were unable to answer fundamental questions related to analgesic routes, actions, and side effects and could not conduct a competent assessment.

Despite an International Association for the Study of Pain publication (Charlton, 2005) that delineates suggested nursing curricula content, no effort on a national or international level has been made to integrate standard pain content into the curricula as there has been for topics such as end-of-life care, genetics, and care of older adults. Perhaps integral to having pain content added to the already-full curricula is having pain content added to National Council Licensure Examinations as a core competency required for licensure.

For those nurses already practicing, many states have balked at requiring mandatory education in pain for relicensure. Thus, education-based opportunities for improving knowledge in pain assessment and management falls to organizations that employ nurses. According to revised language in the Joint Commission standards that went into effect January 1, 2009, organizations are responsible to educate all registered nurses, advanced practice nurses, and doctors in pain assessment and pain management (Joint Commission, 2008). This clearly poses an opportunity to correct previous shortcomings in training nurses about pain.

Research-Based Opportunities for Improvement

Many opportunities arise to strengthen research that is relevant to pain management nursing. Increasingly, nurses are using methodologies, interdisciplinary teams, and standardized outcome measures in a way that facilitates their inclusion in major journals and in important systematic reviews. In recent years, nursing research has been strengthened by improved methods, larger sample sizes, and validated measures developed to measure phenomena of interest to nurses (Brown, 2009). Nurse researchers are also strengthening the scientific base by appropriately using trustworthy qualitative methods to explore clinical problems that are not yet quantifiable.

Despite many successful programs of research advancing the art and science of pain management nursing, many important researchable questions remain for nurses to investigate, including the following:

- Evaluation and treatment of pain in low-birth-weight babies.
- Control of perioperative pain in the opioid-tolerant patient.
- Evaluation of pain in developmentally disabled individuals.
- The best strategy for assessing and treating pain in people with an addiction disorder.
- Modification of social, cultural, and environmental factors influencing pain.
- Establishment of safety and efficacy profiles for analgesics used for older adults.
- Relative potency (in analgesic terms) of nondrug pain control methods.
- Analgesic prescribing patterns (a comparison of nurse practitioners to physicians).
- Nursing care of chronic pain patients admitted to hospitals for acute pain flare-ups.
- Quality of pain control as a nurse-sensitive outcome.

Hundreds if not thousands of important research questions need to be answered. A key opportunity includes the need to develop a prioritized research agenda for pain management nursing that can guide university or college faculty, scholars, and funding agencies as they conduct, advise, and support young investigators.

Another major opportunity to improve pain management nursing entails the need to narrow the gap between research and practice. In general areas of nursing, that gap is 17 years from the time of publication until findings are used in practice. This gap was the impetus behind the federally funded clinical practice guidelines written in 1992 and 1994 for acute pain and cancer pain, respectively (Acute Pain Management Guideline Panel, 1992; Jacox et al., 1994). Bridging that gap is even more difficult today, with more than half a million new articles published each year. Over the past year, on average, 2,000 articles a month have been catalogued by PubMed on the subject of pain. It is unrealistic to expect that practicing professionals can stay apprised of this immense literature base, including identifying the most relevant new information, critically reviewing it, synthesizing it, and translating the implications to practice. Thus, ongoing systematic reviews, position papers, and evidence-based clinical guidelines are becoming important tools to help bridge this gap.

A lot of attention has been paid by the Centers for Medicare & Medicaid Services and the Joint Commission in looking at so-called nurse-sensitive outcomes. These outcome studies have set the stage for refusing to reimburse organizations for costly but preventable clinical problems like acquired infections, falls, and dermal ulcers. The literature implies that pain is an important nurse-sensitive outcome, but it currently lacks the research basis needed to attract the attention of these standard-setters. Nurse opinion leaders from around the world believe the quality of pain relief varies based on the number and skill mix of nurses in a given setting (Van den Heede, Clarke, Sermeus, Vleugels, & Aiken, 2007). That research supports the opinion that better pain management is provided in settings with better nurse staffing and higher education levels, but it has yet to influence regulators, payers, and policy makers.

Public Policy-Based Opportunities for Improvement

Opportunities for improving the way in which pain is assessed and managed extend from the bedside to the boardrooms. Problems with fragmentation, gaps, and duplications in services in the American health care delivery system have long been known. Many helpful approaches to treating pain have been abandoned, partly because the reimbursement structure rather than patient need drives health care decisions. For example, unimodal, interventional pain management programs that produce partial, temporary benefit for a limited number of conditions have flourished, while more effective multidisciplinary, multimodal treatment programs have all but disappeared (Loeser, 2005). Insurers routinely deny payment for integrated chronic pain management programs that can be effectively led by nurses (Wells-Federman, Arnstein, & Caudill-Slosberg, 2002), despite evidence that they cut health care costs for years after payers realize a return on their investment (Friedman, Myers, Sobel, Caudill, & Benson, 1995; Lorig, Mazonson, & Holman, 1993).

Pain management nurses represent a valuable resource for meeting many complex needs of patients with severe or chronic pain. Constraints placed by organizational culture, regulations, or reimbursement policies interfere with fully using the clinical expertise and caring capacity of nurses. An opportunity exists to promote better access to these valuable and necessary services for patients and their families with life-altering pain. In addition, because all nurses are accountable for the assessment and management of pain, a clear, consistent interpretation of that role component is needed, which then must be aligned with the expectations of those who employ, educate, regulate, and receive nursing care services.

This important work has begun in many regards as the scope and standards of practice for pain management nursing (American Society for Pain Management Nursing and American Nurses Association, 2005) have been published, and a growing number of state boards of nursing have issued statements and regulatory guidance pertaining to the pain management role in general, as well as specific pain-related activities (including advocacy) that are within the scope of nursing practice. The National Council of State Boards of Nursing (2007) has responded to the need to address key issues. These include the obligation of all nurses to safely and effectively treat pain, with additional guidance for managing patients who require opioid treatment to function properly.

Achieving consensus and implementing changes at the board of nursing level has additional challenges now that established medicine has declared "turf wars" to actively restrict the practice and payment for services not provided by medical doctors. In an important case, an advanced practice nurse, fully educated, deemed competent, credentialed, and practicing within the scope of nursing practice established by the state of Louisiana, was ordered to stop treating patients with chronic pain. Providing an injection into a painful muscle was deemed the practice of medicine. The Louisiana State Board of Nursing was reprimanded for extending the scope of practice to include procedures conventionally done by physicians without first going through the state's Board of Medical Examiners (Percy, 2006).

Another key opportunity to improve public policy relates to finding balance between using opioids when medically necessary and restricting access of these medicines to those who would divert or abuse them. With more than 2 million first-time users of opioids obtained without a prescription in 2005, the problem of nonmedical use of these medically necessary analgesics is a serious societal problem. Prescription opioids now account for more overdose deaths than heroin, and concerns about their misuse or abuse cannot be ignored (Katz et al., 2008). Regulatory attempts to curtail the growth of this problem have affected the thousands of professionals who prescribe, dispense, or administer these medications, as well as the millions of patients who need to take them for legitimate medical purposes.

The legal tenor in recent years has convinced many that the war on drugs has been transformed to a war on pain patients and those who treat them. The fear that patients using opioids or professionals prescribing opioids are considered guilty until proven innocent is largely unfounded. The media, however, take every opportunity to characterize carelessness involving these drugs as criminal acts. The Federation of State Medical Boards has delineated guidelines that protect physicians prescribing opioids (Fishman, 2007); however, no such protections have been adopted for nurses with prescriptive authority.

Trends and Future Assumptions

Medical Advances

Medical science continues to expand its capacity to forestall death. As a result, people are living longer but increasingly spend their final years with daily, unrelenting pain (Desbiens et al., 1997; Looi & Audisio, 2007; National Center for Health Statistics, 2006). Pain is emerging as a more formidable foe than death, whose conquest will demand stretching of the limits of our technology and ability to provide compassionate care. The number of surgical interventions being performed is constantly increasing, as is the prevalence of chronic diseases like arthritis, diabetes, and cancer—diseases associated with painful syndromes. As science better defines the physiology of acute and inflammatory pain, as well as the pathophysiological changes associated with chronic pain, new treatments and therapeutic targets are emerging. Consumer demand is driving industry to develop well-tolerated, effective pain relievers. The global pain pharmaceutical market is expected to grow by 25% in the next 5 years, with nonopioid options expected to command a major portion of this market (Visiongain, 2007).

Current therapies are limited to a few physiological targets. The first-line target, a cyclooxygenase blocker that prevents prostaglandin synthesis, is limited by undesired effects exerted on the gastrointestinal, hematological, renal, and cardiovascular systems. Other targets focus on inhibitory nerve components (opioid, norepinephrine, serotonin, and γ-aminobutyric acid [GABA] receptors). Emerging targets include other precursors to prostaglandins that are being examined with the hope of greater efficacy and lower toxicity than current options.

Researchers are studying new drugs called p38 inhibitors that block cyclooxygenase-2, other proinflammatory cytokines such as tumor necrosis factor and interleukins, or both, thereby preventing the transduction of pain. Genetically engineered opioids that target specific receptor subtypes are being investigated, as are drugs that inactivate specific sodium channels, proteins, amino acids, neuropeptides, neurotransmitters, and receptors known to transmit pain. Exciting developments in agents that are active on the *N*-methyl-D-aspartate (NMDA) receptor hold promise not only to treat stubborn pain but also to prevent and treat tolerance or opioid-induced hyperalgesia.

Targets also include nonneuronal cells in the central nervous system, like the microglia that contribute to central sensitization and chronic pain. Blocking the up-regulation or hastening the down-regulation of these cells holds promise to effectively treat pain syndromes now considered incurable. As the basic science identifies a plethora of additional molecular targets involved the development of abnormal pain states, uncertainty exists about whether using a single "magic bullet" or hitting multiple targets simultaneously will result in the safest, most efficacious treatment (Basbaum, 2005).

In addition to the investigation of novel drugs, scientists continue trying to perfect existing drugs or use them in a novel way. New drug delivery systems, with more topical, transcutaneous, or transmucosal options, may have advantages of providing safer, quicker, or better analgesia. Some products in development will have a duration of action measured in weeks rather than in hours. New abuse-deterrent formulations and those with imbedded radiofrequency identifiers will aid in curtailing the abuse or diversion of those products.

Given the multiplicity of key brain structures and diverse mechanisms that drive the perception of pain, the challenge to develop new products is a formidable one. For example, neuroplastic changes associated with the development of chronic pain are a maladaptive variation of the same process that is required for learning and memory (Arnstein, 1997). Thus, new therapies conceivably could be developed to halt chronic pain-producing neuroplasticity but also could have the unfortunate side effect of producing an Alzheimer's or Wernicke's psychosis-like impairment of these higher brain functions. With the remarkable advances in brain imaging technology, however, it may become possible to target the functioning of a single misfiring brain cell or prevent cortical reorganization believed responsible for phantom pains by using novel approaches like virtual reality or mirror therapy (Brodie, Whyte, & Niven, 2007).

Technological Advances

Technologies will likely advance as well in the area of gene therapy. Despite much being known about the genetic basis of certain diseases, difficulty in delivering the genetically based therapy to the biological target has been a serious limiting factor. Stockholm-based Diamyd Medical is investigating a promising therapy for chronic pain. The approach uses a deactivated version of herpes simplex virus with a high affinity for nerve cells to deliver genes that stimulate endogenous opioid production for 3 months or longer (Rice, 2008).

As patients become more technologically savvy, electronic devices will increasingly be used to educate patients, monitor their progress, and facilitate communication with professionals. The use of electronic pain diaries in research and clinical practice is already providing patients and the professional team with real-time information organized in a way that supports decisions about optimal treatment strategies (Gaertner, Elsner, Pollmann-Dahmen, Radbruch, & Sabatowski, 2004). Websites like Reliefinsite.com offer free or "premium" pain diaries to facilitate access to this important information. Other websites are being developed to help patients become the experts in their disease and their response to treatments. The prototypes developed to date customize individualized logs to help patients track their pain while cataloguing all tests, results, and treatments tried. Additional features allow patients to find new research or seek advice related to their condition or primary concern.

The future will certainly have better, user-friendly technologies in health care organizations. These will help track a patient's diagnostic and therapeutic history, as well as help identify and monitor patients at risk for opioid-induced respiratory depression. The problems inherent in monitoring devices include their invasive nature and the lack of sensitivity or specificity that results in false alarms or delayed identification of serious problems. Future systems will be less invasive and more reliable, such as mattress coverings that detect the strength of the heartbeat and the tidal volume of gas exchanged with respirations.

Despite anticipated exponential growth in technologies, there may be, perhaps to a greater extent, the need for personal contact and compassionate care. The demand for complementary and alternative medical therapies will likely continue. Pain management nurses will need to be knowledgeable and develop skills in these techniques as a way to engage patients in self-care while enhancing their sense of control. Some technologies will aid in making these interpersonal contacts, such as communication-related technologies and those that bridge cultural and linguistic gaps in our increasingly multicultural, multilingual society.

Prescription monitoring programs will evolve into useful tools available at the point of care to help guide therapy and aid in the identification of drug crimes. An estimated 7 million opioid units (e.g., pills, patches) are stolen and diverted each year from pharmacies and other health care settings (Gaertner et al., 2004). The use of electronic tracking devices should reduce criminal access to these medications and better direct them to patients with a legitimate medical need for pain relief.

Nursing Advances

Despite remarkable advances in health care technologies, the most important components of pain management nursing remain the knowledge, skill, and compassion of the nurse at the bedside. This role will be better defined and recognized as an essential professional accountable for many aspects of patient assessment, pain treatments, and refinement of treatment plans. Nurses will have an acknowledged accountability for quality pain management, rather than an outdated view of the nurse as an instrument of the prescriber. Thus, high degrees of uncontrolled pain will no longer be dismissed as the fault of an irresponsible prescriber but rather will be seen as a clinical problem that the nurse must act to resolve. The depth and breadth of knowledge needed to practice pain management nursing will need to be expanded to include a working knowledge of the principles of pain, emotional distress, palliative care, addiction medicine, and care for specific populations.

Increasingly, policies and procedures that help guide nursing practice are being kept on electronic "bookshelves," which facilitates access and the process of distributing updates. New intranet search engines (such as those created by Google) will allow nurses to customize their searches and receive alerts when documents are revised. With these electronic resources, links can be imbedded to call up key points, patient education guides, recent literature, position papers, and practice guidelines. Links to videos can also be imbedded so that a 2-minute neurological examination is available at the fingertips wherever a nurse needs to review it.

Organizational Improvement Advances

Health care organizations are being transformed into high-reliability groups. Strategies like Six Sigma, Toyota Lean, and rapid tests of change that helped other industries enhance quality process and outcomes are being tailored to the needs of health care. Organizations are being held accountable for identifying and fixing root causes of problems they experience, especially surrounding the occurrence of sentinel events. As technology advances and different clinical and administrative systems can interface, real-time data will track quality and be used to proactively improve processes and outcomes.

The importance of leadership, teamwork, and communication systems that enhance the safety and efficacy of care is increasingly evident. Data about pain management need to be displayed consistently on unit- and departmental-quality dashboards to make them more visible and hold staff accountable for documenting this aspect of practice. Failure to reassess pain or to document pain reassessments may be related to intrinsic (knowledge or skill deficits) or extrinsic (time pressures or workload) variables. Systems such as electronic documentation systems will be tailored to support the timely entry of data so that decisions about ongoing pain treatment can be based on up-to-date information.

Vision of the Preferred Future for Pain Management Nursing

Given the many opportunities for improvement and the current challenges facing pain management nursing, the situation is destined to change for better or worse. An optimistic vision of the preferred future is presented here, knowing quite well that many successes and challenges will be encountered with the dedicated efforts of many pain management nurses striving for optimal pain control. Whenever professionals work together to resolve complex issues, a clear vision of the desired outcome is needed, because "hope is not a method."

Interdisciplinary Team Synchronization

For optimal success, pain management nursing will require strong interprofessional teamwork, communication, and collaboration to promote safe, effective, patient-focused care. Synchronization of the interdisciplinary team based on patient-centered shared goals and coordinated treatment activities will be the norm. Intimidating and disruptive behaviors by any team member, as well as passive activities (e.g., refusing to perform a duty or return phone calls), undermine the team's ability to provide safe, effective pain control. These violations in professional codes of conduct will no longer be ignored, regardless of seniority, clinical discipline, or revenue-generating capacity. Structured processes for identifying and dealing with disruptive professionals that any patient, family member, or professional can initiate will be in place to promote the environment of care needed for optimal pain management.

Integrated Information Systems and Decisional Support

Clinical information systems will play a major role in supporting patient care. As always, patient assessment lays the foundation for the treatment plan. With integrated clinical information systems, the patient's history, diagnostic reports, and treatment responses will be part of the same database as the clinical documentation and active orders. The system would also have information about the patient's functional genetic polymorphisms that can help guide the selection of drugs and doses that will in the short term promote safe, effective pain relief with the least risk of side effects and in the long term prevent at-risk patients from developing chronically painful conditions (Stamer & Stuber, 2007; Reyes-Gibby et al., 2007).

This system will provide a link between recent literature or practice guidelines and individualized patient information. Rather than standardized "evidence-based practice," the preferred "evidence-informed decision making" will facilitate a treatment planning process tailored to the individual. The system will also have the ability to generate timely reminders or alerts when decisions or actions are needed. For example, if pain were entered into the electronic record at a level of 5 or greater on a 0-10 scale, this would trigger inquiry about additional aspects of the pain (description, location, progression over time, exacerbation, and relief patterns) that could be integrated with other clinical information (medical diagnosis and medication administration record) already recorded to provide decisional support to the nurse. Actions advised can be simple, such as prompting the nurse to administer an available as-needed analgesic, obtain psychosocial insights about what may be amplifying pain, or follow a pattern of failed responses to generate a consult order (Lang et al., 2006).

Safety Enhancement Systems

Electronic systems can be tools to minimize medication administration or other treatment errors through the use of timing alerts and barcode confirmation of the right patient, medication, and dose. Safety will be enhanced by systems that eliminate shortcut strategies or workarounds in high-risk areas of practice. Smart infusion pumps will contain the hospital's drug library information and have guardrails in place to prevent common types of medication errors. Formulas entered into the pump will help discriminate dosing protocols for opioid-naïve patients from those for patients who are opioid tolerant until the response to the medications can be determined and safely adjusted.

Built-in barcode readers (or other unique identifiers) will ensure a match exists among the treatment order, the patient, and the actual treatment provided. Automatic identification (Auto-ID) features identify both the patient and the clinician during pump operation, and data are recorded and transmitted to the medical record. Imbedded in infusion pumps will be hard-stops to prevent incorrect or unsafe practices. In addition to being integrated to communicate with provider-order-entry systems, opioid infusion pumps will be linked to monitoring systems capable of detecting hypoventilation or hypotension. If established physiological thresholds indicating potential harm are crossed, the pump will stop the infusion, trigger an alarm, and alert the nurse to check the patient.

Clarity of the Pain Management Nurses' Role and Responsibility

Despite all the technological advances, the clinician at the bedside will remain the final and most important ingredient in promoting safe, effective pain treatment. The value-added contribution of nurses is clear and easy to explain. Internationally accepted descriptions of the role and responsibility of all nurses will be written and widely distributed. The current classification systems of nursing diagnoses, nursing interventions, and nursing outcomes will be revised for inclusion in the 11th edition of the *International Classification of Diseases (ICD-11),* with an anticipated release date in 2012 by the World Health Organization.

At the organizational level, there will be clearly articulated job descriptions, performance evaluations, and quality-indicating dashboards to delineate and monitor the accountability each nurse has for assessing and satisfactorily managing pain. Minimum standards of nursing care and guidelines detailing best practices will be aligned with national position papers and clinical practice guidelines. Credentialed pain management nurses will be employed in settings where pain is commonly experienced or historically difficult to treat. These nurses will have job descriptions that permit a higher level of independent functioning aligned with their credentials and skill sets to optimize patient and family access to needed biopsychosocial interventions known to relieve pain. At the state level, a mechanism will be created for convening an ad hoc multidisciplinary panel of experts (e.g., a pain commission or advisory council) to develop and review proposed legislation promoting balanced policies that take into account both the needs of patients with severe pain and the need to protect the public from problems related to drug trafficking, drug misuse, and addiction disorders. This group, which will include at least one nurse, will also educate policy makers about the negative impacts on patient care caused by current or proposed laws.

For advanced practice nurses, the preferred future will achieve uniformity of prescriptive authority, including the independent authority to prescribe schedule II opioid analgesics. Many nurse leaders believe that nurse practitioners who are educationally prepared at the doctorate level will foster this parity; however, the research-derived evidence of nurse practitioners' knowledge, skill, and trustworthiness in regard to prescribing opioids is the most influential factor contributing to that authority being granted.

Summary

Nurses are uniquely positioned professionals with the knowledge, skills, and compassion to solve the mysteries of pain one patient at a time. Given the opportunity to work directly with patients and families over time, pain management nurses can understand the unique physical, mental, social, spiritual, and environmental factors contributing to the complexity of pain and its relief. If, as Wall suggested, pain is a "drive," nurses are capable of deciphering what the unmet need is and either meeting it or advocating with the health care team that realistic needs be met. Although a long-range goal is to integrate this knowledge into all aspects of health care, no substitute exists for the valued knowledge, skill, and compassion that define pain management nurses.

References

Acute Pain Management Guideline Panel. (1992). Acute pain management: Operative or medical procedures and trauma. Clinical Practice Guideline. (AHCPR Publication No. 92-0032). Rockville, MD: Agency for Health Care Policy and Research, Public Health Service, U.S. Department of Health and Human Services.

American Academy of Pediatrics & Canadian Paediatric Society. (2006). Policy statement: Prevention and management of pain in the neonate. An update. *Pediatrics, 118*(5), 2231–2241.

American Society of Anesthesiologists. (2006). Practice guidelines for the perioperative management of patients with obstructive sleep apnea. *Anesthesiology, 104*(5), 1081–1093.

American Society for Pain Management Nursing & American Nurses Association. (2005). *Pain management nursing: Scope and standards of practice.* Silver Spring, MD: Nursingbooks.org.

Arnstein, P. M. (1997). The neuroplastic phenomenon: A physiologic link between chronic pain and learning. *Journal of Neuroscience Nursing, 29*(3), 179–186.

Basbaum, A. (2005). The future of pain therapy: Something old, something new, something borrowed, something blue. In H. Merskey, J. D. Loseser, & R. Dubner (Eds.), *The paths of pain, 1975–2005* (pp. 513–532). Seattle: IASP Press.

Bernabei, R., Gambassi, G., Lapane, K., Landi, F., Gatsonis, C., Dunlop, R., Lipsitz, L., Steel, & K., Mor, V. (1998). Management of pain in elderly patients with cancer: SAGE Study Group. Systematic assessment of geriatric drug use via epidemiology. *Journal of the American Medical Association, 279,* 1877–1882.

Brodie, E. E., Whyte, A., & Niven, C. A. (2007). Analgesia through the looking-glass? A randomized controlled trial investigating the effect of viewing a "virtual" limb upon phantom limb pain, sensation and movement. *European Journal of Pain, 11*(4), 428–436.

Brown, S. J. (2009). *Evidence-based nursing: The research-practice connection.* Sudbury, MA: Jones and Bartlett.

Charlton, J. E. (Ed.). (2005). *Core curriculum for professional education in pain* (3rd ed.). Seattle: IASP Press. Retrieved October 26, 2008, from http://www.iasp-pain.org/AM/Template.cfm?Section=Home&Template=/CM/HTMLDisplay.cfm&ContentID=2307#TOC.

Desbiens, N. A., Mueller-Rizner, N., Connors, A. F., Jr., Hamel, M.B., Wenger, N.S. (1997). Pain in the oldest—old during hospitalization and up to one year later. *Journal of the American Geriatrics Society, 45,* 1167–1172.

Fishman, S. M. (2007). *Responsible opioid prescribing: A physician's guide.* Dallas: Federation of State Medical Boards of the United States.

Friedman, R., Myers, P., Sobel, D., Caudill, M. A., & Benson, H. (1995). Behavioral medicine, clinical health psychology and cost offset. *Health Psychology, 14*(6), 509–518.

Gaertner, J., Elsner, F., Pollmann-Dahmen, K., Radbruch, L., & Sabatowski, L. (2004). Electronic pain diary: A randomized crossover study. *Journal of Pain and Symptom Management, 28*(3), 259–267.

Hurley, R. W., & Adams, M. C. (2008). Sex, gender, and pain: can overview of a complex field. *Anesthesia and Analgesia, 107*(1), 309–317.

Institute for Safe Medication Practices. (2008). *ISMP's list of high-alert medications.* Retrieved March 28, 2008, from http://www.ismp.org/tools/highalertmedications.pdf.

Jacox, A., Carr, D. B., Payne, R., Berde, C.B., Breibart, W. Cain, J.M., Chapman, C.R., Cleeland, C.S., Ferrell, B.T., Finley, R.S., Hester, N.O., Stratton Hill, C., Leak, W.D., Lipman, A.G., Logan, C.L., McGarvey, C.L., Miaskowski, C.A., Mulder, D.S., Paice, J.A., Shapiro, B.S., Silberstein, E.B., Smith, R.S., Stover, J., Tsou, C.V., Vecchiarelli, L., & Weissman, D.E. (1994). *Management of cancer pain.* Clinical Practice Guideline, No. 9. (AHCPR Publication No. 94-0592). Rockville, MD: Agency for Healthcare Policy and Research, Public Health Service, U.S. Department of Health and Human Services.

Joint Commission. (2008). *2009 accreditation requirements.* Retrieved October 26, 2008, from http://www.jointcommission.org/Standards/SII/.

Katz, N., Fernandez, K., Chang, A., Benoit, C., Butler, F. (2008). Internet-based survey of nonmedical prescription opioid use in the United States. *Clinical Journal of Pain, 24*(6), 528–535.

Kehlet, H., & Dahl, J. B. (1993). The value of "multimodal" or "balanced analgesia" in postoperative pain treatment. *Anesthesia and Analgesia, 77,* 1048–1056.

Lang, N. M., Hook, M. L., Akre, M. E., Kim, T. Y., Berg, K., Lundeen, S. P., Hagel, M.E., Ela, S.E. (2006). Translating knowledge-based nursing into referential an executable applications in an intelligent clinical information system. In C. A. Weaver, C. W. Delaney, P. Weber, & R. Carr (Eds.), *Nursing and informatics for the 21st century: An international look at practice, trends and the future* (pp. 291–303). Chicago: HIMMS Press.

Loeser, J. D. (2005). Multidisciplinary pain management. In H. Merskey, J. D. Loseser, & R. Dubner (Eds.), *The paths of pain, 1975–2005* (pp. 503–511). Seattle: IASP Press.

Looi, Y., & Audisio, R. (2007). A review of the literature on post-operative pain in older cancer patients. *European Journal of Cancer, 43*(15), 2222–2230.

Lorig, K. R., Mazonson, P. D., & Holman, H. R. (1993). Evidence suggesting that health education for self-management in patients with chronic arthritis has sustained health benefits while reducing health care costs. *Arthritis and Rheumatism, 36*(4), 439–46.

Maclean, S., Obispo, J., & Young, K. D. (2007). The gap between pediatric emergency department procedural pain management treatments available and actual practice. *Pediatric Emergency Care, 23*(2), 87–93.

Macrae, W. A. (2001). Chronic pain after surgery. *British Journal of Anaesthesia, 87*(1), 88–98.

Maheshwari, A. V., Boutary, M., Yun, A. G., Sirianni, L. E., & Dorr, L. D. (2006). Multimodal analgesia without routine parenteral narcotics for total hip arthroplasty. *Clinical Orthopaedics and Related Research, 453,* 231–238.

McCaffery, M. (1968). *Nursing practice theories related to cognition, bodily pain, and man-environment interactions.* Los Angeles: University of California at Los Angeles, Students' Store.

McCaffery, M., & Pasero, C. (1999). *Pain clinical manual* (2nd ed.). St. Louis: Mosby.

National Center for Health Statistics. (2006). *Chartbook on trends in the health of Americans.* Hyattsville, MD: Author. Retrieved April 24, 2008, from http://www.cdc.gov/nchs/data/hus/hus06.pdf.

National Council of State Boards of Nursing. (2007). *Regulatory implications of pain management.* Chicago: Author. Retrieved October 25, 2008, from https://www.ncsbn.org/05_18_07_Pain_Statement.pdf.

Percy, L. (2006). Louisiana court rules on conflicts between nursing and medical board opinions. *American Society of Anesthesiologists Newsletter, 70*(7). Retrieved October 25, 2008, from http://www.asahq.org/Newsletters/2006/07-06/stateBeat07_06.html.

Perkins, F. M., & Kehlet, H. (2000). Chronic pain as an outcome of surgery: A review of predictive factors. *Anesthesiology, 93,* 1123–1133.

Plaisance, L., & Logan, C. C. (2005). Nursing students' knowledge and attitudes regarding pain. *Pain Management Nursing, 7*(4), 167–175.

Pletcher, M. J., Kertesz, S. G., Kohn, M. A., & Gonzales, R. (2008). Trends in opioid prescribing by race/ethnicity for patients seeking care in U.S. emergency departments. *Journal of the American Medical Association, 299*(1), 70–78.

Reuben, S. S., & Buvanendran, A. (2007). Preventing the development of chronic pain after orthopedic surgery with preventive multimodal analgesia techniques. *Journal of Bone and Joint Surgery, 89,* 1343–1358.

Reyes-Gibby, C. C., Shete, S., Rakvag, T., Bhat SV, Skorpen F, Bruera E, Kaasa S, Klepstad P. Pain. 2007. Exploring joint effects of genes and clinical efficacy of morphine for cancer pain. *Pain, 130,* 25–30.

Rice, J. (2008). *Gene therapy for chronic pain: Researchers use gene therapy to stop pain signals before they reach the brain.* Technology Review (MIT Publication). Retrieved September 20, 2008, from http://www.technologyreview.com/Biotech/20118/?a=f.

Rivara, F. P., Mackenzie, E. J., Jurkovich, G. J., Nathens, A.B., Wang, J., & Scharfstein, D.O. (2008). Prevalence of pain in patients 1 year after major trauma. *Archives of Surgery, 143*(3), 282–287.

Simons, S. H., van Dijk, M., Anand, K. S., Roofthooft, D., van Lingen, R.A., & Tibboel, D. (2003). Do we still hurt newborn babies? A prospective study of procedural pain and analgesia in neonates. *Archives of Pediatrics & Adolescent Medicine, 157*(11), 1058–1064.

Stamer, U. M., & Stuber, F. (2007). Genetic factors in pain and its treatment. *Current Opinions in Anaesthesiology, 20,* 478–484.

Van den Heede, K., Clarke, S. P., Sermeus, W., Vleugels, A., & Aiken, L. H. (2007). International experts' perspective on the state of the nurse staffing and patient outcomes literature. *Journal of Nursing Scholarship, 39*(4), 290–297.

Visiongain. (2007). *Global pain pharmaceutical market analysis and forecasts: 2007–2022.* Retrieved September 21, 2008, from http://www.visiongain.com/report_license.aspx?rid=232.

U.S. Food and Drug Administration. (2007). *FDA announces important changes and additional warnings for COX-2 selective and non-selective non-steroidal anti-inflammatory drugs (NSAIDs).* Retrieved March 28, 2008, from http://www.fda.gov/cder/drug/advisory/COX2.htm.

Wall, P. (1999). *Pain: The science of suffering.* London: Weidenfeld & Nicolson (Orion).

Wells-Federman, C., Arnstein, P. M., & Caudill-Slosberg, M. A. (2002). Nurse-led pain-management program: Effect on self-efficacy, pain intensity, pain-related disability and depressive symptoms in chronic pain patients. *Pain Management Nursing, 3*(5), 141–153.

Index

A

D

E

F

G

I

J

K

L

M

O

S

T

U

V

W

Y

Z